Atlas of Metabolic Diseases

Atlas of Metabolic Diseases

Second edition

William L. Nyhan, MD PhD
Professor of Pediatrics
Department of Pediatrics
Division of Biochemical Genetics
University of California, San Diego
USA

Bruce A. Barshop, MD PhD
Professor of Pediatrics
Department of Pediatrics
Division of Biochemical Genetics
University of California, San Diego
USA

and

Pinar T. Ozand, MD PhD
Head, Section of Inborn Errors of Metabolism
Department of Pediatrics, MBC #58
King Faisal Specialist Hospital and Research Centre
Riyadh
Saudi Arabia

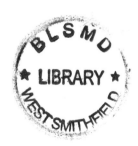

Hodder Arnold

A MEMBER OF THE HODDER HEADLINE GROUP

First published in Great Britain in 2005 by
Hodder Education, a member of the Hodder Headline Group,
338 Euston Road, London NW1 3BH

http:// at www.hoddereducation.com

Distributed in the United States of America by
Oxford University Press Inc.,
198 Madison Avenue, New York, NY10016
Oxford is a registered trademark of Oxford University Press

British Library Cataloguing in Publication Data
A catalogue record for this book is available from the British Library

Library of Congress Cataloging-in-Publication Data
A catalog record for this book is available from the Library of Congress

ISBN 0 340 809701

1 2 3 4 5 6 7 8 9 10

Commissioning Editor: Jo Koster
Development Editor: Dan Edwards
Project Editor: Naomi Wilkinson
Production Controller: Jo Walker
Cover Design: Sarah Rees
Indexers: Indexing Specialists (UK) Ltd

Typeset in 10/12 pts Minion by Charon Tec Pvt. Ltd, Chennai, India
www.charontec.com
Printed and bound in Italy by Printer Trento

What do you think about this book? Or any other Hodder Arnold title?
Please visit our website at www.hoddereducation.com

Contents

Contributors

Chapter 110
Deborah Marsden MBBS, FACMG
Assistant Professor, Harvard Medical School
Children's Hospital Boston
Boston, MA
USA

Chapter 112
Aida I. Al Aqeel MD FRCP_{Lond., Edin.} **FACMG**
Consultant Pediatric Metabolist
Geneticist and Endocrinologist
Riyadh Armed Forces Hospital
Riyadh
Saudi Arabia

Preface

This book is designed as a source of practical information of use in the diagnosis and management of patients with inherited diseases of metabolism. We have kept the focus, as did Garrod, on the inborn errors. This permits a unity of theme. At the same time, the reality is that genetically-determined human variation in metabolism leads to an enormous variety of clinical expression crossing most of the boundaries of clinical subspecialty.

We want this book to be helpful to physicians at the bedside, in the intensive care unit and in the clinics and offices, as well as to biochemical geneticists and clinical chemists involved in laboratory diagnosis. The atlas format has permitted us to include very many illustrations of patients. Metabolic pathways have been shown with a reductionist or high power view of just that area most relevant to each disease. In addition, the chapters deal with individual diseases. There are introductory chapters to the organic acidemias, the disorders of the urea cycle, the disorders of fatty acid oxidation, the lactic acidemias, the glycogenoses and the mucopolysaccharidoses which provide some general considerations of these areas of metabolism and permit us to avoid some redundancy. With these exceptions each chapter represents defective activity of a single enzyme. Mutations in a single gene can lead to a very large family of different variant enzymes and accordingly very different clinical phenotypes. In general, we have considered this variation in each chapter, with emphasis on the most common expression. In three instances we have given variants separate treatments. There is historical precedent for separate consideration of the Hurler disease from the Scheie and Hurler-Scheie variants and for the separate consideration of mucolipidoses II and III. In the first edition we had chapters for complete deficiency of hypoxanthine guanine phosphoribosyltransferase (HPRT) and the other variants; now that chapter has been divided into two halves.

The rates of discovery of new or previously unrecognized diseases in this field are enormous. In the 1980s we saw for the first time descriptions of many of the currently known disorders of fatty acid oxidation; in the 1990s we saw the numbers of known discrete mitochondrial DNA mutations increase rapidly. Some of these diseases are turning out to be relatively common. Medium-chain acyl CoA dehydrogenase (MCAD) deficiency occurs in approximately 10 000 births, and most patients have the same mutation. On the other hand, although it is clear that in the aggregate the inherited diseases of metabolism make up a sizeable portion of human morbidity and mortality, each individual disease tends to be rarely encountered. Even an expert may find years have elapsed since he last saw a patient with a given disorder, reviewed the literature and ordered it in a way that would help with diagnosis or treatment. It helps to have the relevant information in one place for ready retrieval. This atlas serves that purpose for us. We are hopeful that it will do the same for our readers.

The advent of molecular biologic approaches to genetics and the increasing exploration of the human genome have changed forever the scope of human genetics and the manner in which it is practiced. In the Atlas we have endeavored to seek a balance among the molecular biology and the nature of mutation, the enzymology and intermediary metabolism and clinical practice. Our focus is on the clinician. Algorithms are provided for the logical workup of a patient with lactic acidemia, and disorders of fatty acid oxidation and a systematic approach to the diagnosis of a patient with hyperammonemia.

Medical genetics is now officially recognized in many countries among clinical and laboratory specialties. Trainees preparing themselves for board examinations might want to read the Atlas from cover to cover. We hope that in addition to medical geneticists, pediatricians, neurologists, internists, pathologists and all those who interact with patients with these disorders will find the Atlas of assistance in their practices.

The field is moving so rapidly it is an experience to keep current in any disease. There is much in this book that is new, different or virtually unique. Certainly, the pictures are for us a resource. Novel mechanisms of disease have been explored. The many enzyme defects in the congenital disorders of glycosylation are becoming known and with this knowledge recognition of some quite different phenotypes. Mutations have now been identified in the genes for the very strange ethylmalonic aciduria whose petechial exacerbations lead regularly to treatment for meningococcemia. The discovery of this gene, ETHE1 by homozygosity mapping illustrates the powerful new influence of molecular biology and the data provided by the human genome project in this field. The function of this mitochondrial protein remains to be determined. Similarly the Sanjad-Sakati and Al Aqeel-Sewairi syndromes, while not metabolic in the old sense were included because they are illustrations of the way in which new molecular techniques are uncovering novel mechanisms of disease. In the Sanjad-Sakati syndrome a phenotype of endocrineopthy and dysmorphic features is caused by mutations in a tubulin-specific chaperone E (TBLE) which is required for proper folding of α-tubulin, the first example to be discovered in human disease resulting from mutation inducing defective folding and assembly of the building blocks of microtubules. In the Al Aqeel-Sewairi syndrome the discovery of mutations in the matrix metalloproteinase (MMP-2) gene not only elucidates this vanishing bone syndrome, but has relevance to many disease processes, such as arthritis, tumor invasion and metastasis.

In the glutamylribose-5-phosphate storage disease the molecule that accumulates and must be detected to identify the disease does not get out of the brain. In I-cell disease and pseudohurler polydystrophy the basic defect is in the processing of lysosomal enzymes to permit their recognition and entry into cellular lysosomes. The fascinating and novel mechanism uncovered in the multiple sulfatase deficiency defect is in an enzyme which catalyzes a posttranslational change of a cysteine moiety in each of the sulfatase enzymes to an aminooxopropionic acid moiety, which change normally converts inactive sulfatase proteins to catalytically-active enzymes.

Among the challenges for diagnosis and management highlighted in this volume are the disorders of fatty acid oxidation and the lactic acidemias and mitochondrial disease. The latter include the acronymic disorders resulting from mitochondrial DNA mutation and the Pearson syndrome, which may present in infancy as a pure hematologic disorder. It also includes the newly discovered deficiency of DNA polymerase, which results in a mitochondrial DNA depletion syndrome. The newly recognized disorders of creatine synthesis are a challenge for diagnosis. They are sometimes suspected when the urine is analyzed for organic acids and amino acids, and everything is high, because we base our analyses per mole of creatinine. They may be elegantly demonstrated by nuclear magnetic resonance spectroscopy (NMRS).

The chapter was written by Deborah Marsden, a former fellow at UCSD, now on the faculty at Harvard.

The Atlas was generated by our experience with patients with metabolic disease. We are grateful to the many physicians who have referred these patients to us and to those who have shared their illustrations with us. We are appreciative of the help of many of our fellows and colleagues who have helped us care for and study these patients. They include Drs. Nadia Sakati, Richard Hass, Fred Levine, Robert Naviaux, Jon Wolff and Karen McGowan.

Original artwork was done by Mrs. Frances Bakay and The Office of Learning Resources at UCSD. Images of tandem mass spectrometry were recovered by Mr. Jon Gangoiti of the Biochemical/Genetics Laboratory at UCSD. We are particularly indebted to the work of many: Mrs. Lilia Fernandez, Ms. Sandra Hoffert, Ms. Susan Allen and Ms. Linh Vuong, a medical student at UCSD, for the conversion of handwritten pages into polished typed electronic manuscript. The majority of the text was expertly typed by Ms. Debra Lin, a student at UCSD.

William L. Nyhan
La Jolla, California
2005

Organic acidemias

Introduction

The inborn errors of organic acid metabolism represent a spectrum of disorders, most of them relatively recently recognized. Many of them produce life-threatening illness very early in life. The variety of metabolic pathways involved is indicated in Figure 1.1. They should be suspected in any patient with metabolic aciduria, and certainly when there is an anion gap (Table 1.1).

A number of these disorders are on the catabolic pathways for the branched-chain amino acids, or other amino acids, but the site of the enzymatic defect is sufficiently removed from the step at which the amino group is lost that the amino acids do not accumulate, and thus these disorders are not detected by methods of amino acid analysis. They remained largely unrecognized until the development of methods of detection, particularly gas chromatography-mass spectrometry (GCMS) [1], that were of sufficient generality not to depend on a single functional group for detection. Quantitative organic analysis is an important aspect of this methodology. Tandem mass spectrometry (MS/MS) [2] (Table 1.2) has added another important method of detection of organic acids as their carnitine esters; this methodology has made these diseases subjects for neonatal screening.

Gas chromatography-mass spectrometry has been the basis for monitoring levels of relevant metabolites in the process of management. Therapeutic intervention, including cofactor or other dosage and dietary restriction, are dependent on accurate knowledge of the concentrations of those compounds that accumulate behind the block. Tandem mass spectrometry may also serve this purpose, but experience with its use except for diagnosis has not been reported. In general, therapeutic efficacy is best when concentrations of accumulated metabolite(s) are kept at the lowest achievable level. This is seldom zero except in cofactor responsive inborn errors, such as biotin-responsive multiple carboxylase deficiency (Chapters 5, p. 36, and 43, p. 279). More commonly a plateau level of metabolite is achieved, at which further restriction of metabolite intake leads to catabolism and an increase in metabolite accumulation, as well as impairment of weight gain and negative nitrogen balance. In disorders in which the organic acid is a product of amino acid metabolism, such as methylmalonicaciduria, we also measure concentrations of amino acids in plasma,

and, while our patients have levels of the precursor amino acids much lower than those usually recommended as normal, we keep them above those at which weight gain stops or nitrogen balance becomes negative [3]. We maintain intake between such floor levels and a ceiling at which the plateau is exceeded and metabolite levels rise.

Quantification of organic acid analysis is essential for management; it may also be important in diagnosis. For instance, the presence of hydroxyisovalerate, hydroxypropionate and methylcitrate may suggest a diagnosis of multiple carboxylase deficiency, but these compounds are also found in propionic acidemia. The two are readily distinguished by quantification. In multiple carboxylase deficiency the amounts of hydroxyisovalerate are large and those of the other compounds small, while in propionic acidemia, the reverse is found.

Other methodology has been applied to the detection of organic acids. Nuclear magnetic resonance (NMR) spectrometry has become available for these purposes as the resolution of the machines has improved considerably [4]. The ability to test urine or other biological fluids without complex sample preparation raises the possibility of much more rapid diagnosis. Wider applicability should reduce the cost of diagnostic procedures. The application of MS/MS [2,5] to the detection of organic acidemias is of particular benefit in emergencies, for it shortens the time required for diagnosis.

Organic acid analysis and the occurrence of unique metabolites has led to highly accurate, rapid methods of prenatal diagnosis by GCMS of the amniotic fluid, especially with selected ion monitoring and stable isotope dilution internal standards [6]. Most experience is with analysis for methylcitrate and methylmalonic acids in the prenatal diagnosis of propionic acidemia and methylmalonicacidemia. Methodology is also available for the prenatal diagnosis of orotic aciduria [7], hepatorenal tyrosinemia [8], holocarboxylase synthetase deficiency [9], galactosemia [10], mevalonic acidemia [11], glutaric CoA dehydrogenase deficiency [12] and 4-hydroxybutyric aciduria [13].

Analysis of the organic acids of the urine may detect the presence of a disorder of neurotransmitter function, although the diagnosis is usually made by analysis of neurotransmitters or their products in cerebrospinal fluid (CSF) [14]. A patient with neonatal hypoglycemia and metabolic acidosis developed

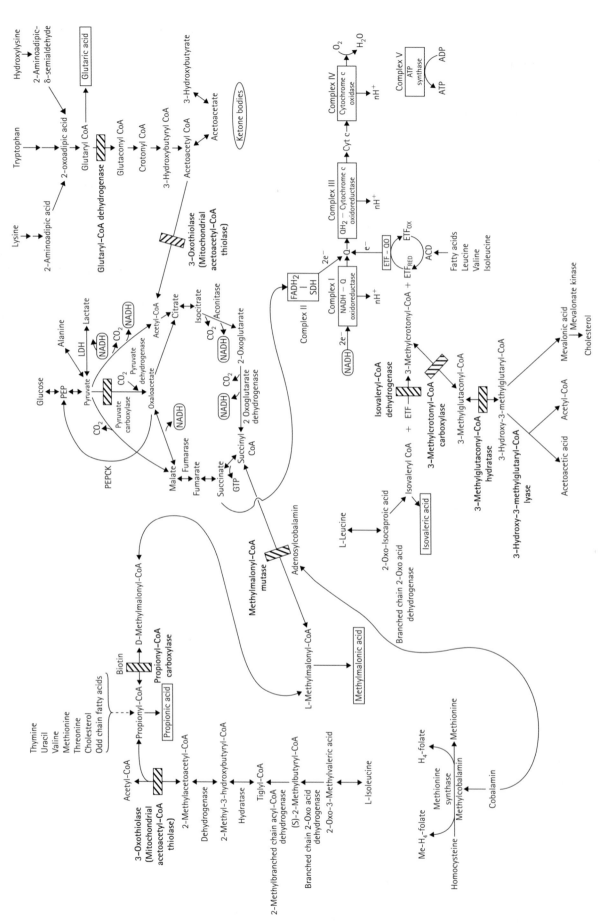

Figure 1.1   *Metabolic interrelations of relevance to the organic acidemias. Many of these disorders are characterized by the accumulation of CoA esters. Many present with lactic acidemia.*

dystonia, oculogyric crises and hypothermia at eight months was found on organic acid analysis of the urine to have increased levels of vanillactic acid neonatally and later vanillpyruvic acid and acetylvanillalanine. Levels of these compounds in CSF were very high, while those of 5-hydroxyindolacetic acid and homovanillic acid were low. Enzyme assay revealed nearly undetectable aromatic L-amino acid decarboxylase activity.

Organic acid analysis is often confounded by the presence of compounds arising from intestinal bacterial metabolites, pharmacologic agents, nutritional supplements or nutritional deficiency. A compendium of metabolites found on organic acid analysis in inborn errors of metabolism and in other situations has been published by Kumps *et al.* [15]. Some of the common confounding metabolites are shown in Table 1.3.

Table 1.1   *Mnemonic for the differential diagnosis of metabolic acidosis with an elevated anion gap (DIMPLES)*

D	Diabetic ketoacidosis
I	Inborn error of metabolism, iron, isoniazid
M	Methanol, metformin
P	Paraldehyde, phenformin
L	Lactic acidemia
E	Ethanol, ethylene glycol
S	Salicylates, solvents, strychnine

The mnemonic has been written as MUDPILES or MUDPIES, including U for uremia, but in clinical practice uremia tends to be recognized as early as the acidosis, making this unnecessary; the latter form leaves out lactic acidemia, an important omission. The current form highlights metabolic causes of acidosis.

Organic acid analysis is commonly ordered on patients during illness, and many illnesses are accompanied by ketosis with its elevated excretion of acetoacetate and 3-hydroxybutyrate. Accompanying ketosis are increases in the excretion of 3-hydroxyisovalerate, 3-hydroxyisobutyrate and dicarboxylic acids including long chain 3-hydroxy compounds. In this way the pattern may be mistaken for long chain 3-hydroxyacyl CoA dehydrogenase (LCHAD) deficiency (Chapter 42), but of course in LCHAD deficiency ketonuria is inappropriately low. This distinction rules out other disorders of fatty acid oxidation suggested by the dicarboxylic aciduria. In disorders of fatty acid oxidation the ratio of adipic to 3-hydroxybutyric acid is >0.5 [16]. Lactic acidemia and lactic aciduria may also be confusing because of associated increase not only in pyruvic acid, but also the branched chain keto and hydroxy acids, as found in defects of the E3 subunit of the pyruvate dehydrogenase complex (Chapter 50).

Bacterial metabolism in the intestine is another confounding variable, which becomes particularly prominent in malabsorptive syndromes. Among the compounds found in the urine are lactic acid; this is D-lactic acid, but the chromatogram does not distinguish the D from the L forms. Specific enzymatic or other distinction must be made or the patient could be treated with oral neomycin or metronidazile and the urine reassayed. Other compounds resulting from intestinal bacteria are propionate metabolites, including methylmalonate and aromatic compounds such as p-hydroxyphenylacetate, p-hydroxyphenyllactate, phenylacetylglutamine, phenylpropionylglycine, glutarate, benzoate and

Table 1.2   *Acyl carnitine profiles of plasma in the diagnosis of organic acidemias*

Disorder	Acylcarnitine	Control reference*	Patient
Glutaric acidemia	C5DC	0.06	0.46–1.34
Propionic acidemia	C3	1.30	6.50–60.10
Methylmalonic acidemia	C3 Methylmalonyl	1.30 0.06	13.00–90.50 0.12–0.94
2-Oxothiolase	C5:1 C5OH	0.04 0.06	0.14–0.72 0.12–0.30
Isovaleric	C5	0.80	52.96–60.47
Methylcrotonyl-CoA carboxylase (incl. maternal)	C5 C5OH	0.22 0.06	15.52–18.38 >0.8
Multiple carboxylase deficiency – holocarboxylase synthetase and biotinidase deficiencies	C5:1	0.04	
Isobutyryl-CoA dehydrogenase deficiency	C4	0.32	
2-Methylbutyryl-CoA dehydrogenase deficiency	C5	0.22 (<0.4)	1.4–2.4
Malonic aciduria	C3DC		
2-Methyl-3-hydroxybutyryl-CoA dehydrogenase deficiency	C5OH C5:1	1.06	

Adapted from Vreken *et al.* [2] and other sources
* 95th percentile of the reference range. Abbreviations include DC- dicarboxylic acid.

Table 1.3 *Some organic acids found in the urine in the absence of inherited metabolic disease*

Compound	Situation	Inborn error in which found
Adipic acid	Gelatin; Fasting-ketosis	Disorders of fatty acid oxidation
3-Hydroxyadipic acid	Fasting	LCHAD deficiency
N-Acetyltyrosine	Parenteral solutions	Tyrosinemia
Phenylacetylglutamine; phenylacetate; phenyllactate; phenylpyruvate	Intestinal bacteria; treatment of urea cycle defects with phenylacetate or phenylbutyrate	Phenylketonuria
4-Hydroxyphenylacetate; -lactate; or -pyruvate	Intestinal bacteria	Tyrosinemia; hawkinsinuria
2-Hydroxyisocaproate	Short bowel syndrome (D-form)	Maple syrup urine disease (MSUD)
3-Hydroxyisovalerate	Ketosis; lactic acidemia	Multiple carboxylase deficiency; isovaleric acidemia, 3 Methylcrotonyl-CoA carboxylase deficiency
Methylmalonic acid	B_{12} deficiency; intestinal bacteria	Methylmalonic acidemia; transcobalamin II deficiency
5-Hydroxyhexanoic acid	MCT ingestion; ketosis	MCAD deficiency; multiple acyl CoA dehydrogenase deficiency
2-Ketoglutaric acid	Urinary tract infection; infancy	2-Ketoglutaryl CoA dehydrogenase deficiency
Glycolic acid	Ethylene glycol poisoning	Hyperoxaluric type I; 4-Hydroxybutyric aciduria
Oxalic acid	Intestinal malabsorption; idiopathic; pyridoxine deficiency; rhubarb, spinach and other vegetables; ethylene glycol; ascorbic acid; methoxyflurane	Hyperoxalurias
5-Oxyproline (pyroglutamic acid)	Nonenzymatic conversion from glutamine in stored sample; vigabatrin; abnormal glycine metabolism; iron oxoprolinate.	Pyroglutamic aciduria; hawkinsinuria; cystinosis
Vanillactic acid	Bananas; neuroblastoma; carbidopa	L-Amino acid decarboxylase deficiency
Furane derivatives: Dicarboxylate; Furoylglycine; 5-Hydroxymethyl-2-furoate	Heated sugars	

hippurate. Bacterial urinary tract infection also produces D-lactic aciduria; increased excretion of 2-oxoglutarate is characteristic; succinate and 3-hydroxypropionate may also be increased.

The administration of valproic acid yields a number of its metabolites, which may cause confusion, but their recognition permits understanding of the secondary effects the drug has on many areas of metabolism. Organic acids found in patients receiving the drug include 3-hydroxyisovalerate, 5-hydroxyhexanoate, p-hydroxyphenylpyruvate, hexanoylglycine, tiglylglycine, isovalerylglycine and a variety of dicarboxylic acids.

Dicarboxylic aciduria is also a prominent result of the intake of medium chain triglyceride which is found increasingly in infant feeding. 5-Hydroxyhexanoate may serve as a clue, but other medium chain dicarboxylic acids, adipic, suberic and sebacic are found. Large quantities of adipic acid are found in the urine of children eating gelatin.

References

1 Hoffmann G, Aramaki S, Blum-Hoffmann E *et al*. Quantitative analysis for organic acids in biological samples: Batch isolation followed by gas chromatographic-mass spectrometric analysis. *Clin Chem* 1989;**38**:587.

2 Vreken P, van Lint AEM, Bootsma AH *et al*. Rapid diagnosis of organic acidemias and fatty acid oxidation defects by quantitative electrospray tandem-MS acylcarnitine analysis in plasma, in *Current Views of Fatty Acid Oxidation and Ketogenesis: From Organelles to Point Mutations*, (ed. Quant and Eaton, Kluwer Academic), Plenum Publishers, New York, 1999:327–7.

3 Nyhan WL. Disorders of propionate metabolism, in *Inherited Diseases of Amino Acid Metabolism: Recent Progress in the Understanding, Recognition and Management*, (eds Bickel H and Wachtel U), Thieme Inc., New York, 1985:363–82.

4 Lehnert W, Hunkler D. Possibilities of selective screening for inborn errors of metabolism using high-resolution 1H-FT-NMR spectrometry. *Eur J Pediatr* 1986;**145**:260.

5 Ozand PT, Rashed M, Gascon GG *et al*. (1994) Unusual presentations of propionic acidemia. *Brain Dev* 1994;**16**:46.

6   Sweetman L, Naylor G, Ladner T *et al.* Prenatal diagnosis of propionic and methylmalonic acidemia by stable isotope dilution analysis of methylcitric and methylmalonic acids in amniotic fluids, in *Stable Isotopes*, (eds Schmidt H-L, Forstel H and Heinzinger K), Elsevier Scientific Publishing Co., Amsterdam, The Netherlands, 1982:287–93.

7   Jakobs C, Sweetman L, Nyhan WL *et al.* Stable isotope dilution analysis of orotic acid and uracil in amniotic fluid. *Clin Chim Acta* 1984;**143**:123.

8   Jakobs C, Sweetman L, Nyhan WL. Chemical analysis of succinylacetone and 4-hydroxyphenylacetate in amniotic fluid using selective ion monitoring. *Prenat Diagn* 1984;**4**:187.

9   Jakobs C, Sweetman L, Nyhan WL, Packman S. Stable isotope dilution analysis of 3-hydroxyisovaleric acid in amniotic fluid: Contribution to the prenatal diagnosis of inherited disorders of leucine catabolism. *J Inherit Metab Dis* 1984;**7**:15.

10 Jakobs C, Warner TB, Sweetman L, Nyhan WL. Stable isotope dilution analysis of galactitol in amniotic fluid: an accurate approach to the prenatal diagnosis of galactosemia. *Pediatr Res* 1984;**18**:714.

11 Gibson KM, Hoffmann G, Nyhan WL *et al.* Mevalonic aciduria: Family studies in mevalonate kinase deficiency, an inborn error of cholesterol biosynthesis. *J Inherit Metab Dis* 1987;**10**:282.

12 Baric I, Wagner L, Feyh P *et al.* Sensitivity and specificity of free and total glutaric acid and 3-hydroxyglutaric acid measurements by stable-isotope dilution assays for the diagnosis of glutaric aciduria type I. *J Inherit Metab Dis* 1999;**22**:867.

13 Gibson KM, Aramaki S, Sweetman L *et al.* Stable isotope dilution analysis of 4-hydroxybutyric acid: An accurate method for quantification in physiological fluids and the prenatal diagnosis of 4-hydroxybutyric aciduria. *Biomed Environ Mass Spectrom* 1990;**19**:89.

14 Abdenur JE, Aheling NG, van Crucha AC *et al.* Aromatic L-amino acid decarboxylase (AADC) deficiency: Unusual neonatal presentation and new findings in organic acid analysis (OA). *Am J Hum Genet* 2002;**71**:424.

15 Kumps A, Duez P, Mardens Y. Metabolic, nutritional, iatrogenic, and artifactual sources of urinary organic acids: a comprehensive table. *Clin Chem* 2002;**48**:708.

16 Treacy E, Pitt J, Eggington M, Hawkins R. Dicarboxylic aciduria, significance and prognostic indications. *Eur J Pediatr* 1994;**153**:918.

Propionic acidemia

MAJOR PHENOTYPIC EXPRESSION

Recurrent episodes of ketosis, acidosis and dehydration, progressive to coma; neutropenia, thrombocytopenia; osteoporosis; hyperglycinemia; propionic acidemia; methylcitraturia; and deficiency of propionyl CoA carboxylase.

INTRODUCTION

A patient with propionic acidemia was reported in 1961 [1] as having hyperglycinemia, a disorder of amino acid metabolism. Its most prominent feature was recurrent attacks of ketoacidosis. Analysis of the amino acids of blood and urine revealed very large quantities of glycine. Attacks were related to the intake of protein, and it was shown that ketonuria resulted regularly from the administration not of glycine, but of branched-chain amino acids and threonine and methionine [1,2]. The discovery of a group of patients with hyperglycinemia who had none of these characteristics led us to the term nonketotic hyperglycinemia (Chapter 27, p. 183) to distinguish them from the original group that we called ketotic hyperglycinemia. The discovery of methylmalonic acidemia in a group of patients who displayed the ketotic hyperglycinemia syndrome [3,4,5] led initially to the thought that all these patients had methylmalonic acidemia. However, study of our initial patient and his sister, by Rosenberg and colleagues [6], indicated that neither excreted methylmalonic acid, and that they had propionic acidemia as a result of defective activity of propionyl CoA carboxylase (Figure 2.1). This enzyme is the first step in the pathway of propionate metabolism in which propionyl CoA, the product of the metabolism of isoleucine, valine, threonine and methionine is converted to methylmalonyl CoA acid, then to succinyl CoA and oxidation in the citric acid cycle.

The enzyme is composed of 2 subunits, α and β in an $\alpha 4$ $\beta 4$ heteropolymeric complex. The apoenzyme is activated by the covalent binding of biotin to the ε amino group of lysine

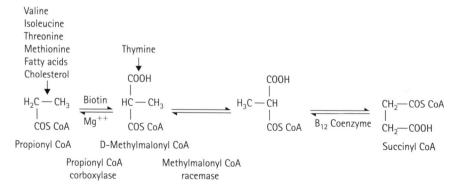

Figure 2.1 *Metabolism of propionic acid. Propionyl CoA carboxylase is the site of the defect in propionic acidemia.*

of the α subunit. cDNA clones have been isolated for the α and β genes [7]. The α gene is on chromosome 13 and the β gene on chromosome 3. The nature of a number of mutations has been defined [8–10].

CLINICAL ABNORMALITIES

Patients with propionic acidemia usually present first with life-threatening illness very early in life (Figure 2.2). Many patients, in fact most of those reported, have died in the course of one of these episodes of illness. Patients with metabolic disease, which presents this way in the neonatal period, may appear to have sepsis, ventricular hemorrhage or some other catastrophic process. It is likely that most patients die undiagnosed. A typical episode is heralded by ketonuria. The initial symptom is often vomiting, and some patients have had such impressive vomiting that they have been operated on with a diagnosis of pyloric stenosis [1,11,12]. Massive ketosis leads to acidosis and dehydration. Lethargy is progressive to coma. Unless the patient is treated vigorously, often with intubation, and assisted ventilation, as well as very large quantities of fluid and electrolytes (and often despite these efforts) the outcome is inevitably death [13]. Presentation of a gravely ill infant can be with hypothermia.

Ketotic episodes are recurrent. They often follow infection, and, furthermore, at least in infancy, the untreated patient appears to be unusually susceptible to infection. We have seen a number of patients in whom septicemia, especially with klebsiella, has been documented (Figure 2.2). Initial presentations in some patients may mimic an immunodeficiency disease. Episodes are also related to diet; patients are intolerant of the usual dietary quantities of protein. A recurrent pattern of illness follows admission to hospital, correction of acidosis and a period of no protein intake, after which the patient appears well. Feeding of the usual quantity of protein is reinitiated and the patient sent home, where ketosis recurs as soon as toxic quantities of intermediates have reaccumulated.

Clinical chemistry reveals dramatic acidosis during the acute episodes. Arterial pH values as low as 6.9 may be seen, and the serum bicarbonate maybe as low as 5 mEq/L or less. There is an anion gap. This to some extent reflects the propionic acidemia, and there is lactic acid accumulation as well, but most of the acidosis results from accumulation of 3-hydroxybutyrate and acetoacetate. Symptomatic hypoglycemia may occur.

Some neonatal presentations of propionic acidemia are with hyperammonemia and coma, suggesting a disorder of the urea cycle; ammonia levels well over 1000 μM are not unusual. Most other patients have typical ketoacidosis at this time, but some do not, making the differential diagnosis difficult. The presence of neutropenia and thrombocytopenia may provide a clue to the presence of an organic academia and some infants have pancytopenia (Figure 2.3). Amino acid analysis reveals the typical elevation of glycine, as well as of glutamine in the hyperammonemic patient. Interestingly, episodes of recurrent illness after infancy almost never lead to clinically significant elevation of ammonia.

Infants with propionic acidemia are impressively hypotonic, and this may lead to delay in achieving developmental milestones even in patients that are ultimately developmentally normal. Our initial patient was mentally retarded and microcephalic [14]. Many of these patients have been retarded [15,16]. Despite mild to moderate cognitive impairment, focal neurologic abnormalities appear to be rare [16]. Atrophy has

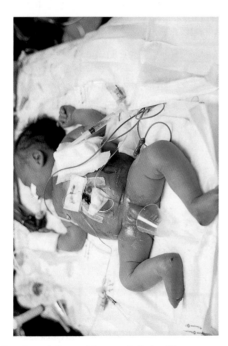

Figure 2.2   *C., an infant with overwhelming illness.*

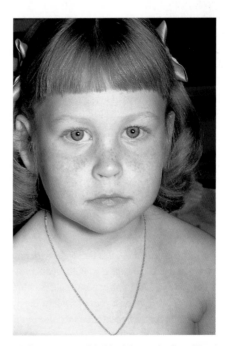

Figure 2.3   *L.S., a 4-year-old girl with propionic acidemia. Despite a neonatal presentation, she was 18 years old at most recent evaluation and was normal cognitively.*

been observed on MRI of the brain [16]. Seizures and abnormalities of the EEG have been observed, as has cerebral atrophy. Of 11 early onset patients reported by Surtees *et al* [17] all died; ages at death ranged from 6 days to 8 years. No patient had an IQ greater than 60. Among nine patients with later onset (6 weeks to 24 months) two died and all had IQs greater than 60.

We have thought that the cognitive and neurologic sequelae in this disease were more likely consequences of repeated overwhelming illness early in life, with attendant shock and diminished perfusion of the brain, than of the metabolic abnormality directly. This was consistent with experience with patients treated promptly and effectively who went on to develop normally into their teens (Figure 2.3) and with a few adult patients (Figure 2.4). The sister of the first patient was diagnosed prior to the development of any symptoms, and protein restriction was initiated immediately and carried out effectively [18]. Despite the occurrence of ketoacidosis with infection she developed normally and was intellectually fine at most recent report at over 30 years of age. Some of the patients of Surtees *et al* [17] were of normal intelligence. One was diagnosed presymptomatically because his brother, whose onset was at 13 months, had the disease, and the presymptomatically diagnosed brother was alive and of normal intelligence and neurologic examination at 1 year of age. Hyperammonemia

over 200 µM was found in four of the early onset group and only one of the late onset group, the brother of the presymptomatically diagnosed patient. Kuhara *et al* [19] reported an asymptomatic 15-year-old boy who had been diagnosed presymptomatically because of an affected sibling.

Nevertheless, a small population of patients with propionic acidemia have had a virtually exclusively neurologic presentation, sometimes without much ketoacidosis. Hypertonia may follow hypotonia or hypotonia may persist (Figure 2.5). Choreoathetosis and dystonic posturing have been observed. Deep tendon reflexes are exaggerated, and the Babinski response may be present.

In two patients with an exclusively neurologic presentation [20] the life-threatening episodes of ketoacidosis that usually serve as alerting signals were absent. In addition, hyperammonemia was prominent in late infancy in one and as late as 15 years in the other. Hypotonia, spastic quadriparesis and choreoathetosis were major manifestations. One patient displayed self-injurious behavior with mutilation of his lower lip (Figure 2.6). Choreoathetosis, pyramidal tract signs and dystonia have also been reported in other patients [19] including an infant who did not have ketoacidosis or hyperammonemia [21].

An infant who presented with a pure hyperammonemia picture without ketoacidosis is shown in Figure 2.7. MRI of the brain revealed extensive atrophy (Figure 2.8). An unusual patient [22] was diagnosed at 31 years of age after admission to a psychiatric hospital where he was admitted for bizarre behavior and studied further because of involuntary movements. We have observed MRI evidence of hypodense myelin, along with areas of increased signal in the basal ganglia [20]. We have also encountered a metabolic stroke in an 8-year-old

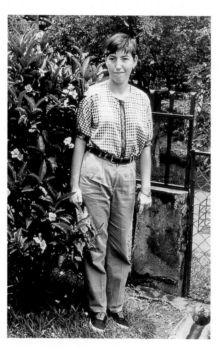

Figure 2.4 *K.Z., a 22-year-old Costa Rican girl with propionic acidemia. Two previous siblings had died with identical symptoms to those that she presented with in the early months of life. One sibling was operated on for pyloric stenosis, but at surgery, the pylorus was deemed normal. The patient's presentation included multiple episodes of metabolic ketoacidosis requiring admission to hospital following diagnosis at 2 years. There were no further admissions for acidotic imbalance. Since this picture was taken we have been informed that she died.*

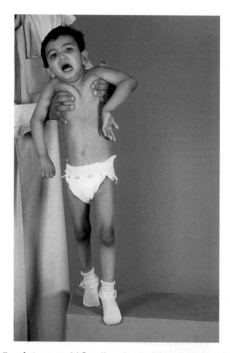

Figure 2.5 *A 4-year-old Saudi patient with propionic acidemia who was still impressively hypotonic.*

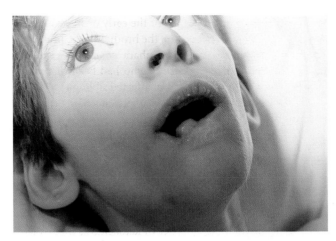

Figure 2.6   *A 20-year-old man with propionic acidemia who presented with severe impairment of cognitive function, spastic quadriparesis and a mutilated lip that led to his referral as a patient with Lesch-Nyhan disease. HPRT assay was normal and metabolic exploration led to the diagnosis.*

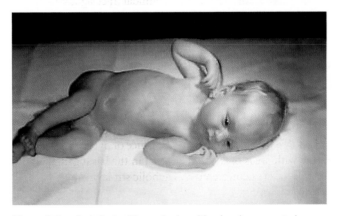

Figure 2.7   *An infant with propionic acidemia who presented acutely at 20 days of age in coma with a blood ammonia of 450 μmol/L and no ketoacidosis. A brother had died at 40 days after an identical clinical presentation.*

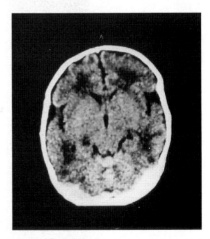

Figure 2.8   *MRI of the brain of the infant in Figure 2.7, illustrating extensive cerebral atrophy. (Illustration and Figure 2.8 were kindly provided by Dr. I. Baric of the University Hospital Center, Zagreb, Croatia.)*

patient with propionic acidemia in which there was virtually complete infarction of the basal ganglia followed by death [23,24]. We have been informed about a similar patient who did not die but remained in a vegetative state. A 15-year-old diagnosed neonatally suddenly developed a stroke of the basal ganglia from which he ultimately recovered [25]. Assessment of cerebral vessels showed no abnormality. Treatment with L-DOPA appeared to be beneficial.

Patients with propionic acidemia also regularly have neutropenia at the time of diagnosis. It is responsive to treatment and may reappear with recurrent metabolic imbalance. Transient thrombocytopenia is seen in infancy. Rarely there may be anemia [26]. These hematological effects mirror the effects of propionyl CoA on marrow cell development, and they respond to metabolic control. Chronic moniliasis occurs in this syndrome, as well as in methylmalonic acidemia. This problem reflects the effect of propionyl CoA on T cell number and function and particularly their response to candida [27,28]. Osteoporosis is a regular concomitant of this disease and may be so severe that pathological fractures occur [2]. Diminished bone density may be documented even in patients maintained in excellent metabolic control.

Acute and recurrent pancreatitis has been observed as a complication of this disease [23], as well as other organic acidemias. In these patients vomiting and abdominal pains are associated with elevated levels of amylase and lipase.

For reasons that are not clear patients have been observed who have no symptoms of disease, at least to the time of the report at teenage, despite documentation of virtually no enzyme activity and ascertainment through symptomatic siblings [19,29]. Infants with propionic acidemia tend to resemble each other and those with methylmalonic acidemia (Figure 2.9). Characteristic facial features are: frontal bossing; widened depressed nasal bridge, and an appearance of wide-set eyes; epicanthal folds, and a long filtrum with upward curvature of the lips. In addition, the nipples may be hypoplastic or inverted (Figure 2.10). Neuropathologic findings [30,31] in patients dying in the neonatal period have been those of spongy degeneration of the white matter. In patients dying later, abnormalities in the basal ganglia were prominent [24,30]. These included gross shrinkage and marbling, as well as microscopic neuronal loss and gliosis.

GENETICS AND PATHOGENESIS

Propionic acidemia is inherited as an autosomal recessive trait. The enzymatic site of the defect is propionyl CoA carboxylase [32,33]. Activity in the extracts of leukocytes and fibroblasts is very low, usually less than 5 percent of control (Table 2.1). Studies with somatic cell hybrids have provided evidence of two complementation groups, PccA and PccBC, which correspond to abnormalities in the α and β subunits, respectively [34–38]. The BC group contains two subgroups, B and C, in which intragroup complementation is thought to

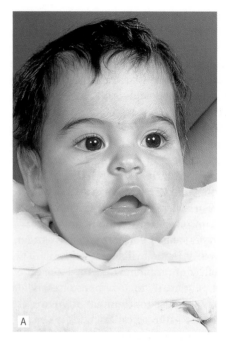

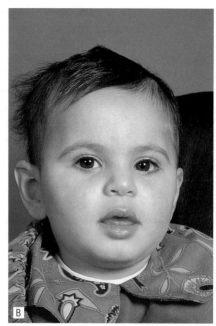

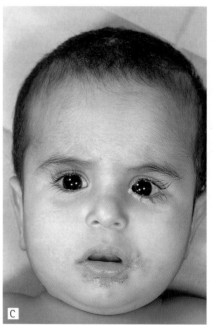

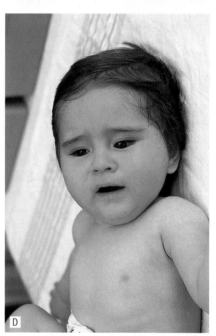

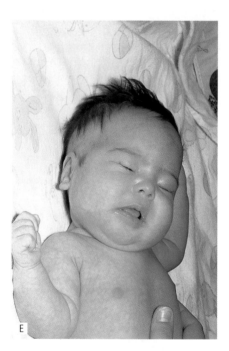

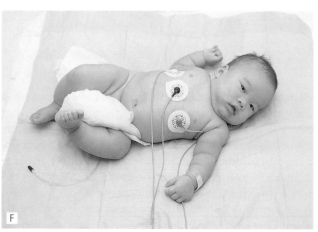

Figure 2.9   *(A–F). Faces of eight different patients with propionic acidemia. Similarities in facial appearance are evident despite considerable ethnic differences. The patients were: A–C, three Saudi Arabs, D and E, two Hispanics, and F, one Asian.*

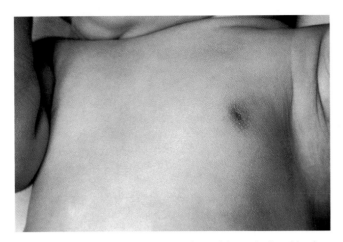

Figure 2.10   *Inverted nipples in a patient with propionic acidemia.*

Table 2.1   *Propionyl CoA carboxylase activity (pmol ^{14}C bicarbonate fixed/mg protein per minute) in patients with propionic acidemia*

	Lymphocytes	
	Normal	Patients
Mean (+/−SD)	232 (+/−87)	10 (+/−9)
(Range)	(160–447)	(0–36)
n	45	23
	Fibroblasts	
	Normal	Patients
Mean (+/−ISE)	294 (+/−94)	15 (+/−17)
(Range)	(128–537)	(0–51)
n	36	10

be interallelic. Patients in the A subgroup have mutations in the A gene for the α chain, and those in the BC groups have mutations in the B gene for the β chain.

Heterozygosity is not reliably determined by assay of the enzyme in cultured fibroblasts. A positive indicates heterozygosity, but a negative may not be consistent with its absence. Heterozygotes for the PccA group display approximately 50 percent of control activity of the enzyme, but those of the PccBC group are not distinguishable from normal [34].

Immunochemical assay of the PccA group has revealed many with little or no α chain of the enzyme [35] and other studies indicated an absence of α chain mRNA; these cells lack the β subunit which is thought to have been degraded while β chain mRNA was present [39]. This is consistent with the expression of 50 percent of activity in heterozygotes. Cells of the BC groups may contain immunoprecipitable α subunits but lack β subunits [40,41]. The normal activity in BC heterozygotes is thought to result from a five-fold greater synthesis of β subunits than α units. The amount of residual carboxylase activity measured in patients is thought to reflect the activity of other carboxylases on the substrate.

The cDNAs for the α [42,43] and β [44] subunits have been cloned, and the genes have been mapped, respectively, to chromosomes 13q32 [45] and 3q13.3-22 [46]. The tetrapeptide sequence, Ala-Met-Lys-Met in the amino acid sequence of the α chain deduced from the gene [7] appears to be a universal feature of the binding site of all carboxylases.

A number of mutations has been defined at the level of the DNA [10,44,47–49]. Among mutations in the A gene, nonsense and splicing mutations, which cause exon skipping and deletions, have led commonly to an absence of mRNA [50]. Among point mutations in this gene, abolition of biotin binding was common [51,52]. Among mutations in the B gene, there have been a number of missense mutations, such as C to T change, that changed an arginine at residue 410 of the β subunit to a tryptophan [48], which was common in Japanese patients; and an insertion/deletion (1218del14ins12) with a frame shift and a stop codon, that has been common in Caucasian cell lines studied [10,47]. A frequent mutation in Spanish patients was 1170insT [53]. However, the 1218del14ins12 was found in 31 percent of Spanish and 44 percent of Latin American alleles [9,53].

Prenatal diagnosis has been accomplished by measurement of activity of propionyl CoA carboxylase in cultured amniotic fluid cells [54] or chorionic villus cells [55] or fixation of ^{14}C propionate in amniocytes [56]. It is more rapidly accomplished by the direct gas chromatography/mass spectrometry (GC/MS) assay of methylcitric acid in amniotic fluid [57], a method which obviates the error always implicit in cell culture approaches – that those cells ultimately analyzed are maternal, not fetal [58]. It has also been accomplished by measurement of propionylcarnitine in amniotic fluid. In those families in which the mutation is known, it may be made by assay of the DNA, ideally with oligonucleotide probes.

There are a number of biochemical consequences of the defective activity of propionyl CoA carboxylase, many of which have direct relevance to the pathogenesis of the clinical manifestations of the disease. The immediately apparent consequence (Figure 2.1) is the inability to catabolize four essential amino acids: isoleucine, valine, threonine, and methionine. These amino acids are responsible for the toxicity of protein ingested in amounts greater than required for growth, and they were shown in the initial studies [1,2] to induce ketonuria when administered individually.

Patients with propionic acidemia have elevated concentrations of glycine in the blood and urine. This was the first of the biochemical abnormalities to be recognized [1]. It occurs along with abnormal ketogenesis, also in methylmalonic acidemia (Chapter 3), in isovaleric acidemia (Chapter 7), and in 3-oxothiolase deficiency (Chapter 17).

The mechanism of hyperglycinemia appears to be an inhibition by propionyl CoA of the synthesis of the glycine-cleaving enzyme leading to defective oxidation of glycine [59]. The hyperglycinemia of propionic acidemia is usually readily differentiated from nonketotic hyperglycinemia by the occurrence of episodes of ketosis. However, we have observed overwhelming illness without ketosis in a patient with propionic acidemia

[60]. It is for this reason that all hyperglycinemic infants should be assessed for a possible diagnosis of propionic acidemia before a diagnosis of nonketotic hyperglycinemia is made.

When propionyl CoA accumulates, other metabolic products are found in the blood and urine. The predominant compound is 3-hydroxypropionic acid; others include tiglic acid, tiglyglycine, butanone and propionylglycine. In addition, the unusual metabolite methylcitrate is formed by condensation of propionyl CoA and oxaloacetic acid [61]. This compound is an end product of metabolism and is very stable, resistant to conditions of shipment and bacterial contamination. In our hands, it is the most reliable chemical indicator of the presence of this disorder. It is useful in prenatal diagnosis as well as the initial diagnosis. Odd chain fatty acids may accumulate in body lipids as a consequence of synthesis from propionyl CoA. They may be demonstrated and quantified in erythrocytes [62]. 3-Ureidopropionate is found in the urine [63], a consequence of propionate inhibition of ureidopropionase. The manifestations of patients with inherited deficiency of this enzyme of pyrimidine metabolism are reminiscent of those of propionic acidemic patients with changes in the basal ganglia, and there is *in vitro* evidence that ureidopropionate is neurotoxic [64].

Abnormal ketogenesis is a major cause of morbidity and mortality in this disease. It could result from a variety of mechanisms. Propionic acid is an inhibitor of mitochondrial oxidation of succinic and α-ketoglutaric acid, and propionyl CoA is an inhibitor of succinate: CoA ligase, and malate dehydrogenase [65]. Carnitine prevents this, consistent with its role in therapy. Carnitine is depleted in these patients, because it forms the propionylcarnitine ester, which is excreted in the urine. Analysis for propionylcarnitine has also been used for diagnosis, and has been effectively explored in prenatal diagnosis [66]. The accumulation of propionyl CoA, and its condensation with oxalacetate to form methylcitrate depletes oxalacetate and so acetylCoA, deprived of substrate with which to condense to form citrate, condenses with itself to form acetoacetate.

The hyperammonemia observed in infants with propionic acidemia is a consequence of the inhibition of the urea cycle at the carbamylphosphate synthetase (CPS) step by propionyl CoA. This results from a competitive inhibition of N-acetylglutamate synthetase [67].

The obligatory biotin cofactor has led to the possibility that some patients with propionic acidemia are biotin responsive [68]. Nevertheless, no patient has been shown to be clinically responsive to biotin. Most patients whom we have tested by assessing the conversion of ^{13}C-propionate to [13]CO$_2$ *in vivo*, before and after biotin, have shown no evidence of response [69]. The one patient in whom there was a small response had no clinical response to a course of treatment with biotin.

TREATMENT

The cornerstone of treatment is the dietary restriction of the intake of all of those amino acids whose metabolism takes

them through propionyl CoA to the amounts that are required for growth and no more. We have provided these amino acids in the form of a standard cow milk formula whose amino acid content is known. We have made up the rest of the calories in fat and carbohydrate [70–72]. It is not necessary to supply a mixture of the other amino acids, although this approach has regularly been employed; it is certainly indicated if an individual amino acid becomes limiting. It is possible to manage such a patient by supplementing just that amino acid. Treatment must be monitored from time to time with quantitative assays of the relevant metabolites in the urine.

We also assess growth in weight, nitrogen balance and the concentrations of amino acids in blood. We aim for an intake of protein below that at which plateau levels of amino acids rise and above the levels required for positive nitrogen balance, and growth and height [72]. The quantification of urinary urea [73] is a useful adjunct to the therapy. It may be useful to monitor erythrocyte concentrations of odd chain fatty acids [74]. We teach our parents to test for ketones in the urine using ketostix. Ideally, the urine is tested daily in infancy. Thereafter, it can be done at intervals, with special attention to periods of intercurrent infection.

The addition of carnitine to the therapeutic management of infants with this disease has had a major impact on management [75–79]. Patients are all carnitine-depleted in the absence of treatment. Treatment increases the excretion of carnitine esters, which should promote detoxification. It also substantially reduces the propensity for ketogenesis as tested by fasting [79]. Concomitantly, it has seemed that our patients tolerate the catabolism of infection better, and require less frequent admission to hospital. Doses generally employed have been from 60 to 100 mg/kg, although ketogenesis is less with 200 mg/kg. Doses higher than this usually produce diarrhea, but, otherwise, toxicity has not been encountered. Much higher doses can be employed parenterally without producing diarrhea.

Experience has indicated that the anabolic properties of human growth hormone have decreased the propensity for catabolism in these patients [80]. Certainly there is improvement in growth, lean body mass and mineralization of bone, as well as decrease in adiposity.

The treatment of the acute episode of ketoacidosis requires vigorous attention to supportive therapy. We use very large amounts of parenteral fluid and electrolytes, along with high doses of intravenous carnitine (Table 2.2). Fasting has been demonstrated [81] to increase the excretion of urinary metabolites of propionate, presumably from the oxidation of odd chain fatty acids stored in lipid. Consistent with this, studies of sources of propionate in patients with propionic acid and methylmalonic acidemia by means of ^{13}C-propionate turnover [82] indicated about 30 percent of propionate production not accounted for, suggesting that this much might come from propionate stored in lipid. Data are not available for propionate turnover in infants and children not subjected to overnight fast, which these authors had shown to increase excretion of urinary metabolites of propionate. The avoidance of fasting is

Table 2.2 *Management of the acute episode of ketoacidosis in propionic acidemia*

	Intravenous		
Water mL/kg	NaHCO$_3$ mEq/L	Glucose %	Carnitine mg/kg
200	200	5	300

recommended in this disorder. This is also an argument for the inclusion of glucose in the infusion solution; larger amounts may be beneficial. In a conscious patient without intestinal intolerance, cornstarch or polycose by mouth or nasogastric tube may be useful.

Neonatal hyperammonemia may require treatment with intravenous sodium benzoate and or phenylacetate (Chapter 28), or hemodialysis. Parenteral mixtures of amino acids in which the concentration of isoleucine, valine, threonine and methionine are reduced or absent, may be useful, especially in the patient with intestinal abnormalities [83]. Insulin may be a useful adjunct [84]. The efficacy of growth hormone in the acute episode has not been assessed. As the serum concentration of bicarbonate returns to normal the concentration in the infusion fluid may be gradually reduced.

Studies of propionate production before and after treatment with metronidazole in three patients with propionic acidemia and three with methylmalonic acidemia [82] indicated that a mean of 22 percent could be attributed to formation of propionate by intestinal bacteria. However, the data were quite variable. In the patient with methylmalonic acidemia with the lowest level of methylmalonate excretion in the urine, the excretion after metronidazole was little changed, and the propionate turnover changed only from 46 to 41 μmol/kg/hr, which does not seem significant. Similarly, these authors reported an average reduction of excretion of propionate metabolites of 41 percent in nine patients with disorders of propionate metabolism treated with metronidazole [85].

In our experience, results have been quite variable as measured by change in metabolite excretion following treatment with oral neomycin or metronidazole even in the same patient, suggesting that the intestine may be colonized by varying clones or groups of organisms, which do or do not make propionate. The reported [85] data are consistent with this in that two patients with low levels of metabolites excreted had barely appreciable changes after metronidazole from 1.9 to 1.6 μmol/kg/hr total metabolites and 4.0 to 2.9 even thought the percentage decreases were 16 and 29 percent. A trial of antibiotic treatment is always worthwhile, and it is especially indicated by a change in excretion in a patient whose pattern is well known. We prefer to start with neomycin because it is not absorbed. We have used a dose of 50 mg/kg. Metronidazole has been used in doses of 10 to 20 mg/kg.

Transplantation of the liver has been employed in propionic acidemia [86–87]. As overall results of the procedure in children have improved, the results in propionic acidemia

have become more encouraging. The metabolic abnormality is not corrected but there may be a five-fold decrease in methylcitrate excretion, and there may be a major reduction in propensity to ketoacidosis.

References

1. Childs B, Nyhan WL, Borden MA, *et al*. Idiopathic hyperglycinemia and hyperglycinuria, a new disorder of amino acid metabolism. *Pediatrics* 1961;**27**:522.
2. Childs B, Nyhan WL. Further observations of a patient with hyperglycinemia. *Pediatrics* 1964;**33**:403.
3. Oberholzer VC, Levin B, Burgess EA, Young WF. Methylmalonic aciduria: An inborn error of metabolism leading to chronic metabolic acidosis. *Arch Dis Child* 1967;**42**:492.
4. Stokke O, Eldjarn L, Norum KR, *et al*. Methylmalonic aciduria: A new inborn error of metabolism which may cause fatal acidosis in the neonatal period. *Scand J Clin Lab Invest* 1967;**20**:313.
5. Rosenberg LE, Lilljeqvist A-C, Hsia YE. Methylmalonic aciduria: An inborn error leading to metabolic acidosis, long-chain ketonuria and intermittent hyperemia. *N Eng J Med* 1968;**278**:1319.
6. Hsia YE, Scully KJ, Rosenberg LE. Defective propionate carboxylation in ketotic hyperglycinaemia. *Lancet* 1969;**1**:757.
7. Lamhonwah A-M, Barankiewicz TJ, Willard HF, *et al*. Isolation of cDNA clones coding for the α and β chains of human propionyl-CoA carboxylase: Chromosomal assignments and DNA polymorphisms associated with PCCA and PCCB genes. *Proc Natl Acad Sci USA* 1986;**83**:4864.
8. Richard E, Desviat LR, Perez-Cerda C, Ugarte M. Three novel splice mutations in the PCCA gene causing identical exon skipping in propionic acidemia patients. *Hum Genet* 1997;**101**:93.
9. Rodriguez-Pombo P, Hoenicka J, Muro S, *et al*. Human propionyl-CoA carboxylase beta subunit gene–Exon-intron definition and mutation spectrum in Spanish and Latin American propionic acidemia. *Am J Hum Genet* 1998;**63**:360.
10. Lamhonwah AM, Troxel CE, Schuster S, Gravel RA. Two distinct mutations at the same site in the PCCB gene in propionic acidemia. *Genomics* 1990;**8**:249.
11. Nyhan WL. Patterns of clinical expression and genetic variation in inborn errors of metabolism, in *Heritable Disorders of Amino Acid Metabolism*, (ed. WL Nyhan), J Wiley & Sons, New York;1974:3–14.
12. Nyhan WL. Introduction, in *Abnormalities in Amino Acid Metabolism in Clinical Medicine* (ed. WL Nyhan), Appleton-Century-Crofts, E. Norwalk, CT;1984:3–18.
13. Hommes FA, Kuipers JRG, Elema JD, *et al*. Propionic acidemia, a new inborn errors of metabolism. *Pediatr Res* 1968;**2**:519.
14. Nyhan WL, Sakati NA. Propionic acidemia, in *Diagnostic Recognition of Genetic Disease* (eds WL Nyhan and NA Sakati), Lea & Febiger, Philadelphia;1987:36–41.
15. Wolf B, Hsia YE, Sweetman L, *et al*. Propionic acidemia: A clinical update *J Pediatr* 1981;**99**:835.
16. North KN, Korson MS, Gopal YR, *et al*. Neonatal-onset propionic acidemia; Neurologic and developmental profiles, and implications for management. *J Pediatr* 1995;**126**:916.
17. Surtees RAH, Matthews EE, Leonard JV. Neurologic outcome of propionic acidemia. *Ped Neurol* 1992;**8**:333.
18. Brandt IK, Hsia YE, Clement DH, Provence SA. Propionic acidemia (ketotic hyperglycinemia): Dietary treatment results in normal growth and development. *Pediatrics* 1974;**53**:391.
19. Kuhara T, Inoue Y, Matsumoto I. Urinary acid profiles of asymptomatic propionyl CoA carboxylase deficiency. *J Pediat* 1988;**113**:787.

20 Nyhan W, Bay C, Webb E, *et al.* Neurologic nonmetabolic presentation of propionic acidemia. *Arch Neurol* 1999;**56**:1143.

21 Ozand PT, Rashed M, Gascon GG, *et al.* Unusual presentations of propionic acidemia. *Brain Dev* 1994;**16**:(suppl) 46.

22 Sethi KD, Ray R, Roesel RA, *et al.* Adult-onset chorea and dementia with propionic acidemia. *Neurology* 1992;**39**:1343.

23 Haas RH, Marsden DL, Capistrano-Estrado S, *et al.* Acute basal ganglia infarction in propionic acidemia. *J Child Neurol* 1995;**10**:18.

24 Hamilton RL, Haas RH, Nyhan WL, *et al.* Neuropathology of propionic acidemia: A report of two patients with basal ganglia lesions. *J Child Neurol* 1995;**10**:25.

25 Burlina AP, Baracchini C, Carollo C, Burlina AB. Propionic acidaemia with basal ganglia stroke: Treatment of acute extrapyramidal symptoms with L-DOPA. *J Inherit Metab Dis* 2001;**24**:596.

26 Sweetman L, Nyhan WL, Cravens J, *et al.* Propionic acidaemia presenting with pancytopenia in infancy. *J Inherit Metab Dis* 1979;**2**:65.

27 Yu A, Sweetman L, Nyhan WL. The pathogenetic mechanism of recurrent mucocutaneous candidiasis in a patient with methylmalonic acidemia (MMA). *Clin Res* 1981;**29**:124A.

28 Muller S, Falkenberg N, Monch E, Jakobs C. Propionic acidemia and immune deficiency. *Lancet* 1980;**1**:551.

29 Wolf B, Paulsen EP, Hsia YE. Asymptomatic propionyl CoA carboxylase deficiency in a 13-year-old girl. *J Pediatr* 1979;**95**:563.

30 Harding BD, Leonard JV, Erdohazi M. Propionic acidaemia: a neuropathological study of two patients presenting in infancy. *Neuropathol Appl Neurobiol* 1991;**17**:133.

31 Nyhan WL, Chisolm JJ, Edwards RO. Idiopathic hyperglycinemia III Report of a second case. *J Pediatr* 1963;**62**:540.

32 Hsia YE, Scully KJ, Rosenberg LE. Human propionyl CoA carboxylase: Some properties of the partially purified enzyme in fibroblasts from controls and patients with propionic acidemia. *Pediatr Res* 1979;**13**:746.

33 Wolf B, Hsia YE, Rosenberg LE. Biochemical differences between mutant propionyl-CoA carboxylases from two complementation groups. *Am J Hum Genet* 1978;**30**:455.

34 Wolf B Rosenberg LE. Heterozygote expression in propionyl coenzyme A carboxylase deficiency: Differences between major complementation groups. *J Clin Invest* 1978;**62**:931.

35 Saunders M, Sweetman L, Robinson B, *et al.* Biotin-responsive organic aciduria: Multiple carboxylase defects and complementation studies with propionic acidemia in cultured fibroblasts. *J Clin Invest* 1979;**64**:1695.

36 Gravel RA, Lam KF, Scully KJ, Hsia YE. Genetic complementation of propionyl-CoA carboxylase deficiency in cultured human fibroblasts. *Am J Hum Genet* 1977;**29**:378.

37 Wolf B, Willard HF, Rosenberg LE. Kinetic analysis of genetic complementation in heterokaryons of propionyl-CoA carboxylase-deficient human fibroblasts. *Am J Hum Genet* 1980;**32**:16.

38 Lamhonwah AM, Lam KF, Tsui F, *et al.* Assignment of the α and β chains of human propionyl-CoA carboxylase to genetic complementation groups. *Am J Hum Genet* 1983;**35**:889.

39 Lamhonwah AM, Gravel RA. Propionic-acidemia: Absence of alpha chain mRNA in fibroblasts from patients of the pccA complementation group. *Am J Hum Genet* 1987;**41**:1124.

40 Kalousek F, Orsulak MD, Rosenberg LE. Absence of cross reacting material in isolated propionyl CoA carboxylase deficiency: Nature of residual carboxylating activity. *Am J Hum Genet* 1983;**35**:409.

41 Ohura T, Kraus JP, Rosenberg LE. Unequal synthesis and differential degradation of propionyl-CoA carboxylase subunits in cells from normal and propionic acidemia patients. *Am J Hum Genet* 1989;**45**:33.

42 Lamhonwah AM, Mahuran D, Gravel RA. Human mitochondrial propionyl-CoA carboxylase: Localization of the N-terminus of the pro- and mature

α chains in the deduced primary sequence of a full length cDNA. *Nucleic Acids Res* 1989;**17**:4396.

43 Stankovics J, Ledley FD. Cloning of functional alpha propionyl-CoA carboxylase and correction of enzyme deficiency in pccA fibroblasts. *Am J Hum Genet* 1993;**52**:144.

44 Ohura T, Ogasawara M, Ikeda H, *et al.* The molecular defect in propionic acidemia: exon skipping cause by an 8-bp deletion from an intron in the PCCB allele. *Hum Genet* 1993;**92**:397.

45 Kennerknecht I, Suormala T, Barbi G, Baumgartner ER. The gene coding for the alpha-chain of human propionyl-CoA carboxylase maps to chromosome band 13q32. *Hum Genet* 1990;**86**:238.

46 Kraus JP, Williamson CL, Firgaira FA, *et al.* Cloning and screening with nanogram amounts of immunopurified mRNAs: cDNA cloning and chromosomal mapping of cystathionine beta-synthase and the beta subunit of propionyl-CoA carboxylase. *Proc Natl Acad Sci USA* 1986;**83**:2047.

47 Tahara T, Kraus JP, Rosenberg LE. An unusual insertion/deletion in the gene encoding the beta-subunit of propionyl-CoA carboxylase is a frequent mutation in Caucasian propionic acidemia. *Proc Natl Acad Sci USA* 1990;**87**:1372.

48 Tahara T, Kraus JP, Ohura T, *et al.* Three independent mutations in the same exon of the PCCB gene: Differences between Caucasian and Japanese propionic acidemia. *J Inherit Metab Dis* 1993;**16**:353.

49 Ohura T, Miyabashi S, Narisawa K, Tada K. Genetic heterogeneity of propionic acidemia: analysis of Japanese patients. *Hum Genet* 1991;**87**:41.

50 Campeau E, Dupuis L, Leclere D, Gravel RA. Detection of a normally rare transcript in propionic acidemia patients with mRNA destabilizing mutations in the PCCA gene. *Hum Mol Genet* 1999;**8**:107.

51 Campeau E, Dupuis L, Leon-del-Rio A, Gravel R. Coding sequence mutations in the alpha subunit of propionyl-CoA carboxylase in patients with propionic acidemia. *Mol Genet Metab* 1999;**67**:1.

52 Leon-del-Rio A, Gravel RA. Sequence requirements for the biotinylation of carboxyl-terminal fragments of human propionyl-CoA carboxylase alpha subunit expressed in *Escherichia coli*. *J Biol Chem* 1994;**269**:22964.

53 Hoenicka J, Muro J, Rodriguez-Pombo P, *et al.* Prevalence of the novel mutation A497V in the PCCB gene in spanish propionic acidemia patients from a small village. *Medizinesche Genetik* 1997;**9**:4311.

54 Gompertz D, Goodey PA, Thom H, *et al.* Prenatal diagnosis and family studies in case of propionic acidemia. *Clin Genet* 1975;**8**:244.

55 Sweetman FR, Gibson KM, Sweetman L, Nyhan WL. Activity of biotin-dependent and GABA metabolizing enzymes in chorionic villus samples: Potential for 1st trimester prenatal diagnosis. *Prenat Diagn* 1986;**6**:187.

56 Willard HF, Ambani LM, Hart AC, *et al.* Rapid prenatal and postnatal detection of inborn errors of propionate, methylmalonate, and cobalamin metabolism: A sensitive assay using cultured cells. *Hum Genet* 1976;**34**:277.

57 Naylor G, Sweetman L, Nyhan WL, *et al.* Isotope dilution analysis of methylcitric acid in amniotic fluid for the prenatal diagnosis of propionic and methylmalonic acidemia. *Clin Chim Acta* 1980;**107**:175.

58 Buchanan PD, Kahler SG, Sweetman L, Nyhan WL. Pitfalls in the prenatal diagnosis of propionic acidemia. *Clin Genet* 1980;**18**:177.

59 Hillman RE, Sowers LH, Cohen JL. Inhibition of glycine oxidation in cultured fibroblasts by isoleucine. *Pediatr Res* 1973;**7**:945.

60 Wadlington WB, Kilroy A, Ando T, *et al.* Hyperglycinemia and propionyl CoA carboxylase deficiency and episodic severe illness without consistent ketosis. *J Pediatr* 1975;**86**:707.

61 Ando T, Rasmussen K, Wright M, Nyhan WL. Isolation and identification of methylcitrate, a major metabolic product of propionate in patients with propionic acidemia. *J Biol Chem* 1972;**247**:2200.

62 Wendel U, Eissler A, Sperl W, Schadewaldt P. On the differences between urinary metabolite excretion and odd-numbered fatty acid production

in propionic and methylmalonic acidaemias. *J Inherit Metab Dis* 1995;**18**:584.

63 Van Gennip AH, Van Lenthe H, Abeling NGGM, *et al.* Inhibition of β-ureidopropionase by propionate may contribute to neurological complications in patients with propionic acidemia. *J Inher Metab Dis* 1997;**20**:379.

64 Kolker S, Okun JG, Horster F, *et al.* 3-Ureidopropionate contributes to the neuropathology of 3-ureidopropionase deficiency and severe propionic aciduria: a hypothesis. *J Neurosci Res* 2001;**66**:666.

65 Stumpf DA, McAfee J, Parks JK, Equren L. Propionate inhibition of succinate: CoA ligase (GDP) and the citric acid cycle in mitochondria. *Pediatr Res* 1980;**14**:1127.

66 Van Hove JLK, Chace DH, Kahler SG, Millington DS. Acylcarnitines in amniotic fluid: Application to the prenatal diagnosis of propionic acidaemia. *J Inherit Metab Dis* 1993;**16**:361.

67 Coude FX, Sweetman L, Nyhan WL. Inhibition by propionyl CoA of N-acetylglutamate synthetase in rat liver mitochondria. *J Clin Invest* 1979;**64**:1544.

68 Barnes ND, Hull D, Balgobin L, Gompertz D. Biotin-responsive propionic acidemia. *Lancet* 1970;**2**:244.

69 Barshop BA, Yoshida I, Ajami A, *et al.* Metabolism of 1-^{13}C-propionate in vivo in patients with disorders of propionate metabolism. *Pediatr Res* 1991;**30**:15.

70 Nyhan WL, Fawcett N, Ando T, *et al.* Response to dietary therapy in B$_{12}$ unresponsive methylmalonic acidemia. *Pediatrics* 1973;**51**:539.

71 Ney DN, Bay C, Saudubray JM, *et al.* An evaluation of protein requirements in methylmalonic acidaemia. *J Inher Metab Dis* 1985;**8**:132.

72 Nyhan WL. Disorders of propionate metabolism. In *Inherited Diseases of Amino Acid Metabolism. Recent Progress in the Understanding, Recognition and Management, International Symposium on Heidelberg, 1984.* (eds H Bickel and U Wachtel), Georg Thiem Verlag Thieme, Inc., Stuttgart/New York, 1985:363–82.

73 Saudubray JM. Use of new diagnostic technology in the management of inborn errors of metabolism, in *Proc. V1 International Congress of Inborn Errors of Metabolism (Milan, Italy),* 1994:28.

74 Wendel U, Baumgartner RE, Van Der Meer SB, Spaapen LJM. Accumulation of odd-numbered long chain fatty acids in fetuses and neonates with inherited disorders of propionate metabolism. *Pediatr Res* 1991;**29**:403.

75 Roe CR, Bohan TP. L-carnitine therapy in propionic acidemia. *Lancet* 1982;**1**:1411.

76 Chalmers RA, Roe CR, Stacey TE, Hoppel CL. Urinary excretion of L-carnitine and acylcarnitines by patients with disorders of organic acid metabolism: evidence for secondary insufficiency of L-carnitine. *Pediatr Res* 1984;**18**:1325.

77 Roe CR, Hoppel CL, Stacey TE, *et al.* Metabolic response to carnitine in methylmalonic aciduria: An effective strategy for elimination of propionyl groups. *Arch Dis Child* 1983;**58**:916.

78 Roe CR, Millington DS, Maltby DA, *et al.* L-carnitine enhances excretion of propionyl coenzyme A as propionyl carnitine in propionic acidemia. *J Clin Invest* 1984;**73**:1785.

79 Wolf JA, Thuy LP, Haas R, *et al.* Carnitine reduces fasting ketogenesis in patients with disorders of propionate metabolism. *Lancet* 1986;**1**:289.

80 Marsden D, Barshop BA, Capistrano-Estrada S, *et al.* Anabolic effect of human growth hormone: management of inherited disorders of catabolic pathways. *Biochem Med Metab Biol* 1994;**52**:145.

81 Thompson GN, Chalmers RA. Increased urinary metabolite excretion during fasting in disorders of propionate metabolism. *Pediatr Res* 1990;**27**:413.

82 Thompson GN, Walter JH, Bresson JL, *et al.* Sources of propionate in inborn errors of metabolism. *Metabolism* 1990;**39**:1133.

83 Nyhan WL, Rice-Asaro M, Acosta P. Advances in the treatment of amino acid and organic acid disorders, in *Treatment of Genetic Diseases,* Desnick RJ (ed. RJ Desnick), Churchill Livingstone, New York, 1991:45–67.

84 Kalloghlian A, Gleispach H, Ozand PT. A patient with propionic acidemia managed with continuous insulin infusion and total parenteral nutrition. *J Child Neurol* 1992;**7** Suppl:S88.

85 Thompson GN, Chalmers RA, Walter JH, *et al.* The use of metronidazole in management of methylmalonic and propionic acidaemias. *Eur J Pediatr* 1990;**149**:792.

86 Kuhara T. Diagnosis of inborn errors of metabolism using filter paper urine, urease treatment, isotope dilution and gas chromatography–mass spectrometry. *J Chromatogr B:Biomed Sci Appl* 2001;**758**:3.

87 Leonard JV, Walter JH, McKiernan PJ. The management of organic acidaemias: The role of transplantation. *J Inherit Metab Dis* 2001;**24**:309.

Methylmalonic acidemia

MAJOR PHENOTYPIC EXPRESSION

Recurrent episodes of ketosis, acidosis, vomiting, and dehydration; anorexia, failure to thrive; hepatomegaly; osteoporosis; neutropenia; thrombocytopenia; hyperglycinemia; elevated concentrations of methylmalonic acid (MMA) in blood and urine; and defective activity of methylmalonyl CoA mutase.

INTRODUCTION

Methylmalonic acidemia represents a family of disorders of the metabolism of branched-chain amino acids in which the activity of methylmalonyl CoA mutase is defective (Figure 3.1). Patients with the inborn error of metabolism were first reported in 1967 by Oberholzer [1] and by Stokke [2] and their colleagues. In 1968, Rosenberg and colleagues [3] first clearly distinguished these patients from those with propionic acidemia (Chapter 2), in whom the clinical presentation is often virtually identical.

Genetic heterogeneity was evident early in the demonstration in that some patients with methylmalonic acidemia were responsive to large doses of vitamin B_{12} while some others were not [4]. The methylmalonyl CoA mutase enzyme has a vitamin B_{12}-derived cofactor, 5'-deoxyadenosylcobalamin. Patients who are B_{12}-responsive clinically have defects in the synthesis of the cofactor. Unresponsive patients have defects in the apoenzyme itself. Complementation studies have indicated the presence of distinct groups (Figure 3.1). Those with apoenzyme defects have been designated mut^- or mut^0 depending on whether they have little or no residual mutase activity. Groups A and B represent defects in 5'-deoxyadenosylcobalamin synthesis. A differential diagnosis of methylmalonic acidemia is shown in Table 3.1.

The cobalamin (Cbl) C and D represent a different type of disorder in which methylmalonic acidemia accompanies elevated concentrations of homocystine and cystathionine in blood and urine [5] (Chapter 4). In these groups defective remethylation of homocysteine to methionine is the consequence of a failure to transform B_{12} to either of the coenzymatically active derivatives, deoxyadenosylcobalamin or methylcobalamin. Cobalamin F disease reflects abnormalities in the transport of cobalamin out of lysosomes, analogous to the defect that causes cystinosis (Chapter 71). Methylmalonic aciduria is also seen in acquired deficiency of B_{12} [6], in pernicious anemia and in transcobalamin II deficiency [7]. In B_{12} deficiency and in intrinsic factor deficiency, the excretion of methylmalonic acid in the urine is a more reliable index of depletion of body stores of cobalamin than the blood level of B_{12}.

All of the methylmalonic acidemias reflect defective activity of methylmalonyl CoA mutase [8]. In inherited defects of the apoenzyme and in abnormalities in coenzyme synthesis, the enzymatic mutase abnormality is evident in tissues, leukocytes and cultured fibroblasts. The gene has been cloned [9] and mapped to chromosome 6 [10].

CLINICAL ABNORMALITIES

Patients with methylmalonic acidemia usually present first with a typical organic acidemia picture of overwhelming illness very early in life [1–3,11–14]. A majority of the reported patients,

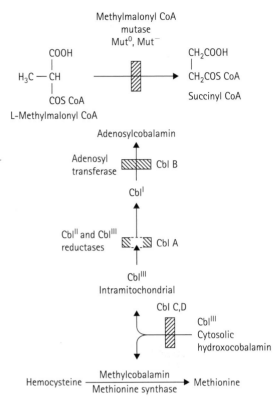

Figure 3.1 *Methylmalonyl CoA mutase, the site of the defect in methylmalonic aciduria. Cobalamin cofactor synthesis is also illustrated in the formation of deoxyadenosylcobalamin, the cofactor for the mutase enzyme and methylcobalamin, the cofactor for methionine synthase. The sites of the defects in the various complementation groups identified are shown as Cbl A, B, and C, D. Mut⁰ represent apoenzyme defects.*

Table 3.1 *Different types of methylmalonic acidemia*

Methylmalonyl CoA mutase deficiency (mut⁰, mut⁻)
Adenosyltransferase deficiency (Cbl B)
Reductase deficiency (Cbl A)
Homocystinuria with methylmalonic acidemia (MMA) (Cbl C, D) (Chapter 4)
B_{12} deficiency (vegan mother – breast feeding) (vegan child)
Pernicious anemia (intrinsic factor deficiency)
Transcobalamin II deficiency
B_{12} transport from lysosome defect (Cbl F)

especially those with apoenzyme defects, have died in such an episode. We believe that many patients die with the disease unrecognized, and that the disease is more common than realized. A typical episode is ushered in with ketonuria and vomiting, followed by acidosis, dehydration and lethargy, leading, in the absence of aggressive treatment, to coma and death.

Episodes of acute illness are recurrent. They may follow even minor infections. Furthermore patients are unusually prone to infection. Episodes are also a consequence of feeding: these patients are intolerant of the usual quantities of dietary protein. More specifically they are intolerant to the amino acids isoleucine, valine, threonine and methionine, all

of which are catabolized through the pathway of propionate and methylmalonate metabolism (see Figure 2.1). Episodic disease may follow a pattern in which the patient is admitted to hospital in extremis, treated vigorously with parenteral fluid and electrolytes, which leads to recovery; oral feedings are reintroduced and, following a sufficient time of ingestion of the usual dietary amounts of protein, another episode of crisis supervenes, and in one of these episodes the patient dies.

During episodes of ketosis, acidosis may be extreme. Arterial pH values as low as 6.9 have been recorded, and the serum bicarbonate is often 5 mEq/L, or less. Ketosis is massive. Hypoglycemia has been observed and has led to seizures during acute episodes [14]. Elevated concentrations of glycine in the blood and urine may be striking, and this may be an early clue to the diagnosis. Concentrations of glycine as high as 1500 μol/L have been observed in the plasma. However, concentrations of glycine may also be normal, even in the same patient. Hyperammonemia may complicate the initial episode in which levels may be as high as in urea cycle defects and lead to deep coma and apnea [15,16]. With development, this propensity to hyperammonemia is lost, and acute episodes after the first year are seldom complicated by hyperammonemia [15].

Failure to thrive may be the initial presentation in this disease, and failure of linear growth may be striking (Figures 3.2–3.4). Developmental failure may parallel the inability to increase weight, height and head circumference. Anorexia is severe, and usually requires tube feeding (Figure 3.3). In addition to the fact that the ketoacidotic episode is often ushered in with vomiting, these patients vomit frequently in infancy, and this may contribute to failure to thrive.

A variety of skin lesions may be seen (Figure 3.5). Most often this is a manifestation of moniliasis. Mucocutaneous moniliasis may also be reflected in cracking and erythema at the angles of the mouth and the eyes [17] (Figure 3.3).

Patients with methylmalonic acidemia have a striking resemblance to each other, especially in infancy (Figure 3.6). The characteristic face includes a high forehead, broad nasal bridge, epicanthal folds, a long smooth filtrum and a triangular mouth. A few have had other minor anomalies [14]. A recent patient of ours had inverted nipples. A patient reported [18] had multiple defects at birth including cardiac septal defects, hydronephrosis and an appearance of Sotos syndrome.

Neurological manifestations of methylmalonic acidemia are varied. In infancy and childhood these features appear to be more consequences of the physiology of the acute episode of shock and diminished cerebral perfusion or hypoglycemia, and especially hyperammonemia with or without cerebral edema, than the metabolic abnormality itself [19]. Developmental retardation is evident in most patients in infancy, but in some this may be more apparent than real evidence of severe chronic disease and extreme hypotonia, both of which interfere with motor development. Catch-up has been observed in patients successfully treated, and the IQ may be normal [14,19].

Neurological abnormality is more common in patients with apoenzyme defects than those with defects in cobalamin synthesis [20,21,22]; however, abnormalities in central nervous

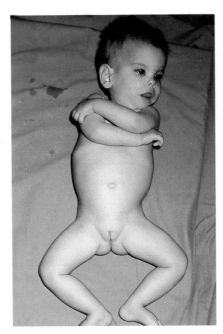

Figure 3.2   *L.G., a 14-month-old girl with methylmalonic acidemia. The size, that of a 3-month-old infant, reflects the severe failure to thrive characteristic of this disorder. The frog-leg position illustrates the marked hypotonia.*

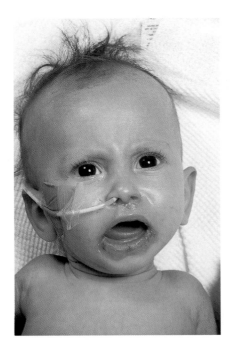

Figure 3.4   *This infant with methylmalonic acidemia had also failed to thrive and was anorexic. She also had alopecia.*

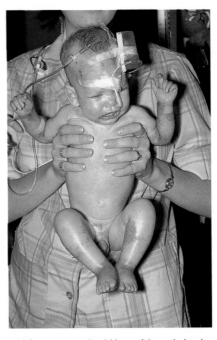

Figure 3.3   *M.E., a 13-month-old boy with methylmalonyl CoA mutase deficiency who also failed to gain in weight, height, or head circumference since 3 months of age. The nasogastric tube is typical, indicating the extreme anorexia. The bright red erythematous lesions are the characteristic monilial infection of the infant in poor metabolic control.*

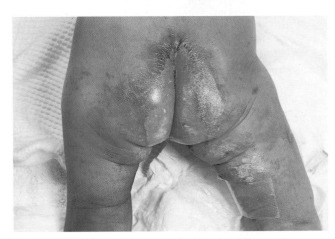

Figure 3.5   *The same infant had a florid perineal dermatitis.*

system function may be seen in any patient with methylmalonic acidemia (Figures 3.7–3.9). Dystonia and weakness profound enough to lead to a wheelchair-bound state has been observed in methylmalonic acidemia [23]. This has been

associated with neuroradiologic evidence of abnormality in the basal ganglia, which has frequently been encountered in disorders of propionate metabolism [24–26]. In patients imaged by computerized tomography (CT) or magnetic resonance imaging (MRI), specific lesions are regularly seen in the basal ganglia (Figures 3.8–3.9) [24–29], even in patients with no relevant clinical findings. Lesions in the globus pallidus are regularly seen in mut^0 and mut^- patients, but they are also seen in cobalamin-responsive patients [24–30]. At the extreme a syndrome of metabolic stroke has been reported with what looks like infarction of the basal ganglia, especially the globus pallidus, and acute dystonia [23,25,31]. Decreased white matter attenuation on CT and high T2 signal on MRI may be seen early [23,30,32]. This may progress to cerebral atrophy and spastic quadriparesis [23]. Some patients have had convulsions, and abnormalities of the electroencephalogram

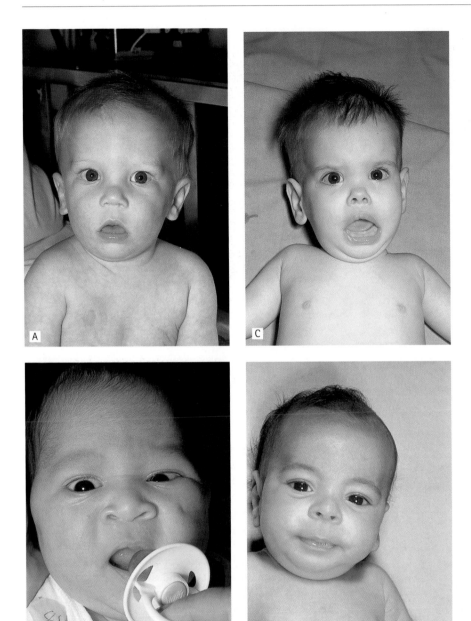

Figure 3.6   *A, B, C, and D: Composite picture of four patients with methylmalonic acidemia highlighting the similarity of the facial features. A high forehead, broad nasal bridge and wide-appearing eyes with epicanthal folds and a long smooth filtrum were characteristic. In some the nose was upturned. In some the mouth is triangular. The patient in 3.6 (C) had had a preauricular skin tag which was removed.*

(EEG) are more common [12,23]. In one patient, who died at six days of age with hyperammonemic coma and ketoacidosis, there was a burst suppression pattern [33]. Neuropathology in this patient revealed diffuse gliosis in the white matter, Alzheimer type II cells, and cerebellar hemorrhage.

In some patients abnormal neurologic signs increased with age [22,23]. Among patients surviving longer, late effects, including central nervous system abnormalities are becoming apparent [22]. We have reported a mut^0 young adult who developed weakness in her teens and became wheelchair-bound. She had acute involuntary spasms of the legs and more general spasms resembling myochymia. Cognitive function was not impaired. Among late effects, blindness developed in a 21-year-old two months before he died; he had been in a wheelchair but rode horses and could drive a yacht and farm equipment before developing optic atrophy [34].

Some patients have hepatomegaly. Liver function tests are normal. Renal functional impairment has been reported [1], and we have observed chronic renal tubular acidosis [35]. Hyperuricemia is usually present, a consequence of competition for its renal tubular excretion. Urate nephropathy and renal failure have been reported [36]. Tubulointerstitial nephritis has

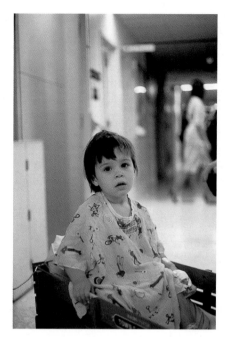

Figure 3.7 *T.J., a boy with B₁₂-responsive methylmalonic acidemia of the cbl A type. He had only the initial severe acidotic episode, but his behavior was sufficiently unusual that he had been characterized as autistic.*

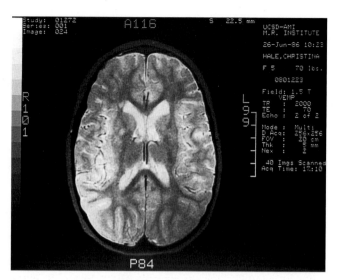

Figure 3.9 *MRI scan of C.H., a patient with methylmalonyl CoA mutase deficiency. There was a diffuse pattern of abnormal signal intensity in the cerebral hemispheres and focal areas of abnormal signal in the basal ganglia.*

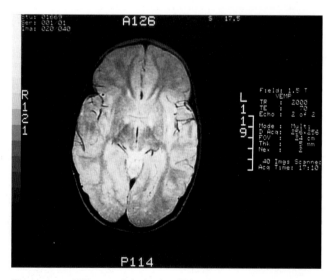

Figure 3.8 *MRI scan of the brain of T.J. revealed increased intensity of T2 signal in the basal ganglia.*

been reported in four biopsied patients of 15 reported with renal disease [37]. End stage renal disease requiring dialysis and/or transplantation has been observed, as another late complication [22,38,39].

Pancreatitis has recently been reported [40] in a variety of organic acidemias. Among the patients, methylmalonic acidemia was particularly prominent. Five of nine patients had methylmalonic acidemia; of these, two died. One of our adult patients with mut⁰ disease died of acute hemorrhagic pancreatitis.

Transient thrombocytopenia has been observed in infancy. Neutropenia is a regular occurrence except in the case of successful treatment and reduction in the accumulation of methylmalonic acid in body fluids. Anemia may occur, especially in the first month of life. Recurrent infections are common.

Chronic moniliasis is highly relevant to metabolic control. High levels of methylmalonate and other intermediates that accumulate when patients are out of control inhibit the maturation of hematopoietic cells and also of T cells, so the T-cell number is low. The response of T cells to Candida is also specifically altered when levels are high [17]. When metabolite levels are lowered by treatment, skin lesions disappear and T-cell responsiveness to Candida returns. Osteoporosis has been found regularly and we have observed femoral and tibial fractures.

Patients with B₁₂ responsiveness, in both the CblA and CblB complementation groups not only had milder disease, they presented later than those with mut⁰ or mut⁻ disease [20,41]. Some 80 percent of mut⁰ patients presented within the first week of life; 42 percent and 33 percent of CblA and CblB patients presented this early. The mut⁰ patients were predominantly dead or severely impaired at follow up. Most died within two months of diagnosis. Most of the CblA and CblB patients were alive at follow up.

At least four successful pregnancies have been reported in women with methylmalonic acidemia [42,43] despite evidence of renal impairment. One was mut⁻ and one B₁₂-responsive. As predicted, levels of MMA decreased dramatically as the fetus grew [43]. These experiences documented that MMA is not teratogenic.

Some patients with MMA have been clinically normal. Presumably these individuals are mut⁻ variants with a considerable level of activity *in vivo*. So-called benign methylmalonic acidemia has been reported in at least nine clinically normal individuals [44,45], eight of them identified through routine neonatal screening [44]. Some of these patients may excrete quite large amounts of MMA. In the Quebec program of screening neonatal urine for MMA [45] a follow up study of 122 individuals with MMA excretion over 1400 mmol/mol creatinine indicated that MMA excretion had resolved by 1 year of age in 65 and in 10 more over 15 months to 7 years; so a majority were transient. The rest were: 13 symptomatic and 22 asymptomatic. MMA levels in blood and urine were appreciably higher in the symptomatic patients. Careful study of the asymptomatic patients revealed one to be mut⁻ and the rest undiagnosed. All of the asymptomatic patients were found to be clinically and cognitively normal at follow-up. Programs of neonatal screening are turning up patients with MMA in appreciably greater numbers than were evident from experience with illness presentations. In the California pilot study of screening by tandem mass spectrometry (MS/MS), a newborn population screened of 309 074 yielded eight methylmalonic acidemic patients. This prevalence rate of 1 in 32 000 represented the third most common disorder detected and the only prevalent organic acidemia. Some of these patients might represent those who might have died undiagnosed, but some of them are likely to represent more benign disease. Clues from the Quebec study [45] indicated that the benign patients are likely to have no urinary metabolites of propionate, such as hydroxypropionate or methylcitrate, and many excrete malonic acid in amounts of 60–227 mmol/mol creatinine.

In addition to the differential diagnosis of methylmalonic acidemia shown in Table 3.1, p. 19, there are a number of patients of variable, atypical phenotype in whom the molecular nature of the disease has not been defined [46,47]. Most have had appreciably lower levels of MMA than in a classic patient and activities of the mutase enzyme are normal. Treatment with B_{12} had no effect, and protein restriction may not decrease the excretion of MMA. Some, but not all have also excreted malonic acid. These patients have not had a crisis of ketoacidotic metabolic imbalance. They have usually been investigated because of failure to thrive or developmental delay. Some have had athetoid movements, myopathy, ophthalmoplegia or pyramidal tract signs [46]. Two siblings developed renal tubular acidosis with hypercalciuria, one of whom developed nephrocalcinosis [47].

GENETICS AND PATHOGENESIS

Each of the forms of methylmalonic acidemia is determined by a rare autosomal recessive gene. Complementation studies [48,49] have indicated that there are at least four distinct forms of methylmalonic acidemia (Figure 3.1). Furthermore,

the mut apoenzyme defect group is heterogeneous. Mut⁰ patients have no activity of the enzyme, while mut⁻ patients have a spectrum of residual activity. Heterozygote detection by enzyme analysis may be unreliable. Screening of infants, 3–4 weeks of age, for methylmalonic aciduria was instituted in Massachusetts, and the data indicated an incidence of 1:48 000 [50]. Such a study would not include infants dying in the neonatal period, so the prevalence of 1:32 000 encountered in the Californian MS/MS trial may well be more accurate. In southern Japan screening of newborn urine by gas chromatography-mass spectrometry (GCMS) yielded a prevalence of 1:5000 [51].

Prenatal detection of methylmalonic acidemia has been accomplished by assay of the activity of methylmalonyl CoA mutase in cultured amniotic cells [52]. The diagnosis has also been made chemically by assay of the maternal urine for methylmalonic acid [53], but this may not be reliable until quite late in pregnancy. Rapid, efficient chemical diagnosis can be made by direct analysis of the amniotic fluid for methylcitric acid or methylmalonic acid using stable isotope dilution methodology and GCMS [54–57]. In a family in which the mutation is known, its determination can be used for prenatal diagnosis, and for heterozygote detection. An infant with defective deoxyadenosylcobalamin synthesis was diagnosed prenatally and effectively treated with cobalamin prenatally [58].

The diagnosis of methylmalonic acidemia is most readily made by assay of the urine for MMA (Figures 3.10, 3.11). Screening tests are now seldom used, and the diagnosis is usually made by organic acid analysis of the urine with GCMS. The amounts of methylmalonic acid excreted are enormous. Excretion of a gram a day by a tiny infant is not unusual. Normal individuals excrete less than 5 mg per 24 hours, amounts that are undetectable in the usual assays. A comparison of the amounts of methylmalonate excreted in patients with various forms of methylmalonic aciduria is shown in Table 3.2.

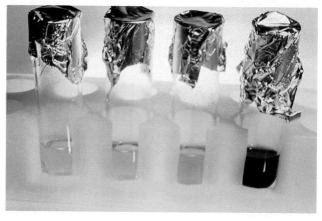

Figure 3.10 *Colorimetric test of urine for methylmalonic acid. The dark green color which develops in the presence of p-nitroaniline has been used for screening.*

Methylmalonic acid, undetectable in the plasma of normal individuals, is present in patients in concentrations of 200 to 2500 μmol/L. The concentrations of methylmalonic acid in the cerebrospinal fluid (CSF) may equal that of the plasma. In patients with cobalamin deficiency, concentrations in CSF tend to be much higher than in plasma [59]. Propionic acid also accumulates in the plasma of patients with methylmalonic acidemia [60], and 3-hydroxypropionate [61] and methylcitrate [62] are found in the urine. The administration of isoleucine, threonine, valine or methionine results in the formation of methylmalonic acid [61].

The diagnosis of methylmalonic acidemia is increasingly made by MS/MS, not only in programs of newborn screening,

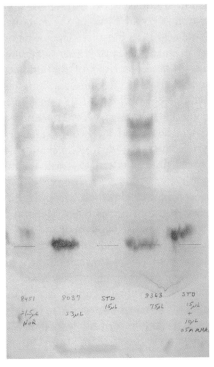

Figure 3.11 *High voltage electrophoresis of the urine. The amino acids have been separated and stained with ninhydrin and then the paper was overstained with Fast Blue B giving a purple band at the origin in the presence of methylmalonic acid. Numbers 8037 and 8363 were patients with mut⁰ methylmalonic acidemia.*

Table 3.2 *Excretion of methylmalonic acid*

Clinical status	Amount excreted mmol/mol creatinine
Normal	0–2
Mut⁰; presentation	3000–13 000
Mut⁰; steady-state	200–2000
B₁₂-responsive; presentation	2000
B₁₂-responsive; steady-state	90–300
B₁₂-deficient infant	4500–5700
Transcobalamin II deficiency	600
Cobalamin C, D	270
Atypical-normal mutase	200

but by quantitative analysis of acylcarnitine profiles of plasma (Chapter 1). Answers are more rapidly available in emergency situation than by GCMS of urinary methylmalonate. The quantification of urinary methylmalonate remains the best approach to monitoring the effectiveness of therapy. Electrospray MS/MS of urine in positive and negative modes has been reported as a rapid approach to diagnosis of a variety of inborn errors of metabolism [63]. Separation of succinic and methylmalonic acids was not achieved, but the disparity in amounts excreted in illness indicated utility in the diagnosis of methylmalonic acidemia. An LC-MS/MS method with a deuterated internal standard has been reported [64] that is rapid and accurate and correlated well with GCMS in the analysis of the same samples; it can be used for plasma or urine. Methodology for the analysis of MMA is of broad applicability in addition to the diagnosis and management of inborn errors of metabolism, because elevated plasma concentration of MMA that responds to B₁₂ is the best indicator of tissue deficiency of cobalamin [65].

All patients with MMA have defective activity of methylmalonylCoA mutase (Figure 3.1, p. 19), the enzyme that catalyzes the conversion of methylmalonylCoA to succinylCoA (see Figure 2.1, p. 8). This enzyme lies on the direct degradative pathway for isoleucine, valine, threonine and methionine. All of these amino acids have been shown to be major sources of methylmalonate in these patients. On the other hand, lipids, although metabolizable via this pathway, do not contribute in measurable fashion to urinary methylmalonic acid [66].

Apoenzyme defect was first demonstrated in liver of four patients who died, by measuring the conversion of ³H-methylmalonylCoA to ³H-succinylCoA [8]. In the mut⁰ group, mutase activity in cultured fibroblasts or tissues is undetectable even in the presence of adenosylcobalamin [67–69]. In the mut⁻ group some residual activity is present. Heterogeneity has been demonstrated in the mut⁰ group because some patients are CRM-negative, and some have reduced amounts of cross-reactive material (CRM) [70]. Some patients in the mut⁻ group may have much later and much milder clinical presentations. Enzyme activity of 2 to 75 percent of control was associated with CRM of 20–100 percent of control [70]. In studies of labeled enzyme synthesis some mut⁰ patients made unstable enzyme, which disappeared, while most made no detectable enzyme [71]. All mut⁻ patients made detectable newly synthesized enzyme.

The study of fibroblasts of patients with B₁₂-sensitive methylmalonic aciduria [72] clarified the nature of these disorders. The content of deoxyadenosylcobalamin is reduced, and the cells cannot convert ⁵⁷Co-hydroxycobalamin to ⁵⁷Co-deoxyadenosylcobalamin [73].

A simplified test for the overall enzymatic block at the mutase step is to test the conversion by cultured fibroblasts of ¹⁴C-propionate to ¹⁴CO₂ [74]. Assessment of ¹⁴C-MMA oxidation permits distinction of MMA from propionic acidemia. The extrapolation of this assay to the incorporation of ¹⁴C-propionate into acid precipitable material has simplified the procedure [75]. This has been employed in studies of complementation among the inherited methylmalonic acidemias. Patients responsive to B_{12} were promptly subfractioned into two complementation groups, designated Cbl A and Cbl B [48,49,76,77]. The Cbl A variants appear to have a defect in CblIII reductase (Figure 3.1, p. 19) because they synthesize deoxyadenosylcobalamin normally from ^{57}Cohydroxycobalamin and adenosine triphosphate (ATP) under reducing conditions which bypass CblIII reductase [73]. In the Cbl B variants, deoxyadenosylcobalamin synthesis is defective under these conditions, and the defect has been shown to be in the adenosyltransferase [78,79]. Patients with defects in cobalamin synthesis generally present later than those with apoenzyme defects, and most survive the illness once diagnosed. Among the Cbl A patients a clinical response to B_{12} is regularly seen, while in Cbl B patients only half respond to B_{12} with a decrease in the amounts of methylmalonic acid in body fluids, suggesting that there is a complete block in the adenosyltransferase in the unresponsive patients.

In the patients with the combined abnormalities of methylmalonic acidemia and homocystinuria the activity of N^5-methyltetrahydrofolate-homocysteine-methyltransferase (methionine synthase) is deficient as well as methylmalonylCoA mutase. Methionine synthase activity is restored by the addition of methylcobalamin [72,78,80]. Thus a defect not yet identified leads to diminished synthesis of both methylcobalamin and deoxyadenosylcobalamin. Patients fall into two complementation groups: CblC and D (Chapter 4).

The cDNA for methylmalonyl CoA mutase was originally obtained from human cDNA hepatic libraries; it was used as a clone to localize the gene to human chromosome 6q12-21.2 [9,10]. A highly informative restriction fragment length polymorphism (RFLP) at this locus, a HindIII polymorphism, is useful for heterozygote detection, prenatal diagnosis and linkage analysis. A relatively small number of mutations has been identified [81,82].

Four mutations in mut$^-$ cells, all of which exhibited interallelic complementation, clustered near the carboxyl terminus of the protein. These missense mutations (R664W, G648D, G630E and G626C) (respectively, arginine to tryptophan, and glycine to aspartic acid, glutamic acid and cysteine) were close to another mutation (G717V) (glycine to valine) in the region that appears likely to be the cobalamin binding domain. The enzyme in these cells could be stimulated in vitro by very high concentrations of hydroxycobalamin. The enzyme specified by G717V mutation was shown to have a very high Km for adenosylcobalamin. The enzyme bearing the G648D mutation also had a high Km. It is of interest that six of seven mutations described in this area involved substitution for a glycine residue, suggesting altered secondary or tertiary structure [83]. Among mut^0 patients mutations near the amino terminal of the protein eliminated enzyme activity entirely [84,85]. G717V has been observed to be common in black Americans [83,84]. Among Japanese, E117X was found in every patient reported [86]. At least one mutation has been reported, an N terminal deletion which interfered with processing of the enzyme, such that it was not taken up by the mitochondria [87]. Gene transfer has been employed [86] as a substitute for complementation in the distinction of mut from Cbl phenotypes. Transfer of a normal mutase cDNA clone corrected activity as measured by ^{14}C-propionate assay. Transfer into Cbl fibroblasts had no effect on activity.

TREATMENT

Patients with methylmalonic acidemia should first be tested for responsiveness to B_{12}. This is important, for a majority of those responding have survived while the majority of the unresponsive, who were detected as a result of ketoacidotic illness have not survived [20] or have survived with major neurologic disability.

In patients with B_{12}-responsive methylmalonic acidemia, excretion of methylmalonic acid in the urine is significantly decreased by the administration of pharmacological doses of cyanocobalamin [3,88]. We continue to employ the method of admission to the general clinical research center (GCRC) and measurement of total MMA excretion for five days, the first two control days and the next three reflecting daily injection of 1 mg of hydroxocobalamin or cyanocobalamin. This method continues to elucidate the true status in patients in whom the results of casual specimens under varying conditions in the clinic or in acute admission to hospital are confusing.

The correlation of B_{12} responsiveness with prognosis is clear [20]; with prognosis all but four of 25 children who responded to B_{12} were alive, while 11 of 20 who did not respond to B_{12} died. The first B_{12}-responsive patient was well at 9 years when reported [89], and was 14 at most recently reported follow-up.

Those who respond are treated with B_{12} in doses sufficient to keep concentrations of methylmalonic acid minimal. B_{12}-responsive patients may do very well with modest protein restriction, growing and developing normally over the long term and tolerating childhood illnesses [90]. Most Cbl A patients can be expected to respond clinically to B_{12}, while about half of the Cbl B patients respond [20]; mut^0 and most mut$^-$ patients have not responded despite in vitro evidence of responsiveness.

Patients who do not respond to B_{12} are treated with a diet designed to keep the precursors of methylmalonic acid at a manageable level [14,91]. This is complicated because isoleucine, threonine, methionine and valine are all essential for normal growth and development. Therefore, optimal therapy consists of a diet containing the minimal requirements of these amino acids for optimal growth and no more. The rest of the calories can be made up of a diet containing fat and carbohydrate, with or without other amino acids. The amount of protein necessary to accomplish this must be individualized. Under conditions of limited intake of protein, caloric intake must be generous. We have found that alanine supplementation is useful in this disorder and may replace mixture of amino acids [92]. The management of such a patient is not easy. It requires enormous commitment on the part of parents, physicians and nutritionists. Furthermore treatment must be monitored by periodic quantitative assay concentrations of methylmalonic acid to ensure optimal control, and of plasma amino acids to ensure the avoidance of protein malnutrition. Nevertheless, it may be successful. The reward in normal development may be high. In 25 years of experience with 66 patients with methylmalonic acidemia, Saudubray and colleagues [93] pointed out that 29 of 50 B_{12}-unresponsive patients died, most of them prior to 1985, and only three after 1985. Of 21 living patients most were judged to have had good or very good results. Treatment after 1985 reflected very rigid restriction of protein [91,93], the addition of carnitine and the use of metronidazole [94,95]. Not only was survival improved, but the number and severity of metabolic decompensations were decreased [93].

Propionic acid is synthesized by intestinal bacteria, and this may be an important source of propionate and methylmalonate in these patients [95]. Treatment with neomycin or metronidazole may reduce levels of propionic and methylmalonic acids in body fluids [94–98]. Doses of metronidazole have ranged from 10 to 20 mg/kg per day and have been divided into three doses. Neomycin has been used in a dose of 50 mg/kg. Other antibiotics such as bacitracin, paromycin, clindamycin or vancomycin may be useful in acute situations. Lincomycin was not effective [96]. In our experience intermittent antibacterial therapy has been useful, suggesting that clonal populations of propionate-forming bacteria may be intermittently present in some patients. An effect of antibiotic treatment on metabolite accumulation may be especially useful during a crisis of metabolic decompensation. A sudden increase in methylmalonic acid excretion unaccompanied by dietary change or stimulus for catabolism may suggest a bacterial source and an argument for neomycin or metronidazole.

An increase in the excretion of metabolites of propionate during fasting suggests the mobilization of odd-chain fatty acids from lipid stores [99,100]. The therapeutic implication is the avoidance of fasting and the use of intravenous calories when the oral route is not available.

In the management of the acute ketoacidotic crisis a program of aggressive fluid and electrolyte therapy is essential as set out for propionic acidemia (Chapter 2). In addition, in MMA advantage can be taken of the very effective excretion of methylmalonate by the kidney [99], which is much more efficient than peritoneal dialysis, by aggressive intravenous hydration (150–200 mL per kilogram of water containing 10 percent glucose and initially isotonic $NaHCO_3$ until the acidosis is corrected). Anabolism may be promoted by the use of insulin and glucose, or the acute use of growth hormone. Vomiting may be relieved with ondansetron (0.15 mg/kg over 15 min IV; up to 3 times qd).

Carnitine has been a useful adjunct to chronic maintenance therapy, removing propionyl groups as carnitine ester [101,102] and diminishing the propensity of these patients to

abnormal ketogenesis [103]. We have found parenteral carnitine in doses of 300 mg/kg very useful in the acute crisis.

Human growth hormone may be useful in adjunctive therapy in this and other organic acidemias [104]. Promotion of anabolism may diminish the propensity for catabolism, and thus the acute catabolic response to infection, stress or protein intake. In our hands protein requirements have increased without increase in metabolite excretion. Growth has been rewarding as well as increase in lean body mass and decrease in adipose tissue.

The fact that so many patients with mut^0 disease die in infancy and that survivors have so often had major retardation of mental development [20,21] has led to consideration of transplantation of liver [22,26,105,106]. Our experience [22] has indicated that liver transplantation does not halt or reverse relentless progression to renal failure. Most such patients will have had evidence of renal impairment at the time liver transplantation is considered. It makes sense to treat such a patient with combined transplantation of liver and kidney [105]. That decision is not so clear in the case of an infant.

Our experience with liver transplantation also indicates that the procedure does not stop the progression of late onset neurologic disease [22] although it completely does away with recurrent attacks of ketoacidotic metabolic imbalance. High concentration of methylmalonic acid in the CSF does not decrease with liver transplantation [107,108]. It is of interest that high CSF concentrations of methylmalonic acid have also been observed in patients with cobalamin deficiency [109]. Transplantation of the liver also did not prevent the occurrence of infarction of the basal ganglia during an episode of pneumonia unassociated with metabolic imbalance [110].

In a novel approach to the treatment of hyperammonemia in the acute crisis of infantile methylmalonic acidemia Gebhart and colleagues [111] used carbamylglutamtate, an activator of carbamylphosphate synthetase that has been used to treat N-acetylglutamate synthetase deficiency [112]. Hyperammonemia was successfully reversed in the patient treated.

References

1 Oberholzer VG, Levin B, Burgess EA, Young WF. Methylmalonic aciduria: an inborn error of metabolism leading to chronic metabolic acidosis. *Arch Dis Child* 1967;**42**:492.

2 Stokke O, Eldjarn L, Norum KR, *et al.* Methylmalonic acidemia: a new inborn error of metabolism which may cause fatal acidosis in the neonatal period. *Scand J Clin Lab Invest* 1967;**20**:313.

3 Rosenberg LE, Lilljeqvist A-C, Hsia YE. Methylmalonic aciduria: an inborn error leading to metabolic acidosis, long chain ketonuria and intermittent hyperglycinemia. *N Engl J Med* 1968;**278**:1319.

4 Rosenberg LE, Lilljeqvist A-C, Hsia YE. Methylmalonic aciduria: metabolic block localization and vitamin B_{12} dependency. *Science* 1968;**162**:805.

5 Mudd SH, Levy HL, Abeles RH. A derangement in B_{12} metabolism leading to homocystinemia, cystathioninemia and methylmalonic aciduria. *Biochem Biophys Res Commun* 1969;**35**:1121.

6 Higginbottom MC, Sweetman L, Nyhan WL. A syndrome of methylmalonic aciduria, homocystinuria, megaloblastic anemia and neurologic abnormalities in a vitamin B12-deficient breast-fed infant of a strict vegetarian. *N Engl J Med* 1978;**299**:317.

7 Barshop BA, Woff J, Nyhan WL, *et al*. Transcobalamin II deficiency presenting with methylmalonic aciduria and homocystinuria and abnormal absorption of cobalamin. *Am J Med Genet* 1990;**35**:222.

8 Morrow G, Barness LA, Cardinale GJ, *et al*. Congenital methylmalonic acidemia: enzymatic evidence for two forms of the disease. *Proc Natl Acad Sci* 1969;**63**:191.

9 Ledley FD, Lumetta M, Nguyen PN, *et al*. Molecular cloning of l-methylmalonyl-CoA mutase: gene transfer and analysis of mut cell lines. *Proc Natl Acad Sci USA* 1988;**85**:3518.

10 Ledley FD, Lumetta MR, Zoghbi HY, *et al*. Mapping of human methylmalonyl CoA mutase (MUT) locus on chromosome 6. *Am J Hum Genet* 1988;**42**:839.

11 Rosenblatt DS, Fenton WA. Inborn errors of cobalamin metabolism, in *Chemistry and Biology of B12*, (ed. R. Banerjee), Wiley, New York, 1999:367.

12 Lindblad B, Lindblad BS, Olin P, *et al*. Methylmalonic acidemia: a disorder associated with acidosis, hyperglycinemia and hyperlactatemia. *Acta Paediatr Scand* 1968;**57**:417.

13 Morrow G, Barness LA, Auerbach VH, *et al*. Observations on the coexistence of methylmalonic acidemia and glycinemia. *J Pediatr* 1969;**74**:680.

14 Nyhan WL, Fawcett N, Ando T, *et al*. Response to dietary therapy in B12 unresponsive methylmalonic acidemia. *Pediatrics* 1973;**51**:539.

15 Cathlineau L, Briad P, Ogier H, *et al*. Occurrence of hyperammonemia in the course of 17 cases of methylmalonic acidemia. *J Pediatr* 1978;**99**:279.

16 Packman S, Mahoney MJ, Tanaka K, Hsia YE. Severe hyperammonemia in a newborn infant with methylmalonyl-CoA mutase deficiency. *J Pediatr* 1978;**92**:769.

17 Yu A, Sweetman L, Nyhan WL. The pathogenetic mechanism of recurrent mucocutaneous candidiasis in a patient with methylmalonic acidemia (MMA). *Clin Res* 1981;**29**:124A.

18 Choy YS, Pertiwi AKD, Zabedah Y, Noor Farizah I. Methylmalonic acidemia – associated birth defects and atypical presentations. *J Inherit Metab Dis* 2002;**25**:47 (Suppl.)

19 Shevell MA, Matiaszuk N, Ledley FD, Rosenblatt DS. Varying neurological phenotypes among mut^0 and mut$^-$ patients with methylmalonyl CoA mutase deficiency. *Am J Med Genet* 1993;**45**:619.

20 Matsui SM, Mahoney MJ, Rosenberg LE. The natural history of the inherited methylmalonic acidemias. *N Engl J Med* 1983;**308**:857.

21 Nicolaides P, Leonard J, Surtees R. Neurological outcome of methylmalonic acidaemia. *Arch Dis Child* 1998;**78**:508.

22 Nyhan WL, Gargus J, Boyle K, *et al*. Progressive neurologic disability in methymalonic acidemia despite transplantation of the liver. *Eur J Pediat* 2002;**161**:377.

23 Thompson GN, Christodoulou J, Danks DM. Metabolic stroke in methylmalonic acidemia. *J Pediatr* 1989;**115**:499.

24 Korf B, Wallman JK, Levy HL. Bilateral lucency of the globus pallidus complicating methylmalonic acidemia. *Ann Neurol* 1986;**20**:364.

25 Heidenreich R, Natowicz M, Hainline BE, *et al*. Acute extrapyramidal syndrome in methylmalonic acidemia: metabolic stroke involving the globus pallidus. *J Pediatr* 1988;**113**:1022.

26 Brismar J, Ozand PT. CT and MR of the brain in disorders of the propionate and methylmalonate metabolism. *Am J Neuroradiol* 1994;**15**:1459.

27 de Sousa C, Piesowicz AT, Brett EM, Leonard JV. Focal changes in the globi pallidus associated with neurological dysfunction in methylmalonic acidaemia. *Neuropediatrics* 1989;**20**:199.

28 Roodhooft AM, Baumgartner ER, Martin JJ, *et al*. Symmetrical necrosis of the basal ganglia in methylmalonic acidaemia. *Eur J Pediatr* 1990;**149**:582.

29 Yamaguchi K, Hirabayashi K, Honma K. Methylmalonic acidemia: brain lesions in a case of vitamin B$_{12}$ non-responsive (mut^0) type. *Clin Neuropathol* 1995;**12**:216.

30 Andreula CF, Deblasi R, Carella A. CT and MRI studies of methylmalonic acidemia. *Am J Neuroradiol* 1991;**12**:410.

31 Bousounis DP. Methylmalonic aciduria resulting in globus pallidus necrosis. *Ann Neurol* 1988;**24**:302.

32 Nyhan WL, Wulfeck, BB, Tallal P, Marsden DL. Metabolic correlates of learning disability, in *Research in Infant Assessment*, (ed. NW. Paul), March of Dimes Birth Defects Foundation, White Plains, NY, 1989: Birth Defects: Original Article Series, Vol. 25 (No. 6) 153.

33 Dave P, Curless RG, Steinman L. Cerebellar hemorrhage complicating methylmalonic and propionic acidemia. *Arch Neurol* 1984;**41**:1293.

34 Sheldon B, Sheldon K, Sheldon P, Sheldon J. Memory of Andrew M. Sheldon, MMA. *OAA Newsletter* 2003;**13**:19.

35 Wolff JA, Strom C, Griswold W, *et al*. Proximal renal tubular acidosis in methylmalonic acidemia. *J Neurogenetics* 1985;**2**:31

36 Broyer M, Guesry P, Burgess E-A, *et al*. Acidemie methylmalonique avec nephropathie hyperuricemique. *Arch Franc Pediatr* 1974;**31**:543.

37 Rutledge SL, Geraghty M, Mroczek E, *et al*. Tubulointerstitial nephritis in methylmalonic acidemia. *Pediatr Nephrol* 1993;**7**:81.

38 Walter JH, Michalski A, Wilson WM, *et al*. Chronic renal failure in methylmalonic acidaemia. *Eur J Pediatr* 1989;**148**:344.

39 Gonwa TA, Mai ML, Melton LB, *et al*. End-stage renal disease (ESRD) after orthotopic liver transplantation (OLTX) using calcineurin-based immunotherapy: risk of development and treatment. *Transplantation* 2001;**72**:1934.

40 Kahler SG, Sherwood WG, Woolf D, *et al*. Pancreatitis in patients with organic acidemias. *J Pediatr* 1994;**124**:239.

41 Shevell MI, Matiaszuk N, Ledley FD, Rosenblatt DS. Varying neurological phentypes among mut^0 and mut$^-$ patients with methylmalonylCoA mutase deficiency. *Am J Med Genet* 1993;**45**:619.

42 Lind S, Westgren M, Angelin B, von Dobeln U. Successful pregnancy in a young woman with methylmalonic acidaemia and a two-year follow-up of the child. *J Inherit Metab Dis* 2002;**25**:48 (Suppl.)

43 Deodato F, Rizzo C, Boenzi S, *et al*. Successful pregnancy in a woman with mut$^-$ Methylmalonic acidaemia. *J Inherit Metab Dis* 2002;**25**:133.

44 Ledley FD, Levy HL, Shih VE, *et al*. Benign methylmalonic aciduria. *N Engl J Med* 1984;**311**:1015.

45 Sniderman LC, Lambert M, Giguere R, *et al*. Outcome of individuals with low-moderate methylmalonic aciduria detected through a neonatal screening program. *J Pediatr* 1999;**134**:675.

46 Mayatepek E, Hoffmann GF, Baumgartner R, *et al*. Atypical vitamin B$_{12}$-unresponsive methylmalonic aciduria in sibship with severe progressive encephalomyelopathy: a new genetic disease? *Eur J Pediatr* 1996;**155**:398.

47 Dudley J, Allen J, Tizard J, McGraw M. Benign methylmalonic acidemia in a sibship with distal renal tubular acidosis. *Pediatr Nephrol* 1998;**12**:564.

48 Gravel RA, Mahoney MJ, Ruddle FH, Rosenberg LE. Genetic complementation in heterokaryons of human fibroblasts defective in cobalamin metabolism. *Proc Natl Acad Sci USA* 1975;**72**:3181.

49 Willard HF, Mellman IS, Rosenberg LE. Genetic complementation among inherited deficiencies of methylmalonyl-CoA mutase activity: evidence for a new class of human cobalamin mutant. *Am J Hum Genet* 1978;**30**:1.

50 Coulombe JT, Shih VE, Levy HL. Massachusetts metabolic disorders screening program. II. Methylmalonic aciduria. *Pediatrics* 1981;**67**:26.

51 Yoshida I. 2001;Personal communication.

52 Morrow III G, Schwarz RH, Hallock JA, Barness LA. Prenatal detection of methylmalonic acidemia. *J Pediatr* 1970;**77**:120.

53 Mahoney MJ, Rosenberg LE, Lindblad B, *et al.* Prenatal diagnosis of methylmalonic aciduria. *Acta Paediatr Scand.* 1975;**64**:44.

54 Naylor G, Sweetman L, Nyhan WL, *et al.* Isotope dilution analysis of methylcitric acid in amniotic fluid for the prenatal diagnosis of propionic and methylmalonic acidemia. *Clin Chim Acta* 1980;**107**:175.

55 Trefz FK, Schmidt H, Tauscher B, *et al.* Improved prenatal diagnosis of methylmalonic acidemia: mass fragmentography of methylmalonic acid in amniotic fluid and maternal urine. *Eur J Pediatr* 1981;**137**:261.

56 Zinn AB, Hine DG, Mahoney MJ, Tanaka K. The stable isotope dilution method for measurement of methylmalonic acid: a highly accurate approach to the prenatal diagnosis of methylmalonic acidemia. *Pediatr Res* 1982;**16**:740.

57 Sweetman L, Naylor G, Ladner T, *et al.* Prenatal diagnosis of propionic and methylmalonic acidemia by stable isotope dilution analysis of methylcitric and methylmalonic acids in amniotic fluids, in *Stable Isotopes* (eds HL Schmidt and K Fšrstel), Elsevier Scientific Publishing Co., Amsterdam, The Netherlands, 1982:287.

58 Ampola MG, Mahoney JJ, Nakamura E, Tanaka K. Prenatal therapy of a patient with vitamin B$_{12}$-responsive methylmalonic acidemia. *N Engl J Med* 1975;**293**:313.

59 Stabler SP, Allen RH, Barrett RE, *et al.* Cerebrospinal fluid methylmalonic acid levels in normal subjects and patients with cobalamin deficiency. *Neurology* 1991;**41**:1627.

60 Ando T, Rasmussen K, Nyhan WL, *et al.* Propionic acidemia in patients with ketotic hyperglycinemia *J Pediatr* 1971;**78**:827.

61 Ando T, Rasmussen K, Nyhan WL, Hull D. 3-hydroxy-propionate: significance of oxidation of propionate in patients with propionic acidemia and methylmalonic acidemia. *Proc Natl Acad Sci USA* 1972;**69**:2807.

62 Ando T, Rasmussen K, Wright JM, Nyhan WL. Isolation and identification of methylcitrate, a major metabolic product of propionate in patients with propionic acidemia. *J Biol Chem* 1972;**247**:2200.

63 Pitt JJ, Eggington M, Kahler SG. Comprehensive screening of urine samples for inborn errors of metabolism by electrospray tandem mass spectrometry. *Clin Chem* 2002;**48**:1970.

64 Magera MJ, Helgeson JK, Matern D, Rinaldo P. Methylmalonic acid measured in plasma and urine by stable-isotope dilution and electrospray tandem mass spectrometry. *Clin Chem* 2000;**46**:1804.

65 Bolann BJ, Solli JD, Schneede J, *et al.* Evaluation of indicators of cobalamin deficiency defined as cobalamin-induced reduction in increased serum methylmalonic acid. *Clin Chem* 2000;**46**:1744.

66 Wolff JA, Sweetman L, Nyhan WL. The role of lipid in the management of methylmalonic acidemia: administration of linoleic acid does not increase excretion of methylmalonic acid. *J Inherit Metab Dis* 1985;**8**:100.

67 Morrow G, Mahoney MJ, Mathews C, Lebowitz J. Studies of methylmalonyl Coenzyme A carboxymutase activity in methylmalonic acidemia. I. Correlation of clinical, hepatic and fibroblast data. *Pediatr Res* 1975;**9**:641.

68 Willard HF, Rosenberg LE. Inherited deficiency of human methylmalonyl CoA mutase activity: reduced affinity of mutant apoenzyme for adenosylcobalamin. *Biochem Biophys Res Commun* 1977;**78**:927.

69 Willard HF, Rosenberg LE. Inherited methylmalonyl CoA mutase apoenzyme deficiency in human fibroblasts: evidence for allelic heterogeneity, genetic compounds, and co-dominant expression. *J Clin Invest* 1980;**65**:690.

70 Kolhouse JF, Utley C, Fenton WA, Rosenberg LE. Immunochemical studies on cultured fibroblasts from patients with inherited methylmalonic acidemia. *Proc Natl Acad Sci USA* 1981;**78**:7737.

71 Fenton WA, Hack AM, Kraus JP, Rosenberg LE. Immunochemical studies of fibroblasts from patients with methylmalonyl-CoA mutase apoenzyme deficiency: detection of a mutation interfering with mitochondrial import. *Proc Natl Acad Sci USA* 1987;**84**:1421.

72 Mahoney MJ, Rosenberg LE, Mudd SH, Uhlendorf BW. Defective metabolism of vitamin B$_{12}$ in fibroblasts from patients with methylmalonic aciduria. *Biochem Biophys Res Commun* 1971;**44**:375.

73 Rosenberg LE, Lilljeqvist AC, Hsia YE, Rosenbloom FM. Vitamin B$_{12}$-dependent methylmalonic aciduria: defective metabolism in cultured fibroblasts. *Biochem Biophys Res Commun.* 1969;**37**:607.

74 Willard HF, Ambani LM, Hart AC, *et al.* Rapid prenatal and postnatal detection of inborn errors of propionate, methylmalonate, and cobalamin metabolism a sensitive assay using cultured cells. *Hum Genet* 1976;**34**:277.

75 Morrow G, Revsin B, Mathews C, Giles H. A simple rapid method for prenatal detection of defects in propionate metabolism. *Clin Genet* 1976;**10**:218.

76 Morrow G, Barness LA, Cardinale GJ. Congential methylmalonic acidemia: enzymatic evidence for two forms of disease. *Proc Natl Acad Sci USA* 1975;**72**:2799.

77 Mahoney MJ, Hart AC, Steen VD, Rosenberg LE. Methylmalonic acidemia: Biochemical heterogeneity in defects of 5'-deoxyadenosylcobalamin synthesis. *Proc Natl Acad Sci USA* 1975;**72**:2799.

78 Fenton WA, Rosenberg LE. Genetic and biochemical analysis of human cobalamin mutants in cell culture. *Ann Rev Genet* 1978;**12**:223.

79 Fenton WA, Rosenberg LE. The defect in the cbl B class of human methylmalonic acidemia: deficiency of cobalamin adenosyltransferase activity in extracts of cultured fibroblasts. *Biochem Biophys Res Commun* 1981;**98**:283.

80 Mudd SH, Uhlendorf BW, Hinds KR, Levy HL. Deranged B$_{12}$ metabolism: studies of fibroblasts grown in tissue culture. *Biochem Med* 1970;**4**:215.

81 Jansen R, Kalousek F, Fenton WA, *et al.* Cloning of full-length methylmalonyl-CoA mutase: gene transfer and analysis of mut cell lines. *Proc Natl Acad Sci USA* 1988;**85**:3618.

82 Crane AM, Ledley FD. Clustering of mutations in methylmalonyl CoA mutase associated with mut$^-$ methylmalonic acidemia. *Am J Hum Genet* 1994;**55**:42.

83 Crane AM, Jansen R, Andrews E, Ledley FD. Cloning and expression of a mutant methylmalonyl Coenzyme A mutase with altered cobalamin affinity that causes mut$^-$ methylmalonic aciduria. *J Clin Invest* 1992;**89**:385.

84 Jansen R, Ledley FD. Heterozygous mutations at the mut locus in fibroblasts with mut^0 methylmalonic acidemia identified by PCR cDNA cloning. *Am J Hum Genet* 1990;**47**:808.

85 Ledley FD, Crane AM, Lumetta M. Heterogeneous alleles and expression of methylmalonyl CoA mutase in *mut* methylmalonic acidemia. *Am J Hum Genet* 1990;**47**:808.

86 Wilkemeyer MG, Crane AM, Ledley FD. Differential diagnosis of *mut* and *cbl* methylmalonic aciduria by DNA-mediated gene transfer in primary fibroblasts. *J Clin Invest* 1991;**87**:915.

87 Fenton WA, Hack AM, Kraus JP, Rosenberg LE. Immunochemical studies of fibroblasts from patients with methylmalonyl-CoA mutase apoenzyme deficiency: Detection of a mutation interfering with mitochondrial import. *Proc Natl Acad Sci USA* 1987;**84**:1421.

88 Lindblad B, Lindstrand K, Svenberg B, Zetterstrom R. The effect of cobamide coenzyme in methylmalonic acidemia. *Acta Paediatr Scand* 1969;**58**:178.

89 Hsia YE, Scully K, Lilljeqvist AC, Rosenberg LE. Vitamin B$_{12}$-dependent methylmalonic aciduria. *Pediatrics* 1970;**46**:497.

90 Morrow III G, Burkel GM. Long-term management of a patient with vitamin B$_{12}$-responsive methylmalonic acidemia. *J Pediatr* 1980;**96**:425.

91 Ney DN, Bay C, Saudubray J-M, *et al.* An evaluation of protein requirements in methylmalonic acidaemia. *J Inherit Metab Dis* 1985;**8**:132.

92 Kelts DG, Ney D, Bay C, *et al.* Studies on requirements for amino acids in infants with disorders of amino acid metabolism. I. Effects of alanine. *Pediatr Res* 1985;**19**:86.

93 Van der Meer SB, Poggi F, Spada M, *et al*. Clinical outcome of long-term management of patients with vitamin B$_{12}$-unresponsive methylmalonic acidemia. *J Pediatr* 1994;**125**:903.

94 Thompson GN, Chalmers RA, Walter JH, *et al*. The use of metronidazole in the management of methylmalonic and propionic acidemias. *Eur J Pediatr* 1990;**149**:792.

95 Walter JH, Thompson GN, Leonard JV, *et al*. Contribution of amino acid catabolism to propionate production in methylmalonic acidemia. *Lancet* 1989;**1**:1298.

96 Snyderman S, Sansaricq C, Norton P, *et al*. The use of neomycin in the treatment of methylmalonic acidemia. *Pediatrics* 1972;**50**:925.

97 Koletzko B, Bachmann C, Wendel U. Antibiotic therapy for improvement of metabolic control in methylmalonic aciduria. *J Pediatr* 1990;**117**:99.

98 Thompson GN, Walter JH, Bresson JL, *et al*. Sources of propionate in inborn errors of propionate metabolism. *Metab Clin Exper* 1990;**39**:1133.

99 Saudubray JM, Ogier H, Charpentier C, *et al*. Neonatal management of organic acidurias. Clinical update. *J Inherit Metab Dis* 1984;**7**:1.

100 Thompson GN, Chalmers RA. Increased urinary metabolite excretion during fasting in disorders of propionate metabolism. *Pediatr Res* 1990;**27**:413.

101 Roe CR, Hoppel CL, Stacey TE, *et al*. Metabolic response to carnitine in methylmalonic aciduria. *Arch Dis Child* 1983;**58**:916.

102 Chalmers RA, Roe CR, Stacey TE, Hoppel CL. Urinary excretion of L-carnitine and acylcarnitines by patients with disorders of organic acid metabolism: evidence for secondary insufficiency of L-carnitine. *Pediatr Res* 1984;**18**:1325.

103 Wolff JA, Carroll JE, Thuy LP, *et al*. Carnitine reduces fasting ketogenesis in patients with disorders of propionate metabolism. *Lancet* 1986;**1**:289.

104 Marsden D, Barshop BA, Capistrano-Estrada S, *et al*. Anabolic effect of human growth hormone: management of inherited disorders of catabolic pathways. *Biochem Med Metabol Biol* 1994;**52**:145.

105 Burdelski M, Ullrich K. Liver transplantation in metabolic disorders: summary of the general discussion. *Eur J Pediatr* 1999;**158**:S95.

106 Van't Hoff WG, McKiernan PJ, Surtees RAH, Leonard JV. Liver transplantation for methylmalonic acidemia. *Eur J Pediatr* 1999;**158**:S70.

107 Kaplan P, Mazur AM, Palmieri M, Berry GT. Liver transplantation for methylmalonic acidopathy (MMA disease) is not curative: cerebral production of methylmalonic acid (MMA) is significant in the pathogenesis of disease. *Am J Hum Genet* 1999;**65**:A238, Abstract #1324.

108 Nyhan WL. Unpublished data.

109 Van Asselt DZ, Karlietis MH, Poels PJ, *et al*. Cerebrospinal fluid methylmalonic acid concentrations in neurological patients with low and normal serum cobalamin concentrations. *Acta Neurol Scand* 1998;**97**:413.

110 Chakrapani A, Sivakumar P, McKiernan PJ, Leonard JV. Metabolic stroke in methylmalonic acidemia five years after liver transplantation. *J Pediatr* 2002;**140**:261.

111 Gebhardt B, Vlaho S, Fischer D, *et al*. N-carbamylglutamate enhances ammonia detoxification in a patient with decompensated methylmalonic aciduria. *Mol Genet and Metab* 2003;In press.

112 Bachman C, Colombo JP, Jaggi K. N-acetylglutamate synthetase (NAGS) deficiency: diagnosis, clinical observation and treatment. *Adv Exp Med Biol* 1982;**153**:313.

4

Methylmalonic aciduria and homocystinuria (cobalamin C and C disease)

MAJOR PHENOTYPIC EXPRESSION

Megaloblastic anemia; failure to thrive; developmental delay; excretion of homocystine and methylmalonic acid; and defective activities of both methylmalonyl CoA mutase and methionine synthase.

INTRODUCTION

Patients with methylmalonic aciduria and homocystinuria have defective metabolism of cobalamin to both cofactors, methylcobalamin and deoxyadenoxylcobalamin. Accordingly, the activities of methionine synthase and methylmalonyl CoA mutase are defective (see Figure 4.1). Patients with impaired synthesis of methylcobalamin and deoxyadenosylcobalamin fall into two distinct complementation groups designated Cbl C and Cbl D. Another group of patients designated Cbl F have defective transport of free cobalamin out of lysosomes. The differential diagnosis of methylmalonic acidemia and homocystinuria is given in Table 4.1.

The molecular natures of the early steps in cobalamin metabolism that lead to Cbl C and Cbl D have not been defined.

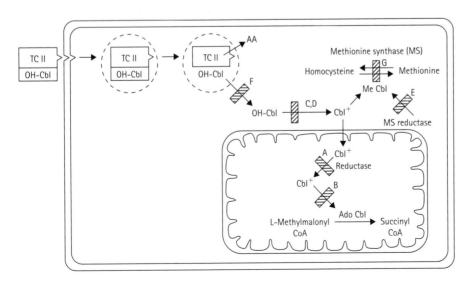

Figure 4.1 *Cobalamin transport and metabolism sites of the defects in complementation groups A to G.*

Table 4.1 *Differential diagnosis: methylmalonic acidemia and homocystinuria*

Disorder	Methylmalonic aciduria	Homocystinuria	Methionine increase	Serum B$_{12}$ low
Cobalamin (Cbl) C	+	+	0	0
Cobalamin (Cbl) D	+	+	0	0
MMA mutase apoenzyme (Mut,$^{0-}$)	+	0	0	0
Cystathionine synthase	0	+	+	0
Methylene tetrahydrofolate reductase	0	+	0($\downarrow$)	0
Cobalamin (Cbl) E, G	0	+	0	0
Cobalamin (Cbl) F	+	0	0	0
B$_{12}$ deficiency	+	+	0	+
Gastrointestinal surgery	+	±	0	+
Autoimmune-multiple endocrine deficiency antibody to parietal cells	+	±	0	+
TC II deficiency	+	±	0	+
Cobalamin enterocyte malabsorption- Immerslund-Grassbeck	+	±	0	+

CLINICAL ABNORMALITIES

The clinical manifestations of Cbl C disease, which is the most common, are those of megaloblastic anemia and failure-to-thrive [1,2] (Figure 4.2). Death may occur within the first 6 months of life [1,3], and there may be overwhelming illness starting in the first days of life. Some patients have seizures; some have microcephaly. Lethargy and/or irritability are prominent. Patients may be difficult to feed. Patients with onset later than the early months of life have had predominantly neurologic presentations. Anorexia, irritability or fatigue may be seen, as well as myelopathy or dementia. Hematologic examination is like that of pernicious anemia with hypersegmented polymorphonuclear leukocytes, and sometimes thrombocytopenia, as well as the megaloblastic anemia. An unrelated patient [4] had severe mental retardation and megaloblastic anemia; he died at 7 years of age. As the numbers of patients recognized with cobalamin C disease has increased, clinical heterogeneity has become apparent [5]. Retinal degeneration has been reported [6] as well as pigmentary retinopathy, which may aid in the clinical diagnosis. Another infant presented at 8 months of age with hypotonia, failure to thrive and macrocytic anemia [7]. He did not appear to see or hear, and visual and auditory evoked potential were abnormal. Infants with neonatal onset who survive the initial episode, may have metabolic decompensation during intercurrent illness, as in other organic acidemias. A 30-year-old patient was reported [8] who presented first at 12 years of age with fatigue, ataxia and mild incontinence, indicating involvement of the spinal cord. Seven years later she developed peripheral nerve disease. A relapsing-remitting course suggested multiple sclerosis. At 24 she had deep vein thrombosis and lost the ability to walk. Six months later she required intensive care. A 34-year-old sister with the same metabolic defect was well. Neither had hematologic abnormalities. A small group of neonates with methylmalonic

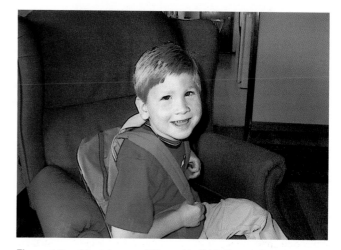

Figure 4.2 *J.A., a 4-year-old boy with Cbl C disease. He looked quite good. His MRIs are shown in Figures 4.3 and 4.4.*

acidemia and homocystinuria of the Cbl C group have presented with microangiopathy, anemia and a hemolytic uremic syndrome. All have died early in life [9].

Cutaneous manifestations consistent with a diagnosis of acrodermatitis enteropathica were reported in two infants with Cbl C diseases [10]. Lesions were erythematous, superficially erosive, desquamative and hyperkeratotic. There was associated cheilosis and perioral erosions. Lesions of this type have been attributed to nutritional deficiency in many inborn errors under treatment, but these patients presented with skin lesions at 9 days and 19 days, before nutritionally restrictive therapy had begun. On the other hand both had very low levels of methionine in plasma: 10 μmol/L and 1 μmol/L; so this could still represent deficiency of an essential amino acid.

Among those with Cbl C disease surviving early infancy neurological manifestations have been prominent. Mental retardation has been the rule [11]. Microcephaly, nystagmus, visual impairment and retinopathy have been prominent

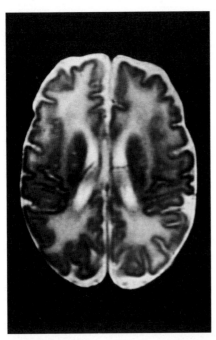

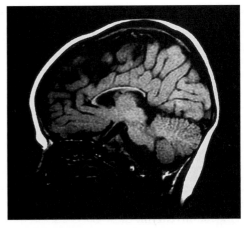

Figure 4.4   *MRI of the brain of the same patient at 23 months. By this time there was extensive paucity of myelination and diffuse atrophy. The corpus callosum was very thin. Neurologic progression occurred despite therapy with hydroxocobalamin. (Images were kindly provided by Dr. G.M. Enns of Stanford University.)*

Figure 4.3   *MRI of the head of a 5-week-old infant with Cbl C disease. Abnormal signal was consistent with white matter disease. (Images were kindly supplied by Dr. G.M. Enns of Stanford University.)*

features. Progressive neurodegenerative disease was reported [12] despite early treatment with hydroxocobalamin and improvement in the concentrations of metabolites. She had presented at nine days of life and was treated with hydroxocobalamin within the next two weeks [10]. She developed choreoathetosis and brisk reflexes at 13 months and seizures at 15 months. Acute stroke with coma has also been observed in this disease [13], although not with the frequency seen in cystathionine synthase deficiency.

Neuroimaging [14,15] revealed MR evidence of diffuse edema and dysmyelination of white matter at presentation, and volume loss of white matter with time, and communication hydrocephalus (Figures 4.3, 4.4). EEG may show epileptiform abnormalities [15]. Evoked responses display increased latency and prolonged conduction [7,15]. In the patient with the neurodegenerative picture, there was prominent involvement of the globus pallidus on magnetic resonance imaging (MRI) and clear evidence of progression. Neurologic progression and cerebral atrophy were observed despite therapy with hydroxocobalamin. The neonatal MRI was normal; that of 1 year revealed white matter loss and ventricular enlargement and normal basal ganglia. At 15 months both globi were hyperintense. Lesions in the basal ganglia have been observed in methylmalonic acidemia of the mut^0 and mut$^-$ types, and in Cbl A and Cbl B disease, and in propionic acidemia. We have also observed similar involvement of the globi pallidi in transcobalamin II deficiency. Multiple small infarcts of the basal ganglia were found in the basal ganglia of a patient with Cbl C disease who died at 22 months [9].

Only two patients have been reported with Cbl D disease: brothers, neither of whom was anemic [2]. The older one was

mentally retarded, and psychotic, and had abnormalities of cerebellar and spinal cord function, including ataxia. His 2-year-old affected brother appeared well at report at 2 years of age. Thromboembolic complications may be observed, as in cystathionine synthase deficiency (Chapter 22).

Five patients have been reported with Cbl F disease [16,17]. Deep tendon reflexes were accentuated, and there was an intention tremor. The first two presented within the first two weeks of life with stomatitis, failure to thrive and hypotonia [6]. Seizures [16,18] were observed, as was developmental delay. There were no hematologic abnormalities in the first patient, but macrocytosis, hypersequenced polymorphonuclear leukocytes and even pancytopenia have been observed. One infant died suddenly despite a good biochemical response to cobalamin.

GENETICS AND PATHOGENESIS

Each of the Cbl group diseases is transmitted in an autosomal recessive fashion. In each the activity of methionine synthase is deficient, and so is that of methylmalonyl-CoA mutase (Figure 3.1, p. 19). Methionine synthase activity has been demonstrated to be restored by the addition of methylcobalamin [19,20]. The fundamental defect in Cbl C and D disease has not yet been delineated, but it appears to be a step in cobalamin processing so early that the formation of methylcobalamin and deoxyadenosyl cobalamin is altered. In Cbl F disease the defect has been identified in the transport step in which cobalamin in lysosomes, once TCII is split off, is normally transported out of the lysosome to begin cofactor synthesis [18]. The transporter defect is analogous to those of sialic acid storage disease and of cystine storage disease (cystinosis) (Chapter 71).

Table 4.2 *Pathological biochemistry of the urine in Cbl C and D diseases (mmol/mol creatinine)*

Metabolite	Pathological (Cbl C&D)	Normal
Urinary methylmalonate	50–700	0–2
Urinary 3-hydroxypropionate	6–30	0–24
Urinary methylcitrate	30–6	0–5
Urinary homocystine	0.08–80	0–0.01

Methionine synthase activity is deficient in Cbl E and G diseases. This enzyme catalyzes the transfer of a methyl of 5-methyltetrahydrofolate to homocysteine. Mutations in the gene coding for this enzyme cause Cbl G disease. In Cbl E disease the mutations are in the gene for methionine synthase reductase which maintains the synthase in its reduced state (Chapter 22).

In the presence of defective cofactor synthesis, methylmalonate and homocystine accumulate. The amounts are distinctly less than in methylmalonyl CoA mutase deficiency or cystathionine synthase deficiency (Table 4.2). The diagnosis is usually made by organic analysis of the urine, which detects methylmalonate, the most abundant metabolite. Methylcitrate and 3-hydroxypropionate are also identified in this way. Screening tests for methylmalonate (Chapter 3, pp. 23 and 24) are also positive, and the diagnosis may first be suspected in this way. Quantitative assay of the urinary amino acids reveals elevated amounts of homocystine. It is important for this purpose to employ fresh urine.

The amounts of homocystine are not large, and this compound is unstable in urine at room temperature. Also, proteinuria may lead to binding of homocystine, which would then be precipitated out and removed from the analysis when the urine is acidified. Screening the urine with the cyanide nitroprusside test is also positive (Chapter 22). Some patients have had hypomethioninemia and cystathioninuria [10,21]. Homocysteine may be found in the plasma by assay for total homocysteine. Regardless of the method homocystine is not found in some patients with Cbl C, and even in Cbl F disease [16].

Once the biochemical diagnosis is made, complementation analysis is performed with cultured fibroblasts incubated with ^{14}C-propionate to determine the specific Cbl complementation group [22]. Studies of the uptake of [57]Co-cyanocobalamin uptake by fibroblasts indicated deficiency in the process of conversion to hydroxycobalamin and the conversion of either to methylcobalamin and deoxyadenoxylcobalamin in patients with Cbl C and D disease [19,22]. Uptake was normal in other forms of homocystinuria and methylmalonic acidemia. Conversion to methylcobalamin and deoxyadenosyl cobalamin was demonstrated to be deficient [19,22]. Cells of patients with Cbl C utilize CN-Cbl poorly and cannot convert CN-Cbl to OH-Cbl [20,23]. This could indicate a defect at cobalamin (III) reductase, catalyzing the reduction of trivalent cobalt prior to alkylation. Concentrations of B_{12} in the serum may be elevated [7].

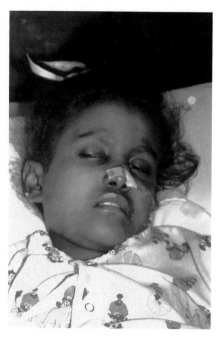

Figure 4.5 *A 12-year-old girl with the Immerslund-Grasbeck B_{12} intestinal absorptive defect [27]. She was bed-ridden, semicomatose, demented, and required intragastric feeding. She had anemia for years, but developed paraparesis at 10 years. The urine had increased levels of homocystine and methylmalonate. Schilling test was abnormal with and without intrinsic factor. Treatment with hydroxocobalamin led to a remarkable improvement.*

The biochemical picture of methylmalonic acidemia and homocystinuria and the acute hematological and clinical neurologic picture of Cbl C disease have been encountered in the exclusively breast-fed infants of strict vegan mothers [24,25] as well as in the breast fed infants of mothers with subclinical pernicious anemia and in TCII deficiency [26]. It is also seen in the Immerslund-Grasbeck defect in ileal absorption of the B_{12}-intrinsic factor complex [27] (Figures 4.5, 4.6). Problems in the differential diagnosis of patients with methylmalonic acidemia were highlighted by a patient who died of mutase deficiency, ultimately diagnosed when a sibling was found to have the disease, but not before the mother was incarcerated for homicide because a commercial clinical laboratory misidentified the propionic acid in the blood as ethylene glycol [28]. This experience points up the importance of quantification and identification by gas chromatography-mass spectrometry (GCMS) as opposed to identification based on elution times in gas chromatography.

TREATMENT

Treatment of all Cbl C disease has largely been unsatisfactory. Most patients have died or been severely handicapped. The documented poor uptake of labeled cyanoB_{12} by fibroblasts [22] indicated that these patients should be treated with

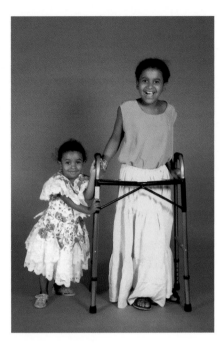

Figure 4.6 *The same patient was able to walk with crutches or a walker after four months of treatment. On the left her 3-year-old sister was found to have severe anemia and was found to have the same disease. Treatment with hydroxocobalamin cured the anemia and prevented neurologic disease [27].*

hydroxycobalamin. Large doses, 1.5 mg intramuscularly (IM) qd have been employed [29,30]. Significant decreases in urinary methylmalonate have been observed, and similar effects were observed in plasma homocysteine. Growth rates have become normal. Reversion to normal of abnormal visual and auditory evoked potentials have been reported [7]. Treatment with hydroxocobalamin has also been reported in Cbl E disease to resolve homocystinuria, methylmalonic aciduria, hypomethioninemia, megaloblastic anemia and failure to thrive [31].

Supplemental uses of betaine, carnitine, and folate have been recommended. The fact that creatine synthesis from guanidinoacetate requires methyl groups provided by the conversion of methionine to homocysteine led to the finding that concentrations of guanidinoacetate are high and those of creatine lower in five patients with Cbl C disease [32]. This raises the possibility that treatment with creatine may be helpful.

References

1 Mudd SH, Levy HL, Abeles RH. A derangement in B_{12} dependency leading to homocystinemia, cystathioninemia and methylmalonic aciduria. *Biochem Biophys Res Commun* 1969;**35**:121.

2 Goodman SI, Moe PG, Hammond KB, *et al*. Homocystinuria with methylmalonic aciduria: two cases in sibship. *Biochem Med* 1970;**4**:500.

3 Mahoney MJ, Hart AC, Steen VD, Rosenberg LE. Methylmalonic acidemia: biochemical heterogeneity in defects of 5′-deoxyadenosylcobalamin synthesis. *Proc Natl Acad Sci* 1975;**72**:2799.

4 Dillon MJ, England JM, Gompertz D, *et al*. Mental retardation, megaloblastic anemia, methylmalonic aciduria and abnormal homocysteine metabolism due to an error in vitamin B_{12} metabolism. *Clin Sci Molec Med* 1974;**47**:43.

5 Mitchell GA, Watkins D, Melancon SB, *et al*. Clinical heterogeneity in cobalamin C variant of combined homocystinuria and methylmalonic aciduria. *J Pediatr* 1986;**108**:410.

6 Robb RM, Dowton SB, Fulton AB, Levy HS. Retinal degeneration in vitamin B_{12} disorder associated with methylmalonic aciduria and sulfur amino acid abnormalities. *Am J Ophthalmol* 1984;**97**:691.

7 Mamlok RJ, Isenberg JN, Rassin DK. A cobalamin metabolic defect with homocystinuria, methylmalonic aciduria and macrocytic anemia. *Neuropediatrics* 1986;**17**:94.

8 Baumgartner EF, Fowler B, Gold R. Hereditary defect of cobalamin metabolism (cbl C) of juvenile onset with neurological features resembling multiple sclerosis. *Proc Int Soc Inborn Errors of Metab*, Milan,1994.

9 Geraghty MT, Perlman EJ, Martin LS, *et al*. Cobalamin C defect associated with hemolytic-uremic syndrome. *J Pediatr* 1992;**120**:934.

10 Howard R, Frieden IJ, Crawford D, *et al*. Methylmalonic acidemia, cobalamin C type, presenting with cutaneous manifestations. *Arch Dermatol* 1997;**133**:1563.

11 Rosenblatt DS, Aspler AL, Shevell MI, *et al*. Clinical heterogeneity and prognosis in combined methylmalonic aciduria and homocytinuira (cbl C). *J Inherit Met Dis* 1997;**20**:528.

12 Enns GM, Barkovich AJ, Rosenblatt DS, *et al*. Progressive neurological deterioration and MRI changes in Cbl C methylmalonic acidaemia – treated with hydroxocobalamin. *J Inherit Metab Dis* 1999;**22**:599.

13 Polanco Y, Polanco FMMA, Cbl C at age 6½. *OAA Newsletter* 2002;**12**:2.

14 Rossi A, Cerone R, Biancheri R, *et al*. Early-onset combined methylmalonic aciduria and homocystinuria: neuroradiologic findings. *Am J Neuroradiol* 2001;**22**:554.

15 Biancheri R, Cerone R, Schiffino MC, *et al*. Cobalamin (cbl) C/D deficiency: clinical neurophysiological and neuroradiologic findings in 14 cases. *Neuropediatrics* 2001;**32**:14.

16 Rosenblatt DS, Laframboise R, Pichette J, *et al*. New disorder of vitamin B_{12} metabolism (cobalamin F) presenting as methylmalonic aciduria. *Pediatrics* 1985;**78**:51.

17 Shih VE, Axel SM, Tewksbury JC, *et al*. Defective lysosomal release of vitamin B_{12} (cblF): A hereditary metabolic disorder associated with sudden death. *Am J Med Genet* 1989;**33**:555.

18 Watkins GA, Rosenblatt PS. Failure of lysosomal release of vitamin B_{12}: a new complementation group causing methylmalonic aciduria (cbl F). *Am J Hum Genet* 1986;**39**:404.

19 Mahoney MJ, Rosenberg LE, Mudd SH, Uhlendorf BW. Defective metabolism of vitamin B_{12} in fibroblasts from patients with methylmalonicaciduria. *Biochem Biophys Res Commun* 1971;**44**:375.

20 Mudd SH, Uhlendorf BW, Hinds KR, Levy HL. Deranged B_{12} metabolism: studies of fibroblasts grown in tissue culture. *Biochem Med* 1970;**4**:215.

21 Levy HL, Mudd SH, Shulman JD, *et al*. A derangement in B_{12} metabolism associated with homocystinemia, cystathioninemia, hypomethionimia and methylmalonic aciduria. *Am J Med* 1970;**48**:390.

22 Willard HF, Mellman IS, Rosenberg LE. Genetic complementation among inherited deficiencies of methylmalonyl-CoA mutase activity: Evidence for a new class of human cobalamin mutant. *Am J Hum Genet* 1978;**30**:1.

23 Mellman I, Willard HF, Youngdahl-Turner P, Rosenberg LE.Cobalamin coenzyme synthesis in normal and mutant human fibroblasts: Evidence for a processing enzyme activity deficient in cbl C cells. *J Biol Chem* 1979;**254**:11847.

24 Higginbottom MC, Sweetman L, Nyhan WL. A syndrome of methylmalonic aciduria, homocystinuria, megaloblastic anemia and neurologic abnormalities in a vitamin B_{12}-deficient breast-fed infant of a strict vegetarian. *N Engl J Med* 1978;**299**:317.

25   Kuhne T, Bubl R, Baumgartner R. Maternal vegan diet causing infantile neurological disorder due to vitamin B_{12} deficiency. *Eur J Pediatr* 1991;**150**:205.

26   Barshop BA, Wolff J, Nyhan WL, *et al*. Transcobalamin II deficiency presenting with methylmalonic aciduria and homocystinuria and abnormal absorption of cobalamin. *Am J Med Genet* 1990;**35**:222.

27   Al Essa M, Sakati NA, Dabbagh O, *et al*. Inborn error of vitamin B_{12} metabolism: a treatable cause of childhood dementia/paralysis. *J Child Neurol* 1998;**13**:239.

28   Shoemaker JD, Lynch RE, Hoffmann JW, Sly WS. Misidentification of propionic acid as ethylene glycol in a patient with methylmalonic acidemia. *J Pediatr* 1992;**120**:417.

29   Cooper BA, Rosenblatt PS. Inherited defects of vitamin B_{12} metabolism. *Ann Rev Nutr* 1987;**7**:291.

30   Andersson HC, Shapira E. Biochemical and clinical response to hydroxocobalamin versus cyanocobalamin treatment in patients with methylmalonic acidemia and homocystinuria (cbl C). *J Pediatr* 1998;**132**:121.

31   Tuchman M, Kelly P, Watkins D, Rosenblatt DS. Vitamin B_{12}-responsive megaloblastic anemia, homocystinuria, and transient methylmalonic aciduria in Cbl E disease. *J Pediatr* 1988;**113**:1052.

32   Bodamer O. Creatine metabolism and Cbl C. *Organic Acidemia Association Newsletter* 2002;**12**:11.

5

Multiple carboxylase deficiency/holocarboxylase synthetase deficiency

---

MAJOR PHENOTYPIC EXPRESSION

Erythematous, scaly eruption; alopecia; episodic, potentially lethal attacks of vomiting, ketosis, acidosis, and dehydration progressive to coma; lactic acidemia; organic aciduria including 3-methylcrotonylglycine, 3-hydroxyisovaleric acid, methylcitric acid and 3-hydroxypropionic acid; defective activity of the propionyl CoA, 3-methylcrotonyl-CoA and pyruvate carboxylases; and defective activity of holocarboxylase synthetase (Figure 5.1).

INTRODUCTION

The first patient described with this disorder [1] was recognized as having an abnormality of leucine metabolism by the identification of 3-methylcrotonylglycine and 3-hydroxyisovaleric acid in the urine. When we found that methylcitric and hydroxypropionic acids were also excreted by the same patient [2], enzymatic analysis revealed defective activity of propionyl CoA carboxylases [3] as well as 3-methylcrotonyl CoA carboxylase [4]. The third mitochondrial carboxylase, pyruvate carboxylase, was also shown to be defective in activity [5]. The disorder was then renamed multiple carboxylase deficiency (Figure 5.2) It is now clear that there are two distinct disorders in which there is multiple carboxylase deficiency: holocarboxylase synthetase (HCS) deficiency [6] (Figure 5.1), which was the defect in the initial patient, and biotinidase deficiency (Chapter 6).

The gene for holocarboxylase synthetase has been cloned and assigned to chromosome 21q22 [7,8]. The nature of the mutation was defined in two Japanese patients: a one-base deletion, 1delG1067, which results in a premature termination; and a missense mutation, T997C, which changes a leucine to a proline. These mutations were found in a number of Japanese mutant alleles. Expression of the L237P mutation yielded an enzyme with decreased activity [9]. Examination

of European and Middle Eastern populations has revealed a variety of mutations, none of them common [10]. Expression yielded activity ranging from 1 to 14 percent of control.

Among the most rewarding features of the disease is the exquisite sensitivity of most variant enzymes to treatment of the patient with biotin, which converts an otherwise uniformly fatal disease to completely normal health.

CLINICAL ABNORMALITIES

Patients with HCS deficiency generally present in the first days or months of life with overwhelming illness identical to those of propionic acidemia (Chapter 2) or other classic organic acidemia [1,11–16]. In seven patients in whom the enzyme defect was documented [14], the age of onset of clinical symptoms varied from the first day of life to 18 months [17]. Most patients presented before 6 weeks of age, but it is clear that patients with an abnormal holocarboxylase synthetase can present at any age from 1 day to 6 years of age [18,19]. The initial impression that the two forms of multiple carboxylase deficiency could be differentiated by the age of onset has not held up, although those with holocarboxylase

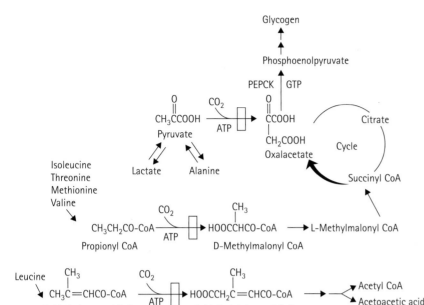

Figure 5.1 *Pyruvate carboxylase, propionyl CoA carboxylase and 3-methylcrotonyl carboxylase. The activities of each are deficient in multiple carboxylase deficiency.*

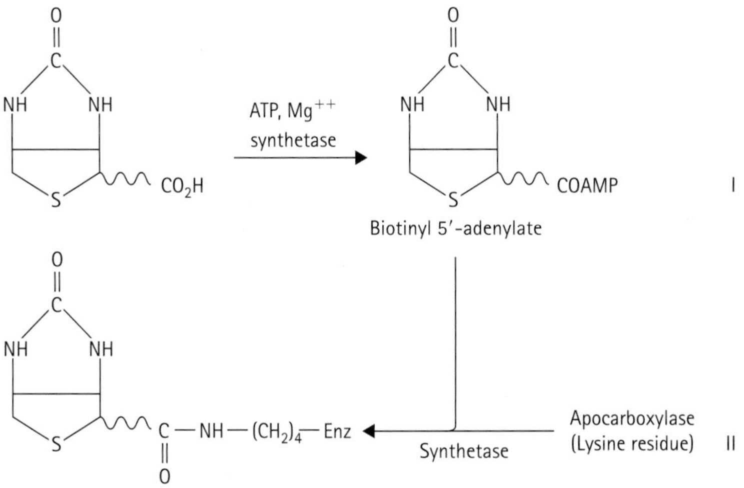

Figure 5.2 *Holocarboxylase synthetase.*

synthetase abnormalities [20] have generally presented within the first six weeks of life, while those with biotinidase deficiency have generally presented after 6 months of age.

In the acute episode of illness the infant has massive ketosis and metabolic acidosis with an anion gap. There may be tachypnea or Kussmaul breathing. Concentrations of ammonia in the blood may be elevated. The episode may progress to dehydration, deep coma, and, unless vigorously treated, death. There is documentation of a number of patients who have died of this disease [11–21]. In fact the initial episode may be lethal within hours of birth [11].

The classic patient with this disease was J.R. [1] in whom all the initial studies were done [1–5,22] and the defect in the HCS enzyme worked out [6,14]. He had had recurrent episodes of vomiting from birth. An erythematous skin rash appeared at 6 weeks of age. At 5 months he developed rapid respirations, vomiting and unresponsiveness, and was found to have ketosis and metabolic acidosis.

The manifestations of the disease in the skin are memorable (Figure 5.3). An erythematous eruption usually involves the entire body. Some patients have died before the development of skin lesions, and now patients are being treated before the development of cutaneous lesions, but cutaneous features are an integral part of the untreated disease. The lesions are bright red, scaly or desquamative. Intertriginous areas may be exudative. Complicating infection with monilia is common. The differential diagnosis of the skin disease includes acrodermatitis enteropathica, seborrheic dermatitis and ichthyosis. The dermatosis is identical to that of clinical biotin deficiency [23]. Varying degrees of alopecia (Figure 5.4), an unusual manifestation in childhood, are associated, including alopecia totalis (Figure 5.4); eyelashes, eyebrows and lanugo hair are absent as well as the hair of the head. The differential diagnosis of alopecia includes:

- multiple carboxylase deficiency (HCS and biotinidase deficiencies)

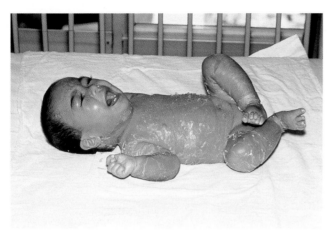

Figure 5.3   *A.F. at 9 months of age. He had a bright red scaly eruption. Alopecia was not prominent during this relapse.*

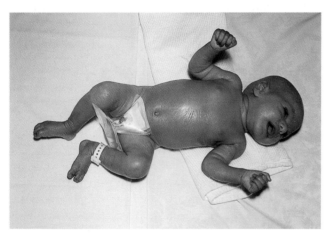

Figure 5.4   *M.Z. at 3-months-of-age. The scaly eruption was erythematous and present throughout the body. He had almost complete alopecia of the scalp, except for a small amount of occipital hair, but there were sparse eyebrows and eyelashes.*

- biotin deficiency
- cartilage hair hypoplasia
- an(hypo)hidrotic ectodermal dysplasia
- trichorhexis nodosa – argininosuccinic aciduria
- vitamin D receptor abnormalities.

Persistent vomiting may lead to failure to thrive. Neurologic abnormalities are not integral features of the disease; they appear to be related more to the effects of the initial, or repeated, episodes of illness in which there might be diminished perfusion of the brain or hyperammonemia, and the neurologic examination may be normal despite a hyperammonemic episode [24]. Hypotonia has been observed, as well as hypertonia and irritability [25,26]. Athetoid movements and opisthotonus have been described [27], as has 'cerebral palsy' [28]. There may be abnormalities of the electroencephalogram (EEG), and abnormalities of computed tomography (CT) or magnetic resonance imaging (MRI) scans, particularly in the white matter. An infant was reported [29]

to have subependymal cysts, seen on cranial ultrasound and MRI, which disappeared following six months of treatment with biotin.

Patients have disordered immunologic function of both T and B cells [11]. A diminution in the number of circulating T lymphocytes has been observed along with a diminution in their *in vitro* response to Candida in a patient with a history of bacteremia [25].

GENETICS AND PATHOGENESIS

The disorder is transmitted as an autosomal recessive trait. Both males and females are affected, and siblings of uninvolved parents have been observed. Consanguinity has been documented [1,11,26]. Fibroblast cultures from two unrelated individuals were studied using the complementation assay for propionic acidemia [5]. They failed to complement each other, but they did complement mutants for all of the other groups studied, such as propionic acidemia. Heterozygote detection has not been possible by enzyme analysis, but in a family in which the mutation is known it should not be demanding.

The metabolic hallmark of this disease is the excretion of 3-methylcrotonylglycine and 3-hydroxyisovaleric acid along with elevated amounts of lactic acid in the blood and urine. Thus the first clinical chemical clue to the disease may be the documentation of lactic acidemia. Organic acid analysis at the time of acute acidosis also reveals methylcitric and 3-hydroxypropionic acids. The organic acidemia may be quite variable, particularly if first studied after intensive therapy with parenteral fluid and electrolytes and resolution of the acidosis. The excretion of 3-hydroxyisovaleric acid is virtually always greater than that of 3-methylcrotonylglycine [11,20,27]; but occasionally, the proportion of these values was reversed [1]. The excretion of 3-hydroxyisovaleric may be as high as 200 times normal [2]. The lactic aciduria may be enormous. These patients may also excrete tiglylglycine in the urine [11].

The lactic acidosis may be striking [15]. In an infant with lactic acidosis it is important to consider this possibility and to assay the organic acids in the urine; if organic acid analysis is not promptly available, a trial of biotin therapy is warranted (with the urine saved for analysis).

The activities of the carboxylases (Figure 5.2) may be measured in leukocyte extracts or in fibroblasts, as well as in tissues. In patients with holocarboxylase synthetase deficiency we have found levels of activity ranging from 0.4 to 53 percent of control (Table 5.1). In parallel studies of propionyl CoA and 3-methylcrotonyl CoA carboxylases in fibroblasts, their kinetic properties were normal [3]. The levels of activity of these enzymes are dependent on the concentrations of biotin in the medium. Activity of all of the carboxylases is markedly deficient when fibroblasts are grown in 6 nmol biotin/L. Carboxylases are normal when the cells are grown in 100 nmol biotin/L.

Table 5.1   *Carboxylase activity in holocarboxylase synthetase deficiency*

	Normal range pmol/min mg/protein		Patient data % of control	
	Leukocyte	Fibroblast	Leukocyte	Fibroblast
Propionyl CoA carboxylase	160–447	128–537	12–43	0.7–52
3-Methylcrotonyl CoA carboxylase	62–288	71–250	15–34	04.47
Pyruvate carboxylase	7–14	96–362	29–53	2–60

The fundamental defect is in holocarboxylase synthetase (EC 6.3.4.10) [6,14] (Figure 5.2). This is a complex enzyme which activates biotin to form D-biotinyl-5′-adenylate, and then catalyzes the attachment of the biotin to an ε-amino group of a lysine residue of the newly synthesized apocarboxylase enzyme. The covalent binding to biotin conveys enzymatic activity and holocarboxylase status to the apocarboxylase protein, which is inactive prior to this conversion.

To date all but one patient studied has had altered Km for biotin; the normal Km is 1–6 nmol/L, and values in 16 patient cells have ranged from 9 to 12 nmol/L. The maximum velocity (Vmax) at saturation concentrations of biotin may be normal or reduced. There appears to be some correlation between the age of onset and severity of illness and the degree of elevation of the Km for biotin of holocarboxylase synthetase [14]. A patient with 70 times normal Km for biotin presented in the first few hours of life [12] and a previous sibling had died in the neonatal period [11]. Patients in whom the Km values for biotin of holocarboxylase synthetase were 20 to 45 times normal presented between one day of life and 7 weeks. A patient with a Km for biotin only three times normal presented at 8 months of age. The Km for biotin was not elevated in the enzyme coded for by the L237P mutation [9]; the Vmax for this enzyme was 4.3 percent of the control mean.

The initial enzymatic step, the biotinyl–AMP (adenosine monophosphate) synthetase reaction, has now been found to be deficient in each of the fibroblast lines studied [30]. In four patients studied, activity ranged from 0.3 to 8 percent of controls. This makes for a much simpler assay than that currently available for the whole reaction, in which the substrate for the synthetase is an apocarboxylase carefully purified from the liver of biotin-deficient rats.

The cDNA for holocarboxylase synthetase [7] codes for a protein of 726 amino acids [7,31]; amino acids 445–701 have homology with related enzymes in *E. coli* and yeast. Among the mutations identified a number are in this domain considered to bind biotin, for instance R508W, G518E, and V550M [32]. This is consistent with the clinical biotin responsiveness of six patients. However, patients with mutations outside this area, like those with the L237P mutation have also responded to biotin.

Prenatal diagnosis has been accomplished by the demonstration of biotin-responsive deficiencies of carboxylases in cultured amniocytes. It has also been demonstrated by assay of the activity of holocarboxylase synthetase [33]. Prenatal diagnosis has also been made by the direct assay of methylcitric acid in the amniotic fluid by stable isotope dilution and selected ion monitoring using gas chromatography-mass spectrometry (GCMS), as in propionic acidemia (Chapter 2). However, the concentrations of 3-hydroxyisovaleric acid in the amniotic fluid of patients with HCS deficiency are higher and its quantification is more reliable [34]. This is the best chemical method for the rapid prenatal diagnosis of this disorder and may unequivocally indicate an affected fetus. However, we have encountered the situation in which the results of this assay were equivocal, in which case assay of holocarboxylase synthetase gave the correct diagnosis [35]. Prenatal diagnosis has been carried out by enzyme assay of amniocytes [33,35] and chorionic villus material [36]. In each case a markedly elevated Km for biotin was diagnostic. In a family in which the mutation is known molecular methods may be used for prenatal diagnosis.

TREATMENT

All patients observed to date have been exquisitely sensitive to treatment with exogenous biotin. None have had acute attacks of ketoacidosis while taking biotin. The initial dose employed was 10 mg/day, and most patients have responded nicely to this dose. Nevertheless, heterogeneity in this condition may be manifest in the level of responsiveness to biotin. In some patients small amounts of metabolites, present when the dose was 10 mg of biotin per day in the urine, disappeared when it was increased to 40 mg/day [25,33]. Another patient, though clinically well when receiving as little as 1 mg of biotin per day, had elevated excretions of metabolites and activities of the carboxylases in leukocytes that were only 4 to 16 percent of normal when the dose was 20 mg of biotin per day [37]. A patient with a very high Km for biotin [14] continued to have skin lesions, large excretions of metabolites and subnormal activities of carboxylases in lymphocytes when receiving doses of biotin as high as 60 mg per day. Another patient required 100 mg per day before skin lesions resolved, and the relevant organic acids were present in small amounts in the urine, even on this regimen [18]. When provided with adequate amounts of biotin none of the patients have required dietary restriction of protein, although moderate restriction in the less responsive patients could well decrease the accumulation of metabolites.

The clinical response to treatment is dramatic. Ketosis and acidosis disappear along with hyperammonemia. Levels of lactic and pyruvic acid in the blood become normal [38]. Lethargy, hypotonia and ataxia disappear [2]. The skin lesions disappear in virtually all patients, and the hair grows. Abnormalities of the EEG and CT scan have been documented to disappear [12]. At the same time persisting neurologic abnormalities, such as developmental delay [18,26] and dilated ventricles [12] once developed would not be expected to regress.

Few pharmacokinetic data have been assembled, but blood levels of biotin approximating 100 ng/mL have been reported in a 3-month-old infant receiving 10 mg of biotin per day [39]. Urinary excretion varied between 2 and 4 mg/g creatinine. In a 2-year-old receiving the same dose, plasma levels as high as 703 ng/mL were observed [26], and in a neonate a level of 660 ng/mL was found following a dose of 20 mg per day [25]. These values exceed the range of the altered Km for biotin in the patients studied and provide a potentially elegant correlation of the kinetics of each variant enzyme and the clinical pharmacology of biotin.

The biochemical response to treatment is striking; the levels of organic acid metabolites often decrease to normal, but it may remain possible to continue to detect 3-hydroxyisovaleric acid in the urine [20,23]. The activities of the carboxylases in leukocytes usually become normal within a few days of the initiation of therapy.

Prenatal therapy with biotin has been successfully pursued in at least four pregnancies at risk [33,35,36,40]. In most, the affected fetus was diagnosed prenatally [33,35,36]. The dose of biotin to the mother was 10 mg per day and levels of biotin in maternal serum were very high. There were no ill effects in the mother or fetus. At birth, assay of holocarboxylase synthetase in cultured skin fibroblasts indicated that infants were affected, but they were clinically well and had levels of urinary organic acids that were normal (Figure 5.5). Prenatal treatment in this condition appears prudent, because birth itself may be sufficiently catabolic that an affected infant may become irreversibly moribund within hours of birth [11]; and certainly death following ketoacidosis and disseminated intravascular coagulation has been recorded even after initiation of biotin therapy [41]. An infant, in whom treatment was carried out prenatally without diagnosis, then suspended while fibroblast cultures were established and an enzymatic diagnosis made, developed severe ketoacidosis, lactic academia and shock, but did respond to biotin therapy [40].

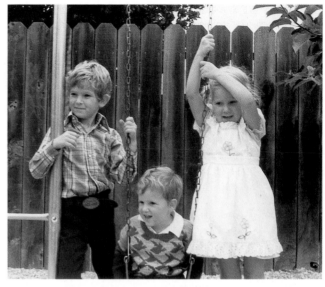

Figure 5.5   *Prenatal diagnosis of holocarboxylase synthetase. J.W., the boy on the left, presented with typical neonatal ketoacidosis, but was diagnosed promptly and treated with biotin and has not had a further episode. His sister, on the right, was diagnosed and treated prenatally and has never had symptoms of multiple carboxylase deficiency. The brother in the middle was normal.*

References

1   Gompertz D, Draffan GH, Watts JL, Hull D. Biotin-responsive 3-methylcrotonylglycinuria. *Lancet* 1971;**2**:22.

2   Sweetman L, Bates SP, Hull D, Nyhan WL. Propionyl-CoA carboxylase deficiency in a patient with biotin responsive 3-methylcrotonylglycinuria. *Pediatr Res* 1977;**11**:1144.

3   Weyler W, Sweetman L, Maggio DC, Nyhan WL. Deficiency of propionyl-CoA carboxylase in a patient with methylcrotonylglycinuria. *Clin Chim Acta* 1977;**76**:321.

4   Gompertz D, Goodey PA, Bartlett K. Evidence for the enzymatic defect in 3-methylcrotonylglycinuria. *FEBS Lett* 1973;**32**:13.

5   Saunders M, Sweetman L, Robinson B, *et al*. Biotin-responsive organic aciduria. Multiple carboxylase defects and complementation studies with propionic acidemia in cultured fibroblasts. *J Clin Invest* 1979;**64**:1695.

6   Burri BJ, Sweetman L, Nyhan WL. Mutant holocarboxylase synthetase. Evidence for the enzyme defect in early infantile biotin-responsive multiple carboxylase deficiency. *J Clin Invest* 1981;**68**:1491.

7   Suzuki Y, Aoki Y, Ishida Y, *et al*. Isolation and characterization of mutations in the holocarboxylase synthetase cDNA. *Nature Genet.* 1994;**8**:122.

8   Zhang XX, Leon-Del-Rio A, Gravel RA, Eydoux P. Assignment of holocarboxylase synthetase gene (HLCS) to human chromosome band 21q22.1 and to mouse chromosome band 16C4 by *in situ* hybridization. *Cytogenet Cell Genet* 1997;**76**:179.

9   Aoki Y, Suzuki Y, Li X, *et al*. Characterization of mutant holocarboxylase synthetase (HCS): a Km for biotin was not elevated in a patient with HCS deficiency. *Pediatr Res* 1997;**42**:849.

10   Aoki Y, Li X, Sakamoto O, *et al*. Identification and characterization of mutations in patients with holocarboxylase synthetase deficiency. *Hum Genet* 1999;**104**:1443.

11   Sweetman L, Nyhan WL, Sakati NA, *et al*. Organic aciduria in neonatal multiple carboxylase deficiency. *J Inherit Metab Dis* 1982;**5**:49.

12 Wolf B, Hsia E, Sweetman L, *et al.* Multiple carboxylase deficiency: clinical and biochemical improvement following neonatal biotin treatment. *Pediatrics* 1981;**68**:113.

13 Bartlett K, Ng H, Dale G, *et al.* Studies on cultured fibroblasts from patient with defects of biotin-dependent carboxylation. *J Inherit Metab Dis* 1981;**4**:183.

14 Burri BJ, Sweetman L, Nyhan WL. Heterogeneity of holocarboxylase synthetase in patients with biotin-responsive multiple carboxylase deficiency. *Am J Hum Genet* 1985;**37**:326.

15 Briones P, Ribes A, Vilaseca MA, *et al.* A new case of holocarboxylase synthetase deficiency. *J Inherit Metab Dis* 1989;**12**:329.

16 Michalski AJ, Berry GT, Segal S. Holo-carboxylase synthetase deficiency: 9-year follow-up of a patient on chronic biotin therapy and a review of the literature. *J Inherit Metab Dis* 1989;**12**:312.

17 Suormala T, Fowler B, Jakobs C, *et al.* Late-onset holocarboxylase synthetase-deficiency: Pre- and post-natal diagnosis and evaluation of effectiveness of antenatal biotin therapy. *Eur J Pediatr* 1998;**157**:570.

18 Suormala T, Fowler B, Duran M, *et al.* Five patients with a biotin-responsive defect in holocarboxylase formation: Evaluation of responsiveness to biotin therapy *in vivo* and comparative biochemical studies *in vitro. Pediatr Res* 1997;**41**:666.

19 Sherwood WG, Saunders M, Robinson BH, *et al.* Lactic acidosis in biotin-responsive multiple carboxylase deficiency caused by holocarboxylase synthetase deficiency of early and late onset. *J Pediat* 1982;**101**:546.

20 Sweetman L. Two forms of biotin-responsive multiple carboxylase deficiency. *J Inher Metab Dis* 1981;**4**:53.

21 Roth K, Cohn R, Yandrasitz J, *et al.* Beta-methylcrotonic aciduria associated with lactic acidosis. *J Pediatr* 1976;**88**:229.

22 Gompertz D, Draffan GH. The identification of tiglylglycine in the urine of a child with 3-methylcrotonyl-glycinuria. *Clin Chim Acta* 1972;**37**:405.

23 Sweetman L, Surh L, Baker H, Peterson RM, Nyhan WL. Clinical and metabolic abnormalities in a boy with dietary deficiency of biotin. *Pediatrics* 1981;**68**:553.

24 Dabbagh O, Brismar J, Gascon GG, Ozand PT. The clinical spectrum of biotin-treatable encephalopathies in Saudi Arabia. *Brain Dev* 1994;**16**:(Suppl) 72.

25 Packman S, Sweetman L, Baker H, Wall S. The neonatal form of biotin-responsive multiple carboxylase deficiency. *J Pediat* 1981;**99**:418.

26 Leonard JV, Seakins JWT, Bartlett K, *et al.* Inherited disorders of 3-methylcrotonyl CoA carboxylation. *Arch Dis Child* 1981;**56**:53.

27 Gompertz D, Bartlett K, Blair D, Stern CMM. Child with a defect in leucine metabolism associated with 3-hydroxyisovaleric aciduria and 3-methylcrotonylglycinuria. *Arch Dis Child* 1973;**48**:975.

28 Livne M, Gibson KM, Amir N, *et al.* Holocarboxylase synthetase deficiency: A treatable metabolic disorder masquerading as cerebral palsy. *J Child Neurol* 1994;**9**:170.

29 Squires L, Betz B, Umfleet J, Kelley R. Resolution of subependymal cysts in neonatal holocarboxylase synthetase deficiency. *Dev Med Child Neurol* 1997;**39**:267.

30 Morita J, Thuy LP, Sweetman L. Deficiency of biotinyl-AMP synthetase activity in fibroblasts of patients with holocarboxylase synthetase deficiency. *Mol Genet Metab* 1989;**64**:250.

31 Leon-Del-Rio A, Leclerc D, Akerman B, *et al.* Isolation of a cDNA encoding human holocarboxylase synthetase by functional complementation of a biotin auxotroph of *Escherichia coli. Proc Natl Acad Sci USA* 1995;**92**:4626.

32 Dupuis L, Leon-Del-Rio A, Leclerc D, *et al.* Clustering of mutations in the biotin-binding region of holocarboxylase synthetase in biotin-responsive multiple carboxylase deficiency. *Hum Mol Genet* 1996;**5**:1011.

33 Packman S, Cowan MJ, Golbus MS, *et al.* Prenatal treatment of biotin-responsive multiple carboxylase deficiency. *Lancet* 1982;**1**:1435.

34 Jakobs C, Sweetman L, Nyhan WL, Packman S. Stable isotope dilution analysis of 3-hydroxyisovaleric acid in amniotic fluid: contribution to the prenatal diagnosis of inherited disorders of leucine catabolism. *J Inher Metab Dis* 1984;**7**:15.

35 Thuy LP, Belmont J, Nyhan WL. Prenatal diagnosis and treatment of holocarboxylase synthetase deficiency. *Prenat Diagn* 1999;**19**:108.

36 Thuy LP, Jurecki E, Nemzer L, Nyhan WL. Prenatal diagnosis of holocarboxylase synthetase deficiency by assay of the enzyme in chorionic villus material followed by prenatal treatment. *Clin Chim Acta* 1999;**284**:59.

37 Narisawa K, Arai N, Igarashi Y, *et al.* Clinical and biochemical findings on a child with multiple biotin-responsive carboxylase deficiencies. *J Inherit Metab Dis* 1982;**5**:67.

38 Charles BM, Hosking G, Green A, *et al.* Biotin-responsive alopecia and developmental regression. *Lancet* 1979;**2**:188.

39 Gaudry M, Munnich A, Ogier H, *et al.* Deficient liver biotinidase activity in multiple carboxylase deficiency. *Lancet* 1983;**2**:397.

40 Roth KS, Yang W, Allan L, *et al.* Prenatal administration of biotin in biotin-responsive multiple carboxylase deficiency. *Pediatr Res* 1982;**16**:126.

41 Roth KS, Yang W, Foreman JW, *et al.* Holocarboxylase synthetase deficiency: a biotin-responsive organic acidemia. *J Pediat* 1980;**96**: 845.

6

Multiple carboxylase deficiency/biotinidase deficiency

MAJOR PHENOTYPIC EXPRESSION

Seizures, ataxia, hypotonia, alopecia, periorificial cutaneous eruption, episodic metabolic acidosis, hearing loss, loss of vision, developmental delay; lactic acidemia, propionic acidemia, excretion of 3-methylcrotonylglycine, 3-hydroxyisovaleric acid, methylcitric acid and 3-hydroxypropionic acid in urine; and defective activity of biotinidase.

INTRODUCTION

Biotinidase deficiency is a form of multiple carboxylase deficiency in which the fundamental defect is an inability to cleave biocytin (Figures 6.1 and 6.2), and this leads to defective activity of propionylCoA carboxylase, 3-methylcrotonylCoA carboxylase and pyruvate carboxylase [1]. Multiple carboxylase deficiency is also caused by defective activity of holocarboxylase synthetase [2] (Chapter 5). In earlier literature biotinidase deficiency was referred to as the later infantile form of multiple carboxylase deficiency [1,3] to distinguish it from the usual neonatal presentation of holocarboxylase synthetase deficiency. However, it is now clear that the latter disorder can present later and the former earlier; the way to distinguish them unambiguously is by enzyme analysis.

Biotin, as a vitamin, cannot be synthesized by humans; but in addition to dietary sources it is synthesized by intestinal microflora. There are dietary sources of free biotin, but covalently bound biotin must ultimately be acted upon by biotinidase to make biotin available from either dietary, intestinal bacterial or recycled sources (Figure 6.1). Biotin is an intrinsic cofactor for each of the carboxylase enzymes, which are synthesized as inactive apoenzymes and must be linked with biotin in the holocarboxylase synthetase reaction (Chapter 5) to become active holoenzymes.

The cDNA for biotinidase has been cloned [4], and the gene has been mapped to chromosome 3p25 [5]. At least 21 mutations were found [6] in 37 children with profound, symptomatic deficiency of biotin. Two were common, accounting for over half of the alleles studied, one a deletion/insertion delG98-G104: insTCC (G98:d7i3) which results in a frame shift and premature termination and the other R538C, a substitution of T for C at nucleotide 1612, only five amino acids from the carboxy terminus of the enzyme. Variants with partial deficiency of biotinidase deficiency have the mutation D444H, which appears to be a polymorphism, in compound with a mutation causing profound deficiency when homozygous on the other allele [7,8].

CLINICAL ABNORMALITIES

Biotinidase deficiency presents with a median age of 3 months or as late as 10 years of age. Symptoms may begin in the neonatal period. Initial symptoms may be dermatologic [9] or seizures [10]. Early infantile seizures may be myoclonic.

The cutaneous lesions tend to be patchy [10–14] (Figures 6.3–6.11, p. 45) in contrast to the total body eruption seen in holocarboxylase synthetase deficiency. However, there may be severe generalized involvement of the skin with redness and

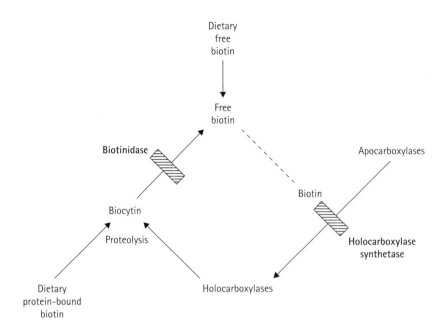

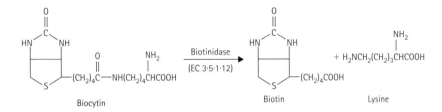

Figure 6.1   *Pathways of metabolism of biotin. Biotin is an essential cofactor for all carboxylase enzymes. Attachment to the inactive newly synthesized apocarboxylase is catalyzed by holocarboxylase synthetase. Biotin is recycled through the activity of biotinidase, and this enzyme would also be required to release biotin bound to protein in the intestine.*

Figure 6.2   *The biotinidase reaction in which biocytin is cleaved to generate biotin and lysine.*

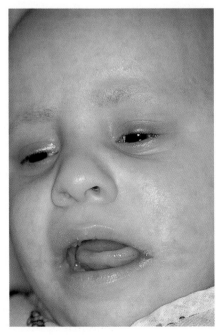

Figure 6.3   *F.E., a 27-month-old Saudi Arabian girl with biotinidase deficiency. She lost all scalp hair and eyebrows at 20 days, but it returned; scalp hair disappeared at 8 months. In addition, she had reddened dermatitis about the eyes and mouth, with cracking at the corners of the lips.*

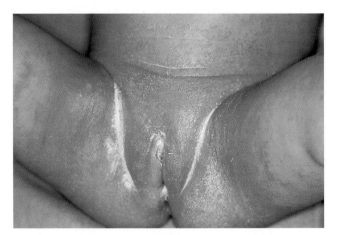

Figure 6.4   *F.E. There was also extensive perineal dermatitis. In addition, she had spastic quadriparesis.*

desquamation [12]. Skin lesions are associated with periorificial cracking, and there may be blepharoconjunctivitis or keratoconjunctivitis of sufficient severity to lead to admission to hospital. Corneal ulceration may occur. Perioral stomatitis is regularly seen, and there may be glossitis. There may also be perineal dermatitis [12] (Figure 6.4). One of our patients had carried a clinical diagnosis of acrodermatitis enteropathica for many years. Anhidrotic ectodermal dysplasia has also

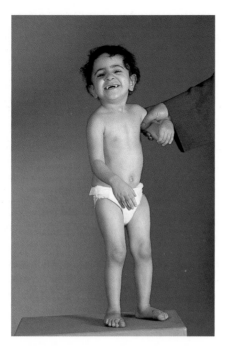

Figure 6.5   *F.E. after six months of treatment with biotin. She had lost the spastic quadriparesis, had no dermatitis and abundant hair.*

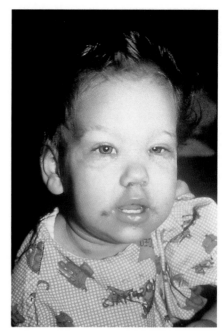

Figure 6.7   *R.R., a girl with biotinidase deficiency, illustrating the periorificial lesions that led to a diagnosis of acrodermatitis enteropathica. The hair was sparse. (Illustration was kindly provided by Dr. Seymour Packman, University of California, San Francisco.)*

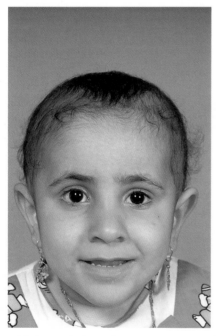

Figure 6.6   *F.E. six months later, illustrating the return of the alopecia following noncompliance with biotin therapy. She again responded to treatment but had essentially total loss of hearing.*

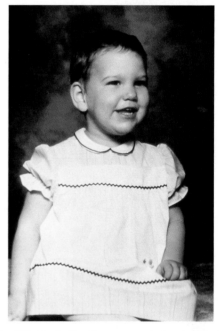

Figure 6.8   *R.R., illustrating the response to treatment with biotin. (Illustration was kindly provided by Dr. Seymour Packman, University of California, San Francisco.)*

been considered in the differential diagnosis of this disorder. The eruption may appear seborrheic. Mucocutaneous candidiasis is a frequent concomitant. The alopecia may be progressive to alopecia totalis (Figure 6.10) [10], but it is usually less than total (Figures 6.7 and 6.11), and may be simply a sparseness of cranial hair, eyebrows or lashes.

In initial experience the diagnosis was made in each patient because of the occurrence of typical episodes of acidosis, ketosis and organic aciduria [3]. Severe, life-threatening acidosis may be seen [13], along with coma, hypothermia, massive

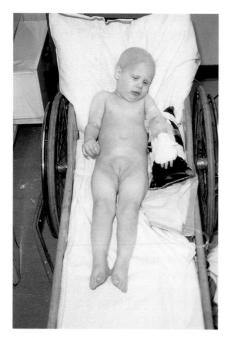

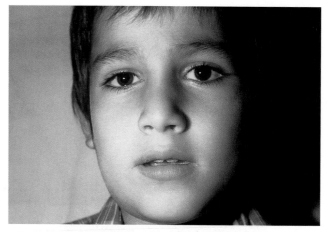

Figure 6.11 *C.G., illustrating the complete reversal of the cutaneous lesions and the alopecia after treatment with biotin. He had significant hearing loss and pale optic discs. (Illustration kindly provided by Dr. E. Zammarchi, Dipartimento di Pediatria, Clinica Pediatrica 1, University of Florence, Florence, Italy.)*

Figure 6.9 *J. Ro, a patient with biotinidase deficiency. In addition to the skin lesions and the alopecia, incapacitating neurologic disease made her bedridden. (Illustration was kindly provided by Dr. Jess Thoene.)*

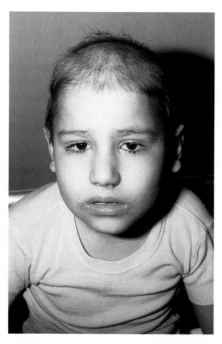

Figure 6.10 *C.G., a boy with biotinidase deficiency, illustrating the characteristic lesions about the mouth and eyes and the alopecia. (Illustration kindly provided by Dr. E. Zammarchi, Dipartimento di Pediatria, Clinica Pediatrica 1, University of Florence, Florence, Italy.)*

hypotonia and absent reflexes [15]. There may be chronic compensated acidosis with serum concentrations of bicarbonate in the range of 15 mEq/L [10]. Episodic acidosis may be seen at times of acute infection [11].

Neurological manifestations are major features of biotinidase deficiency. Ataxia is a prominent feature and may be so profound as to interfere with walking [10]. Ataxia may also be intermittent [14]. There may be associated intention tremor. Seizures occur in over 70 percent of patients and may be the only obvious symptom [16,17]; so testing for biotinidase deficiency is warranted in any patient with unexplained seizures. Seizures may be generalized or myoclonic. They may be frequent, or intermittent, or they may occur only with fever. Infantile spasms may be the initial presenting feature of the disease [18]. In one study [17] of 78 children, 55 percent had seizures; and of these, seizures were the presenting complaint in 70 percent. Seizures were poorly controlled with anticonvulsant medication in 40 percent, but in 75 percent they disappeared after treatment with biotin. This experience, like other responses to biotin in multiple carboxylase deficiencies, can be one of the most striking and rewarding in medicine. Development may be delayed [10,12]. Hypotonia has also been observed in over half of the patients [3]. Two patients developed acute severe hypotonia at 10 months in which there was loss of head control [19,20]. The neurologic decline of Leigh syndrome has been described in a number of patients [12,21–23]. Stridorous or labored breathing and apnea have been seen in these patients [21], followed by psychomotor regression or bulbar symptoms [22]. Deep tendon reflexes may be brisk. Death from the disease has been reported at 9 months and at 3 years of age [14].

Neurosensory abnormalities involving the optic and auditory nerves have been observed in a considerable number of patients, often as late manifestations [3,24–29]. Loss of visual function is associated with optic atrophy [3,24,28]. It appears to be more common in patients in whom diagnosis and treatment is delayed [30]. Neurosensory hearing loss seems to follow the same pattern [3,25]. Among 33 children diagnosed because of symptoms, and none treated from birth, 76 percent had

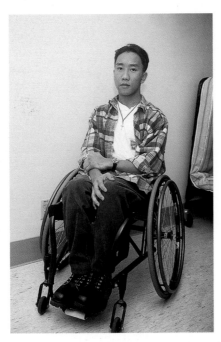

Figure 6.12   *F.M., an 18-year-old man with biotinidase deficiency who presented at 13 years with spastic diplegia and loss of vision. Vision improved with biotin, but optic discs were white and he remained wheelchair-dependent.*

hearing loss [31]. A patient diagnosed at 10 months of age and treated with 10 mg of biotin per day [19,26] subsequently developed sensorineural hearing loss and severe myopia with progressive retinal epithelial dysplasia and optic atrophy. Treatment with biotin does not necessarily prevent these optic and auditory manifestations, but the authors of the report [31] were not aware of hearing loss in any infants diagnosed via newborn screening and treated from the neonatal period. Many of the neurological features of disease disappear in response to treatment with biotin, as do the cutaneous and metabolic features; but sensorineural abnormalities involving the optic and auditory nerves are persistent. Since most of these patients have been treated for some time before these lesions are detected, the question has been raised that they might be a consequence of treatment with biotin; however, this seems unlikely because these complications have never been encountered in patients with holocarboxylase synthetase deficiency who have been treated with biotin from an earlier age, sometimes with higher doses. Furthermore, these abnormalities have been observed in a number of patients prior to the initiation of treatment with biotin [27,32].

An unusual late-onset presentation has been described [27,33–35] in patients with spastic paraparesis studied at 13 and 15 years of age (Figure 6.12). In each there was progressive optic atrophy. In one boy the first symptom was acute loss of vision during an intercurrent infection [31]. In this patient there was improvement in visual acuity, and disappearance of pyramidal tract signs in the lower limbs after months of treatment with biotin [33]. In the other [27] there was considerable improvement in both areas but he was still quite spastic

and essentially wheelchair bound. Acute loss of vision, optic atrophy and spastic paraparesis developed in one patient at 10 years of age [34].

Immunodeficiency has been reported [13], and there have been abnormalities in the function of both T and B cells. In two patients with extensive chronic mucocutaneous candidiasis responses to Candida antigen *in vitro* and *in vivo* were absent. In one there was a deficiency of IgA and no antibody response to immunization with pneumococcal polysaccharide; in the other, the percentage of circulating T lymphocytes was abnormally low. In this family two previous siblings had died at 8 and 39 months of age of what appeared to be the same disease [13,36]. An unrelated patient was reported [37] to have impaired lymphocyte-suppressing activity *in vitro* that improved on treatment with biotin and fatty acids. Deficiency of biotin in guinea pigs has been associated with decreased numbers of T and B lymphocytes [38]. All of these immunologic problems disappear with biotin treatment. One patient was initially thought to have severe combined immunodeficiency and treated with bone marrow transplantation, but manifestations persisted until treatment with biotin was initiated [39].

The electroencephalograph (EEG) is often normal in biotinidase deficiency, but among children with seizures there were 16 abnormal EEGs [17]. Diffuse slowing or convulsive activity has been observed, and usually the EEG has rapidly become normal with biotin treatment [40]. Visual evoked potentials (responses) (VEP, VER) have been abnormal in a number of patients [41,42], returning promptly to normal with biotin treatment. In a 13-year-old boy with optic atrophy and spastic paraparesis [27], positron emission tomography (PET) showed a low relative metabolic rate for glucose in temporal and occipital lobes, which became normal following treatment.

Neuroimaging studies have been highly variable. Calcification of the basal ganglia was reported in a 26-month-old infant [43]. Magnetic resonance imaging (MRI) and computed tomography (CT) evidence of white matter lucency indicative of delayed myelination and diffuse atrophy have been reported [44,45].

The neuropathology has been characterized by atrophy and neuronal loss in the cerebellum [14]. Atrophy of the superior vermis has been associated with virtually complete disappearance of the layer of Purkinje cells. In addition there was moderate gliosis in the white matter and a subacute necrotizing myelopathy. The histopathologic picture of subacute necrotizing encephalopathy has been reported in a patient with the clinical picture of Leigh syndrome [22]. There was rarefaction and spongy degeneration in the subcortical white matter, the midbrain, pons and medulla.

GENETICS AND PATHOGENESIS

Biotinidase deficiency is transmitted in an autosomal recessive pattern. Siblings of uninvolved parents have been observed and consanguinity has been documented [15,20]. Parents of patients display about 50 percent of normal activity of biotinidase consistent with heterozygosity [46]. Biotinidase activity is detectable in normal amniocytes, so that prenatal diagnosis of biotinidase deficiency should be possible, but this has not yet been reported, although prenatal assay of the enzyme in amniocytes and chorionic villi has yielded evidence of normal fetuses and a heterozygote [47,48]. In a family in which the mutation is known, molecular analysis would appear to be the method of choice for prenatal diagnosis, and carrier detection.

Metabolic abnormalities in biotinidase deficiency include lactic acidemia, in the presence or absence of recurrent episodes of ketoacidosis. For this reason testing for biotinidase deficiency is of interest in any patient with unexplained lactic acidemia. In young infants there may be hyperammonemia during acute episodes of illness. The characteristic organic aciduria consists of the excretion of 3-methylcrotonylglycine, 3-hydroxyisovaleric acid, 3-hydroxypropionic acid and 2-methylcitric acid [3,9]. Some patients with otherwise typical phenotypes and enzyme deficiency have been reported not to have organic aciduria [3,49,50]. Elevated concentrations of lactate and pyruvate have been reported in the cerebrospinal fluid (CSF) [51], as was reversion to normal with treatment. In fact, an elevated cerebrospinal fluid concentration of lactate may occur in the absence of hyperlactic acidemia [22,40,51,52]. The CSF to plasma ratio of lactic acid may be as high as 3.7 [52]. The concentration of 3-hydroxyisovaleric acid may also be higher in CSF than in plasma [52].

The diagnosis is made by the assay of biotinidase (Figure 6.2, p. 43) in serum [1,46]. The enzyme has also been shown to be deficient in the liver. Methods available for biotinidase include the cleavage of N-biotinyl-3-aminobenzoate [46], of biotinyl-^{14}C-p-aminobenzoic acid [53] or of the ^{14}C-labeled natural substrate N-biotinyllysine [54] and a sensitive fluorimetric method with biotinyl-6-aminoquinoline [55], which has advantages for kinetic and other studies over the release of p-aminobenzoate followed by diazotization in the Bratton-Marshall reaction. Values obtained with the various assays have been quite similar. In the original assay [3,46] the mean was 5.80 and the range 4.30–7.54 nmol/min/mL, whereas values obtained in patients ranged from undetectable to 0.18 nmol/min/mL. Small amounts of biotinidase activity are detectable in normal fibroblasts, while none was found in patient fibroblasts.

Wolf and colleagues have developed a simple colorimetric test for biotinidase deficiency that can be employed with spots of blood dried on filter paper, and they have demonstrated that the test is suitable for incorporation into a statewide program of neonatal screening [48,56]. Two infants with the disease were identified among the first 81 243 infants screened. This led to the discovery of two more patients who were previously undiagnosed siblings. By now millions of newborns have been screened throughout the world, and the yield of known patients has resulted in an estimate of frequency of biotinidase deficiency of one in 60 000 births [57].

Patients have been classified as profoundly or partially deficient on the basis of phenotype, the presence or absence of immunoreactive enzyme – cross-reacting material (CRM) – and the isoform pattern of sodium dodecylsulfate (SDS)-immuno blots [58]. Most patients were CRM-positive and had normal kinetics of the enzyme. In one variant patient with late onset disease [34] the plasma biotinidase enzyme displayed biphasic kinetics with two different low values for Vmax and two Km values. It is clear that there is a population of patients with partial deficiency identified by newborn screening who are biochemically different from those who have come to attention because of symptomatic disease.

The cloning of the gene for biotinidase and the identification of the nature of mutation promises correlation of phenotype with genotype, but so far this is far from clear. The relatively common R538C mutation involves a CpG dinucleotide, a likely place for mutation [6], and this and the G98:d7i3 cause severe disease. On the other side, compounds of the D444H with a variety of mutations including T404I and C594delC are associated with partial deficiency [59]. Patients with late onset disease, spastic paresis and optic problems had mutations L215F, R538C, V457M and G98:d7i3, which are usually found in infantile onset severe disease [35].

The immediate consequence of biotinidase deficiency is that levels of biotin in blood, urine and tissues are low [10]. The low level may be more dramatically evident in the urine than in the blood. These observations initially suggested a defect in the absorption or transport of biotin [60,61] or its excessive renal excretion [62]. Increased renal clearance of biotin may be observed [60] in the biotin-deficient state, which reverts to normal on repletion with biotin [61], but increased renal clearance of biotin has been found when plasma biotin levels were normal [63,64]. Interruption of treatment with biotin led to a more rapid fall in plasma biotin and greater renal loss of biotin in patients than controls.

Biocytin has been detected in the urine of patients with biotinidase deficiency [65]. This compound is not detectable in normal urine. The levels of biocytin were considerably higher than the levels of biotin when the patients were not being treated with biotin. If the normal renal clearance of biotin at half that of creatinine is a reflection of renal reabsorption, the increased clearance of biotin in biotinidase deficiency might be caused by an inhibition of biotin reabsorption by the elevated amounts of biocytin. Biocytin could compete with biotin as substrate for holocarboxylase synthetase, increasing the concentration of biotin needed for effective holocarboxylase synthesis. It is also possible that elevated levels of biocytin are directly toxic, but there is no evidence for this as yet. A specific high performance liquid chromatography (HPLC) method for biocytin has been developed [66]. In patients prior to treatment, levels of biocytin in urine ranged from 6.2 to 28.8 nmol/mmol creatinine. During therapy, levels increased 1.3- to 4-fold, but increase in dosage to 200 mg per day in a patient did not change the excretion of biocytin from the level observed with 10 mg per day. Other derivatives of biotin were found in the urine and tentatively identified as bis-norbiotin and oxidation products.

The low tissue stores of biotin that result from biotinidase deficiency lead to deficient activity of carboxylases (Figure 5.2, p. 37) and this of course results in the lactic acidemia and the accumulation of the other organic acid metabolites. Activities of carboxylases were found to be more severely compromised in brain than in liver and kidney [22], which would be consistent with the higher levels of lactate and 3-hydroxyisovalerate found in CSF.

Activities of carboxylases in freshly isolated lymphocytes are low. On the other hand, activities of each of the carboxylases in cultured fibroblasts are normal whether cells are cultivated in high or low concentrations of biotin [11,67–69]. This is typical of biotinidase deficiency and was used to distinguish these patients from those with holocarboxylase synthetase deficiency in whom fibroblasts display lower activity of carboxylases when grown in media containing low concentrations of biotin [70]. A rapid diagnostic method for distinguishing holocarboxylase synthetase abnormalities from biotinidase deficiency is the assay of the activity of carboxylases in freshly isolated lymphocytes in the presence and absence of preincubation with biotin [69]. Of course direct assay of the relevant enzyme is diagnostic. Activity of holocarboxylase synthetase is normal in patients with biotinidase deficiency.

Biotinidase in human and rat brain is much lower than in other tissues, and biotin levels in brain are depleted in biotinidase deficiency earlier and more severely than in other tissues [22,50]. This inefficient recycling of biotin would make the brain more dependent on transfer of biotin than other tissues, and thus more susceptible to deficiency. This would be consistent with the preferential elevation of lactate and 3-hydroxyisovalerate in the CSF and the occasional absence of organic aciduria, as well as the concomitance of CSF accumulation in patients with neurological symptoms. Pyruvate carboxylase may be predominantly affected by biotinidase deficiency in the brain. Neurological symptomatology could be the result of the toxic effect of local accumulation of lactate and organic acids. These observations are consistent with the fact that sometimes abnormalities of the central nervous system are the first manifestations of the disease. It is of interest that high CSF concentrations of lactate and 3-hydroxyisovalerate are not seen in holocarboxylase synthetase deficiency, where central nervous system abnormalities are not expected except as a result of a catastrophic event. Concentrations of 3-hydroxyisovalerate in the CSF were high in a patient with isolated deficiency of 3-methylcrotonyl CoA carboxylase, and this patient had severe neurologic abnormalities, indicating that this compound as well as lactate may be toxic to brain.

TREATMENT

Patients are effectively treated with relatively small doses of biotin. The dose most commonly employed is 10 mg/day, but as little as 5 mg/day has been effective [11]. The organic aciduria and virtually all of the clinical manifestations of the disease disappear promptly after the initiation of treatment. However, auditory and optic nerve losses are not reversed [10,13,17,25,35,71,72]. Presymptomatic treatment in a patient diagnosed by assay of cord blood because the disease had previously been diagnosed in a sibling has been followed by completely normal development, including vision and hearing for 14 months [73]. In one patient, oral and cutaneous administration of unsaturated fatty acids was followed by remission of alopecia and cutaneous lesions [74], suggesting that a deficiency of acetyl CoA carboxylase required for fatty acid synthesis is involved in the pathogenesis of these manifestations.

References

1 Wolf B, Grier RE, Parker WD, et al. Deficient biotinidase activity in late onset multiple carboxylase deficiency. N Engl J Med 1983;308:161.

2 Burri BJ, Sweetman L, Nyhan WL. Mutant holocarboxylase synthetase: evidence for the enzyme defect in early infantile biotin-responsive multiple carboxylase deficiency. J Clin Invest 1981;68:1491.

3 Wolf B, Grier RE, Allen RJ, et al. Phenotypic variation in biotinidase deficiency. J Pediatr 1983;103:233.

4 Cole H, Reynolds TR, Lockyer J, et al. Human serum biotinidase: cDNA cloning sequence and characterization. J Biol Chem 1994;269:6566.

5 Cole H, Weremowicz H, Morton CC, Wolf B. Localization of serum biotinidase (BTD) to human chromosome 3 in band p25. Genomics 1994;22:662.

6 Pomponio RJ, Hymes J, Reynolds TR, et al. Mutations in the human biotinidase gene that cause profound biotinidase deficiency in symptomatic children: molecular biochemical and clinical analysis Pediatr Res 1997;42:840.

7 Norrgard KJ, Pomponio RJ, Swango KL, et al. Double mutation (A171T and D444H) is a common cause of profound biotinidase deficiency in children ascertained by newborn screening in United States. Hum Mutat 1998;11:410.

8 Swango KL, Demirkol M, Huner G, et al. Partial biotinidase deficiency is usually due to the D444H mutation in the biotinidase gene. Hum Genet 1998;102:571.

9 Sweetman L. Two forms of biotin-responsive multiple carboxylase deficiency. J Inherit Metab Dis 1981;4:53.

10 Thoene J, Baker H, Yoshino M, Sweetman L. Biotin-responsive carboxylase deficiency associated with subnormal plasma and urinary biotin. N Engl J Med 1981;304:817.

11 Bartlett K, Ng H, Leonard JV. A combined defect of three mitochondrial carboxylases presenting as biotin-responsive 3-methylcrotonyl glycinuria and 3-hydroxyisovaleric aciduria. Clin Chim Acta 1980;100:183.

12 Dabbagh O, Brismar J, Gascon GG, Ozand PT. The clinical spectrum of biotin-treatable encephalopathies in Saudi Arabia. Brain Dev. 1994;16:72.

13 Cowan MJ, Wara DW, Packman S, et al. Multiple biotin-dependent carboxylase deficiencies associated with defects in T-cell and B-cell immunity. Lancet 1979;2:115.

14 Sander JE, Malamud N, Cowan MJ, et al. Intermittent ataxia and immunodeficiency with multiple carboxylase deficiencies: A biotin-responsive disorder. Ann Neurol. 1980;8:544.

15 Munnich A, Saudubray JM, Ogier H, et al. Deficit multiple des carboxylases. Une maladie metabolique vitamino-dependante curable par la biotine. Arch Fr Pediatr. 1981;38:83.

16 Schubiger G, Caflish U, Baumgartner R, et al. Biotinidase deficiency: clinical course and biochemical findings. J Inherit Metab Dis 1984;7:129.

17 Salbert BA, Pellock JM, Wolf B. Characterization of seizures associated with biotinidase deficiency. *Neurol* 1993;**43**:1351.

18 Kalayci O, Coskun T, Tokatli A, *et al*. Infantile spasms as the initial symptom of biotinidase deficiency. *J Pediatr* 1994;**124**:103.

19 Charles BM, Hosking G, Green A, *et al*. Biotin-responsive alopecia and developmental regression. *Lancet* 1979;**2**:118.

20 Keeton BR, Moosa A. Organic aciduria: Treatable cause of floppy infant syndrome. *Arch Dis Child* 1981;**51**:636.

21 Mitchell G, Ogier H, Munnich A, *et al*. Neurological deterioration and lactic acidemia in biotinidase deficiency. A treatable condition mimicking Leigh's disease. *Neuropediatrics* 1986;**17**:129.

22 Baumgartner ER, Suormala TU, Wick H, *et al*. Biotinidase deficiency: A cause of subacute necrotizing encephalomyelopathy (Leigh syndrome). Report of a case with a lethal outcome. *Pediatr Res* 1989;**26**:260.

23 Dionisi-Vici C, Bachmann C, Graziani MC, Sabetta G. Laryngeal stridor as a leading symptom in a biotinidase-deficient patient case report. *J Inherit Metab Dis* 1988;**11**:312.

24 DiRocco M, Superti-Furga A, Caprino D, Oddino N. Letter: Phenotypic variability in biotinidase deficiency. *J Pediatr* 1984;**104**:964.

25 Wolf B, Grier RE, Heard GS. Hearing loss in biotinidase deficiency. *Lancet* 1983;**2**:1365.

26 Taitz LS, Green A, Strachan I, *et al*. Biotinidase deficiency and the eye and ear. *Lancet* 1983;**1**:918.

27 Lott IT, Lottenberg S, Nyhan WL, Buchsbaum MJ. Cerebral metabolic change after treatment in biotinidase deficiency. *J Inherit Metab Dis* 1993;**16**:399.

28 Campana G, Valentini G, Legnaioli MI, *et al*. Ocular aspects of biotinidase deficiency: Clinical and genetic original studies. *Ophthalmic Paediatr Genet* 1987;**8**:125.

29 Salbert BA, Astruc J, Wolf B. Ophthalmologic findings in biotinidase deficiency. *Ophthalmologica* 1993;**206**:177.

30 Leonard JV, Daish P, Naughten ER, Bartlett K. The management and long term outcome of organic acidaemias. *J Inherit Metab Dis* 1984;**7**:13.

31 Wolf B, Spencer R, Gleason T. Hearing loss is a common feature of symptomatic children with profound biotinidase deficiency. *J Pediatr* 2002;**140**:242.

32 Thuy LP, Zielinska B, Zammarchi E, *et al*. Multiple carboxylase deficiency due to deficiency of biotinidase. *J Neurogenet* 1986;**3**:357.

33 Ramaekers VT, Brab M, Rau G, Heimann G. Recovery from neurologic deficits following biotin treatment in a biotinidase Km variant. *Neuropediatrics* 1993;**24**:98.

34 Ramaekers VT, Suormala TM, Brab M, *et al*. A biotinidase Km variant causing late onset bilateral optic neuropathy. *Arch Dis Child* 1992;**67**:115.

35 Wolf B, Pomponio RJ, Norrgard KJ, *et al*. Delayed-onset profound biotinidase deficiency. *J Pediatr* 1998;**132**:362.

36 Williams ML, Packman S, Cowan MJ. Alopecia and periorificial dermatitis in biotin-responsive multiple carboxylase deficiency. *J Am Acad Derm* 1983;**9**:97.

37 Fischer A, Munnich A, Saudubray JM, *et al*. Biotin-responsive immunoregulatory dysfunction in multiple carboxylase deficiency. *J Clin Immun* 1982;**2**:35.

38 Petrelli F, Moretti P, Campanati G. Studies on the relationships between biotin and the behaviour of B and T lymphocytes in the guinea pig. *Experientia* 1981;**37**:1204.

39 Hurvitz H, Ginat-Israeali T, Elpeleg ON, *et al*. Biotinidase deficiency associated with severe combined immunodeficiency. *Lancet* 1989;**2**:228.

40 Fois A, Cioni M, Balestri P, *et al*. Biotinidase deficiency: metabolites in CSF. *J Inherit Metab Dis* 1986;**9**:284.

41 Collins JE, Nicholson NS, Dalton N, Leonard JV. Biotinidase deficiency: early neurological presentation. *Dev Med Child Neurol* 1994;**36**:263.

42 Taitz LS, Leonard JV, Bartlett K. Long-term auditory auditory and visual complications of biotinidase deficiency. *Early Hum Dev* 1985;**11**:325.

43 Schulz PE, Seiner SP, Belmont JW, Fishman MA. Basal ganglia calcifications in a case of biotinidase deficiency. *Neurol* 1988;**38**:1326.

44 Bousounis DP, Camfield PR, Wolf B. Reversal of brain atrophy with biotin treatment in biotinidase deficiency. *Neuropediatrics* 1993;**24**:214.

45 Ginat-Israeli T, Hurvitz H, Klar A, *et al*. Deteriorating neurological and neuroradiological course in treated biotinidase deficiency. *Neuropediatrics* 1993;**24**:103.

46 Wolf B, Grier RE, Allen RJ, *et al*. Biotinidase deficiency: the enzymatic defect in late-onset multiple carboxylase deficiency. *Clin Chim Acta* 1983;**131**:273.

47 Pomponio RJ, Hymes J, Pandya A, *et al*. Prenatal diagnosis of heterozygosity for biotinidase deficiency by enzymatic and molecular analyses. *Prenat Diagn* 1998;**18**:117.

48 Chalmers RA, Mistry J, Docherty PW, Stratton D. First trimester prenatal exclusion of biotinidase deficiency. *J Inherit Metab Dis* 1994;**17**:751.

49 Swick HM, Kien CL. Biotin deficiency with neurologic and cutaneous manifestations but without organic aciduria. *J Pediatr* 1983;**103**:265.

50 Wolf B, Heard GS, Jefferson LG, *et al*. Clinical findings in four children with biotinidase deficiency detected through a statewide neonatal screening program. *N Engl J Med* 1985;**313**:16.

51 Di Rocco M, Superti-Furga A, Durand P, *et al*. Different organic acid patterns in urine and in cerebrospinal fluid in a patient with biotinidase deficiency. *J Inherit Metab Dis* 1984;**7**:119.

52 Duran M, Baumgartner ER, Suormala TM, *et al*. Cerebrospinal fluid organic acids in biotinidase deficiency. *J Inherit Metab Dis* 1993;**16**:513.

53 Wolf B, Secor McVoy J. A sensitive radioassay for biotinidase activity: deficient activity in tissues of serum biotinidase-deficient individuals. *Clin Chim Acta* 1983;**135**:275.

54 Thuy LP, Zielinska B, Sweetman L, Nyhan WL. Determination of biotinidase activity in human plasma using (14C) biocytin as substrate. *Ann NY Acad Sci* 1985;**447**:434.

55 Wastell H, Dale G, Bartlett K. A sensitive fluorimetric rate assay for biotinidase using a new derivative of biotin biotinyl-6-aminoquinoline. *Anal Biochem* 1984;**140**:69.

56 Heard GS, Wolf B, Jefferson KG, *et al*. Newborn screening for biotinidase deficiency: results of a one-year pilot study. *J Pediatr* 1986;**108**:40.

57 Wolf B. Worldwide survey of neonatal screening for biotinidase deficiency. *J Inherit Metab Dis* 1991;**14**:923.

58 Hart PS, Hymes J, Wolf B. Biochemical and immunological characterization of serum biotinidase in profound biotinidase deficiency. *Am J Hum Genet* 1992;**50**:125.

59 Funghini S, Donati MA, Pasquini E, *et al*. Two new mutations in children affected by partial biotinidase deficiency ascertained by newborn screening. *J Inherit Metab Dis* 2002;**25**:328.

60 Thoene JG, Lemons R, Baker H. Impaired intestinal absorption of biotin in juvenile multiple carboxylase deficiency. *N Engl J Med* 1983;**308**:639.

61 Thoene J, Wolf B. Biotinidase deficiency in juvenile multiple carboxylase deficiency. *Lancet* 1983;**2**:398.

62 Baumgartner R, Suormala T, Wick H, Geisert J. Renal loss of biotin: a cause of biotin-responsive multiple carboxylase deficiency. *Pediatr Res* 1982;**16**:695.

63 Baumgartner R, Suormala T, Wick H, *et al*. Biotinidase deficiency: factors responsible for increased biotin requirement. *J Inherit Metab Dis* 1985;**8**:59.

64 Baumgartner R, Suomala T, Wick H, *et al*. Biotinidase deficiency associated with renal loss of biocytin and biotin. *Ann NY Acad Sci* 1985;**447**:272.

65 Bonjour JP, Bausch J, Suormala T, Baumgartner ER. Detection of biocytin in urine of children with congenital biotinidase deficiency. *Intl J Vitam Nutr Res* 1984;**54**:223.

66   Suormala TM, Baumgartner ER, Bausch J, *et al.* Quantitative determination of biocytin in urine of patients with biotinidase deficiency using high-performance liquid chromatography (HPLC). *Clin Chim Acta* 1988;**177**:253.

67   Bartlett K, Ng H, Dale G, *et al.* Studies on cultured fibroblasts from patient with defects of biotin-dependent carboxylation. *J Inherit Metab Dis* 1981;**4**:183.

68   Leonard JV, Seakins JWT, Bartlett K, *et al.* Inherited disorders of 3-methylcrotonyl-CoA carboxylation. *Arch Dis Child* 1981;**56**:53.

69   Packman S, Caswell NW, Baker H. Biochemical evidence for diverse etiologies in biotin-responsive multiple carboxylase deficiency. *Biochem Gen* 1982;**20**:17.

70   Sweetman L, Bates SP, Hull D, Nyhan WL. Propionyl CoA carboxylase deficiency in a patient with biotin-responsive 3-methylcrotonylglycinuria. *Pediatr Res* 1977;**11**:1144.

71   Suormala T, Wick H, Bonjour JP, Baumgartner ER. Rapid differential diagnosis of carboxylase deficiencies and evaluation for biotin-responsiveness in a single blood sample. *Clin Chim Acta* 1985;**145**: 151.

72   Munnich A, Saudubray J-M, Cotisson A, *et al.* Biotin-dependent multiple carboxylase deficiency presenting as a congenital lactic acidosis. *Eur J Pediatr* 1981;**137**:203.

73   Wallace SJ. Biotinidase deficiency: presymptomatic treatment. *Arch Dis Child* 1985;**60**: 574.

74   Munnich A, Saudubray JM, Coude FX, *et al.* Fatty acid-responsive alopecia in multiple carboxylase deficiency. *Lancet* 1980;**1**:1080.

Isovaleric acidemia

7

MAJOR PHENOTYPIC EXPRESSION

Episodic overwhelming illness with vomiting, ketosis, acidosis and coma; characteristic odor; neutropenia and thrombocytopenia; isovaleric acidemia; urinary excretion of isovalerylglycine and 3-hydroxyisovaleric acid; C5 and C5/C3 acylcarnitine profile; and deficiency of isovaleryl CoA dehydrogenase.

INTRODUCTION

Isovaleric acidemia was first described in 1966 by Tanaka and colleagues [1,2]. It was the unusual odor that led to the recognition of the disorder as an inborn error of metabolism [1,2]. The smell, that of typical volatile, short-chain organic acid, was so recognized by two chemists, L.B. Sjostrim and D. Tokendall, in the original patients. It was then documented as isovaleric acid by gas chromatography. The molecular defect is in the enzyme, isovaleryl CoA dehydrogenase [3] (Figure 7.1). The gene has been localized to chromosome 15q12–15 [4,5]. Mutations have been reported, including missense point mutations, deletions, and mutations that result in novel processing of this mitochondrial enzyme, such as a variant that causes an mRNA splicing error deleting exon 2 and producing a truncated protein that fails to interact properly with receptors for import into mitochondria [6–9].

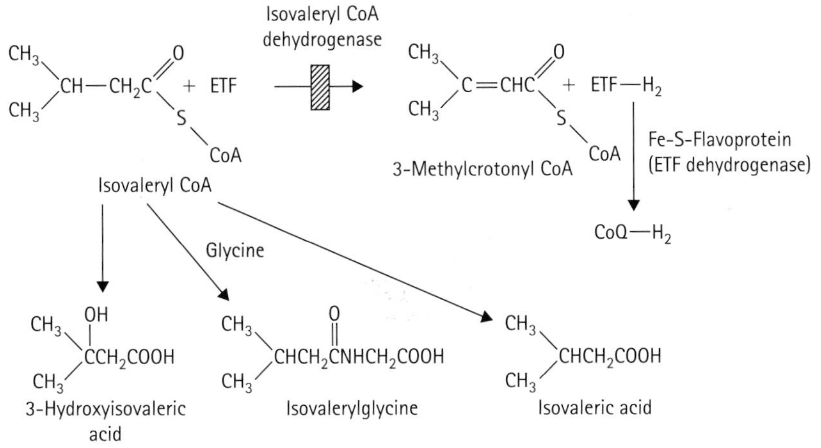

Figure 7.1 *Isovaleryl CoA dehydrogenase, the site of the molecular defect in isovaleric acidemia. The characteristic urinary metabolites in this disease are isovalerylglycine and 3-hydroxyisovaleric acid.*

CLINICAL ABNORMALITIES

Patients with isovaleric acidemia present usually with an organic acidemia picture of acute overwhelming illness in the first days or weeks of life [10–16] (Figures 7.2, 7.3). The onset is usually with vomiting, but the infant may progress directly to a deep coma. Hypothermia may be present. There may be convulsions, either focal or generalized [13]. Analysis of the urine usually reveals massive ketonuria, and electrolyte analysis indicates a metabolic acidosis. There may be prominent hyperammonemia early in infancy [13–16]. Hypocalcemia may be present [10,13]. It has been estimated that more than half of the patients die during the first episode very early in life, but the numbers of patients reported are quite small, and the proportion of patients dying undiagnosed early in life may be considerably greater. Intraventricular hemorrhage, cerebral edema and cerebellar hemorrhage have been described [13,15,17,18]. Vomiting may be so severe that a diagnosis of pyloric stenosis is suspected. Five infants have been treated surgically during the neonatal period, four undergoing pyloromyotomy [2,11, 19–21]; the fifth was thought to have a duodenal band [10].

The characteristic odor of isovaleric acid may alert the physician to the diagnosis. It has been popularized as the odor of sweaty feet, but it does not smell a bit like most locker rooms. It is a pungent, rather unpleasant odor. It can permeate a laboratory working with samples from an acutely ill patient. It was first recognized in the special care nursery when an isolette was opened to examine the baby. It is also important to remember that the odor may be absent at the time it would be most useful, during the acute illness of the first episode. These babies are often born in one hospital, lapse into coma, are treated with parenteral fluids to correct the acidosis or with exchange transfusion for the hyperammonemia and then transported to a neonatal intensive care unit. By this time, the odor may be undetectable. In some patients the odor has never been detected, even after the diagnosis was known [22] (Figure 7.4).

Patients who survive the initial episode may have recurrent attacks following infection or surgery in which there is acidosis, ketosis and coma much like the initial episode. Vomiting or ataxia may be an initial symptom. The odor may return. The presentation may suggest a diagnosis of Reye syndrome. Hyperglycemia may occasionally be found as it may in any infant overwhelmingly ill, and this in the presence of massive ketosis can lead to a mistaken diagnosis of diabetes mellitus [23,24]. Treatment with insulin is potentially dangerous in such a patient.

An occasional patient has a more indolent, milder intermittent form presenting first, later in the first year, or later [21]. Episodic disease is associated with intercurrent infection or unusual intake of protein. Episodes decrease in frequency

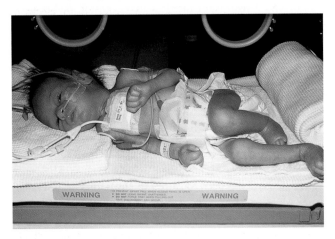

Figure 7.2   *A.A.D. An infant with isovaleric acidemia in the incubator. A nasogastric tube was in place.*

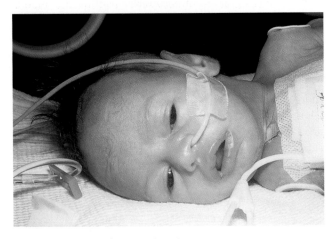

Figure 7.3   *A.A.D. Close-up of the face.*

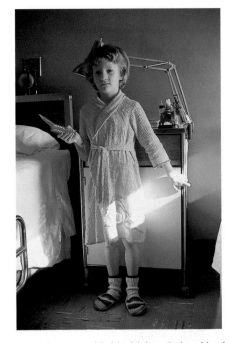

Figure 7.4   *T.M. A 7-year-old girl with isovaleric acidemia. She was somewhat microcephalic. The first years of life were characterized by recurrent episodes of acidosis, dehydration and coma.*

with age, probably as a consequence of decreased frequency of infection. The acute neonatal disease and the chronic, intermittent form of the disease may occur in the same family.

Pancreatitis, both acute and chronic, has been reported as a complication of isovaleric acidemia [25]. In three patients, the initial presentation was with pancreatitis. In pediatric patients with pancreatitis investigation for organic acidemia is prudent.

Hematological abnormalities may be prominent, especially in infancy. Leukopenia and thrombocytopenia are common, and in some infants anemia and a picture of pancytopenia [10, 13–16,26–28]. These abnormalities may be encountered during the initial or later attacks. The majority of patients surviving the initial episode are developmentally normal (Figure 7.5), but some are mildly retarded [2,12,19,21,27,29–31] and some severely so [28,31] and microcephalic [31,32]. Hypotonia is common early. Later there may be ataxia, tremor, dysmetria, extrapyramidal movements and brisk deep tendon reflexes [28,29]. One of the original patients had an unsteady gait as a teenager and was a mildly retarded adult, but had an uneventful pregnancy and a normal infant [33]. The electroencephalogram (EEG) may reveal slow wave dysrhythmia. Among our patients a 5-year-old with truncal ataxia had mild slowing, while her neurologically-normal affected sister had a normal EEG. Magnetic resonance imaging (MRI) may be normal, or may show extensive atrophy in an infant with near fatal neonatal illness and cardiac arrest [31]. Neuropathology of the infant dying in the acute episode may show cerebellar edema with herniation [13]. Spongiform changes may be seen in the white matter [10,34–36], but less prominently than in other organic acidemias or nonketotic hyperglycinemia [36]. Histology of the liver may be that of fatty change [36].

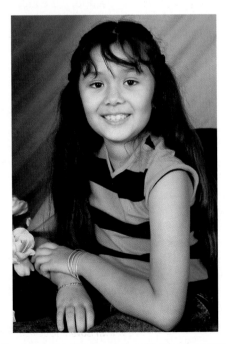

Figure 7.5 *A.H. A girl with isovaleric acidemia whose course has been entirely benign following the initial episode.*

GENETICS AND PATHOGENESIS

Isovaleric acidemia is an autosomal recessive disease. Heterozygote detection has been carried out by assay of the conversion of leucine-2-^{14}C to CO_2 in fibroblasts [12,35, 37,38]. Prenatal diagnosis has been approached in the same manner [37]. An accurate method for the gas chromatographic-mass spectrometric analysis of 3-hydroxyisovaleric acid [39] or isovalerylglycine permits rapid prenatal diagnosis via direct detection in the amniotic fluid [40]. Isovalerylglycine appears to be the metabolite of choice; it has been diagnostic as early as 12 weeks of gestation. Prenatal diagnosis has also been made by the incorporation of labeled isovaleric acid in chorionic villus material [41].

Assay of the enzyme in fibroblasts of a series of patients revealed considerable heterogeneity and residual activity, as much as 13 percent of the control level [38,42–44]. The enzyme may also be assayed in leukocytes. The assay is not generally available. Isovaleryl CoA dehydrogenase is made as a 45 KDa [45] subunit precursor and processed to a 43 KDa during import into the mitochondria and then assembled as a tetramer. It is a flavine adenine dinucleotide (FAD) containing enzyme, whose electrons are transferred to electron transfer flavoprotein (ETF) and transmitted to coenzyme Q of the electron transport chain by ETF dehydrogenase [46].

The gene has been located on chromosome 15q14–15 [47]. Complementation studies of 12 patients revealed a single group, comprising acute neonatal and chronic, intermittent patients [48]. A number of different types of mutation have been defined [8]. Of two missense mutations, one led to a leucine to proline change at position 13. These mutations lead to mature and precursor proteins of normal size. A single base deletion at position 1179 led to a frameshift and addition of eight amino acids and then a termination leading to a smaller precursor protein. A number of mutations have led to abnormal splicing of the RNA [8] including the deletion of exon 2, and the synthesis of a protein 20 amino acids smaller which was processed normally into mitochondria [6,8].

The immediate consequence of the enzyme defect is the elevated concentration of isovaleric acid in the blood. 3-Hydroxyisovaleric acid is also prominent [49]. These elevations are especially true in the acute episode. However, methods for the detection of volatile short-chain acids like isovaleric acid are considerably less than perfect, and mistakes have been made in which the diagnosis of isovaleric acidemia was missed [50]. The way in which the diagnosis has usually been securely made is by the identification of large amounts of isovalerylglycine in the urine [22,51,52]. This compound is very stable and is present in the urine even at times of remission and excellent general health. Amounts in the urine may be as great as 3 g per day (2000–9000 mmol/mol creatinine) (normal 0–2), whereas in normal individuals less than 2 mg are found. A simple screening test has been developed [53], but today most patients are detected by organic acid analysis.

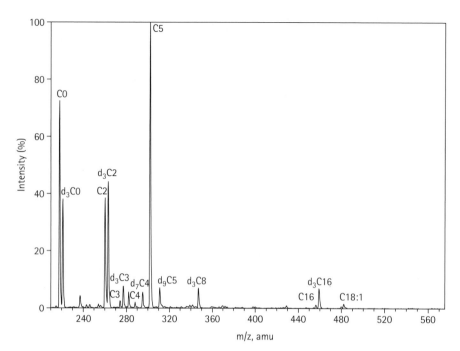

Figure 7.6 *Acylcarnitine profile of the blood plasma of a patient with isovaleric acidemia. C5 is isovalerylcarnitine. (Illustration provided by Jon Gangoiti of UCSD.)*

Analysis of organic acids at the time of acute attack reveals the presence of 4-hydroxyisovaleric acid, mesaconic acid and methylsuccinic acid [18,54], as well as isovalerylglycine and 3-hydroxyisovaleric acid. Lactic acid, acetoacetic acid and 3-hydroxybutyric acid are also found in large amounts in the urine. Isovalerylglucuronide has also been identified in the urine [55], and probably represents an additional detoxification pathway. Similarly, isovalerylcarnitine (Figure 7.6) has been identified in the urine [56], and this provides another approach to the diagnosis. After the acute attack has resolved organic acid analysis usually reveals only isovalerylglycine. Isovalerylglycine can also be identified by nuclear magnetic resonance (NMR) spectroscopy [22,57].

With the advent of tandem mass spectrometry we can expect the diagnosis to be made increasingly by the analysis of acylcarnitine profiles either in blood spots on filter paper in programs of neonatal screening or in plasma of ill patients. An isolated elevation of C5 acylcarnitine is likely isovalerylcarnitine. 2-Methylbutyrylcarnitine is also C5; its elevation in multiple acyl CoA dehydrogenase deficiency is accompanied by C4, but isolated 2-methylbutyryl CA dehydrogenase deficiency must be distinguished by the presence of 2-methylbutyrylglycine in the urine or by enzyme assay. In isovaleric acidemia the ratio of C5 to C3 is useful [58].

TREATMENT

The acute episode should be treated vigorously with parenteral solutions of fluid and electrolytes containing sodium bicarbonate and glucose. The initial episode, especially if complicated by hyperammonemia, may require exchange transfusions or dialysis or the use of benzoate or phenylacetate to promote waste nitrogen elimination. Intravenous carnitine may alleviate hyperammonemia and carnitine deficiency, and it may promote the excretion of isovalerylcarnitine. The administration of exogenous glycine may be helpful in the acute episode [59]. Doses employed have approximated 250 mg/kg/day.

Glycine is also employed in chronic therapy [32,60]. It has been reported to prevent the increase in accumulation of isovaleric acid that follows an oral load of leucine [61]. A dose of 800 mg per day has been recorded for an infant [59]. In an approach to optimal use of glycine supplementation, quantification of isovalerylglycine excretion was studied [62] in two patients with disease of different severity. Different doses were employed, and one was challenged with leucine. Interestingly, the patient with the milder disease excreted much more isovalerylglycine, suggesting that disease severity may be a function of the efficiency of glycine conjugation. Doses up to 600 mg/kg appeared to be useful especially at times when isovaleric acid accumulation might be highest; doses up to 250 mg/kg might be adequate under baseline healthy conditions of dietary restriction.

Carnitine may become depleted in isovaleric acidemia. Patients tend to have low levels of free-carnitine in plasma and increased losses of esterified carnitine in urine [63–66]. Supplementation restores plasma free carnitine to normal and increases urinary excretion of isovalerylcarnitine. Studies with isotopically-labeled carnitine showed that administered carnitine rapidly enters mitochondrial pools and esterifies with available acyl compounds [56]. Comparison of oral and intravenous use indicated an oral bioavailability of only 15 percent; intravenous use is required in acute episodic illness. Oral dosage of 100 mg/kg appears adequate for chronic use. There have been conflicting results of studies to determine whether glycine or carnitine is more effective in removing isovalerylCoA [64,67,68]. It appears prudent to employ both in long term management.

The cornerstone of long-term therapy is the restriction of the dietary intake of leucine [27]. Our approach to the treatment of organic acidemia is to provide whole protein containing the offending amino acid required for growth and little more. Our experience with isovaleric acidemia is that the provision of protein can be somewhat more liberal than in other organic acidemias such as propionic acidemia (Chapter 2) or methylmalonic acidemia (Chapter 3).

In studies of stable isotopically labeled leucine, more than 90 percent of the excreted metabolites of leucine were produced by endogenous metabolism when the whole leucine-containing protein intake was 0.75 g/kg [69]. Nutritional therapy, as well as glycine supplementation should be monitored by quantification of the excretion of isovalerylglycine. Determinations of the concentration of amino acids in plasma ensures against any one or more amino acids reaching concentrations that would be limiting for growth. Mixtures of amino acids lacking leucine may be employed to increase amino acid nitrogen or nonleucine essential amino acids. Supplementation with alanine may accomplish a similar goal [70].

References

1 Tanaka K, Budd MA, Efron ML, Isselbacher KJ. Isovaleric acidemia: A new genetic defect of leucine metabolism. *Proc Natl Acad Sci* 1966;**56**:236.

2 Budd MA, Tanaka K, Holmes LB, *et al.* Isovaleric acidemia: Clinical features of a genetic defect of leucine metabolism. *N Engl J Med* 1967;**277**:3211.

3 Rhead WR, Tanaka K. Demonstration of a specific mitochondrial isovaleryl CoA dehydrogenase deficiency in fibroblasts from patients with isovaleric acidemia. *Proc Natl Acad Sci* 1980;**77**:580.

4 Tanaka K. Isovaleric acidemia: Personal history clinical survey and study of the molecular basis. *Prog Clin Biol Res* 1990;**321**:273.

5 Parimoo B, Tanaka K. Structural organization of the human isovaleryl-CoA dehydrogenase gene. *Genomics* 1993;**15**:582.

6 Vockley J, Nagao M, Parimoo B, Tanaka K. The variant human isovaleryl-CoA dehydrogenase gene responsible for type II isovaleric acidemia determines an RNA splicing error leading to the deletion of the entire second coding exon and the production of a truncated precursor protein that interacts poorly with mitochondrial import receptors. *J Biol Chem* 1992;**267**:2494.

7 Matsubara Y, Ito M, Glassberg R, *et al.* Nucleotide sequence of messenger RNA encoding human isovaleryl coenzyme A dehydrogenase and its expression in isovaleric acidemia fibroblasts. *J Clin Invest* 1990;**85**:1058.

8 Vockley J, Parimoo B, Tanaka K. Molecular characterization of four different classes of mutations in the isovaleryl-CoA dehydrogenase gene responsible for isovaleric acidemia. *Am J Hum Genet* 1991;**49**:147.

9 Vockley J, Anderson BD, Willard JM, *et al.* Abnormal splicing of IVD RNA in isovaleric acidemia caused by amino acid altering point mutations in the IVD gene: A novel molecular mechanism for disease. *Am J Hum Genet* 1998;**63**:A14.

10 Newman CGH, Wilson BDR, Callagham P, Young L. Neonatal death associated with isovaleric acidemia. *Lancet* 1967;**2**:439.

11 Spirer Z, Swirsky-Fein S, Zakut V, *et al.* Acute neonatal isovaleric acidemia: A report of two cases. *Israel J Med Sci* 1976;**11**:1055.

12 Saudubray J-M, Sorin M, Depondt E, *et al.* Acidemie isovalerique: Etude et traitement chez trois freres. *Arch Franc Ped* 1976;**33**:795.

13 Fischer AQ, Challa VR, Burton BK, McLean WT. Cerebellar hemorrhage complicating isovaleric acidemia: A case report. *Neurology* 1981;**31**:746.

14 Wilson WG, Audenaert SM, Squillaro EJ. Hyperammonaemia in a preterm infant with isovaleric acidemia. *J Inherit Metab Dis* 1984;**7**:71.

15 Mendiola JJ, Robotham JL, Liehr JG, Williams JC. Neonatal lethargy due to isovaleric acidemia and hyperammonemia. *Tex Med* 1984;**80**:52.

16 Beauvais P, Peter MO, Barbier B. [Neonatal form of isovaleric acidemia: Apropos of a new case.] *Arch Franc Pediatr* 1985;**42**:531.

17 Berry GT, Yudkoff M, Segal S. Isovaleric acidemia: Medical and neurodevelopmental effects of long-term therapy. *J Pediatr* 1988;**113**:58.

18 Truscott RJW, Malegan D, McCairns E, *et al.* New metabolites in isovaleric acidemia. *Clin Chim Acta* 1981;**110**:187.

19 Lehnert W, Schenck W, Niederhof H. Isovaleric acidemia kombiniert mit hypertrophischer Pylorusstenose. *Klin Paediat* 1979;**191**:477.

20 Nyhan WL. Introduction in *Abnormalities in Amino Acid Metabolism in Clinical Medicine* (ed. WL Nyhan), Appleton Century Crofts Norwalk Conn, 1984:3–18.

21 Ichiba Y, Sato K, Yuasa S. Report of a case of isovaleric acidemia. *J Japanese Pediatr Soc* 1979;**83**:480.

22 Ando T, Klingberg WD, Ward AN, *et al.* Isovaleric acidemia presenting with altered metabolism of glycine. *Pediatr Res* 1971;**5**:478.

23 Williams KM, Peden VH, Hillman RE. Isovaleric acidemia appearing as diabetic ketoacidosis. *Am J Dis Child* 1981;**135**:1068.

24 Attia N, Sakati N, Al Ashwal A, *et al.* Isovaleric acidemia appearing as diabetic ketoacidosis. *J Inherit Metab Dis* 1996;**19**:85.

25 Kahler SG, Sherwood WG, Woolf D, *et al.* Pancreatitis in patients with organic acidemias. *Pediatrics* 1994;**124**:239.

26 Kelleher J, Yudkof M, Hutchinson R, *et al.* The pancytopenia of isovaleric acidemia. *Pediatrics* 1980;**65**:1023.

27 Levy HL, Erickson A, Lott IT, Kurtz DJ. Isovaleric acidemia. Results of family study and dietary treatment. *Pediatrics* 1973;**52**:83.

28 Guibaud P, Divry P, Dubois Y, *et al.* Une observation d'acidemie isovalerique. *Arch Franc Ped* 1973;**30**:633.

29 Rousson R, Guibaud P. Long term outcome of organic acidurias: survey of 105 French cases (1967–1983). *J Inherit Metab Dis* 1984;**7**:10.

30 Dodelson de Kremer R, Depetris de Boldini C, Paschini de Capra A, *et al.* Variacion en la expresion fenotupica de la acidemia isovalerica en pacientes argentinos. Observaciones de un prolongado seguimiento. *Medicina (BAires)* 1992;**52**:131.

31 Nyhan WL, Barshop B. Unpublished experience.

32 Krieger I, Tanaka K. Therapeutic effects of glycine in isovaleric acidemia. *Pediatr Res* 1976;**10**:25.

33 Shih VE, Aubry RH, DeGrande G, *et al.* Maternal isovaleric acidemia. *J Pediatr* 1984;**105**:77.

34 Malan C, Neethling AC, Shanley BC, *et al.* Isovaleric acidemia in two South African children. *S Afr Med J* 1977;**51**:980.

35 Spirer Z, Swirsky-Fein S, Zakut V, *et al.* Acute neonatal isovaleric acidemia: a report of two cases. *Israel J Med Sci* 1975;**11**:1005.

36 Shuman RM, Leech RW, Scott CR. The neuropathology of the nonketotic and ketotic hyperglycinemias: three cases. *Neurology* 1978;**28**:139.

37 Blaskovics ME, Ng WG, Donnell GN. Prenatal diagnosis and a case report of isovaleric acidemia. *J Inherit Metab Dis* 1978;**1**:9.

38 Shih VE, Mandell R, Tanaka K. Diagnosis of isovaleric acidemia in cultured fibroblasts. *Clin Chim Acta* 1973;**48**:437.

39 Jakobs C, Sweetman L, Nyhan WL, Packman S. Stable isotope dilution analysis of 3-hydroxyisovaleric acid in amniotic fluid: Contribution to the prenatal diagnosis of inherited disorders of leucine catabolism. *J Inherit Metab Dis* 1984;**7**:15.

40 Hine DG, Hack AM, Goodman SI, Tanaka K. Stable isotope dilution analysis of isovalerylglycine in amniotic fluid and urine and its application for the prenatal diagnosis of isovaleric acidemia. *Pediatr Res* 1986;**20**:222.

41 Kleijer WJ, Van Der Kraan M, Huijmans JGM, *et al*. Prenatal diagnosis of isovaleric acidaemia by enzyme and metabolite assay in the first and second trimesters. *Prenat Diagn* 1995;**15**:527.

42 Rhead WJ, Hall CL, Tanaka K. Novel tritium release assays for isovaleryl CoA dehydrogenases. *J Biol Chem* 1981;**256**:1616.

43 Hyman DB, Tanaka K. Isovaleryl-CoA dehydrogenase activity in isovaleric acidemia fibroblasts using an improved tritium release assay. *Pediatr Res* 1986;**20**:59.

44 Frerman FE, Goodman SI. Fluorometric assay of acyl CoA dehydrogenases in normal and mutant fibroblasts. *Biochem Med* 1985;**33**:38.

45 Ikeda Y, Fenton WA, Tanaka K. *In vitro* translation and posttranslational processing of four mitochondrial acyl-CoA dehydrogenases. *Fed Proc* 1984;**43**:2024.

46 Ikeda Y, Keese SM, Fenton WA, Tanaka K. Biosynthesis of four rat liver mitochondrial acyl-CoA dehydrogenases: *in vitro* synthesis import into mitochondria and processing of their precursors in a cell-free system and in cultured cells. *Arch Biochem Biophys* 1987;**252**:662.

47 Kraus JP, Matsubara Y, Barton D, *et al*. Isolation of cDNA clones coding for rat isovaleryl-CoA dehydrogenase and assignment of the gene to human chromosome 15. *Genomics* 1987;**1**:264.

48 Dubiel B, Dabrowski C, Wetts R, Tanaka K. Complementation studies of isovaleric acidemia and glutaric aciduria type II using cultured skin fibroblasts. *J Clin Invest* 1983;**72**:1543.

49 Tanaka K, Orr JC, Isselbacher KJ. Identification of 3-hydroxyisovaleric acid in the urine of a patient with isovaleric acidemia. *Biochim Biophys Acta* 1968;**152**:638.

50 Ando T, Nyhan W, Bachmann C, *et al*. Isovaleric acidemia: Identification of isovalerate isovalerylglycine and 3-hydroxyisovalerate in urine of a patient previously reported as having butyric and hexanoic acidemia. *J Pediatr* 1973;**82**:243.

51 Tanaka K, Isselbacher KJ. The isolation and identification of N-isovaleryl-glycine from urine of patients with isovaleric acidemia. *J Biol Chem* 1967;**242**:2966.

52 Tanaka K, West-Dull A, Hine DG, *et al*. Gas-chromatographic method of analysis for urinary organic acids II: Description of the procedure and its application to diagnosis of patients with organic acidurias. *Clin Chem* 1980;**26**:1847.

53 Ando T, Nyhan WL. A simple screening method for detecting isovaleric acidemia. *Clin Chem* 1970;**16**:420.

54 Lehnert W, Niederhof H. 4-Hydroxyisovaleric acid: A new metabolite in isovaleric acidemia. *Eur J Pediatr* 1981;**136**:281.

55 Hine DG, Tanaka K. The identification and the excretion pattern of isovaleryl glucuronide in the urine of patients with isovaleric acidemia. *Pediatr Res* 1984;**18**:508.

56 Van Hove JL, Kahler SG, Millington DS, *et al*. Intravenous L-carnitine and acetyl-L-carnitine in medium-chain acyl-coenzyme. A dehydrogenase deficiency and isovaleric acidemia. *Pediatr Res* 1994;**35**:96.

57 Lehnert W, Hunkler D. Possibilities of selective screening for inborn errors of metabolism using high-resolution 1H-FT-NMR spectrometry. *Eur J Pediatr* 1986;**145**:260.

58 Vreken P, van Lint AEM, Bootsma AH, *et al*. Rapid diagnosis of organic acidemias and fatty acid oxidation defects by quantitative electrospray tandem-MS acyl-carnitine analysis in plasma in *Current Views of Fatty Acid Oxidation and Ketogenesis: From Organelles to Point Mutations* (ed. Quant PA and Eaton S) Kluwer Academic/Plenum Publishers, New York, 1999:327–337.

59 Cohn RM, Yudkoff M, Rothman R, Segal S. Isovaleric acidemia: Use of glycine therapy in neonates. *N Engl J Med* 1978;**299**:966.

60 Yudkoff M, Cohn RM, Puschak R, *et al*. Glycine therapy in isovaleric acidemia. *J Pediatr* 1978;**92**:813.

61 Levy HL, Erickson AM. Isovaleric acidemia in *Heritable Disorders of Amino Acid Metabolism* (ed. WL Nyhan) John Wiley and Sons Inc., New York, 1974: 81–97.

62 Naglak M, Salvo R, Madsen K, *et al*. The treatment of isovaleric acidemia with glycine supplement. *Pediatr Res* 1988;**24**:9.

63 Roe CR, Millington DS, Maltby DA, *et al*. L-carnitine therapy in isovaleric acidemia. *J Clin Invest* 1984;**74**:2290.

64 De Sousa C, Chalmers RA, Stacey TE, *et al*. The response to L-carnitine and glycine therapy in isovaleric acidemia. *Eur J Pediatr* 1986;**144**:451.

65 Chalmers RA, Roe CR, Stacey TE, Hoppel CL. Urinary excretion of L-carnitine and acylcarnitines by patients with disorders of organic acid metabolism: Evidence of secondary insufficiency of L-carnitine. *Pediatr Res* 1984;**18**:1325.

66 Stanley CA, Hale DE, Whiteman DEH, *et al*. Systemic carnitine (carn) deficiency in isovaleric acidemia. *Pediatr Res* 1983;**17**:296a.

67 Fries MH, Rinaldo P, Schmidt-Sommerfeld E, *et al*. Isovaleric acidemia: Response to a leucine load after three weeks of supplementation with glycine L-carnitine and combined glycine-carnitine therapy. *J Pediatr* 1998;**129**:449.

68 Itoh T, Ito T, Ohba S, *et al*. Effect of carnitine administration on glycine metabolism in patients with isovaleric acidemia: Significance of acetylcarnitine determination to estimate the proper carnitine dose. *Tohoku J Exp Med* 1996;**179**:101.

69 Millington DS, Roe CR, Maltby DA, Inoue F. Endogenous catabolism is the major source of toxic metabolites in isovaleric acidemia. *J Pediatr* 1987;**110**:56.

70 Wolff JA, Kelts DG, Algert S, *et al*. Alanine decreases the protein requirements of infants with inborn errors of amino acid metabolism. *J Neurogenet* 1985;**2**:41.

Glutaric aciduria (type I)

MAJOR PHENOTYPIC EXPRESSION

Megalencephaly; acute encephalitis-like crises; neurodegenerative disorder with spasticity, dystonia, choreoathetosis, ataxia and dyskinesia; seizures, increased signal on imaging of caudate and putamen and frontotemporal atrophy; glutaric aciduria and 3-hydroxyglutaric aciduria; and deficient activity of glutaryl CoA dehydrogenase.

INTRODUCTION

Glutaric aciduria was first described by Goodman *et al.*[1] in two siblings who began at 3 and 7 months of age to have a neurodegenerative disorder characterized by opisthotonos, dystonia and spasticity. One had a chronic compensated metabolic acidosis in which the serum bicarbonate concentration ranged from 7.5 to 15.7 mEq/L. It has now become apparent that macrocephaly is a prominent, often the initial, manifestation in infancy [2,3].

The cause of this disease is deficiency in the activity of glutaryl CoA dehydrogenase. This enzyme is on the pathway for the catabolism of lysine, hydroxylysine and tryptophan (Figure 8.1). This pathway is also the site of the defect in 2-oxoadipic aciduria (Chapter 15).

The disorder provides an argument for organic acid analysis in patients with dystonic cerebral palsy [4] and with megalencephaly. Diagnostic difficulty in infancy is highlighted by the fact that glutaric aciduria may be absent, even at times of acute neurologic decompensation [3,5]. Some patients are identified by the presence of 3-hydroxyglutaric acid rather than glutaric acid in the urine [6,7]. Analysis of organic acids in the cerebrospinal fluid [5,8] or enzyme assay may be required for diagnosis. The presence of glutarylcarnitine in blood or urine may also be diagnostic, and this forms the basis for neonatal screening [9,10].

Glutaryl CoA dehydrogenase has been mapped to chromosome 19p13.2 [11]. The gene contains 11 exons over 7 kb [12]. Nearly 100 mutations have been identified, and most patients are heterozygous for two different mutations [13]. Mutations common in inbred populations are 1VS1 + 56 > T mutation in Indians in Island Lake, Canada [14] and A421V in the Old Order Amish in Lancaster County, Pennsylvania [12].

CLINICAL ABNORMALITIES

Megalencephaly may be present at birth [3] and may necessitate cesarean section, or it may develop in the first weeks or months of life [2,3]. By 6 months, head circumference may be well above the 98th percentile [2], or 2 to 5 SD above the mean [3]. At this time, magnetic resonance (MRI) or computed tomography (CT) may reveal only increased signal intensity in the white matter, especially in the putamen and caudate. Some patients may have frontotemporal atrophy early. The neuroradiological studies are usually ordered to rule out hydrocephalus, and they do. Macrocephaly is not found in every patient, but in a series of 11 infants [3] it was present in all but two, and these two never had an acute encephalopathic crisis. A real clue to early diagnosis is the crossing of percentiles for head growth; this acceleration is maximal at 3–9 months.

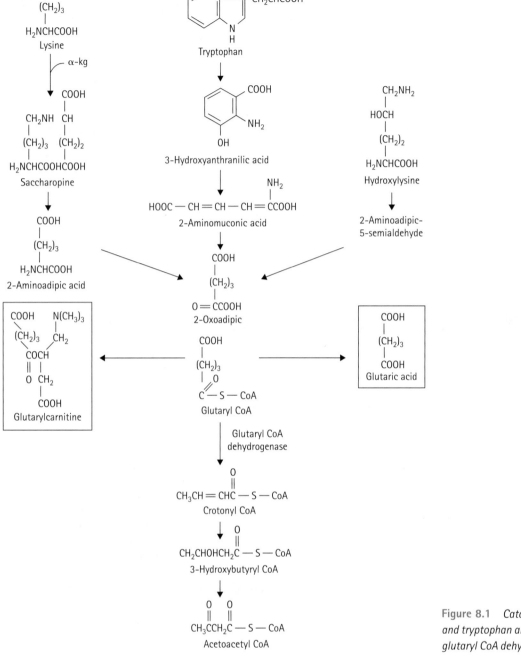

Figure 8.1 *Catabolic pathways for lysine and tryptophan and the site of the defect in glutaryl CoA dehydrogenase.*

Patients with or without macrocephaly develop normally until the initial neurologic presentation, which may be at 2 to 37 months. The mean age of onset of the encephalopathic episode is 14 months. However, it is now clear that many of these infants considered to be presymptomatic may have hypotonia, jitteriness, irritability or vomiting. Most present with an acute encephalopathic episode, often preceded by an infection and often accompanied by fever, so that an initial diagnosis of encephalitis is commonly made. The episode is characterized by acute loss of functions such as head control, sucking and swallowing reflexes, and the ability to sit, pull to standing or grasp toys [15]. Examination reveals profound hypotonia. There may be dystonic or athetoid movements and stiffness. There may be convulsions and paroxysmal abnormalities of the electroencephalograph (EEG). An increase in cerebrospinal fluid (CSF) concentration of protein may further suggest a diagnosis of encephalitis [16]. Recovery from the acute episode is slow and incomplete, leaving some evidence of developmental deficiency and dystonia or dyskinesia [17–23] (Figures 8.2–8.11).

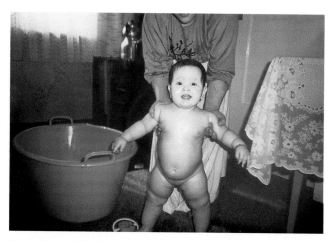

Figure 8.2   *S.S., an 8-month-old infant with glutaric aciduria. She was macrocephalic from birth, but seemed otherwise well prior to encephalopathic crisis. (Illustration kindly provided by Dr. Georg Hoffmann of the University of Heidelberg. A black and white version was published in Pediatrics [3].)*

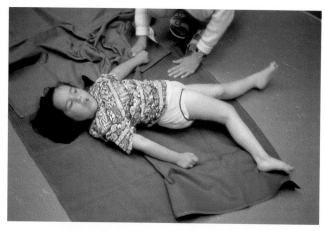

Figure 8.4   *J.S. was an unrelated patient with glutaric aciduria who had been macrocephalic at birth. She had not yet had an encephalopathic crisis by 2 years of age. However, by 5 years of age after an encephalopathic crisis, she was neurologically devastated. (Illustration kindly provided by Dr. Georg Hoffmann of the University of Heidelberg.)*

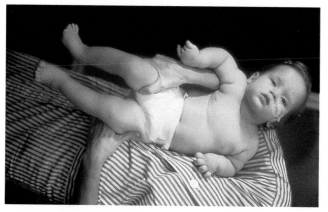

Figure 8.3   *S.S. at 14 months, after encephalopathic crisis. (Illustration kindly provided by Dr. Georg Hoffmann of the University of Heidelberg. A black and white version was published in Pediatrics [3].)*

There may be hypotonia, grimacing, opisthotonos, rigidity, clenched fists, or tongue-thrusting. There may be repeated episodes associated with catabolic situations, in which each is followed by further evidence of neurologic deterioration. Cognitive function is initially spared, but progressive impairment may occur. Some patients do not have acute episodes; instead the course is one of slow neurologic degeneration. The ultimate picture of spastic, dystonic cerebral palsy and mental deficiency is the same. On the other hand, the course may be quite variable, even among siblings; for instance, one sib at 4 years could not sit, while his 8-year-old brother was doing well in school [17]. At the other extreme two asymptomatic homozygous individuals have been observed [18,24], but these patients also had neuroradiographic evidence of frontotemporal atrophy. We have studied [6] siblings with pronounced dystonia who were intellectually normal and had normal MRI scans of the brain.

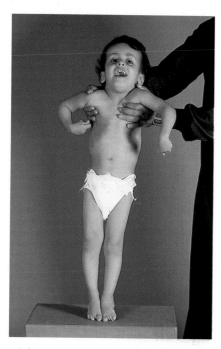

Figure 8.5   *A.S., an 18-month-old boy with glutaric aciduria illustrating the dystonic posturing and facial grimacing. He had developed normally until an initial episode at 7 months during which the CSF protein was 500 mg/dL.*

Profuse sweating is another common manifestation [3]. Some patients have had repeated episodes of unexplained fever (hyperpyrexic crises), irritability, ill-temper, anorexia and insomnia. Some have had hepatomegaly. Death in a Reye-like syndrome has been reported [19]. Death usually occurs before the end of the first decade [17,20–22].

Episodes of metabolic imbalance, ketoacidosis, or hypoglycemia that characterize most organic acidurias do not occur

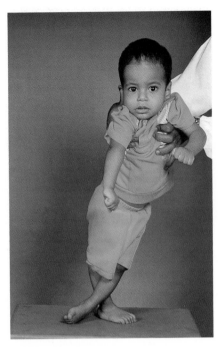

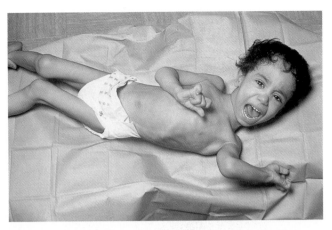

Figure 8.8   *F.Q.O.M., a 15-month-old boy with glutaric aciduria. Dystonic posturing was associated with athetoid movements of the hands.*

Figure 8.6   *A.T., a 15-month-old boy with glutaric aciduria. He was dystonic and the legs scissored.*

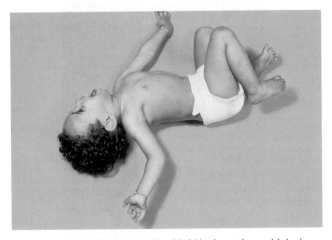

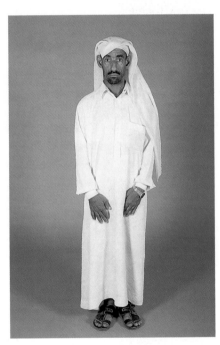

Figure 8.7   *A.M. This 20-month-old girl had spastic quadriplegia and oposthotonic posturing of the head.*

Figure 8.9   *A 47-year-old Saudi man with glutaric aciduria. He came to attention because of a cousin with the disease and severe dystonia, chorea and opisthotonus. This man, her uncle, had some dystonia of the hands on intention or excitement and imperfect gait. He had glutaric aciduria and the classic MS/MS findings. The mutation was found by Dr. S. Goodman of the University of Colorado: a leucine 179 arginine that has not been reported in another family. Two children in this family were diagnosed as having the disease but have had no neurological abnormalities.*

in this disorder. Low levels of bicarbonate may be seen chronically [1] or during acute episodes of illness [3], but in some patients they have always been normal [21,22]. Rarely there may be ketosis, hypoglycemia, hyperammonemia and elevated levels of transaminases in the blood during the acute episodes [16,18,19–25].

An unusual clinical occurrence is rhabdomyolysis, as seen in disorders of fatty acid oxidation [26]. The patient reported had three episodes, the last one fatal. Levels of creatine kinase ranged from 78 000 to 189 000 IU.

Neuroradiographic findings are characteristically fronto-temporal atrophy on CT or MRI with increased CSF-containing spaces in the sylvian fissures and anterior to the temporal lobes [3,18,25,27–30] (Figures 8.12–8.14). This may be manifest

in utero or may occur in infancy antedating neurologic symptoms [3]; or it may develop after the first encephalopathic episode. In these latter patients the initial abnormal finding may be decreased attenuation in the cerebral white matter on CT or increased signal intensity on MRI of the basal ganglia [2], but enlargement of the sylvian fissure may be seen prior to the changes in the basal ganglia [25]. Reduced density in

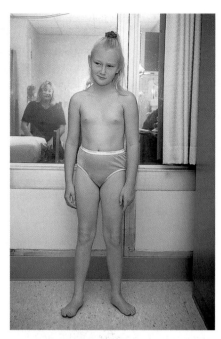

Figure 8.10 *A 9-year-old girl with glutaryl CoA dehydrogenase who excreted 3-hydroxyglutaric acid [6]. Photographed walking, she illustrated a wide-based, dystonic gait.*

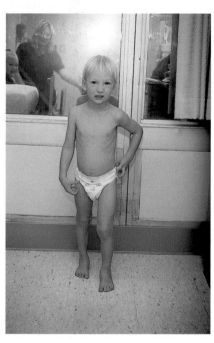

Figure 8.11 *Her 3-year-old brother displayed dystonic grimacing, athetoid posturing of the arms and hands, and a somewhat broad gait.*

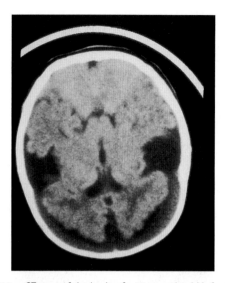

Figure 8.12 *CT scan of the brain of a 13-month-old infant with glutaric aciduria. The patient was presymptomatic, but there was extensive frontotemporal atrophy. (Illustration kindly provided by Dr. Georg Hoffmann of the University of Heidelberg.)*

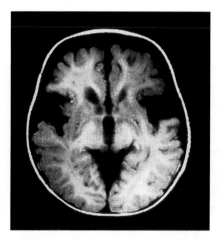

Figure 8.13 *MRI scan of the patient in Figure 8.5, illustrating extreme loss of volume and the pattern of frontotemporal atrophy. (Illustration kindly provided by Dr. Georg Hoffmann of the University of Heidelberg.)*

the caudate has been found by ultrasound [3]. Subdural collections of fluid have been observed in a number of patients [25,30] (Figure 8.15). There may be hygromas, or actual subdural hematomas [31–33], because of rupture of bridging veins stretched by the enlargement of these spaces. These occurrences have given rise to a suspicion of child abuse. Retinal hemorrhages may add to this suspicion. Certainly this disease is not the most common cause of this syndrome of non-accidental trauma, but it is reasonable to be sure to exclude glutaric aciduria in any such patient without other obvious signs of trauma.

The neuropathology [28,34,35] is that of extensive striatal neurotoxicity. There is neuronal loss and astrocytic proliferation in the caudate nucleus and the putamen, and in some in the globus pallidus. Changes tend to be more extensive in older patients [35]. Prominent spongiform change is seen predominantly in the white matter. Despite the cortical atrophy reported on imaging studies, neuronal loss was not found in the cortex. There may be microvesicular lipid in the liver.

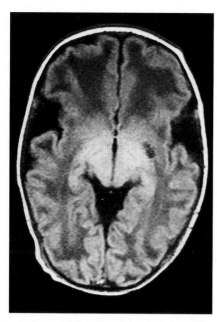

Figure 8.14   *CT scan of the brain of a 3-week-old with glutaric aciduria, illustrating the early occurrence of frontotemporal atrophy. (Illustration kindly provided by Dr. Georg Hoffmann of the University of Heidelberg.)*

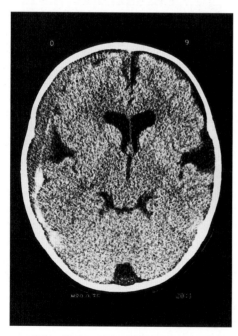

Figure 8.15   *CT scan of the same patient at 9 months, illustrating the development of a chronic subdural hematoma. (Illustration kindly provided by Dr. Georg Hoffmann of the University of Heidelberg.)*

GENETICS AND PATHOGENESIS

The site of the molecular defect is in glutaryl CoA dehydrogenase (Figure 8.1, p. 58). Activity is most commonly measured

in fibroblast or leukocyte lysates in which residual activity is virtually undetectable [18,36,37]. The disease is transmitted as an autosomal recessive trait. Intermediate activities of the enzyme have been documented in leucocytes and fibroblasts of heterozygotes [18], and consanguinity has been observed [16,17].

The enzyme (EC 1.3.99.7) is a flavoprotein mitochondrial dehydrogenase. Its electrons are transferred to ubiquinone in interactions with the electron transfer flavoprotein (ETF) and its dehydrogenase (ETF:ubiquinione oxidoreductase). Flavin adenine dinucleotide (FAD) is bound to the enzyme. Paper chemistry would indicate that glutaconyl CoA was an intermediate in the reaction, but if so it must remain bound to the enzyme because the only products of labeled substrate are crotonyl CoA and CO_2 [38,39].

The cDNA for the enzyme has been cloned and sequenced. There are 11 exons. The gene has been mapped to chromosome 19p13.2 [11]. The mutation (IV1 + 5GtoT) that has been found in homozygous Indians in Manitoba, in a population in which glutaric aciduria is common in a splicing mutation [24]. The G to T transversion in intron 1 at position +5 changes a donor splice site to Ggtcatt, which permits variable splicing, some normal but most using a cryptic donor site 26 bases upstream and leading to a deletion of 26 base pairs, removing eight amino acids and causing a translational frame shift. Variable amounts of normal and truncated mRNA in varying individuals would determine variable phenotypes. In the Amish population, in which glutaric aciduria is also common, a C to T change at 1298 changes the alanine at 421 to valine [12].

The most common mutation in the broader population was C1240 to T, which changed arginine at 402 to tryptophan (R402W). This mutation was found in 30 percent of alleles in Spain and in 40 percent of those in Germans [40,41]. Expression of various mutations in *E. coli* led to enzyme activities ranging from less than 17 percent of normal activity to 20 percent in the Amish mutation.

Correlations between genotype and clinical severity have been elusive, possibly because neurologic impairment is related to the occurrence of encephalopathic crises rather than any other clinical, biochemical or molecular feature. However, certain mutations have correlated well with high excretion of glutaric and 3-hydroxyglutaric acids, and others have been found in patients with low excretion [40]. In the former group the most frequent mutations were R402W and A293T resulting from a G913A change in exon 8. These mutations were found in the low excretor group only in heterozygosity, especially in combination with R227P or V400M, which together accounted for over half of the mutant alleles in the low excretor group [40,42]. Among eight families identified in Israel, six were of Muslim origin and two nonAskenazi Jews, and eight previously unidentified mutations were found including a 1 bp deletion at 1173 [43]. The siblings with 3-hydroxyglutaric aciduria [6] were compounds of R227P and E365K.

Defective enzyme activity leads to glutaric aciduria, the feature by which the diagnosis is usually made. The amounts reported may be massive: 850–1700 mmol/mol creatinine [1] and 900–1200 mmol/mol creatinine [3]. Normal levels of glutaric acid in urine range from 0.6 to 4 mmol/mol creatinine. However, patients with smaller amounts (80–200 mmol/mol creatinine [3] have been observed, and many patients have been reported in whom glutaric acid and other characteristic metabolites were not found in the urine [4]. Metabolites in the urine have also been observed intermittently [44]. The other characteristic metabolites found in the urine are 3-hydroxyglutaric and glutaconic acids [16]; amounts are usually less than those of glutaric acid. On the other hand, we have seen children with documented deficiency of the enzyme in whom only 3-hydroxyglutaric was found in the urine, in the absence of accumulation of glutaric acid [6]. Excretion of glutaconic acid may exceed that of 3-hydroxyglutaric acid only in an acute ketotic episode when the urine also contains 3-hydroxybutyric, acetoacetic, adipic, suberic and sebacic acids [20].

Levels of glutaric acid in plasma have ranged from 3 to 60 μmol/L [3], but normal levels have also been recorded. Glutaric acid is undetectable in normal plasma or CSF. In patients, levels of glutaric acid in the CSF have ranged from 20 to 40 μmol/L [3,5]. The CSF may be the only fluid in which elevated levels are found [5]. Glutaric acid concentrations have been found to be elevated in all tissues examined [29].

Measurement of bound glutaric acid by organic acid analysis following mild alkaline hydrolysis may indicate the diagnosis in patients with normal urinary glutaric acid [45]. This is probably a reflection of the excretion of glutarylcarnitine, which may be detected by tandem mass spectrometry [45].

The analysis of glutarylcarnitine in blood spots has been incorporated into most programs of expanded neonatal screening [10]. There are cautions about the possibility of false negatives. An infant with glutaric aciduria was missed on a neonatal screen [9]. Actually there was glutarylcarnitine on the initial spot, but a repeat was normal, and the patient was only identified after developing dystonia at 11 months during an intercurrent infection. That state has since increased the sensitivity of the screen for this disease by adjusting the signal ratio cut off, and now recommends a complete workup for any positive rather than a repeat. With time amounts of acylcarnitines may decrease as carnitine stores are depleted. In addition patients with mutations that put them in the low excretor group [40] have been tested for glutarylcarnitine in blood spots and all gave negative results even in the presence of carnitine supplementation.

Diagnostic confusion is symbolized by the fact that classic patients may excrete no elevated glutaric acid at all, and 3-hydroxyglutaric excretion may be normal. On the other side of the coin elevated excretion of glutaric acid (100–150 mmol/mol creatinine) has been reported [46] in a patient found not to have glutaryl CoA dehydrogenase deficiency; antibiotic treatment abolished the glutaric aciduria; so the source must have been intestinal bacteria. An additional confounder is ketosis, which has been reported [47] to cause significant increases in the excretion of 3-hydroxyglutaric acid in the urine of patients who did not have glutaryl CoA dehydrogenase deficiency. In two patients with glutaryl CoA dehydrogenase and no elevation of glutarylcarnitine in the blood, there was a sizeable excretion of glutarylcarnitine in the urine [48].

Most patients have low concentrations of free-carnitine in plasma and elevated levels of esterified carnitine, especially in urine [3,18,45]. Low muscle carnitine has been reported [18], even in an asymptomatic patient.

The incidence of the disorder is not known, although it has been estimated at one in 30 000 in Sweden [49]. Increased frequency of the disease has been observed in Ojibway Indians in Manitoba [50] and in the Amish of Lancaster County, Pennsylvania [51]. Carrier detection has been improved by assay of the enzyme in cultured interleukin-2-dependent leukocytes [52], but there was still some overlap between controls and obligate heterozygotes. Molecular analysis for mutation is the most reliable method of carrier detection. Prenatal diagnosis has been made by the detection of increased amounts of glutaric acid [53] in amniotic fluid, as well as by assay of the enzyme in cultured amniocytes. Molecular analysis for mutation is the most reliable method of prenatal diagnosis. The value of prenatal diagnosis has been questioned [18] on the basis of the existence of asymptomatic homozygotes, but these individuals had frontotemporal atrophy, and studies of intellectual function were not reported.

Considerable attention has been devoted to pathogenesis and the extraordinary vulnerability of the striatum, particularly the caudate and putamen. It has seemed likely that the accumulation of metabolites and something about the catabolic response to acute infection are relevant to neuronal damage. The similarity of structures of glutaric and glutamic acids, and the fact that glutaric and 3-hydroxyglutaric acids inhibit glutamate decarboxylase of brain [54] has led to an excitotoxic theory of neuronal damage in this disease. In striatal slice cultures 3-hydroxyglutaric acid induced neuronal degeneration by activation of N-methyl-D-aspartate (NMDA) receptors [55]. Convulsions and striatal neuronal damage were caused in rats by direct striatal injection of 3-hydroxyglutaric acid [56].

TREATMENT

Treatment with carnitine and the prompt, vigorous intervention in intercurrent illness with the provision of energy from glucose, water and electrolytes appears increasingly likely to prevent striatal degeneration [57]. A protocol we have employed (Table 8.1) was derived from the large experience of Morton with the glutaric aciduria of the Amish. Some have added insulin to the regimen, and it is likely that we will as well. The initial dose for chronic oral carnitine administration approximates 100 mg/kg, and we adjust dosage dependent on intestinal tolerance and urinary carnitine ester excretion.

Implicit in programs of neonatal screening is the expectation that treatment will prevent encephalopathic neuronal

Table 8.1   *Management of acute imbalance in glutaric acidemia I*

Time hr		mL/kg
0–1	IV bolus 5% dextrose in Ringer lactate + 2 mEq/kg NaHCO$_3$	20
1–24	IV 12.5% dextrose 20 mEq/L KCl, 50 mEq/L NaHCO$_3$, 50 mEq/L NaCl	140
	For vomiting 0.15 mg/kg Zofran IV, may repeat in 4–8 hr. Alternative Kytril 10 μg/kg IV	
	Calorimetry – provide CHO at least 1.5 × BMR	

damage. Experience to date suggests that this is the case [10]. The occurrence of frontotemporal atrophy at birth implies restriction of any postnatal therapeutic effects, but there is even evidence that this may improve [15]. Hoffmann has written [15] that current therapy prevents brain degeneration in over 90 percent of infants treated prospectively, while more than 90 percent of untreated affected patients will develop severe neurologic disability. Experience from the same group [58] indicates that some genotypes may lead to acute encephalopathy despite adherence to all of the current mainstays of treatment. An infant homozygous for E365K experienced such an episode and despite treatment was left with a dystonic, dyskinetic movement disorder and characteristic striatal lesions on MRI [58].

A diet low in tryptophan and lysine will decrease in the excretion of glutaric acid in urine to one-third or more [1,3,20,59] of the usual values, but clinical improvement resulting from diet alone has been little or none. Riboflavin, as the coenzyme of the dehydrogenase, has appeared logical, and 100–300 mg/day have been used [60,61], but also without clear evidence of therapeutic effect. Low concentrations of gamma amino butyric acid (GABA) in the basal ganglia led to the use of the GABA analog 4-amino-3-(4-chlorphenyl) butyric acid (baclofen, Lioresal); results have usually not been impressive, but improvement was reported in two of three patients in a double-blind controlled study given 2 mg/kg per day [9]. Valproic acid has been recommended, but most feel this drug is contraindicated [3]. Improvement has been reported clinically and in concentrations of GABA in the CSF following vigabatrine in doses of 35–50 mg/kg [62].

References

1   Goodman SI, Markey SP, Moe PG, *et al.* Glutaric aciduria: a 'new' disorder of amino acid metabolism. *Biochem Med* 1975;**12**:12.

2   Iafolla AK, Kahler SG. Megalencephaly in the neonatal period as the initial manifestation of glutaric aciduria type I. *J Pediatr* 1989:**114**:1004.

3   Hoffmann GF, Trefz FK, Barth PG, *et al.* Glutaryl-CoA dehydrogenase deficiency: a distinct encephalopathy. *Pediatrics* 1991;**88**:1194.

4   Hauser SE, Peters H. Glutaric aciduria type I: an underdiagnosed cause of encephalopathy and dystonia-dyskinesia syndrome in children. *J Paediatr Child Health* 1998;**34**:302.

5   Campistol J, Ribes A, Alvarez L, *et al.* Glutaric aciduria type I: unusual biochemical presentation. *J Pediatr* 1992;**121**:83.

6   Nyhan WL, Zschocke J, Hoffmann G, *et al.* Glutaryl-CoA dehydrogenase deficiency presenting as 3-hydroxyglutaric aciduria. *Mol Genet Metab* 1999;**66**:199.

7   Baric I, Wagner L, Feyh P, *et al.* Sensitivity and specificity of free and total glutaric acid and 3-hydroxyglutaric acid measurements by stable-isotope dilution assays for the diagnosis for glutaric aciduria type I. *J Inherit Metab Dis* 1999;**22**:867.

8   Hoffman GF, Meier-Augenstein W, Nyhan WL. Physiology and pathophysiology of organic acids in cerebrospinal fluid. *J Inherit Metab Dis* 1993;**16**:648.

9   Smith WE, Millington DS, Koever DD, Lesser PS. Glutaric academia type I missed by newborn screening in an infant with dystonia following promethazine administration. *Pediatrics* 2001;**107**:1184.

10   Soufi S, Rashed MS, Al Essa M, *et al.* Glutaric academia type 1: first Saudi patient diagnosed by tandem mass spectrometry-based neonatal screening. *Ann Saudi Med* 1998;**18**:160.

11   Greenberg CR, Duncan AMV, Gregory CA, *et al.* Assignment of human glutaryl-CoA dehydrogenase (GCDH) to the short arm of chromosome 19 (19p132) by *in situ* hybridization and somatic cell hybrid analysis. *Genomics* 1994;**21**:289.

12   Biery BJ, Stein DE, Morton DH, Goodman SI. Gene structure and mutations of glutaryl-coenzyme A dehydrogenase: Impaired association of enzyme subunits due to an A421V substitution causes glutaric academia (type I) in the Amish. *Am J Human Genet* 1996;**59**:1006.

13   Goodman SI, Stein DE, Schlesinger S, *et al.* Glutaryl-CoA dehydrogenase mutations in glutaric academia (type 1): Review and report of thirty novel mutations. *Hum Mutat* 1998;**12**:141.

14   Greenberg CR, Reimer D, Singal R, *et al.* A G-to-T transversion at the +5 position of intron 1 in the glutaryl-CoA dehydrogenase gene is associated with the Island Lake variant of glutaric academia type 1. *Hum Mol Genet* 1995;**4**:493.

15   Hoffmann GF, Zschocke J. Glutaric aciduria type I: from clinical biochemical and molecular diversity to successful therapy. *J Inherit Metab Dis* 1999;**22**:381.

16   Coates R, Rashed M, Rahbeeni Z, *et al.* Glutaric aciduria type 1 first reported Saudi patient. *Ann Saudi Med* 1994;**114**:316.

17   Gregersen N, Brandt NJ, Christensen E, *et al.* Glutaric aciduria: clinical and laboratory findings in two brothers. *J Pediatr* 1977;**90**:740.

18   Amir N, Elpeleg OBN, Shalev RS, Christensen E. Glutaric aciduria type I: enzymatic and neuroradiologic investigations of two kindreds. *J Pediatr* 1989;**90**:983.

19   Goodman SI, Norenberg M, Shikes RH, *et al.* Glutaric aciduria: biochemical and morphologic considerations. *J Pediatr* 1977;**90**:746.

20   Floret D, Divry P, Dingeon N, Monnet P. Acidurie glutarique: une nouvelle observation. *Arch Fr Pediatr* 1979;**36**:462.

21   Brandt NJ, Brandt S, Christensen E, *et al.* Glutaric aciduria in progressive choreo-athetosis. *Clin Genet* 1978;**13**:77.

22   Kyllerman M, Steen G. Intermittently progressive dyskinetic syndrome in glutaric aciduria. *Neuropediatrics* 1977;**8**:397.

23   Dunger DB, Snodgrass GJAI. Glutaric aciduria type I presenting with hypoglycemia. *J Inherit Metab Dis* 1984;**7**:122

24   Amir N, Elpeleg O, Shalev RS, Christensen E. Clinical heterogeneity and neuroradiologic features. *Neurology* 1987;**37**:1654.

25   Yager JY, McClarty BM, Seshia SS. CT-scan findings in an infant with glutaric aciduria type I. *Dev Med Child Neurol* 1988;**30**:808.

26   Wilson CJ, Collins JE, Leonard JV. Recurrent rhabdomyolysis in a child with glutaric aciduria type I. *J Inherit Metab Dis* 1999;**22**:663.

27   Hoffman GF, Trefz FK, Barth PG, *et al.* Macrocephaly: an important indication for organic acid analysis. *J Inherit Metab Dis* 1991;**14**:329.

28 Brismar J, Ozand PT. CT and MRI of the brain in glutaric acidemia type I: a review of 59 published cases and a report of 5 new patients. *Am J Neuroradiol* 1995;**16**:675.

29 Leibel RL, Shih VE, Goodman SI, *et al*. Glutaric acidemia: a metabolic disorder causing progressive choreoathetosis. *Neurology* 1980;**30**:1163.

30 Osaka H, Kimura S, Nezu A, *et al*. Chronic subdural hematoma as an initial manifestation of glutaric aciduria type-1. *Brain Dev* 1993;**15**:125.

31 Muntau AC, Röschinger W, Pfluger T, *et al*. Subdurale Hygrome und Hämatome im Säuglingsalter als Initialmanifestation der glutarazidurie Typ I: Folgenschwere Fehldiagnose als Kindesmiβhandlung. *Monatsschr Kinderh* 1997;**145**:646.

32 Drigo P, Burlina AB, Battistella PA. Subdural hematoma and glutaric aciduria type I. *Brain Dev* 1993;**15**:460.

33 Woefle J, Kreft B, Emons D, Haverkamp F. A diagnostic pitfall. *Pediatr Radiol* 1996;**26**:779.

34 Chow CW, Haan EA, Goodman SI, *et al*. Neuropathology in glutaric acidemia type I. *Acta Neuropath* 1988;**76**:590.

35 Soffer D, Amir N, Elpeleg ON, *et al*. Striatal degeneration and spongy myelinopathy in glutaric acidemia. *J Neurol Sci* 1992;**107**:199.

36 Goodman SI, Kohlhoff JG. Glutaric aciduria: inherited deficiency of glutaryl CoA dehydrogenase activity. *Biochem Med* 1975;**13**:138.

37 Hyman DB, Tanaka K. Specific glutaryl-CoA dehydrogenating activity is deficient in cultured fibroblasts from glutaric aciduria patients. *J Clin Invest* 1984;**73**:778.

38 Lenich AC, Goodman SI. The purification and characterization of glutaryl-coenzyme. A dehydrogenase from porcine and human liver. *J Biol Chem* 1986;**261**:4090.

39 Besrat A, Polan CE, Henderson LM. Mammalian metabolism of glutaric acid. *J Biol Chem* 1969;**244**:1461.

40 Busquets C, Merinero B, Christensen E, *et al*. Glutaryl-CoA dehydrogenase deficiency in Spain: evidence of two groups of patients genetically and biochemically distinct. *Pediatr Res* 2000;**48**:315.

41 Zschocke J, Quak E, Guldberg P, Hoffmann GF. Mutation analysis in glutaric aciduria type I. *J Med Genet* 2000;**37**:177.

42 Christensen E, Ribes A, Busquets C, *et al*. Compound heterozygotes with R227P mutation on one allele in the glutaryl-CoA dehydrogenase gene is associated with no or very low glutarate excretion. *J Inherit Metab Dis* 1997;**20**:383.

43 Anikster Y, Shaag A, Joseph A, *et al*. Glutaric aciduria type I in the Arab and Jewish communities in Israel. *Am J Hum Genet* 1999;**59**:1012.

44 Hellstrom B. Progressive dystonia and dyskinesia in childhood a review of some recent advances. *Acta Paediatr Scand* 1982;**71**:177.

45 Ribes A, Riudor E, Briones P, *et al*. Significance of bound glutarate in the diagnosis of glutaric aciduria type I. *J Inherit Metab Dis* 1992;**15**:367.

46 Wendel U, Bakkeren J, de Jong J, Bongaerts G. Glutaric aciduria mediated by gut bacteria. *J Inherit Metab Dis* 1995;**18**:358.

47 Pitt J, Carpenter K, Wilcken B, Boneh A. 3-Hydroxyglutarate excretion is increased in ketotic patients: implications for glutaryl-CoA dehydrogenase deficiency testing. *J Inherit Metab Dis* 2002;**25**:83.

48 Tortorelli S, Cuthbert CD, Tauscher A, *et al*. The clinical significance of urine glutarylcarnitine for the biochemical diagnosis of glutaric acidemia type I. Abstract of the Annual Meeting of the SIMD. *Genet Med* May/June 2003;**56**. Abs.45.

49 Kyllerman M, Steen G. Glutaric aciduria. A 'common' metabolic disorder? *Arch Fr Pediatr* 1980;**37**:279.

50 Haworth JC, Booth FA, Coddle E, *et al*. Phenotypic variability in glutaric aciduria type I: report of fourteen cases in five Canadian Indian kindreds. *J Pediatr* 1991;**118**:51.

51 Morton DH, Bennett MJ, Seargeant LED, *et al*. Glutaric aciduria type I: a common cause of episodic encephalopathy and spastic paralysis in the Amish of Lancaster County Pennsylvania. *Am J Med Genet* 1991;**41**:89.

52 Seargeant LED, Coddle E, Dialing LA, *et al*. Carrier detection in glutaric aciduria type I using interleuken-2-independent cultured lymphocytes. *J Inherit Metab Dis* 1992;**15**:733.

53 Goodman SI, Gallegos DA, Pullin CJ, *et al*. Antenatal diagnosis of glutaric acidemia. *Am J Hum Genet* 1980;**32**:695.

54 Stokke O, Goodman SI, Moe PG. Inhibition of brain glutamate decarboxylase by glutarate glutaconate and β-hydroxyglutarate: explanation of the symptoms in glutaric aciduria. *Clin Chim Acta* 1976;**66**:411.

55 Ullrich K, Flott-Rahmel B, Schluff P, *et al*. Glutaric aciduria type I: Pathomechanisms of neurodegeneration. *J Inherit Metab Dis* 1999;**22**:392.

56 de Mello CF, Kölker S, Ahlemeyer B, *et al*. Intrastriatal administration of 3-hydroxyglutaric acid induces convulsions and striatal lesions in rats. *Brain Res* 2001;**1**:70.

57 Hoffmann GF, Athanassopoulos S, Burlina AB, *et al*. Clinical course early diagnosis treatment and prevention of disease in glutaryl-CoA dehydrogenase deficiency. *Neuropediatrics* 1996;**27**:115.

58 Kölker S, Ramaekers VT, Zschocke J, Hoffmann GF. Acute encephalopathy despite early therapy in a patient with homozygosity for E365K in the glutaryl-coenzyme. A dehydrogenase gene. *J Pediatr* 2001;**138**:277.

59 Brandt NJ, Gregersen N, Christensen E, *et al*. Treatment of glutaryl-CoA dehydrogenase deficiency (glutaric aciduria). *J Pediatr* 1979;**94**:669.

60 Bennett MJ, Marlow N, Pollitt RJ, Wales JKH. Glutaric aciduria type I: biochemical investigations and postmortem findings. *Eur J Pediatr* 1986;**145**:403.

61 Lipkin PH, Roe CR, Goodman SI, Batshaw ML. A case of glutaric acidemia type I: effect of riboflavin and carnitine. *J Pediatr* 1988;**112**:62.

62 Francois B, Jaeken J, Gillia P. Vigabatrin in the treatment of glutaric aciduria type I. *J Inherit Metab Dis* 1990;**13**:352.

3-Methylcrotonyl CoA carboxylase deficiency/
3-methylcrotonyl glycinuria

MAJOR PHENOTYPIC EXPRESSION

Reye-like episodes of ketoacidosis, hypoglycemia, hyperammonemia and coma; seizures, failure to thrive; excretion of 3-methylcrotonyl glycine and 3-hydroxyisovaleric acid; and deficiency of 3-methylcrotonyl CoA carboxylase. An increasing population of asymptomatic individuals, mostly adult women discovered because of elevated 3-hydroxyisovaleryl-carnitine detected in the neonatal screening blood spots of their infants.

INTRODUCTION

3-Methylcrotonyl CoA carboxylase (EC 6.4.1.4) deficiency (Figure 9.1) is a disorder of leucine catabolism in which elevated quantities of 3-hydroxyisovaleric acid and 3-methylcrotonyl glycine are found in the urine. The disorder is often referred to as isolated 3-methylcrotonyl CoA carboxylase deficiency, to distinguish it from multiple carboxylase deficiency,

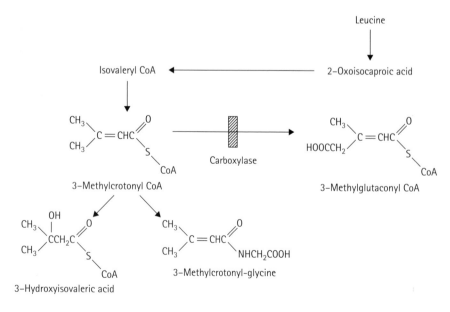

Figure 9.1   *3-Methylcrotonyl CoA carboxylase, the site of the defect in 3-methylcrotonyl CoA carboxylase deficiency. The formation of the key metabolites results from hydration to 3-hydroxyisovaleric acid and conjugation with glycine.*

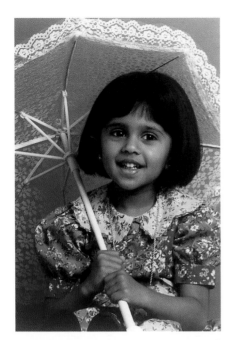

Figure 9.2   *N.B., a 4-year-old girl with 3-methylcrotonyl CoA carboxylase deficiency. Her appearance and behavior have been quite normal for age. Her height was at the 25th percentile for age and the weight just below the 5th percentile. Muscle tone was reduced. She had always been a very fussy eater and ate very little. (Illustration was kindly provided by Dr. Vivian Shih and the parents of the patient.)*

as early reports and the majority of subsequent patients with 3-methylcrotonyl glycinuria have had biotin-responsive multiple carboxylase deficiency as a consequence of deficiency of holocarboxylase synthetase (Chapter 5) or biotinidase (Chapter 6) [1,2]. No patients with the isolated disorder have to date been responsive to biotin. The disease was considered to be rare [3–11], until the development of programs of neonatal screening began turning up so many patients that this disorder is being considered the most common of the organic acidemias [12]. In most instances it is the mother, not the newborn, that has 3-methylcrotonyl CoA carboxylase deficiency. The gene has been cloned, and mutations have been defined.

CLINICAL ABNORMALITIES

The classic presentation of this disease has been relatively late in infancy between 1- and 3-years-of-age, with an acute episode consistent with a diagnosis of Reye syndrome [11,13]. The episode is classic for organic acidemia in that there is massive ketosis and systemic acidosis, leading to lethargy, coma and even a fatal outcome [9]. Hypoglycemia may be prominent, symptomatic and life-threatening [6,11]. Death has also occurred from cerebral edema and cardiac arrest. There may be hyperammonemia and elevated levels of transaminases in blood. There may be microvesicular and macrovesicular deposition of fat in the liver [8,9].

The onset of the initial episode maybe with vomiting or convulsions. Between episodes, vomiting is uncommon, and most patients appear completely well. Patients have noted subjectively that protein restriction led to general improvement, as well as a decrease in the number of exacerbations [3]. One patient had a neonatal onset of focal seizures and hypotonia, developed some developmental retardation and died in status epilepticus [14]. Hypotonia is commonly observed, and patients have been designated as having familial hypotonia and carnitine deficiency [13].

A number of patients have displayed quite a variety of clinical manifestations. One had chronic vomiting and failure to thrive. The onset of vomiting followed a graduation from human milk to conventional cow's milk-based formula at 3 weeks of life. In addition to vomiting, there was chronic diarrhea, numerous upper respiratory infections, a respiratory syncitial virus-induced bronchiolitis and chronic mucocandidiasis. He had severe gastroesophageal reflux. Nevertheless, the existence of so many previously undiagnosed adults with the disease suggests that the general prognosis is good. Also, most patients, once over the initial episode, have been intellectually normal [5]. An increasing number of patients have been asymptomatic or very mildly symptomatic. Initially there were patients diagnosed because they were siblings of patients, and many never expressed symptoms of the disease [15,16].

A sizeable number of recent patients have been adults discovered because their newly born infants failed the neonatal screening test for 3-hydroxyisovaleryl-carnitine [12,17,18]. Some of these women have had myopathy or weakness, and carnitine deficiency, which could have been responsible for this symptomology [12]. Some also had elevated levels of uric acid and transaminases in the blood and histologic evidence of lipid deposits in the liver. These observations suggest that some of the nonspecific manifestations in earlier patients may have been unrelated to the underlying metabolic disorder. Nevertheless, the importance of the diagnosis is that any patient, regardless of even asymptomatic status, is at risk of the development, with the stress of infection, surgery, or a high protein load, of a typical Reye-like episode, which could be life threatening. A patient, who developed feeding difficulties and failure to gain weight at 11 weeks, later developed seizures, spasticity, and fatal metabolic acidosis [19]. Another patient [20] had a metabolic stroke during an episode of hypoglycemia and metabolic imbalance coincident with a febrile illness. Following diagnosis and treatment she was stable for five years of follow-up, but hemiparesis and developmental delay remained. This adds to the list of metabolic diseases in which stroke-like episodes occur (Appendix).

GENETICS AND PATHOGENESIS

The genetics of this disorder are autosomal recessive. Prenatal diagnosis should be possible by the assay of the enzyme in amniocytes or chorionic villus material [9,21] or the direct

GCMS determination of 3-hydroxyisovaleric acid in amniotic fluid [22]. Heterozygote detection may not be reliable, but values in fibroblasts, such as 21 percent and 42 percent of control activity have been found in parents [9].

The molecular defect is in 3-methylcrotonyl CoA carboxylase (Figure 9.1). The diagnosis should be confirmed by the assay of the enzyme in leukocytes or cultured fibroblasts [3,9,21]. The other carboxylases for propionyl CoA and pyruvate should also be assayed, and so should biotinidase, because the distinction from multiple carboxylase deficiency is so important. A trial of biotin may be of interest, even though a responsive patient with the isolated disease has yet to be discovered. The amounts of residual activity in fibroblasts may range from 0.05–3 percent in a single family [9], and as much as 12 percent [3]. Lymphocyte values may be much higher, approximately 46 percent of control in a patient in whom the mean fibroblast level was 10 percent [3]. Cultivation of cells in different levels of biotin does not affect activity. The enzyme has been purified from bovine kidney and rat liver and is an oligomer with two protein α and β subunits, like propionyl CoA carboxylase [23,24]. Complementation studies [18] have shown clearly the presence of different A and B groups.

The genes for the α and β subunits have been cloned and sequenced independently by 3 different groups [17,18,25]. The A gene is located on chromosome 3q25–28 and has 19 exons. The B gene, on chromosome 5q12–13, has 17 exons. The genes encode proteins of 725 and 563 amino acids, respectively. A number of mutations has been defined: 7 mutant alleles in the A gene and 14 mutant alleles in the B gene. Genotype-phenotype correlations were made difficult by the fact that some individuals with no detectable enzyme activity have been asymptomatic. Yet some mutations are consistent with structural activity information on the enzyme. A missense mutation M325R led to absence of labeled biotin attachment to the α subunit [18]. A missense mutation in the A gene and two in the B gene involved nonconservative substitutions of residues that are highly conserved in man, plants, and fungi. Construction of a null A gene in Aspergillus abolished the ability of this organism to grow on leucine as a sole carbon source [18].

The accumulation of 3-methylcrotonyl CoA behind the block leads to the excretion of 3-hydroxyisovaleric acid and 3-methylcrotonylglycine (Table 9.1). The amounts are quite variable; usually but not always [3], the levels of the former are higher than the latter. Varying levels of the glycine conjugate, 3-methylcrotonylglycine, in different patients may reflect varying efficiency of glycine-N-acylase. Hydroxyisovalerylglycine has not been detected, presumably because the hydroxy acid is a poor substrate for glycine-N-acylase. Supplementation with glycine has been reported [20] not to increase the excretion of 3-methylcrotonylglycine. 3-Hydroxyisovalerylcarnitine has been identified in the urine [26] and identified as a product of leucine, and its occurrence in the blood has provided the basis for programs of neonatal screening. The identification of this carnitine ester provides evidence for the intramitochondrial origin of 3-hydroxyisovaleric acid via crotonase

Table 9.1   *Urinary excretion of the key metabolites*

Metabolite	Range of excretion (mmol/mol creatinine)
3-Hydroxyisovaleric acid	100–60 000
3-Methylcrotonylglycine	70–5200

catalyzed conversion from 3-methylcrotonyl CoA and hydrolysis of the CoA ester. This contrasts with the microsomal origin of the compound in isovaleric acidemia in which 3-hydroxyisovalerylcarnitine is not found. It is important that 3-hydroxypropionic and methylcitric acids are not found in the urine. At the time of acute ketotic illness, 3-hydroxybutyric acid, acetoacetic acid and dicarboxylic acids are found on organic acid analysis. 2-Oxoglutaric acid excretion may be elevated, and 3-methylcrotonylglutamic acid has been found [10].

Concentrations of free carnitine in the blood may be very low, and the excretion of carnitine esters is high.

The development of tandem mass spectrometry and assay of carnitine esters of CoA containing organic acids has led to highly effective programs of expanded neonatal screening [27,28]. These programs have given for the first time, reliable data on the prevalence of 3-methylcrotonyl CoA carboxylase deficiency. It is another metabolic disease that appears to be common in the Amish-Mennonite populations of the US. [12]. An incidence in the population of North Carolina was reported as 1 in 52 000 [27]. In Australia incidences of 1 in 27 000 [25] and 1 in 110 000 [29] have been reported. The incidence in Bavaria was 1 in 30 000 [30].

TREATMENT

The modest restriction of the intake of protein and a modest supplement of carnitine (100 mg/kg) is adequate to prevent most further evidence of disease, once the diagnosis is made. Generally, the protein intake prescribed has been from 1.3 to 2.0 g/kg/d [5,8,20]. A protein-free source of calories, vitamins and minerals, such as 80.56 (Mead Johnson) or Prophree (Ross) may be useful. Alternatively, low protein intake may be supplemented by a leucine-free medical food (Analog, Maxamaid XLeu, SHS) [31,32]. Computer programs are available [31] to aid in the preparation of diets. Recommended intake of leucine has ranged from 60–100 mg/kg in infants under 6 months, 30–60 mg/kg in children over 7 years. Carnitine therapy should be designed to restore plasma concentrations of free-carnitine and to achieve maximum excretion of carnitine esters, within the range of intestinal intolerance.

The acute ketoacidotic episode is treated as in classical organic acidemia with large amounts of water and electrolyte containing bicarbonate (Chapter 2) and intravenous carnitine (300 mg/kg). If prolonged parenteral nutrition is required, formulations are available that exclude leucine [33]. These can be supplemented with standard parenteral solutions of amino acids, so that total restriction of any individual amino acid is not pursued for more than a few days.

References

1 Sweetman L, Nyhan WL. Inheritable biotin-treatable disorders and associated phenomena. *Annu Rev Nutr* 1986;**6**:317.

2 Leonard JV, Seakins JW, Bartlett K, *et al.* Inherited disorders of 3-methylcrotonyl CoA carboxylation. *Arch Dis Child* 1981;**56**:53.

3 Tuchman M, Berry SA, Thuy LP, Nyhan WL. Partial methylcrotonyl-coenzyme. A carboxylase deficiency in an infant with failure to thrive gastrointestinal dysfunction and hypertonia. *Pediatrics* 1993;**91**:664.

4 Finnie MDA, Cottral K, Seakins JWT, Sweden W. Massive excretion of 2-oxoglutaric acid and 3-hydroisovaleric acid in a patient with deficiency of 3-methylcrotonyl-CoA carboxylase. *Clin Chim Acta* 1976;**95**:513.

5 Beemer FA, Bartlett K, Duran M, *et al.* Isolated biotin-resistant 3-methylcrotonyl-CoA carboxylase deficiency in two sibs. *Eur J Pediatr* 1982;**138**:351.

6 Bartlett K, Bennett MJ, Hill RP, *et al.* Isolated biotin-resistant-3-methylcrotonyl CoA carboxylase deficiency presenting with life-threatening hypoglycemia. *J Inherit Metab Dis* 1984;**7**:182.

7 Tsai MY, Johnson DD, Sweetman L, Berry SA. Two siblings with biotin-resistant 3-methylcrotonyl-coenzyme. A carboxylase deficiency. *J Pediatr* 1989;**115**:110.

8 Layward EM, Tanner MS, Politt RJ, Barlett K. Isolated biotin-resistant 3-methylcrotonyl-CoA carboxylase deficiency presenting as a Reye syndrome-like illness. *J Inherit Metab Dis* 1989;**12**:339.

9 Kobori JA, Johnston K, Sweetman L. Isolated 3-methylcrotonyl CoA carboxylase deficiency presenting as a Reye-like syndrome. *Pediatr Res* 1989;**25**:142A.

10 Rolland MO, Divry P, Zabot MT, *et al.* Isolated 3-methylcrotonyl-CoA carboxylase deficiency in a16-month-old child. *J Inherit Metab Dis* 1991;**14**:838.

11 Gitzelmann R, Steinmann B, Niederwieser A, *et al.* Isolated (biotin-resistant) 3-methylcrotonyl-CoA carboxylase deficiency presenting with life-threatening hypoglycemia. *J Inherit Metab Dis* 1987;**10**:290.

12 Gibson KM, Bennett MJ, Naylor EW, Morton DH. 3-Methylcrotonyl-coenzyme A carboxylase deficiency in Amish/Mennonite adults identified by detection of increased acylcarnitines in blood spots of their children. *J Pediatr* 1998;**132**:519.

13 Elpeleg ON, Hawkin S, Barash V, *et al.* Familial hypotonia of childhood caused by isolated 3-methylcrotonyl-coenzyme A carboxylase deficiency. *J Pediatr* 1992;**121**:407.

14 Bannwart C, Wermuth B, Baumgartner R, *et al.* Isolated biotin-resistant 3-methylcrotonyl-CoA carboxylase presenting as a clinically severe form in a newborn with fatal outcome. *J Inherit Metab Dis* 1992;**15**:863.

15 Mourmans J, Bakkersen J, de Jong J, *et al.* Isolated (biotin-resistant) 3-methylcrotonyl-CoA carboxylase deficiency: four sibs devoid of pathology. *J Inherit Metab Dis* 1995;**18**:643.

16 Pearson MA, Aleck KA, Heidenreich RA. Benign clinical presentation of 3-methylcrotonylglycinuria. *J Inherit Metab Dis* 1995;**18**:640.

17 Holzinger A, Roschinger W, Lagler F, *et al.* Cloning of the human MCCA and MCCB genes and mutations therein reveal the molecular cause of 3-methylcrotonyl-CoA: carboxylase deficiency. *Hum Molec Genet* 2001;**10**:1299.

18 Gallardo ME, Resviate LR, Rodriguez JM, *et al.* The molecular basis of 3-methylcrotonylglycinuria, a disorder of leucine catabolism. *Am J Hum Genet* 2001;**68**:334.

19 Finnie MD, Cottrall K, Seakins JW, Snedden W. Massive excretion of 2-oxoglutatic acid and 3-hydroxyisovaleric acid in a patient with a deficiency of 3-methylcrotonyl-CoA carboxylase. *Clin Chim Acta* 1976;**73**:513.

20 Steen C, Baumgartner ER, Duran M, *et al.* Metabolic stroke in isolated 3-methylcrotonyl-CoA carboxylase deficiency. *Eur J Pediatr* 1999;**158**:730.

21 Weyler W, Sweetman L, Maggio DC, Nyhan WL. Deficiency of propionyl-CoA carboxylase in a patient with methylcrotonylglycinuria. *Clin Chim Acta* 1977;**76**:321.

22 Jakobs C, Sweetman L, Nyhan WL, Packman S. Stable isotope dilution analysis of 3-hydroxyisovaleric acid in amniotic fluid: contribution to the prenatal diagnosis of inherited disorders of leucine catabolism. *J Inherit Metab Dis* 1984;**7**:15.

23 Lau EP, Cochran BC, Munson L, Fall RR. Bovine kidney-3-methylcrotonyl-CoA and propionyl-CoA-carboxylases: each enzyme contains non-identical subunits. *Proc Natl Acad Sci USA* 1979;**76**:214.

24 Oei J, Robinson BH. Simultaneous preparation of the three biotin-containing mitochondrial carboxylases from rat liver. *Biochim Biophys Acta* 1985;**840**:1.

25 Baumgartner MR, Almashanu S, Sourmala T, *et al.* The molecular basis of human 3-methylcrotonyl-CoA carboxylase deficiency. *J Clin Invest* 2001;**107**:95.

26 van Hove JLK, Rutledge SL, Nada MA, *et al.* 3-Hydroxyisovalerylcarnitine in 3-methylcrotonyl-CoA carboxylase deficiency. *J Inherit Metab Dis* 1995;**18**:92.

27 Smith WE, Muenzer J, Frazier D, *et al.* Evaluation of elevated hydroxyisovalerylcarnitine in the newborn screen by tandem mass spectrometry. *Am J Hum Genet* 2000;**67**:(suppl 2) 292.

28 Ranieri E, Gerace R, Barlett B, *et al.* The introduction of tandem mass spectrometry in to the South Australian neonatal screening program: benefits and costs. *J Inherit Metab Dis* 2000a;**23**:(suppl 1:006) (poster).

29 Wilcken B, Wiley V, Carpenter K. Two years of routine newborn screening by tandem mass spectrometry (MSMS) in New South Wales Australia. *J Inherit Metab Dis* 2000;**23**:(suppl 1:007) (poster).

30 Roscher A, Liebl B, Fingerhut R, Olgemoller B. Prospective study of MS-MS newborn screening in Bavaria Germany: interim results. *J Inherit Metab Dis* 2000;**23**:(suppl 1:008).

31 Acosta PB. *The Ross Metabolic Formula System Nutrition Support Protocols.* Ross Laboratories, Columbus Ohio;1989: Appendices A G and I.

32 Elsas LJ II, Acosta PB. Nutrition support of inherited metabolic diseases. In *Modern Nutrition in Health and Disease* 7th ed (eds ME Shils and VR Young). Lea and Febiger, Philadelphia, 1988:1337–79.

33 Nyhan WL, Rice-Asaro M, Acosta P. Advances in the treatment of amino acid an organic acid disorders in *Treatment of Genetic Diseases* (ed. RJ Desnick). Churchill Livingstone, New York, 1991:45–67.

3-Methylglutaconic aciduria

MAJOR PHENOTYPIC EXPRESSION

3-Methylglutaconic aciduria is heterogeneous. At least three distinct disorders have been recognized. The molecular defect has been defined in all three.

I. Retardation of speech and mental development, fasting hypoglycemia, metabolic acidosis, excretion of 3-methylglutaconic acid, 3-methylglutaric acid and 3-hydroxyisovaleric acid, and defective activity of 3-methylglutaconyl CoA hydratase. The gene is known as AUH; it was previously shown to code for an AU specific RNA-binding protein; it is now known to have 3-methylcrotonyl CoA hydratase activity.

II. Barth syndrome of cardiomyopathy, neutropenia, recurrent infections, shortness of stature, excretion of 3-methylglutaconic and 3-methylglutaric acids, normal activity of 3-methylglutaconyl CoA hydratase, and an X-linked pattern of inheritance. This mitochondrial disease is caused by mutations in the tafazzin gene (TAZ).

III. Costeff syndrome of optic atrophy and progressive neurodegenerative disease, excretion of 3-methylglutaconic and 3-methylglutaric acids, normal activity of 3-methylglutaconyl CoA hydratase, and mutation in the OPA3 gene.

A fourth or unspecified group of patients with 3-methylglutaconic aciduria appears to be heterogeneous.

INTRODUCTION

3-Methylglutaconic aciduria is a relatively common finding in the analysis of the organic acids of the urine. The organic aciduria was linked to a single defined molecular entity, with the discovery of the enzyme deficiency in 3-methylglutaconic acid hydratase [1,2]. The disease has now been reported in eight patients in seven families [1–7]. A second form of 3-methylglutaconic aciduria, first described by Kelley *et al.* [8] is the X-linked disorder known as Barth syndrome in which congenital myopathy and retardation of growth are associated with neutropenia [9]. The third group of patients is the Costeff optic atrophy syndrome in which mutation in the OPA3 gene has been defined [10,11]. Another group of patients has been referred to as "unspecified" [12] or "unclassified", in whom manifestations referable to the central nervous system have been prominent. This group of patients is clearly heterogeneous. A classification [3] is shown in Table 10.1. Methylglutaconic aciduria may be a general marker of mitochondrial electron transport abnormality. It is also seen in

Table 10.1 *Classification of 3-methylglutaconic aciduria*

Type	Disorder
I	3-Methylglutaconyl-CoA hydratase deficiency
II	X-linked cardiomyopathy and neutropenia
III	Costeff Iraqui-Jewish optic atrophy syndrome [10,11]
IV	Unspecified
	1. Pearson syndrome and mitochondrial DNA deletions [30,31]
	2. Mitochondrial ATP synthase deficiency [32]
	3. Progressive encephalopathy [12,33–43]
	4. Neonatal lactic acidosis, ketosis, hypoglycemia [44–46]

the hyperammonemia of neonatal carbamyl phosphate synthetase deficiency.

I. 3-METHYLGLUTACONYL CoA HYDRATASE DEFICIENCY

Clinical abnormalities

3-Methylglutaconic aciduria due to deficiency of 3-methyl-glutaconyl CoA hydratase activity has been described in a small number of patients with a variety of phenotypes, but commonalities include episodic hypoglycemia and acidosis, usually following infection, and developmental retardation. The first two siblings described [1] had retardation of speech development. The 7-year-old proband also had some delay in motor development, a short attention span and nocturnal enuresis. He had had a single episode of unexplained unconsciousness, which lasted much of a day. Fasting for 18 hours was followed by symptomatic hypoglycemia and a mild metabolic acidosis. His 5-year-old brother had speech development that ranged from the second to the fourth year level and no other abnormalities. He did not develop hypoglycemia on fasting. An unrelated patient [3] developed mild hyperchloremic acidosis during an episode of bronchiolitis at 4 months of age. A Chinese boy had microcephaly and retardation of speech, and he developed a Reye-like episode of hypoglycemic, acidotic, hyperammonemic coma [4]. A patient who required cardiopulmonary resuscitation at birth, and had an episode of acidosis at 6 months, had delayed development, and dystonic paraparesis [7]. Another had neonatal vomiting and irritability and by 1 year had episodic crying, hepatomegaly, poor feeding and self-injurious behavior [6]. A prematurely born infant had hypotonia, delayed development and seizures [7]. A patient with atrophy in the basal ganglia had severely delayed development, spastic quadriparesis and dystonia [5].

Genetics and pathogenesis

The disorder is autosomal recessive. The first two patients were Moroccans living in the Netherlands, but there was no known consanguinity.

Organic acid analysis of the urine has revealed large amounts of 3-methylglutaconic acid, 3-methylglutaric acid and 3-hydroxyisovaleric acid [1,3,7]. 3-Methylglutaric acid may be absent except during intercurrent illness [3]. The amounts of 3-methylglutaconic acid excreted ranged from 250 to 1150 mmol/mol creatinine (normal <6). Two isomers are found. The amounts of 3-hydroxyisovaleric acid ranged from 50 to 400 mmol/mol creatinine (normal <16). This reflects reversal of the carboxylase reaction (Figure 10.1) followed by hydration. The elevated amounts of 3-hydroxyisovaleric acid assist in the distinction of this disorder from other causes of 3-methylglutaconic aciduria. Hydration of 3-methylglutaconic acid itself yields 3-methylglutaric acid; amounts in the urine range from 5–20 mmol/mol creatinine. The excretion of each compound was increased by increasing the intake of protein, decreased by restriction of protein intake, and markedly increased by the administration of 100 mg/kg of leucine. The excretion of 3-hydroxy-3-methylglutaric acid was not increased and remained unchanged by these manipulations.

These observations led [1] to the hypothesis that the fundamental defect was in the activity of 3-methylglutaconyl CoA hydratase (Figure 10.1). This was proven when an assay was developed which documented the molecular defect in the hydratase in fibroblasts derived from the original patients [2]. The substrate 3-methylglutaconyl CoA was synthesized from 3-methylcrotonyl CoA and ^{14}C-labeled bicarbonate

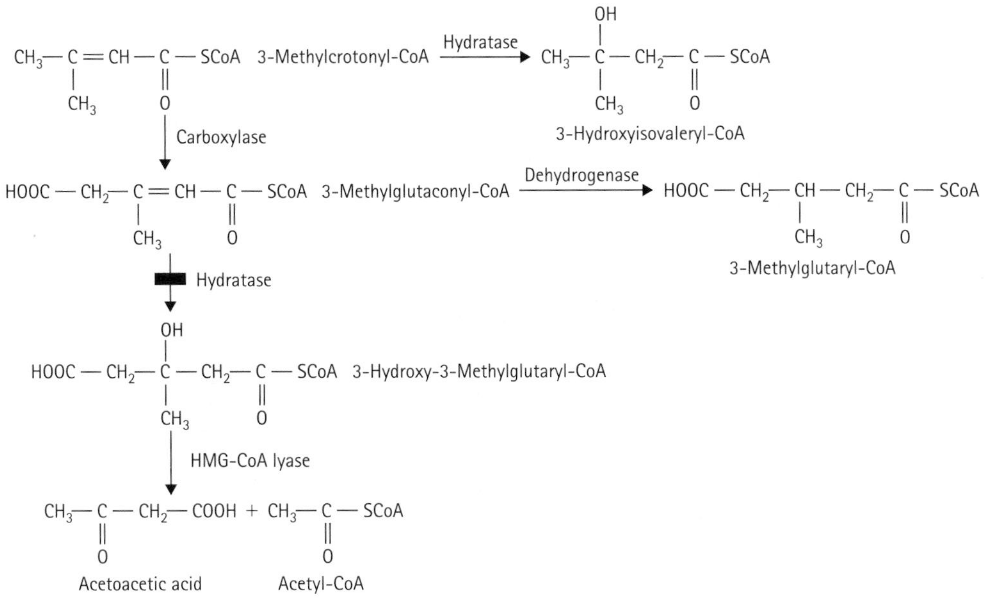

Figure 10.1 *Metabolic interrelations of 3-methylglutaconyl CoA, the source of 3-methylglutaconic acid in the urine. The hydratase is illustrated, the molecular defect identified. The majority of patients reported have not had defective hydratase activity.*

using 3-methylcrotonyl CoA carboxylase and in the assay the products and precursor were separated using high performance liquid chromatography. The activity found in the patients was 2–3 percent of the control level. A coupled assay has been developed [13] in which cell extracts are incubated with 3-methylcrotonyl CoA, adenosine triphosphate (ATP) and $NaH^{14}CO_3$ for the *in situ* generation of labeled 3-methylglutaryl CoA. Activity in fibroblast extracts of three patients was 4 percent of the control fibroblast mean, while in lymphoblasts of the third patient the activity was 17 percent of the mean of seven control lymphoblast lines [3,7]. Heterozygote detection and prenatal diagnosis should be possible by enzyme analysis, but neither has been documented. Prenatal diagnosis should also be possible by gas chromatography/mass spectrometry (GCMS) analysis for 3-hydroxyisovaleric and 3-methylgutaconic acids in amniotic fluid [14,15] or of tandem mass spectrometry (MS/MS) analysis for 3-methylglutaconylcarnitine [6].

The gene for this disease was identified by heterologous expression in *E. coli* after recognition that the gene AUH (GenBank accession numbers NM-001498 and NT-008476) recognized originally as coding for an AU-specific RNA binding protein contained a hydratase motif with considerable sequence identity with crotonase [16]. High activity of the specific hydratase was found. Sequence analysis of one of the original patients of Duran *et al.* [1] revealed a nonsense mutation C589T leading to R197X a termination before a glutamate important in catalysis. In another patient homozygous for 1VS8-1G→71A, a consensus sequence of a splice acceptor site, leads to skipping of exon 9.

Treatment

Restriction of the dietary intake of leucine decreased the excretion of 3-methylglutaconic acid and 3-hydroxyisovaleric acid to normal levels [1]. Therefore nutritional management appears prudent. Carnitine deficiency has been documented [6], and carnitine should serve to remove accumulated CoA esters. Improvement with carnitine therapy has been reported [6,7].

II. BARTH SYNDROME, X-LINKED CARDIOMYOPATHY AND NEUTROPENIA

More than 30 patients have been reported with this syndrome in which there is 3-methylglutaconic aciduria, but the activity of the hydratase is normal [8,11].

Clinical abnormalities

The major clinical manifestation in these patients is cardiomyopathy [11,17]. Patients may present at birth or within the first few weeks of life usually with congestive failure and are found to have dilated cardiomyopathy. The cardiac disease is severe and may be lethal within the first year. With medical management and with age the cardiomyopathy may improve, and echocardiography may show some evidence of left ventricular hypertrophy or fibroelastosis, although autopsies have not shown prominent fibroelastosis.

Postnatal retardation of growth may be severe, but in those surviving to 2-years-of-age, deceleration of growth has ceased, and patients have grown along curves paralleling but 3–4.5 standard deviation (SD) below the normal curve. Response to exogenous human growth hormone may be disappointing. In one patient a normal adult height was achieved.

Hypotonia and weakness of muscles are the only abnormal neurologic findings: The Gower sign is positive (Figure 10.2). Muscle biopsy has revealed mild lipid infiltration or nonspecific mitochondrial abnormalities. Facial myopathy may produce a characteristic appearance [18]. Cognitive function is usually normal, but mild learning disability has been observed.

Chronic cyclic neutropenia is variable but persistent. The absolute neutrophil count usually ranges from 0 to $1100/mm^3$. Susceptibility to infection may be a problem, and patients have died of documented or suspected sepsis and of pneumonia. There may be chronic diarrhea or recurrent apthous ulcers. Neutrophil counts have responded to infection by rising, but often after the patient was sufficiently ill to be admitted to hospital. Response to granulocyte colony stimulating factor (GCSF) may be good. Frequency and severity of infections also decrease with age [17].

Genetics and pathogenesis

Pedigrees are those of an X-linked recessive disease of the male.

The key metabolites are 3-methylglutaconic, 3-methylglutaric acid and 2-ethylhydracrylic acid. The combined excretion of the first two compounds ranged from 29 to

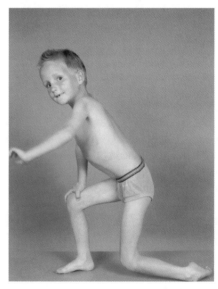

Figure 10.2 *A boy with Barth syndrome illustrating the Gower sign. (Illustration was kindly provided by Prof. Dr. Barth of The Netherlands.)*

108 mmol/mol creatinine [8,11,17]. These levels were about one tenth of those seen in hydratase deficiency. In this disorder the activity of the hydratase was normal [11]. In contrast to hydratase deficiency the excretion of 3-hydroxyisovaleric acid is normal. The excretion of 2-ethylhydracrylic (2-ethyl-3-hydroxypropionic acid) ranged from 2 to 37 mmol/mol creatinine (normal <3). This might suggest an abnormality in the degradation of isoleucine. Isoleucine loading increased its excretion and that of lactic acid [8]. The excretion of these organic acids in the urine was not changed by leucine loading or leucine restriction [8]. Lactic acid in the blood may be normal or mildly elevated.

In one patient the plasma concentration of carnitine was low, and episodic hypoglycemia was responsive to carnitine supplementation [8].

Cholesterol levels were low in a number of patients [11] suggesting an abnormality of cholesterol biosynthesis. Activities of the first four enzymes of the pathway as well as the incorporation of ^{14}C-acetate into ^{14}C-cholesterol in fibroblasts were normal [8]. If that pathway were blocked the so-called mevalonic shunt pathway could recycle 3-methylcrotonic acid as a source of 3-methylglutaconic acid. Alternatively, 3-methylglutaric acid could reflect disordered fatty acid oxidation, as could the excretion of 2-ethylhydracrylic acid. Cardiolipin, a phospholipid component of the inner mitochondrial membrane, involved in electron transport chain function, is deficient in fibroblasts of patients [9].

In biopsied muscle studies of the electron transport chain deficiencies of complex I and IV were revealed [17,18,19]. In fibroblasts there was deficiency of complex I [20].

The gene, tafazzin, was found by linkage analysis to be at Xq28 and linked to the DX55 marker [21,22], and the gene G4.5 in this region, which is expressed at high level in cardiac and skeletal muscle, was found to be mutated in Barth syndrome [22,23]. Nine mutations, four of which produced a stop codon were found in patients and heterozygous mothers. Four missense mutations were found in exon 8. Correlations of genotype and phenotype have not been possible.

Treatment

Restriction of protein intake has been employed [8]. Carnitine supplementation may be useful. Cholesterol supplementation has been followed by some decrease in the excretion of 3-methylglutaconic and 3-methylglutaric acids, but the changes were not great. Successful heart transplantation has been carried out in one patient.

III. COSTEFF SYNDROME

Clinical abnormalities

A distinct phenotype observed in Iraqi (Baghdadi) Jews has been referred to as Costeff syndrome, Behr syndrome or optic atrophy plus syndrome [24–27]. Optic atrophy is a prominent manifestation, and may be associated with nystagmus. Onset is often infantile but may be late, from 6–37 years-of-age. In addition, these patients have ataxia, choreiform movements and extrapyramidal signs with spasticity, which may develop later in patients with early onset optic atrophy. Rigidity may be prominent. Cognitive development is impaired. Life span appears to be normal.

Metabolites found in the urine are 3-methylglutaconic acid and 3-methylglutaric acid. There is no elevation of 2-ethyl-3-hydroxypropionic acid or 3-hydroxyisovaleric acid [25,27]. 3-Methylglutaconic acid is excreted in 10–200 mmol/mol creatinine; amounts of 3-methylglutaric acid are smaller. The activity of 3-methylglutaconyl CoA hydratase is normal.

Genetics and pathogenesis

Transmission is autosomal recessive. The gene was mapped to chromosome 19q13.2-13.3 [28]. The gene, OPA3, was isolated in a search for candidate genes between two polymorphic markers [10]. One of four clones studied could not be amplified from the cDNA of patients, while control cDNA yielded an expected band. The gene has two exons. Among patients a homozygous G to C change was found at the −1 position of intron 1 in the 3′ acceptor splice site [10]. The cDNA was found to be expressed widely, prominently in skeletal muscle and kidney and, within the brain, cortex, medulla and cerebellum. Lack of mRNA in patients was associated in the patients studied with early-onset optic atrophy and a movement disorder beginning in adolescence. The protein product, whose function is unknown, is predicted to be 20 KDa and to contain a mitochondrial targeting peptide.

Heterozygotes are readily ascertained by a screening assay for the mutation [10]. Carrier frequency of the founder mutation in OPA3 was 1–10 in this isolate, which represents the original middle eastern Jewish gene pool derived from the approximately 120 000 Jews exiled to Babylon in 586 BC. This population also carries high gene frequencies for the MEFV gene for familial Mediterranean fever, the common mutation in factor XI and autosomal dominant psuedocholinesterase deficiency. Prenatal diagnosis should be possible by mutational analysis.

Treatment

Effective treatment has not been reported. A trial of coenzyme Q was ineffective [29].

IV. UNSPECIFIED

1. Associated with Pearson syndrome (Chapter 56)

Four patients have been reported in whom the Pearson syndrome of aplastic anemia has been associated with lactic acidemia and 3-methylglutaconic aciduria [30].

CLINICAL ABNORMALITIES

Patients with Pearson syndrome present with failure to thrive and anemia. There may be vomiting and diarrhea. Alopecia has been described. Episodic acidosis and electrolyte imbalance may complicate chronic lactic acidemia. Hematologic findings include anemia, neutropenia and thrombocytopenia. Multiple transfusions may be required. Pancreatic insufficiency is a component of the syndrome. Some patients have had a renal Fanconi syndrome. In patients surviving infancy and childhood retinopathy and tremor may develop along with increased T2 signal in the MRI of the brain and a clinical Kearns-Sayre syndrome (Chapter 55).

GENETICS AND PATHOGENESIS

The Pearson syndrome is a mitochondrial disease in which there is maternal inheritance of site-specific deletions [31]. In the patients with 3-methylglutaconic aciduria heteroplasmy was demonstrated and deletions of 5 to 5.9 Kb in mt DNA [30].

Analysis of the organic acids of the urine revealed 3-methylglutaconic acid in amounts ranging from 32–80 mmol/mol creatinine. The excretion of 3-methylglutaric acid was 22 mmol/mol creatinine and undetectable in the others. In addition, the urinary pattern included elevated amounts of lactic acid, pyruvic acid, and 3-hydroxybutyric acid. 2-Oxoglutaric acid, fumaric acid, malic acid and 2-methyl-3-hydroxybutyric acid were found to be elevated in some patients. The occurrence of 3-methylglutaconic aciduria in this syndrome and in ATP synthase deficiency is consistent with the fact 3-methylglutaconic aciduria is a marker for abnormality in the mitochondrial respiratory chain.

TREATMENT

One patient was treated with dichloroacetate [30].

2. ATP synthase deficiency

A single patient has been described in whom 3-methylglutaconic aciduria has been associated with ATP synthase deficiency [32].

CLINICAL ABNORMALITIES

The patient presented with respiratory distress and severe metabolic acidosis at 15 hours of life. Episodic crises of lactic acidosis in the first year were precipitated by infection or fasting. At 4 months she was found to have hypertrophic cardiomyopathy. Gross motor and mental development were retarded. Magnetic resonance imaging revealed hypoplasia at the corpus callosum and slight cerebral atrophy. ATP synthase deficiency has previously been observed in hypertrophic cardiomyopathy.

GENETICS AND PATHOGENESIS

The patient was the daughter of Yugoslavian gypsies in whom there was no known consanguinity. Transmission was thought to be autosomal recessive. Thorough investigation of mtDNA failed to reveal abnormalities in the genes that code for portions of ATP synthase.

Deficiency of ATP synthase was demonstrated in mitochondria isolated from muscle [32]. Mitochondrial respiratory rate was reduced in the presence of a number of substrates, but restored by an uncoupler. Activity of 3-methylglutaconyl CoA hydratase was normal. The patient had intermittent lactic acidosis and a fasting blood concentration of 3.4 mmol/L. The cerebrospinal fluid (CSF) lactic acid was 5.0 mmol/L. The blood lactate:pyruvate ratio was increased to 28.6. The excretion of 3-methylglutaconic acid ranged from 91 to 284 mmol/mol creatinine. The excretion of 3-methylglutaric acid ranged from 20 to 83 mmol/mol creatinine.

TREATMENT

Acidosis was controlled with $NaHCO_3$ and parenteral glucose.

3. Encephalopathy

CLINICAL ABNORMALITIES

There remains a considerable group of heterogeneous patients with 3-methylglutaconic aciduria in whom neurologic manifestations are predominant and hydratase activity is normal [12,33] (Table 10.1) (Figures 10.3–10.8). Among the patients described [34–39] progressive neurological deterioration followed some months of normal development. In one [34]

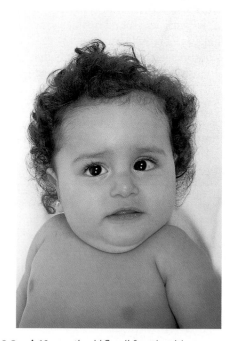

Figure 10.3   *A 10-month-old Saudi female with 3-methylglutaconic aciduria. She presented with severe acidosis and hypoglycemia on the third day of life. Blood sugar was zero, and she had seizures. At 9 months she had little evidence of development, cortical fisting and increased deep tendon reflexes. EEG was abnormal and MRI revealed atrophy. Parents were first cousins.*

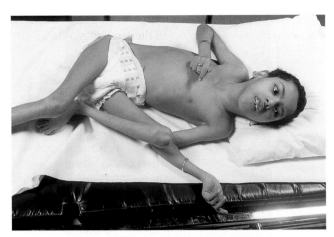

Figure 10.4 *A 10-year-old girl with 3-methylglutaconic aciduria who had presented with neonatal acidosis and hypoglycemia. She had microcephaly, global developmental delay, rigidity and spastic quadriplegia. Hips were dislocated, and contractures had developed. Babinski responses were positive. A brother had the same disease. Reprinted with permission from* Brain Dev *[33].*

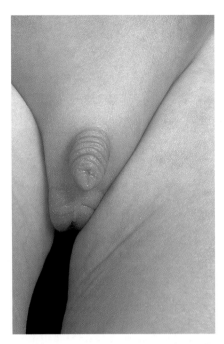

Figure 10.6 *The 7-month-old boy also had a micropenis and bilateral cryptorchidism. Reprinted with permission from* Brain Dev *[33].*

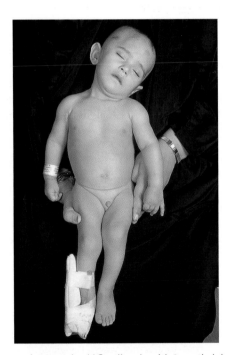

Figure 10.5 *A 7-month-old Saudi male with 3-methylglutaconic acidura who had a pure neurologic presentation without neonatal acidosis, although the blood concentration of lactic acid at 7 months was 4.6 mmol/L. He had severe developmental delay, tonic posturing and myoclonic jerks. Muscle tone was increased, deep tendon reflexes brisk, and he had sustained ankle clonus and bilateral Babinski responses. Reprinted with permission from* Brain Dev *[33].*

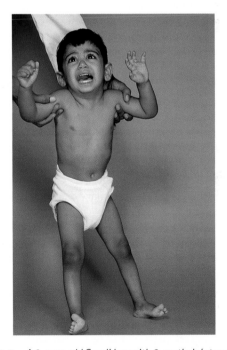

Figure 10.7 *A 3-year-old Saudi boy with 3-methylglutaconic aciduria who presented at two years with rigidity and loss of acquired milestones. He had dystonic posturing and choreoathetoid movements. Muscle tone and deep tendon reflexes were increased and the Babinksi responses positive. MRI revealed atrophy and infarction of the lentiform nuclei and caudate.*

growth in length, weight and head circumference ceased at 9 months and by 3 years she was judged to be at a 4-month development level. She had hypotonia, bizarre posturing of the right arm, self-mutilative behavior and an abnormal electroencephalogram (EEG). In this patient the 3-methylglutaconic

aciduria was later reported [1] to have disappeared. Two siblings [37] developed spastic paraparesis, choreoathetosis, optic atrophy, neurogenic impairment of hearing and dementia. Despite the severity of the clinical manifestations the

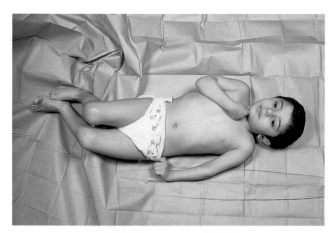

Figure 10.8   *A 27-month-old Saudi boy with 3-methylglutaconic aciduria. He began to deteriorate at 18 months and lost acquired milestones. He had choreoathetosis and dystonia. None of the patients in Figs 10.3 and 10.7 had optic atrophy. Reprinted with permission from Brain Dev [33].*

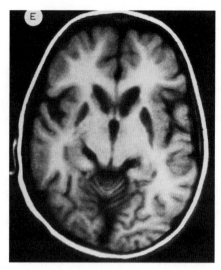

Figure 10.9   *MRI of the brain of a 4-year-old boy with 3-methylglutaconic aciduria with dystonic neurologic disease and optic atrophy. Atrophy was prominent especially in the posterior fossa, and there were bilateral slit-like low intensity (T_1) lesions in the lentiform and caudate nuclei. Reprinted with permission from Al Aqeel et al., Brain Dev [33].*

amounts of 3-methylglutaconic acid in the urine were usually 10 to 50 times less than those found in 3-methylglutaconyl CoA hydratase deficiency. 3-Hydroxyisovaleric acid was not found in the urine.

Two unrelated infants developed a picture of failure to thrive after developing normally for 3–4 months and then underwent regression in psychomotor development [39]. They developed marked hypotonia, spastic paraparesis, optic atrophy and signs of hepatic damage. Deafness has occurred in some patients [33,39,40]. Many have had seizures, both grand mal and myoclonic. In some patients, global involvement of the nervous system began very early and developmental milestones were never achieved [33]. Some have had prominent extrapyramidal signs. About 25 percent of patients have had dysmorphic features [33] including cryptorchidism and micropenis (Figure 10.6). Many have died in infancy or early childhood. Despite some elevation of lactic acid in blood and CSF most have not had clinical acidosis.

Neuroradiological studies [41](Figure 10.9) revealed global atrophy and prominent lesions in the basal ganglia. Cerebellar atrophy was particularly evident in those with neonatal acidosis. One had symmetrical hypodensity on CT scan of the basal ganglia [42]. Brainstem auditory evoked responses (BAER) and visual evoked responses (VER) may be absent [43].

A subgroup of patients has presented with major early neonatal acidosis or hypoglycemia or both [44–46]. Pyramidal tract signs and seizures were common along with spastic quadriplegia and optic atrophy. In addition two adult women have been reported with 3-methylglutaconic aciduria in whom there were no clinical abnormalities [47].

Genetics and pathogenesis

Inheritance appears to be autosomal recessive. Affected males and females have been observed, as has consanguinity (Figure 10.3).

The common biochemical characteristic of this group of patients is the 3-methylglutaconic aciduria. Amounts have generally ranged from 25 to 70 mmol/mol creatinine, but levels as high as 1600 mmol/mol creatinine have been observed [12,33,35]. Amounts of 3-methylglutaric acid are lower, and 3-hydroxyisovalerate excretion is not elevated [35]. Some have also had increased amounts of pyruvic acid and 2-oxoglutaric acid and other citric acid cycle intermediates. Hydratase activity is normal. Fasting was followed by normal ketogenesis [39]. One patient had hypermethioninemia [42], and excretion of 3-methylglutaconic acid increased following a 100 mg/kg methionine load. Fasting led to metabolic acidosis and lactic acidemia.

Treatment

No effective therapy has been reported. 3-Methylglutaconic aciduria reverted to normal when the patient was given a methionine-restricted diet, but there was no clinical improvement [42].

References

1   Duran M, Beemer FA, Tibosch AS, *et al*. Inherited 3-methylglutaconic aciduria in two brothers – another defect of leucine metabolism. *J Pediatr* 1982;**101**:551.

2   Narasawa K, Gibson KM, Sweetman L, *et al*. Deficiency of 3-methylglutaconyl CoA hydratase in two siblings with 3-methylglutaconic aciduria. *J Clin Invest* 1986;**77**:1148.

3   Gibson KM, Lee CF, Wappner RS. 3-Methylglutaconyl-coenzyme-A hydratase deficiency: a new case. *J Inherit Metab Dis* 1992;**15**:363.

4 Hou JW, Wang TR. 3-Methylglutaconic aciduria presenting as Reye syndrome in a Chinese boy. *J Inherit Metab Dis* 1995;**18**:645.

5 Shoji Y, Takashi T, Sawaish Y, *et al.* A severe form of 3-methylglutaconic aciduria type I. *Proc 39th Meeting Jap Inherit Metab Dis* 1996;48.

6 Jooste S, Erasmus E, Mienie LJ, *et al.* The detection of 3-methyl-glutarylcarnitine and a new dicarboxylic conjugate 3-methyl-glutaconylcarnitine in 3-methylglutaconic aciduria. *Clin Chim Acta* 1994;**230**:1.

7 Gibson KM, Wappner RS, Jooste S, *et al.* Variable clinical presentation in three patients with 3-methylglutaconyl-coenzyme A hydratase deficiency. *J Inherit Metab Dis* 1998;**21**:631.

8 Kelley FI, Cheatham JP, Clark BJ, *et al.* X-Linked dilated cardiomyopathy with neutropenia growth retardation and 3-methylglutaconic aciduria. *J Pediatr* 1991;**119**:738.

9 Vreken P, Valianpour F, Nijtmans LG, *et al.* Defective remodeling of cardiolipin and phosphatidylglycerol in Barth syndrome. *Biochem Biophys Res Commun* 2000;**279**:378.

10 Costeff H, Elpeleg O, Apter N, *et al.* 3-Methylglutaconic aciduria in 'optic atrophy plus'. *Ann Neurol* 1993;**33**:103.

11 Anikster Y, Kleta R, Shaag A, *et al.* Type III 3-methylglutaconic aciduria (optic atrophy plus syndrome or Costeff optic atrophy syndrome): Identification of the OPA3 gene and its founder mutation in Iraqi Jews. *Am J Hum Genet* 2001;**69**:1218.

12 Gibson KM, Sherwood WG, Hoffmann GF, *et al.* Phenotypic heterogeneity in the syndromes of 3-methylglutaconic aciduria. *J Pediatr* 1991; **118**:885.

13 Narisawa K, Gibson KM, Sweetman L, Nyhan WL. 3-Methylglutaconyl-CoA hydratase 3-methylcrotonyl-CoA carboxylase and 3-hydroxy-3-methylglutaryl-CoA lyase deficiencies: A coupled enzyme assay useful for their detection. *Clin Chim Acta* 1989;**184**:57.

14 Jakobs C, Sweetman L, Nyhan WL, Packman S. Stable isotope dilution analysis of 3-hydroxyisovaleric acid in amniotic fluid: Contribution to the prenatal diagnosis of inherited disorders of leucine catabolism. *J Inherit Metab Dis* 1984;**7**:15.

15 Chitayat D, Chemke J, Gibson KM, *et al.* 3-Methylglutaconic aciduria: A marker for as yet unspecifiec disorders and the relevance of prenatal diagnosis in a "new" type ("type 4"). *J Inherit Metab Dis* 1992;**15**:204.

16 Ijlst L, Loupatty FJ, Ruiter JPN, *et al.* 3-Methylglutaconic aciduria type I is caused by mutation AUH. *Am J Hum Genet* 2002;**71**:1463.

17 Barth PG, Scholte HR, Berden JA. An X-linked mitochondrial disease affecting cardiac muscle skeletal muscle and neutrophil leukocytes. *J Neurol Sci* 1983;**62**:327.

18 Christodoulou J, McInnes RR, Jay V, *et al.* Barth syndrome: Clinical observations and genetic linkage studies. *Am J Med Genet* 1994;**50**:255.

19 Carragher F, Kirk J, FitzPatrick D, *et al.* 3-Methylglutaconic aciduria and reduced activity of mitochondrial respiratory chain enzymes in a patient with Barth syndrome. *J Inherit Metab Dis* 1998;**21**:78.

20 Barth PS, Van Den Bogert C, Bolhuis PA, *et al.* X-linked cardioskeletal myopathy and neutropenia (Barth syndrome): Respiratory-chain abnormalities in cultured fibroblasts. *J Inherit Metab Dis* 1996;**19**:157.

21 Ades LC, Gedeon AK, Wilson MJ, *et al.* Barth syndrome: Clinical features and confirmation of gene localization to distal Xq28. *Am J Med Genet* 1993;**45**:327.

22 Bione S, Adamo P, Mestrini E, *et al.* A novel X-linked gene G45 is responsible for Barth syndrome. *Nat Genet* 1996;**12**:385.

23 Johnston J, Kelley RI, Feigenbaum A, *et al.* Mutation characterization and genotype-phenotype correlation in Barth syndrome. *Am J Hum Genet* 1997;**61**:1053.

24 Costeff HI, Gadoth N, Apter N, *et al.* A familial syndrome of infantile optic atrophy movement disorder and spastic paraplegia. *Neurology* 1989;**39**:595.

25 Zeharia A, Elpeleg ON, Makumel M, *et al.* 3-Methylglutaconic aciduria: A new variant. *Pediatrics* 1992;**89**:1080.

26 Elpeleg ON, Costeff H, Joseph A, *et al.* 3-Methylglutaconic aciduria in the Iraqi-Jewish "optic atrophy plus" (Costeff) syndrome. *Dev Med Child Neurol* 1994;**36**:167.

27 Sheffer RN, Zlotogora J, Elpeleg ON, *et al.* Behr's syndrome and 3-methylglutaconic aciduria. *Am J Ophthalmol* 1992;**114**:494.

28 Nystuen A, Costeff H, Elpeleg ON, *et al.* Iraqi-Jewish kindreds with optic atrophy plus (3-methylglutaconic aciduria type 3) demonstrate linkage disequilibrium with the CTG repeat in the 3′ untranslated region of the myotonic dystrophy protein kinase gene. *Hum Mol Genet* 1997;**6**:563.

29 Anikster Y, Kleta R, Shaag A, *et al.* Type III 3-methylglutaconic aciduria (optic atrophy plus syndrome or Costeff optic atrophy syndrome): Identification of the OPA3 gene and its founder mutation in Iraqi Jews. *Am J Hum Genet* 2001;**69**:1218.

30 Gibson KM, Bennett MJ, Mize CE, *et al.* 3-Methylglutaconic aciduria: Neonatal onset with lactic acidosis. *J Inherit Metab Dis* 1992;**121**:940.

31 Rotig A, Cormier V, Koll F, *et al.* Site-specific deletions of the mitochondrial genome in the Pearson marrow-pancreas syndrome. *Genomics* 1991;**10**:502.

32 Holme E, Greter J, Jacobson CE, *et al.* Mitochondrial ATP-synthase deficiency in a child with 3-methylglutaconic aciduria. *Pediatr Res* 1992;**32**:731.

33 Aqeel AA, Rashed M, Ozand PT, *et al.* 3-Methylglutaconic aciduria: Ten new cases with a possible new phenotype. *Brain Dev* 1994;**16**:23.

34 Robinson BH, Sherwood WG, Lampty M, Lowden JA. β-Methylglutaconic aciduria. *J Clin Invest* 1986;**77**:1148.

35 Gibson KM, Nyhan WL, Sweetman L, *et al.* 3-Methylglutaconic aciduria: A phenotype in which activity of 3-methylglutaconyl-coenzyme A hydratase is normal. *Eur J Pediatr* 1988;**148**:76.

36 Chitayat D, Chemke J, Gibson KM, *et al.* 3-Methylglutaconic aciduria: A marker for as yet unspecified disorders and the relevance of prenatal diagnosis in a 'new' type (type 4). *J Inherit Metab Dis* 1992;**15**:204.

37 Greter J, Harberg B, Steen G, Soderhjelm U. 3-Methylglutaconic aciduria: Report on a sibship with infantile progressive encephalopathy. *Eur J Pediatr* 1978;**129**:231.

38 Haan EA, Scholem RD, Pitt JJ, *et al.* Episodes of severe metabolic acidosis in a patient with 3-methylglutaconic aciduria. *Eur J Pediatr* 1987;**146**:484.

39 Hagberg B, Hjalmarson O, Lindstedt S, *et al.* 3-Methylglutaconic aciduria in two infants. *Clin Chim Acta* 1983;**134**:9.

40 Bakkeren JAJM, Sengers RCA, Ruitenbeek W, Trijbels JMF. 3-Methylglutaconic aciduria in a patient with a disturbed mitochondrial energy metabolism. *Eur J Pediatr* 1992;**151**:313.

41 Brismar J, Ozand PT. CT and MR of the brain in the diagnosis of organic acidemias: Experience from 107 patients. *Brain Dev* 1994;**16**:104.

42 Di Rocco M, Caruso U, Moroni I, *et al.* 3-Methylglutconic ciduria and hypermethioninaemia in a child with clinical and neuroradiological findings of Leigh disease. *J Inherit Metab Dis* 1999;**22**:93.

43 Stigsby B, Yarworth S, Rahbeeni Z, *et al.* Neurophysiologic correlates of organic acidemias: A survey of 107 patients. *Brain Dev* 1994;**16**:125.

44 Elpeleg ON, Meiron D, Barash V, *et al.* 3-Methylglutaconic aciduria with persistent metabolic acidosis and 'uncoupling episodes'. *J Inherit Metab Dis* 1990;**13**:235.

45 Divry P, Vianey-Liaud C, Mory O, Ravussin JJ, 3-Methylglutaconic aciduria: Neonatal onset with lactic acidosis. *J Inherit Metab Dis* 1987;**10**:286.

46 Largilliere C, Vallee L, Cartigny B, *et al.* 3-Methylglutaconic aciduria:neonatal onset with lactic acidosis. *J Inherit Metab Dis* 1989;**12**:333.

47 Kuhara T, Matsumoto I, Saiki K, *et al.* 3-Methylglutaconic aciduria in two adults. *Clin Chim Acta* 1992;**207**:151.

3-Hydroxyisobutyric aciduria

MAJOR PHENOTYPIC EXPRESSION

Recurrent episodes of ketoacidosis; failure to thrive; lactic acidemia; 3-hydroxyisobutyric aciduria; 2-ethyl-3-hydroxy-propionic aciduria; and defective oxidation of valine and β-alanine.

INTRODUCTION

3-Hydroxyisobutyric aciduria is an inborn error of the metabolism of valine (Figure 11.1) which was described in 1991 [1] in a report of a patient who had a typical organic acidemia phenotype with recurrent episodes of vomiting, ketosis and acidosis, leading to dehydration and admission to hospital, where vigorous resuscitation with large amounts of water and electrolytes were required. He had lactic acidemia and hyperalaninemia. Organic acid analysis of the urine revealed large amounts of 3-hydroxyisobutyric acid and 2-ethyl-3-hydroxypropionic acid. Loading with valine reproduced the

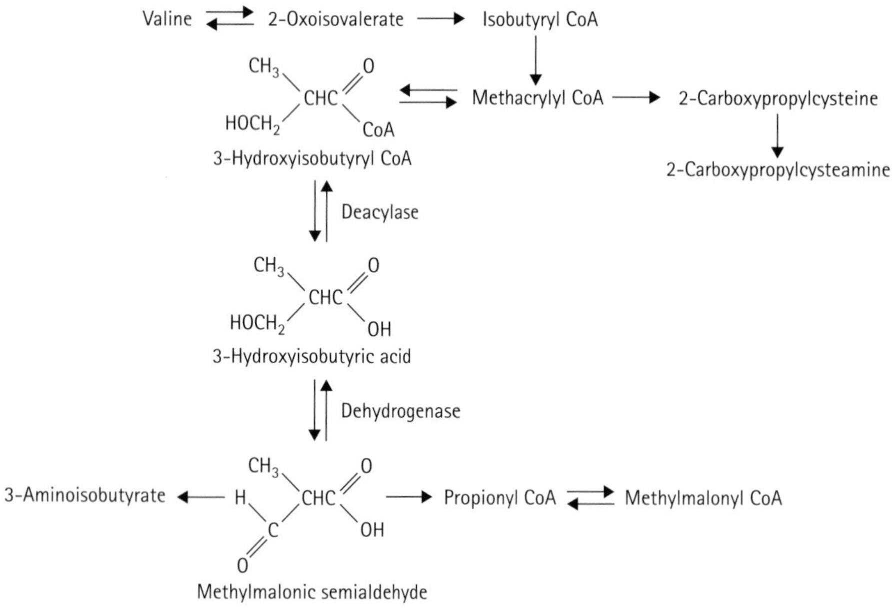

Figure 11.1   *The pathway for the catabolism of valine. 3-hydroxyisobutyric acid is normally converted to methylmalonic semialdehyde, which is converted to propionyl CoA.*

clinical illness. Cultured fibroblasts were defective in the conversions of ^{14}C-valine and ^{14}C-β-alanine to ^{14}CO$_2$ [2]. These observations and the excretion of 2-ethyl-3-hydroxy-propionate suggest a fundamental defect in a semialdehyde dehydrogenase active on methylmalonic semialdehyde, malonic semialdehyde and ethylmalonic semialdehyde.

Another patient with 3-hydroxyisobutyric acidemia who had malformations, massive acidosis and hypotonia [3] was found to have defective activity of 3-hydroxyisobutyryl CoA deacylase [4]. 3-Hydroxyisobutyric aciduria and 3-aminoiso-butyric aciduria has been reported along with hypermethi-oninemia in an apparently healthy baby [5].

In the catabolic pathway for valine, following transamina-tion to the oxoacid and the action of the branched-chain oxoacid dehydrogenase, the product is (S)-isobutyryl CoA. The next reaction, catalyzed by 2-methyl branched-chain acyl CoA dehydrogenase, forms (S)-methacryly CoA, which is converted in a hydratase reaction to 3-hydroxyisobutyryl CoA. 3-Hydroxyisobutaryl CoA deacylase catalyzes the conversion to (S)-3-Hydroxyisobutyric acid, and a dehydro-genase to (S)methylmalonic semialdehyde, while methyl-malonic semialdehyde dehydrogenase catalyzes conversion to propionyl CoA. The rest of the pathway is shared with isoleucine metabolism, as well as that of threonine and methionine. The dehydrogenase is reversible. So, hydroxy-isobutyrate can be formed from the semialdehyde. The semi-aldehyde can also undergo spontaneous keto-enol tautomerism producing a mixture of S- and R-methylmalonic semialdehy-des and hydroxyisobutyric acids. Methylmalonic semialde-hyde dehydrogenase is active against malonic semialdehyde (Figure 11.2), but it is not active against ethylmalonic semialdehyde [6].

CLINICAL ABNORMALITIES

The patient reported by Ko and colleagues [1] (Figure 11.3) had shortness of stature and anorexia. At birth he had been small for gestational age. He had other features of the Silver-Russel syndrome, including a small, triangular face with a long philtrum, fifth finger clinodactyly, bilateral simian creases and bilateral syndactyly of the second and third toes. Hypospadias and cryptorchidism were repaired surgically. He had a systolic ejection murmur and an electrocardiogram

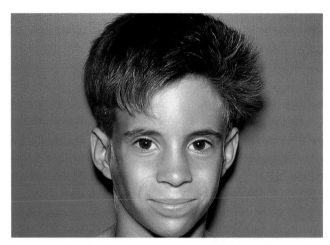

Figure 11.3   *S.B., a 12-year-old boy with 3-hydroxyisobutyric aciduria. He had the phenotype of the Silver-Russel syndrome; with shortness of stature, a triangular-shaped face, a long philtrum, fifth finger clinodactyly, bilateral simian palmar creases and bilateral syndactyly of second and third toes.*

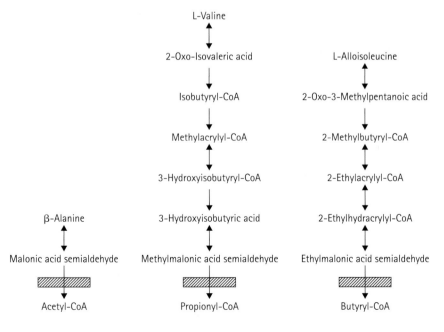

Figure 11.2   *Block in the pathways for β-alanine, valine and alloisoleucine that would account for deficient oxidation of valine and β-alanine, along with the excretion of large amounts of 2-ethyldracryllic acid in the urine. The data suggest a fundamental defect in a single semialdehyde dehydrogenase.*

(ECG) consistent with myocardial hypertrophy, but the echocardiogram was normal. He was difficult to feed, anorexic and vomited frequently. Gavage feedings were required in the neonatal period. He avoided eating protein-containing foods and disliked milk, meat and eggs. Early development was slow, but by 10 years his IQ was 100.

His first episode of acidosis was at 3 years of age and was associated with a serum bicarbonate concentration of 8 mmol/L and a grand mal convulsion. The electroencephalogram (EEG) remained abnormal, but there were no abnormal neurologic findings. He had multiple repeated episodes of vomiting, Kussmaul respirations, lethargy and ketoacidosis, requiring admission to hospital and parenteral fluid therapy. On at least one occasion hypoglycemia was observed.

The steady-state concentration of lactate in the blood was 2 mmol/L and that of pyruvate 0.14 mmol/L. The concentration of alanine was 730 mmol/L. During an episode of acute ketoacidosis the lactate was 6.8 and the pyruvate 0.33 mmol/L.

Another of our patients had repeated episodes of life-threatening acidosis, requiring admission to intensive care, and persistent lactic acidemia. His physical features were consistent with those of Williams syndrome, but the deletion in chromosome 7 was not present.

Another patient with 3-hydroxyisobutyric aciduria had massive acidosis, hypotonia and malformations [7]. 3-Hydroxyisobutyric aciduria was reported in twins who developed infantile spasms at 5 months [8]. One died at 4 years with seizures and disseminated intravascular coagulopathy following an acute febrile infection illness. The other had static encephalopathy, microcephaly and seizures. Another pair of male twins, monozygotic, had 3-hydroxyisobutyric aciduria and congenital dysgenesis of the brain and intracerebral calcifications [9]. They died at four and 18 days of respiratory failure. Calcifications were visible on computed tomography (CT) scan in the frontal and subependymal regions and over the lateral ventricles. The brains had an hourglass shape and smooth cortical outlines with lissencephaly, pachygyria, polymicrogyria, agenesis of the corpus callosum and a smooth interface of gray and white matter. The cerebellum was hypoplastic. There were only four layers of neurons, laminar heterotopia and cystic arteries in the white matter. Dysmorphic features included triangular or myopathic facies, short sloping forehead, malar hypoplasia, long prominent philtrum and micrognathia. There were bilateral Sidney lines, clinodactyly of the fourth and fifth toes and cortical thumbs.

An apparently healthy infant has been reported with 3-hydroxyisobutyric aciduria [5]. The male infant had episodes of vomiting and diarrhea at 3 weeks and 9 months, and he had persistent hypermethioninemia. Concentrations of methionine ranged from 1200 to 1600 μmol/L while the infant was receiving breast milk. A low methionine diet led to some reduction in levels, but levels as high as 1200 were also seen despite the diet. The development of the infant was normal at 4 years of age [10].

Two consanguineous siblings were reported with increased excretion of 3-hydroxybutyrate, 3-hydroxypropionate and 2-ethylhydracrylate, and increased plasma β-alanine [11]. They both had failure to thrive, microcephly and cataracts, but so did six siblings who did not share the biochemical abnormalities.

GENETICS AND PATHOGENESIS

The genetics of this condition, or conditions, are not clear. The fact that all of those in whom sex has been specified were male raises the possibility of X-linked recessive transmission, but an autosomal recessive mode is as likely.

The molecular nature of the disorder is not clear either. Most available information is on the patterns of metabolites found in body fluids. The unifying feature in all patients is the excretion of 3-hydroxyisobutyric acid in the urine. Our reported patient [1] excreted 180–390 mmol/mol creatinine under ordinary conditions. Normal individuals excrete less than 33 mmol/mol creatinine. This patient also excreted 19–85 mmol/mol creatinine of 2-ethyl-3-hydroxypropionate, and 500 to 30 000 mmol/mol creatinine of lactate. The blood lactate ranged from 2 to 6.8 mmol/L.

A key finding was the response to valine loading, which led to a typical ketoacidotic attack in which there was vomiting, sweating, hypoglycemia and acidosis (Figure 11.4). Urinary

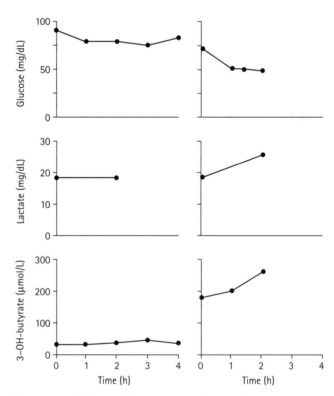

Figure 11.4 *Effects of valine and isoleucine on plasma concentrations of glucose, lactic acid and 3-hydroxybutyric acid. Following isoleucine the patient was asymptomatic. After valine he became acutely ill, hypoglycemic, lactic acidemic and ketotic. The serum concentration of bicarbonate was 10 mmol/L.*

excretion of lactic acid and 3-hydroxybutyric acid rose. Loading with isoleucine was uneventful. Each loading test was conducted with 100 mg/kg of the amino acid; blood was obtained at 0, 1, 2 and 4 hours and urine was collected for 24 hours in 8-hour aliquots. The valine load led to a massive increase in the excretion of 3-hydroxyisobutyrate (Figure 11.5). Over 30 percent of the administered valine was excreted as 3-hydroxyisobutyrate. The excretion of 3-aminoisobutyrate also rose after valine. There was excellent direct correlation of the degree of ketosis as reflected in 3-hydroxybutyrate excretion, as well as the excretion of urinary lactate and the excretion of 3-hydroxyisobutyrate (Figure 11.6).

Lactic acid excretion was elevated in all of the patients reported except for the normal, hypermethioninemic infant [5,10].

The infant with malformations reported by Mienie et al. [7] also excreted abnormal amounts of 3-hydroxypropionic acid and 3-hydroxyisovaleric acid, as well as 2-ethyl-3-hydroxypropionic acid; each of these compounds increased with valine loading, as did the 3-hydroxyisobutyric acid. S-2-carboxypropylcysteine was also detected in the urine of this patient. Methylmalonic semialdehyde was not detected in any of these patients, nor was β-alanine. In our patient the excretion of 3-aminoisobutyric acid and its plasma concentration rose after valine. In contrast, the hypermethioninemic infant [5,10] had very large excesses in the excretion of 3-aminoisobutyric acid, β-alanine, 2-hydroxymethylbutyric acid and 3-hydroxypropionic acid. Loading with valine increased the excretion of 3-hydroxyisobutyric acid, but not that of aminoisobutyric acid, although the plasma level increased. Excretion of 2-ethyl-3-hydroxypropioniate was also elevated. Loading with thymine, as expected, increased the excretion of 3-aminoisobutyric acid. The aminoisobutyric aciduria in this patient could be a coincidental finding as aminoisobutyric aciduria is quite a common but harmless variation. The concentration of free carnitine was elevated in our patient [1], and the excretion of esterified carnitine was increased.

The metabolic pattern in this infant reported by Pollitt et al. [10] was postulated to result from defective metabolism of methylmalonic, malonic and ethylmalonic semialdehydes (Figure 11.2). Evidence for this has been obtained by study of the oxidation of ^{14}C-valine and ^{14}C-β-alanine in intact cultured fibroblasts [2]. The oxidation of valine was 8 percent of control and that of β-alanine was 26 percent. Similar results have been obtained in our second patient. Defective oxidation of valine was also demonstrated in fibroblasts of the hypermethioninemic infant [12]. An assay for methylmalonic semialdehyde dehydrogenase in fibroblast extracts confirmed deficiency, but the nature of the assay with 1-^{14}C-β-alanine precluded assessment of residual activity. Activity of 3-hydroxyisobutyrate dehydrogenase was normal in our index patient [2].

Prenatal diagnosis by enzyme assay has not yet been attempted. It should be possible by determining conversion of ^{14}C-valine or β-alanine to ^{14}CO$_2$ by cultured amniocytes

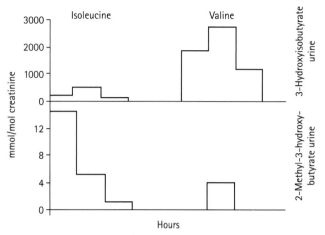

Figure 11.5 *The effects of valine and isoleucine on the urinary excretion of 3-hydroxyisobutyric acid and 2-methyl-3-hydroxybutyric acid. During the 24 hours after administration the patient excreted 35 percent of the administered valine, most of it as 3-hydroxyisobutyric acid. Aminobutyrate excretion also increased.*

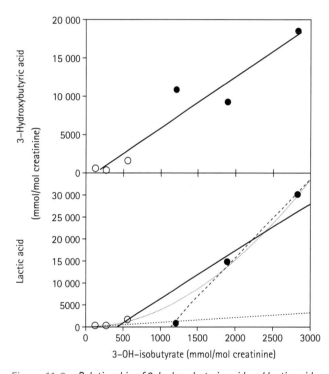

Figure 11.6 *Relationship of 3-hydroxybutyric acid and lactic acid with 3-hydroxyisobutyric excretion. Hollow circles: values following isoleucine challenge; filled circles: following valine challenge. Top: excretion of 3-hydroxybutyrate; line shows fit for y = 6.74 x − 786 (r = 0.958). Bottom: excretion of lactate; solid line shows fit for y = 10.7 x − 4432 (r = 0.935); dotted curve shows y = 0.00455 x² − 2.16 x; dashed lines show y = 1.01 x + 10.7 and y = 17.74 x − 2.16 x; dashed lines show y = 1.01 x + m10.7 and y = 17.74 x − 200 28. The excretion of 3-hydroxybutyrate (a measure of ketosis) and that of lactate correlated positively with the excretion of 3-hydroxyisobutyrate (r = 0.958 and 0.935, respectively).*

or chorionic villus cells. 3-Hydroxyisobutyric acid was found to be elevated in the amniotic fluid of affected twins [9]. A stable isotope gas chromatography/mass spectrometry (GCMS) method for hydroxyisobutyric acid in amniotic fluid should be possible.

Differential diagnosis – related disorder

3-Hydroxyisobutyryl CoA deacylase deficiency was described in a male infant with multiple malformations who died at 3 months of age [3,4]. The condition is of particular interest because the key intermediate is a highly reactive compound that has been shown to be teratogenic in rats [13].

The key compounds found in the urine of the patient were 2-carboxylpropylcysteine and 2-carboxypropylcysteamine (Figure 11.1, p. 78), adducts that could result from addition of cysteine across the double bond of methacryl-CoA. They can be detected by high-voltage electropheresis of the amino acids of the urine and shown to be sulfur-containing by iodoplatinate staining. The cysteine adduct was also found in the urine of the patient of Mienie et al. [7].

Methylmalonic semialdehyde dehydrogenase deficiency has been described [14] in a boy found initially via an elevated concentration of methionine in newborn screening. The value was over 1000 μmol/L. At 4 years of age his development was judged to be normal. Loading with valine increased 3-hydroxybutyric acid excretion. Incubation of fibroblasts with ^{14}C-valine led to no production of ^{14}CO$_2$, with ^{14}C-β-alanine to very little as compared with control cells. Examination of the plasma and urine revealed elevated quantities of β-alanine, 3-hydroxypropionic acid, (R)- and (S)-3-aminoisobutyric acid, (R)- and (S)-3-hydroxyisobutyric acid and (S)-2-hydroxymethylbutyric acid. Direct enzymatic assay of methylmalonate semialdehyde dehydrogenase is difficult because the semialdehyde substrate is not commercially available and very unstable. The gene has been localized to chromosome 14q24.3. Mutational analysis in the index patient revealed homozygosity for G1336A, which changed a highly conserved glycine at 446 to arginine.

TREATMENT

The clear evidence of valine intolerance makes restriction of the intake of protein prudent. This and the administration of carnitine were followed by considerable improvement in our patient. The addition of human growth hormone led to further improvement [15], considerable increase in protein tolerance and intake without increase in 3-hydroxyisobutyrate excretion, and a rewarding increment in growth. The patient has not had a ketoacidotic episode requiring admission to hospital for years.

References

1   Ko F-J, Nyhan WL, Wolff J, et al. 3-Hydroxyisobutyric aciduria: an inborn error of valine metabolism. Pediatr Res 1991;**30**:322.
2   Gibson KM, Lee CF, Bennett MJ, et al. Combined malonic methylmalonic and ethylmalonic acid semialdehyde dehydrogenase deficiencies: an inborn error of β-alanine l-valine and l-alloisoleucine metabolism? J Inherit Metab Dis 1993;**16**:563.
3   Truscott RJW, Malegan D, McCairns E, et al. Two new sulphur-containing amino acids in man. Biomed Mass Spectrom 1981;**8**:99.
4   Brown GK, Hunt SM, Scholem R, et al. b-Hydroxyisobutyryl coenzyme A deacylase deficiency: a defect in valine metabolism associated with physical malformations. Pediatrics 1982;**70**:532.
5   Congdon PJ, Haigh D, Smith R, et al. Hypermethioninaemia and 3-hydroxyisobutyric aciduria in an apparently healthy baby. J Inherit Metab Dis 1981;**4**:79.
6   Goodwin GW, Rougraff PM, Davis EJ, Harris RA. Purification and characterization of methylmalonate-semialdehyde dehydrogenase from rat liver: identity to malonate dehydrogenase. J Biol Chem 1989;**264**:14965.
7   Mienie LJ, Erasmus E. Biochemical studies on a patient with a possible 3-hydroxyisobutyratedehydrogenase deficiency. Fifth International Congress of Inborn Errors of Metabolism 1990;OC27.
8   Brewster M, Goodman S, Rhead W, et al. Valine-related 3-hydroxyisobutyric aciduria in twins. Proc Soc Inherit Metab Dis 1991;p 8.
9   Chitayat D, Meagher-Villemure M, Mamer OA, et al. Brain dysgenesis and congenital intracerebral calcification associated with 3-hydroxyisobutyric aciduria. J Pediatr 1992;**121**:86.
10 Pollitt RJ, Green A, Smith R. Excessive excretion of β-alanine and of 3-hydroxypropionic R- and S-3-aminobutyric R- and S-3-hydroxyisobutyric and S-2-(hydroxymethyl) butyric acids probably due to a defect in the metabolism of the corresponding malonic semialdehydes. J Inherit Metab Dis 1985;**8**:75.
11 Allen JT, Brown AY, Hamilton-Shields J, et al. Two cases of 3-hydroxyisobutyric aciduria with multiple clinical abnormalities. J Inherit Metab Dis 1998;**21**:A106.
12 Gray RGF, Pollitt RJ, Webley J. Methylmalonic semialdehyde dehydrogenase deficiency: demonstration of defective valine and β-alanine metabolism and reduced malonic semialdehyde dehydrogenase activity in cultured fibroblasts. Biochem Med Metab Biol 1987;**38**:121.
13 Singh RR, Lawrence WH, Autian J. Embryonic-fetal toxicity and teratogenic effects of a group of methacrylate esters in rats. J Dent Res 1972;**51**:1632.
14 Chambliss KL, Gray RGF, Rylance G, et al. Molecular characterization of methylmalonate semialdehyde dehydrogenase deficiency. J Inherit Metab Dis 2000;**23**:497.
15 Marsden D, Barshop BA, Capistrano-Estrada S, et al. Anabolic effect of human growth hormone: management of inherited disorders of catabolic pathways. Biochem Med Metab Biol 1994;**52**:145.

Malonic aciduria

MAJOR PHENOTYPIC EXPRESSION

Patients have been described with and without deficiency of malonyl CoA decarboxylase. Each may have a variable phenotype. Both display developmental delay, seizures, episodic metabolic acidosis with ketosis, hyperammonemia, hypoglycemia and lactic acidemia, and a pattern of organic aciduria in which methylmalonic acid, citric acid cycle intermediates, 3-hydroxy-3-methylglutaric acid and dicarboxylic acids are dominated by malonic aciduria.

INTRODUCTION

Malonic acid is a potent inhibitor of many metabolic pathways as well as playing its classic role as an inhibitor of succinic acid dehydrogenase in the citric acid cycle (Figures 12.1 and 12.2). Its accumulation might be expected to disrupt the metabolism of many compounds. Succinic aciduria has been reported in malonyl CoA decarboxylase deficiency [1,2], a disorder described in patients with metabolic acidosis and a propensity for hypoglycemia. Hypoglycemia might be expected to result from that fact that malonyl CoA is an inhibitor of pyruvate carboxylase [3]. It could also result, along with dicarboxylic aciduria, from abnormality in fatty acid oxidation, a consequence of the fact that malonyl CoA is an inhibitor of carnitine palmitoyl transferase I [4], an enzyme necessary for the effective transport of long-chain fatty acids across the mitochondrial membrane to where the enzymes of β-oxidation are situated. Inhibition of glutaryl CoA dehydrogenase by malonyl CoA has also been reported [2], and this would be expected to lead to accumulation of glutaric acid and the hydroxyglutaric acids. Methylmalonic acid accumulation would be expected because malonyl CoA is an inhibitor of methylmalonyl CoA mutase [5].

Malonic aciduria with normal activity of malonyl CoA decarboxylase has been reported [6] in patients from the Middle East. The gene for malonyl CoA decarboxylase has been cloned, and two different mutations have been identified in homozygotes [7].

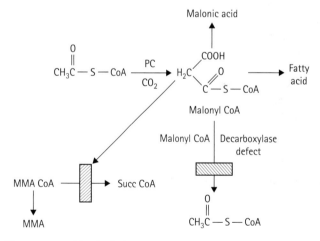

Figure 12.1   *Metabolic interrelations. The structure of malonyl CoA and the mechanism for methylmalonic aciduria in malonic aciduria. The site of the defect in malonyl CoA decarboxylase deficiency is shown.*

CLINICAL ABNORMALITIES

The clinical picture of malonic aciduria with normal activity of the decarboxylase was illustrated by a patient reported at 3 years of age [6] who was strikingly dystonic, frequently in opisthotonos, and who had spastic tetraplegia with hypertonicity, fisted thumbs, increased deep tendon reflexes,

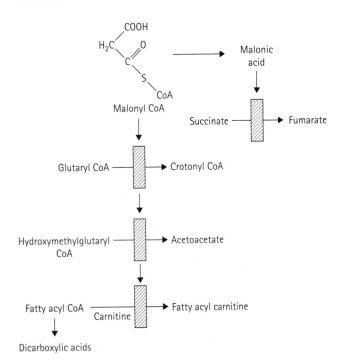

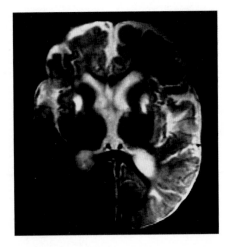

Figure 12.3   *MRI scan of the brain of Patient 1 at 3 years of age.*

Figure 12.2   *Metabolic interrelations. The metabolic milieu in malonic aciduria.*

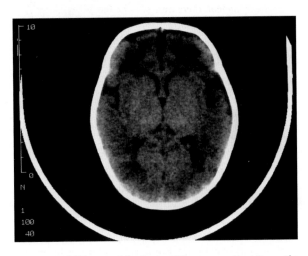

Figure 12.4   *MRI scan of the brain of the same patient 2 months later. There was massive progression of the atrophy, especially in the frontal area, with major increase in the size of the interhemispheric fissure. Increased signal in this T_2 image was prominent in the basal ganglia, and there was widespread deep white matter change. An area of increased signal in the right occipital area would be consistent with an infarct.*

a crossed adductor response, ankle clonus and bilaterally positive Babinski responses. He could not sit, stand or walk. Developmental testing with the Bayley scales at the age of 2 years 7 months adjudged his mental and motor age to be 6 months. Physical development was also retarded. His height of 76 cm at 3 years was well below the 5th percentile and at the 50th percentile for 12 months. His weight of 8.8 kg was at the 50th percentile for 8 months. His head circumference of 48 cm was at the 2 standard deviation (SD) line. He had myoclonic seizures, visualized as spike discharges on electroencephalogram (EEG) and generalized background slow waves.

Metabolic acidosis is a prominent clinical feature of the disease. It may be a cause of early infantile death. One of the three patients was admitted because of ketoacidosis, hypoglycemia and lactic acidosis at 5 months and died [6]. Another had his first episode at 9 months. It was characterized by massive ketosis, lactic acidosis and hyperammonemia. The concentration of uric acid in the blood was elevated, and that of cholesterol was low. Cutaneous and oral monoliasis was observed in one patient [6].

Neuroimaging (Figures 12.3–12.5) revealed a striking and progressive picture. Hypodense myelin was seen as early as the second week of life (Figure 12.5). Frontotemporal atrophy and increasing ventricular size was documented on computed tomography (CT) and magnetic resonance imaging (MRI). Bilateral hypodense lesions were seen in the basal ganglia on CT and there was increased signal intensity in T2 weighted images on MRI in the putamen and caudate and in the periventricular white matter. Later cystic lesions appeared in the putamen and the deep white matter of the cerebral hemispheres.

Patients with malonyl CoA decarboxylase deficiency have also presented with developmental delay, hypotonia and seizures. They have also had hypoglycaemia, metabolic acidosis and lactic acidemia. In addition a number have had hypertrophic cardiomyopathy [1,2,8–11]. The disease may be fatal in the neonatal period [12].

GENETICS AND PATHOGENESIS

The occurrence of the consanguinity in both malonyl CoA decarboxylase deficiency and in malonic aciduria with

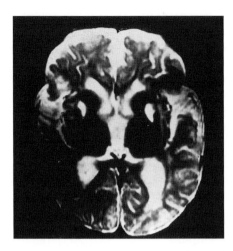

Figure 12.5   *CT scan of Patient 2. There was already evidence of frontotemporal atrophy; the interhemispheric fissure was particularly prominent. There were symmetrical areas of hypodensity in the frontal deep white matter.*

Table 12.1   *Organic acids (mmol/mol creatinine) of the urine in three patients with malonic aciduria*

Acid	Patient 1	Patient 2	Patient 3	Upper limit of normal
Malonic	1671	266	173	2
Lactic	1167	29	11	25
Pyruvic	83			12
Methylmalonic	264	108	29	2
3-Hydroxypropionic	41	0		10
3-Hydroxybutyric	622	0	16	3
Acetoacetic	0			2
3-Hydroxyisovaleric	209	0	10	46
Succinic	630			57
2-Oxoglutaric	543			152
Aconitic	276	69		47
Malic	171	37		5
Fumaric	140	0		2
3-Hydroxy-3-methylglutaric	604			36
3-Methylglutaconic	160	0	10	9
Adipic	193	35	38	12
3-Hydroxyadipic	101		88	13
Glutaric	70	0	11	2
2-Hydroxyglutaric	50	63	34	16
3-Hydroxyglutaric	32	0		3
Suberic	35	0	12	2
Sebacic	35	0		2
Ethylmalonic	35	0		7
Octenedioic	30	0		7
Hydroxydecanedioic	87		20	2

The sample from patient 1 was from the first admission in ketoacidosis.
(Reprinted with kind permission from *Brain Dev* [6].)

normal activity of this enzyme indicates autosomal recessive modes of transmission.

The most consistent and striking feature of the metabolic abnormalities is the excretion of very large amounts of malonic acid (Table 12.1). The first patient studied displayed malonic aciduria at every assay over a year of study. The amounts at the time of an acute acidotic episode were considerably higher than after a year of relative metabolic health, when the levels approximated those seen in the other two patients. Patient 2 was the 2-week-old brother of the first patient diagnosed before the development of acidotic symptoms, but already spastic. The third patient was 5 months of age and severely acidotic. Similar amounts of malonic acid were found in the urine in malonyl CoA decarboxylase deficiency [1,2,8]. A low fat high carbohydrate diet led to normal levels of malonic acid excretion.

Lactic aciduria was also very pronounced at the time of acute illness in the first patient in Table 12.1. This was mirrored in a lactic acidemia of 12.3 mmol/L, which subsided slowly following the acute metabolic acidosis. 3-Hydroxybutyric aciduria and 3-hydroxyisovaleric aciduria were also concomitants of ketosis. All three patients had methylmalonic aciduria, and Patient 1 also excreted 3-hydroxypropionic acid. Elevated excretion of 3-hydroxy-3-methylglutaric (HMG) acid was sufficiently high that fibroblasts were assayed for the activity of HMG-CoA lyase; the activity was normal. Citric acid cycle intermediates that accumulated included 3-oxoglutaric, aconitic and fumaric acids, as well as succinic acid. Disordered fatty acid oxidation was indicated by the excretion of adipic, glutaric and other dicarboxylic acids, as well as hydroxy-dicarboxylic acids. In malonyl CoA decarboxylase deficiency methylmalonic acid is also excreted regularly [1,2,8]. Amounts ranged from 30 to 300 mmol/mol creatine. Amounts are not always less than those of malonic acid.

The activity of mitochondrial malonyl CoA decarboxylase in cultured fibroblasts was normal in the group of patients shown

in Table 12.1. The activity of glutaryl CoA dehydrogenase was also normal, as were pyruvate carboxylase, propionyl CoA carboxylase and biotinidase. In the other group there is deficient activity of malonyl CoA decarboxylase in fibroblasts and lymphocytes [1,2,8].

Malonylcarnitine (C3-DC) concentration is elevated up to 14 times the upper limit in controls (0.25 μm) in stable patients with malonyl CoA decarboxylase deficiency [13]. This disorder should be detectable in programs of expanded neonatal screening. C50H, 3-hydroxyisovalerylcarnitine, the marker for 3-methylcrotonyl-CoA carboxylase deficiency, may also be found in malonic aciduria [14]. The C3-DC and the organic acids of the urine would permit differentiation of the disorders, and others in which C50H is elevated.

TREATMENT

Acute management of the ketoacidosis and hypoglycemia is with the administration of liberal quantities of parenteral fluids containing electrolytes and glucose.

It is not clear that chronic management influences the progression of the neurologic disease or the atrophy of the brain. Treatment appears to be followed by diminished recurrence of episodes of ketoacidosis. Diets employed have been moderately restricted in both lipid and protein and high in carbohydrate. Supplementation with carnitine seems reasonable. Treatment with clonazepam has been followed by control of seizures. The regimen employed in Patient 1 in Table 12.1 also included riboflavin, niacin and baclophen.

References

1 Brown GK, Scholem RD, Bankier A, Danks DM. Malonyl coenzyme A decarboxylase deficiency. *J Inherit Metab Dis* 1984;**7**:21.

2 Haan EA, Scholem RD, Croll HB, Brown GK. Malonyl coenzyme A decarboxylase deficiency. Clinical and biochemical findings in a second child with a more severe enzyme defect. *Eur J Pediatr* 1986;**144**:567.

3 Scrutton MC, Utter MF. Pyruvate carboxylase IX. Some properties of the activation by certain acyl derivatives of coenzyme A. *J Biol Chem* 1967;**242**:1723.

4 McGarry JD, Mannaerts GP, Foster DW. Properties of malonyl CoA in the regulation of hepatic fatty acid oxidation and ketogenesis. *J Clin Invest* 1977;**60**:265.

5 Babior BM, Woodams AD, Brodie JD. Cleavage of coenzyme B12 by methylmalonyl CoA mutase. *J Biol Chem* 1973;**248**:1445.

6 Ozand P, Nyhan WL, Aqueel A, Christodoulo J. New organic acidemias: malonic aciduria. *Brain Dev* 1994;**16**:7.

7 FitzPatrick DR, Hill A, Tolmie JL, *et al.* The molecular basis of malonyl-CoA decarboxylase deficiency. *Am J Hum Genet* 1999;**65**:318.

8 MacPhee GB, Logan RW, Mitchell JS, *et al.* Malonyl coenzyme A decarboxylase deficiency. *Arch Dis Child* 1993;**69**:433.

9 Matalon R, Michaels K, Kaul R, *et al.* Malonic aciduria and cardiomyopathy. *J Inherit Metab Dis* 1993;**16**:571.

10 Yano S, Sweetman L, Thorburn DR, *et al.* A new case of malonyl coenzyme A decarboxylase deficiency presenting with cardiomyopathy. *Eur J Pediatr* 1997;**156**:382.

11 Gibson KM, Cohen J, Waber L, Bennett MJ, Fatal infantile malonyl-CoA decarboxylase (MACAD) deficiency in a patient with malonic aciduria and hypertrophic cardiomyopathy. *Am J Hum Genet* 1998;**63**:A267.

12 Buyukgebiz B, Jakobs C, Scholte HR, *et al.* Fatal neonatal malonic aciduria. *J Inherit Metab Dis* 1998;**21**:76.

13 Santer R, Lassker U, Fingerhut R, *et al.* Tandem mass spectrometric (TMS) detection of malonyl carnitine (C3-DC) in patients with malonyl CoA decarboxylase deficiency (MCDD). *J Inherit Metab Dis* 2002;**25**: (Suppl 1) 53.

14 Van Hove JL, Rutledge SL, Nada MA, *et al.* 3-Hydroxyisovalerylcarnitine in 3-methylcrotonyl-CoA carboxylase deficiency. *J Inherit Metab Dis* 1995;**18**:592.

D-2-hydroxyglutaric aciduria

MAJOR PHENOTYPIC EXPRESSION

Developmental delay, macrocephaly, seizures, vomiting, cerebral atrophy, and D-2-hydroxyglutaric aciduria.

INTRODUCTION

D-2-hydroxyglutaric aciduria is an organic aciduria in which the clinical phenotype is emerging [1–7]. There are at least two phenotypes, severe and mild [7], but there is probably a spectrum [6]. The metabolic defect has not yet been identified; nor are its sources and metabolic products clear (Figure 13.1). 2-Hydroxyglutaric aciduria is identifiable by systems of gas chromatography/mass spectrometry (GCMS) organic acid analysis of the urine, but it is critical that the optical isomeric form be determined, because D-2-hydroxyglutaric aciduria and L-2-hydroxyglutaric aciduria (Chapter 14) are quite distinct diseases.

D-2-hydroxyglutaric acid was first reported in 1980 by Chalmers and colleagues [8]; the patient was normal except for the presence of protein-losing enteropathy. This and the absence of elevation of the compound in the blood suggested the possibility of an enteric bacterial metabolism for the compound in that patient. Patients with neurologic abnormalities and accumulation of D-2-hydroxyglutaric acid in body fluids have been reported since 1993 [1–7].

CLINICAL ABNORMALITIES

Developmental retardation appears to be a common feature of the disease [1–7]. Of 17 patients assembled [7] it was severe in 10, and there were early-onset manifestations: at 7 months, one [1] could not sit or roll and did not fix or follow; another [3] was cortically blind. Most of the patients classified as severe [7] had little evidence of mental development. Among the patients with milder presentations mental retardation and hypotonia were the rule, although the younger sister of one patient appeared by 3 years to have only speech delay, and both sisters were dysmorphic, suggesting the possibility of another etiology for the mental retardation [1].

The first symptom may be vomiting. In three patients [1,7] it was sufficiently severe that a diagnosis of pyloric stenosis was made and a pyloromyotomy performed. Metabolic diseases that may present in the neonatal period as pyloric stenosis [7,9] or similar surgical disease include (Appendix):

- D-2-hydroxyglutaric aciduria
- Propionic acidemia [9]
- Methylmalonic acidemia [9]
- Galactosemia [9]
- Ketothiolase deficiency [9]
- Ethylmalonic acidemia [9]
- Isovaleric acidemia [9]
- Phenylketonuria [9].

Macrocephaly may be another early symptom [1] (Figure 13.2). At 7 months, the head circumference in one patient at 47 cm was in the fiftieth percentile for 19 months. This patient also had chronic subdural collections of fluid. Macrocephaly

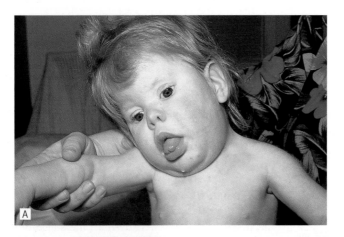

Figure 13.1   *D-2-hydroxyglutaric acid and pathways potentially involved in its synthesis and metabolism.*

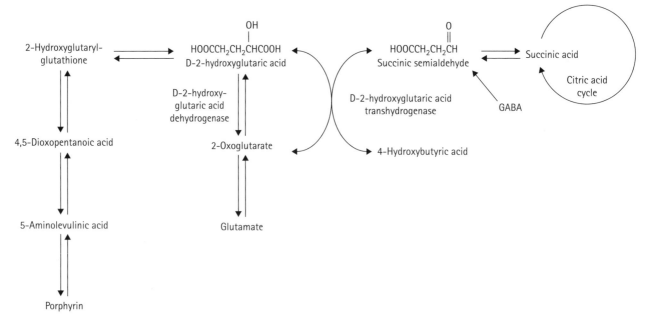

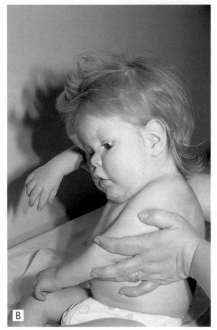

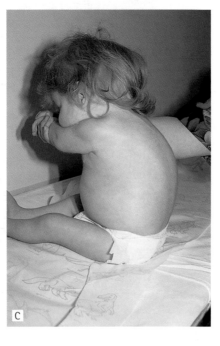

Figure 13.2   *A. F., a 19-month-old patient with D-2-hydroxyglutaric aciduria. (a) She had macrocephaly, deeply recessed orbits, epicanthal folds, a wide nasal bridge and an upturned nose. There were micrognathia and a carp-shaped mouth. (b) She could not sit without support. There was frontal and occipital bossing. (c) The curvature of the spine is an index of the marked hypotonia even when supported while sitting.*

was also present in three of the patients classified as mild [7]; and four of the severe patients become microcephalic. Macrocephaly and subdural collections of fluid are also characteristic of glutaric aciduria resulting from glutaryl CoA dehydrogenase deficiency [10] (Chapter 8), and these diseases should be considered (Appendix) before a diagnosis of non-accidental trauma is made.

Involuntary movements described have included chorea, dystonic posturing and episodic opisthotonic arching and extensor posturing [1,3,7]. Hypotonia has been observed in a number of patients [1,3,4,7], but there may also be hypertonia. Irritability and lethargy have been observed. Spasticity increased deep tendon reflexes and positive Babinski responses have been present [1,7]. Seizures may be grand mal and myoclonic; some were of neonatal onset; and electroencephalogram (EEG) abnormalities [1,3] included hypsarrhythmia [1]. The concentration of protein in the cerebrospinal fluid may be increased [1].

Cardiomyopathy was found in five of the severely affected patients in three of whom it was clinically symptomatic. It was dilated in four and hypertrophic in one. In two patients cardiomegaly was evident only by ultrasound, and in the other three severe patients imaging was not performed. One patient had a ventricular septal defect and one a mild coarctation of the aorta and hypertrophy of the left ventricle. A patient with severe disease displayed respiratory distress and died at 10 months of cardiogenic shock as a result of cardiomyopathy [11]. Other patients have had stridor or apnea, and one required tracheostomy [6].

A variety of dysmorphic features have been noted in patients with this disease, including plagiocephaly, asymmetric ears, transverse palmar creases, epicanthal folds, a frontal upsweep of the hair and coarse features [1].

Imaging of the central nervous system with magnetic resonance (MR) or computed tomography (CT) has regularly revealed cerebral atrophy with consistent enlargement of the lateral ventricles [1,3,4,6,7]. Early MRI showed subependymal cysts and delayed cerebral maturation, as exemplified by poor development of gyri, or poor operculation or myelination [6,7]. Subdural effusions have been found in four patients [7]. One 14-month-old developed acute left-sided hemiparesis and a right middle cerebral artery infarction, and later a left striatal infarction, and finally infarction of the left anterior, middle and posterior cerebral arteries followed by disappearance of the left hemisphere [6]. Another patient had multiple aneurisms of the middle cerebral arteries bilaterally. A patient with severe disease who died at 10 months had on MRI increased T2 signal in the substantia nigra, candate and thalamus, lesions similar to those of patients with mitochondrial disease [11]. Another infant had absence of the corpus callosum [12]. This patient also had multiple intracranial hemorrhages; he also had a variant C667T substitution in the methylene tetrahydrofolate reductase gene. Absence of the corpus callosum was also reported in two other patients with D-2-hydroxyglutaric aciduria [13,14].

GENETICS AND PATHOGENESIS

The genetic transmission of the disorder appears to be autosomal recessive. Affected offspring of normal parents have been observed [1,3,15], as has consanguinity [8]. Prenatal diagnosis of an affected fetus has been made by the analysis of D-2-hydroxyglutaric acid in amniotic fluid by selective ion monitoring by GCMS with stable isotope dilution internal standard [15].

The biochemical hallmark of the disease is the accumulation of D-2-hydroxyglutaric acid in body fluids. The compound is readily detected and quantified by organic acid analysis of the urine. The identification as the D-form is accomplished by chemical ionization GCMS of the O-acetyl-di-2-butyl ester [15]. Urinary excretion of D-2-hydroxyglutaric acid ranged from 18 (this patient also recorded a level of 1072) to 7076 mmol/mol creatinine [1,2,6]. Control individuals excreted 3 to 17 mmol/mol creatinine. In our patient, the concentration in the cerebrospinal fluid (CSF) of 313 mol/L was slightly higher than that of the plasma (283 μmol/L) [1], while in another patient [2,3] the plasma concentration of 62 μmol/L was slightly greater than that of the CSF (25 mol/L). Overall the CSF level was higher than that of the plasma in all but one patient [7].

Excretion of L-2-hydroxyglutaric acid was normal in all but 1 patient [7]. There was no relationship between the level of D-2-hydroxyglutaric acid in urine, plasma or CSF and the severity of disease, although the highest levels were seen in severe patients [7]. One patient with severe disease had intermittently normal and high levels of excretion [11].

Excretion of 2-oxoglutaric acid ranged from 404 to 862 mmol/mol creatinine [1], amounts similar to those reported in 2-oxoglutaric aciduria [16]. This was found in other patients [7], and other citric acid cycle compounds were up in some, usually to a lesser level [7]. The excretion of this compound normally decreases with age, and decrease toward normal has been observed in two patients [2,4] while their excretion of D-2-hydroxyglutaric acid remained high. Elevated concentrations of 4-aminobutyric acid (GABA) were found in the CSF in almost all of the patients studied [7]. Levels of 20 and 28 μmol/L were reported [1,3]. One patient had an increased amount of glycine in the urine. Decreased levels of carnitine have been found in many patients, but many have been receiving valproate [7]. Acylcarnitine profiles have been normal, but one had multiple elevations, as seen in multiple acylCoA dehydrogenase deficiency, but without excretion of glutaric and ethylmalonic acids. Increased levels of lactic acid in the urine were found in a few patients [7,11].

In studies of cultured fibroblasts [17], the media in which cells derived from patients with D-2-hydroxyglutaric aciduria contained 5 to 30 times the control concentration of D-2-hydroxyglutaric acid.

D-2-hydroxyglutaric acid is a metabolic intermediate in a variety of pathways (Figure 13.1). The simplest conversion from 2-oxoglutarate is catalyzed by D-2-hydroxyglutaric acid dehydrogenase (EC 1.1.99.6). This has been postulated as the site of the defect [8]. The same reaction is catalyzed by a transhydrogenase and in the exchange 4-hydroxybutyric acid is converted to succinic semialdehyde [18]. Succinic semialdehyde is the immediate catabolic product of 4-aminobutyric (GABA) and thus interference with this pathway and accumulation of GABA would be expected to have neurologic consequences, as in the case of GABA transaminase deficiency [19]. The product 4-hydroxybutyric acid is also neuropharmacologically active, as illustrated by patients with 4-hydroxybutyric aciduria which is due to succinic semialdehyde dehydrogenase deficiency (Chapter 16). The elevated levels of GABA in the CSF in patients with D-2-hydroxyglutaric aciduria would be consistent with abnormalities in this pathway. Levels of 4-hydroxybutyric acid were not elevated in any of the patients studied. 2-Hydroxyglutaric acid is formed from lysine, at least in microbial metabolism, via 2-aminoadipic acid [20], but it is not known whether this compound is the d- or l-form.

In patients with multiple acylCoA dehydrogenase deficiency (glutaric aciduria type II) (Chapter 45), 2-hydroxyglutaric acid excretion is elevated, and it is the D-isomer that is predominant [21]. This raises the possibility that an electron transport related dehydrogenase is the site of the defect in D-2-hydroxyglutaric aciduria. Of course, in glutaric aciduria type II, any hydroxyl acid accumulated might lead to the formation of D-2-hydroxyglutaric aciduria in the presence of 2-oxoglutarate in a transhydrogenase reaction [18]. Exogenous D-2-hydroxyglutaric acid was reported [11] to inhibit cytochrome c oxidase activity in fibroblasts *in vitro*, but electron transport chain activity in the fibroblasts of patients was normal, including cytochrome oxidase. D-2-hydroxyglutaric acid was also found to inhibit *in vitro* the activity of cytochrome oxidase in rat brain fractions [11].

TREATMENT

Approaches to treatment have not been developed.

References

1   Nyhan WL, Shelton GD, Jakobs C, *et al.* D-2-hydroxyglutaric aciduria. *J Child Neurol* 1995;**10**:132.

2   Gibson KM, Craigen W, Herman GE, Jakobs C. D-2-hydroxyglutaric aciduria in a newborn with neurologic abnormalities: a new metabolic disorder? *J Inherit Metab Dis* 1993;**16**:490.

3   Craigen WJ, Sekul EA, Levy MI, *et al.* D-2-hydroxyglutaric aciduria in a neonate with seizures and central nervous system dysfunction. *Pediatr Neurol* 1994;**10**:49.

4   Loonen MCB, Huijmans JGM, Duran M, *et al.* D-2-hydroxyglutaric aciduria. *Proc Eur Fed Child Neurol Soc* Bern; June 23–26, 1993.

5   Huijmans JGM, Duran M, de Klerk JBC, *et al.* Phenotypic and biochemical variation of 2-hydroxyglutaric aciduria. *Proc 31st SSIEM Ann Symp* Manchester UK; September 7–10 1993, Poster 43.

6   van der Knaap MS, Jakobs C, Hoffmann GF, *et al.* D-2-hydroxyglutaric aciduria: Further clinical delineation. *J Inherit Metab Dis* 1999;**22**:404.

7   van der Knaap MS, Jakobs C, Hoffmann GF, *et al.* D-2-hydroxyglutaric aciduria: Biochemical marker or clinical disease entity? *Ann Neurol* 1999;**45**:111.

8   Chalmers RA, Lawson AM, Watts RW, *et al.* D-2-hydroxyglutaric aciduria: case report and biochemical studies. *J Inherit Metab Dis* 1980;**3**:11.

9   Nyhan WL. Abnormalities in amino acid metabolism in *Clinical Medicine* (WL Nyhan). Appleton Century Crofts, Norwalk Conn, 1984:5.

10 Hoffman GF, Trefz FK, Barth PG, *et al.* Glutaryl–CoA dehydrogenase deficiency: a distinct encephalopathy. *Pediatrics* 1991;**88**:1194.

11 Wajner M, Vargas CR, Funayama C, *et al.* D-2-hydroxyglutaric aciduria in a patient with a severe clinical phenotype and unusual MRI findings. *J Inherit Metab Dis* 2002;**25**:28.

12 Wang X, Jakobs C, Bawle EV. d2-Hydroxyglutaric aciduria with absence of corpus callosum and neonatal intracranial haemorrhage. *J Inherit Metab Dis* 2003;**26**:92.

13 Amiel J, De Lonlay P, Francannet C, *et al.* Facial anomalies in d-2-hydroxglutaric aciduria. *Am J Med Genet* 1999;**86**:124.

14 Baker NS, Sarnat HB, Jack RM, *et al.* D-2-hydroxyglutaric aciduria: hypotonia cortical blindness seizures cardiomyopathy and cylindrical spirals in skeletal muscle. *J Child Neurol* 1997;**12**:31.

15 Gibson KM, TenBrink HJ, Schor R, *et al.* Stable isotope dilution analysis of d- and l-2-hydroxyglutaric acid: application to the detection and prenatal diagnosis of d- and l-2-hydroxyglutaric aciduria. *Pediatr Res* 1993;**34**:277.

16 Kohlschutter A, Behbehani A, Lagenbeck U, *et al.* A familial progressive neurodegenerative disease with 2-oxoglutaric aciduria. *Eur J Pediatr* 1982;**138**:32.

17 Struys EA, Verhoeven NM, Roos B, Jakobs C. Disease-related metabolites in culture medium of fibroblasts from patients with d-2-hydroxyglutaric aciduria L-2-hydroxyglutaric aciduria and combined D/L-2-hydroxyglutaric aciduria. *Clin Chem* 2003;**49**:1133.

18 Kaufman EE, Nelson T, Fales HM, Levin DM. Isolation and characterization of a hydroxy-acid–oxoacid transhydrogenase from rat kidney mitochondria. *J Biol Chem* 1988;**263**:16872.

19 Gibson KM, Sweetman L, Nyhan WL, *et al.* Demonstration of 4-aminobutyric acid aminotransferase deficiency in lymphocytes and lymphoblasts. *J Inherit Metab Dis* 1985;**8**:204.

20 Kopchick JJ, Hartline RA. α-Hydroxyglutarate as an intermediate in the catabolism of α-aminoadipate by *Pseudomonas putida. J Biol Chem* 1979;**254**:3259.

21 Goodman SI, Reale M, Berlow S. Glutaric acidemia type II: a form with deleterious intrauterine effects. *J Pediatr* 1983;**102**:411.

14

L-2-hydroxyglutaric aciduria

MAJOR PHENOTYPIC EXPRESSION

Ataxia, hypotonia, tremor, psychomotor retardation, seizures; rarely neonatal expression with apnea; cerebellar atrophy; and L-2-hydroxyglutaric aciduria.

INTRODUCTION

L-2-Hydroxyglutaric aciduria was first described by Duran and colleagues [1] in 1980 in a 5-year-old Moroccan boy with psychomotor retardation. A survey of eight patients including this one by Barth in 1992 [2], and a later report by Barth and colleagues [3], established the usual phenotype of mental retardation and cerebellar signs with onset after the first year of life. At least 40 patients are known [4]. Imaging of the central nervous system has revealed abnormal loss of subcortical white matter and cerebellar atrophy [2,3]. We have recently [4] reported a patient with a much more severe phenotype who presented with disease that was rapidly fatal by 28 days of life. L-2-Hydroxyglutaric acid (Figure 14.1) was found in increased concentrations in the urine, blood and cerebrospinal fluid. The concentration in the cerebrospinal fluid (CSF) was greater than that of the plasma. The enzymatic defect has not yet been defined.

CLINICAL ABNORMALITIES

Patients have generally appeared well for the first year [3]. Delay in walking, abnormal gait, delay in speech and febrile seizures have been the presenting complaints in seven of 12 patients [3]. In four patients learning disability in school first

$$HOOC - CH_2 - CH_2 - \overset{\displaystyle OH}{\underset{\displaystyle |}{CH}} - COOH$$

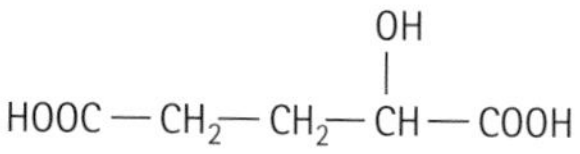

Figure 14.1 *The structure of L-2 hydroxyglutaric acid. Sources of L-2-hydroxyglutaric acid are not known.*

called attention to the disease. In one, cerebellar signs at 10 years of age were the first evidence of disease recognized.

Cerebellar manifestations were prominent in all but one of the patients summarized by Barth *et al.* [3]. Ataxia, dysarthria and dysmetria were present. Mental retardation was observed in all. Seizures were prominent in half of 10 patients (Figure 14.2). They were either febrile or nonfebrile grand mal seizures. Spasticity has been observed [5].

Progressive deterioration was documented in one patient [5] after a number of years of relative stability; by 16 years she was unable to walk and had repeated seizures. Progression was also reported in two patients by Divry and colleagues [6], who emphasized ataxia, brisk tendon reflexes and positive Babinski as extrapyramidal signs and first reported macrocephaly in both patients. Macrocephaly was also observed in three Australian patients of Serbian, Iranian and Iraqi parents [7]; one demonstrated rapid neurological deterioration over 5 months and died; the others did not. One had strabismus and myopia.

A very different clinical picture was exemplified by a female patient who was limp at birth and had poor respiratory effort

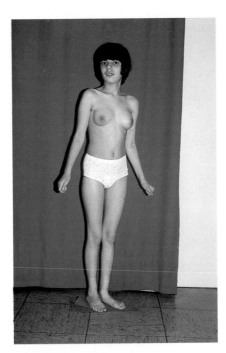

Figure 14.2　*A girl with L-2-hydroxyglutaric aciduria. She was slightly delayed in her early development. At 2-years-of-age she developed grand mal seizures and progressive ataxia. By 9-years-of-age pyramidal signs were evident. (This illustration and Figures 3 and 4 were kindly provided by Dr. Georg Hoffmann of the University of Heidelberg, Germany.)*

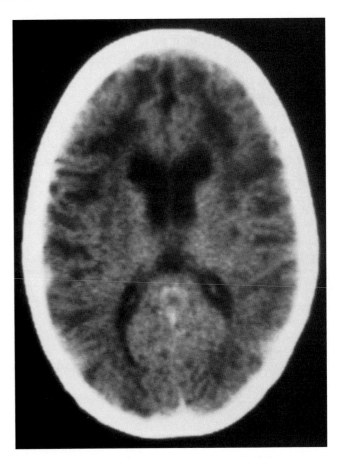

Figure 14.3　*CT scan of the brain of a 2-year-old with L-2-hydroxyglutaric aciduria illustrating cerebellar atrophy and increased size of the ventricles.*

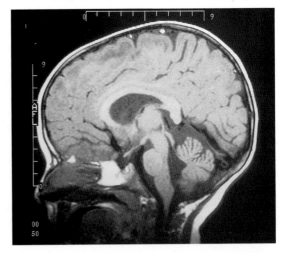

Figure 14.4　*A 3-year-old with L-2-hydroxyglutaric aciduria had pronounced atrophy of the cerebellum.*

and bradycardia [4]. Initial pO$_2$ was 18, and Apgar scores at 1, 5 and 10 minutes were 3, 6 and 8, respectively. At 80 minutes there was profound apnea and cyanosis requiring assisted ventilation. Episodic seizures began on day 2, and the electroencephalograph (EEG) revealed a burst suppression pattern and focal epileptogenic activity. Moro, grasp and suck reflexes were absent. She died on day 28 after the withdrawal of life support.

Imaging of the central nervous system (Figures 14.3 and 14.4) in the older patients [3,5] by magnetic resonance (MR) or computed tomography (CT) scan revealed loss of substance in the subcortical white matter and cerebellar atrophy and increased ventricular size. On MRI, there was decreased signal on T1 and increased signal on T2 in subcortical areas. The caudate nuclei were atrophic, and there were signal changes in the putamen. In the cerebellum, folial atrophy involved the vermis particularly, and there were signal changes in the dentate nuclei. Magnetic resonance spectroscopy showed abnormalities in the gray as well as white matter [5], indicating neuronal loss and neurodegeneration. The pattern on neuroimaging has been stated to be unique among neurodegenerative disorders [3]. A parasellar arachnoid cyst was observed in one patient [6]. In the infant with the rapidly fatal presentation, CT scan at one day of age revealed hypodense cerebellar white matter [4]. By two weeks, this had become more hypodense, and the cerebellum was small. In one patient calcifications were observed in the frontal lobe [8].

Neuropathology has been reported only in the infant who died at 28 days [4]. The brain stem and cerebellum were disproportionately small. The most striking changes were in the neocerebellum. The folia were small and illustrated patchy dropout of Purkinje cells. There was striking astrocytosis of the white matter in an olivopontocerebellar distribution.

GENETICS AND PATHOGENESIS

The disease is autosomal recessive in transmission [3]. Many families have had more than one affected offspring, and males and females have been similarly affected. A number of families have been consanguineous [3,6,7].

Organic analysis of the urine is the usual method of detection; although analysis of the cerebrospinal fluid [9] also can serve in case finding. Gas chromatography/mass spectrometry (GCMS) reveals a large quantity of 2-hydroxyglutaric acid. It is essential to determine the optical configuration of the compound identified because D-2-hydroxyglutaric aciduria (Chapter 13) is a different disease. A stable isotope dilution, internal standard, selected ion monitoring, GCMS method has been developed [8] in which the D- and L-acids are separated as the O-acetyl-di-2-butyl esters. In 13 patients, the concentrations of L-2-hydroxyglutaric acid in the urine were 1283 ± 676 mmol/mol creatine (range 332–2742). In control subjects the range was 1.3 to 19. In patients the cerebrospinal fluid concentrations may be greater than that of the plasma [3] or about equal [8]. The CSF concentration was $62 \pm 30\,\mu$mol/L (range 34–100) while that of the plasma was $47 \pm 13\,\mu$mol/L (range 27–62). The control ranges were 0.3–2.3 and 0.5–$10\,\mu$mol, respectively.

Prenatal diagnosis is feasible using this method. The normal amniotic fluid concentration of L-2-hydroxyglutaric acid is 3.1–$5.2\,\mu$mol/L [8].

Elevated concentrations of lysine have been observed in plasma and CSF [3,6], or only in CSF [6,8]; but loading with L-lysine did not increase excretion of L-2-hydroxyglutaric acid. In the infant with rapidly fatal disease, concentrations of lysine were normal [9].

Abnormalities in concentrations of carnitine or dicarboxylic acids have not been found [3]. Levels of pipecolic acid were normal [3]. The increased concentration of 2-hydroxyglutaric acid in the CSF indicates endogenous origin and suggests direct involvement in pathogenesis.

There are no clues to the nature of the molecular defect. There was no difference in the conversion of ^{14}C-2-oxoglutaric acid to L-2-hydroxyglutaric acid in fibroblasts of patients and controls [3]. L-2-hydroxyglutaric acid is not degraded by a peroxisomal oxidase yielding H_2O_2. L-2-hydroxyglutaric acid dehydrogenase is active in the presence of nicotinamide-adenine dinucleotide (NAD) in mammalian (including human) liver [10]. The enzyme is expressed only in liver.

TREATMENT

Information on treatment is not available.

References

1   Duran M. L-2-hydroxyglutaric aciduria: an inborn error of metabolism? *J Inherit Metab Dis* 1980;**3**:109.

2   Barth PG. L-2-hydroxyglutaric acidemia: a novel inherited neurometabolic disease. *Ann Neurol* 1992;**32**:66.

3   Barth PG, Hoffmann GF, Jaeken J, *et al*. L-2-hydroxyglutaric acidemia: clinical and biochemical findings in 12 patients and preliminary report on L-2-hydroxyacid dehydrogenase. *J Inherit Metab Dis* 1993;**16**:753.

4   Chen E, Nyhan WL, Jakobs C, *et al*. L-2-Hydroxyglutaric aciduria: first report of severe neurodegenerative disease and neonatal death; neuropathological correlations. *J Inherit Metab Dis* 1996;**19**:335.

5   Hanefeld F, Kruse B, Bruhn H, Frahm J. *In vivo* proton magnetic resonance spectroscopy of the brain in a patient with L-2-hydroxyglutaric academia. *Pediatr Res* 1994;**35**:614.

6   Divry P, Jakobs C, Vianey-Saban C, *et al*. L-2-hydroxyglutaric aciduria: two further cases. *J Inherit Metab Dis* 1993;**16**:5.

7   Wilcken B, Pitt J, Heath D, *et al*. L-2-hydroxyglutaric aciduria: three Australian cases. *J Inherit Metab Dis* 1993;**16**:501.

8   Gibson KM, ten Brink HJ, Schor DS, *et al*. Stable-isotope dilution analysis of D- and L-2-hydroxyglutaric acid: application to the detection and prenatal diagnosis of D- and L-2-hydroxyglutaric acidemias. *Pediatr Res* 1993;**34**:277.

9   Hoffman GF, Meier-Augenstein W, Stockler S, *et al*. Physiology and pathophysiology of organic acids in cerebrospinal fluid. *J Inherit Metab Dis* 1993;**16**:648.

10 Jansen GA, Wanders RJA. L-2-hydroxyglutarate dehydrogenase: identification of a novel enzyme activity in rat and human liver. Implications for L-2-hydroxyglutaric academia. *Biochim Biophys Acta* 1993;**1225**:53.

2-oxoadipic aciduria

MAJOR PHENOTYPIC EXPRESSION

Not clear. May be no clinical disease.

INTRODUCTION

Individuals with 2-oxoadipic aciduria have usually been found because of the presence of aminoadipic aciduria, detected by qualitative chromatography on paper or thin layer; high-voltage electrophoresis; quantitative column chromatography; or the amino acid analyzer [1]. 2-Oxoadipic aciduria was recognized by thin layer chromatography of the dinitrophenylhydrazone [1] and proven by gas chromatography/mass spectrometry (GCMS) [1,2]. Deficiency of 2-oxoadipic acid dehydrogenase leads to accumulation of 2-oxoadipic acid, 2-hydroxyadipic acid and 2-aminoadipic acid (Figure 15.1). These compounds were initially reported in the urine of two patients with mental retardation [1,2]. Any relationship would appear to represent ascertainment bias, because two asymptomatic siblings have had the same urinary metabolites as their siblings [2,3]. Three normal siblings detected by newborn screening have also been reported [4]. It is possible that this is a metabolic marker without clinical consequences. It is also possible that this might be a disorder that produces transient effects early in life, as in the case of hawkinsinuria. As in hawkinsinuria intermittent acidosis may be a characteristic in infancy.

We have studied a patient who presented with a typical organic acidemia phenotype of acute ketoacidosis who was found to have 2-oxoadipic aciduria and 2-aminoadipic aciduria which disappeared by 2 years 7 months years of age and went on to have Kearns-Sayre disease and be shown to have the

usual deletion in mitochondrial DNA [5]. This may be another example of the ability of abnormalities in oxidative phosphorylation to mimic other disorders of metabolism.

CLINICAL ABNORMALITIES

The first patient reported [1] was described at 14 months, at which time motor and mental development were quite retarded. There was striking hypotonia and edema of the dorsa of the hands and feet. The infant had been a collodion baby at birth [6] and later developed ichthyosiform erythroderma. He had a convulsion on the first day of life, but there were no others and the electroencephalogram (EEG) was normal. At 14 months there was evident dilatation of the ventricular system and slight retardation bone age. Analysis of the phenotype was complicated by the fact that the mother and her brother were retarded, and the father was unknown. An intermittent acidosis and an intermittently positive 2,4-dinitrophenylhydrazine test of the urine led to further testing which revealed the unusual spot of 2-aminoadipic acid on thin layer chromatography. The second patient [2] had slow development and at 34 months had an IQ of 25 and was self-abusive. He had always been difficult to feed and had no speech. His sister was normal. A third child with aminoadipic aciduria was markedly retarded at 6 years. He also had hypotonia and dysphagia. It is not known whether or not he had

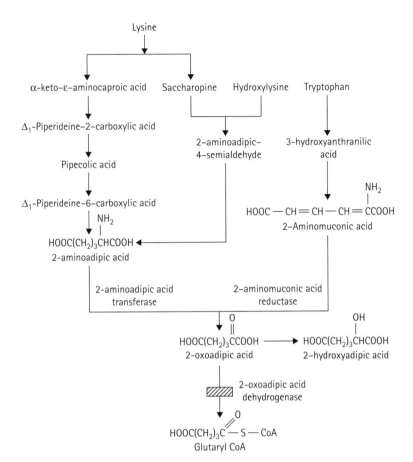

Figure 15.1 *Metabolic pathways and site of the defect in 2-oxoadipic aciduria.*

ketoaciduria. A fourth patient [3], with aminoadipic aciduria, was studied at 9 years [7]. His psychomotor development had been slow and his IQ ranged from 81 to 86. He was hypotonic and had hypoplasia of the distal phalanges of the toes. His brother was normal. Three other patients [8–11] had developmental delay or learning disability, and one of them was ataxic.

The metabolic phenotype most readily demonstrated is the aminoadipic aciduria. Amounts of aminoadipic acid reported have included 0.52 [1] to 1.49 [2] mmol/24 hours in infants 14 and 34 months of age, and 0.99–2.48 mmol/24 hours in a 9-year-old [3]. A 6-year-old excreted 90–324 mmol/mol creatinine. Plasma concentrations have ranged from 34 to 62 mol/L. 2-Aminoadipic acid was not detected in cerebrospinal fluid. 2-Oxoadipic acid was excreted at the level of 151 mmol/mol creatinine [1], or 1.45, [1] 0.68 and 2.45 mmol/L[2]. Serum levels of 34 μmol/L and 58 μmol/L have been reported [2].

Organic acid analysis also revealed the presence of 2-hydroxyadipic acid in the urine [1], as well as increased amounts of 3-hydroxybutyric, glutaric, 1,2-butenedicarboxylic and 2-hydroxyglutaric acids. Glutaric acid would be expected to arise from spontaneous decarboxylation of 2-oxoadipic acid. 2-Oxoglutaric acid was excreted at an elevated level [1], but in the other patient [2] and his sibling the excretion of 2-oxoglutarate was reported to be normal.

GENETICS AND PATHOGENESIS

It is likely that transmission is autosomal recessive, in view of a number of families with affected siblings demonstrating the metabolic features. In one family [1] the mother excreted an elevated amount of 2-aminoadipic acid, but considerably less than any of the patients, suggesting heterozygosity.

Dietary studies in which the protein intake was reduced, and the intake of lysine was varied from 0 to 390 mg/kg per day documented a very close relationship between the intake of lysine and the urinary excretion of 2-aminoadipic acid [1,7]. An acute oral load of 100 mg/kg of lysine was followed by high and prolonged increase in the concentration of lysine in plasma and marked increases in the levels of 2-aminoadipic acid in plasma and urine. A compensated metabolic acidosis was present for 24 hours. Tryptophan loading also led to oxoadipic aciduria [7].

The accumulations of 2-aminoadipic and 2-oxoadipic acid appear to result from defective activity of 2-oxoadipic acid dehydrogenase, but direct enzymatic analysis has not been accomplished. Degradative studies in fibroblasts were consistent with this hypothesis [12]. Patient-derived fibroblasts were unable to convert 2-aminoadipic-1-^{14}C or 2-oxoadipic-1-^{14}C to ^{14}CO$_2$. ^{14}C-labeled glutaric acid was oxidized normally.

The enzyme 2-oxoadipic dehydrogenase has not been separated from 2-oxoglutaric dehydrogenase. Electrons are thought to be transferred via nicotinamide adenine dinucleotide (NADH): ubiquinone oxidoreductase (complex I), which would provide an avenue for oxoadipic aciduria in disorders of the respiratory electron transport chain.

TREATMENT

There is no experience reported with treatment, but it is clear that a lowered intake of lysine will reduce the amounts of the relevant compounds in the urine. It is not at all clear that treatment is justified. In an infant diagnosed early, especially if acidotic, treatment might be prudent.

References

1   Przyrembel H, Bachmann D, Lombeck I, *et al.* Alpha-ketoadipic aciduria a newborn error of lysine metabolism; biochemical studies. *Clin Chim Acta* 1975;58:257.

2   Wilson RW, Wilson CM, Gates SC, Higgins JV. α-Ketoadipic aciduria: a description of a new metabolic error in lysine-tryptophan degradation. *Pediatr Res* 1975;9:522.

3   Fischer MH, Gerritsen T, Opitz JM. α-aminoadipic aciduria a non-deleterious inborn metabolic defect. *Humangenetik* 1974;24:265.

4   Wilcken B. Personal communication quoted in Goodman SI, Frerman FE. Organic acidemias due to defects in lysine oxidation: 2-ketoadipic acidemia and glutaric acidemia in *The Metabolic and Molecular Bases of Inherited Disease* (eds CR Scriver, AL Beaudet, WS Sly, D Valle) McGraw Hill New York;2001: 2195.

5   Barshop BA, Nyhan WL, Naviaux RK, *et al.* Kearns-Sayre syndrome presenting as 2-oxoadipic aciduria. *Mol Genet Metab* 2000;69:64.

6   Bremer HJ, Wadman SK, Przyrembel H, *et al.* α-ketoadipic aciduria – a new inborn defect of lysine degradation. Proceedings of the 12th Meeting of the Society for the Study of Inborn Errors of Metabolism Heidelberg 1974 in *Inborn Errors of Calcium and Bone Metabolism* (eds H Bickel, J Stern) Medical and Technical Publishing Co., Lancaster; 1976: 271.

7   Fischer MH, Brown RR. Tryptophan and lysine metabolism in alpha-aminoadipic aciduria. *Am J Med Genet* 1980;5:35.

8   Lorman S, Lowenthal A. α-aminoadipic aciduria in an oligophrenic child. *Clin Chim Acta* 1974;57:97.

9   Casey RE, Zeleski WA, Philp M, *et al.* Biochemical and clinical studies of a new case of α-aminoadipic aciduria. *J Inherit Metab Dis* 1978;1:129.

10   Duran M, Beemer FA, Wadman SK, *et al.* A patient with α-ketoadipic and α-aminoadipic aciduria. *J Inherit Metab Dis* 1984;7:61.

11   Vianey-Liaud C, Divry P, Cotte J, Teyssier G. α-aminoadipic and α-ketoadipic aciduria: detection of a new case by a screening program using two dimensional thin layer chromatography of amino acids. *J Inherit Metab Dis* 1985;8:(Suppl 2) 133.

12   Wendel U, Rudiger HW, Przyrembel H, *et al.* Alpha-ketoadipic aciduria: degradation studies with fibroblasts. *Clin Chim Acta* 1975;58:271.

4-hydroxybutyric aciduria

MAJOR PHENOTYPIC EXPRESSION

Mental retardation, ataxia, hypotonia, hyporeflexia, convulsions, hyperkinetic behavior or lethargy bordering on narcolepsy, macrocephaly, excretion of 4-hydroxybutyric acid in the urine, and deficiency of succinic semialdehyde dehydrogenase.

INTRODUCTION

4-Hydroxybutyric aciduria [1,2] is a metabolic disorder that serves as a model for conditions in which the metabolic block causes the accumulation of a compound of established neuropharmacologic activity. 4-hydroxybutyric acid was once developed as an intravenous anesthetic in order to obtain an analogue of 4-aminobutyric acid (GABA), which would cross the blood–brain barrier. However, on testing in animals it was found to produce convulsions [3–5] and thus it never came to human trials. The first patient with 4-hydroxybutyric aciduria was described by Jakobs and colleagues [1] in 1981. Thirty-one patients in 21 families were studied by 1983 [2,6,7]. A recent report [8] of experience with 23 patients emphasized the importance and difficulty of organic acid analysis in the diagnosis of this disorder.

Among disorders of GABA metabolism 4-hydroxybutyric aciduria has been more frequently encountered, probably because the key intermediate 4-hydroxybutyric acid is detectable by analysis of organic acids [2]. The fundamental defect is in the activity of the succinic semialdehyde dehydrogenase (EC 1.2.1.24) (Figure 16.1). In the reaction catalyzed by this enzyme, the product of GABA transamination is normally converted to succinic acid and hence to oxidation via the citric acid cycle [9] 4-hydroxybutyric acid is converted via β-oxidation into 3,4-dihydroxybutyric acid and thereafter to its keto acid, to glycolaldehyde and glycolic acid [10].

The genes for rat and human semialdehyde dehydrogenase have been cloned [11,12]. The locus for the human gene is chromosome 6p22 [12,13]. Mutation analysis has elucidated two exon-skipping mutations at consensus splice sites in four patients in two families [13].

CLINICAL ABNORMALITIES

Retardation of psychomotor development is a common feature of patients with 4-hydroxybutyric aciduria and may be severe (Figures 16.2, 16.3). Most have had delayed development of speech [8]. The first patient presented at 20 months of age with retardation of motor development [1] (Figure 16.4). He could not stand, walk, or speak. He had had brief convulsions between 6 and 12 months. He was ataxic and hypotonic but not weak. The electroencephalograph (EEG) was diffusely abnormal, and computed tomography (CT) scan revealed cerebral atrophy. Bone age was retarded. At 5 years of age his condition was described as stable, without deterioration [14]. He still had no speech and an ataxic gait.

Nonprogressive ataxia and hypotonia have been recognized as characteristic of this syndrome [2,8,14–18] along with relatively mild mental retardation. Two siblings, first seen at 9 and 11 years-of-age, had moderate ataxia and intention tremor (Figure 16.5). Their speech was mildly dysarthric. The girl was hypotonic, but her brother was not. Deep tendon

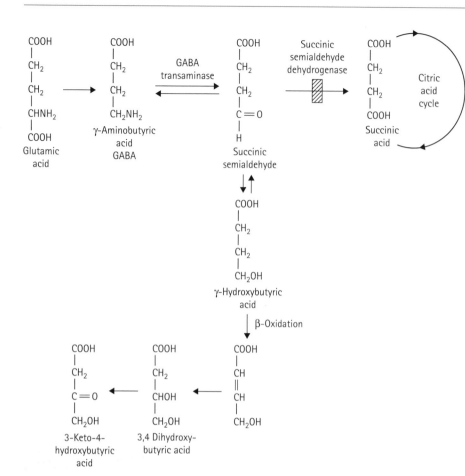

Figure 16.1   *Succinic semialdehyde dehydrogenase, the site of defect in 4-hydroxybutyric aciduria, and the formation and metabolism of 4-hydroxybutyric acid.*

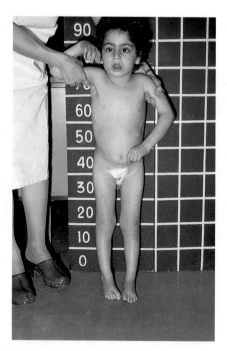

Figure 16.2   *B.R., a 4-year-old boy with 4-hydroxybutyric aciduria. He was mentally retarded and was later admitted to an institution. (Illustration was kindly provided by Dr. Priscille Divry, Hopital Debrousse, Lyon, France.)*

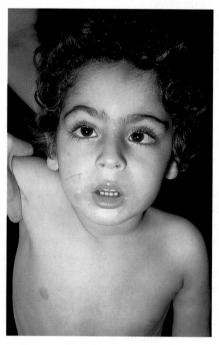

Figure 16.3   *Close-up view of the patient in Figure 16.2. (Illustration kindly provided by Dr. Priscille Divry, Hopital Debrousse, Lyon, France.)*

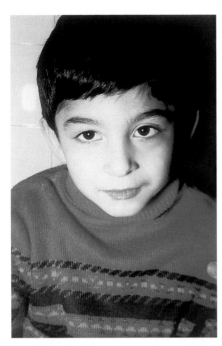

Figure 16.4 *S.B., the index patient with 4-hydroxybutyric aciduria (Case report). (Illustration kindly provided by Dr. Dietz Rating, now of the University of Heidelberg, Germany.)*

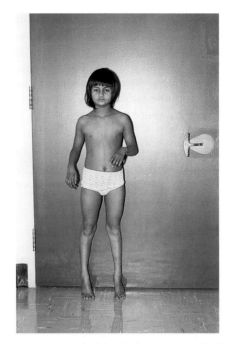

Figure 16.6 *A 9-year-old with 4-hydroxybutyric aciduria. Her extreme hyperkinetic behavior had led to treatment with thioridazine, which ultimately led to the dyskinesia illustrated.*

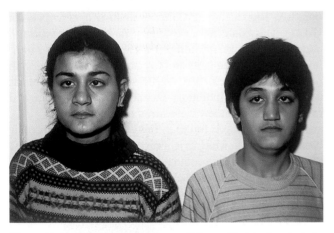

Figure 16.5 *R.F. and R.M., Lebanese siblings with 4-hydroxybutyric aciduria. (Illustration was kindly provided by Dr. Deitz Rating, Heidelberg, Germany.)*

reflexes were difficult to elicit. Two years later, the ataxia in both of these children had improved considerably. Another patient was mentally retarded and markedly hypotonic and ataxic, and no improvement was noted with time. At 6 years-of-age, he could hardly stand and could not walk. Seizures began before 1 year-of-age. Sensory examination was normal in all of the children. Seizures occurred in slightly less than half of recently reported patients [8]. Hypotonia was observed in 74 percent. Optokinetic nystagmus has been described [8]. Both microcephaly and macrocephaly have been observed. One patient underwent a pyloromyotomy [8].

Extremes of activity have been observed in different patients or families. Extremely hyperkinetic behavior has been the

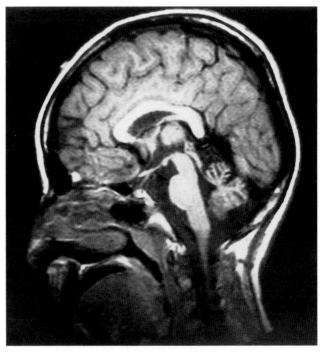

Figure 16.7 *MRI scan of the brain of a patient with 4-hydroxybutyric aciduria, illustrating cerebral atrophy.*

characteristic mode for some patients [15,16] (Figure 16.6). Others, such as a pair of siblings we have studied, were lethargic and somnolent to a degree that suggested narcolepsy. Some have been thought to be autistic [16]. Ataxia has been observed to resolve with age [19].

Magnetic resonance imaging (MRI) of the brain may be normal [15] or may reveal cerebral atrophy (Figure 16.7). One patient had a normal MRI, followed by symmetric lesions in the globus pallidus, thalamus and brainstem four years later [8].

A possibility of two groups of phenotypes was suggested [8] by some patients whose early development was normal. Even so ultimate disease was not mild.

GENETICS AND PATHOGENESIS

4-Hydroxybutyric aciduria is an autosomal recessive disorder. In seven of 21 families of probands, the parents were consanguineous [1,2,6,14]. Intermediate levels of enzyme activity have been found in parents [17,18].

Prenatal diagnosis of an affected fetus has been accomplished [20] by gas chromatography/mass spectrometry (GCMS) assay of the concentration of 4-hydroxybutyric acid in amniotic fluid. Enzyme activity was absent in fetal brain, liver and kidney [21]. Succinic semialdehyde dehydrogenase is also measurable in chorionic villus samples [22], providing another avenue for prenatal diagnosis.

The molelcular defect in 4-hydroxybutyric aciduria is in the enzyme succinic semialdehyde hydrogenase (EC 1.2.1.2) (Figure 16.1) [7,18,22,23]. Succinic semialdehyde is the product of the transamination of GABA and is normally converted to succinic acid. When succinic semialdehyde accumulates, it is reduced to 4-hydroxybutyric acid. The enzyme is active in lymphocytes freshly isolated from peripheral blood and in cultured lymphoblasts [7,17,22,23]. Accumulation of labeled succinic semialdehyde has been demonstrated in patients' lymphocytes following incubation with ^{14}C-labeled GABA, and there was no evidence of further metabolism to succinic acid [7]. Direct assay of the enzyme with ^{14}C-labeled succinic semialdehyde yielded activity that approximated 4 percent of the control level in one patient [22] and was undetectable in another [18]. In another [16] it was as high as 21 percent in lymphocytes.

Although clinical expression has been highly variable with quite mild and severe or even fatal disease, the degree of phenotypic variation has not correlated with the amount of residual enzyme activity [2] even when monitored by a whole cell assay in which levels of activity tend to be higher [24,25].

The cDNA for succinic acid semialdehyde dehydrogenase has been isolated from E. coli [26,27]. Characterization of the human gene was accomplished following purification of the mammalian enzyme. Studies of the nature of mutation have begun [13,28]. Three splicing errors have led to losses of exon 8, 9, and part of 4. In addition an insertion, a deletion, 4 nonsense mutations and a number of missense mutations have been reported [28]. Information is not sufficient to consider genotype-phenotype correlation.

The immediate consequence of the metabolic block is the accumulation of 4-hydroxybutyric acid. This compound has been found in large amounts in the urine in all of the studied patients [1,2,14,29]. Its nature was documented by GCMS. In the index patient [1], the amounts excreted varied from 170 to 340 mmol/mol creatinine. Concentrations in urine have ranged from 2 fold to 500 fold the normal level [30,31]. Succinic semialdehyde may be found in the urine, but the amounts are small. They ranged from 5 to 10 mmol/mol creatinine in one patient [1]. The ratio of 4-hydroxybutyric acid to succinic semialdehyde approximated 35 times. 3,4-Dihydroxybutyric acid has also been found regularly in the urine, and what appeared to be its 3-keto analogue.

Increased concentrations of 4-hydroxybutyric acid are also found in the cerebrospinal fluid (CSF) [1,2,6,29] and in the plasma. In the index patient, the concentration in the cerebrospinal fluid was 600 μm/L, approximately 60 percent of the levels found in the plasma [1], and in the second patient it was 350 μm/L, almost three times that of the plasma [6]. Overall elevations have ranged from 100 fold to 1200 fold [30,31]. 4-Hydroxybutyric acid is not readily detected in the CSF of control individuals. Quantification of this compound, even in patients, may be spuriously low. A stable isotope dilution, internal standard method [30] has revealed consistently higher levels and would be best for prenatal diagnosis. Administration of glutamic acid increased the plasma concentration of 4-hydroxybutyric acid [6]. GABA has also been found in increased concentration in the CSF. The level of 654 pm/mL [1] was over six times the control mean.

Among patients with 4-hydroxybutyric aciduria, concentrations have been higher in younger and lower in older patients [30,31]. This could reflect changing ratios of brain mass to body mass with age. It could provide an explanation for somnolence in young patients and hyperactivity or aggression in older patients. It has been suggested that 4-hydroxybutyric acid might bind to inhibitory sites at high concentration and to excitatory sites at low concentrations [2].

Other compounds found in the urine of patients include dicarboxylic acids, which might suggest a disorder of fatty acid oxidation [32,33]. They could result from secondary inhibition of mitochondrial fatty acid oxidation. 4,5-Dihydroxyhexanoic acid identified in the urine of these patients [32] has not been found in other metabolic diseases, and so may be a specific marker for this disease. It could arise from the condensation of a 2-carbon moiety with succinic semialdehyde. The occurrence of 3-hydroxypropionic acid and glycine in the urine of some patients might suggest a diagnosis of a disorder of propionate metabolism. Identification of the key compound 4-hydroxybutyric acid should avoid any confusion. Glycine would be a product of glycolic acid, which can be formed from β-oxidation of 4-hydroxybutyric acid [34].

TREATMENT

Treatment has been undertaken with vigabatrine (γ-vinyl-GABA), which is an irreversible inhibitor of GABA transaminase [2,16,35,36]. Cerebellar signs were reported in five of six patients treated [2]. Doses employed have included 1.5 g/d in a 30 kg patient [16] in whom alertness appeared to improve and hypotonia to decrease. Long-term efficacy remains to be established. At least one patient was reported not to improve. Patients should be closely monitored because the drug may be expected to increase levels of GABA in the central nervous system and, as indicated by GABA transaminase deficiency, this would be expected to cause neurologic disease. Several treated patients have developed seizures [37]. Methylphenidate may decrease daytime somnolence [38].

References

1. Jakobs C, Bojasch M, Monch E, et al. Urinary excretion of gamma-hydroxybutyric acid in a patient with neurological abnormalities. The probability of a new inborn error of metabolism. *Clin Chim Acta* 1981;**111**:169.

2. Jakobs C, Jaeken J, Gibson KM. Inherited disorders of GABA metabolism. *J Inherit Metab Dis* 1993;**16**:704.

3. Labroit H, Jouany J, Gerard J, Fabiani F. Report of a clinical and experimental study. Sodium 4-hydroxybutyrate a metabolite substrate with central inhibitory activity. *Presse Med* 1960;**68**:1867.

4. Godschalk M, Dzoljic MRI, Bonta IL. Slow wave sleep and a state resembling absence epilepsy induced in the rat by gamma-hydroxybutyrate. *Eur J Pharmacol* 1977;**44**:105.

5. Snead OC. Gamma-hydroxy-butyrate in the monkey I. Electroencephalographic behavioral and pharmacokinetic studies. *Neurology* 1978;**28**:638.

6. Divry P, Baltassat P, Rolland MO, et al. A new patient with 4-hydroxybutyric aciduria a possible defect of 4-aminobutyrate metabolism. *Clin Chim Acta* 1983;**129**:303.

7. Gibson KM, Sweetman L, Nyhan WL, et al. Succinic semialdehyde dehydrogenase deficiency: an inborn error of gamma-aminobutyric acid metabolism. *Clin Chim Acta* 1983;**133**:33.

8. Gibson KM, Christensen E, Jakobs C, et al. The clinical phenotype of succinic semialdehyde dehydrogenase deficiency (4-hydroxybutyric aciduria): case reports of 23 new patients. *Pediatrics* 1997;**99**:567.

9. Roberts E, (ed). *Inhibition in the Neuron System and γ-Aminobutyric Acid.* Pergamon Press, New York;1960.

10. Walkenstein SS, Wiser R, Gudmundsen C, Kimmel H. Metabolism of 4-hydroxybutyric acid. *Biochim Biophys Acta* 1964;**86**:640.

11. Chambliss KL, Claudle DL, Hinson DD, et al. Molecular cloning of the mature NAD(+)-dependent succinic semialdehyde dehydrogenase from rat and human: cDNA isolation evolutionary homology and tissue expression. *J Biol Chem* 1995;**270**:461.

12. Trettel F, Malaspina P, Jodice C, et al. Human succinic semialdehyde dehydrogenase: molecular cloning and chromosomal localization. *Adv Exp Med Biol* 1997;**414**:253.

13. Chambliss KL, Hinson DD, Trette F, et al. Two exon skipping mutations as the molecular basis of succinic semialdehyde dehydrogenase deficiency (4-hydroxybutyric aciduria) *Am J Hum Genet* 1998;**63**:399.

14. Rating D, Hanefeld F, Siemes H, et al. 4-hydroxybutyric aciduria: a new inborn error of metabolism I. Clinical review. *J Inherit Metab Dis* 1984;**7**:92.

15. Gibson KM, Hoffmann G, Nyhan WL, et al. 4-Hydroxybutyric aciduria in a patient without ataxia or convulsions. *Eur J Pediatr* 1988;**147**:529.

16. Uziel G, Bardelli P, Pantaleoni C, et al. 4-Hydroxybutyric aciduria: clinical findings and Vigabatrin therapy. *J Inherit Metab Dis* 1993;**16**:520.

17. Gibson KM, Sweetman L, Nyhan WL, et al. Demonstration of 4-aminobutyric acid amiotransferase deficiency in lymphocytes and lymphoblasts. *J Inherit Metab Dis* 1985;**8**:204.

18. Gibson KM, Sweetman L, Jansen I, et al. Properties of succinic semialdehyde dehydrogenase in cultured human lymphoblasts. *J Neurogenet* 1985;**2**:111.

19. Hodson AK, Gibson KM, Jakobs C. Developmental resolution of ataxia in succinic semialdehyde dehydrogenase deficiency. *Ann Neurol* 1990;**28**:438.

20. Jakobs C, Ogier H, Rabier D, Gibson KM. Prenatal detection of succinic semialdehyde dehydrogenase deficiency (4-hydroxybutyric aciduria). *Prenat Diagn* 1993;**13**:150.

21. Chambliss KL, Lee CF, Ogier H, et al. Enzymatic and immunologic demonstration of normal and defective succinic semialdehyde dehydrogenase activity in fetal brain liver and kidney. *J Inherit Metab Dis* 1993;**16**:523.

22. Sweetman FR, Gibson KM, Sweetman L, et al. Activity of biotin-dependent and GABA metabolizing enzymes in chorionic villus samples: potential for 1st trimester prenatal diagnosis. *Prenat Diagn* 1986;**6**:187.

23. Gibson KM, Nyhan WL, Jaeken J. Inborn errors of GABA metabolism. *Bio Essays* 1986;**4**:24.

24. Pattarelli PP, Nyhan WL, Gibson KM. Oxidation of [U-^{14}C] succinic semialdehyde in cultured human lymphoblasts: measurement of residual succinic semialdehyde dehydrogenase activity in 11 patients with 4-hydroxybutyric aciduria. *Pediatr Res* 1988;**24**:455.

25. Gibson KM, Lee CF, Chambliss KL, et al. 4-Hydroxybutyric aciduria: Application of a fluorometric assay to the determination of succinic semialdehyde dehydrogenase activity in extracts of cultured human lymphoblasts. *Clin Chim Acta* 1991;**196**:219.

26. Marek LE, Henson JM. Cloning and expression of the *Escherichia coli* K-12 GAD gene. *J Bacteriol* 1988;**170**:991.

27. Bartsch K, von Johnn-Marteville A, Schulz A. Molecular analysis of two genes of the *Escherichia coli* gab cluster: nucleotide sequence of the glutamate: succinic semialdehyde transaminase gene (gabT) and characterization of the succinic semialdehyde dehydrogenase gene (gabD). *J Bacteriol* 1990;**172**:7035.

28. Hogema BM, Jakobs C, Oudejans CBM, et al. Mutation analysis in succinic semialdehyde dehydrogenase (SSADH) deficiency (4-hydroxybutyric aciduria). *Amer J Hum Genet* 1999;**65**:A238.

29. Jakobs C, Kneer J, Rating D, et al. A new inborn error of metabolism: gamma-hydroxybutyric aciduria – biochemical findings. *J Inherit Metab Dis* 1984;**7**:92.

30. Gibson KM, Aramaki S, Sweetman L, et al. Stable isotope dilution analysis of 4-hydroxybutyric acid: an accurate method for quantification in physiological fluids and the prenatal diagnosis of 4-hydroxybutyric aciduria. *Biomed Environ Mass Spectrom* 1990;**19**:89.

31. Jakobs C, Smit LME, Kneer J, et al. The first adult case with 4-hydroxybutyric aciduria. *J Inherit Metab Dis* 1990;**13**:341.

32. Brown GK, Cromby CH, Manning NJ, Pollitt RJ. Urinary organic acids in succinic semialdehyde dehydrogenase deficiency: evidence of a-oxidation of 4-hydroxybutyric acid interaction of succinic semialdehyde with pyruvate dehydrogenase and possible secondary inhibition of mitochondrial β-oxidation *J Inher Metab Dis* 1987;**10**:367.

33. Ishiguro Y, Kajita M, Aoshiima T, et al. The first case of 4-hydroxybutyric aciduria in Japan *Brain Dev* 2001;**23**:128.

34. Vamecq J, Draye J-P, Poupaert JH. Studies on the metabolism of glycolyl-CoA. *Biochem Cell Biol* 1990;**68**:846.

35. Jakobs C, Michael T, Jaeger E, et al. Further evaluation of Vigabatrin therapy in 4-hydroxybutyric aciduria. *Eur J Pediatr* 1992;**151**:466.

36. Howells D, Jakobs C, Kok RM, et al. Vigabatrin therapy in succinic semialdehyde dehydrogenase deficiency. *Mol Neuropharmacol* 1992;**2**:181.

37. Gibson KM, Hoffmann GF, Hodson AK, et al. 4-Hydroxybutyric acid and the clinical phenotype of succinic semialdehyde dehydrogenase deficiency an inborn error of GABA metabolism. *Neuropediatrics* 1998;**29**:14.

38. Daly DM, Hodson A, Gibson KM. Central auditory processing in a patient with SSADH deficiency. *Soc Neurosci Absts* 1991;**17**:(Part I) 892.

Mitochondrial acetoacetyl-CoA thiolase (3-oxothiolase) deficiency

MAJOR PHENOTYPIC EXPRESSION

Acute episodes of ketosis and acidosis, vomiting, lethargy, urinary excretion of 2-methyl-3-hydroxybutyric acid, tiglyglycine and 2-methylacetoacetic acid, deficiency of mitochondrial acetoacetyl CoA thiolase (2-methylacetoacetic acid 3-oxothiolase).

INTRODUCTION

The disease was first reported in 1971 [1] as a disorder of isoleucine metabolism because of the excretion of large amounts of 2-methyl-3-hydroxybutyric and 2-methylacetoacetic acids in the urine and their increase in response to the administration of protein or isoleucine [2,3]. Since then, more than 30 patients have been reported [4].

These patients have been characterized by the occurrence of multiple episodes of massive ketosis. They have been differentiated as defects in ketolysis [5] from ketoacidotic disorders such as propionic acidemia, methylmalonic acidemia and isovaleric acidemia where the mechanism appears to be excessive production of acetoacetate. There could be elements of overproduction in this disease too, for the block (Figure 17.1) is just prior to the formation of propionyl CoA, and CoA-containing intermediates accumulate behind the block as far as tiglyl CoA. On the other hand, a major peripheral role for the mitochondrial acetoacetyl CoA thiolase, which is deficient in this disease, is in the utilization of acetoacetyl CoA and its conversion to acetyl CoA (Figure 17.2).

The molecular defect is in the mitochondrial short chain-length-specific thiolase, 2-methylacetoacetyl CoA thiolase (EC 2.3.1.9) [6,7,8]. The products of this enzymatic cleavage are acetyl CoA and propionyl CoA (Figure 17.1). The cDNA has been cloned [9] and the gene is located on chromosome 11 at q22.3–23.1 [10]. A number of mutations have been defined [4,11,12].

CLINICAL ABNORMALITIES

Among the patients reported [1,2,8,13–26] there has been considerable heterogeneity, but a unifying feature is the occurrence of episodes of acute illness in which there is massive ketosis and acidosis. Episodes may be ushered in by vomiting. At least one patient [17] underwent pyloromyotomy. There may be associated lethargy, coma, hyperventilation and dehydration. This is a life-threatening illness, and death has been reported [2,4,16]. Many have had siblings who died early in life. A few patients have had neonatal onsets, but most have presented first in late infancy or childhood. Twenty-one of 26 patients presented before 25 months-of-age [26].

Episodes of acute illness are induced most commonly by intercurrent infection or other cause of catabolism such as appendectomy [15]. They can also be induced by the intake of

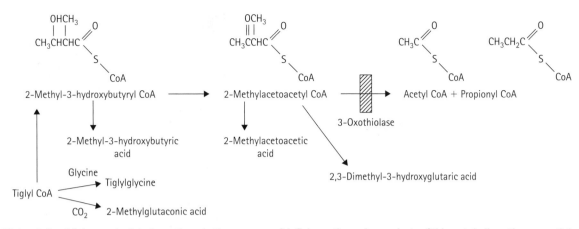

Figure 17.1   *3-Oxothiolase and related reactions. In the presence of deficiency the major products of this metabolic pathway are tiglyglycine and 2-methyl-3-hydroxybutyric acid.*

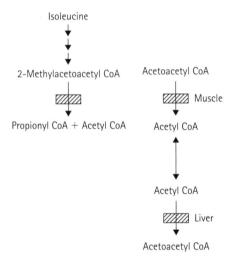

Figure 17.2   *The multiple roles of mitochondrial acetyl CoA thiolase. In addition to its place in the catabolism of isoleucine, it is involved in ketone body synthesis in liver and in its utilization in peripheral tissues.*

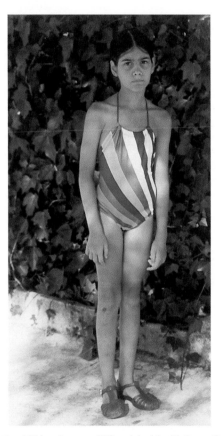

Figure 17.3   *M.M., a 7-year-old Spanish girl with 3-oxothiolase deficiency. She had many episodes of severe ketoacidosis and was developmentally delayed. Gait was spastic on the right side, and Babinski response was positive on the right.*

protein. During episodes of acute illness patients often require admission to hospital and parenteral fluid therapy containing alkali. During acidosis concentrations of sugar in the blood may be elevated. Hyperglycemia and ketoacidosis may lead to a diagnosis of diabetes mellitus and the administration of insulin. Another problem of differential diagnosis was raised by experience with a 1-year-old girl who presented with vomiting, ketosis and severe acidosis [16] and was initially thought to have salicylate intoxication. This impression was heightened by the colorimetric test of the blood for salicylates, which gave an abnormally high reading because of cross-reaction with acetoacetic acid. Fortunately, organic acid analysis was also carried out, providing the diagnosis. Blood ammonia and lactate are usually not elevated. Levels of carnitine are low [11].

Most patients have no other clinical manifestations besides the episodic ketoacidosis. Specifically, intellectual development may be normal [1,2,4,6,15,18]. In fact, one patient had been asymptomatic at report at 36 years [6]; a total of three have not

experienced ketoacidotic episodes. Congestive cardiac myopathy has been reported [17,27]. This might be a consequence of carnitine deficiency. Seizures have been observed especially in the acute episode. Another patient had abdominal pain during the acute episode [8]. A number have developed mental retardation (Figure 17.3), or speech problems [2,13,14,18].

In four recently reported patients, all had significant neurological abnormality, and in each development was slow prior

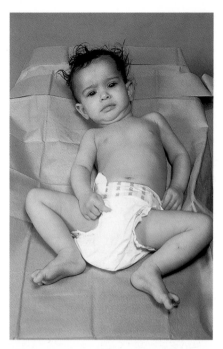

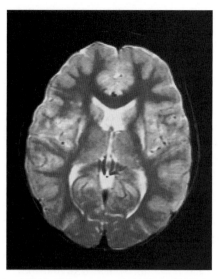

Figure 17.6   *M.M.S. MRI scan revealed bilateral high intensity T2 lesions in the lentiform nuclei. The nuclei were reduced in volume bilaterally.*

Figure 17.4   *M.A.S., a 9-month-old infant with 3-oxothiolase deficiency [24]. Hypotonia was impressive and motor development delayed.*

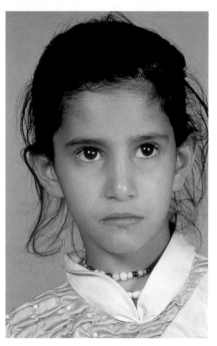

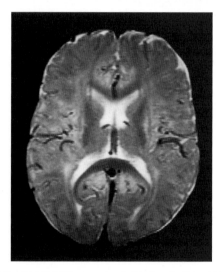

Figure 17.7   *M.A.S. MRI scan revealed lesions in the white matter of the external capsule.*

Figure 17.5   *M.M.S., the 7-year-old sister of M.A.S. She had marked impairment of motor skills.*

Some patients have been reported as mild examples of the disease [28,29]. Actually a majority of patients have done well once diagnosed. The frequency of attacks diminishes by age. In the most recent assembly of experience with patients worldwide [4], the latest attack was at 10 years of age. In addition to the three patients with no episodes, 11 had only one. Only 12 of 26 patients had recurrent episodes of ketoacidosis.

to the initial acidotic episode [25] (Figures 17.4, 17.5). All had severe degrees of central hypotonia. Some patients were ataxic [4,15,21]. Others had severe headaches. MRI scans revealed high intensity T2 lesions in the posterior lateral putamina (Figures 17.6, 17.7). This appearance is unusual enough to suggest the diagnosis [25].

Concentrations of amino acids are usually normal, but three patients have had hyperglycinuria [13–15]. This is reminiscent of propionic acidemia, as were the neutropenia, thrombocytopenia and hyperglycinemia in one of them, a 12-week-old girl [13], who developed episodes of lethargy and vomiting. The increased quantities of 3-hydroxybutyric acid in this disease have been reported to induce fetal hemoglobin and may ameliorate a coexisting β-thalassemia.

The diagnostic feature of this disorder is the organic aciduria. 2-Methyl-3-hydroxybutyric acid and 2-methylacetoacetic acid and tiglylglycine are the key metabolites. They are found regularly in the urine of these patients and occur in only trace amounts in normal urine. In general the amounts of 2-methyl-3-hydroxybutyric acid are considerably greater than those of 2-methylacetoacetic acid; the latter may even be undetectable. 2-Methyl-3-hydroxybutyric acid may be found in the urine in concentrations of 200 to 1000 mmol/mol of creatinine under normal circumstances, increasing at times of acute illness and in response to the administration of protein or of isoleucine to as high as 14 400 mmol/mol creatinine [2,15,6,18]. Normal individuals excrete less than 10 mmol/mol creatinine. Tiglylglycine is excreted in amounts up to 7000 mmol/mol creatinine [6,18,30] but some patients do not normally excrete tiglylglycine. In one of our patients [18], none of these metabolites were present in urine assayed in the absence of acute ketosis.

Organic acid analysis during ketosis can, however, be confusing. Key metabolites can be masked at the time of the acute ketosis. In addition severe ketosis may lead in anyone to the excretion of 3-hydroxy acids, including 2-methyl-3-hydroxy-butryric acid in amounts as high as 200 mmol/mol creatinine, as well as 3-hydroxyisovaleric acid [31]. During ketosis we have also observed 2-methyl-3-hydroxybutryic acid and 2-methylacetoacetic acid in the urine of patients with propionic academia [32]. Therefore, it is important in the assessment of any nondiabetic patient who develops acute acidosis and massive ketosis to carry out analysis of the organic acids of the urine after successful treatment of the ketosis, as well as at the time of the acute illness. Patients with propionic acidemia can be clearly distinguished by the excretion of 3-hydroxy-propionic acid and methylcitric acid. Some patients with 3-oxothiolase deficiency may not be distinguishable from anyone else with ketosis until the ketosis has subsided. Among the organic acidemias this is the disorder most likely to be missed by organic acid analysis. It may be necessary to administer an isoleucine load in the absence of ketosis in order to clarify the organic aciduria of this condition. We have employed a single dose of 100 mg/kg of isoleucine for this purpose. Others [2,6,14,15] have given 3 doses of 75 mg/kg per day for 2 days. In 8 hours following 100 mg/kg our patients have excreted up to 1000 to 4000 mmol/mol creatinine of 2-methyl-3-hydroxyisobutyric acid or tiglyglycine [33].

In addition to these metabolites, butanone may also be found in the urine in this disorder [2,14,15], and

(E)-2-methylglutaconic acid appears also to be a characteristic metabolite [34]. It is thought to result from carboxylation of tiglyl CoA catalyzed by 3-methylcrotonyl CoA carboxylase. 2,3-Dimethyl-3-hydroxyglutaric acid has also been identified in the urine of a patient with this disease [3]. It is thought that this compound results from accumulated 2-methylacetoacetyl CoA in the reaction catalyzed by 3-methyl-3-hydroxyglutaryl CoA synthase. A similar reaction in propionic acidemia with propionyl CoA as substrate instead of the usual acetyl CoA yields 3-ethyl-3-hydroxyglutaric acid [3]. Adipic acid and other dicarboxylic acids may be found during ketosis. A characteristic acylcarnitine profile has also been observed via tandem mass spectroscopy (MS/MS) [35] (Figure 17.8). The MS/MS diagnosis is made on the basis of tiglylcarnitine and 2-methyl-3-hydroxybutyrylcarnitine in the blood.

GENETICS AND PATHOGENESIS

The disorder is autosomal recessive (Figure 17.9). Consanguinity has been reported [2,25], but it has been rare among families reported [4]. A method for the analysis of 2-methyl-3-hydroxybutyric acid in amniotic fluid [36] should be useful in the rapid prenatal diagnosis of the disorder. Prenatal diagnosis should also be possible by assay of the enzyme in cultured amniocytes. Heterozygosity has been determined by assay of the enzyme in cultured fibroblasts [6,37], but it may not be reliable in distinguishing an individual heterozygote from normal. In one family the mother and brother of the patient were heterozygotes, but the father was found on enzyme assay to be a homozygote [4,6,11].

The enzymatic defect in the mitochondrial acetoacetyl CoA thiolase can be demonstrated by assay of the oxidation

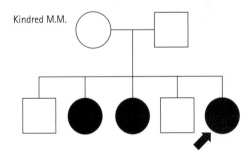

Figure 17.9   *The family of the patient shown in Figure 17.3. The two previously affected siblings had died at 13 and 21 months.*

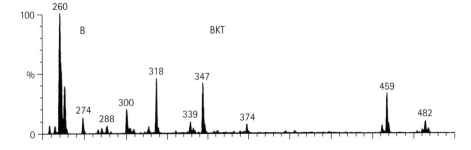

Figure 17.8   *Tandem mass spectrometric profile of acyl carnitine esters in the blood of a patient with 3-oxothiolase deficiency (BKT). The key compounds were tiglylcarnitine m/z 300 and 2-methyl-3-hydroxybutyrlcarnitine (m/z 318). (Reprinted with permission from* Pediatric Research *[29].)*

of ^{14}C-isoleucine by cultured fibroblasts [3,17,38–40], or by the conversion of tritiated tiglyl CoA into propionic acid [3]. Assay of the activity of the K$^+$ dependent acetoacetyl CoA-3-ketothiolase with acetoacetyl CoA as the substrate has revealed as much as 12 percent of normal activity [6]. Most patients have no demonstrable enzyme activity and no immunoreactive cross-reacting material (CRM) protein [4].

There are three 3-oxothiolases in mammalian tissues, two of them mitochondrial and one cytoplasmic [7]. The cytoplasmic enzyme is involved in the synthesis of 3-oxoacyl compounds. The other mitochondrial enzyme (EC 2.3.1.16) has a very broad range of substrates against which it is active (for example, 3-oxohexanoyl CoA), while the enzyme that is defective in this disorder has a high degree of substrate specificity, restricted to acetoacetyl CoA and 2-methylacetoacetyl CoA. A further distinctive property of this enzyme is its enhancement by potassium ions of its activity against acetoacetyl CoA [7]. It is the only enzyme with appreciable activity towards 2-methylacetoacetyl CoA. Thus when homogenates derived from patients are tested using 2-methylacetoacetyl CoA as substrate virtually no activity has been observed; in the presence of acetoacetyl CoA a depressed level of activity is found, reflecting the activities of the cytoplasmic and the nonspecific mitochondrial thiolase. Activation of cleavage of acetoacetyl CoA by potassium is not seen, providing further evidence of deficiency of the short-chain-length-specific mitochondrial thiolase (EC 2.3.1.9). The K$^+$-stimulated activity against the 2-methyl-acetoacetyl CoA has been 0–4 percent of control [8,14,18,24,25]. A patient with a less severe phenotype had 7 percent of control activity [18], but in general enzyme activity has not correlated with clinical severity. A coupled assay for fibroblast extracts in which NaH^{14}C0$_3$ is fixed ultimately to methylmalonyl CoA [38] revealed activity of 2 percent of controls in five patients and 20 percent of control in the milder patient [18].

The enzyme in liver is a 176 kD tetramer of four identical subunits. A precursor enzyme is imported into the mitochondria where a leader peptide is removed to release the tetrapeptide. Immunochemical studies of the enzyme protein have revealed considerable heterogeneity, including no evidence of enzyme by immunoblot or by pulse chase and evidence of an unstable protein by the presence of detectable protein following a 1 hour pulse that was gone after a 6 hour chase [39,40].

Complementation analysis of seven patients with thiolase deficiency, in which the conversion of ^{14}C-labeled isoleucine to glutamate and aspartate of cell protein was the measure of activity, revealed evidence of three complementation groups [41]. Assessment of the degradative pathways of isoleucine by study of the incorporation of ^{14}C-2-methylbutyrate into macromolecules in intact cells revealed low activity in nine patients with clinically severe phenotypes [42], and over 30 percent of control activity in patients with milder disease.

The gene has now been cloned and sequenced [4,10,43–46]. The cDNA is 1518 bp in 12 exons and encodes a 427 amino acid precursor protein. The sequence is of a 33 residue leader sequence and a 394 amino acid mature enzyme of 41 385

molecular weight. In a study of four patients the length of the mRNA was normal. The amounts of mRNA were reduced in two and normal in two [45]. Many patients to date have been compounds of two mutations. For instance, in a German family a G to A mutation at position 1138 led to a change from alanine to threonine at amino acid 347 of the mature enzyme [46]; this is a highly conserved region of the enzyme. This allele was inherited from one parent; the mutation in the other parent led to no mRNA expression. In another family a G to A mutation at 547 led to a glycine to arginine change at position 150; the other allele in this patient was altered at a splice site leading to skipping of exon 8 [10]. This individual was the asymptomatic father of a patient with severe attacks of the ketoacidosis [5] who received the G to A 547 mutation from his father and an AG to CG transition at a splice site in exon 10 that led to skipping of exon 11 [11].

In a series of 26 patients there were 45 independent chromosomes and 30 different mutations. Only five were homozygous mutant. Expression analysis and the nature of mutation indicated that 24 of the mutations coded for absent activity. Only a minority of mutations led to appreciable residual activity. This would be expected to lead to a milder clinical phenotype, as was seen in one of the homozygotes who had the G145E mutation. The extensive heteroallelic nature of mutation was associated with a general absence of genotype/phenotype correlation. Mutant siblings had different clinical phenotypes. *In vitro* evidence of residual activity in fibroblasts was a better predictor of relatively mild disease. An absence of tiglylglycine in the urine suggests the presence of residual activity *in vitro* and was often associated with mild disease. Its absence does not exclude a severe phenotype, but its presence is a useful predictor of severe disease.

TREATMENT

The considerable heterogeneity in the severity of clinical presentation indicates that there should be individual programs of treatment. Nevertheless, it would appear prudent to restrict the intake of isoleucine in any patient with this disorder. Long fasting should be avoided [26], especially during intercurrent febrile illness or intestinal upset. In this situation intravenous glucose is indicated and may abort a ketoacidotic crisis.

The acute acidotic attack should be treated with copious amounts of water and electrolytes (Chapter 2, pp. 14 and 15). Carnitine is useful intravenously in the acute situation and orally long-term in order to esterify and remove tiglyl CoA and the other accumulated CoA esters.

DIFFERENTIAL DIAGNOSIS – RELATED DISORDERS OF KETOLYSIS

Patients have been observed in whom the clinical picture and pattern of excretion of 2-methyl-3-hydroxybutyric acid and

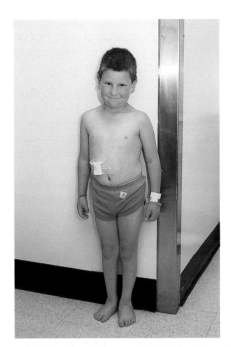

Figure 17.10   *Z.M., a boy with repeated episodes of vomiting and ketoacidosis, along with tiglyglycinuria and 2-methyl-3-hydroxybutyric aciduria which increased on administration of isoleucine, consistent with 3-oxothiolase deficiency. However, assay of the enzyme revealed normal activity. The incorporation of 1-^{14}C-2-methylbutyrate into macromolecules was 24 percent of control; in a series of patients with 3-oxothiolase deficiency the range was 2–31 percent of control.*

tiglylglycine are typical of 3-oxothiolase deficiency but the activity of the thiolase enzyme is normal (Figure 17.10). The patient illustrated was studied by Iden and colleagues [42] in their assessment of the pathway from ^{14}C-2-methylbutyrate to macromolecules, and an abnormality was demonstrated in the pathway that was equivalent to the milder patients with thiolase deficiency, indicating the presence of a defect in the pathway not yet identified.

Cytosolic acetoacetyl CoA thiolase deficiency has been reported in two patients with hypotonia and delayed development [47,48]. One was also ataxic and choreic. One patient had elevated levels of acetoacetate in blood and urine [48] the other did not; but had elevated levels of lactate and pyruvate and a low lactate to pyruvate ratio [47]. Abnormalities were found in the cytosolic thiolase, and the synthesis of cholesterol from acetate was reduced. Ketosis was reduced by restriction of fat intake, but there was no clinical improvement.

Succinyl CoA:3-oxoacid CoA transferase deficiency has been reported in patients [49–51] who presented with ketoacidosis in infancy and had repeated episodes of ketoacidosis with infections. Two patients died, as had four siblings. Activity of the transferase enzyme in fibroblasts was deficient, virtually completely in the patients who died [50,52] and 20 percent of control in the survivor. This enzyme catalyzes the conversion of acetoacetic acid to acetoacetyl CoA. It is thus a key enzyme in the utilization of acetoacetate and

3-hydroxybutyrate formed in liver and transported in the blood to peripheral tissues. The organic acid analysis of the urine revealed only 3-hydroxybutyrate, acetoacetate and 3-hydroxyisovaleric, all consistent with ketosis. The diagnosis may be suspected by the persistence of ketosis in the steady-state fed condition.

References

1   Daum RS, Lamm PH, Mamer OA, Scriver CR. A "new" disorder of isoleucine catabolism. *Lancet* 1971;**2**:1289.
2   Daum RS, Scriver CR, Mamer OA, *et al.* An inherited disorder of isoleucine catabolism causing accumulation of α-methylacetoacetate and α-methyl-β-hydroxybutyrate and intermittent metabolic acidosis. *Pediatr Res* 1973;**7**:149.
3   Pollitt RJ. The occurrence of substituted 3-methyl-3-hydroxyglutaric acids in urine in propionic acidemia and in β-ketothiolase deficiency. *Biomed Mass Spectrom* 1983;**4**:253.
4   Fukao T, Scriver CR, Kondo N, *et al.* The clinical phenotype and outcome of mitochondrial acetoacetyl-CoA thiolase deficiency (β-ketothiolase or T2 deficiency) in 26 enzymatically proved and mutation-defined patients. *Mol Genet Metab* 2001;**72**:109.
5   Saudubray JM, Specola N. Ketolysis defects: in *Inborn Metabolic Diseases* (eds Fernandes J, Saudubray J-M, Tada K) Springer-Verlag, Berlin; 1990:411.
6   Schutgens RBH, Middleton B, Blijj JF, *et al.* Beta-ketothiolase deficiency in a family confirmed by in vitro enzymatic assays in fibroblasts. *Eur J Pediatr* 1982;**139**:39.
7   Middleton B. The oxoacyl-coenzyme A thiolases of animal tissues. *Biochem J* 1973;**132**:717.
8   Middleton B, Bartlett K. The synthesis and characterization of 2-methyl-acetoacetyl coenzyme A and its use in the identification of the site of the defect in 2-methyl-acetoacetic and 2-methyl-3-hydroxybutyric aciduria. *Clin Chim Acta* 1983;**128**:291.
9   Fukao T, Yamaguchi S, Nagasawa H, *et al.* Molecular cloning of cDNA for human mitochondrial acetoacetyl-CoA thiolase and molecular analysis of 3-ketothiolase deficiency. *J Inherit Metab Dis* 1990;**13**:757.
10   Masuno M, Kano M, Fukao T, *et al.* Chromosome mapping of the human mitochondrial acetoacetyl-CoA thiolase gene to band 11q223-q231 by fluorescence *in situ* hybridization. *Cytogenet Cell Genet* 1992;**60**:121.
11   Fukao T, Yamaguchi S, Orii T, *et al.* Identification of three mutant alleles of the gene for mitochondrial acetoacetyl-Coenzyme A thiolase. *J Clin Invest* 1992;**89**:474.
12   Fukao T, Yamaguchi S, Orri T, *et al.* Molecular basis of 3-ketothiolase deficiency: Identification of an AG to AC substitution at the splice acceptor site of intron 10 causing exon 11 skipping. *Biochim Biophys Acta* 1992;**1139**:184.
13   Robinson JP, Feigin RD, Tenenbaum SM, Hillman RE. Hyperglycinemia with ketosis due to a defect in isoleucine catabolism. *Pediatrics* 1972;**50**:890.
14   Hillman RE, Keating JP. Ketothiolase deficiency as a cause of the ketotic hyperglycinemia syndrome. *Pediatrics* 1974;**53**:221.
15   Gompertz D, Saudubray JM, Charpentier C, *et al.* A defect in isoleucine metabolism associated with α-methyl-β-hydroxybutyric acid and α-methylacetoacetic aciduria. Quantitative *in vivo* and *in vitro* studies. *Clin Chim Acta* 1974;**57**:269.
16   Robinson BH, Sherwood G, Taylor J, *et al.* Acetoacetyl CoA thiolase deficiency. A cause of severe ketoacidosis in infancy simulating salicylism. *J Pediatr* 1979;**95**:228.
17   Henry CG, Strauss AW, Keating JP, Hillman RE. Congestive cardiomyopathy associated with β-ketothiolase deficiency. *J Pediatr* 1981;**99**:754.

18   Middleton B, Bartlett K, Romanos A, *et al*. 3-Ketothiolase deficiency. *Eur J Pediatr* 1986;**144**:586.

19   Hartlage P, Eller G, Carter L, *et al*. Mitochondrial acetoacetyl-CoA thiolase deficiency. *Biochem Med Metab Biol* 1986;**36**:198.

20   Saudubray JM, Specola N, Middleton B, *et al*. Hyperketotic states due to inherited defects of ketolysis. *Enzyme* 1987;**38**:80.

21   Halvorsen S, Stokke O, Jellum E. A variant form of 2-methyl-3-hydroxybutyric and 2-methylacetoacetic aciduria. *Acta Paediatr Scand* 1979;**68**:123.

22   Hiyama K, Sakura N, Matsumoto T, Kuhara T. Deficient beta-ketothiolase activity in leukocytes from a patient with 2-methylacetoacetic aciduria. *Clin Chim Acta* 1986;**155**:189.

23   Leonard JV, Middleton B, Seakins JWT. Acetoacetyl CoA thiolase deficiency presenting as ketotic hypoglycemia. *Pediatr Res* 1987;**21**:211.

24   Middleton B, Gray RGF, Bennett MJ. Two cases of beta-ketothiolase deficiency: a comparison. *J Inherit Metab Dis* 1984;**7**:131.

25   Ozand PT, Rashed MR, Gascon GG, *et al*. 3-Ketothiolase deficiency: a review and four new patients with neurologic symptoms. *Brain Dev* 1994;**16**:(suppl) 38.

26   Sovik O. Mitochondrial 2-methylacetoacetyl-CoA thiolase deficiency: an inborn error of isoleucine and ketone body metabolism. *J Inherit Metab Dis* 1993;**16**:46.

27   Henry GC, Strauss AW, Keating JP, Hillman RE. Congestive cardiomyopathy associated with beta-ketothiolase deficiency. *J Pediatr* 1981;**99**:754.

28   Gibson KM, Feigenbaum ASJ. Phenotypically mild presentation in a patient with 2-methylacetoacetyl-coenzyme A (beta-keto) thiolase deficiency. *J Inherit Metab Dis* 1997;**20**:712.

29   Sebetta G, Bachmann C, Giardini O, *et al*. Beta-ketothiolase deficiency with favourable evolution. *J Inherit Metab Dis* 1987;**10**:405.

30   Merinero B, Perez-Cerda C, Garcia MJ, *et al*. Two siblings with different clinical conditions. *J Inherit Metab Dis* 1987;**10**:(suppl 2) 276.

31   Landaas S. Accumulation of 3-hydroxyisobutyric acid 2-methyl-3-hydroxybutyric acid and 3-hydroxyisovaleric acid in ketoacidosis. *Clin Chim Acta* 1975;**64**:143.

32   Sweetman L, Weyler W, Nyhan WL, *et al*. Abnormal metabolites of isoleucine in a patient with propionyl-CoA carboxylase deficiency. *Biomed Mass Spectrom* 1978;**5**:198.

33   Aramaki S, Lehotay D, Sweetman L, *et al*. Urinary excretion of 2-methylacetoacetate 2-methyl-3-hydroxybutyrate and tiglylglycine after isoleucine loading in the diagnosis of 2-methylacetoacetyl-CoA thiolase deficiency. *J Inherit Metab Dis* 1991;**14**:63.

34   Duran M, Bruinvis L, Ketting D, *et al*. The identification of (E)-2-methylglutaconic acid a new isoleucine metabolite in the urine of patients with β-ketothiolase deficiency propionic acidemia and methylmalonic academia. *Biomed Mass Spectrom* 1982;**9**:1.

35   Rashed MR, Ozand PT, Bucknall M, Little D. Diagnosis of inborn errors of metabolism from blood spots by acylcarnitines and amino acids profiling using automated electrospray tandem mass spectrometry. *Pediatr Res* 1995;**38**:324.

36   Jakobs C, Sweetman L, Nyhan WL. Hydroxy acid metabolites of branched-chain amino acids in amniotic fluid. *Clin Chim Acta* 1984;**140**:157.

37   Middleton B. Identification of heterozygotes for the defect of mitochondrial 3-ketothiolase causing 2-methyl-3-hydroxy-butyric aciduria. *J Inherit Metab Dis* 1987;**10**:(suppl 2) 270.

38   Gibson KM, Lee CF, Kamali V, Sovik O. A coupled assay detecting defects in fibroblast isoleucine degradation distal to enoyl-CoA hydratase: application to 3-oxothiolase deficiency. *Clin Chim Acta* 1992;**205**:127.

39   Nagasawa H, Yamaguchi S, Orii T, *et al*. Heterogeneity of defects in mitochondrial acetoacetyl-CoA thiolase biosynthesis in fibroblasts from four patients with 3-ketothiolase deficiency. *Pediatr Res* 1989;**26**:145.

40   Yamaguchi S, Orii T, Sakura N, *et al*. Defect in biosynthesis of mitochondrial acetoacetyl-coenzyme A thiolase in cultured fibroblasts from a boy with 3-ketothiolase deficiency. *J Clin Invest* 1988;**81**:813.

41   Sovik O, Saudubray JM, Munnich A, Sweetman L. Genetic complementation of analysis of mitochondrial 2-methylacetoacetyl-CoA thiolase deficiency in cultured fibroblasts. *J Inherit Metab Dis* 1992;**15**:359.

42   Iden P, Middleton B, Robinson B, *et al*. 3-Oxothiolase activities and [^{14}C]-2-methylbutanoic acid incorporation in cultured fibroblasts from 13 cases of suspected 3-oxothiolase deficiency. *Pediatr Res* 1990;**28**:518.

43   Yamaguchi S, Fukao T, Nagasawa H, *et al*. 3-Ketothiolase deficiency: Molecular heterogeneity of the enzyme defect and cloning of the cDNA: in Fatty Acid Oxidation: Clinical Biochemical and Molecular Aspects Prog *Clin Biol Res* 1990;**321**:673.

44   Fukao T, Kamijo K, Osumi T, *et al*. Molecular cloning and nucleotide sequencing of cDNA encoding the entire precursor of rat mitochondrial acetoacetyl-CoA thiolase. *J Biochem* 1989;**106**:197.

45   Fukao T, Yamaguchi S, Kano M, *et al*. Molecular cloning and sequence of the complementary DNA encoding human mitochondrial acetoacetyl-coenzyme A thiolase and study of the variant enzymes in cultured fibroblasts from patients with 3-ketothiolase deficiency. *J Clin Invest* 1990;**86**:2086.

46   Fukao T, Yamaguchi S, Tomatsu S, *et al*. Evidence for a structural mutation (347Ala to Thr) in a German family with 3-ketothiolase deficiency. *Biochem Biophys Res Commun* 1991;**179**:124.

47   De Groot CJ, Luit-De Haan G, Hulstaert CE, Hommes FA. A patient with severe neurologic symptoms and acetoacetyl-CoA thiolase deficiency. *Pediatr Res* 1977;**11**:1112.

48   Bennett MJ, Hosking GP, Smith MF, *et al*. Biochemical investigations on a patient with a defect in cystosolic acetoacetyl-CoA thiolase associated with mental retardation. *J Inherit Metab Dis* 1984;**7**:125.

49   Cornblath M, Gingell RL, Fleming GA, *et al*. A new syndrome of ketoacidosis in infancy. *J Pediatr* 1971;**79**:413.

50   Spence MW, Murphy MG, Cook HW, *et al*. Succinyl-CoA: 3-ketoacid CoA-transferase deficiency. A "new" phenotype? *Pediatr Res* 1973;**7**:394.

51   Middleton B, Day R, Lombers A, Saudubray JM. Infantile ketoacidosis associated with decreased activity of succinyl- CoA: 3-ketoacid CoA-transferase. *J Inherit Metab Dis* 1987;**10**:(suppl 2) 273.

52   Tildon JT, Cornblath M. Succinyl-CoA: 3-ketoacid CoA transferase deficiency. *J Clin Invest* 1972;**51**:493.

PART 2

Disorders of amino acid metabolism

Albinism

MAJOR PHENOTYPIC EXPRESSION

Absence of normal pigmentation in the skin and hair, translucent irides, hypopigmented ocular fundus, nystagmus, photophobia, misdirection of optic chiasmatic fibers, and in the classic form of oculocutaneous albinism, absent activity of tyrosinase in the melanocytes.

INTRODUCTION

Oculocutaneous albinism represents a group of genetically determined diseases that affect a considerable population. It was recognized by Garrod [1] in 1908 as an inborn error of metabolism in which he postulated a defect in an intracellular enzyme of melanin synthesis. Albinism is found in fish, birds and mammals, including all human races. The primary defect maybe restricted to the pigment cell (melanocyte) system or may involve many cell types, among them the melanocytes. The melanocytes are specialized cells in which the biosynthesis of melanin occurs in the melanosomes. The cells arise from melanoblasts that develop early in embryogenesis in the neural crest and the neuroectoderm. Melanocytes migrate to the choroid, iris and retina and to the skin where melanosomes are transported to keratinocytes and hair producing pigment.

Melanin is a product of the metabolism of tyrosine (Figure 18.1) [2]. The first two steps, the conversions to dihydroxyphenylalanine (DOPA) and DOPAquinone, are catalyzed by the same enzyme, tyrosinase (EC 1.14.18.1), a copper-containing oxidase expressed only in melanocytes. The remaining steps of melanogenesis can proceed nonenzymically. Melanin exists in nature as a polymer of high molecular weight. Only part of the repeating structure is illustrated in Figure 18.1. The entire transformation takes place in the melanosome. There are two major melanin pigments: eumelanin, the black or brown coloration; and pheomelanin, the red or yellow (Figures 18.1, 18.2). Each is produced subsequent to the formation of DOPAquinone [3,4]. The pheomelanin pathway begins with cysteinyl-DOPA followed by ring closure and polymerization. Both types of melanin may be synthesized in a single melanocyte, and mixtures of the two types of melanin may occur. Melanogenesis is stimulated by ultraviolet light and by melanocyte-stimulating hormone. In human albinos the melanocytes are present in normal number and appearance, and they contain melanosomes. These organelles appear ultrastructurally normal, but they do not contain melanin pigment.

Oculocutaneous albinism is characterized not only by hypopigmentation but by some distinctive optic abnormalities in addition to the lack of pigment which permits visualization of choroidal vessels with the ophthalmoscope and transillumination of the globe. The fovea is hypoplastic, foveal reflex reduced or absent, and visual acuity low. Nystagmus is regularly observed, as are head posturing designed to reduce the movement of the eyes. The abnormal decussation of the optic nerve fibers at the chiasm is an impressive anatomic concomitant of albinism that is present in a variety of mammals as well as humans [5,6]. In normal individuals, all fibers projecting from the nasal retina cross at the chiasm to the contralateral side of the brain, while the temporal fibers remain and terminate on the ipsilateral side of the brain. In albinism, fibers from the foveal and temporal retina cross to

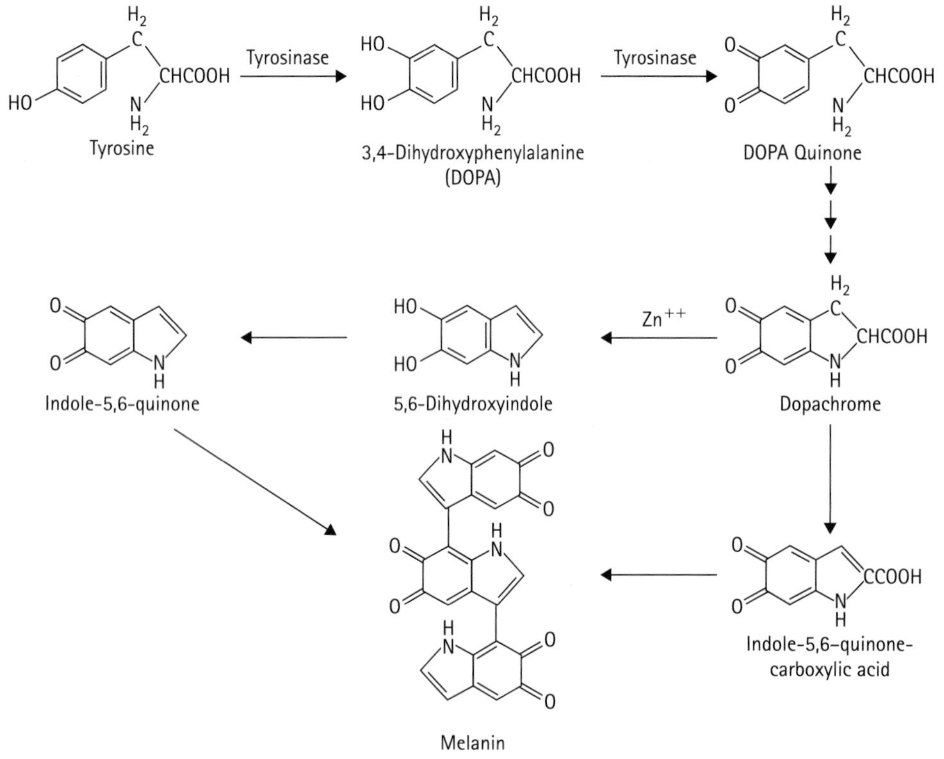

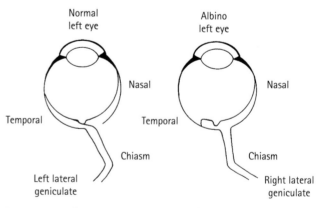

Figure 18.1 *The formation of eumelanin from tyrosine. The rate limiting steps is the hydroxylation of tyrosine. Eumelanin is the pigment responsible for the appearance of the black Labrador Retriever.*

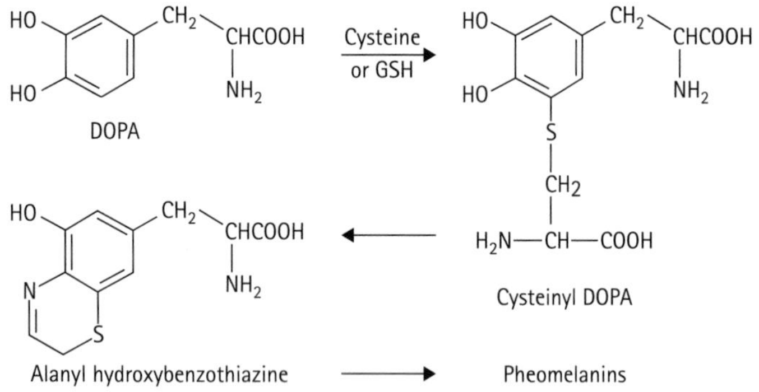

Figure 18.2 *The formation of pheomelanin from DOPA. Abbreviations include DOPA, dihydroxyphenylalanine, and GSH, glutathione. Pheomelanin is the pigment responsible for the appearance of the Golden Retriever.*

the contralateral side (Figure 18.3). This routing alteration can be detected by visual evoked responses [5]. The abnormal projection is not a result of the altered pigmentation because it has been shown that a majority of retinal ganglion fibers are present in normally pigmented cats heterozygous for tyrosine negative albinism [6]. In addition there is foveal hypoplasia. Patients with albinism also have abnormal pigment in the inner ear and they display abnormal brain-stem-evoked responses (BAER) [7]; and they may be more sensitive to drug-or noise-induced hearing loss.

Albinism is clinically and genetically heterogeneous. Oculocutaneous albinism is distinguished from ocular albinism in which only the eye is included. In oculocutaneous albinism a number of specific types have been distinguished (Table 18.1). The molecular biology of this group of disorders has advanced appreciably. To date the variation identified has been allelic and transmission has been autosomal recessive. Ocular albinism may be autosomal or X-linked (Table 18.2).

Oculocutaneous albinism (OCA1 and OCA3) is caused by mutations in two genes (TYR and TYRP1) which code for

Figure 18.3 *Schematic representation of the decussation of temporal fibers in normal and albino eye.*

two proteins with very similar amino acid sequences, tyrosinase and tyrosinase-related protein. These are homologues of the mouse genes, albino (*o*) and brown (*b*). A third human member of the tyrosinase gene family (DCT) is homologous

Table 18.1 *Oculocutaneous albinism*

Disorder common name	Classification	Protein	Gene	Skin color	Hair color	Skin tanning	Pigmented Nevi-freckles	Eye color	Nystagmus	Other
Tyrosinase Negative	OCA1A	Tyrosinase	TYR	Pink-white	White	0	0	Gray-blue; red reflex	+	Visual acuity reduced
Minimal Pigment OCA, Yellow OCA, Platinum OCA, Temperature-sensitive OCA	OCA1B	Tyrosinase		White at birth; cream or tan later	White at birth; blond to brown later	Possible	+	Blue in infancy, darkens in some with age	+	Visual acuity reduced
Tyrsinase-positive	OCA2	P protein	P	White-yellow, darkens with age. Caucasian: yellow-blond. African-American: yellow to dark yellow	Hypopigmented	0	+	Blue, hazel	+	
Brown, Rufous	OCA3	Tyrosine-related proteins	TYRP1	Light brown; reddish brown	Beige to light brown; red to mahogany	+	0	Blue-gray to light brown, red-brown hazel	+	Africans and New Guineans
Orthologue of murine under white (uw)	OCA4	MATP (membrane associated transporter protein)	MATP (AIM1)	Similar to OCA2	Hypopigmented	0	0	Hypopigmented	+	Visual acuity reduced
Hermansky-Pudlak		HPS membrane proteins	HPS1 HPS2 HPS3 HPS4	Creamy	White, blond, red, brown	0	++	Blue-gray to brown, age-dependent	+	Platelet abnormalities
Chediak-Higashi Syndrome		LYST membrane protein	CHS1	Creamy to gray	Light brown to blond-silver gray metallic sheen		+	Blue-brown	+/-	Giant lysosomal granules, pancytopenia, malignancy
Griscelli Disease	GS1	Nyosin type 5A GTPase, Rab27a	MYO5A		Silver-gray sheen					GS1-Neurologic; GS2-Immuno-deficiency, hemophagocytosis
	GS2		Rab27a							
Cross Syndrome				Pink to pink-white	White to light blond		+	Gray-blue		Oligophrenia, micro-ophthalmia, athetosis, gingival fibrosis

Table 18.2 *Ocular albinism*

Type	Fundal pigment	Visual acuity	Nystagmus	Melanosomes	Mapping	Gene	Protein
X-linked ocular albinism OA1 (Nettleship Falls)	Male 0 Female mosaic	20/50 20/400	+	Abnormal, giant and normal	Xp22.2–22.3	OA1	Membrane protein
X-linked ocular albinism OA2 (Forsius-Eriksson) (Aland Island eye disease)	Male 0 Female normal	Moderate myopia	+	Normal	Xq12–21		
X-linked ocular albinism and sensorineural deafness	Male 0 Female normal	Moderate myopia	+	Macromelanosomes	Xq		
Autosomal recessive ocular albinism	0–+	20/100	+	Normal	?		
Ocular albinism-Lentigenes-Deafness-Sensorineural syndrome Autosomal dominant	0	20/200	+	Macromelanosomes	?		

to the mouse slaty (*slt*) locus; it codes for tyrosinase-related protein 2, for which a human disease has not been described.

There have been major advances in the molecular biology of oculocutaneous albinism, notably in the understanding of the tyrosinase gene. The gene (TYR) is located on chromosome 11q14-q21 [8]. The gene contains five exons [9]; exon 1 contains 273 codons in over half of the coding region. Six different polymorphic sites have been identified in the gene, and they have been used to develop molecular haplotypes useful in population studies on the origin of mutation [10]. A number of mutations have been identified [10,11]. Most are missense mutations, but there are nonsense mutations, splice site mutations and frameshifts [10] and at least one deletion of the entire gene [12].

Tyrosinase-positive oculocutaneous albinism, OCA2, has been mapped to chromosome 15q11.2-q12 [13]. The locus was found to be linked to loci D15510 and D15513 in the area deleted in the Prader-Willi and Angelman syndromes. This region is homologous to that of the *p* pink-eyed dilute locus in the mouse [14]. This established the P human gene that maps to 15q11.q2.13 as a candidate for the OCA2 gene. A patient with Prader-Willi syndrome and OCA2 was found to have two deletions in the P locus [15]. More recently, members of an original Maryland isolate of OCA2 were found to be homozygous for a 2.7 kb deletion in the P gene [16]. This gene appears to have an African origin [16]. A number of point mutations have been found in the P gene in patients with OCA2. The gene product of the P protein functions in ion transport into the melanosome and maintenance of its acid pH [17,18].

Two mutations have been found in the TYRP1 gene in OCA3, a stop codon (S166X) [19] and a deletion (1104delA) [20]. These two mutations accounted for nearly all of the individuals with OCA3 studied.

In OCA-4 mutation has been found in the gene on chromosome 5p, which codes for a membrane-associated transport protein (MATP), which has also been referred to as AIM-1 (antigen in melanoma).

Cutaneous hypopigmentation occurs in a number of disorders. When it is localized to areas in the skin and hair it is referred as piebaldism. There may be a white forelock, which is often triangular in shape with the apex pointing backward. The white area always includes the skin beneath the forelock. There may be other patches of depigmented hair. Lack of pigment in the skin tends to be ventral in distribution, occurring in patches over the anterior trunk or extremities. This condition is inherited in an autosomal dominant fashion [21]. The defective gene is the KIT gene on chromosome 4q12, which codes for the tyrosine kinase receptor for mast cells growth factor, and a number of mutations have been delineated [22]. Waardenburg syndrome, in which partial albinism is associated with deafness, heterochromia iridis and lateral displacement of medial canthi (telecanthi) (WSI), is also dominant; types 1 and 3 are due to mutations in the PAX3 homeobox transcription factor gene on chromosome 2q35 [23] type 2 is due to mutation in the MITF gene on chromosome 3p12-14 for the bHLH transcription factor involved in melanocyte survival. Hypopigmentation is also seen in the Prader-Willi and Angelman syndromes [24,25], in which there are deletions in chromosome 15q11.2-q12, a region to which the P gene, which is defective in OCA2, has been mapped [13,26].

CLINICAL ABNORMALITIES

Tyrosinase-negative oculocutaneous albinism – OCA1

Patients with mutations in the tyrosinase gene and abnormality of melanocyte tyrosinase in classic oculocutaneous

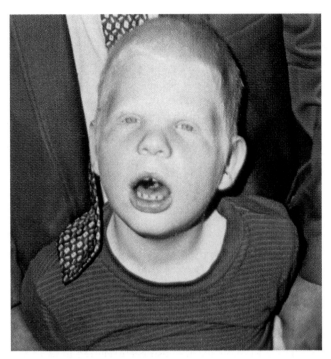

Figure 18.4   *T.G., oculocutaneous albinism. OCA1. This boy was one of two brothers, both albino and both severely retarded. The intelligence of patients with all forms of oculocutaneous albinism is usually normal. He had snow-white hair and pink-red skin. The irides were pale and gray, and there was a pupillary red reflex.*

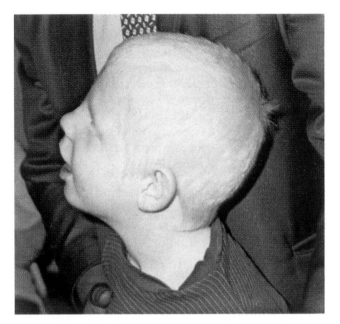

Figure 18.5   *T.G. The lateral projection illustrates the white eyelashes.*

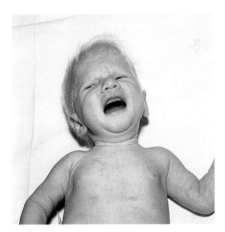

Figure 18.6   *C.B. This boy with oculocutaneous albinism also had coarctation of the aorta.*

albinism have a total absence of pigment in the skin, hair and eyes (Table 18.1). There is considerable heterogeneity dependent on the amount of residual tyrosinase activity, but all patients with OCA1 have hypopigmentation at birth.

OCA1A

In these patients the hair is snow-white or milk-white and the skin has a pink or reddish hue (Figures 18.4–18.6). No pigmented areas, such as freckles develop in the skin. The iris is blue or gray, and the pupils display a red reflex at all ages. No visible pigment can be seen in the fundus. Patients with this form of albinism have severe nystagmus and photophobia [27]. They squint even in moderate light. Strabismus is common. Visual acuity is reduced and gets worse with age [27]. Many are legally blind.

Tyrosinase activity in hair roots is absent. Studies of tyrosinase *in vitro* can be assessed autoradiographically following incubation with ^{14}C-labeled tyrosine [28], or by visualizing pigment formation directly following incubation with substrate quantities of tyrosine or DOPA [29]. Tests may be performed using hair follicles, which can be incubated directly following careful plucking of the hair. Infants and children may have immature development of the pigment system. Therefore, it is recommended that the testing of hair roots be done after 2 years-of-age. Electron microscopy of the skin or hair roots reveals melanosomes of normal appearance. They do not function to produce melanin in the absence of tyrosinase.

OCA1B

OCA1B variants are the result of mutations that code for tyrosinase enzymes with a certain amount of residual activity. These leaky mutations lead to a phenotype with some pigment; the older terms yellow, minimal pigment, and temperature sensitive OCA (Table 18.1) are now recognized as part of a spectrum of variation in the gene. These patients have also been referred to as having Amish albinism [30]. The minimal pigment designation group reflected the development of a minimal amount of pigment in the irides in the first 10 years of life [31]. The yellow color is that of pheomelanin, which is produced preferentially when DOPAquinone is in small supply, because of the high affinity of the compound for sulfhydryl compounds, leading to cysteinyl DOPA and pheomelanin. The patients may have considerable pigment and may resemble more the tyrosinase positive OCA2 albino. Affected individuals have generalized albinism and are quite white at birth, indistinguishable from OCA1A, but over the first few years they develop relatively normal skin pigmentation and yellow or blond hair. The irides are blue in infancy but may develop a tan pigment or freckles with age. Ocular manifestations, such as nystagmus, decreased visual acuity, retinal hypopigmentation and red reflex, are persistent in adult life. In these patients the tyrosinase response of the hair bulbs may be confusing, but is usually negative [32].

An interesting OCA1B variant was referred to as temperature-sensitive oculocutaneous albinism [32,33]. Pigment at birth is no different from OCA1A, while later, certainly by puberty, a pattern of pigment develops which is related to temperature. The hair of the arms becomes a light red-brown and that of the legs, a darker brown, while the scalp and the axillary hair remain white. The skin does not tan. Tyrosinase activity in hair bulbs was found to be temperature sensitive. Above 35°C, the activity was defective. This was consistent with the phenotypic development of pigmentation in the cooler extremity areas of the body. This pattern is similar to that of the Siamese cat and the Himalayan mouse.

Tyrosinase-positive oculocutaneous albinism – OCA2

In this form of albinism there is some color in the hair and irides at birth and changes to yellow or even red with age [34–36]. The skin is white or cream colored. In Blacks, it is usually easy to distinguish this yellow-haired, yellow-skinned phenotype (Figure 18.7) from that of the tyrosinase negative.

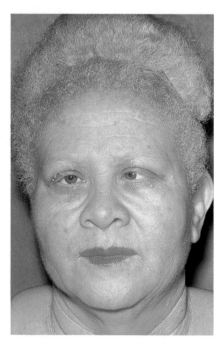

Figure 18.7 *O.C. Black female with albinism. There was a certain amount of pigment in the face, and the hair was yellow.*

In Caucasians there is more overlap; the skin may be pink. Pigmented nevi and freckles are common in the tyrosinase positive albinos. There may be lentigines, but the skin does not tan. The iris color may be blue-gray early, but brown pigment increases with age, especially at the pupillary border. Nystagmus and photophobia are usually less severe than in tyrosinase negative patients. Strabismus, central scotomata and partial aniridia maybe observed.

Incubation of hair bulbs with tyrosine yields microscopically discernible pigment [34,37]. The ultrastructure of the melanocyte is normal.

TYRP1-Related oculocutaneous albinism – OCA3

OCA3 was originally referred to as brown oculocutaneous albinism (Table 18.1), because cultured melanocytes from a patient produced small quantities of a brown, rather than black, melanin. This entity found in Africans and New Guineans, has been related to the Brown (*b*) locus in mice. It has also been linked to the TYRP2 human gene that codes for the TYRP 1 protein, precipitable with tyrosinase antisera and DHICA (dihydroindole-quinonoid carboxylic acid) oxidase activity. The gene was mapped to chromosome 9p, and a mutation found in the proband, a ΔA368 in exon 6, a one base-pair shift that leads to premature termination at 384 [19,38,39,40]. What had been called rufous, or red OCA was found to map to the same locus, and 50 percent of South Africans with this phenotype had the deletion ΔA1104. Individuals with red hair and reddish-brown skin have also been called xanthous albinos. Among the South Africans, patients had hazel or brown irides [41]. Many do not have the nystagmus, strabismus or foveal hypoplasia of OCA, and optic nerve misrouting has not been demonstrated [41].

OCA4 – Orthologue of mouse under white gene – MATP

Patients with OCA4 were originally thought to have OCA2. They have typical hypopigmentation of skin and hair. Optic nerve misrouting leads to nystagmus, strabismus and low visual activity.

GENETICS AND PATHOGENESIS

All forms of oculocutaneous albinism are transmitted as autosomal recessive traits [42,43]. In groups of albinos there is a high level of parental consanguinity. It was clear early on that more than one gene was involved because in offspring of the mating of two albinos, a number were reported to be normal [44]. These observations indicated that not only was there more than one gene, which was also indicated by data on tyrosinase positive and negative albinism, but that some genes were not allelic.

Sequence analysis in OCA1 yielded an additional cytosine in exon 2 in a Japanese subject in 1989 [11] that led to a premature termination and a truncated protein. Now more than a hundred different mutations have been reported in OCA1, most of them in Caucasian individuals [10,12,45].

Most of the mutations identified have been in OCA1A, in which there is no residual enzyme activity. Expression studies have also revealed no activity [46]. Many are compounds of two different mutations, and in a moderate number the second mutation has not been identified. Among Caucasian populations, the two most frequent mutations were P81L, a proline-to-leucine change [47], and T373K, a threonine-to-lysine [48].

The P81L mutation abolished an Hae111 restriction site, permitting rapid screening. A G47D mutation was found in exon 1, a single haplotype, in 11 of 12 families studied in Puerto Rico consistent with a common founder [49]. This type of OCA1 is homologous to temperature-sensitive albinism of the Siamese cat and the Himalayan mouse. In fact, the mutation in the mouse has been found (a histidine to an arginine) on codon 420 [50], only two from the site of human mutation. Two frequent mutations in Japanese populations have been R77Q, an arginine to glutamine change and a single base insertion at codon 310, insC 929 [51]. Missense mutations have tended to cluster in four domains of the gene [10]. Two have been in putative copper binding sites and a third at the amino terminal of the peptide.

In OCA1B, in which the enzyme has 5–10 percent residual activity, three mutations have been reported [10,52]. In the Amish, in whom this phenotype was first described a P406L, proline-to-leucine alteration was found [52], and affected individuals were homozygous. Other mutations include V275F and R403S, respectively a valine-to-phenylalanine and arginine-to-serine change, the former in a compound with P81L [53]. Among patients studied to date the pigmentary phenotype correlated only modestly with the genotype or the measured activity of tyrosinase in hair bulbs, but even among homozygous individuals for P406L there are varying phenotypes; so there must be other factors influencing pigmentation.

A temperature-sensitive variant has been found, R422Q, an arginine-to-glutamine alteration [33,54]. Expression of the mutation and hair bulb studies indicated that tyrosinase enzyme is inactive above 35°C.

In OCA2 the 2.7 Kb deletion of exon 7 in the P gene found in the original African-American family [16] is the most common mutation [55], reaching allele frequencies as high as 90 percent in Africa [56]. A full spectrum of other mutations has been observed, missense, frameshift, splice-site and deletion [57]. Albinism is also prevalent in American Indians. In the Navajo OCA2 is caused by a 122.5 Kb deletion of the P gene [58]. This mutation was not found in other American Indian albinos, or in any other ethnic group. Both break points were in long interspersed nucleotide elements (LINEs); they were oppositely oriented and not homologous in sequence, suggesting a mechanism of nonhomologous end joining (NHEJ) in causing the deletion. The P gene is in an area rich in repetitive

sequences; chromosomal rearrangements leading to the Angelman and Prader-Willi syndrome are in this area.

Gene modification has recently been demonstrated in OCA2 [59]. Variation in the melanocortin receptor (MC1R) is associated with red hair in the normal population. In eight probands with OCA who had red hair at birth all had mutations in the P gene; in six of eight who continued to have red hair after birth there were mutations in the MC1R gene. It is not possible to assay for function of the P protein. Polymorphisms may be distinguished from pathogenic mutations by transfection of murine melanocytes that are P-deficient [60].

In patients with OCA3 the 1104delA mutation was found in 50 percent of 19 patients with rufous albinism [20]. The S116X mutation was found in 45 percent [19]. These mutations appear to determine a relatively mild phenotype, and sibs compoundly heterozygous for these two mutations had even more pigment, resembling individuals with OCA2 [61].

Mutation has also been identified in OCA4. In a Turkish patient homozygous G to A transition in the splice acceptor site of exon 2 would be expected to lead to skipping of exon 2 [61].

Albinism is common among genetic diseases. OCA2 is the most common type of albinism worldwide; it occurs in 1 in 3900 South African Bantus [13]. OCA1 has been estimated at 1 in 39 000 in US Caucasians and 1 in 28 000 in US Blacks. It is common in American Indians [62,63].

Differential diagnosis

In the Chediak-Higashi syndrome [64] (Table 18.1) tyrosinase-positive oculocutaneous pigment dilution is associated with giant peroxidase-positive lysosomal granules in the leukocytes, neutropenia, thrombocytopenia, folic acid deficient anemia, neurologic abnormalities and susceptibility to infections and to lymphoma or leukemia. The melanocytes contain giant melanosomes. Visual evoked potentials reveal misrouted optic fibers. The CHS1 gene, which codes for the LYST transmembrane protein has been found to contain frameshift and nonsense mutations in patients with this disease. mRNA levels are reduced [65].

In the Hermansky-Pudlak syndrome [66,67], universal albinism and all of the ocular characteristics of albinism are associated with bleeding, platelet abnormalities and large pigment-containing reticuloendothelial cells with storage of ceroid, pulmonary fibrosis and granulomatous colitis. It is common in Puerto Rico. In this population there is a common 16bp duplication in the HPS1 gene on chromosome 10q; homozygous individuals have restrictive fibrotic pulmonary disease [68]. A number of other mutations observed lead to truncated proteins. In two patients, siblings, mutations have been observed in the HPS2 gene on chromosome 5q [69]. Actually there are also patients with mutations on HSP3 and HSP4 genes, the latter on chromosome 12 [70]. The latter patients have a severe Hermansky-Pudlak phenotype, like that of HSP1; and melanocytes from HSP4 patients are also deficient in HSP1, indicating interaction between the two proteins.

In the Cross syndrome, hypopigmentation is associated with a relative deficiency of melanosomes and with micro-ophthalmia, cataracts, gingival fibromatosis and cerebral abnormalities [71]. In the Griscelli syndrome [72], silver-gray hair and scattered areas of hypo- and hyperpigmentation are associated with neutropenia, thrombocytopenia and recurrent bacterial infections.

Large clusters of pigment are distributed unevenly in the hair shaft. Distinct groups of patients have either a neuro-logic disorder in which there is severe developmental delay (GS1) or an immunologic disease (GS2). In GS1, patients have mutations in the myosin 5A gene (MYO5A) that encodes a myosin Va motor protein [73]. Patients with GS2 have immunologic deficiency and hemophagocytosis; they have mutations in the small GTPase Rab27a. Both the GS1 and GS2 genes map to the same chromosmal 15q21.1 region. A third form (GS3) has been related to mutation in the melanophilin gene that codes a member of the Rab effector family [73]. The phenotype was restricted to hypopigmenta-tion. The three GS proteins form a complex involved in melanosome transport. A defect in any one leads to identical dilution of pigment.

In ocular albinism (Table 18.2, p. 114) the pigmentary abnormality is confined to the eyes and does not affect the hair or skin. The iris is light blue but may develop pigment with age, while the retina does not. Head nodding is usually confined to infancy. Nystagmus may also improve with age. Photophobia is usually severe and visual acuity reduced. In the X-linked disorder, heterozygous females may display a mosaic pattern of pigment in the fundus and translucent iri-des [74]. Diagnosis may be made by electron microscopic identification of macromelanosomes in skin or hair bulbs. In a less severe form of ocular hypopigmentation, females may not have the mosaic retinal pattern [75]. A considerable vari-ety of mutations has been reported, including deletion of the entire gene [76,77]. Autosomal recessive and dominant forms have been reported [78]. None has been defined on a molec-ular basis.

TREATMENT

Avoidance of solar radiation, by the use of hats and long sleeves and pants and the use of sun screens with an SPF rating of 25 or more, is important because of the risk of developing skin cancer, including malignant melanoma [79]. Tinted glasses are helpful for the photophobia. Surgery for strabismus may be cosmetically advantageous, but it does not improve vision, which is a consequence of the anomalous decussation of the optic tracts in the brain. Corrective eyeglasses improve visual acuity. A national organization of albinism and hypopigmen-tation (NOAH) (www.albinism.org) provides information and meetings for patients and families to interact. A booklet *Facts About Albinism* is available from the University of Minnesota (www.cbc.umn.edu/iac).

References

1 Garrod AE. Inborn errors of metabolism The Croonian lectures. Lecture II. *Lancet* 1908;**2**:73.
2 Lerner AB, Fitzpatrick TB. Biochemistry of melanin formation. *Physiol Rev* 1950;**30**:91.
3 Prota G. Some new aspects of eumelanin chemistry. *Prog Clin Biol Res* 1988;**256**:101.
4 Thody AJ, Higgins EM, Wakamatsu K, *et al.* Pheomelanin as well as eumelanin is present in human epidermis. *J Invest Dermatol* 1991;**97**:340.
5 Creel D, O'Donnell FE, Witkop CJ. Visual system anomalies in human ocular albinos. *Science* 1978;**201**:931.
6 Leventhal AG, Vitek DJ, Creel DJ. Abnormal visual pathways in normally pigmented cats that are heterozygous for albinism. *Science* 1985;**229**:1395.
7 Creel DJ, Garber SR, King RA, Witkop CJ Jr. Auditory brainstem anomalies in human albinos. *Science* 1980;**209**:1253.
8 Barton DE, Kwon BS, Francke U. Human tyrosinase gene mapped to chromosome 11 (q14-q21) defines second region of homology with mouse chromosome 7. *Genomics* 1988;**3**:17.
9 Giebel LB, Strunk KM, Spritz RA. Organization and nucleotide sequences of the human tyrosinase gene and a truncated tyrosinase-related segment. *Genomics* 1991;**9**:435.
10 Oetting WS, King RA. Molecular basis of Type 1 (tyrosinase-related) oculocutaneous albinism: mutations and polymorphisms of the human tyrosine gene. *Hum Mutat* 1993;**2**:1.
11 Tomita Y, Takeda A, Okinaga S, *et al.* Human oculocutaneous albinism caused by a single base insertion in the tyrosinase gene. *Biochem Biophys Res Commun* 1989;**164**:990.
12 Oetting WS, King RA. Molecular basis of albinism: Mutations and polymorphisms of pigmentation genes associated with albinism. *Hum Mutat* 1999;**13**:99.
13 Ramsay M, Colman MA, Stevens G, *et al.* The tyrosinase-positive oculocutaneous albinism locus maps to chromosome 15q112-q12. *Am J Hum Genet* 1992;**51**:879.
14 Rinchik EM, Bultman SJ, Horsthemke B, *et al.* A gene for the mouse pink-eyed dilution locus and for human type II oculocutaneous albinism. *Nature* 1993;**361**:72.
15 Lee S-T, Nicholls RD, Bundey S, *et al.* Mutations of the P gene in oculocutaneous albinism ocular albinism and Prader-Willi syndrome plus albinism. *N Engl J Med* 1994;**330**:529.
16 Durham-Pierre D, Gardner JM, Nakatsu Y, *et al.* African origin of a common mutation of the human P gene in African American tyrosinase positive oculocutaneous albinism (OCA2). *Nat Genet* 1994;**7**:176.
17 Puri N, Brilliant MH. The function of the pink-eyed dilution protein [Abstract]. *Pigment Cell Res* 1998;**11**:174.
18 Bhatnagar V, Anjaiah S, Puri N, *et al.* pH of melanosomes of B16 murine melanoma is acidic: Its physiological importance in the regulation of melanin biosynthesis. *Arch Biochem Biophys* 1993;**307**:183.
19 Boissy RE, Zhao H, Oetting WS, *et al.* Mutation in and lack of expression of tyrosinase-related protein-1 (TRP-1) in melanocytes from an individual with brown oculocutaneous albinism: A new subtype of albinism classified as "OCA3". *Am J Hum Genet* 1996;**48**:1145.
20 Manga P, Kromberg JG, Box NF, *et al.* Rufous oculocutaneous albinism in southern African blacks is caused by mutations in the TYRP1 gene. *Am J Hum Genet* 1997;**61**:1095.
21 Jimbow K, Fitzpatrick TB, Szabo G, Hori Y. Congenital circumscribed hypomelanosis: A characterization based on electron microscopic study of tuberous sclerosis nevus depigmentosus and piebaldism. *J Invest Dermatol* 1975;**64**:50.

22 Spritz RA, Holmes SA, Ramesar R, *et al*. Mutations of the KIT (mast/stem cell growth factor receptor) proto-oncogene account for a continuous range of phenotypes in human piebaldism. *Am J Hum Genet* 1992;**51**:1058.

23 Tassabehji M, Read AP, Newton VE, *et al*. Waardenburg's syndrome patients have mutations in the human homologue of the Pax-3 paired box gene. *Nature* 1992;**355**:635.

24 Wiesner GL, Bendel CM, Olds DP, *et al*. Hypopigmentation in the Prader-Willi syndrome. *Am J Hum Genet* 1992;**40**:431.

25 King RA, Wiesner GL, Townsend D, White JG. Hypopigmentation in Angelman syndrome. *Am J Med Genet* 1992;**46**:40.

26 Brilliant MH. The mouse pink-eyed dilution locus: a model for aspects of Prader-Willi syndrome Angelman syndrome and a form of hypomelanosis of Ito. *Mamm Genome* 1992;**3**:187.

27 Witkop CJ Jr, Hill CW, Desnick SJ, *et al*. Ophthalmologic biochemical platelet and ultrastructural defects in the various types of oculocutaneous albinism. *J Invest Dermatol* 1973;**60**:443.

28 Kukita A, Fitzpatrick TB. Demonstration of tyrosinase in melanocytes of the human hair matrix by autoradiography. *Science* 1955;**121**:893.

29 King RA, Witkop CJ. Hairbulb tyrosinase activity in oculocutaneous albinism. *Nature* 1976;**263**:69.

30 Nance WE, Tuckson CE, Witkop CJ. Amish albinism a distinctive autosomal recessive phenotype. *Am J Hum Genet* 1970;**22**:579.

31 King RA, Wirstschafter JD, Olds DP, Brumbaugh JA. Minimal pigment: a new type of oculocutaneous albinism. *Clin Genet* 1982;**29**:42.

32 King RA, Olds DP. Hair bulb tyrosinase activity in oculocutaneous albinism: suggestions for pathway control and block location. *Am J Med Genet* 1985;**20**:49.

33 King RA, Townsend D, Oetting WS, *et al*. Temperature-sensitive tyrosinase associated with peripheral pigmentation in oculocutaneous albinism. *J Clin Invest* 1991;**87**:1046.

34 Kugelman TP, Van Scott EJ. Tyrosine activity in melanocytes of human albinos. *J Invest Dermatol* 1961;**37**:73.

35 Witkop CJ, Nance WE, Rawls RF, White JG. Autosomal recessive oculocutaneous albinism in man: Evidence for genetic heterogeneity. *Am J Hum Genet* 1970;**22**:55.

36 Nance WE, Witkop CJ, Rawls RF. Genetic and biochemical evidence for two forms of oculocutaneous albinism in man. *Birth Defects* 1971;**7**:125.

37 King RA, Witkop CJ. Detection of heterozygotes for tyrosinase-negative oculocutaneous albinism by hairbulb tyrosinase assay. *Am J Hum Genet* 1977;**29**:1643.

38 Murty VVVS, Bouchard B, Mathew S, *et al*. Assignment of the human *TYRP* (brown) locus to chromosome region 9q23 by nonradioactive *in situ* hybridization. *Genomics* 1992;**13**:227.

39 Box NF, Wyeth JR, Mayne CJ, *et al*. Complete sequence and polymorphism study of the human TYRP1 gene encoding tyrosinase-related protein 1. *Mamm Genome* 1998;**9**:50.

40 Manga P, Kromberg J, Box N, *et al*. Rufous oculocutaneous albinism is caused by mutations of the TRP1 gene of chromosome 9p [Abstract]. *Brazil J Genet* 1996;**19**:180.

41 Kromberg JG, Castle DJ, Zwane EM, *et al*. Red or rufous albinism in southern Africa. *Ophthalmic Pediatr Genet* 1990;**11**:229.

42 Hogen LT. The genetic analysis of familial traits. *J Genet* 1931;**25**:97.

43 Frenk E, Calme A. Hypopigmentation oculo-cutanée familiar transmission dominante du trouble de la formation des m lanosomes. *Schweiz Med Wochenschr* 1977;**107**:1964.

44 Trevor-Roper PD. Albinism. *Proc Roy Soc Med Soc Ophthal* 1963;**56**:21.

45 Oetting WS, Fryer JP, King RA. Mutations in brief: Mutations of the human tyrosinase gene associated with tyrosinase-related oculocutaneous albinism. (OCA1) *Hum Mutat* 1998;**12**:433.

46 Tripathi RK, Hearing VJ, Urabe K, *et al*. Mutational mapping of the catalytic activities of human tyrosinase. *J Biol Chem* 1992;**267**:23707.

47 Giebel LB, Strunk KM, King RA, *et al*. A frequent tyrosinase gene mutation in classic tyrosinase-negative (Type IA) oculocutaneous albinism. *Proc Natl Acad Sci USA* 1990;**87**:3255.

48 Spritz RA, Strunk KM, Giebel LB, King RA. Detection of mutations in the tyrosinase gene in a patient with Type IA oculocutaneous albinism. *N Engl J Med* 1990;**322**:1724.

49 Oetting WS, Witkop CJ Jr, Brown SA, *et al*. A frequent tyrosinase gene mutation associated with Type 1-A (Tyrosinase-negative) oculocutaneous albinism in Puerto Rico. *Am J Hum Genet* 1993;**52**:17.

50 Kwon BS, Halaban H, Chintamaneni C. Molecular basis of mouse Himalayan mutation. *Biochem Biophys Res Commun* 1989;**161**:252.

51 Matsunaga J, Dakeishi M, Shimizu H, Tomita Y. R278TER and P431L mutations of the tyrosinase gene exist in Japanese patients with tyrosinase-negative oculocutaneous albinism. *J Dermatol Sci* 1996;**13**:134.

52 Giebel LB, Tripathi RK, Strunk KM, *et al*. Tyrosinase gene mutations associated with Type IB ('yellow') oculocutaneous albinism. *Am J Hum Genet* 1991;**48**:1159.

53 Tripathi RK, Strunk KM, Giebel LB, *et al*. Tyrosinase gene mutations in Type 1 (tyrosinase-deficient) oculocutaneous albinism define two clusters of missense substitutions. *Am J Med Genet* 1992;**43**:865.

54 Giebel LB, Tripathi RK, King RA, Spritz RA. A tyrosinase gene missense mutation in temperature-sensitive Type 1 oculocutaneous albinism. *J Clin Invest* 1991;**87**:1119.

55 Spritz RA, Fukai K, Holmes SA, Luande J. Frequent intragenic deletion of the P gene in Tanzanian patients with Type II oculocutaneous albinism (OCA2). *Am J Hum Genet* 1995;**56**:1320.

56 Puri N, Durham-Pierre D, Aquaron R, *et al*. Type 2 oculocutaneous albinism (OCA2) in Zimbabwe and Cameroon: Distribution of the 27-kb deletion allele of the P gene. *Hum Genet* 1997;**100**:651.

57 Lee S-T, Nicholls RD, Schnur RE, *et al*. Diverse mutations of the P gene among African-Americans with Type II (tyrosinase-positive) oculocutaneous albinism (OCA2). *Hum Mol Genet* 1994;**3**:2047.

58 Yi Z, Garrison N, Cohen-Barak O, *et al*. A 1225-kilobase deletion of the P gene underlies the high prevalence of oculocutaneous albinism Type 2 in the Navajo population. *Am J Hum Genet* 2003;**72**:62.

59 King RA, Willaert RK, Schmidt RM, *et al*. MC1R mutations modify the classic phenotype of oculocutaneous albinism Type 2 (OCA2). *Am J Hum Genet* 2003;**73**:638.

60 Sviderskaya EV, Bennett DC, Ho L, *et al*. Complementation of hypigmentation in *p*-mutant (*pink-eyed Dilution*) mouse melanocytes by normal human *P* cDNA and defective complementation by OCA2 mutant sequences. *J Invest Dermatol* 1997;**108**:30.

61 Newton JM, Cohen-Barak O, Hagiwara N, *et al*. Mutations in the human orthologue of the mouse *underwhite* gene (*uw*) underlie a new form of oculocutaneous albinism OCA4. *Am J Hum Genet* 2001;**69**:981.

62 Witkop CJ, Niswander JD, Bergsma DR, *et al*. Tyrosinase positive oculocutaneous albinism among the Zuni and the Brandywine triracial isolate: Biochemical and clinical characteristics and fertility. *Am J Phys Anthropol* 1972;**36**:397.

63 Park KC, Chintamaneni CH, Halaban R, *et al*. Molecular analyses of a tyrosinase-negative albino family. *Am J Hum Genet* 1993;**52**:406.

64 Windhorst DB, Clickson AS, Good RA. Chediak-Higashi syndrome hereditary gigantism of cytoplasmic organelles. *Science* 1966;**151**:81.

65 Barbosa MDFS, Barat FJ, Tchernev VT, *et al*. Identification of mutations in two major mRNA isoforms of the Chediak-Higashi syndrome gene in human and mouse. *Hum Mol Genet* 1997;**6**:1091.

66 Hermansky F, Pudlak P. Albinism associated with hemorrhagic diathesis and unusual pigmented reticular cells in the bone marrow: report of two cases with histochemical studies. *Blood* 1959;**14**:162.

67 Witkop CJ Jr, White JG, King RA. Oculocutaneous albinism: in *Heritable Disorders of Amino Acid Metabolism* (ed Nyhan WL). J Wiley and Sons Inc., New York;1974:177.

68 Gahl WA, Brantly M, Kaiser-Kupfer MI, *et al.* Genetic defects and clinical characteristics of patients with a form of oculocutaneous albinism (Hermansky-Pudlak syndrome). *N Engl J Med* 1998;**338**:1258.

69 Gahl WA, Dell'Angelica E, Shotelersuk V, Bonifacino JS. A human disorder due to mutant b3A subunit of adaptor complex-3: Failed vesicle formation in brothers with Hermansky-Pudlak syndrome (HPS) [Abstract]. *Am J Hum Genet* 1998;**63**:A2.

70 Anderson PD, Huizing M, Gahl WA. Hermansky-Pudlak syndrome Type-4 (HPS-4); clinical and molecular characteristics. *J Invest Med* 2004;S100 [Abstract].

71 Cross HE, McKusick VA, Breen W. A new oculocerebral syndrome with hypopigmentation. *J Pediatr* 1967;**70**:3.

72 Griscelli C, Durandy A, Guy-Grand D, *et al.* A syndrome-associated partial albinism and immunodeficiency. *Am J Med* 1978;**65**:691.

73 Ménasché G, Ho CH, Sanal O, *et al.* Griscelli syndrome restricted to hypopigmentation results from a melanophilin defect (GS3) or a MYO5A F-exon deletion (GS1). *J Clin Invest* 2003;**112**:450.

74 Nettleship E. On some hereditary diseases of the eye. *Trans Ophthalmol Soc UK* 1909;**29**:59.

75 Forsius H, Eriksson AW. Ein neues Augensyndrom mit X-chromosomaler Transmission Eine Sippe mit Fundusalbinismus Foveahypoplasie Nystagmus Myopie Astigmatismus und Dyschromatopsie. *Klin Monatsble Augenheilkd* 1964;**144**:447.

76 Schnur RE, Gao M, Wick PA, *et al.* OA1 mutations and deletions in X-linked ocular albinism. *Am J Hum Genet* 1998;**62**:800.

77 Tijmes NT, Bergen AAB, de Jong PTVM. Paucity of signs in X-linked ocular albinism with a 700-kb deletion spanning the OA1 gene. *Br J Ophthalmol* 1998;**82**:457.

78 O'Donnell FE, King RA, Green WR, Witkop DJ Jr. Autosomal recessively inherited ocular albinism. *Arch Ophthalmol* 1978;**96**:1621.

79 Young TE. Malignant melanoma in an albino. *Arch Path* 1975;**64**:186.

Alkaptonuria

MAJOR PHENOTYPIC EXPRESSION

Dark deposits of pigment in the sclerae, cartilage and skin, early osteoarthritis; dark urine, homogentisic aciduria, and defective activity of homogentisic oxidase.

INTRODUCTION

Alkaptonuria was recognized by Garrod [1,2] as an inborn error of metabolism, around the beginning of the twentieth century. In fact, it was out of his studies of patients with alkaptonuria and their families that he conceived the idea that inborn errors of metabolism result from alterations, each in a single enzyme that is itself the consequence of a single genetic event. This was the first enunciation of what came to be known as the one-gene-one-enzyme hypothesis [3].

Alkaptonuria, or the excretion of urine which darkens on exposure to oxygen, is the result of the excretion of large amounts of homogentisic acid. The material precipitated by Boedeker [4] as the lead salt was identified by Wolkow and Baumann [5] as 2,5-dihydroxyphenylacetic acid and named homogentisic acid, as a similar structure to gentisic acid, 2,5-dihydroxyphenylbenzoic acid. Homogentisic acid is a normal intermediate in the catabolism of the aromatic amino acids, phenylalanine and tyrosine (Figure 19.1). It accumulates because of a defective activity of homogentisic acid oxidase [6]. This enzyme, which in mammalian systems is found only in liver and kidney, has been shown to be defective in both tissues in alkaptonuria. It catalyzes the conversion of homogentisic acid to maleylacetoacetic acid, which is ultimately converted to fumaric and acetoacetic acids. The gene for homogentisic acid oxidase has been cloned and mapped to chromosome 3q21-23 [7–9]. The gene contains 14 exons over 60 kb of genomic DNA. A number and variety of mutations have been identified, as well as a number of polymorphisms [10–12]. A promising therapy involves treatment with 2-(2-nitro-4-trifluoromethylbenzoyl)-1,3-cyclohexanedione, or NTBC (nitisinone) [13,14]. This herbicide inhibits 4-hydroxyphenylpyruvate dioxygenase, the enzyme that produces homogentisic acid. NTBC successfully treats tyrosinemia type I (Chapter 26). It should be even more effective in alkaptonuria.

CLINICAL ABNORMALITIES

The urine of an alkaptonuric individual usually appears normal when passed. It turns dark on standing, but most people do not leave their urine standing around to be observed, so most individuals live many years, usually well into adulthood, without recognizing that they are alkaptonuric. The addition of alkali to the urine will cause the pigment to appear more rapidly (Figure 19.2) [4]. Infants have been recognized because their cloth diapers, which had been washed with an alkaline soap or detergent, turned black or brown when they became wet with urine. Cloth diapers are seldom used today, and instead we have observed a reddish discoloration from alkaptonuric urine in disposable diapers (Figure 19.3).

In some patients the diagnosis is suggested by a positive test for urinary-reducing substance, a feature that was also

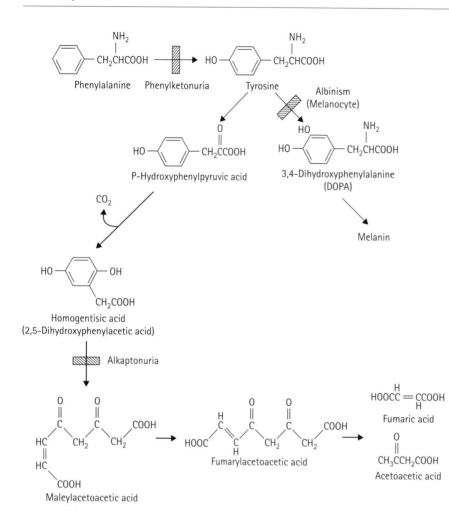

Figure 19.1   *Aromatic amino acid metabolism. The site of the defect in alkaptonuria is in the homogentisic acid oxidase.*

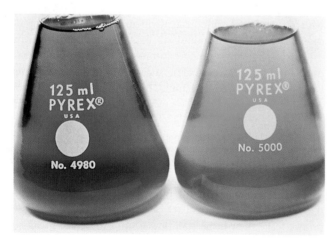

Figure 19.2   *Alkaptonuric urine. The flask on the right contains fresh urine darkened somewhat; the flask on the left to which sodium hydroxide was added contains a black suspension.*

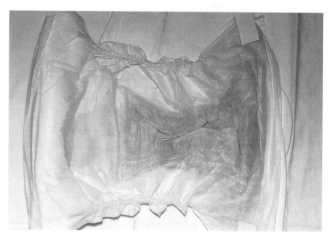

Figure 19.3   *Diaper of an infant with alkaptonuria. Cloth diapers washed in detergent turn black on contact with alkaptonuric urine. We find that disposable diapers like this one become pink or red.*

recognized in 1859 [4]. The urine does not contain glucose, and so laboratories that test urine only with glucose oxidase will miss this opportunity to find alkaptonuria. Homogentisic acid reduces the silver in a photographic emulsion, and alkaptonuric urine may be used to develop a photograph, providing a dramatic qualitative and even quantitative test for the disease

[15,16]. Homogentisic acid may be identified by paper chromatography, and there is a specific enzymatic analysis that permits quantification [17]. We more often find it first on analysis of the urine for organic acids [18], and we have developed an high performance liquid chromatography (HPLC) method for the quantitation of homogentisic acid and

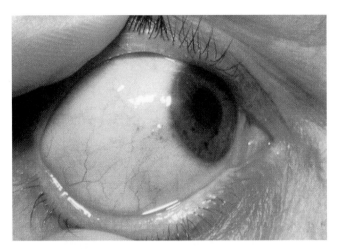

Figure19.4   *Ochronotic pigment in the sclera.*

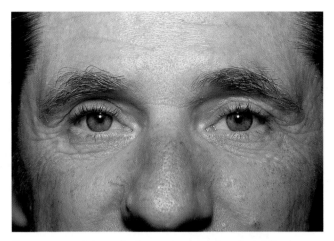

Figure 19.6   *Ochronotic pigment has been deposited diffusely over the nose of this 52-year-old man.*

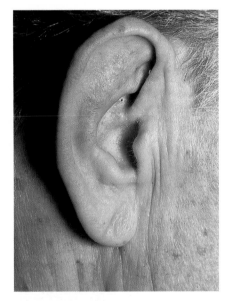

Figure 19.5   *Ochronotic pigment in the cartilage of the ear.*

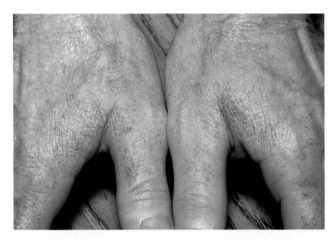

Figure 19.7   *The same patient had fine, stippled pigment over the dorsum of his hands.*

its products [19]. An adult with alkaptonuria excretes as much as 4–8 g of homogentisic acid daily [20]. The compound is excreted so efficiently that little is found in the plasma, although the amounts found by stable isotope internal standard gas chromatography mass spectrometry are considerably higher than those of normal plasma [21].

Patients with alkaptonuria have no symptoms as children or young adults. With age they develop pigmentation of the sclerae or cartilage of the ear (Figures 19.4, 19.5). The condition of widespread deposition of pigment in alkaptonuria was first called ochronosis by Virchow [22] because the gray, blue or black pigment appeared ochre under the microscope. These pigment deposits should be visible by 30 years-of-age. Actually, deposition may be widespread throughout the cartilage and fibrous tissue of the body [23–27]. Pigment may be seen at surgery and of course the diagnosis may become apparent first in this way with the rapid formation of pigment on exposure of tissues to air [28]. Pigment may be seen

in the buccal mucosa and the nails. There may be deposits in the skin (Figures 19.6, 19.7), leading to areas of dusky coloration of the skin. In addition to those shown, the cheeks, forehead, axillae and genital regions may be involved. The sweat may be dark and the cerumen brown or black.

The benign early course of these patients contrasts sharply with the severity of the ochronotic arthritis that develops early in adult life (Figure 19.8) [14,22,23,24,29–31]. The roentgenographic picture is of severe osteoarthritis (Figures 19.9, 19.10), developing much earlier than in nonalkaptonuric individuals. Some clinical features are reminiscent of rheumatoid arthritis, because there are acute periods of inflammation. Early symptoms may be in the hip or knee – large weight-bearing joints, but back pain is often the earliest complaint [14]. Limitation of motion is seen early. Ultimately, marked limitation of motion is the rule, and ankyloses are common. The arthritis has been noted to be earlier in onset and greater in severity in males although the incidence in the two sexes is equal [32].

The roentgenographic appearance may be pathognomonic (Figures 19.9, 19.10) [23,33]. The intervertebral disks

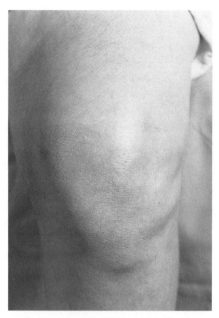

Figure 19.8 *Knee of patient A.B. with ochronotic arthritis.*

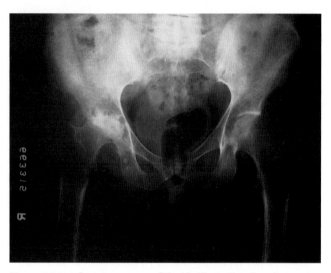

Figure 19.9 *Roentgenogram of the hip illustrating the advanced, early onset osteoarthritis characteristic of this disease.*

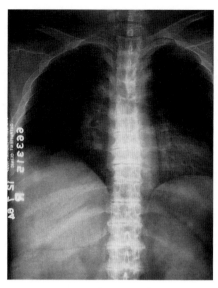

Figure 19.10 *Roentgenogram of the osteoarthritic spine in the patient with alkaptonuria resembles bamboo.*

Calcification of the ear cartilage is another roentgenographic characteristic of the disease.

Torn muscles or tendons indicate connective tissue disease [14], and thickening of the Achilles tendon is characteristic. Many have effusions of joints or the suprapatellar bursa. Urinary tract calculi are common late findings, appearing at a mean of 64 years [14]. Calculi in the prostate are very common in men over 60 [14].

Patients with alkaptonuria have a high incidence of heart disease [35]. Mitral and aortic valvulitis may be seen at autopsy. Aortic dilation or calcification of the aortic and mitral valve are common [14]. Myocardial infarction is a common cause of death, and there may be coronary artery calcification [14].

Index of the inflammatory nature of the disease is elevated sedimentation rate ranging from 55–110 mm/hr [14]. Levels of osteocalcin are elevated in some patients, representing the formation of new bone [14], and urinary collagen N-telopeptide, an index of bone resorption is also elevated.

GENETICS AND PATHOGENESIS

Alkaptonuria is inherited as an autosomal recessive trait [35]. Consanguinity was originally noted by Garrod [1], and subsequently by others [36]. Heterozygote detection should be possible by assay of the enzyme in biopsied liver, but this has not been done. Cloning of the gene for homogentisic acid oxidase in man [7,8] and the homologous gene in the mouse on chromosome 16 [9] have permitted molecular studies in patients with alkaptonuria.

A majority of patients have represented compounds of two different mutations. In one series [14] mutations were defined in 90 percent of alleles tested. Most have been missense, but nonsense mutations and intronic mutations resulting in frame shift have been observed. Mutations have been

undergo marked degeneration. There may be rupture of an intervertebral disc. The disc spaces become narrow and calcium is deposited. There is a variable degree of fusion of the vertebral bodies. The bamboo-like appearance (Figure 19.10) is diagnostic of ochronotic arthritis. In contrast to rheumatoid disease, there is little osteophyte formation or calcification of the intervertebral ligaments. Mean decrement in height approximates 8 cm [14]. In contrast to osteoarthritis, the large joints at the hip and shoulder are most commonly involved in ochronosis, whereas the sacroiliac joint may be uninvolved. In the involved joints there are degenerative osteoarthritic changes, occasional free intra-articular bodies [34], and calcification of the surrounding tendons. The arthritis of this disease is disabling. The patient may become bedridden or chairbound.

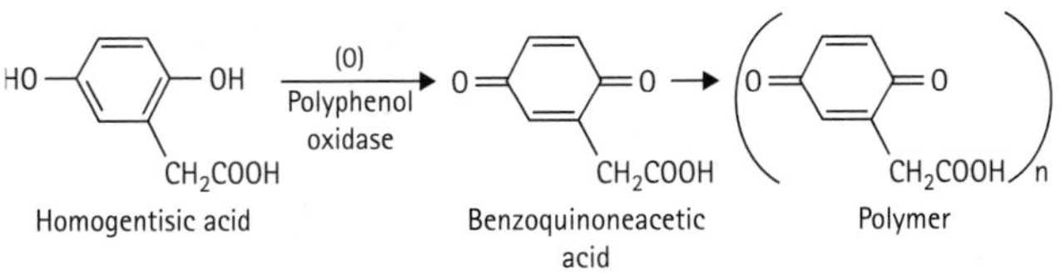

Figure 19.11 *The oxidation of homogentisic acid to benzoquinone-acetic acid which precedes formation of the black polymer. Benzoquinone acetic acid is a highly reactive compound. This or a polymeric form may bind to macromolecules in connective tissue.*

identified in every exon but 14. There has been some clustering in exons 7 to 10 [12]. One mutation (M368V) has been observed in at least one allele in 14 patients [14]. Correlation between genotype and phenotype has not been apparent. In a highly consanguineous Turkish population, a frequent mutation was R225H [37] which has also been found in Spanish patients; different haplotypes suggest that this results from a propensity to mutation at a CpG dinucleotide.

Abnormality in the gene determines very low activity of homogentisic acid oxidase [17]. The defective enzyme has also been documented in autopsied kidney [38]. In normal individuals intravenously administered ^{14}C -labeled homogentisic acid is oxidized rapidly to $^{14}CO_2$, while in alkaptonuric individuals 90 percent is excreted unchanged in the urine [39].

The arthritis and other ochronotic elements of the disease are thought to result from the binding of highly reactive oxidation products of homogentisic acid to cartilage and other tissues. Homogentisic acid is oxidized to benzoquinone-acetic acid and ultimately to the polymeric ochronotic pigment (Figure 19.11). The reaction is catalyzed by an oxidase present in mammalian skin and cartilage [40]. Benzoquinone-acetic acid and p-quinones in general form 1,4 addition products with sulfhydryl and amino groups [41].

TREATMENT

For many years no treatment has been successful in reducing the accumulation of homogentisic acid or interfering with its late effects on tissues. We have shown that it is possible to reduce the formation of homogentisic acid by reducing the intake of phenylalanine and tyrosine, and this is relatively easy in an infant [19]. However, compliance with a rather difficult diet would be a major problem in this disorder in which the symptoms are so many years in the future. Dietary reduction also reduced the excretion of homogentisic acid in a 45-year-old, but the authors judged it impractical [42]. Another approach was to employ reducing agents, such as ascorbic acid, in an attempt to prevent the oxidation of homogentisic acid to benzoquinone-acetic acid. It has been reported that the administration of vitamin C did not reduce the levels of homogentisic acid in alkaptonuric urine [43], but the authors felt that there was a significantly reduced tendency of the patient's urine to darken on standing. Homogentisic acid

inhibits the growth of cultured human articular chondrocytes. Ascorbic acid prevents this effect, and also prevents the binding of ^{14}C-homogentisic acid to connective tissues in rats [44]. We have more recently demonstrated that treatment of alkaptonuric patients with ascorbic acid was associated with a complete disappearance of benzoquinoneacetic acid from the urine. Similar results were reported by Mayatepek *et al.* [42]. Long-term experience with ascorbic acid therapy is not yet available.

The potential therapy with NTBC represents an advance toward rational therapy because the compound inhibits the enzyme directly before homogentisic acid in the pathway of tyrosine catabolism (Figure 19.1). Extensive experience in hepatorenal tyrosinemia (Chapter 26) indicated its surprising safety. Theoretical toxicity would be the reproduction of symptoms of oculocutaneous tyrosinemia (Chapter 25, p. 179 and 180) and photophobia and corneal crystals have been observed in infants with hepatorenal tyrosinemia treated with NTBC [13]. In experience with two adults [14] in whom diet was not modified 0.7 to 1.4 mg qd reduced urinary homogentisic acid excretion to 0.13 and 1.4 g per day. Plasma levels of tyrosine rose to 719 and 1288 μmol/L. There were no ocular symptoms and slit lamp examination was normal, but the trials were stopped.

Arthritis, once developed, may require orthopedic treatment. In one series [14] 50 percent of patients underwent surgical replacement of at least a hip, knee or shoulder.

References

1 Garrod AE. The incidence of alkaptonuria: a study in chemical individuality. *Lancet* 1902;**2**:1616.

2 Garrod AE. *Inborn Errors of Metabolism*. Oxford University Press, London;1923.

3 Beadle GW, Tatum EL. Genetic control of biochemical reactions in neurospora. *Proc Natl Acad Sci USA* 1941;**27**:499.

4 Boedeker C. Ueber das Alcapton: ein Bietrag zur Frage: Welche Stoffe des Harns Konnen Kupferreduction bewirken? *Z Rat Med* 1859;**7**:130.

5 Wolkow M, Baumann E. Uber das Wesen der Alkaptonurie. *Z Physiol Chem* 1891;**15**:228.

6 La Du BN, Zannoni VG, Laster L, Seegmiller JE. The nature of the defect in tyrosine metabolism in alcaptonuria. *J Biol Chem* 1958;**230**:251.

7 Pollak MR, Chou Y-HW, Cerda JJ, et al. Homozygosity mapping of the gene for alkaptonuria to chromosome 3q2. *Nat Genet* 1993;**5**:201.

8 Janocha S, Wolz W, Srsen S, et al. The human gene for alkaptonuria (AKU) maps to chromosome 3q. *Genomics* 1994;**19**:5.

9 Montagutelli X, Lalouette A, Coude M, et al. aku a mutation of the mouse homologous to human alkaptonuria maps to chromosome 16. *Genomics* 1994;**19**:9.

10 Fernandez-Canon JM, Granadino B, Beltran-Valero de Bernabe D, et al. The molecular basis of alkaptonuria. *Nat Genet* 1996;**14**:19.

11 Granadino B, Beltran-Valero de Bernabe D, Fernandez-Canon JM, et al. The human homogentisate 12-dioxygenase (HGO) gene. *Genomics* 1997;**43**:115.

12 Beltran-Valero de Bernabe D, Granadino B, Chiarelli I, et al. Mutation and polymorphism analysis of the human homogentisate 12-dioxygenase gene in alkaptonuria patients. *Am J Hum Genet* 1998;**62**:776.

13   Anikster Y, Nyhan WL, Gahl WA. NTBC in alkaptonuria. *Am J Hum Genet* 1998;**63**:920.

14   Phornphutkul C, Introne WJ, Perry MB, *et al.* Natural history of alkaptonuria. *N Engl J Med* 2002;**347**:2111.

15   Fishberg EH. The instantaneous diagnosis of alkaptonuria on a single drop of urine. *JAMA* 1942;**119**:882.

16   Neuberger A. Studies on alcaptonuria I. The estimation of homogentisic acid. *Biochem J* 1947;**41**:431.

17   Seegmiller JE, Zannoni VG, Laster L, La Du BN. An enzymatic spectrophotometric method for the determination of homogentisic in plasma and urine. *J Biol Chem* 1961;**236**:774.

18   Hoffmann G, Aramaki S, Blum-Hoffmann E, *et al.* Quantitative analysis for organic acids in biological samples: batch isolation followed by gas chromatographic/mass spectrometric analysis. *Clin Chem* 1989;**38**:587.

19   Wolff JA, Barshop B, Nyhan WL, *et al.* Effects of ascorbic acid in alkaptonuria: alterations in benzoquinone acetic acid and an ontogenic effect in infancy. *Pediatr Res* 1989;**26**:140.

20   Neuberger A, Rimington C, Wilson JMG. Studies on alcaptonuria II. Investigations on a case of human alcaptonuria. *Biochem J* 1947;**41**:438.

21   Deutsch JC, Santhosh-Kumar CR. Quantitation of homogentisic acid in normal human plasma. *J Chromatogr B Biomed Appl* 1996;**677**:147.

22   Virchow R. 1866 Ein Fall von allgemeiner Ochronose der Knorpel und knopfelähnlichen Theile. *Arch Pathol Anat* **37** 212.

23   Bunim JJ, McGuire JS, Jr Hilbish TF, *et al.* Alcaptonuria clinical staff conference at the National Institutes of Health. *Ann Int Med* 1957;**47**:1210.

24   O'Brien WM, La Du BN, Bunim JJ. Biochemical pathological and clinical aspects of alcaptonuria ochronosis and ochronotic arthropathy. *Am J Med* 1963;**34**:813.

25   Cooper PA. Alkaptonuria with ochronosis. *Proc R Soc Med* 1951;**44**:917.

26   Minno AM, Rogers JA. Ochronosis: report of a case. *Ann Intern Med* 1957;**46**:179.

27   Osler W. Ochronosis: the pigmentation of cartilages sclerotics and skin in alkaptonuria. *Lancet* 1904;**1**:10.

28   Rose GK. Ochronosis. *Br J Surg* 1957;**44**:481.

29   O'Brien WM, La Du BN, Bunim JJ. Biochemical pathologic and clinical aspects of alcaptonuria: ochronosis and ochronotic arthropathy. *Am J Med* 1963;**34**:813.

30   Yules JH. Ochronotic arthritis: report of a case. *Bull N Engl Med Center* 1957;**16**:168.

31   O'Brien WM, Banfield WG, Sokoloff L. Studies on the pathogenesis of ochronotic arthropathy. *Arthritis Rheum* 1961;**4**:137.

32   Harrold AJ. Alkaptonuric arthritis. *J Bone Joint Surg* (Br) 1956;**38**:532.

33   Pomeranz MM, Friedman LJ, Tunick IS. Roentgen findings in alkaptonuric ochronosis. *Radiology* 1941;**37**:295.

34   Sutro CJ, Anderson ME. Alkaptonuric arthritis: cause for free intraarticular bodies. *Surgery* 1947;**22**:120.

35   Hogben L, Worrall RL, Zieve I. The genetic basis of alkaptonuria. *Proc R Soc Edinb* (Biol) 1932;**52**:264.

36   Khachadurian A, Abu Feisal K. Alkaptonuria: report of a family with seven cases appearing in four successive generations with metabolic studies in one patient. *J Chron Dis* 1958;**7**:455.

37   Uyguner O, Goicoechea de Jorge E, Cefle A, *et al.* Molecular analysis of the HGO gene mutations in Turkish alkaptonuria patients suggest that the R58fs mutation originated from Central Asia and was spread throughout Europe and Anatolia by human migrations. *J Inherit Metab Dis* 2003;**26**:17.

38   Zannoni VG, Seegmiller JE, La Du BN. Nature of the defect in alkaptonuria. *Nature* 1962;**193**:952.

39   Lustberg TJ, Schulman JD, Seegmiller JE. Metabolic fate of homogentisic acid-1-[14]C (HGA) in alkaptonuria and effectiveness of ascorbic acid in preventing experimental ochronosis. *Arthritis Rheum* 1969;**12**:678.

40   Zannoni VG, Lomtevas N, Goldfinger S. Oxidation of homogentisic acid to ochronotic pigment in connective tissue. *Biochim Biophys Acta* 1969;**177**:94.

41   Stoner R, Blivaiss BB. Homogentisic acid metabolism: a 14 addition reaction of benzoquinone-1-acetic acid with amino acids and other biological amines. *Fed Proc* 1965;**24**:656.

42   Mayatepek E, Kallas K, Anninos A, Muller E. Effects of ascorbic acid and low-protein diet in alkaptonuria. *Eur J Pediatr* 1998;**157**:867.

43   Sealock RR, Gladstone M, Steele JM. Administration of ascorbic acid to an alkaptonuric patient. *Proc Soc Exp Biol Med* 1940;**44**:580.

44   Lustberg TJ, Schulman JD, Seegmiller JE. Decreased binding of ^{14}C-homogentisic acid induced by ascorbic acid in connective tissue of rats with experimental alcaptonuria. *Nature* 1970;**228**:770.

Phenylketonuria

MAJOR PHENOTYPIC EXPRESSION

Mental retardation, blue eyes, blond hair, fair skin, eczematous rash, vomiting in infancy, seizures, hyperactivity, unusual odor, positive urinary ferric chloride test, hyperphenylalaninemia and deficiency of phenylalanine hydroxylase.

INTRODUCTION

Phenylketonuria (PKU) is a disorder of aromatic amino acid metabolism in which phenylalanine cannot be converted to tyrosine (Figure 20.1). The defective enzyme, phenylalanine hydroxylase, is expressed only in liver. This disease is a model for a public health approach to the control of inherited disease since dietary treatment is effective in preventing mental retardation. Routine neonatal screening programs have been most effective in the developed countries of the world. For these reasons, the full blown picture of the classic disease is rarely observed today in these countries. Nevertheless, it does occur, and it is important that it be recognized.

The disorder was discovered by Folling [1] who tested the urine of two siblings, brought to him by their mother, by the addition of ferric chloride and noted the deep green color that results from the presence of phenylpyruvic acid (Figures 20.1, 20.2). The term phenylketonuria was first proposed by Penrose [2] who recognized the disease as the first in which there was a chemical cause of mental retardation. The site of the molecular defect in the phenylalanine hydroxylase reaction was discovered by Jervis [3] who found that the conversion of phenylalanine to tyrosine could not be carried out *in vitro* by the preparations of liver obtained from patients with PKU. The gene coding for phenylalanine hydroxylase has been identified and found to have 13 exons on chromosome 12, and a large number of mutations have been identified [4,5].

A few mutant alleles account for a majority of human mutant chromosomes. Eight mutations have resulted in more than two-thirds of European mutant alleles.

CLINICAL ABNORMALITIES

The most important and sometimes the only manifestation of PKU is mental retardation (Figures 20.3–20.8). The intelligence of all but one percent of untreated patients is very low, with intelligence quotients usually under 50 [6,7]. A few patients with untreated PKU have had borderline intelligence.

Phenylketonuric infants appear normal at birth. Retardation of development may not be evident for months. Vomiting may be a prominent early symptom. It may be severe enough to suggest a diagnosis of pyloric stenosis, and pyloromyotomy has been performed on such patients [8,9]. Irritability, an eczematoid rash (Figure 20.3), and an unusual odor may also be observed very early in life. The odor of the phenylketonuric patient is that of phenylacetic acid (Figure 20.1). It has variously been described as mousy, barny, wolflike or musty. Currently the odor is most often noted in patients with disorders of urea cycle treated with sodium phenylacetate, and in these circumstances it may be pervasive.

Patients with PKU are often quite good looking children. They are fair-haired, fair-skinned and blue-eyed in over 90 percent of the cases [4] (Figures 20.4, 20.5). However, there is

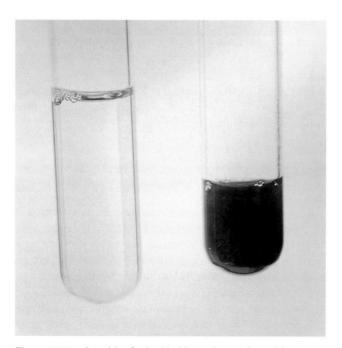

Figure 20.1 shows the chemical structures in the metabolism of phenylalanine, with Phenylalanine, Tyrosine, Phenylpyruvate, Phenylacetate, O-Hydroxyphenylpyruvate, Phenyllactate, Phenylacetylglutamine, and O-Hydroxyphenylacetate labeled.

Figure 20.1   Metabolism of phenylalanine. The site of the defect in PKU is in phenylalanine hydroxylase. The compounds that accumulate as a consequence of the block are shown below.

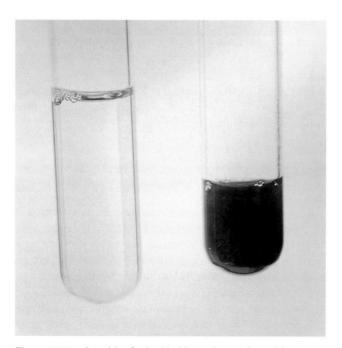

Figure 20.2   *A positive ferric chloride test in a patient with untreated PKU.*

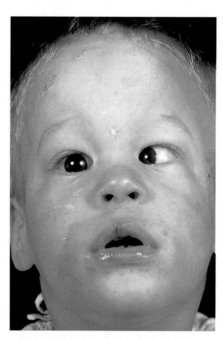

Figure 20.3   *The face of this patient with PKU illustrates the rather subtle eczematoid rash. The brown eyes remind us that all patients with this disease do not have blue eyes. In addition, he had epicanthal folds and a left internal strabismus.*

no amount of pigment in skin, hair or irides that excludes the diagnosis. In a family the pigmentation of the untreated affected child is less than that of unaffected members (Figure 20.7). The dermatitis is usually mild (Figure 20.3), and it is absent in three-quarters of the patients, but it may be a bothersome symptom. Patients may complain of intractable itching in the absence of visible cutaneous lesions. Sclerodermatous skin has been reported [10] in an infant with PKU.

Neurological manifestations are not usually prominent, but about a third of the patients may have all of the signs of cerebral palsy [11]. They are spastic, hypertonic and have increased deep tendon reflexes. Only about five percent have these manifestations to a severe degree. They may have contractures and limitation of mobility. Hyperactivity is common

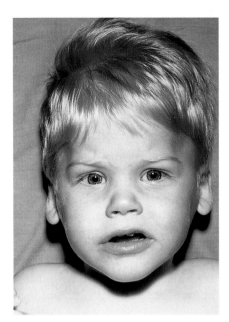

Figure 20.4   *L.S. This patient was diagnosed as having PKU at 10 months-of-age. The eyes were blue, the skin fair and the hair blond.*

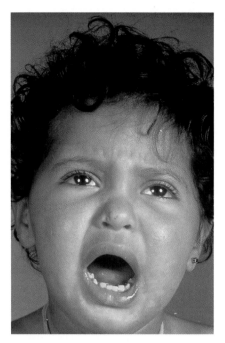

Figure 20.6   *A.D. A Saudi Arabian infant with classic PKU. Routine neonatal screening had not yet been initiated in that country at the time of diagnosis.*

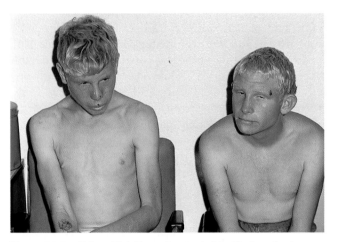

Figure 20.5   *B.A. and L.A. Severely retarded, institutionalized brothers with untreated PKU. They were quite fair of hair and skin.*

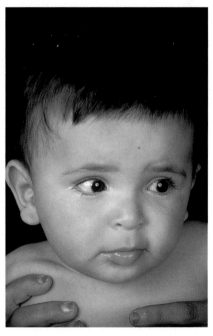

Figure 20.7   *E.Q. Another Saudi infant with classic PKU was considerably less pigmented than expected.*

(Figure 20.8), and there may be abnormalities of gait. Another one-third of the patients have very mild neurological signs such as a unilateral Babinski response or hyperactive deep tendon reflexes. Another third of untreated patients have no neurological signs except for mental retardation.

Seizures occur in about a fourth of the patients [7]. They are usually neither prominent nor difficult to manage. Nevertheless, about 80 percent have electroencephalograph (EEG) abnormalities [12]. Hyperactivity and behavior problems are common. Purposeless movements, rhythmic rocking, stereotypy, tremors and athetosis may be seen. Somatic development tends to be normal, but stature may be short. Patients treated from the neonatal period are of normal stature. Some patients have minor malformations [13]. These include widely

spaced incisor teeth, pes planus, partial syndactyly, and epicanthus (Figure 20.3). Congential heart disease appears to be more common in PKU than in the general population [14]. Some patients have microcephaly [11]. It has been calculated that in the absence of treatment a patient may lose 50 IQ points in the first year of life [15]. In the past a majority of patients with untreated PKU required institutional care (Figure 20.5).

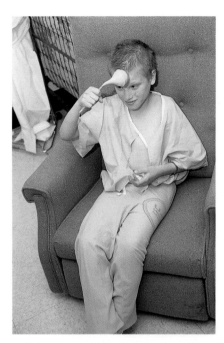

Figure 20.8   *This 10-year-old boy was found in a Romanian orphanage. A diagnosis of PKU was made at the age of 7 years. He had not been treated. He was very hyperactive and had seizures. His hair was blond, but his eyes hazel. He was hypertonic and had a rapid unusual limping gait, in which he leaned forward to the left, toe-walked, swinging his right arm and keeping the left at his side.*

GENETICS AND PATHOGENESIS

Phenylketonuria is transmitted by an autosomal recessive gene on chromosome 12q22–24.1. The gene for human phenylalanine hydroxylase has been cloned. Hundreds of different alleles have been discovered over 90 percent of which cause disease [16,17], but only five are responsible for most human disease; the rest are rare. Almost two thirds are missense mutations; 13 percent are small deletions; 12 percent splicesite mutations; six percent nonsense mutations; and one percent small insertions. Large deletions are rare.

Restriction enzyme polymorphism permitted heterozygote detection and prenatal diagnosis in the approximately 75 percent of families in which relevant polymorphism was identified [18]. Affected fetuses have been diagnosed prenatally in this way. Restriction fragment length polymorphism (RFLP) exists in or near the phenylalanine hydroxylase gene that permits assessment of the transmission of alleles within a family. A composite family of RFLPs on an allele is referred to as an RFLP haplotype. Some 50 haplotypes have been described for the phenylalanine hydroxylase locus. Once the mutation in the phenylalanine hydroxylase gene is known, mutational analysis may be used for prenatal diagnosis and for heterozygote detection. This provides a practical argument for seeking the precise molecular diagnosis. In the best studied Northern European population eight mutations have resulted in 64 percent of the mutant phenylalanine hydroxylase chromosomes [4,5]. Two mutations, in each of which there was zero enzyme activity and cross-reacting material (CRM), accounted for 46 percent; these were an arginine to tryptophan change in amino acid residue 408 (R408W) of exon 12 and a splicing mutation of intron 12. A number of the abnormal alleles identified have involved cytosine-phosphate-guanine (CpG) dinucleotides, which are known to be highly mutable.

Expression of the mutant genes and assessment of enzyme activity *in vitro* has permitted correlations of phenotype with genotype [4]. Correlations with pretreatment concentrations of phenylalanine, and phenylalanine tolerance and the response to oral loading with protein were quite strong. The R408W mutation expressed 100 percent of mRNA but less than one percent of enzyme activity and immunoreactive hydroxylase protein [4,19]. Arginine to glutamine mutations in exon 5 and 7 were associated with variant phenotypes.

Different mutations have been found in other populations. Most of these have been missense mutations such as the one that leads to complete inactivation of the enzyme in Northern African Jews [20]. A few deletions have been observed, such as the 22 bp deletion in exon 6 in an Arab family [21]. The primary effect of mutation in the gene is defective activity of the enzyme. This has been demonstrated by liver biopsy [22] in which activity correlated well with *in vitro* expression analysis of the mutant gene. Correlations were also excellent in eight patients tested *in vivo* with deuterated phenylalanine [23]. Analysis of genotpye-phenotype correlations in an assembly of 365 patients reported [24] revealed a predominantly predictable or consistent phenotypic degree of severity in the majority. However, there were a number of genotypes that were associated with inconsistent phenotypes – both classic PKU and the variant hyperphenylalaninemia in patients with the same genotype. In a head to head comparison between a mutation $311C{\rightarrow}A$ (A104D), associated with mild hyperphenylalaninemia, and $470G{\rightarrow}A$ (R157N), with classic PKU, *in vitro* expression studies and *in vivo* ^{13}C-phenylalanine metabolism [25] indicated quite different impacts of mutation on enzyme function and physical properties. The severe mutation coded for a protein that was degraded faster than the milder variant.

The incidence of classic PKU has become clear from experience with the screening programs around the world. The incidence in the United States is approximately 1:10 000. Approximately 1 in 50 is a carrier of the gene. Heterozygosity has been demonstrated by assay of the enzyme in liver, and of course, by mutational analysis.

Phenylalanine hydroxylase, the defective enzyme in PKU, has a tetrahydrobiopterin cofactor that is required for the hydroxylation of phenylalanine. In the hydroxylase reaction a quinonoid dihydrobiopterin is formed. The reduction of this compound to reform tetrahydrobiopterin is catalyzed by dihydropteridine reductase [26,27]. The quinonoid oxidation product is unstable and unless it is promptly reduced it forms the 7,8-dihydrobiopterin and is no longer a substrate for dihydropteridine reductase, but it can be reduced by dihydrofolate reductase in the presence of the reduced form of nicotinamide-adenosine dinucleotide phosphate (NADPH).

The synthesis of biopterin begins with guanosine triphosphate and proceeds through reduced neopterin (α-D-erythro-7,8-dihydroneopterin triphosphate) to a dihydro-precursor of tetrahydrobiopterin [28–30].

Three isozymes of phenylalanine hydroxylase have been found in liver [31]. The three isozymes have identical molecular weights and kinetic constants but differ in charge [31,32]. In classic PKU all three isozymes are missing. Immunochemical study of phenylalanine hydroxylase from phenylketonuric human liver has revealed no cross-reacting material using antibody that reacted with normal hepatic enzyme [33]. The activity of phenylalanine hydroxylase in classic PKU has been reported as undetectable [3, 34–37].

In the presence of a defect in phenylalanine hydroxylase the first compound that accumulates is phenylalanine itself. In classic PKU, the plasma concentration of phenylalanine is virtually always above 1200 μmol/L. It is transaminated (Figure 20.1) to form phenylpyruvic acid, the phenylketone for which the disease was named. There is a roughly linear relationship between the concentrations of phenylalanine in the blood and the urinary excretion of phenylpyruvic acid [38]. This is the compound that is responsible for the positive ferric chloride ($FeCl_3$) test. A deep green color is seen on the addition of 10 percent ($FeCl_3$) to the urine of patients with untreated PKU (Figure 20.2). Phenylpyruvic acid is subsequently converted to phenyllactic acid, phenylacetic acid, and phenylacetylglutamine. Phenylpyruvate is also hydroxylated in the ortho position, ultimately yielding orthohydroxyphenylacetic acid. These are not abnormal metabolites, but normal ones that occur in abnormal amounts in PKU. It is current theory that it is this abnormal chemical milieu in which the patient with PKU lives that produces the mental retardation and other manifestations of the disease.

There are a variety of secondary effects of the accumulation of phenylalanine and its metabolites. Decreased pigmentation has been related to the inhibition of tyrosinase by phenylalanine. Decreased levels of 5-hydroxytryptamine (serotonin) appear to be due to inhibition of 5-hydroxytryptophan decarboxylase by phenylpyruvic, phenyllactic and phenylacetic acids. Decreased amounts of epinephrine, norepinephrine and dopamine are presumably caused by inhibition of dopamine decarboxylase. The metabolites that accumulate in PKU also inhibit glutamic acid decarboxylase in brain, and this would decrease levels of 4-aminobutyric acid (GABA). Studies of protein synthesis and turnover *in vivo* via continuous infusion of ^{13}C-leucine have revealed no abnormality in PKU [39].

DIAGNOSIS

The diagnosis of PKU should be made in the neonatal period. This is accomplished by the routine screening of all infants for an elevated concentration of phenylalanine in the blood. It is generally carried out on discharge from hospital after the initiation of protein-containing feedings. A drop of blood collected from the heel on filter paper is analyzed for phenylalanine by the bacterial inhibition method developed by Guthrie [40], or by a quantitative determination of the concentration of phenylalanine. This is now incorporated into expanded programs of screening employing tandem mass spectrometry. A positive screening test is usually repeated. A second positive is followed up with quantitative assay of the concentrations of phenylalanine and tyrosine in the blood confirming the phenylalaninemia and excluding transient tyrosinemia of the newborn, a common cause of a positive screening test. In the presence of an elevated concentration of phenylalanine and normal or reduced tyrosine, the patient may be admitted to hospital, where protein and phenylalanine intake are carefully monitored and fresh urine specimens collected. Patients with classical PKU ingesting a normal diet display a very rapid rise of plasma phenylalanine to levels well over 1800 μmol/L. A concentration of 1200 μmol/L or more is diagnostic of PKU. Patients with classic PKU also excrete the metabolites phenylpyruvic acid and ortho-hydroxyphenylacetic acid in the urine. Cofactor abnormalities (Chapter 21) can be ruled out at that time. A protocol for the management of the newborn detected by a positive screening test is given in Table 20.1.

The diagnosis of PKU is often challenged [41] with dietary phenylalanine 90–110 days after diagnosis and again after one year of age [15]. A conventional challenge in a 3–6-month-old infant is a three-day intake of 24 oz. of evaporated milk:water 1:1 which provides 180 mg/kg of phenylalanine. The challenge can be adjusted to 180 mg/kg of phenylalanine for an older, larger child. In most patients with classic PKU, the challenge yields a sharp rise in the plasma concentration of phenylalanine to 1800–2400 μmol/L in 48 hours at which time the challenge is stopped.

It is important to remember that this challenge was developed for use with infants, and the predominant experience is at the 3-month level. A dose of 180 mg/kg per day of phenylalanine for three days would be a sizable challenge for an older child or adult with PKU. In fact symptomatic hypoglycemia and hyperinsulinemia have been reported in a 15-year-old so challenged [42]. Infants in whom this test did not yield levels higher than 1200 μmol/L [36] were classified as variants. Currently we consider those with levels over 600 μmol/L as having classic PKU (Table 20.1).

It was the widespread screening of infant populations that led to the recognition that not all patients with hyperphenylalaninemia have classic PKU. Some variants represent molecular heterogeneity at the phenylalanine hydroxylase locus specifying variant enzymes with partial activity. Most of the variants have phenylalanine concentrations under 1200 μmol/L, and such infants can tolerate more than 75 mg/kg of phenylalanine per day. A small number of variant patients have been studied by liver biopsy [33,36,43], and in each a substantial defect in phenylalanine hydroxylase activity was demonstrated. Most have had levels of activity that were 10–20 percent of normal.

Transient phenylalaninemia may represent an isolated delay in the maturation of phenylalanine metabolizing enzymes. It is

Table 20.1   *Protocol for PKU and variants*

1. When newborn screen positive: ──────────────▶ Obtain plasma for quantitative amino acids
   Begin low phenylalanine diet

2. Plasma phenylalanine over 340 μmol/L (6 mg/dL). Plasma phenylalanine 150–300 μmol/L (2.5–6 mg/dL)

   Repeat ▼   ▼
   Plasma phenylalanine > 180 μmol/L ◀─── elevated ◀─── Repeat ──────▶ Normal level < 150 μmol/L
                                                                       no further control

3. Exclude cofactor deficiency
   Urinary pterins

                                          Abnormal
   Dihydropteridine reductase ───────────────────────────────▶ CSF BH4, neurotransmitters
                                                               Enzyme diagnosis.
                                                               Treatment with BH4, L-DOPA
                                                               5-OH tryptophan, carbidopa.

4. Exclude transient tyrosinemia
   Tyrosine concentrations high, exceed phenylalanine ──────────────▶ Continue to monitor concentrations and determine
                                                                      transient status.
                                                                      Consider ascorbic acid treatment to accelerate.

5. Phenylalanine elevated; tyrosine low.
   Phenylalanine > 600 μmol/L (10 mg/dL) – Classic PKU ──────────▶ Diet therapy.
   Phenylalanine < 300 μmol/L – Hyperphenylalaninemia ──────────▶ Normal diet.
                                                                  Continue to monitor phenylalanine.
   Phenylalanine 300–600 μmol/L. Hyperphenylalaninemia ─────────▶ Needs some dietary restriction.

6. Initial Dietary Therapy for Classic PKU means delete phenylalanine from diet as follows (phenex-1 or Lofenelac 0.7–1.0 cal/ml).

Plasma Phenylalanine		Delete Phenylalanine for:	Monitor Plasma
(μmol/L)	(mg/dL)	Hours	Quantitative Phenylalanine*
240–605	(4–10)	24	qd
605–1210	(10–20)	48	qd
1210–2420	(20–40)	72	q1–3d
>2420	(>40)	96	q1–3d

   * To prevent phenylalanine deficiency
   When plasma phenylalanine reaches the treatment range phenylalanine is added to the diet.

   Individual amino acid requirements vary. The following are guidelines for initial dietary phenylalanine content dependent on the maximum pretreatment plasma levels:

Plasma Phenylalanine		Dietary Phenylalanine
(μmol/L)	(mg/dL)	mg/kg
<605	(<10)	70
605–1210	(10–20)	55
1210–1815	(20–30)	45
1815–2420	(30–40)	35
>2420	(>40)	25

   Monitor neonatal levels sufficiently frequently to establish a steady state concentration at the desired level while the infant receives a constant intake of phenylalanine and tyrosine.
   Aim to keep plasma phenylalanine between 100 and 300 μmol/L.

7. Monitor thereafter every week until 6 months old;
   q 2 weeks until 1-year-old
   q 4 weeks until 3-years-old
   q 6 months until 12-years-old
   Yearly thereafter.

because of this phenomenon that patients with phenylalaninemia are routinely tested for their dietary tolerance to phenylalanine during the first year of life.

TREATMENT

The treatment of PKU is the provision of a diet sufficiently low in phenylalanine that the serum concentrations are maintained in a reasonable range and metabolites disappear from body fluids. This requires the provision of enough phenylalanine to meet the normal requirements of this essential amino acid for growth. It also requires the frequent quantitative assessment of the concentration of phenylalanine in the blood. Levels recommended as acceptable have ranged from 180 to 900 μmol/L. However, Smith and colleagues [44] have recommended a smaller window between 120 and 300 μmol/L. Their data show a linear relationship between IQ and mean concentration during therapy over 300 μmol/L, but the differences were not clear until levels exceeded 800 μmol/L. Setting the lower level at 120 μmol/L is less secure; patients with long periods below this level appeared to have low IQ levels, only in the early cohort born prior to 1971, and no other lower limit was assessed. We strive to keep levels below 300 μmol/L and find that most patients in steady state do not approach any lower limit areas.

A patient detected in the neonatal period and managed with these guidelines should have an IQ in the normal range. The prevention of clinical disease by the restriction of dietary phenylalanine has provided the strongest evidence for the concept that the clinical manifestations of the disease result from the abnormal chemical milieu that follows the genetic defect. Preparations are now available that facilitate long-term treatment (Lofenalac-Mead-Johnson; Analog XP-Ross) and listings are available of the phenylalanine contents of foods and sources of low-protein products [45].

In the history of the management of the patient with PKU, the issue of termination of the diet has undergone evolution. It was once thought that in most patients with PKU the diet could safely be stopped at five years of age. In a study from Poland, a decrease in IQ was found in most patients with classic PKU after discontinuing the diet [46]. Furthermore, there were difficulties in adaptation problems with performance in school and EEG abnormalities. Similarly, among 47 patients with PKU, treated at the Hospital for Sick Children in London, given a normal diet between the ages of 5 and 15, there was a statistically significant fall in IQ of 5 to 9 points after discontinuing treatment [47]. The change in IQ was uniformly negative and was progressive. Among 21 patients treated at the Universitats-Kinderklinik, Heidelberg, who were given a relaxed low phenylalanine diet rather than a normal diet at about the same time as the London group, there were smaller and nonsignificant falls in IQ. Data from the United States Collaborative Study on 115 children suggested that discontinuing dietary treatment at 6 years of age led to a reduction in IQ [48]. There were significant differences in school performance as measured by the Wide Range Achievement Test.

Actually, the IQ alone may not be the most sensitive criterion on which to base this decision in an individual patient. Other aspects of clinical condition which might benefit from treatment longer than necessary to produce a stable IQ might affect the way a child functions in society. Behavioral abnormalities are common in children with PKU despite early diagnosis and treatment and normal IQ. Mannerisms, hyperactivity and signs of anxiety have been reported in 8-year-old children treated since early neonatal diagnosis, and those whose diet was less strictly controlled were twice as likely to display abnormal behaviors than those more strictly controlled [49]. On the other hand, a study [50] of 586 German 10-year-old PKU patients via a personality questionnaire failed to reveal differences from controls.

If high levels of phenylalanine continue to retard myelinization, one might even expect treatment to be useful well up to puberty, since myelination at least in the formatio reticularis is not finished at 8 years of life. In addition, the effect of high concentrations of phenylalanine on synaptogenesis is not known. Some older patients find that their skin feels better with modest restriction of phenylalanine. In any case the rigidity with which one controls the level of phenylalanine can probably be relaxed after 6 years-of-age, but it is prudent to continue some restriction in the intake of phenylalanine. A study of 25 adults with PKU all of whom had been treated early [51] revealed normal intelligence, but in each patient scores were lower than control siblings in measures of intelligence and attention. Patients were advised to continue dietary restriction for life, but only 10 followed this regimen. Others discontinued treatment before or during adolescence. Intellectual outcome appears to have best been predicted by the presence or absence of early insult to brain, while performance on a test of problem-solving correlated best with concurrent levels of phenylalanine even in adulthood. As patients become older some relaxation of dietary control appears inevitable. In a recent study of 95 patients treated from the neonatal period and assessed at 12 years-of-age best cognition results were those of patients whose phenylalanine values were kept consistently below 900 μM.

Reduced concentrations of carnitine in serum have been found in patients with PKU [52]. This was the case in those less than 2 years of age managed with a restricted diet. In contrast, untreated infants with PKU had normal levels of carnitine as did older patients. The data provide an argument for supplementation with carnitine at least in infants treated for PKU.

Poor linear growth has been observed in some patients with PKU, and this has been thought to result from protein insufficiency. The level of prealbumin has been found [53] to correlate well with protein adequacy in this disease, and the threshold level is 20 mg/dL. Linear growth can be expected to be impaired in patients with levels lower than 20 mg/dL.

Maternal PKU and its production of severe mental retardation in the offspring provides a paradigmatic example of chemical teratogenesis. It is important that the gains of the neonatal screening programs should not be followed by the production of new generations of retarded children of mothers with PKU. On the other hand, the result of dietary treatment of maternal PKU detected in the first or second trimester has not been greatly successful [54]. While the offspring of untreated pregnancies appear usually to be more severely retarded, microcephaly and retardation, as well as congenital heart disease do occur in the offspring of women who are treated in pregnancy. Therapy begun prior to conception is more promising [55].

Male patients with PKU may have low sperm counts and semen volume. A survey of male patients over 18 years in the US identified 40 men who had 64 children but did not yield data on fertility rate [56]. Abnormalities were not identified in live-born offspring that could be related to paternal PKU.

References

1   Folling A. Uber Ausscheidung von Phenylbrenztraubensaure in den Harn als Stoffwechselanomalie in Verbindung mit Imbezillitat Hoppe-Seyler's Z. *Physiol Chem* 1934;**227**:169.

2   Penrose L, Quastel JH. Metabolic studies in phenylketonuria. *J Biochem* 1937;**31**:266.

3   Jervis GA. Phenylpyruvic oligophrenia deficiency of phenylalanine-oxidizing system. *Proc Soc Exp Biol Med* 1953;**82**:514.

4   Okano Y, Eisensmith RC, Butler F, *et al*. Molecular basis of phenotypic heterogeneity in phenylketonuria. *N Engl J Med* 1991;**324**:1232.

5   Scriver CR. Phenylketonuria – genotypes and phenotypes. *N Engl J Med* 1991;**324**:1280.

6   Jervis GA. Phenylpyruvic ologophrenia. *Assoc Res Nerv Ment Dis Proc* 1954;**33**:259.

7   Pitt DB, Dansk DM. The natural history of untreated phenylketonuria. *J Pediatr Child Health* 1991;**27**:189.

8   Partington MW. The early symptoms of phenylketonuria. *Pediatrics* 1961;**27**:465.

9   Centerwall W. Phenylketonuria. *Medical Bulletin Los Angeles Children's Hospital* 1959;**63**:83.

10 Haktan M, Aydin A, Bahat H, *et al*. Progressive systemic scleroderma in an infant with partial phenylketonuria. *J Inherit Metab Dis* 1989;**12**:486.

11 Paine RS. The variability in manifestations of untreated patients with phenylketonuria (phenylpyruvic aciduria). *Pediatrics* 1957;**20**:290.

12 Low NW, Bosma JF, Armstrong MD. Studies on phenylketonuria. *Arch Neurol Psychiatr* 1957;**77**:359.

13 Cowie V. Phenylpyruvic oligophrenia. *J Mental Sci* 1951;**97**:505.

14 Verkerk PH, Van Spronsen FJ, Smith GPA, *et al*. Prevalence of congenital heart disease in patients with phenylketonuria. *J Pediatr* 1991;**119**:282.

15 Koch R, Blaskovics M, Wenz E, *et al*. Phenylalaninemia and phenylketonuria in *Heritable Disorders of Amino Acid Metabolism* (ed. WL Nyhan). John Wiley and Sons, New York;1974:109.

16 Scriver CR, Byck S, Prevost L, *et al*. The phenylalanine hydroxylase locus: A marker for the history of phenylketonuria and human genetic diversity. *Ciba Found Symp* 1996;**197**:73.

17 Scriver CR, Waters PJ, Sarkissian C, *et al*. *PAHdb*: A locus-specific knowledge base. *Hum Mutat* 2000;**15**:99.

18 Woo SLC, Lidsky AS, Guttler F, *et al*. Cloned human phenylalanine hydroxylase gene allows prenatal diagnosis and carrier detection of classical phenylketonuria. *Nature* 1983;**306**:152.

19 Svensson E, Eisensmith RC, Dworniczak B, *et al*. Two missense mutations causing mild hyperphenylalaninemia associated with DNA haplotype 12. *Hum Mutat* 1992;**1**:129.

20 Weinstein M, Eisensmith RC, Abadia V, *et al*. A missense mutation S349P completely inactivates phenylalanine hydroxylase in North Africa Jews with phenylketonuria. *Hum Genet* 1993;**90**:545.

21 Kleiman S, Schwartz G, Woo SLC, Shiloh Y. 122-bp deletion in the phenylalanine hydroxylase gene causing phenylketonuria in an Arab family. *Hum Mutation* 1992;**1**:344.

22 Lyonnet S, Caillaud C, Rey F, *et al*. Molecular genetics of phenylketonuria in Mediterranean countries: a mutation associated with partial phenylalanine hydroxylase deficiency. *Am J Hum Genet* 1989;**44**:511.

23 Trefz RK, Erlenmaier T, Hunneman DH, *et al*. Sensitive *in vivo* assay of the phenylalanine hydroxylating system with a small intravenous dose of heptadeutero L-phenylalanine using high pressure liquid chromatography and capillary gas chromatography/mass fragmentography. *Clin Chim Acta* 1979;**99**:211.

24 Kayaalp E, Treacy E, Waters PJ, *et al*. Human phenylalanine hydroxylase mutations and hyperphenylalaninemia phenotypes: A metanalysis of genotype-phenotype correlations. *Am J Hum Genet* 1997;**61**:1309.

25 Waters PJ, Parniak MA, Hewson AS, Scriver CR. Alterations in protein aggregation and degradation due to mild and severe missense mutations (A104D R157N) in the human phenylalanine hydroxylase gene (PAH). *Hum Mutat* 1998;**12**:344.

26 Kaufman S. Metabolism of phenylalanine hydroxylation cofactor. *J Biol Chem* 1967;**242**:3934.

27 Craine JE, Hall ES, Kaufman S. The isolation and characterization of dihydropteridine reductase from sheep liver. *J Biol Chem* 1972;**247**:6082.

28 Brown GM. The biosynthesis of pteridines. *Adv Enzymol* 1971;**35**:35.

29 Eto I, Fukushima K, Shiota T. Enzymatic synthesis of biopterin from D-erythrodihydroneopterin triphosphate by extracts of kidneys from Syrian golden hamsters. *J Biol Chem* 1976;**251**:6505.

30 Gal EM, Nelson JM, Sherman AD. Biopterin: III Purification and characterization of enzymes involved in the cerebral synthesis of 78-dihypdrobiopterin. *Neurochem Res* 1978;**3**:69.

31 Barranger JA, Geiger PJ, Huzino A, Bessman SP. Isozymes of phenylalanine hydroxylase. *Science* 1972;**175**:903.

32 Tourian A. The unique identity of rat hepatoma phenylalanine hydroxylase. *Biochem Biophys Res Commun* 1976;**68**:51.

33 Friedman PA, Kaufman A, Kang ES. Nature of the molecular defect in phenylketonuria and hyperphenylalaninemia. *Nature* 1972;**240**:157.

34 Bartholome K, Lutz P, Bickel H. Determination of phenylalanine hydroxylase activity in patients with phenylketonuria and hyperphenylalaninemia. *Pediat Res* 1975;**9**:899.

35 Embden G, Baldes K. Uber den Abbau des Phenylalanins im tierischen Organismus. *Biochem Z* 1913;**55**:301.

36 Justice P, O'Flynn ME, Hsia DYY. Phenylalanine hydroxylase activity in hyperphenylalaninemia. *Lancet* 1967;**1**:928.

37 Mitoma C, Auld RM, Udenfriend S. On the nature of enzymatic defect in phenylpyruvic oligophrenia. *Proc Soc Exper Biol Med* 1957;**94**:634.

38 Armstrong MD, Low NL. Phenylketonuria: VII Relation between age serum phenylalanine level and phenylpyruvic acid excretion. *Proc Soc Exper Biol Med* 1957;**94**:142.

39 Thompson GN, Pacy PJ, Watts RWE, Halliday D. Protein metabolism in phenylketonuria and Lesch-Nyhan syndrome. *Pediatr Res* 1990;**28**:240.

40 Guthrie R, Suzi A. A simple phenylalanine method for detecting phenylketonuria in large populations of newborn infants. *Pediatrics* 1963;**12**:338.

41 O'Flynn ME, Holtzman NA, Blaskovics M, *et al*. The diagnosis of phenylketonuria. A report from the Collaborative Study of Children Treated for Phenylketonuria. *Am J Dis Child* 1980;**134**:769.

42 Ziyai F, Wong PWK, Justice P, Michals K. Protein-induced hypoglycemia in a phenylketonuric patient. *J Pediatr* 1978;**92**:681.

43 Kang ES, Kaufman S, Gerald PS. Clinical and biochemical observations of patients with atypical phenylketonuria. *Pediatrics* 1970;**45**:83.

44 Smith I, Beasley MG, Ades AE. Intelligence and quality of dietary treatment in phenylketonuria. *Arch Dis Child* 1990;**65**:472.

45 Acosta PB, Schaeffler GE, Wenz E, Koch R. *PKU – A guide to management.* California State Department of Public Health, Berkeley California;1972.

46 Cabalska B, Duczynska N, Brozymowska J, *et al.* Termination of dietary treatment of phenylketonuria. *Eur J Pediatr* 1977;**126**:253.

47 Smith I, Lobascher ME, Stevenson JE, *et al.* Effect of stopping low-phenylalanine diet on intellectual progress of children with phenylketonuria *Br Med J* 1978;**2**:723.

48 Koch R, Azen CG, Friedman EG, Williamson ML. Preliminary report on the effects of diet discontinuation in PKU. *J Pediatr* 1982;**100**:870.

49 Smith I, Beasley MG, Wolff OH, Ades AE. Behavior disturbance in 8-year-old children with early treated phenylketonuria. *J Pediatr* 1988;**112**:403.

50 Weglage J, Rupp A, Schmidt E. Personality characteristics in patients with phenylketonuria treated early. *Pediatr Res* 1994;**35**:611.

51 Ris MD, Williams SE, Hunt MM, *et al.* Early-treated phenylketonuria: adult neuropsychological outcome. *J Pediatr* 1994;**124**:388.

52 Vilaseca MA, Briones P, Ferre I, *et al.* Controlled diet in phenylketonuria may cause carnitine deficiency. *J Inherit Metab Dis* 1994;**16**:101.

53 Arnold GL, Vladutiu CJ, Kirby RS, *et al.* Protein insufficiency and linear growth restriction in phenylketonuria. *J Pediatr* 2002;**141**:243.

54 Levy HL, Kaplan GN, Erickson AM. Comparison of treated and untreated pregnancies in a mother with phenylketonuria. *J Pediatr* 1982;**100**:876.

55 NIH and National Institute of Child Health and Human Development. *Report of the NIH Consensus Development Conference on Phenylketonuria (PKU): screening and management.* The Institutes, Bethesda Md;2001.

56 Fisch RO, Matalon R, Weisberg S, Michals K. Children of fathers with phenylketonuria: An international survey. *J Pediatr* 1991;**118**:739.

21

Hyperphenylalaninemia and defective metabolism of tetrahydrobiopterin

MAJOR PHENOTYPIC EXPRESSION

Mental retardation, muscular rigidity, dystonic movements, myoclonic seizures, drooling, microcephaly, hyperphenyl-alaninemia, and defective synthesis of tetrahydrobiopterin (BH_4) because of defective activity of GTP cyclohydrolase, or 6-pyruvoyltetrahydropterin synthase, and defective recycling of BH_4 due to deficiency of dihydropteridine reductase and pterin-4α-carbinolamine dehydratase.

INTRODUCTION

The existence of variant forms of hyperphenylalaninemia resulting from abnormalities of cofactor synthesis was predicted with the discovery of biopterin (Figure 21.1) and its role in the phenylalanine hydroxylase reaction [1–4]. The first patients were reported in the 1970s as an outgrowth of the programs of neonatal screening for PKU. A majority of the patients recognized early were diagnosed because they developed progressive cerebral deterioration despite an early neonatal diagnosis of hyperphenylalaninemia and effective dietary control of the levels of phenylalanine in blood.

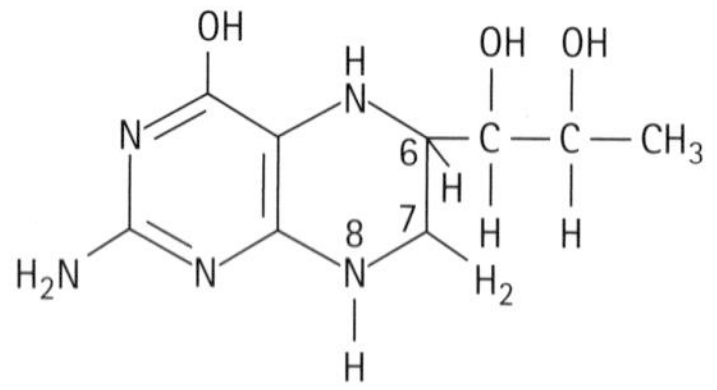

Figure 21.1 *Tetrahydrobiopterin (BH_4), the pteridine cofactor of phenylalanine hydroxylase.*

Patients are now being diagnosed because of the initiation of programs in which all hyperphenylalaninemic infants are being investigated for the possibility of defective metabolism of biopterin. However, it has already been documented that it is possible to miss a patient with abnormal synthesis of BH_4 because early phenylalanine levels may be normal. Therefore, evaluation for a disorder in this pathway should be undertaken in infants with unexplained neurological disease. These disorders, four of which have so far been defined, result from inadequate quantities of BH_4, (Figure 21.1) which derive from defective synthesis of this cofactor or defective recycling. The clinical manifestations of the various disorders are quite similar.

In 1974 Bartholome [2] described a patient who was later found to have a block in the synthesis of BH_4. This patient was initially diagnosed as having PKU, but had a progressive deterioration, although dietary restriction of phenylalanine had been exemplary. In the same year Smith [3] described patients in whom their phenylalaninemia was atypical in that they had a progressive neurological illness despite restriction of the intake of phenylalanine. She postulated a disorder in BH_4 metabolism. In the same year Kaufman and colleagues [4] reported deficiency of dihydropteridine reductase in such a patient.

Phenylalanine hydroxylase requires BH_4 for activity in the hydroxylation to tyrosine [1,2,5]. In the conversion of phenylalanine to tyrosine, BH_4 is oxidized to its hydroxyl compound, 4α-carbinolamine. This is recycled to quinonoid dihydropterin in a reaction catalyzed by 4α-carbinolamine dehydratase (PCD) [6] (EC 4.2.1.96).

The oxidized quinonoid dihydropterin compound must be reduced to form BH_4 before it can again be active as a cofactor (Figure 21.2). The reduction is catalyzed by dihydropteridine reductase (DHPR) [4–7] (EC 1.6.99.7). The quinonoid oxidation product is unstable and, unless it is promptly reduced, it forms a 7,8-dihydrobiopterin, which is no longer a substrate for dihydropteridine reductase.

The synthesis of the tetrahydrobiopterin cofactor is originally from guanosine triphosphate (GTP), and it proceeds through a number of steps in which reduced neopterin triphosphate (7,8-dihydroneopterin triphosphate) is an intermediate [8–10] (Figure 21.3). The first step is the GTP cyclohydrolase I reaction (GTPCH) [11] (EC 3.5.4.16). The next step is the 6-pyruvoyltetrahydropterin synthase (6-PTS) [12,13] (EC 4.6.1.10). Sepiapterin reductase and the reduced form of nicotinamide-adenine dinucleotide phosphate (NADPH) are involved in the conversion of 6PT to BH_4. Aldose reductase and carbonyl reductases may also serve to catalyze this reaction, and this may be why defects in sepiapterin reductase have not been identified as causative of human disease.

The gene has been cloned for DHPR [14,15]. The gene maps to chromosome 4 (p15.3). The gene for GTPCH is on chromosome 14q22.1–22.2. The cDNA for the human enzyme has been cloned [16]. The cDNA for 6-PTS has been cloned [17,18] and mapped to chromosome 11q22.2-23.3 [19]. The gene for PCD has been localized to chromosome 10q22 [20]. Mutations have been identified in the genes for each of the four enzymes defective in human metabolism DHPR [21], PCD [22], GTPCH [23,24] and 6-PTS [18]. These different abnormalities of biopterin metabolism account for less than two percent of patients with hyperphenylalaninemia. Each is inherited in an autosomal recessive fashion.

An international data base [25] includes over 300 patients; over 200 had 6-PTS deficiency, over 100, DHPR deficiency and less than 20 PCD deficiency, or 11 have GTPCH deficiency. Some remain unclassified, indicating the possibility of disorders yet to be identified. In addition to these disorders there are a number of disorders of biopterin metabolism in which hyperphenylalaninemia does not occur, such as dihydroxyphenylalanine (DOPA)-responsive dystonia or Sagawa disease, which results from autosomal dominant mutations in GTPCH [26].

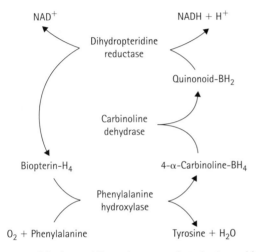

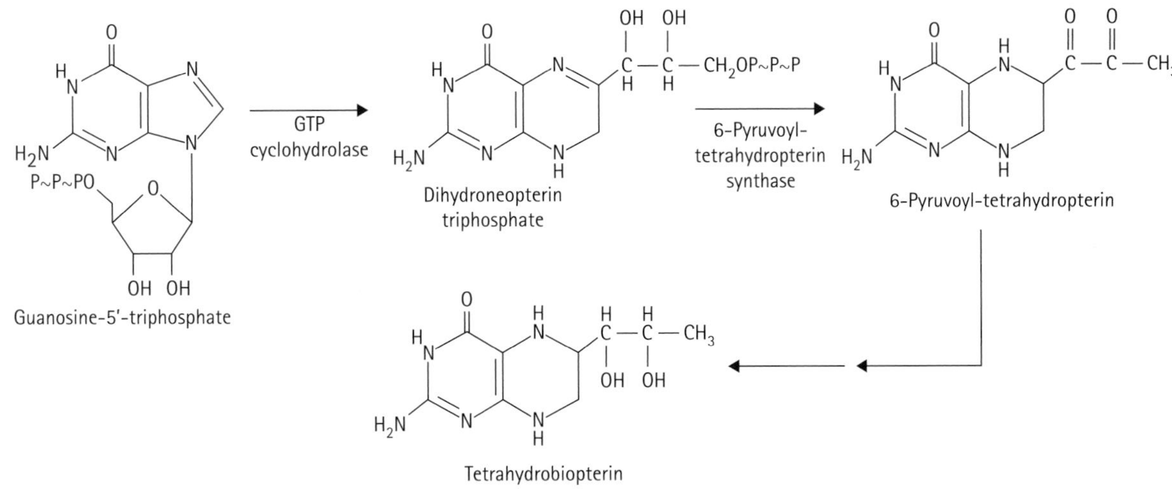

Figure 21.2   *Dihydropteridine reductase and pterin-4α-carbinoline dehydratase, enzymes involved in regeneration of BH_4 following the phenylalanine hydroxylase reaction. Defects in this system lead to defective function of BH_4 in the metabolism of phenylalanine and the neurotransmitters. Abbreviations employed include: BH_4: tetrahydrobiopterin; BH_2: dihydrobiopterin; NAD^+: nicotinamide dinucleotide and NADH, its reduced form.*

Figure 21.3   *Biopterin synthesis; GTP cyclohydrolase I and 6-pyruvoyltetrahydropterin synthase are sites of clinically defective biopterin synthesis.*

CLINICAL ABNORMALITIES

The clinical manifestations in most of these disorders are indistinguishable except for PCD deficiency. These latter patients have a much milder phenotype [22]. They might have been categorized clinically as having mild hyperphenylalaninemia. They were first recognized on the basis of a high urinary neopterin and an unknown compound, which proved to be primapterine, a 7-isomer of biopterin the side chain of which is in the 6 position (Figure 21.1) [27–29].

The classic presentation of abnormality in BH_4 metabolism is of an infant who appears normal at birth, but is found on screening to have an elevated concentration of phenylalanine in blood. A tendency to low birth weight has been observed in patients with defective synthesis, especially with 6-PTS deficiency, but not in reductase deficient patients. Failure to thrive may be impressive. Mild hypotonia may be present early. Some patients have had increased tone early [30], or there may be hypotonia of the trunk and hypertonia of the limbs. Development may be normal for 2 to 3 months; thereafter, a decrease in activity or a loss of head control may herald the onset of a progressive neurological degenerative disease [31,32] (Figures 21.4–21.10). Onset may be with convulsions as early as 3 months of age [33].

Ultimately these patients become hypertonic, especially in the lower extremities [34]. There may be bradykinesia, episodic 'lead pipe' rigidity or 'cog-wheel' rigidity [32]. The picture may be reminiscent of Parkinson disease. A 'stiff baby' syndrome has been described [35] in which torticollis was present and progressive rigidity. Episodes of extensor posturing of the extremities and opisthotonic arching of the back are characteristic. The hands are pronated. Deep tendon reflexes are increased. Clonus is frequently elicited, and the Babinski responses are present [36]. Drooling is a function of difficulty in swallowing and handling secretions. Feeding becomes difficult as well. The patient may be unable to swallow even pureed foods [30]. The typical patient is withdrawn and appears drowsy or expressionless, but irritability is also characteristic. Involuntary movements may be dystonic in nature. There may be oculogyric spasms. Some patients have tremors. Seizures are characteristically myoclonic and myoclonic seizures may be the presenting complaint [32], but

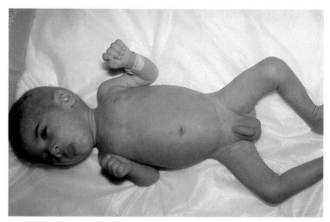

Figure 21.5 *R.M., a severely affected infant with 6-pyruvoyltetrahydropterin synthase (6-PTS) deficiency. He had bradykinesia, rigidity and myoclonus. Color of the skin and eyes were fair. After treatment with BH_4 and biogenic amine precursors, at 9 years-of-age, he was attending normal school with average performance for age and grade.*

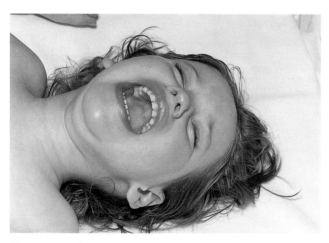

Figure 21.4 *G.H., a 3-year-old girl with defective synthesis of biopterin. The diagnosis was made and biopterin replacement was begun along with 5-hydroxytryptophan, L-DOPA and carbidopa treatments. Nevertheless, she was significantly neurologically impaired. She could sit unassisted and crawl. Muscle tone was decreased and deep tendon reflexes exaggerated. By 6 years-of-age she had a wide-based ataxic gait and drooled frequently.*

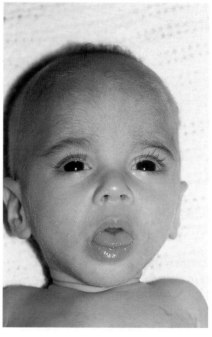

Figure 21.6 *Close-up of the face of R.M.*

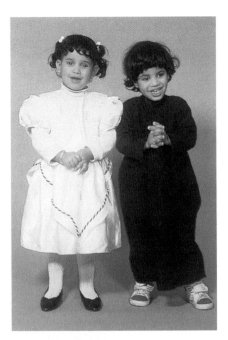

Figure 21.7 *R.M., on the right, 3.5 years later; next to him, his sister who was diagnosed and treated early, was normal neurologically with a normal IQ for age.*

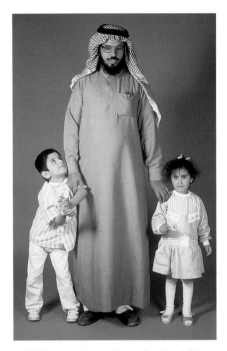

Figure 21.9 *A.M., 2 years later illustrating his ability to stand with a broad gait and posturing. The sister on the left, also affected, appeared normal, having been diagnosed and treated early.*

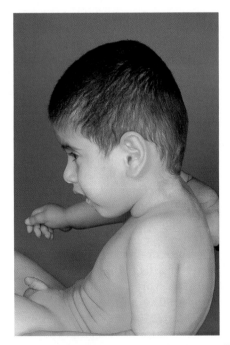

Figure 21.8 *A.M., another patient with 6PTS deficiency, illustrating the hypotonia. Despite late treatment he achieved some milestones.*

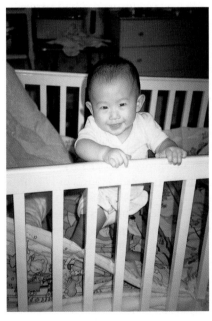

Figure 21.10 *I.T. An infant with defective BH₄ synthesis detected by newborn screening and treated early was developing nicely.*

grand mal seizures may occur as well. The electroencephalograph (EEG) pattern is abnormal. The impairment in intellectual function is usually profound, but there is heterogeneity, and some patients with only mild retardation have been described. These have tended to be younger patients, and progressive deterioration of the IQ has been documented,

for instance from 83 at 20 months to 24 at 11 years of age [33]. Microcephaly may be a consequence, and computed tomography (CT) or magnetic resonance imaging (MRI) scan of brain may reveal cerebral atrophy [37] or lucency of the white matter [38]. Abnormalities of the basal ganglia have been described and a pattern of intracranial calcification similar to that of methotrexate toxicity or folate malabsorption [39,40].

Patients not treated, in whom levels of phenylalanine are not kept from being elevated, may develop the fair hair and skin or relative lack of pigmentation that is characteristic of the patient with PKU [32,36] (Figure 21.5). Some patients have had episodes of hyperthermia without apparent infection [36]. Severe bronchopneumonia may require intensive care [32]. Death occurs often within the first 5 years of life [41]. One patient died of sudden infant death syndrome (SIDS) in hospital [32].

Patients with defective metabolism of BH_4 usually have hyperphenylalaninemia. Most are detected initially in programs of neonatal screening for PKU. However, some patients have had levels more consistent with atypical hyperphenylalaninemia or the variant forms of defective phenylalanine hydroxylase, and at least one patient in whom hyperphenylalaninemia has not been observed has been discovered through the study of siblings of known patients with BH_4 defects [42].

GENETICS AND PATHOGENESIS

Each of the defects in BH_4 metabolism is autosomal recessive. Consanguinity has been reported [36]. The overall frequency has been estimated at 1 in 10^6 births. In some groups higher incidence has been seen. In parts of Italy these defects amount to 10 percent of all patients with hyperphenylalaninemia, in Turkey 15 percent and in Taiwan 19 percent. In Saudi Arabia the figure is 68 percent [32].

Levels of dihydropteridine reductase consistent with heterozygosity have been reported [43] in lymphocytes, lymphoblasts and fibroblasts of parents. Obligate heterozygotes for GTP cyclohydrolase I deficiency were also found to have intermediate levels of activity [44]. In 6-PTS deficiency heterozygotes tended to have quite low levels of enzyme activity and may be symptomatic [45]. Prenatal diagnosis has been carried out in DHPR deficiency by enzyme assay [46,47]. Prenatal diagnosis has most commonly been carried out by the assessment of pterins in amniotic fluid [47,48]. In GTPCH deficiency levels of BH_4 and neopterin in amniotic fluid are very low; in 6-PTS deficiency BH_4 is low and neopterin high; in DHPR deficiency BH_4 is high and neopterin normal or slightly elevated [47–50]. Affected and nonaffected fetuses have been diagnosed in this way in DHPR deficiency [47], in 6-PTS deficiency [47] and in GTPCH deficiency [49]. Molecular diagnosis by restriction fragment length polymorphism (RFLP) analysis in amniocytes has been reported in DHPR deficiency [51].

Four enzymatic defects have been described in this syndrome. DHPR deficiency [4], PCD deficiency [29] and the defects in the synthesis of BH_4, GTPCH deficiency [36,52] and 6-PTS deficiencies [35,53,54].

Each of these defects leads to a situation in which phenylalanine cannot be converted to tyrosine, even though the phenylalanine hydroxylase apoenzyme is normal. Tetrahydrobiopterin is also the cofactor for the hydroxylation of tryptophan and tyrosine. Thus its deficiency interferes with the synthesis of serotonin, dihydroxyphenylalanine (DOPA) and norepinephrine. Data have been obtained that indicate that this is the case, since levels of 5-hydroxyindoleacetic acid, vanillylmandelic acid and homovanillic acid in the urine and cerebrospinal fluids are considerably lower than normal [30,31]. Low levels of dopamine and serotonin have also been documented in the urine [36]. Since it is possible in these disorders to have severe neurological disease in the presence of only mild hyperphenylalaninemia, levels of BH_4 may be relatively more sufficient for phenylalanine hydroxylation than that of tryptophan or tyrosine [30]. Defective neurotransmitter metabolism is doubtless related to the genesis of neurological abnormalities.

6-Pyruvoyltetrahydropterin synthase deficiency

Deficiency of 6-PTS is the most common of the defects in biopterin metabolism, approximating 60 percent of the patients. The majority have had the typical form, but there are a number in whom the presentation is atypical. The typical patients have high levels of neopterin and low biopterin in the urine and cerebrospinal fluid (CSF). These patients have the highest neopterin levels and the highest ratios of neopterin to BH_4 of all the abnormalities in pterin metabolism. The atypical patients have been referred to as peripheral because the CSF is normal, but with time it can become abnormal [55]. Clinical presentation in these patients is milder and response to treatment more satisfactory. A 20 mg/kg load of BH_4 per kilogram leads to a rapid decrease in the plasma concentration of phenylalanine.

The enzyme 6-PTS was formerly called the phosphate eliminating enzyme, because it catalyzes the elimination of inorganic triphosphate from the dihydroneopterin triphosphate product of the cyclohydrolase reaction (Figure 21.3). This is an irreversible step. Markedly deficient activity was demonstrated first in biopsied liver [56]. The enzyme is expressed in erythrocytes, and typical patients have less than 4 percent of control activity [57]. Patients with the atypical, peripheral form have partial activity in erythrocytes ranging from 5 to 23 percent of normal [58–60]. Residual activity does not always correlate with a milder phenotype; typical patients may have activities as high as 20 percent [45,48]. Enzyme deficiency can also be documented in fibroblasts [61] in which activity is about one percent of control levels.

The reading frame of the cDNA for 6-PTS encompasses 435 bp over 6 exons. Twenty-eight mutations have been found distributed throughout all the exons of the gene [18,62,63]. Two were splice site mutations [61]. There were a few deletions, and a majority were point mutations, some producing stop codons. N52S and P87S appear to be common in Asians. Mild hyperphenylalaninemia and dystonia were observed in a patient with a homozygous I114V mutation [64].

GTP cyclohydrolase deficiency

Defects in GTPCH account for about four percent of those with abnormalities in biopterin metabolism. In these patients levels of both neopterin and biopterin are low, but their ratio may be normal [36,44,59,65]. Concentrations of neurotransmitters and their metabolites 5-hydroxyindoleacetic acid and homovanillic acid are low. High concentrations of phenylalanine are corrected with BH_4 loading or replacement.

Defective enzyme activity has been documented in liver, lymphocytes [36,60] and fibroblasts [66]. The human gene has been cloned and found to span 30kb in six exons [16]. A mutation converting methionine to isoleucine at position 211 (M211I) caused deficiency of the enzyme in a patient who was missed on neonatal screening [67]. Missense mutations, such as this and R184H as well as nonsense mutations (Q110X) lead to complete deficiency of the enzyme.

Dihydropteridine reductase deficiency

DHPR deficiency accounts for approximately a third of the patients with defects in biopterin metabolism. Levels of neurotransmitters are low in CSF and urine. These include homovanillic acid (HVA), vanillylmandelic acid (VMA), 3-methoxyhydroxyphenylglycol (MHPG) and 5-hydroxyindoleacetic acid (HIAA); the metabolites of dopamine, norepinephrine, epinephrine and serotonin, respectively [68]. Total urinary pterins are elevated and BH_4 is low.

Deficient activity of the enzyme has been documented in liver, brain and cultured fibroblasts [4]. The enzyme can also be assayed in erythrocytes [69]. Activity is generally very low, and some patients are CRM positive and some CRM negative without correlation with degrees of clinical severity [70–72]. The gene was mapped to chromosome 4p15.31 [73]. The intron/exon structure has been determined for the gene that codes for a 25.7 kD protein [74,75]. A number of mutations have been identified spread throughout the gene. An insertion of an extra codon for threonine between alanine at position 122 and the threonine at residue 123 [21] was an early identification, but accounts for most of the mutations reported [76]. A number of RFLPs has been identified in the gene, which may be useful for prenatal diagnosis and population genetic studies [51,74].

Pterin-4α-carbinolamine dehydratase deficiency

PCD deficiency occurs in about four percent of patients with defective BH_4 metabolism [25]. When the phenylalanine hydroxylation reaction takes place, the carbinolamine intermediate is converted to dihydropterin in a reaction catalyzed by the dehydratase PCD. When PCD is defective, there is a conversion to 7-biopterin (primapterin), and the excretion of this compound is a distinguishing characteristic of this disorder [77,78]. The dehydratase reaction can also proceed nonenzymatically [79], and this could be a reason for the relatively mild phenotype.

PCD is a bifunctional protein with transcriptional function; its gene codes for four exons over 5 kb [80]. Many mutations described have been nonsense mutations, but they have clustered in exon 4 [63].

Diagnosis

Although only two percent of the patients found to have hyperphenylalaninemia have disorders of biopterin metabolism, every patient should be tested for an abnormality of BH_4 because the implications for management and counseling are so different [80].

The diagnosis of these disorders may be made in a number of ways. Among the simplest is the administration of tetrahydrobiopterin [41]. Doses of 2 mg/kg intravenously and 7.5–20 mg/kg orally have been recommended [81]. Administration of BH_4 leads to a prompt decrease to normal in the concentration of phenylalanine in patients with synthesis and reductase defects, and of course no change in the patient with PKU. It is important that the patient be on a diet containing normal amounts of phenylalanine, not the therapeutic diet employed for patients with PKU. A few patients with DHPR defects have been missed using the BH_4 loading test [82,83]. BH_4 is an investigational drug in the US, which makes the paperwork feasible for the treatment of a patient, but not for a diagnostic test. Loading tests, in any case, must be confirmed by analysis of enzyme activity in any abnormality of BH_4 metabolism. The gold standard for the diagnosis of DHPR deficiency is assay of the enzyme.

Currently, routine testing for patients with hyperphenylalaninemia includes the assay of DHPR activity in dried spots on Guthrie cards [43,84,85]. Definitive testing for activity can be accomplished in cultured fibroblasts, lymphoblasts, or freshly isolated lymphocytes. The defect has also been demonstrated in biopsied liver [4,30]. The other test that has become routine for the detection of BH_4 abnormalities in hyperphenylalaninemic infants is the assay of pterin metabolites in the urine.

Pterin metabolites in urine are measured by high performance liquid chromatography (HPLC) [86,87]. The normal values for biopterin and neopterin are 0.4–2.5 and 0.1–5.0 mmol/mol creatinine, respectively, and the proportion of biopterin is 20–80 percent [88]. In those with defective GTPCH, all pterins are low in blood and urine and the ratio is normal [36,52]. In patients with 6PTS deficiency, the concentrations of biopterin are very low and those of neopterin high [81]. In PCD deficiency primapterin is formed in the urine, and BH_4 is low. In patients with DHPR deficiency there is a lack of feedback inhibition, and so there may be massive overproduction of urinary pterins, but the level of BH_4 is always low. On the other hand, patients with DHPR deficiency have been reported in whom urinary pterin analysis was normal [89], indicating further the importance of enzyme analysis in the diagnosis of this condition. The normal plasma BH4 value is 1.4–3.0; that of blood 2.4–6.0 ng/mL [88].

TREATMENT

Patients with defects in pterin metabolism, especially those with abnormalities in BH_4 synthesis should be treated with BH_4 [41,88,90] (Figure 21.11). This compound is available from B. Schircks, Ch 8641, Jona, Switzerland from Suntory, Tokyo, Japan. It is given daily in large doses (2–20 mg/kg) [81,91,92]. BH_4 tablets contain 100 mg BH_4, 100 mg ascorbic acid and 50 mg N-acetylcysteine. Protein intake is also restricted. BH_4 treatment may reduce concentrations of tyrosine in plasma and CSF. Levels may be monitored and supplemental tyrosine (as in PKU formulations) employed if necessary.

In BH_4 synthesis defects a single daily dose of 2–5 mg/kg is usually sufficient to control levels of phenylalanine. In DHPR defects larger doses (20 mg/kg) may be required, and it must be given fractionally through the day. Some patients with DHPR deficiency must be treated with sufficient restriction of phenylalanine intake to maintain normal plasma levels [82,93]. Treatment with DOPA, 5-hydoxytryptophan and carbidopa is introduced slowly and sequentially; steps are 1 mg/kg over days or weeks. DOPA is given in doses of 8–12 mg/kg and 5-hydroxytryptophan 6–9 mg/kg. Carbidopa is 10–20 percent of DOPA in most formulations. In addition to controlling the concentration of phenylalanine, treatment of this condition must correct deficiencies of neurotransmitters. This cannot

be done with BH_4 alone, possibly because of reduced penetration into the brain, although it is clear that it does enter [94,95].

Neutrotransmitter balance is treated with a regimen of biogenic amine precursors including 5-hydroxytryptophan and L-DOPA along with carbidopa [96,97], which inhibits peripheral decarboxylation permitting entry to the central nervous system (CNS), where decarboxylation to serotonin and dopamine takes place. Preparations, such as Sinemet, which combine DOPA and carbidopa may be useful. Measurements of neurotransmitter metabolites and pterins in the cerebrospinal fluid are required in order to determine optimal doses and to monitor the effectiveness of therapeutic regimens. The level of prolactin in serum is elevated in these diseases, which is an index of abnormal dopamine homeostasis, and it may be useful to monitor levels in order to guide therapy [93]. Levels of folate may be low in DHPR deficiency, and DHPR appears to have a role in tetrahydrofolate synthesis [98,99]. Folinic acid has been employed in a dose of 12.5 mg per day [98].

Progressive improvement, with disappearance of myoclonus, involuntary movements and tetraplegia, has been reported following treatment with biogenic amine precursors without BH_4 [4,27], but this would not be recommended. There is evidence that early treatment may prevent progression [32,81], but overall experience indicates that prognosis should be guarded. Many patients have considerable neurological impairment despite therapy. Programs must be individually tailored to meet the needs of the patient.

References

1 Kaufman S. A new cofactor required for the enzymatic conversion of phenylalanine to tyrosine. *J Biol Chem* 1958;**230**:931.

2 Bartholome K. A new molecular defect in phenylketonuria. *Lancet* 1974;**2**:1580.

3 Smith I. Atypical phenylketonuria accompanied by a severe progressive neurological illness unresponsive to dietary treatment. *Arch Dis Child* 1974;**49**:245.

4 Kaufman S, Holtzman NA, Milstein S, *et al.* Phenylketonuria due to a deficiency of dihydropteridine reductase. *N Engl J Med* 1975;**293**:785.

5 Kaufman S. Metabolism of phenylalanine hydroxylation cofactor. *J Biol Chem* 1967;**242**:3943.

6 Lei XD, Kaufman S. Human white blood cells and hair follicles are good sources of mRNA for the pterin carbinolamine dehydratase/dimerization cofactor of HNF for mutation detection. *Biochem Biophys Res Commun* 1998;**248**:432.

7 Craine JE, Hall ES, Kaufman S. The isolation and characterization of dihydropteridine reductase from sheep liver. *J Biol Chem* 1972;**247**:6082.

8 Brown GM. The biosynthesis of pteridines. *Adv Enzymol* 1971;**35**:35.

9 Eto I, Fukushima K, Shioa T. Enzymatic synthesis of biopterin from d-erythro-dihydroneopterin triphosphate by extracts of kidneys from Syrian golden hamsters. *J Biol Chem* 1976;**251**:6505.

10 Gal EM, Nelson JM, Sherman AD. Biopterin: III Purification and characterization of enzymes involved in the cerebral synthesis of 78-dihydrobiopterin. *Neurochem Res* 1978;**3**:69.

11 Burg AW, Brown GM. The biosynthesis of folic acid VIII. Purification and properties of the enzyme that catalyzes the production of formate from carbon 8 of guanosine triphosphate. *J Biol Chem* 1968;**243**:2349.

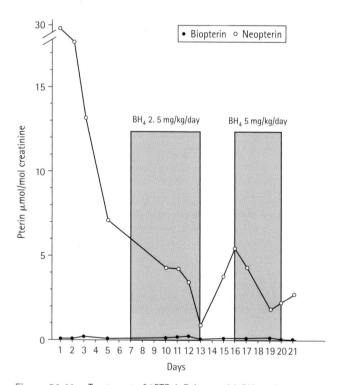

Figure 21.11 *Treatment of 6PTS deficiency with BH₄, reduced the excretion of neopterin in the urine.*

12   Takikawa S, Curtius H-C, Redweik U, Ghisla S. Purification of 6-pyruvoyl tetra-hydropterin synthase from human liver. *Biochem Biophys Res Commun* 1986;**134**:646.

13   Takikawa S-I, Curtius H-C, Redweik U, *et al.* Biosynthesis of tetrahydrobiopterin. Purification and characterization of 6-pyruvoyl-tetrahydropterin synthase from human liver. *Eur J Biochem* 1986;**161**:295.

14   Dahl HHM, Hutchinson W, McAdam W, *et al.* Human dihydropteridine reductase: characterization of a cDNA clone and its use in analysis of patients with dihydropteridine reductase deficiency. *Nucleic Acids Res* 1987;**15**:1921.

15   Lockyer J, Cook RG, Milstein S, *et al.* Structure and expression of human dihydropteridine reductase. *Proc Natl Acad Sci USA* 1987;**84**:3329.

16   Nomura T, Ichinose H, Sumi-Ichinose C, *et al.* Cloning and sequencing of cDNA encoding mouse GTP cyclohydrolase I. *Biochem Biophys Res Commun* 1993;**191**:523.

17   Hatakayema K, Ashida A, Owada M, *et al.* Molecular basis of malignant hyperphenylalaninemia: a mutation in the gene encoding human 6-pyruvoyl-tetra-hydropterin synthase. *First IUBMB Conference*;1992: *Biochemistry of Disease 2-a-05-P7* (Abstr).

18   Oppliger T, Thony B, Leimbacher W, *et al.* Structural and functional consequences of mutations in 6-pyruvoyltetra-hydropterin synthase causing hyperphenyl-alaninemia in man. *SSIEM Symposium* 1995;**37**: P026.

19   Kluge C, Brecevic L, Heizmann CW, *et al.* Chromosomal localization genomic structure and characterization of a single human gene (PTS) and retropseudogene for 6-pyruvoyltetrahydropterin synthase. *Eur J Biochem* 1996;**240**:477.

20   Thony B, Heizmann CW, Mattei MG. Chromosomal location of two human genes encoding tetrahydrobiopterin-metabolizing enzymes: 6-pyruvoyl-tetrahydropterin synthase maps to 11q223-q233 and pterin-4α-carbinolamine dehydratase maps to 10q22. *Genomics* 1994;**19**:365.

21   Howells DW, Forrest SM, Dahl HHM, Cotton RGH. Insertion of an extra codon for threonine is a cause of dihydropteridine reductase deficiency. *Am J Hum Genet* 1990;**47**:279.

22   Citron BA, Kaufman S, Milstien S, *et al.* Mutation in the 4α-carbinolamine dehydratase gene leads to mild hyperphenylalaninemia with defective cofactor metabolism. *Am J Hum Genet* 1993;**53**:768.

23   Ichinose H, Ohye T, Matsuda Y, *et al.* Characterization of mouse and human GTP cyclohydrolase I genes: Mutations in patients with GTP cyclohydrolase I deficiency. *J Biol Chem* 1995;**270**:10062.

24   Thöny B, Blau N. Mutations in the GTP cyclohydrolase I and 6-pyruvoyl-tetrahydropterin synthase genes. *Hum Mutat* 1997;**10**:11.

25   Blau N, Barnes I, Dhondt JL. International database of tetrahydrobiopterin deficiencies. *J Inherit Metab Dis* 1995;**19**:8.

26   Ichinose H, Inagaki H, Suzuki T, *et al.* Molecular mechanisms of hereditary progressive dystonia with marked diurnal fluctuation Segawa's disease. *Brain Dev* 2000;**22**:(Suppl 1) S107.

27   Dhondt J, Guibaud P, Rolland M, *et al.* Neonatal hyperphenylalaninemia presumably caused by a new variant of biopterin synthetase deficiency. *Eur J Pediatr* 1988;**147**:153.

28   Blaskovics M, Guidici T. A new variant of biopterin deficiency. *N Engl J Med* 1988;**319**:1611.

29   Blau N, Curtius H-C, Kuster T, *et al.* Primapterinuria: a new variant of atypical phenylketonuria. *J Inherit Metab Dis* 1989;**12**:(Suppl 2) 335.

30   Brewster TG, Moskowitz HA, Kaufman S, *et al.* Dihydropteridine reductase deficiency associated with severe neurologic disease and mild hyperphenylalaninemia. *Pediatrics* 1979;**63**:94.

31   Smith I, Clayton BE, Wolff OH. New variant of phenylketonuria with progressive neurological illness unresponsive to phenylalanine restriction. *Lancet* 1975;**1**:328.

32   Al Aqeel A, Ozand PT, Gascon G, *et al.* Biopterin-dependent hyperphenylalaninemia due to deficiency of 6-pyruvoyl tetrahydropterin synthase. *Neurology* 1991;**41**:730.

33   Narisawa K, Arai N, Ishizawa S, *et al.* Dihydropteridine reductase deficiency: diagnosis by leukocyte enzyme assay. *Clin Chim Acta* 1980;**105**:335l.

34   Endres W, Niederwieser A, Curtius H-Ch, *et al.* Atypical phenylketonuria due to biopterin deficiency. *Helv Paediatr Acta* 1982;**37**:489.

35   Allen RJ, Young W, Bonacci J, *et al.* Neonatal dystonic parkinsonism a 'stiff baby syndrome' in biopterin deficiency with hyperprolactinemia detected by newborn screening for hyperphenylalaninemia and responsiveness to treatment. *Ann Neurol* 1990;**28**:434.

36   Niederwieser A, Blau N, Wang M, *et al.* GTP cyclohydrolase I deficiency a new enzyme defect causing hyperphenylalaninemia with neopterin biopterin dopamine and serotonin deficiencies and muscular hypotonia. *Eur J Pediatr* 1984;**141**:208.

37   Butler IJ, OöFlynn ME, Seifert WE, Howell RR. Neurotransmitter defects and treatment of disorders of hyperphenylalaninemia. *J Pediatr* 1981;**98**:729.

38   Brismar J, Al Aqeel A, Gascon G, Ozand P. Malignant hyperphenyl-alaninemia: CT and MR of the brain. *Am J Neuroradiol* 1990;**11**:135.

39   Smith I, Leeming RJ, Cavanagh NP, Hyland K. Neurological aspects of biopterin metabolism. *Arch Dis Child* 1986;**61**:130.

40   Gudinchet F, Maeder P, Meuli RA, *et al.* Cranial CT and MRI in malignant phenylketonuria. *Pediatr Radiol* 1992;**22**:223.

41   Danks DM, Schlesinger P, Firgaira F, *et al.* Malignant hyperphenyl-alaninemia – clinical features biochemical findings and experience with administration of biopterins. *Pediatr Res* 1979;**13**:1150.

42   Matalon R. Screening for biopterin defects: experience with 387 patients with hyperphenylalaninemia. Twenty-second meeting of SSIEM, Newcastle, England;September 4–7 1984.

43   Firgaira FA, Cotton RGH, Danks DM. Dihydropteridine reductase deficiency diagnosis by assays on peripheral blood-cells. *Lancet* 1979;**2**:1260.

44   Naylor EW, Ennis D, Davidson AGF, *et al.* Guanosine triphosphate cyclohydrolase I deficiency: early diagnosis by routine urine pteridine screening. *Pediatrics* 1987;**79**:374.

45   Scriver CR, Clow CL, Kaplan P, Niederwieser A. Hyperphenylalaninemia due to deficiency of 6-pyruvoyl tetrahydropterin synthase. Unusual gene dosage effect in heterozygotes. *Hum Genet* 1987;**77**:168.

46   Guardamagna O, Spada M, Ponzone A, *et al.* Prenatal diagnosis of dihydropteridine reductase deficiency in a twin pregnancy. *Pteridines* 1992;**3**:19.

47   Blau N, Niederwieser A, Curtius H-C, *et al.* Prenatal diagnosis of atypical phenylketonuria. *J Inherit Metab Dis* 1989;**12**:295.

48   Blau N, Kierat L, Matasovic A, *et al.* Antenatal diagnosis of tetrahydrobiopterin deficiency by quantification of pterins in amniotic fluid and enzyme activity in fetal and extrafetal tissue. *Clin Chim Acta* 1994;**226**:159.

49   Dhondt JL, Tilmont P, Ringel J, *et al.* Pterins [AU108] analysis in amniotic fluid for the prenatal diagnosis of GTP cyclohydrolase deficiency. *J Inherit Metab Dis* 1990;**13**:879.

50   Niederweiser A, Shintaku H, Hasler T, *et al.* Prenatal diagnosis of 'dihydrobiopterin synthetase' deficiency a variant form of phenylketonuria. *Eur J Pediatr* 1986;**145**:176.

51   Dahl HHM, Wake S, Cotton RGH, Danks DM. The use of restriction fragment length polymorphism in prenatal diagnosis of dihydropteridine reductase deficiency. *J Med Genet* 1988;**25**:25.

52   Dhondt JL, Farriaux JP, Boudha A, *et al.* Neonatal hyperphenylalaninemia presumably caused by guanosine triphosphate cyclohydrolase deficiency. *J Pediatr* 1985;**106**:954.

53   Niederwieser A, Curtius H-Ch, Bettoni O, *et al.* Atypical phenylketonuria caused by 78-dihydrobiopterin synthetase deficiency. *Lancet* 1979;**1**:131.

54   Dhondt JL. Strategy for the screening of tetrahydrobiopterin deficiency among hyperphenylalaninemic patients: 15-years experience. *J Inherit Metab Dis* 1991;**14**:117.

55 Ponzone A, Blau N, Guardamagna O, *et al.* Progression of 6-pyruvoyl-tetrahydropterin synthase deficiency from a peripheral into a central phenotype. *J Inherit Metab Dis* 1990;**13**:298.

56 Niederwieser A, Leimbacher W, Curtius H-C, *et al.* Atypical phenylketonuria with dihydrobiopterin synthetase deficiency: absence of phosphate-eliminating enzyme activity demonstrated in liver. *Eur J Pediatr* 1985;**144**:13.

57 Niederwieser A, Shintaku H, Hasler TH, *et al.* Prenatal diagnosis of 'dihydropterin synthetase' deficiency a variant form of phenylketonuria. *Eur J Pediatr* 1986;**145**:176.

58 Niederwieser A, Shintaku H, Leimbacher W, *et al.* Peripheral tetrahydrobiopterin deficiency with hyperphenyl-alaninemia due to incomplete 6-pyruvoyl tetrahydropterin synthase deficiency or heterozygosy. *Eur J Pediatr* 1987;**146**:228.

59 Dhondt JL, Farriaux JP, Boudha A, *et al.* Neonatal hyperphenylalaninemia presumably caused by guanosine triphosphatecyclohydrolase deficiency. *J Pediatr* 1985;**106**:954.

60 Blau N, Niederwieser A. Guanosine triphosphate cyclohydrolase I assay in human and rat liver using high-performance liquid chromatography of neopterin phosphates and guanine nucleotides. *Anal Biochem* 1983;**128**:446.

61 Oppliger T, Thony B, Kluge C, *et al.* Identification of mutations causing 6-pyruvoyl-tetrahydropterin synthase deficiency in four Italian families. *Hum Mutat* 1997;**10**:25.

62 Romstad A, Guldberg P, Levy HL, *et al.* Singe-step mutation scanning of the 6-pyruvoyl-tetrahydropterin synthase gene in patients with hyperphenylalaninemia. *Clin Chem* 1999;**45**:2102.

63 Blau N, Thony B, Dianzani I. BIOMDB: Database of Mutations Causing Tetrahydrobiopterin Deficiency http://wwwbh4org (accessed October 2004).

64 Hanihara T, Inoue K, Kawanishi C, *et al.* 6-Pyrovoyl-tetrahydropterin synthase deficiency with generalized dystonia and diurnal fluctuation of symptoms: A clinical and molecular study. *Mov Disord* 1997;**12**:408.

65 Coskun T, Karagoz T, Kalkanoglu S, *et al.* Guanosine triphosphate clyclohydrolase I deficiency. A rare cause of hyperphenylalaninemia. *Tur J Pediatr* 1999;**41**:231.

66 Milstein S, Kaufman S, Sakai N. Tetrahydrobiopterin biosynthesis defects examined in cytokine-stimulated fibroblasts. *J Inherited Metab Dis* 1993;**16**:975.

67 Blau N, Ichinose H, Nagatsu T, *et al.* A missense mutation in a patient with guanosine triphosphate cyclo-hydrolase deficiency missed in the newborn screening program. *J Pediatr* 1995;**126**:401.

68 Niederwieser A, Ponzone A, Curtius H-C. Differential diagnosis of tetrahydrobiopterin deficiency. *J Inherit Metab Dis* 1985;**8**:34.

69 Narisawa K, Arai N, Hayakawa H, Tada K. Diagnosis of dihydropteridine reductase deficiency by erythrocyte enzyme assay. *Pediatrics* 1981;**68**:591.

70 Cotton RGH, Jennings I, Bracco G, *et al.* Tetrahydrobiopterin non-responsiveness in dihydropteridine reductase deficiency is associated with the presence of mutant protein *J Inherit Metab Dis* 1986;**9**:239.

71 Ponzone A, Guardamagna O, Bracco G, *et al.* Two mutations of dihydro-pteridine reductase deficiency. *Arch Dis Child* 1988;**63**:154.

72 Firgaira FA, Choo KH, Cotton RGH, Danks DM. Molecular and immunological comparison of human dihydropteridine reductase in liver cultured fibroblasts and continuous lymphoid cells. *Biochem J* 1981;**197**:45.

73 Sumi S, Ishikawa T, Ito Y, *et al.* Probable assignment of the dihydropteridine reductase gene to 4p1531. *Tohoku J Exp Med* 1990;**160**:93.

74 Smooker PM, Howells DW, Cotton RGH. Dihydropteridine reductase deficiency-D – identification of natural mutations and analysis by recombinant expression and *in vivo* protein studies. *Am J Hum Genet* 1991;**49**:(Suppl) A193.

75 Dianzani I, De Santis L, Smooker PM, *et al.* Dihydropteridine reductase deficiency: Physical structure of the QDPR gene identification of two new mutations and genotype-phenotype correlations. *Hum Mutat* 1998;**12**:267.

76 De Sanctis L, Alliaudi C, Spada M, *et al.* Genotype-phenotype correlation in dehydropteridine reductase deficiency. *J Inherit Metab Dis* 2000;**23**:333.

77 Curtius H-Ch, Kuster T, Matasovic A, *et al.* Primapterin anapterin and 6-oxo-primapterin three new 7-substituted pterins identified in a patient with hyperphenyl-alaninemia. *Biochem Biophys Res Commun* 1988;**153**:715.

78 Curtius H-Ch, Matasovic A, Schoedon G, *et al.* 7-Substituted pterins. *J Biol Chem* 1990;**265**:3932.

79 Curtius H-Ch, Adler C, Rebrin I, *et al.* 7-Substituted pterins; formation during phenyalanine hydroxylation in the absence of dehydratase. *Biochem Biophys Res Commun* 1990;**172**:1060.

80 Thony B, Neuheiser F, Blau N, Heizmann CW. Characterization of the human PCBD gene encoding the bifunctional protein pterin-4α-carbinolamine dehydratase/dimerization cofactor for the transcription factor HNF-1 alpha. *Biochem Biophys Res Commun* 1995;**210**:966.

81 Al Aqeel A, Ozand PT, Gascon GG, *et al.* Response of 6-pyruvoyl-tetrahydropterin synthase to deficiency of tetrahydrobiopterin. *J Child Neurol* 1992;**7**:S26.

82 Lipson A, Yu J, O'Halloran M, *et al.* Dihydropteridine reductase deficiency: Non-response to oral tetrahydrobiopterin load test. *J Inherit Metab Dis* 1984;**7**:69.

83 Endres W, Ibel H, Kierat L, *et al.* Tetrahydrobiopterin and 'non-responsive' dehydropteridine reductase deficiency. *Lancet* 1987;**2**:223.

84 Sahota A, Blair JA, Barford PA, *et al.* Neonatal screening for dihydropteridine reductase deficiency. *J Inherit Metab Dis* 1985;**8**:99.

85 Arai N, Narisawa K, Hayakawa H, Taka K. Hyperphenylalaninemia due to dehydropteridine reductase deficiency: Diagnosis by enzyme assay on dried blood spots. *Pediatrics* 1982;**98**:426.

86 Niederwieser A, Curtius HC, Gitzelmann R, *et al.* Excretion of pterins in phenylketonuria and phenylketonuria variants. *Helv Paediatr Acta* 1980;**35**:335.

87 Howells DW, Smith I, Hyland K. Estimation of tetrahydrobiopterin and other pterins in cerebrospinal fluid using reversed-phase high-performance liquid chromatography with electrochemical and fluorescence detection. *J Chromatogr* 1986;**381**:285.

88 Smith I. Disorders of tetrahydrobiopterin metabolism in *Inborn Metabolism Diseases Diagnosis and Treatment* (eds Fernandes J, Saudubray J-M, Tada K) Springer-Verlag, Berlin;1991:183.

89 Blau N, Heizmann CW, Sperl W, *et al.* Atypical (Mild) forms of dihydro-pteridine reductase deficiency: Neurochemical evaluation and mutation detection. *Pediatr Res* 1992;**32**:726.

90 Curtius H-C, Niederwieser A, Viscontini M, *et al.* Atypical phenylketonuria due to tetrahydrobiopterin deficiency. Diagnosis and treatment with tetra-hydrobiopterin dihydrobiopterin and sepiapterin. *Clin Chim Acta* 1979;**93**:251.

91 Ponzone A, Guardamagna O, Dianzani I, *et al.* Catalytic activity of tetrahydrobiopterin in dihydropteridine reductase deficiency and indications for treatment. *Pediatr Res* 1993;**33**:125.

92 Smith I, Hyland K, Kendall B, Leeming R. Clinical role of pteridine therapy in tetrahydrobiopterin deficiency. *J Inherit Metab Dis* 1985;**8**:39.

93 Spada M, Ferraris S, Altare F, *et al.* Monitoring treatment in tetrahydrobiopterin deficiency by serum prolactin. *SSIEM Symposium* 1995;**33**:P029.

94 Kapatos G, Kaufman S. Peripherally administered reduced pterins do enter the brain. *Science* 1981;**212**:955.

95 Hoshiga M, Hatakeyama K, Watanabe M, *et al.* Autoradiographic distribution of [^{14}C]tetrahydrobiopterin and its developmental change in mice. *J Pharmacol Exp Ther* 1993;**267**:971.

96 Bartholome K, Byrd DJ. L-DOPA and 5-hydroxytryptophan therapy in phenylketonuria with normal phenylalanine hydroxylase. *Lancet* 1975;**2**:1042.

97 Endres W. Biopterin deficiency: Therapy of tetrahydrobiopterin deficiencies monotherapy of combined treatment with neurotransmitter precursors in *International Symposium on Recent Progress in the Understanding* *Recognition and Management of Inherited Diseases of Amino Acid Metabolism* (eds Bickel H, Wachtel U) Georg Thieme. Stuttgart;1985:124.

98 Irons M, Levy HL, O'Flynn E, *et al.* Folinic acid therapy in treatment of dihydropteridine reductase deficiency. *J Pediatr* 1987;**110**:61.

99 Pollock RJ, Kaufman S. Dihydropterine reductase may function in tetrahydrofolate metabolism. *J Neurochem* 1978;**31**:115.

22

Homocystinuria

MAJOR PHENOTYPIC EXPRESSION

Ectopia lentis, vascular occlusive disease, malar flush, osteoporosis, accumulation of homocystine and methionine and defective activity of cystathionine synthase.

INTRODUCTION

Homocystinuria was first described in 1962 by Carson, Neill and colleagues [1,2]. The enzymatic defect was identified by Mudd and colleagues [3] two years later. Since then considerable experience has been developed which has defined the clinical phenotype, the abnormal biochemistry and the natural history of the disease [4].

The molecular defect is in the enzyme cystathionine synthase (EC 4.2.1.22) (Figure 22.1). This enzyme is on the metabolic pathway for methionine, and patients may be recognized by an increase in the concentration of methionine in the blood. This property forms the basis for the inclusion of homocystinuria in most programs of routine neonatal screening. In some patients, accumulation of methionine may give a prominent, unpleasant odor. The clinical picture regularly includes many features, like subluxation of the lenses of the eyes, which are characteristic of a disorder of connective tissue. Extreme variability of clinical presentation is a consequence of whether or not there are thrombotic events and if so which areas of the body suffer infarction. Variability also results from the fact that there are two distinct populations of homocystinuric patients, one of which responds to treatment with pyridoxine and one that does not [4].

CLINICAL ABNORMALITIES

Ectopia lentis is a striking and readily recognizable manifestation of the disease. (Figures 22.2–22.5) It may be the only manifestation [4–8], and by 38 years-of-age only three percent of patients have both lenses in place. Dislocation is usually present by 10 years-of-age. The dislocation is said to be usually, but not always, downward – the opposite of the situation in Marfan disease. Its presence may be signaled by iridodonesis, a dancing or shimmering iris. Electron microscopy reveals partially broken zonules, abnormal zonular attachment and a spongy capsular appearance [8]. Complications may include dislocation into the anterior chamber and papillary block glaucoma. Other ocular abnormalities include myopia, optic atrophy, cataracts or retinal detachment [9].

The pigmentation of the iris may be lighter than in family members, and the same may be true for the skin and hair. A pronounced malar flush [10] was first recognized in Ireland, but we have also seen it in patients with considerable cutaneous pigment (Figures 22.2, 22.3). The skin may otherwise have blotchy erythema and pallor, and livido reticularis [11] is particularly common in the distal extremities, which may be quite cold and show other evidence of vascular instability.

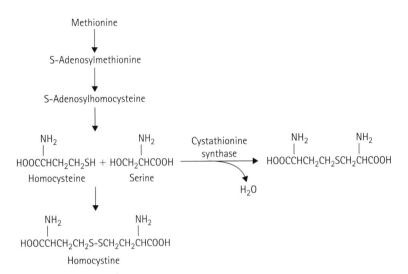

Figure 22.1   *In homocystinuria, the defective enzyme is cystathionine synthase.*

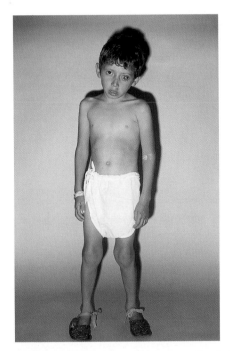

Figure 22.2   *M.G., a 6-year-old boy with homocystinuria. He had short stature and genu valgum.*

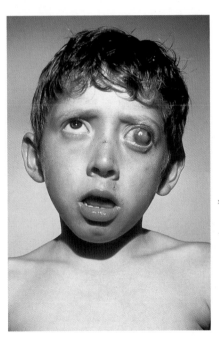

Figure 22.3   *Closer view illustrates M.G.'s eyes. Subluxed lenses had previously been removed bilaterally, after which he developed glaucoma in the left eye. He had fair skin and hair and a pronounced malar flush.*

Skeletal abnormalities are prominent, especially genu valgum (Figure 22.6). Valgus may also be present in the ankles, often along with pes cavus. The feet may be everted. Some patients may be tall and thin and have a marfanoid appearance (Figures 22.7, 22.8), but true arachnodactyly is rare, and some patients have a failure to thrive or shortness of stature. Pectus excavatum or carinatum may be present (Figure 22.8). There is a generalized osteoporosis. This is the most common musculoskeletal change, and fifty percent of patients have osteoporosis by the end of the second decade. Roentgenograms (Figures 22.9–22.11) characteristically reveal platyspondyly. There may be posterior biconcave or fish mouth appearance, and there may be impressive compression fractures or kyphoscoliosis [12,13].

Mental retardation is common but not invariable. This is probably a function of the presence or absence of thrombotic or vascular disease involving the nervous system. In patients responding to pyridoxine the mean IQ was 78, while that of nonresponders was 64 [4]. IQ scores among affected siblings were similar [14]. Seizures occurring in about 20 percent of patients, and abnormalities of the electroencephalogram (EEG), also common, probably also reflect the variable nature of vascular accident in this disease. Many patients have been observed to have typical strokes, with transient or permanent

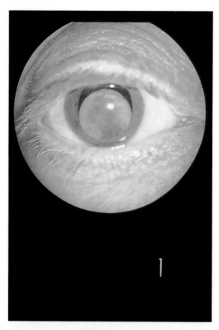

Figure 22.4 *The dislocated lens in homocystinuria is usually downward, while in Marfan syndrome it is upward.*

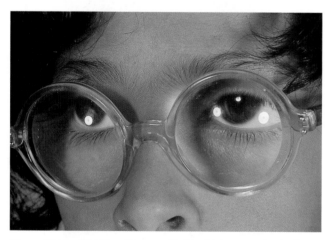

Figure 22.5 *N.M.M., a 10-year-old girl with homocystinuria. She had been found one year previously to have left-sided glaucoma and subluxed lenses bilaterally. The left lens was removed.*

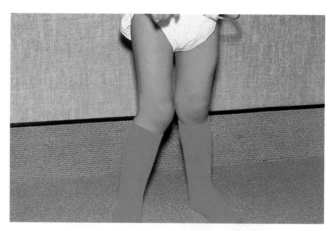

Figure 22.6 *Pronounced genu valgum in a 3-year-old with homocystinuria.*

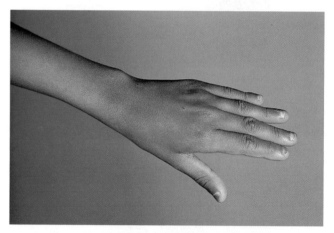

Figure 22.7 *N.M.M. She appeared tall and thin and height was in the 5th percentile. She had long, thin fingers.*

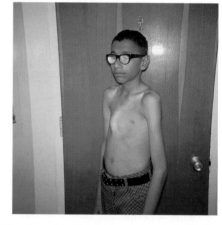

Figure 22.8 *A marfanoid appearance in a patient with homocystinuria. He had a prominent pectus carinatum and very thick corrective lenses.*

hemiplegia. A small number of patients has had dystonia [14–19]. Spasmodic torticollis may usher in ultimately fatal dystonia.

Psychiatric abnormalities have been observed in more than half of one series of 63 patients [14]. Three children were reported to have folate-responsive periodic behavior including rage attacks [20,21]. A 3-year-old had episodic repetitive behavior thought to represent psychomotor seizures [20]. Adults have been diagnosed as schizophrenic or depressed [14], or to have personality disorders.

Neuroimaging by computed tomography (CT) or magnetic resonance imaging (MRI) may be normal until the occurrence of cerebrovascular disease. Evidence of infarction has been obtained in patients presenting with hemiparesis, with or without papilledema. Cerebral venous and dural sinus thrombosis has been demonstrated by CT scan and confirmed by digital subtraction angiography [22].

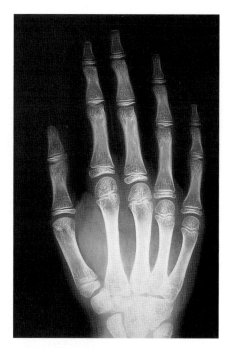

Figure 22.9   *Roentgenogram of the hand of the patient shown in Figures 22.5 and 22.7 illustrates the arachnodactyly.*

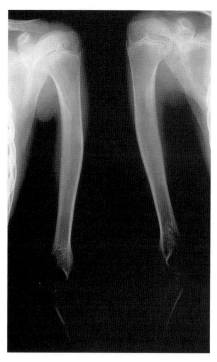

Figure 22.11   *Roentgenogram of the humeri of a 12-year-old girl with homocystinuria revealed osteopenia and lateral bowing.*

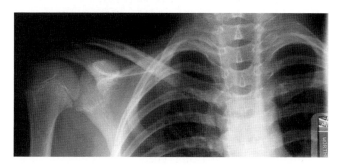

Figure 22.10   *Roentgenogram of the spine of the same patient revealed osteopenia and compression of thoracic vertebrae.*

Neuropathologic study has revealed occlusion of vessels, old and new thrombi, spongy degeneration and neuronal loss [23–25]. In the patient who died at 18 years-of-age with dystonia, the brain was histologically normal [17].

Vascular disease in homocystinuria involves the vessels themselves as well as a tendency of the blood to clot (Figure 22.12). Thromboses may be arterial or venous and may be fatal. Cerebrovascular disease occurred in one-third of 147 patients, and 32 percent of those thromboembolic events were strokes [4]. Ten patients had myocardial infarction. There were 11 percent peripheral arterial occlusions, 51 percent peripheral venous occlusions, and 32 of these patients had pulmonary emboli. Surgery may be especially strongly associated with thromboembolic accidents [26]. Medial degeneration of the vessels and intimal proliferation both narrow vessel lumens, and initial injury is followed by the adherence of unusually sticky platelets. The end result is severe narrowing of the arteries. This may be demonstrated angiographically, as may aneurysmal dilatation [27].

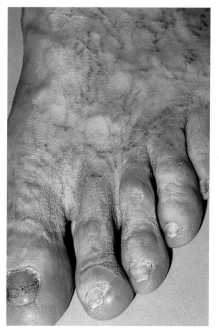

Figure 22.12   *Prominent venous pattern in the feet of a man with homocystinuria.*

GENETICS AND PATHOGENESIS

Deficiency of cystathionine synthase is autosomal recessively transmitted. It occurs with a frequency of one in 50 000 in Ireland and New England and one in 1 million in Japan; overall frequency is between one in 200 000 and 300 000. The defective enzyme may be demonstrated in cultured lympho-cytes and fibroblasts, as well as in tissues such as liver. Ranges of activity are from zero to 10 percent of the control mean. Pyridoxine-responsive patients always have some residual activity, and increased activity of hepatic enzyme has been documented in response to treatment.

The enzyme cystathionine β-synthase is a tetramer of 63 kD [28], which undergoes posttranslational proteolytic increase in activity with decrease in size to 48 kD. It has bind-ing sites for pyridoxal phosphate, as well as homocysteine and serine. S-adenosylmethionine and heme are activators [29,30]. In most patients enzyme size is normal, but exceptions have been encountered [31].

The locus for human cystathionine β-synthase was map-ped to chromosome 21 by Chinese hamster-human cell hybrids [32] and cDNA prepared from immunopurified mRNA [33] was used to verify the locus at the subtelomeric region of chromosome 21q22.3 [34], where it is syntenic with α-A-crystallin. There are 23 exons over some 28 Kb [35], from which the 551 amino acids are encoded by exons 1–14 and 16. Alternate splicing may include exon 15, which is repre-sented in a few mRNA molecules, but the 14 encoded amino acids are not found in the expressed enzyme. There is also alternative splicing among 5 exons (designated -1a to -1e) in the 5′-untranslated region. More than 130 mutations have been identified [36], and the functional consequences in many have been confirmed by expression systems. Among the first to be identified was a G to A change at 919 in exon 8, which converts glycine 307 to serine [37], and this mutation is the leading cause of homocystinuria in Ireland.

Another point mutation in exon 8 is a T to C transition at position 833, causing a substitution of threonine for isoleucine 278, which is the predominant mutation in the Netherlands and in Italy, and is associated with a pyridoxine-responsive phenotype when it is homozygous, and may or may not be when present in a compound heterozygote. The third most frequent alteration is a splice mutation in intron 11, 1224-2 A > C (IVS 11-2 A > C), which results in the skipping of all of exon 12. Interestingly, about half of the point mutations in the coding region originate from deamination of methylcyto-sine in CpG dinucleotides [38], and nearly one quarter of the point mutations are found in exon 3, the most highly con-served region of the gene.

Most patients have been compounds of two different mutant alleles. For instance, a pyridoxine-responsive patient had an I278T mutation, as well as a 135 bp deletion that deleted 45 amino acids from 408 to 453 [39]. This patient had been previously found to have one abnormally small polypeptide subunit [31]. An interesting mutation [40] in a pyridoxine-responsive patient homozygous for G1330A changed aspartate 444 to asparagine and abolished the regula-tory stimulation of activity by S-adenosylmethionine. A gen-eral lack of correlation between genotype and phenotype is exemplified by three siblings with the same molecular defect, one of whom had a single episode of claudication in the calf as his only clinical manifestation, while the other two had

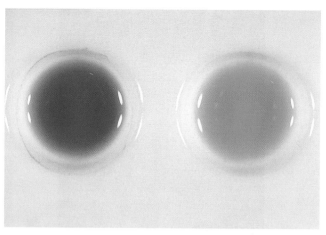

Figure 22.13 *Positive cyanide nitroprusside test on the left indicating the excretion of larger than normal (right) amounts of sulfhydryl-containing amino acid.*

marked defects in intellectual function and changes in the skeleton [41].

Deficiency of the enzyme leads to the accumulation of homocystine and its excretion in large amounts in the urine. Patients generally have elevated concentrations of methion-ine in blood, and newborn screening programs based upon blood methionine levels have been enacted [42]. Screening for urinary homocystine in the past was most readily carried out by using the nitroprusside tests [43,44] (Figure 22.13), which are tests for the excretion of sulfur-containing amino acids, or by staining a paper chromatogram or electrophero-gram with iodoplatinate. The diagnosis can be confirmed by quantification of the amino acids of the urine, where homo-cystine and the mixed disulfide of cysteine and homocystine are found. Since the major portion of homocysteine in plasma is bound to protein [45], the preferred method is to determine total plasma homocyst[e]ine by adding a reducing agent to release bound homocysteine prior to deproteiniza-tion, after which HPLC with detection of a fluorescent thiol reagent [46] or mass spectrometry [47] may be used.

Heterozygosity has been documented by the assay of cys-tathionine synthase in lymphocytes, fibroblasts and liver [3]. Prenatal diagnosis has been accomplished by assay of the enzyme in cultured amniocytes, and affected fetuses have been detected [48,49]. Activity in normal chorionic villus material is so low that prenatal diagnosis by this method is precluded. Neonatal screening programs depend predomi-nantly on screening for elevated concentrations of methion-ine in blood. Clearly they miss a certain number of patients, particularly those who are pyridoxine responsive and thus most amenable to therapy, but they do provide early diagno-sis for some patients.

Heterozygote detection has been carried out by enzyme assay of cultured fibroblasts, but there is overlap between car-rier and controls [50,51]. As many as 90 percent of carriers have been estimated to be detectable by measuring peak plasma levels of homocystine after an overload of methionine [52].

TREATMENT

Pyridoxine responsiveness should be determined in all patients with homocystinuria, and those who respond should be treated. This is the major feature currently determining prognosis [4]. Of six patients treated from the neonatal period, IQ scores ranged from 82 to 110 [4]. It is clear that reduction of levels of homocystine with pyridoxine will prevent thromboembolic events [4]; thromboembolic complications are decreased among those who respond to pyridoxine even in those treated late. Doses have ranged from 100 to 1200 mg/day and should be determined individually. Peripheral neuropathy has occurred in individuals treated with large doses of pyridoxine [53]. Doses up to 500 mg per day appear to be safe. Patients requiring larger doses to reduce levels of homocystine should certainly be monitored with tests of nerve conduction. Folate deficiency should be avoided by concomitant treatment with folate. Dietary therapy is much less effective, but should be employed in B_6-unresponsive patients, especially in infancy where it is easiest to ensure compliance. Concentrations of homocyst[e]ine may also be reduced in B_6-unresponsive patients by treatment with betaine [54]. Doses have ranged from 86 to 280 mg/kg. Especially rigorous therapy to ensure minimal levels of homocystine are warranted in preparation for surgery [4].

Ancillary supportive measures may be necessary. Orthopedic intervention may be required for pes planus and lower extremity valgus. The utility of agents such as bisphosphonates to increase bone mineralization remains to be established. Ectopia lentis may require aphakic contact lenses or spectacles; surgical intervention such as lensectomy may be indicated, and though there is controversy about the utility of implantation given the limited postoperative capsular support [55], intraocular lens implants may be considered.

References

1   Field CMB, Carson NAJ, Cusworth DC, et al. Homocystinuria: A new disorder of metabolism [abstr]. Tenth International Congress of Pediatrics 1962.

2   Carson NA, Neill DW. Metabolic abnormalities detected in a survey of mentally backward individuals in Northern Ireland. Arch Dis Child 1962;37:505.

3   Mudd SH, Finkelstein JD, Irreverre F, Laster L. Homocystinuria: An enzymatic defect. Science 1964;143:1443.

4   Mudd SH, Skovby F, Levy HL, et al. The natural history of homocystinuria due to cystathionine beta-synthase deficiency. Am J Hum Genet 1985;37:1.

5   Spaeth GL, Barber GW. Homocystinuria. In a mentally retarded child and her normal cousin. Trans Am Acad Ophthalmol Otolaryngol. 1965;69:912.

6   Drayer JI, Cleophas AJ, Trijbels JM, et al. Symptoms, diagnostic pitfalls, and treatment of homocystinuria in seven adult patients. Neth J Med 1980;23:89.

7   Wilcken B, Turner G. Homocystinuria in New South Wales. Arch Dis Child 1978;53:242.

8   Michalski A, Leonard JV, Taylor DS. The eye and inherited metabolic disease: a review. J R Soc Med 1988;81:286.

9   Harrison DA, Mullaney PB, Mesfer SA, et al. Management of ophthalmic complications of homocystinuria. Ophthalmology 1998;105:1886.

10 Carson NA, Cusworth DC, Dent CE, et al. Homocystinuria: A new inborn error of metabolism associated with mental deficiency. Arch Dis Child 1963;38:425.

11 Gaull G, Sturman JA, Schaffner F. Homocystinuria due to cystathionine synthase deficiency: enzymatic and ultrastructural studies. J Pediatr 1974;84:381.

12 Schimke RN, McKusick VA, Huang T, Pollack AD. Homocystinuria. Studies of 20 families with 38 affected members. JAMA 1965;193:711.

13 Brenton DP. Skeletal abnormalities in homocystinuria. Postgrad Med J 1977;53:488.

14 Abbott MH, Folstein SE, Abbey H, Pyeritz RE. Psychiatric manifestations of homocystinuria due to cystathionine beta-synthase deficiency: prevalence, natural history, and relationship to neurologic impairment and vitamin B6-responsiveness. Am J Med Genet 1987;26:959.

15 Hagberg B, Hambraeus L, Bensch K. A case of homocystinuria with a dystonic neurological syndrome. Neuropadiatrie 1970;1:337.

16 Davous P, Rondot P. Homocystinuria and dystonia. J Neurol Neurosurg Psychiatry 1983;46:283.

17 Kempster PA, Brenton DP, Gale AN, Stern GM. Dystonia in homocystinuria. J Neurol Neurosurg Psychiatry 1988;51:859.

18 Arbour L, Rosenblatt B, Clow C, Wilson GN. Postoperative dystonia in a female patient with homocystinuria. J Pediatr 1988;113:863.

19 Berardelli A, Thompson PD, Zaccagnini M, et al. Two sisters with generalized dystonia associated with homocystinuria. Mov Disord. 1991;6:163.

20 Murphy JV, Thome LM, Michals K, Matalon R. Folic acid responsive rages, seizures and homocystinuria. J Inherit Metab Dis 1985;8:Suppl 2 109.

21 Freeman JM, Finkelstein JD, Mudd SH. Folate-responsive homocystinuria and 'schizophrenia'. A defect in methylation due to deficient 5,10-methylenetetrahydrofolate reductase activity N Engl J Med 1975;292:491.

22 Schwab FJ, Peyster RG, Brill CB. CT of cerebral venous sinus thrombosis in a child with homocystinuria. Pediatr Radiol 1987;17:244.

23 Carson NA, Dent CE, Field CM, Gaull GE. Homocystinuria: Clinical and pathological review of ten cases. J Pediatr 1965;66:565.

24 Dunn HG, Perry TL, Dolman CL. Homocystinuria. A recently discovered cause of mental defect and cerebrovascular thrombosis. Neurology 1966;16:407.

25 Chou SM, Waisman HA. Spongy degeneration of the central nervous system: Case of homocystinuria. Arch Pathol 1965;79:357.

26 Jackson GM, Grisolia JS, Wolf PL, et al. Postoperative thromboemboli in cystathionine beta-synthase deficiency. Am Heart J 1984;108:627.

27 Wicherink-Bol HF, Boers GH, Drayer JI, Rosenbusch G. Angiographic findings in homocystinuria. Cardiovasc Intervent Radiol 1983;6:125.

28 Skovby F, Kraus JP, Rosenberg LE. Biosynthesis and proteolytic activation of cystathionine beta-synthase in rat liver. J Biol Chem 1984;259:588.

29 Kery V, Bukovska G, Kraus JP. Transsulfuration depends on heme in addition to pyridoxal 5'-phosphate. Cystathionine beta-synthase is a heme protein. J Biol Chem 1994;269:25283.

30 Kery V, Elleder D, Kraus JP. Delta-aminolevulinate increases heme saturation and yield of human cystathionine beta-synthase expressed in Escherichia coli. Arch Biochem Biophys 1995;316:24.

31 Skovby F, Kraus JP, Rosenberg LE. Homocystinuria: biogenesis of cystathionine beta-synthase subunits in cultured fibroblasts and in an in vitro translation system programmed with fibroblast messenger RNA. Am J Hum Genet 1984;36:452.

32 Skovby F, Krassikoff N, Francke U. Assignment of the gene for cystathionine beta-synthase to human chromosome 21 in somatic cell hybrids. Hum Genet 1984;65:291.

33   Kraus JP, Williamson CL, Firgaira FA, *et al*. Cloning and screening with nanogram amounts of immunopurified mRNAs: cDNA cloning and chromosomal mapping of cystathionine beta-synthase and the beta subunit of propionyl-CoA carboxylase. *Proc Natl Acad Sci USA* 1986;**83**:2047.

34   Munke M, Kraus JP, Ohura T, Francke U. The gene for cystathionine beta-synthase [CBS] maps to the subtelomeric region on human chromosome 21q and to proximal mouse chromosome 17. *Am J Hum Genet* 1988;**42**:550.

35   Kraus JP, Oliveriusova J, Sokolova *et al*. The human cystathionine beta-synthase [CBS] gene: complete sequence, alternative splicing, and polymorphisms. *Genomics* 1998;**52**:312.

36   Kraus JP, Kozich V, Janosik M. Cystathionine beta-synthase internet mutation database, http://www.uchsc.edu/cbs/cbsdata/cbsmain.htm (accessed 2004).

37   Gu Z, Ramesch V, Kozich V, *et al*. Identification of a molecular genetic defect in homocystinuria due to cystathionine β-synthase deficiency. *Am J Hum Genet* 1991;**49**:406.

38   Kraus JP, Janosik M, Kozich V, *et al*. Cystathionine beta-synthase mutations in homocystinuria. *Hum Mutat* 1999;**13**:362.

39   Kozich V, Kraus JP. Screening for mutations by expressing patient cDNA segments in *E. coli*: homocystinuria due to cystathionine beta-synthase deficiency. *Hum Mutat* 1992;**1**:113.

40   Kluijtmans LA, Boers GH, Stevens EM, *et al*. Defective cystathionine beta-synthase regulation by S-adenosylmethionine in a partially pyridoxine responsive homocystinuria patient. *J Clin Invest* 1996;**98**:285.

41   de Franchis R, Kozich V, McInnes RR, Kraus JP. Identical genotypes in siblings with different homocystinuric phenotypes: identification of three mutations in cystathionine beta-synthase using an improved bacterial expression system. *Hum Mol Genet* 1994;**3**:1103.

42   Peterschmitt MJ, Simmons, JR Levy HL. Reduction of false negative results in screening of newborns for homocystinuria. *N Engl J Med* 1999;**341**:1572.

43   Thuy LP, Nyhan WL. A screening method for cystine and homocystine in urine. *Clin Chim Acta* 1992;**211**:175.

44   Spaeth GL, Barber GW. Prevalence of homocystinuria among the mentally retarded: evaluation of a specific screening test. *Pediatrics* 1967;**40**:586.

45   Wiley VC, Dudman NP, Wilcken DE. Interrelations between plasma free and protein-bound homocysteine and cysteine in homocystinuria. *Metabolism* 1988;**37**:191.

46   Jacobsen DW, Gatautis VJ, Green R. Determination of plasma homocysteine by high-performance liquid chromatography with fluorescence detection. *Anal Biochem* 1989;**178**:208.

47   Magera MJ, Lacey JM, Casetta B, Rinaldo P. Method for the determination of total homocysteine in plasma and urine by stable isotope dilution and electrospray tandem mass spectrometry. *Clin Chem* 1999;**45**:1517.

48   Fleisher LD, Longhi RC, Tallan HH, *et al*. Homocystinuria: investigations of cystathionine synthase in cultured fetal cells and the prenatal determination of genetic status. *J Pediatr* 1974;**85**:677.

49   Fowler B, Borresen AL, Boman N. Prenatal diagnosis of homocystinuria. *Lancet* 1982;**2**:875.

50   Boers GH, Fowler B, Smals AG, *et al*. Improved identification of heterozygotes for homocystinuria due to cystathionine synthase deficiency by the combination of methionine loading and enzyme determination in cultured fibroblasts. *Hum Genet* 1985;**69**:164.

51   McGill JJ, Mettler G, Rosenblatt DS, Scriver CR. Detection of heterozygotes for recessive alleles. Homocyst[e]inemia: paradigm of pitfalls in phenotypes. *Am J Med Genet* 1990;**36**:45.

52   Clarke R, Daly L, Robinson K, *et al*. Hyperhomocysteinemia: an independent risk factor for vascular disease. *N Engl J Med* 1991;**324**:1149.

53   Bendich A, Cohen M. Vitamin B6 safety issues. *Ann NY Acad Sci* 1990;**585**:321.

54   Wilcken DE, Wilcken B, Dudman NP, Tyrrell PA. Homocystinuria – the effects of betaine in the treatment of patients not responsive to pyridoxine. *N Engl J Med* 1983;**309**:448.

55   Neely DE, Plager DA. Management of ectopia lentis in children. *Ophthalmol Clin North Am* 2001;**14**:493.

23

Homocystinuria due to n(5,10)-methylenetetrahydrofolate reductase

MAJOR PHENOTYPIC EXPRESSION

Variable developmental delay or psychosis, thrombotic vascular disease, homocystinuria, homocysteinemia, normal or low concentrations of methionine and defective activity of methylenetetrahydrofolate (MeFH4) reductase.

INTRODUCTION

Since the initial description in 1972 by Freeman, Mudd and their colleagues [1–3], more than 40 patients have been reported with deficiency of MeFH4 reductase (EC 1.5.1.20) (MIM 236250) [4,5].

One-carbon units, critical for the synthesis of purines, thymidylate, serine and methionine, are transferred from their predominantly glycine and serine sources by way of folic acid intermediates. Entry into the pool is via 5,10-methylene FH4. This compound serves directly the synthesis of thymidylate. It is oxidized to formyl-FH4 for the *de novo* synthesis of purines. In the synthesis of methionine, the methylene, MeFH4 is reduced to 5-methyl-FH4 (Figure 23.1). The reductase reaction involves the conversion of the nicotinamide-adenine dinucleotide (NADPH) cofactor to NADP. The methyl-FH4 product is the donor of the methyl group to homocysteine to form methionine.

Folic acid is pteroylglutamic acid in which pteroic acid is linked by amide formation to one or more molecules of glutamic acid, each linked to the γ carboxyl of the preceding amino acid. Biologically active folic acid molecules are all tetrahydro derivatives (FH4).

The reductase is a cytoplasmic enzyme. It is encoded by a gene on human chromosome 1 at p36.3 [6]. It contains

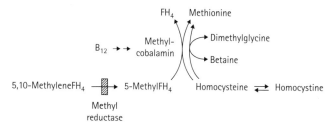

Figure 23.1 *Role of methylene tetrahydrofolate reductase in the metabolism of homocystine and methionine.*

11 exons [7]. The smaller enzyme from *E. coli* has been crystallized [8]. A number of mutations has been identified, most often single base missense substitutions [6,9].

CLINICAL ABNORMALITIES

The clinical pictures have been very different in patients reported (Figures 23.2 and 23.3), as have degrees of severity and ages of onset. Each of the first two patients described [1,2] were sisters who were mildly mentally retarded; the proband's IQ was tested at 11 and 15 years at 60 and 46; her sister's at 60. The sister's behavior was unremarkable, but the proband appeared to be schizophrenic, on the basis of progressive

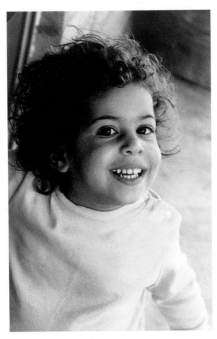

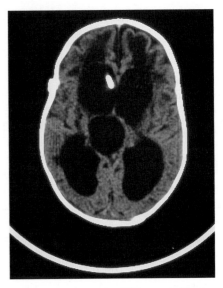

Figure 23.4   *CT scan of the brain of E.E. revealed profound atrophy.*

Figure 23.2   *A.H., a 7-year-old, Caucasian/African American with methylene tetrahydrofolate reductase deficiency. She was quite ill at presentation, but became stable with some residual neurologic abnormalities, including visual defects, hyperactivity and behavioral lability. (Illustration was kindly provided by Dr. R.A. Heidenreich of the University of Arizona.)*

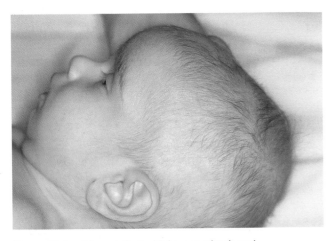

Figure 23.3   *E.E., an infant with homocystinuria and hypomethioninemia (2.4 μmol/L). She developed central apnea of 10 days. Treatment with 15 mg of folinic acid daily permitted discontinuation of artificial ventilation. By 6-months-of-age, she had microcephaly and enopthalmos and had developed no milestone activities.*

depression and withdrawal, feelings of persecution and halluci-nation. She developed anorexia and loss of weight. Psychotic symptoms disappeared following treatment with pyridoxine and folic acid, recurred on discontinuation of the medication and remitted on readministration. Though tall and thin, neither had any of the skeletal or ocular manifestations of cystathionine synthase deficiency. The proband had a tremor and a diffusely slow electroencephalogram (EEG). Brisk deep tendon reflexes and positive Babinski responses were observed during a period of noncompliance with medications. Both sisters later developed progressive peripheral neuropathy.

A different end of the spectrum was exemplified by two patients reported by Narisawa [10,11] in whom there was pro-gression to death within one year, representing an infantile form of the disease. A similar patient was reported by Harpey, Rosenblatt *et al.* [12].

A somewhat different presentation was reported [13] in two siblings who developed infantile spasms at 1 and 18 months-of-age and were severely retarded, but one deterio-rated rapidly and died at 2.5 years. Severe mental retardation in sisters and early death in one were reported by Wendel [14]. The survivor was hypotonic and athetoid and could not sit without support.

The most common presentation is with delayed develop-ment [13–17] (Figure 23.3). One patient was described as hav-ing phenotypic features of Angelman syndrome [17]. A number have been microcephalic [4]. Many have had seizures, and most had abnormal EEGs. A number have had psychiatric abnormalities. Imaging of the brain by computed tomography (CT) or magnetic resonance imaging (MRI) may reveal atro-phy [18] or defective myelination (Figure 23.4).

A myopathic presentation was illustrated by a 16-year-old patient, reported by Shih *et al.* [15], who had proximal mus-cle weakness and a waddling gait and who had episodes in which there were flinging movements of the arms. A similar patient reported by Haan *et al.* [16] had severely retarded mental development, spasticity and seizures. His disease appeared static for seven years but he then experienced rapidly progressive deterioration and died at 7½ years. This patient sucked and fed poorly in the early months but passed the early milestones normally, walking somewhat at 15 months, though never achieving independent walking. He was microcephalic and spastic and had ankle clonus and bilateral Babinski responses. He had a malar flush; ethnically he was a Caucasian Australian. The abnormal EEG displayed slow activity and multifocal epileptiform discharges. Autopsy revealed a small brain with atrophic gyri, poor myelination and extensive gliosis. Abnormalities of gait have been described in most of those able to walk [4].

The occurrence of thrombotic phenomena in this disease, as well as in cystathionine synthase deficiency, indicate that it is homocysteine or homocystine that is responsible for the genesis of the vascular disease. Autopsy revealed multiple thromboses throughout the body, including the dural sinuses and small cerebral vessels, in the patient reported by Wendel [14] and the two autopsied of four affected siblings reported by Wong and colleagues [19]. In a family of six siblings, three had recurrent strokes beginning in their 20s; two died within a year of the onset of symptoms [20]. Two of these patients were described to have marfanoid habitus. None of these patients has had ectopia lentis or osteoporosis. Nor has megaloblastic anemia occurred, and methylmalonic acid was not found in blood or urine.

Onset and diagnosis have occurred from birth or before [13] to adulthood [20]. In one family with two affected siblings, one developed weakness, paresthesias, incoordination and lapses of memory at 15 and was bound to a wheelchair in his early 20s, while his brother was asymptomatic at 37 years [20].

The diagnostic feature is the detection of homocystine in the urine in the absence of elevation of plasma concentrations of methionine. Examination of fresh urine with cyanide-nitroprusside reveals a strongly positive red reaction. Homocystine may be detected on screening by high-voltage electropherogram, or paper or thin layer chromatogram. Quantification of the amino acids of fresh urine reveals elevated quantities of homocystine. Amounts reported have varied from 48 mmol/mol creatinine to 190 mmol/mol creatinine (15–667 µmol/day) [4]. These amounts are appreciably lower than in cystathionine synthase deficiency (Chapter 22). In fact screening spot tests may be normal [21]. Concentrations of total homocysteine (tHcy) have varied from 60–184 µmol/L (normal 4–14) [4,9,20,22,23]. Concentrations of methionine in plasma have been low. Reported values have ranged from 0 to 300 µmol/L [2,4,13,15] but have usually been under 18 µmol/L; a mean of 12 µmol/L was reported [4]. This feature is also different from the picture in cystathionine synthase deficiency (Chapter 22) in which the levels of methionine are usually high. Cystathionine may or may not be present in the urine.

Many patients have had low concentrations of folic acid in plasma [10]. Values reported have included 2, 3 and 6 ng/mL (normal 5 to 21) [2,9,10] in bioassay and 1.0 ng/mL (normal 1.9 to 14) [15] in radioimmunoassay. Folate concentration may also be low in cerebrospinal fluid [10]. B_{12} concentrations are normal. Treatment with folic acid increases concentrations of folic acid and derivatives in the blood, the cerebrospinal fluid

remains devoid of 5-methyl FH4, the only folate derivative actively transported across the blood–brain barrier [10].

GENETICS AND PATHOGENESIS

The disease is inherited as an autosomal recessive trait. Consanguinity has been documented [4,9]. Intermediate levels of enzyme activity have been documented in cultured fibroblasts and lymphocytes of parents [12,24–26]. Activity in control cells varies with time in culture and is greatest at confluence; assay should be done then to avoid misclassifying a normal as heterozygous [24]. Prenatal diagnosis has been made by assay of the enzyme in cultured aminocytes [12,13]. It should also be possible in chorionic villus samples, as the enzyme is active in this tissue [12,27]. If the mutations are known on each allele, prenatal diagnosis and heterozygote detection can be carried out by molecular analysis.

The molecular defect is in the activity of the enzyme N(5,10)-methylenetetrahydrofolate reductase (Figure 23.1). Defective enzyme activity has been documented in liver and cultured fibroblasts [2,24,25], and in freshly isolated lymphocytes [15]. Levels of activity have generally ranged from 1 to 18 percent of control values [2,9,13,24,25] and as low as undetectable in lymphocytes [15].

There is a rough correlation between clinical severity and the level of enzyme activity. Studies in cultured fibroblasts in which the portion of folate present was methyl-FH4 [28] and the synthesis of methionine from labeled formate [29] have provided better correlation with clinical severity than measurements of reductase activity [30]. A screening test for reductase deficiency takes advantage of the fact that *Lactobacillus casei* may utilize methyl-FH4 for growth [31]. Cultured normal fibroblasts can grow in homocystine whereas cells deficient in MeFH4 reductase cannot, providing another screening test [25]. Cells of patients deficient in methionine synthase (cbl C, D, E, F and G) also fail this screening test.

Differing levels of activity as well as different clinical phenotypes in different families are consistent with heterogeneity of the mutations in this disease. This has been supported by studies of heat inactivation [25] in which different patterns of decreased thermostability were observed in two families, while a third with defective activity had a normal pattern of response to heat.

Kang and colleagues have reported thermolabile reductase in adults with no neurologic disease in whom enzyme activity was about 50 percent of control [32]. Termed intermediate hyperhomocysteinemia, this variant has been associated with increased risk for the development of coronary vascular disease [33–35]. Thermolabile enzyme has also been found in patients with early onset disease [36]. A common mutation C677T which converts an alanine 222 to valine conveys thermolability [37]. Patients with TT homozygosity had higher concentrations of Hcy than CC normals or CT heterozotes [38]. In response to cholestyramine utilized in familial hypercholesterolemia to lower cholesterol, Hcy levels increase in CT and TT individuals, and concentrations of folic acid decreased in all [39].

Among the mutations identified [6] a nonsense mutation and a threonine to methionine change were found in early onset patients with severe disease. An arginine to glutamine change, which appears relatively conservative, was found in two patients with late onset neurologic disease and a thermolabile enzyme [20]. Most mutations have occurred in a single family. In general, mutations that lead to virtually complete loss of enzyme activity (0–3 percent of control) are associated with earlier onset and more severe clinical manifestations, while those leading to greater amounts of residual activity lead to later onset and milder symptomatology [6].

In a patient with homocystinuria this disease may be distinguished from cystathionine synthase deficiency by the administration of methionine and assay of sulfate in the urine. In MeFH4 reductase deficiency as much as 65–73 percent is converted to sulfate in 24 hours [9], while only 5–10 percent is formed in cystathionine synthase deficiency.

Levels of neurotransmitters in the cerebrospinal fluid have been observed to be low in patients with this disease [4]. The enzyme does have dihydropteridine reductase activity and it is active in brain [40], providing for a possible role in neurotransmitter synthesis in the central nervous system. A decrease in S-adenosylmethionine has been correlated with demyelination [41].

The differential diagnosis of hyperhomocysteinemia includes not only cystathionine synthase deficiency (Chapter 22) and MeFH4 reductase deficiency, but also cblC and D diseases (Chapter 4), methionine synthase deficiency (cblG) [42] and methionine synthase reductase deficiency (cblE) [43]. Patients with these diseases present early with megaloblastic anemia and developmental delay. The gene (MTR) for methionine synthase is located on chromosome 1p43. A number of mutations have been identified [42] including five deletions, two nonsense mutations, a splice site alteration and a group of missense mutations. The only common mutation P1173L resulted from a C to T transition in a CpG island. In methionine synthase reductase deficiency (cblE) the gene has been mapped to chromosome 5p15.2–15.3, and a number of mutations have been identified [43]. The most common mutation has been a 140 bp insertion between C.903 and 904, having been identified in three unrelated patients. It results from activation of an exon splicing enhancer because of a T to C transition in intron 6. Some normally spliced mRNA is made [42]. Another insertion observed was of 2bp, C.1623-1624 insTA. Folate dependency was documented despite treatment with hydroxocobalamin.

TREATMENT

Methyl-FH4 reductase deficiency is an inborn error of folate metabolism. Therefore, it is reasonable in every patient to assess the possibility of clinical and biochemical responses to exogenous folate.

Varying results have been reported in different families. In the initial patient [2], treatment with 20 mg a day of oral folic acid regularly decreased the excretion of homocystine in the urine by factors of 10- to 20-fold. Initially, she was treated with 300 mg per day of pyridoxine, but the response to folate alone was just as good. Mental function improved, and psychotic symptoms disappeared in this patient with folate treatment.

Homocystine excretion was also greatly reduced by folate treatment in the patient reported by Shih [15], but there was no clinical improvement. The patient reported by Haan et al. [16] did not reduce the excretion of homocystine when folic acid was given, but the dose was only 1 mg per day. B₁₂ was also without effect. This patient deteriorated neurologically when treated with 300 mg a day of pyridoxine, losing abilities to crawl, pull himself up, stand and walk with support. Those abilities returned slowly during the year following cessation of pyridoxine. Intramuscular formyltetrahydrofolate did not improve his clinical state.

In the patient treated by Wong and colleagues [19] no biochemical or clinical improvement occurred following treatment with as much as 60 mg per day of folic acid. Successful treatment may be the exception rather than the rule [4,5,44]. Methyl-FH4 is available as folinic acid, and this has been employed in a number of patients. Failure to improve clinically with either folate or folinic acid was also observed in the patient reported by Singer et al. [3], in whom treatment also failed to elevate the abnormally low cerebrospinal fluid (CSF) concentration of folate.

One objective of therapy might be to give a dose sufficient to raise the CSF level of folate. One patient was reported to respond to a combination of folinic acid, methionine, pyridoxine and cobalamine [12]. Overall experience has been that the disease is resistant to treatment [4]. Cobalamin should be given since subacute combined degeneration of the cord has been observed in a child given methyltetrahydrofolate alone [45].

Betaine also serves as a methyl donor in the synthesis of methionine in a reaction in which it is converted to dimethylglycine. (Figure 23.1) Its administration has been shown to reduce levels of homocystine in cystathionine synthase deficiency, and it should do so as well in MeFH4 reductase deficiency. Several patients have been treated with some success [4,22,23,46–48]. Doses of 2–20 g per day have been employed (20–120 mg/kg) [23]. In two patients treated from the first month of life with betaine and folic acid, cognitive function was normal at 5 years of age [47].

References

1 Freeman JM, Finkelstein JD, Mudd SH, Uhlendorf BW. Homocystinuria presenting as reversible 'schizophrenia'. A new defect in methionine metabolism with reduced methylene-tetrahydrofolate-reductase activity. *Pediatr Res* 1972;**6**:423 (abstr).

2 Freeman JM, Finkelstein JD, Mudd SH. Folate responsive homocystinuria and 'schizophrenia': a defect in methylation due to deficient 510-methylene-tetrahydrofolate reductase activity. *N Engl J Med* 1975;**292**:491.

3   Singer H, Butler I, Rothenberg S, *et al*. Interrelationships among serum folate CSF folate neurotransmitters and neuropsychiatric symptoms. *Neurology* 1980;**30**:419.

4   Erbe RW. Inborn errors of folate metabolism: in *Folates and Pterins,* Vol 3 (Nutritional Pharmacological and Physiological Aspects) (eds RL Blakley, VM Whitehead). John Wiley, New York;1986: 413.

5   Fowler B. Genetic defects of folate and cobalamin metabolism. *Eur J Pediatr* 1998;**157**:S60.

6   Goyette P, Sumner JS, Milos R, *et al*. Human methylenetetrahydrofolate reductase (MTHFR): isolation of cDNA mapping and mutation identification. *Nature Genetics* 1994;**7**:145.

7   Goyette P, Pai A, Milos R, *et al*. Gene structure of human and mouse methylenetetrahydrofolate reductase (MTHFR). *Mamm Genome* 1998;**9**:652.

8   Guenther BD, Sheppard CA, Tran P, *et al*. The structure and properties of methylenetetrahydrofolate reductase from *Escherichia coli* suggest how folate ameliorates human hyperhomocystinemia. *Nat Struct Biol* 1999;**6**:359.

9   Goyette P, Christensen B, Rosenbatt DS, Rozen R. Severe and mild mutations in *cts* for the methylenetetrahydrofolate (MTHFR) gene and description of 5 novel mutations in MTHFR. *Am J Hum Genet* 1996;**59**:1268.

10 Narisawa K, Wada Y, Saito T, *et al*. Infantile type of homocystinuria with N510-methylenetetrahydrofolate reductase defect. *Tohoku J Exp Med* 1977;**121**:185.

11 Narisawa K. Brain damage in the infantile type of 510-methylenetetrahydrofolate reductase deficiency. *Folic Acid Neuro Psychiatry Intern Med* 1979;**35**:391.

12 Harpey JP, Rosenblatt DS, Cooper BA, *et al*. Homocystinuria caused by 510-methylenetetrahydrofolate reductase deficiency: a case in an infant responding to methionine folinic acid pyridoxine and vitamin B$_{12}$ therapy. *J Pediatr* 1981;**98**:275.

13 Christensen E, Brandt NJ. Prenatal diagnosis of 510 methylenetetrahydrofolate reductase deficiency. *N Engl J Med* 1985;**313**:50 (letter).

14 Wendel U, Claussen U, Diekmann E. Prenatal diagnosis for methylenetetrahydrofolate reductase deficiency. *J Pediatr* 1983; **102**:938.

15 Shih VE, Salem MZ, Mudd SH, *et al*. A new form of homocystinuria due to N(510)-methylenetetrahydrofolate reductase deficiency. *Pediatr Res* 1972;**6**:395 (Abstract).

16 Haan EA, Rogers JG, Lewis GP, Rowe PB. 5-10-Methylenetetrahydrofolate reductase deficiency. Clinical and biochemical features of a further case. *J Inherit Metab Dis* 1985;**8**:53.

17 Arn PH, Williams CA, Zori RT, *et al*. Methylenetetrahydrofolate reductase deficiency in a patient with phenotypic findings of Angelman syndrome. *Am J Med Genet* 1998;**77**:198.

18 Sewell AC, Neirich U, Fowler B. Early infantile methylenetetrahydrofolate reductase deficiency: a rare cause of progressive brain atrophy. *J Inherit Metab Dis* 1998;**21**:22 (Abstract).

19 Wong PWK, Justice P, Hruby M. *et al*. Folic acid nonresponsive homocystinuria due to methylenetetrahydrofolate reductase deficiency. *Pediatrics* 1977;**59**:749.

20 Visy JM, LeCoz P, Chadefaux B, *et al*. Homocystinuria due to 510-methylene-tetrahydrofolate reductase deficiency revealed by stroke in adult siblings. *Neurology* 1991;**41**:1313.

21 Fowler B, Jakobs C. Post- and prenatal diagnostic methods for the homocystinurias. *Eur J Pediatr* 1998;**157**:S88.

22 Ronge E, Kjellman B. Long-term treatment with betaine in methylenetetrahydrofolate reductase deficiency. *Arch Dis Child* 1996; **74**:239.

23 Sakura N, Ono H, Homura H, *et al*. Betaine dose and treatment intervals in therapy for homocytinuria due to 510-methylenetetrahydrofolate reductase deficiency. *J Inherit Metab Dis* 1998;**21**:84.

24 Rosenblatt DS, Erbe RW. Methylenetetrahydrofolate reductase in cultured human cells I. Growth and metabolic studies. *Pediatr Res* 1977; **11**:1137.

25 Rosenblatt DS, Erbe RW. Methylenetetrahydrofolate reductase in cultured human cells II. Genetic and biochemical studies of methylenetetrahydrofolate reductase deficiency. *Pediatr Res* 1977;**11**:1141.

26 Wong PWK, Justice P, Berlow S. Detection of homozygotes and heterozygotes with methylenetetrahydrofolate reductase deficiency. *J Lab Clin Med* 1977;**90**:283.

27 Shin YS, Pilz G, Enders W. Methylenetetrahydrofolate reductase and methylenetetrahydrofolate methyltransferase in human fetal tissues and chorionic villi. *J Inherit Metab Dis* 1986;**9**:275.

28 Rosenblatt DS, Cooper BA, Lue-Shing, *et al*. Folate distribution in cultured human cells. Studies on 510-CH2-H4-PteGlu reductase deficiency. *J Clin Invest* 1979;**63**:1019.

29 Boss GR, Erbe RW. Decreased rates of methionine synthesis by methylenetetrahydrofolate reductase-deficient fibroblasts and lymphoblasts. *J Clin Invest* 1981;**67**:1659.

30 Fowler B, Whitehouse C, Wenzel F, Wraith JE. Methionine and serine formation in control and mutant human cultured fibroblasts: evidence for methyl trapping and characterization of remethylation defects. *Pediatr Res* 1997;**41**:145.

31 Cooper BA, Rosenblatt DS. Folate coenzyme forms in fibroblasts from patients deficient in 510-methylenetetrahydrofolate reductase. *Biochem Soc Trans* 1976;**4**:921.

32 Kang S-S, Wong PWK, Susmano A, *et al*. Thermolabile methylenetetrahydrofolate reductase: an inherited risk factor for coronary artery disease. *Am J Hum Genet* 1991;**48**:536.

33 Kang S-S, Wong PWK, Bock H-GO, *et al*. Intermediate hyperhomocysteinemia resulting from compound heterozygosity of methylenetetrahydrofolate reductase mutations. *Am J Hum Genet* 1991;**48**:546.

34 Kang S, Zhou J, Wong P, *et al*. Intermediate homocysteinemia: a thermolabile variant of methylenetetrahydrofolate reductase. *Am J Hum Genet* 1988;**43**:414.

35 Kang SS, Wong PWK, Zhou J, *et al*. Thermolabile methylenetetrahydrofolate reductase in patients with coronary artery disease. *Metabolism* 1988;**37**:611.

36 Hyland K, Smith I, Bottiglieri T, *et al*. Demyelination and decreased S-adenosylmethionine in 510-methylenetetrahydrofolate reductase deficiency. *Neurology* 1988;**38**:459.

37 Frosst P, Blom HJ, Milo R, *et al*. A candidate genetic risk factor for vascular disease: a common methylenetetrahydrofolate reductase mutation causes thermoinstability. *Nat Genet* 1995;**10**:111.

38 Goyette P, Frosst P, Rosenblatt DS, Rozen R. Seven novel mutations in the methylenetetrahydrofolate reductase gene and genotype/phenotype correlations in severe methylenetetrahydrofolate reductase deficiency. *Am J Hum Genet* 1995;**56**:1052.

39 Tonstad S, Refsum H, Ose L, Ueland PM. The C677T mutation in the methylenetetrahydrofolate reductase gene predisposes to hyper-homocysteinemia in children with familial hypercholesterolemia treated with cholestyramine. *J Pediatr* 1998;**132**:365.

40 Burton EG, Sallach HJ. Methylenetetrahydrofolate reductase in rat central nervous system: intracellular and regional distribution. *Arch Biochem Biophys* 1975;**166**:483.

41 Hyland K, Smith I, Bottiglieri T, *et al*. Demyelination and decreased S-adenosylmethionine in 510-methylenetetrahydrofolate reductase deficiency. *Neurology* 1988;**38**:459.

42 Watkins D, Ru M, Hwang H-Y, *et al.* Hyperhomocysteinemia due to methionine synthase deficiency cblG: structure of the *MTR* gene genotype diversity and recognition of a common mutation P1173L. *Am J Hum Genet* 2002;**71**:143.

43 Zavad'àkovà P, Fowler B, Zeman J, *et al.* CblE type of homocystinuria due to methionine synthase reductase deficiency: clinical and molecular studies and prenatal diagnosis in two families. *J Inherit Metab Dis* 2002;**25**:461.

44 Ogier de Baulny H, Gerard M, Saudubray JM, Zittoun J. Remethylation defects: guidelines for clinical diagnosis and treatment. *Eur J Pediatr* 1998;**157**:S77.

45 Clayton PT, Smith I, Harding B, *et al.* Subacute combined degeneration of the cord dementia and Parkinsonism due to an inborn error of folate metabolism. *J Neurol Neurosurg Psychiatry* 1986;**49**:920.

46 Wendel U, Bremer HJ. Betaine in the treatment of homocystinuria due to 510-methylene THF reductase deficiency. *Eur J Pediatr* 1987;**142**:147.

47 Brandt NJ, Christensen E, Skovby FD, Jernes B. Treatment of methylenetetrahydrofolate reductase deficiency from the neonatal period. Proc SSIEM 24th Annual Symposium 1986, Amersfoort, The Netherlands: 23 (Abstract).

48 Holme E, Kjellman B, Ronge E. Betaine for treatment of homocystinuria caused by methylenetetrahydrofolate reductase deficiency. *Arch Dis Child* 1989;**64**:1061.

24

Maple syrup urine disease (branched-chain oxoaciduria)

MAJOR PHENOTYPIC EXPRESSION

Overwhelming illness in the first days of life with lethargy progressive to coma, opisthotonus, and convulsions; recurrent episodes leading to developmental delay; characteristic maple syrup odor, branched-chain amino acidemia and amino-aciduria; branched-chain oxoaciduria; deficiency of branched-chain oxoacid dehydrogenase.

INTRODUCTION

Maple syrup urine disease (MSUD) is a disorder of branched-chain amino acid metabolism in which elevated quantities of leucine, isoleucine, and valine and their corresponding oxoacids accumulate in body fluids [1]. The disease was first described in 1954 by Menkes, Hurst and Craig [2], who observed an unusual odor quite like that of maple syrup in the urine of four infants who died of a progressive encephalopathic disease in the first weeks of life. Elevated quantities of the branched-chain amino acids were found by Westall and colleagues [3] and the oxoacids derived from each of these amino acids were isolated and identified as their 2,4-dinitrophenylhydrazones by Menkes [4]. Defective decarboxylation of ^{14}C-oxoacid was demonstrated in leukocytes by Dancis, Hutzler and Levitz [5].

The fundamental defect is in the activity of the branched-chain oxoacid dehydrogenase multienzyme complex [1,6,7] (Figures 24.1, 24.2); The components are E1, a decarboxylase; E2, an acyl transferase; and E3, a flavoprotein lipoamide dehydrogenase (dihydrolipoyl dehydrogenase). E1 is composed of two proteins in an $\alpha 2\beta 2$ structure. The enzyme complex, which was purified to homogeneity by Reed and colleagues [7], is

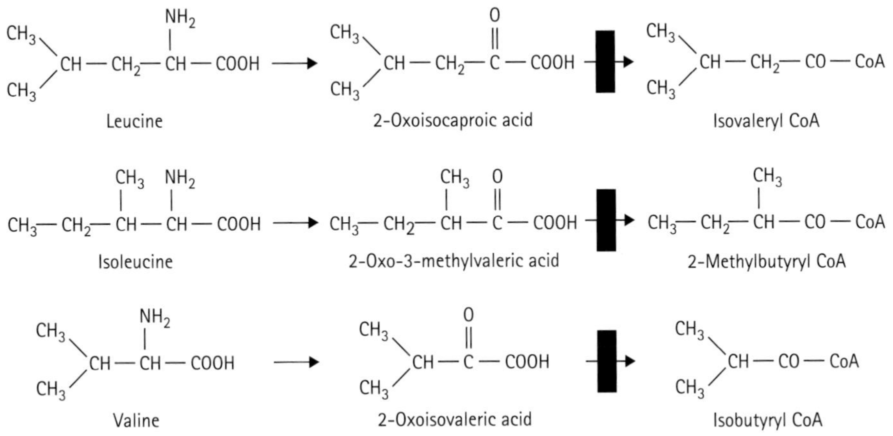

Figure 24.1 *Metabolic pathways in the catabolism of leucine, isoleucine and valine. The site of the defect is shown at the oxo-acid step in each of the three pathways.*

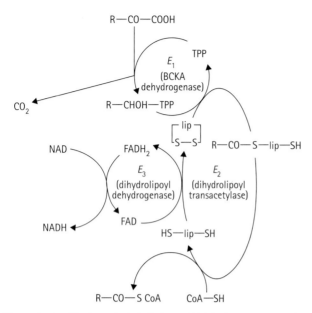

Figure 24.2   *The branched chain ketoacid dehydrogenase complex.*

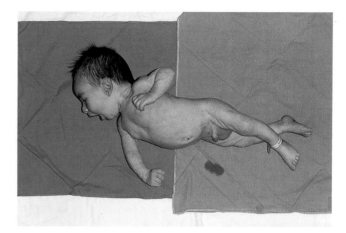

Figure 24.3   *M.B., an 11-day-old infant with maple syrup urine disease. He is shown in the characteristic opisthotonic position. (The illustration was kindly provided by Dr. Havelock Thompson of the University of West Virginia.)*

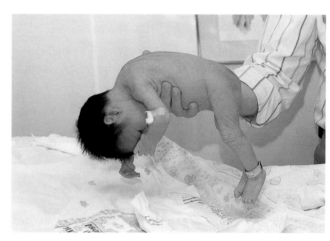

Figure 24.4   *G.V., a 3-week-old infant with maple syrup urine disease who presented with almost pure hypotonia. At this age treatment had begun and tone improved somewhat, but he was still largely flaccid and had no sucking reflex. Tone and sucking became normal as the levels of the branched-chain amino acids were brought to normal.*

analogous to the pyruvate dehydrogenase complex (PDHC) (Chapter 50); in fact the E3 component of the two complexes is the same protein, and in E3 deficiency (Chapter 51) defective activity of each dehydrogenase enzyme results. Expression studies have shown that the complex does not assemble spontaneously; the E1 α and β proteins require chaperonins for folding and assembly [8].

The cDNA of each of the component genes has been cloned. The E1α gene has been localized to chromosome 19q13.1-13.2 [9], E1β to 6p21-22 [10], E2 to 1p31 [10] and E3 to 7q31-32 [11]. Mutations have been identified in each gene. To date, a majority has been in the E1α and E2 genes. The mutation in the Mennonite population in which MSUD is common is a T to A transition that yields a single missense tyrosine to asparagine (Y393N) change at position 393 [12].

CLINICAL ABNORMALITIES

Infants with classic MSUD appear normal at birth, but they usually remain well for only a few days. Vomiting or difficulty to feed may be early symptoms. Usually by the end of the first week they become lethargic, and progressive neurologic deterioration is rapid [12–15]. The cry may be high-pitched. There may be periods of flaccidity, in which deep tendon reflexes and Moro reflex are absent, alternating with hypertonicity. General muscular rigidity is common. The absolutely characteristic picture is of a markedly hypertonic comatose or semicomatose infant in an opisthotonic position (Figure 24.3). Extreme opisthotonus of this degree is very unusual in an infant only a few days old. There may be dystonic extension of the arms, or a decerebrate appearance. Rarely, an infant may present with hypotonia and flaccidity (Figure 24.4). There may be abnormal eye movements. Convulsions occur regularly. These

symptoms proceed to apnea, coma, and death, unless a vigorous therapeutic program is instituted [13]. Cerebral edema, and a picture of pseudotumor cerebri may be seen and has been documented by computed tomography (CT) or magnetic resonance imaging (MRI) scan [16–19].

Rarely, an infant who is not so effectively treated may survive this early phase of the disease, left with prominent neurological abnormalities and profound mental retardation (Figures 24.5–24.7). Any patient with MSUD remains a candidate for further episodes of acute overwhelming illness and coma, any one of which may be fatal or lead to neurologic damage. Episodic illness is often triggered by the catabolic state that accompanies infection. It may also follow dietary indiscretion in which the amount of protein ingested by normal infants or children are consumed. Cerebral edema and

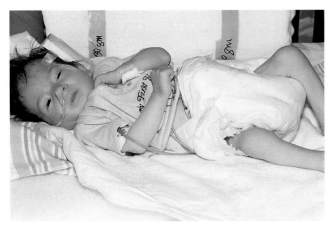

Figure 24.5   *P.C., a Mexican infant with maple syrup urine disease in relapse. She was semi-comatose, hypertonic and had exaggerated deep tendon reflexes and ankle clonus.*

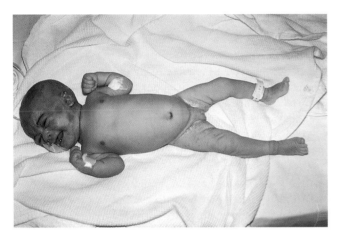

Figure 24.6   *E.S.H., a Saudi infant with maple syrup urine disease. He was quite rigid. The dermatitis reflects the problem of the dietary management of the disease.*

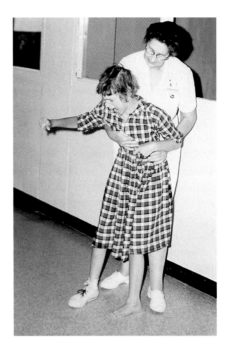

Figure 24.7   *C.H., a teenager with maple syrup urine disease. She was severely retarded and ataxic.*

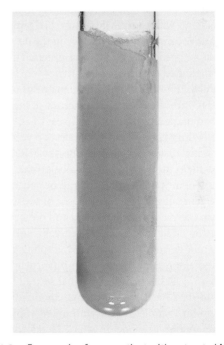

Figure 24.8   *Frozen urine from a patient with untreated MSUD. The odor of maple syrup is concentrated in an oil at the top.*

death has been reported in four infants 3 to 5 years-of-age during therapy for severe metabolic acidosis and dehydration, which occurred with intercurrent infection [17]. Four patients with cerebral edema were documented to have hyponatremia and decreased osmolarity in the serum [19].

The characteristic odor may be detected as soon as neurological symptoms develop. At the same time, it should be pointed out that not every patient with this disease is recognizable by the smell. Infants with this clinical picture should be screened for metabolic disease, whether or not an odor is detected. The odor is particularly likely to be absent in a comatose patient who has not received protein for days and has received copious amounts of parenteral fluid prior to transfer from a referring hospital. The odor may be found in the hair, the sweat, or cerumen. It is usually best appreciated in the urine. Freezing the urine may bring out the smell by concentrating it in an oil that freezes poorly or not at all at the top of the frozen specimen (Figure 24.8). The odor is sweet, malty, or caramel-like. It really does call forth an olfactory image of maple syrup. The odor of the patient with the disease once

appeared provincially North American because of the localized occurrence of maple syrup. Then Mediterraneans and others [20–22] realized that this odor was produced by the ingestion of fenugreek (foenum graecum), from Trigonella by an infant, or by the mother prior to delivery. The compound responsible for the odor was isolated and identified as sotolone (4,5-dimethyl-3-hydroxy-2[5H]-furanone). This compound, derived from isoleucine, has now been isolated from the urine of patients with maple syrup urine disease; as well as from maple syrup itself [23].

Hypoglycemia may be observed in the acute episode of illness but is not common [24,25]. Acidosis is also not a major feature, although the patient may be ketonuric. Pancreatitis has been observed in MSUD, as it has in other organic acidemias [26–28]. One patient with pancreatitis had transitory retinopathy [25].

The electoencephalogram (EEG) of the newborn with MSUD has been described as a comb-like rhythm [28,29] of sharp waves. Later, the EEG may be normal between attacks, when there may be generalized slowing or paroxysmal discharges. A normal EEG may be seen despite abnormalities on CT of the brain and developmental delay [30]. Leucine loading in an asymptomatic adult with MSUD led to EEG abnormalities [31].

Neuroimaging most commonly shows decreased attenuation in white matter consistent with delayed or abnormal myelination [16,29,32,33]. This appearance resolves after some months of successful treatment. In one patient [33], complete resolution of white matter lucency on CT of the brain was seen after 40 days of treatment. Impressively, ventricular size decreased. Generalized lucency of the cerebral white matter has been seen as early as 9 days, despite a restricted diet [34]. In 9 of 10 patients with classic MSUD who had general lucency; there was also localized intense lucency in the deep cerebellar white matter and peduncles and the brain stem. These changes have been attributed to edema [34], but may well be dysmyelination or delayed myelination [25,35]. In one of our patients, MRI at one month showed striking lucency of the white matter which had markedly improved by 1 year of age. In another patient studied first by MRI of the brain at 6 years of age, in whom the initial diagnosis had been late, the MRI was normal except for a slight increase in the ventricular size.

The usual neuropathological finding in patients dying of MSUD is a generalized status spongiosus of the white matter similar to that seen in phenylketonuria and nonketotic hyperglycinemia [36]. The changes have generally been described in infants 9 months to 4.5 years-of-age, but spongiform change was reported along with edema in an infant who died at 12 days of life [37]. Patients in the original series [2] who died at 11 and 14 days had cerebral edema. Spongiform changes and intramyelin vacuoles on electron microscopy have been observed in an animal model in which Hereford calves died of MSUD within the first week of life [38].

A number of variants of branched-chain oxoaciduria has now been described [39]. Each is milder in its clinical presentation than classic MSUD. The first of these to be described [40–44] has been referred to as intermittent branched-chain ketoaciduria. Involved individuals may have no problems except in the presence of some special stress such as infection or surgery. On the other hand, this disorder, too, can be lethal. Patients with no symptoms at all for a period of years can suddenly develop coma, convulsions, and death following an apparently mild infection [43]. More commonly these patients have intermittent bouts of acute ataxia.

A third form has been referred to as intermediate branched-chain ketoaciduria [45–47]. These patients usually presented with mental retardation and hence some symptomatology was considered to be continuous as opposed to intermittent. However in our experience the biochemical abnormality of the accumulation of amino acids and oxoacids in body fluids, in all these patients, including the intermittent form, is always demonstrable, except of course when successfully treated; so the designations intermittent and intermediate are misnomers for what is in fact a spectrum of variants. Some of the patients have had lethargy and problems with feeding from very early. Many have failed to thrive. One patient reported as intermediate [47] presented first with ketoacidosis and coma at the age of 10 months and subsequently responded to dietary therapy with no further episodes and had an IQ of 92; however his dehydrogenase activity was undetectable. Others described as intermittent have had levels of activity indistinguishable from those with classic phenotypes [48,49]. Some have presented with opthalmoplegia [50–53].

Dancis [39] based a classification of variants on protein intolerance. In the classic form of the disease he considered the patients unable to tolerate maintenance requirements of protein and requiring artificial purified amino acid diets for survival. Enzyme levels were 0–2 percent of normal. In the second group, protein tolerance was sufficient to maintain normal growth in infancy or 1.5–2.0 g/kg of protein. Enzyme levels in this group were between 2 and 8 percent of normal. In the third group an unrestricted diet was tolerated. Enzyme activity was between 8 and 16 percent of normal.

Another variant may be distinguished by the fact that the biochemical abnormalities are corrected by the administration of high doses of thiamine [54]. This thiamine-responsive MSUD or thiamine-responsive branched-chain oxoaciduria was originally described in a patient with relatively mild clinical symptomatology who responded to as little as 10 mg of thiamine per day [54]. Patients described to date have all had residual activity of the enzyme [55,56], but doses up to 300 mg per day have been required, and two of them presented with classical clinical disease in infancy [57]. These patients have been quite heterogeneous, and nutritional therapy has been necessary.

A patient with E3 deficiency [57] presented with feeding difficulties in the first week, vomiting and failure to thrive. By 6 weeks severe developmental delay was apparent along with hypotonia and very poor head control. At 8 months he had lactic acidosis (10 mmol/L) and respiratory distress. He died in severe acidosis following liver biopsy at 18 months-of-age. E3 deficiency is considered under Lactic Acidosis (Chapter 51).

GENETICS AND PATHOGENESIS

MSUD is transmitted as an autosomal recessive trait. This is true of each of the variants. Classic MSUD has been seen throughout the world and in all ethnic groups. It is common among the Mennonites of Pennsylvania in whom the incidence is 1 in 760. In the New England screening program an incidence of 1 in 290 000 was encountered [58]. Heterozygote detection by enzymatic assay may not be reliable. Once a mutation is identified in a proband, molecular techniques may be used to establish carrier status. The activity of the enzyme can be measured in cultured amniotic fluid cells, and the disease has been diagnosed prenatally in a substantial number of patients. Mutations can readily be tested for in prenatal diagnosis, especially with allele-specific oligonucleotide probes [12,59].

The molecular defect in MSUD is in the branched chain oxoacid dehydrogenase which catalyzes the decarboxylation of the oxoacids (Figures 24.1, 24.2). Activity is widely distributed in mammalian tissues. The enzyme is located on the inner surface of the inner mitochondrial membrane. Activity can be measured in human liver, kidney and leukocytes, cultured fibroblasts or lymphoblasts and amniotic fluid cells [60–63].

In the reaction, as in case of pyruvate or α-ketoglutarate, there is first a thiamine pyrophosphate (TPP) mediated conversion of the carboxyl group to CO_2 and the formation of a covalently bound enzyme, TPP, substrate complex (Figure 24.2). Next there is an oxidative transfer to the second, lipoic acid-bearing enzyme, liberating TPP after which there is transfer to Coenzyme A, and lipoic acid is regenerated. Regulation of enzyme involves acyl CoA compounds, and activity is stimulated by carnitine [64], presumably by the formation of acylcarnitine esters of acyl CoA compounds and prevention of product inhibition. The enzyme is inhibited by adenosine diphosphate (ADP), a condition under which pyruvate decarboxylation is stimulated. Additional regulation has been demonstrated in a phosphorylation/dephosphorylation cycle in which the dehydrogenase complex is inactivated by a kinase catalyzed phosphorylation and activated through action of the phosphatase.

Measurement of the activity of branched-chain ketoacid decarboxylase *in vitro* in fibroblasts or leukocytes has generally been carried out by studying the conversion of leucine-^{14}C, isoleucine-^{14}C, valine-^{14}C, or α-oxoisocaproic acid-^{14}C to $^{14}CO_2$. In patients with classic MSUD each activity has been virtually nil [6,65]. In contrast, the oxidation of isovaleric acid-^{14}C to $^{14}CO_2$ is normal.

Patients with intermittent branched-chain oxoaciduria and other variants have been found to have residual activity [6,39]. Activity of up to 15–25 percent of the normal level has been observed [47]. A patient with E3 deficiency had defective activity of pyruvate dehydrogenase and 2-oxoglutarate dehydrogenase as well as BKAD [57].

Abnormal activities have been identified in the individual components of the enzyme complex [66], but these assays are demanding, and dissection of the individual components in patients has been facilitated by northern and western blotting with specific antibodies and cDNA probes [66,67]. More recently this dissection has been done by retroviral complementation of dehydrogenase activity using plasmids containing the wild type for each of the three genes E1α, E1β and E2; the one that restored activity identified the mutated gene

[68]. There may be functional deficiency of E1β and lack of immunoreactive protein as a consequence of mutation in E1α [12], consistent with a requirement for protein interactions in assembly and stabilization.

Mutational analysis has identified a number of the MSUD mutations in E1α [69]. The vast majority of these have been missense mutations, and most have been associated with the severe, classic phenotype. The most prevalent mutation, the T to A change found in Mennonites [12] has also been found in other populations [69]. Of three other missense mutations in E1α, one led to a classical phenotype [69], and two were intermediate in Mexican-American patients [70]. The G245R mutation appears to be common in that population. Four E1α mutations are common in Japanese [71]. In the E1β gene most of the mutations have been found in Japanese [71]. An 11 base pair deletion in the mitochondrial target sequence is relatively common [72].

A number of mutations have been found in E2 [68,73–77]. They include single base substitutions [73–76], insertions [70,75], and deletions [74,76,78], and these mutations have led to missense, nonsense, frameshift and internal deletion, as well as exon skipping at splice junctions and coding regions. Many have been compounds of two mutations [73–76]. The E2 gene appears to have a propensity for splicing errors, some induced by large mutations in introns. The original thiamine-responsive patient of Scriver [54] had a 17 base pair insertion in the E2 mRNA [73], resulting from a deletion in intron 4 (77). Many of the E2 variants have been seen in patients with clinical variant phenotypes.

Five missense mutations have been reported in E3 in a single compound patient [77,79]. A G229C mutation is common in Ashkenazi Jews [79].

Defective activity of the dehydrogenase complex leads to elevated concentrations of leucine, isoleucine and valine in the plasma and urine (Table 24.1) [3,14,15]. Patients also excrete the oxoacid products of the transamination of each of these amino acids (Table 24.2), consistent with the site of enzymatic block [14,15,80] (Figure 24.1, p. 159). Isovaleric acid, α-methylbutyric acid and isobutyric acid are not found. Among the amino acids the concentration of leucine is virtually always higher than those of isoleucine and valine [3]. An exception was a variant patient described as valine-toxic [81]. Two other patients were unusual in that most of the branched chain oxoacids were derived from isoleucine [82,83]. The oxoacid analogs of leucine and isoleucine are usually present in much higher quantities than the corresponding hydroxyacids. In contrast 2-hydroxyisovaleric acid is usually present in much higher concentration than its oxoacid. Alloisoleucine is also regularly found [80]. This product of isoleucine accumulation

Table 24.1 *Concentrations of amino acids in plasma in untreated MSUD*

Valine (μmol/L)	Isoleucine (μmol/L)	Leucine (μmol/L)	Alloisoleucine (μmol/L)
500–1800	200–1300	500–5000	Trace–300

Table 24.2 *Organic acids of the urine in MSUD*

Oxo acids (mmol/m creatinine)			Hydroxy acids (mmol/m creatinine)		
2-Oxoisocaproic acid	2-Oxo-3-methylvaleric acid	2-Oxoisovaleric acid	2-Hydroxy-isocaproic acid	2-Hydroxy-3-methylvaleric acid	2-Hydroxy-isovaleric acid
400–4400	500–2500	300–800	3–8	60–400	850–3600

was originally mistaken for methionine in the amino acid analyzer, creating some confusion in the management of early patients. The concentration of alanine in the plasma of these patients is decreased [13]. During illness as the leucine rises, the alanine falls. The molar ratio of leucine to alanine is a more sensitive measure than leucine alone, and may be useful in diagnosis or neonatal screening [19]. In a series of 18 newborns with MSUD the ratio was 1.3 to 12.4 (normal 0.12–0.53).

Measurement of *in vivo* oxidation of 1-^{13}C-leucine by measurement of ^{13}C in leucine and its oxoacid following an oral bolus correlated well with clinical phenotype [84].

Screening for the disease has been carried out by the addition of 2,4-dinitrophenylhydrazine, which produces a yellow precipitate of dinitrophenylhydrazones [85] in the presence of oxoacids. The individual oxoacids are distinguished by gas chromatography/mass spectrometry (GC/MS) of the oximes [86]. The ferric chloride test on the urine may yield a greenish-gray color. Rapid screening for MSUD is now done best by tandem MS, and this forms the basis for all of the neonatal screening programs for this disease. The method is not useful for management because it does not distinguish between leucine and isoleucine, but this is not a problem for screening. The leucine (isoleucine) alanine ratio [19] should be a useful assessment in these programs.

TREATMENT

Emergency treatment of an infant in coma requires prompt reduction of levels of leucine and the other branched-chain amino acids. This has formerly been approached by exchange transfusions, peritoneal dialysis or both; but direct measurements have indicated the removal of small quantities of amino acids in this way [87]. Hemodialysis is doubtless effective, but it is formidable in a young infant and the prospect of repeat dialysis with each respiratory infection in the early years of life is impossible to consider. Recently Saudubray and colleagues [88] have reported on continuous venovenous extracorporeal hemodiafiltration as a more rapid method for the lowering of high levels of leucine. In six neonatal infants and six children with later episodes this approach was begun after 6 hours of conservative management including enteral amino acid mixtures and leucine concentration is over 1700 μmol/L. In each the decrease in leucine was logarithmic and usually reached <1000 μmol/L in 24 hr, while the rate of decrease with enteral therapy after cessation of the diafiltration

was a slower linear fall. Follow-up developmental levels in this series were encouraging; some had quotients over 100 with follow up at as long as 3 to 5 years.

The alternative approach has been to take advantage of the power of the anabolic laying down of accumulated amino acids into protein to lower toxic levels of branched-chain amino acids. This can be accomplished by providing mixtures of amino acids not containing leucine, isoleucine and valine and energy as provided by 10 percent glucose intravenously. Intravenous solutions have been developed for this purpose and shown to be rapidly effective [89–91], but these solutions are not generally available, and very expensive. We have successfully employed 200 mL/kg of 10 percent glucose intravenously and 2 g/kg of amino acid mixture providing 88 Cal/kg. Berry and colleagues [90] have used larger quantities of glucose, requiring a central line and insulin. In a patient who is not vomiting, it is also possible to accomplish this by intragastric drip. Even in the presence of vomiting we have found that provision of enteral amino acid mixtures dripped in minimal volume over 24 hours are usually tolerated [92,93]. Our mixtures contained extra quantities of alanine and glutamine [93] and so do those employed by Morton *et al.* [19]. In their extensive experience the rate of fall of plasma leucine with this approach was consistently greater than those reported for dialysis or hemoperfusion [19]. Commercial mixtures suitable for enteral use in minimal volume for the management of the acute episodes are now available in the US (Complex® MSUD Amino Acid Blend Applied Nutrition Corp., Randolph, NJ). A protocol for acute management is given as Table 24.3.

Wendel and colleagues [94] treated the acute crisis with insulin and glucose as an anabolic approach to therapy. In each episode studied, the introduction of this regime led to reduction in toxic levels of leucine. Studies of the *in vivo* metabolism of ^{13}C-leucine have indicated that protein synthesis is normal and that there is no significant route for disposal of leucine other than protein synthesis [95], providing further argument for anabolic approaches to therapy. In these studies leucine oxidation was undetectable, consistent with what we have found in fibroblasts *in vitro* [96]. We have recently employed enteral anabolic therapy, parenteral insulin and glucose and human growth hormone (Table 24.3).

Chronic management consists of restricting of the intake of each of the three branched-chain amino acids to those essential for growth and no more. This type of dietary management is much more difficult than that of phenylketonuria. It requires very close regulation of an artificial diet and frequent access to an amino acid analyzer. The best results are

Table 24.3 *Management of the acute crisis in maple syrup urine disease*

Stop oral feedings. Begin IV hydration with 10% glucose and maintenance electrolyte.

Begin nasogastric or gastrostomy drip with 2.0–4.0 g/kg of amino acid protein equivalent – lacking leucine, isoleucine and valine.

Complex ® MSUD Amino Acid Blend-Applied Nutrition Corp., Randolph, NJ. – 13 g of mixture provides 10 g of amino acids – 2.0 g/kg = 2.6 g/kg of Complex. This contains 8 Cal/kg. Add H_2O to make 8 mL/kg or 1 Cal/mL to make for minimal volume in a vomiting or potentially vomiting patient, and drip this volume in slowly over 24 hours.

Obtain plasma stat for amino acids at least q 12 hours initially until therapeutic trend established; thereafter at least daily.

Plan to add isoleucine even in the first 24 hours, as hypoisoleucinemia will stop anabolism, lead to catabolism and consequent rise in leucine. A level of 20 mg/kg of added isoleucine is usually sufficient, but if added later even 100 mg/kg may be required. Valine supplementation may also be necessary before a steady-state leucine level is achieved.

In patients needing additional therapy add insulin – 0.1 u/kg per hour. Provide glucose as 10% IV – at least 20 mL/u insulin. Monitor blood sugar and urine – dipstix and adjust.

In patients needing additional therapy add human growth hormone 0.05 mg/kg/24 hr. SQ

Thiamine at 100 mg/kg can be given parenterally at the start of therapy. Patient could be discharged with po allithiamine and later tested to see if thiamine added anything to treatment.

---

seen in those in whom treatment has been initiated earliest. The largest experience with the management of this disease is that of Snyderman [13,97] and Morton [19], and both have written that there can be little doubt about the beneficial effect of therapy in this disorder. Commercial products are available that are useful in the management of this disorder [98] (Ketonex-Ross, MSUD-Mead-Johnson).

In thiamine-responsive MSUD, the doses employed have ranged from 10–300 mg/day [54,56]. It has appeared reasonable to test each patient with larger amounts before deciding that thiamine is not a useful adjunct to therapy. However, this is complicated by data that indicate not more than a few milligrams of an oral dose are absorbed [99]; implying that parenteral administration may be necessary to assess the effects of larger doses. Allithiamine may be useful orally.

The management of intercurrent illness is particularly important in this disease [100], and parents must be taught to be efficient partners in recognition and prompt management. Written protocols or letters to Emergency Room physicians for use when illness occurs in out of town situations are useful adjuncts. A regimen of restriction of leucine intake at the first sign of illness, continuation of other amino acids (including 10 mg/kg of isoleucine and of valine) and the supply of abundant calories particularly as glucose or glucose polymer is useful.

Liver transplantation is an option in the treatment of MSUD [101–105]. Orthotopic liver transplantation was carried out in two patients with the disease for nonmetabolic

reasons. Both had liver failure, one from hepatitis A [101] and the other from intoxication with vitamin A [102]. Both have remained metabolically and neurologically stable without any restriction of protein intake for over two years. A third patient [5,103] was transplanted because of the request of parents concerned with delayed psychomotor development and frequent metabolic decompensation. In each patient, dramatic decrease in plasma levels of branched-chain amino acids occurred immediately, reaching near normal levels in ten hours despite post-transplant catabolic stress. None of the patients had a further episode of metabolic derangement. Whole body stable isotope labeled leucine oxidation was normal in the one patient tested. Another patient has received a liver transplant because of liver failure [105]. At 9 years neurological findings included stupor, dystonia, ataxia, hyperreflexion and positive Babinski signs. Five years following the procedure neurological examination was normal as were plasma amino acid concentrations and calculated brain uptake of neutral amino acids.

References

1   Peinemann F, Danner DJ. Maple syrup urine disease: 1954 to 1993. *J Inherit Metab Dis* 1994;**17**:3.

2   Menkes JH, Hurst PL, Craig JM. New syndrome: progressive infantile cerebral dysfunction associated with unusual urinary substance. *Pediatrics* 1954;**14**:462.

3   Westall RG, Dancis J, Miller S. Maple syrup urine disease – a new molecular disease. *Am J Dis Child* 1957;**94**:571.

4   Menkes JH. Maple syrup urine disease: isolation and identification of organic acids in the urine. *Pediatrics* 1959;**23**:348.

5   Dancis J, Hutzler J, Levitz M. Metabolism of the white blood cells in maple-syrup-urine disease. *Biochim Biophys Acta* 1960;**43**:342.

6   Dancis J, Hutzler H, Snyderman SE, Cox RP. Enzyme activity in classical and variant forms of maple syrup urine disease. *J Pediatr* 1972;**81**:312.

7   Pettit FH, Yeaman SJ, Reed LJ. Purification and characterization of branched chain α-keto acid dehydrogenase complex of bovine kidney. *Proc Natl Acad Sci USA* 1978;**75**:4881.

8   Wynn RM, Song J, Chuang DT. GroEL/GroES promote dissociation/ reassociation cycles of a heterodimeric intermediate during $\alpha_2 \beta_2$ protein assembly. *J Biol Chem* 2000;**275**:2786.

9   Fekete J, Plattner R, Crabb DW, *et al.* Localization of the human gene for the E1 alpha subunit of branched chain keto acid dehydrogenase (BCKDHA) to chromosome 19q131–q132. *Cytogenet Cell Genet* 1989;**50**:236.

10 Zneimer SM, Lau KS, Eddy RL, *et al.* Regional assignment of two genes of the human branched-chain alpha-keto acid dehydrogenase complex: the E1 beta gene (BCKDHB) to chromosome 6p21–22 and the E2 gene (DBT) to chromosome 1p3. *Genomics* 1991;**10**:740.

11 Scherer SW, Otulakowski G, Robinson BH, Tsui LC. Localization of the human dihydrolipoamide dehydrogenase gene (DLD) to 7q31-q32. *Cytogenet Cell Genet* 1991;**56**:176.

12 Matsuda I, Nobukuni Y, Mitsubuchi H, *et al.* A T-to-A substitution in the E1 alpha subunit gene of the branched-chain alpha-ketoacid dehydrogenase complex in two cell lines derived from Mennonite maple syrup urine disease patients. *Biochem Biophys Res Commun* 1990;**172**:646.

13 Snyderman SE. Maple syrup urine disease: in *Heritable Disorders of Amino Acid Metabolism* (ed. WL Nyhan). J Wiley and Sons Inc., New York:1960:17–31.

14 Dancis J, Levitz M, Westall RG. Maple syrup urine disease: branched chain keto-aciduria. *Pediatrics* 1960;**25**:72.

15   Mackenzie DY, Woolf LI. Maple syrup urine disease: inborn error of metabolism of valine leucine and isoleucine associated with gross mental deficiency. *Br Med J* 1959;**1**:90.

16   Mantovani JF, Naidich TP, Prensky AL, *et al.* MSUD: presentation with pseudotumor cerebri and CT abnormalities. *J Pediatr* 1980;**96**:279.

17   Riviello JJ Jr, Rezvani I, DiGeorge AM, Foley CM. Cerebral edema causing death in children with metabolic disease. *J Pediatr* 1991;**119**:42.

18   Mikati MA, Dudin GE, Der Kaloustian VM, *et al.* Maple syrup urine disease with increased intracranial pressure. *Am J Dis Child* 1982;**136**:642.

19   Morton DH, Strauss KA, Robinson DL, *et al.* Diagnosis and treatment of maple syrup disease: a study of 36 patients.*Pediatrics* 2002;**109**:999.

20   Hauser GJ, Chitayat D, Berns L, *et al.* Peculiar odours in newborns and maternal prenatal ingestion of spicy food. *Eur J Pediatr* 1985;**144**:403.

21   Bartley GB, Hilty MD, Anderson BD, *et al.* 'Maple syrup' urine odor due to fenugreek ingestion. *N Engl J Med* 1981;**305**:467.

22   Monastiri K, Limame D, Kaabachi N, *et al.* Fenugreek odour in maple syrup urine disease. *J Inherit Metab Dis* 1997;**20**:614.

23   Podebrad F, Heil M, Reichert S, *et al.* 45-Dimethyl-3-hydroxy-2[5H]-furanone (sotolone) – the odour of maple syrup urine disease. *J Inherit Metab Dis* 1999;**22**:107.

24   Donnell GN, Lieberman E, Shaw KNF, Koch R. Hypoglycemia in maple syrup urine disease. *Am J Dis Child* 1967;**113**:60.

25   Treacy E, Clow CL, Reade TR, *et al.* Maple syrup urine disease: interrelations between branched-chain amino- oxo- and hydroxyacids; implications for treatment associations with CNS demyelination. *J Inherit Metab Dis* 1992;**15**:121.

26   Friedrich CA, Marble M, Maher J, Valle D. Successful control of branched-chain amino acids (BCAA) in maple syrup urine disease using elemental amino acids in total parenteral nutrition during acute pancreatitis. *Am J Hum Genet* 1992;**51**:A350.

27   Kahler SG, Sherwood GW, Woolf D, *et al.* Pancreatitis in patients with organic acidemias. *J Pediatr* 1994;**124**:239.

28   Estivill E, Sanmarti FX, Vidal R, *et al.* (Comb-like rhythm: an EEG pattern peculiar to leucinosis.) *An Esp Pediatr* 1985;**22**:123.

29   Tharp BR. Unique EEG pattern (comb-like rhythm) in neonatal maple syrup urine disease. *Pediatr Neurol* 1992;**8**:65.

30   Verdu A, Lopez Herce J, Pascual Castroviejo I, *et al.* Maple syrup urine disease variant form: presentation with psychomotor retardation and CT scan abnormalities. *Acta Paediatr Scand* 1985;**74**:815.

31   Snyderman SE. Treatment outcome of maple syrup urine disease. *Acta Paediatr Jpn* 1988;**30**:417.

32   Suzuki S, Naito H, Abe T, Nihei K. Cranial computed tomography in a patient with a variant form of maple syrup urine disease. *Neuropediatrics* 1983;**14**:102.

33   Romero FJ, Ibarra B, Rovira M, *et al.* Cerebral computed tomography in maple syrup urine disease. *J Comput Assist Tomogr* 1984;**8**:410.

34   Brismar J, Aqeel A, Brismar G, *et al.* Maple syrup urine disease: findings on CT and MR scans of the brain in 10 infants. *AJNR Am J Neuroradiol* 1990;**11**:1219.

35   Taccone A, Schiaffino MC, Cerone R, *et al.* Computed tomography in maple syrup urine disease. *Eur J Radiol* 1992;**14**:207.

36   Crome L, Dutton G, Ross CF. Maple syrup urine disease. *J Path Bact* 1961;**81**:379.

37   Menkes JH, Philippart M, Fiol RE. Cerebral lipids in maple syrup urine disease. *J Pediatr* 1965;**66**:584.

38   Harper PA, Healy PJ, Dennis JA. Maple syrup urine disease as a cause of spongiform encephalopathy in calves. *Vet Rec* 1986;**119**:62.

39   Dancis J. Variants of maple syrup urine disease: in *Heritable Disorders of Amino Acid Metabolism* (ed. WL Nyhan) J Wiley and Sons Inc., New York;1974:32–36.

40   Morris MD, Lewis BD, Doolan PD, Harper HA. Clinical and biochemical observations on an apparently nonfatal variant of branched-chain ketoaciduria. *Pediatrics* 1961;**28**:918.

41   Kiil R, Rokkones T. Late manifesting variant of branched-chain ketoaciduria. *Acta Paediatr Scand* 1964;**53**:356.

42   Van Der Hort HL, Wadman SK. A variant form of branched-chain ketoaciduria. *Acta Paediatr Scand* 1971;**60**:594.

43   Goedde HW, Langenbeck V, Brackertz D, *et al.* Clinical and biochemical genetic aspects of intermittent branched-chain ketoaciduria. *Acta Paediatr Scand* 1967;**59**:83.

44   Dancis J, Hutzler J, Rokkones T. Intermittent branched-chain ketonuria. Variant maple-syrup-urine disease. *N Eng J Med* 1967;**276**:84.

45   Schulman JD, Lustberg TJ, Kennedy JL, *et al.* A new variant of maple syrup urine disease (branched-chain ketoaciduria). *Am J Med* 1970;**49**:118.

46   Fischer MH, Gerritsen T. Biochemical studies on a variant of branched-chain ketoaciduria in a nineteen-year-old female. *Pediatrics* 1971;**48**:795.

47   Gonzalez Rios MC, Chuang DT, Cox RP, *et al.* A distinct variant of intermediate maple syrup urine disease. *Clin Genet* 1985;**27**:153.

48   Valman HB, Patrick AD, Seakins JW, *et al.* Family with intermittent maple syrup urine disease. *Arch Dis Child* 1973;**48**:225.

49   Dent CE, Westall RG. Studies in maple syrup urine disease. *Arch Dis Child* 1961;**36**:259.

50   Chhabria S, Tomasi LG, Wong PW. Ophthalmoplegia and bulbar palsy in variant form of maple syrup urine disease. *Ann Neurol* 1979;**6**:71.

51   MacDonald JT, Sher PK. Ophthalmoplegia as a sign of metabolic disease in the newborn. *Neurology* 1977;**27**:971.

52   Hurwitz LJ, Carson NA, Allen IV, Chopra JS. Congenital ophthalmoplegia floppy baby syndrome myopathy and aminoaciduria. Report of a family. *J Neurol Neurosurg Psychiatry* 1969;**32**:495.

53   Zee DS, Freeman JM, Holtzman NA. Opthalmoplegia in maple syrup urine disease. *J Pediatr* 1974;**84**:113.

54   Scriver CR, Clow CL, Mackenzie S, Delvin E. Thiamine-responsive maple syrup urine disease. *Lancet* 1971;**1**:310.

55   Duran M, Wadman SK. Thiamine-responsive inborn errors of metabolism. *J Inherit Metab Dis* 1985;**8**:70.

56   Fernhoff PM, Lubitz D, Danner DJ, *et al.* Thiamine response in maple syrup urine disease. *Pediatr Res* 1985;**19**:1011.

57   Munnich A, Saudubray JM, Taylor J, *et al.* Congenital lactic acidosis alpha-ketoglutaric aciduria and variant form of maple syrup urine disease due to a single enzyme defect: dihydrolipoyl dehydrogenase deficiency. *Acta Paediatr Scand* 1982;**71**:167.

58   Naylor EW. Newborn screening for maple syrup urine disease: in *Laboratory Methods for Neonatal Screening* (ed. BL Therrell) American Public Health Association, Washington DC;1993: 115–124.

59   Zhang B, Edenberg HJ, Crabb DW, Harris RA. Evidence for both a regulatory mutation and a structural mutation in a family with maple syrup urine disease. *J Clin Invest* 1989;**83**:1425.

60   Dancis J, Hutzler J, Levitz M. Tissue distribution of branched chain keto-acid decarboxylase. *Biochim Biophys Acta* 1961;**52**:60.

61   Dancis J, Jansen V, Hutzler J, Levitz M. The metabolism of leucine in tissue culture of skin fibroblasts of maple syrup urine disease. *Biochim Biophys Acta* 1963;**77**:523.

62   Elsas LJ, Priest JH, Wheeler FB, *et al.* Maple syrup urine disease: Coenzyme function and prenatal monitoring. *Metabolism* 1974;**23**:569.

63   Wendel U, Rudiger HW, Passarge E, Mikkelsen M. Maple syrup urine disease: rapid prenatal diagnosis by enzyme assay. *Humangenetik* 1973;**19**:127.

64   Aftring RP, May ME, Buse MG. Regulation of branched chain ketoacid metabolism in rat liver: in *Metabolism and Clinical Implications of Branched Chain Amino and Ketoacids* (eds M Walser JR Williamson) Elsevier North Holland Inc., Amsterdam;1981:67–72.

65 Dancis J, Hutzler J, Levitz M. The diagnosis of maple syrup urine disease (Branched-chain ketoaciduria) by the *in vitro* study of the peripheral leukocyte. *Pediatrics* 1963;**32**:234.

66 Indo Y, Akaboshi I, Nobukuni Y, *et al.* Maple syrup urine disease: a possible biochemical basis for clinical heterogeneity. *Hum Genet* 1988;**80**:6.

67 Nobukuni Y, Mitsubuchi H, Ohta K, *et al.* Molecular diagnosis of maple syrup urine disease: screening and identification of gene mutations in the branched-chain α-ketoacid dehydrogenase multienzyme complex. *J Inherit Metab Dis* 1992;**15**:827.

68 Nellis MN, Danner DJ. Gene preference in maple syrup urine disease. *Am J Hum Genet* 2001;**68**:232.

69 Chuang JL, Fisher CR, Cox RP, Chuang DT. Molecular basis of maple syrup urine disease: novel mutations at the E1 alpha locus that impair E1 (alpha 2 beta 2) assembly or decrease steady-state E1 alpha mRNA levels of branched-chain alpha-keto acid dehydrogenase complex. *Am J Hum Genet* 1994;**55**:297.

70 Chuang JL, Davie JR, Chinsky JM, *et al.* Molecular and biochemical basis of intermediate maple syrup urine disease. Occurrence of homozygous G245R and F364C mutations at the E1 alpha locus of Hispanic-Mexican patients. *J Clin Invest* 1995;**95**:954.

71 Nobukuni Y, Mitsubuchi H, Hayashida Y, *et al.* Heterogeneity of mutations in maple syrup urine disease (MSUD): screening and identification of affection E1α and E1β subunits of the branched-chain α-keto-acid dehydrogenase multienzyme complex. *Biochim Biophys Acta* 1993;**1225**:64.

72 Nobukuni Y, Mitsubuchi H, Akaboshi I, *et al.* Maple syrup urine disease: complete defect of the E1-beta subunit of the branched chain alpha-ketoacid dehydrogenase complex due to a deletion of an 11-bp repeat sequence which encodes a mitochondrial targeting leader peptide in a family with the disease. *J Clin Invest* 1991;**87**:1862.

73 Fisher CW, Lau KS, Fisher CR, *et al.* A 17-bp insertion and a Phe215-Cys missense mutation in the dihydrolipoyl transacylase (E2) mRNA from a thiamine-responsive maple syrup urine disease patient WG-34. *Biochem Biophys Res Commun* 1991;**174**:804.

74 Chuang DT, Fisher CW, Lau KS, *et al.* Maple syrup urine disease: domain structure mutations and exon skipping in the dihydrolipoyl transacylase (E2) component of the branched-chain alpha-ketoacid dehydrogenase complex. *Mol Biol Med* 1991;**8**:49.

75 Fisher CW, Fisher CR, Chuang JL, *et al.* Occurrence of a 2-bp (AT) deletion allele and a nonsense (G-to-T) mutant allele at the E2 (DBT) locus of six patients with maple syrup urine disease: multiple exon skipping as a secondary effect of the mutations. *Am J Hum Genet* 1993;**52**:414.

76 Herring WJ, McKean M, Dracopoli N, Danner DJ. Branched chain acyltransferase absence due to an Alu-based genomic deletion allele and an exon skipping allele in a compound heterozygote proband expressing maple syrup urine disease. *Biochim Biophys Acta* 1992;**1138**:236.

77 Chuang DT, Shih VE. Maple syrup urine disease (branched-chain ketoaciduria): in *The Metabolic and Molecular Basis of Inherited Disease* (eds CR Scriver, AL Beaudet, WS Sly, D Valle). 8th ed. McGraw Hill, New York;2001:1971.

78 Mitsubuchi H, Nobukuni Y, Akaboshi I, *et al.* Maple syrup urine disease caused by a partial deletion in the inner E2 core domain of the branched chain alpha-keto acid dehydrogenase complex due to aberrant splicing. A single base deletion at a 5′-splice donor site of an intron of the E2 gene disrupts the consensus sequence in this region. *J Clin Invest* 1991;**87**:1207.

79 Liu TC, Kim H, Arizmendi C, *et al.* Identification of two missense mutations in a dihydrolipoamide dehydrogenase-deficient patient. *Proc Natl Acad Sci USA* 1993;**90**:235.

80 Norton PM, Roitman E, Snyderman SE, Holt Jr LE. A new finding in maple syrup urine disease. *Lancet* 1964;**1**:26.

81 Zipf WB, Hieber VC, Allen RJ. Valine-toxic intermittent maple syrup urine disease: a previously unrecognized variant. *Pediatrics* 1979;**63**:286.

82 Fischer MH, Gerritsen T. Biochemical studies on a variant of branched chain ketoaciduria in a 19-year-old female. *Pediatrics* 1971;**48**:795.

83 Gretter TE, Lonsdale D, Mercer RD, *et al.* Maple syrup urine disease variant. Report of a case. *Cleve Clin Q* 1972;**39**:129.

84 Schadewaldt P, Bodner-Leidecker A, Hammen H-W, Wendel U. Whole-body L-leucine oxidation in patients with variant form of maple syrup urine disease. *Pediatr Res* 2001;**49**:627.

85 Borden M. Methodology –Screening for metabolic diseases: in *Abnormalities in Amino Acid Metabolism in Clinical Medicine* (ed. WL Nyhan) Appleton Century Crofts, Norwalk Connecticut;1984:401.

86 Hoffmann G, Aramaki S, Blum-Hoffmann E, *et al.* Quantitative analysis for organic acids in biological samples: Batch isolation followed by gas chromatographic-mass spectrometric analysis. *Clin Chem* 1989;**38**:587.

87 Saudubray J-M, Ogier H, Charpentier C, *et al.* Neonatal management of organic acidurias: clinical update. *J Inherit Metab Dis* 1984;**7**:2.

88 Jouvet P, Jugie M, Saudubray J-M, *et al.* Combined nutritional support and continuous extracorporeal removal therapy in the severe acute phase of maple syrup urine disease. *Intensive Care Med* 2001;**27**:1798.

89 Nyhan WL, Rice-Asaro M, Acosta P. Advances in the treatment of amino acid and organic acid disorders: in *Treatment of Genetic Diseases* (ed. RJ Desnick) Churchill Livingstone, New York;1991:45.

90 Berry GT, Heidenreich R, Kaplan P, *et al.* Branched-chain amino acid-free parenteral nutrition in the treatment of acute metabolic decompensation in patients with maple syrup urine disease. *N Engl J Med* 1991;**324**:175.

91 Townsend I, Kerr DS. Total parenteral nutrition therapy of toxic maple syrup urine disease. *Am J Clin Nutr* 1982;**36**:359.

92 Parini R, Sereni LP, Bagozzi DC, *et al.* Nasogastric drip feeding as the only treatment of neonatal maple syrup urine disease. *Pediatrics* 1993;**92**:280.

93 Nyhan WL, Rice-Kelts M, Klein J. Treatment of the acute crisis in maple syrup urine disease. *Arch Pediatr Adolesc Med* 1998;**152**:593.

94 Wendel U, Langenbeck U, Lombeck I, Bremer JH. Maple syrup urine disease: therapeutic use of insulin in catabolic states. *Eur J Pediatr* 1982;**139**:172.

95 Thompson GN, Bresson JL, Pacy PJ, *et al.* Protein and leucine metabolism in maple syrup urine disease. *Am J Physiol* 1990;**258**:E654.

96 Yoshida I, Sweeetman L, Nyhan WL. Metabolism of branched-chain amino acids in fibroblasts from patients with maple syrup urine disease and other abnormalities of branched-chain ketoacid dehydrogenase activity. *Pediat Res* 1986;**20**:169.

97 Snyderman SE, Norton PM, Roitman E, Holt Jr LE. Maple syrup urine disease with particular reference to diet therapy. *Pediatrics* 1964;**34**:454.

98 Smith BA, Waisman HA. Leucine equivalency system in managing branched chain ketoaciduria. *J Am Diet Assoc* 1971;**59**:342.

99 Haas RH. Thiamin and the brain. *Ann Rev Nutr* 1988;**8**:383.

100 Dixon MA, Leonard JV. Intercurrent illness in inborn errors of intermediary metabolism. *Arch Dis Child* 1992;**67**:1387.

101 Wendel U, Saudubray JM, Bodner A, Schadewaldt P. Liver transplantation in maple syrup urine. *Eur J Pediatr* 1999;**158**: S60.

102 Merinero B, Perez-Cerda C, Sanz P, *et al.* Liver transplantation (LT) in a Spanish MSUD patient. (abstract). *32nd* Annual Symposium Society for the Study of Inborn Errors of Metabolism, Edinburgh;1994:64.

103 Netter JC, Cossariza G, Narcy C, *et al.* Devenir a moyen terme de deux cas de leucinose: place de la transplantation hepatique dans le traitment. *Arch Pediatr* 1994;**1**:730.

104 Kaplan P, Mazur AM, Smith R, *et al.* Transplantation for maple syrup urine disease (MSUD) and methylmalonic acidopathy (MMA). (abstract) *J Inherit Metab Dis* 1997;**20**:[Suppl 1] 37.

105 Robinson DL, Strauss KA, Puffenberger EG, Morton DH. Effects of liver transplant and bone marrow transplant upon amino acid homeostasis and the neuropathology of maple syrup urine disease. *Am J Hum Genet* 2002;**71**:412.

25

Oculocutaneous tyrosinemia/tyrosine aminotransferase deficiency

---

MAJOR PHENOTYPIC EXPRESSION

Dendritic keratitis, causing lacrimation, photophobia, inflammation, ulcers and scars; keratoses of the palms and soles; hypertyrosinemia; defective activity of hepatic cytoplasmic tyrosine aminotransferase.

INTRODUCTION

Oculocutaneous tyrosinemia was first described in 1967 by Campbell, Buist and Jacinto[1] in a report of a patient with corneal ulcers, erythematous papular lesions on the palms and soles, and severe retardation of mental development. A number of patients has since been reported, and it is clear that mental retardation is not a uniform feature of the disease [2–8]. Patients were described in 1938 by Richner [9] and in 1947 by Hanhart [10] with typical lesions of the eyes and skin, and this came to be known as the Richner-Hanhart syndrome, or keratosis palmaris et plantaris; it appears likely that oculocutaneous tyrosinemia and the Richner-Hanhart syndrome are the same disease, although plasma concentrations of tyrosine are not available for the original patients of Richner and Hanhart. Among the disorders in which elevated concentrations of tyrosine have been reported, this disorder appears to be a true hypertyrosinemia or tyrosine intoxication in the sense that the clinical manifestations are a consequence of the elevated levels of tyrosine. It has been referred to as tyrosinemia type II.

The enzymatic site of the defect in oculocutaneous tyrosinemia is in the hepatic tyrosine aminotransferase (TAT, L-tyrosine-2-oxoglutarate aminotransferase, EC 2.6.1.5) (Figure 25.1). There are two separate tyrosine aminotransferases,

one in the cytosol and the other in the mitochondria. In this disorder it is the cytosolic enzyme that is deficient [11–15]. The activity of the mitochondrial enzyme is normal. The gene for TAT is located on chromosome 16 at q22.1-22.3 [16]. The gene has been cloned and sequenced [17]. A number of mutations has been defined [16–18].

CLINICAL ABNORMALITIES

The most important manifestations of oculocutaneous tyrosinemia are those involving the eye [1,2,19], because they can lead to scarring of the cornea and permanent visual impairment. Ocular manifestations such as lacrimation, photophobia, pain in the eye, or a history of red eyes are usually the initial manifestations of the disease and continue to be the most regularly encountered (Figure 25.2). Ocular symptoms may begin as early as the first day of life [20] and usually within the first years, but onset can be as late as 38 years [21], and documented patients have been asymptomatic [21]. Many patients have had symptoms of the eyes without cutaneous manifestations [5,22–24], but others [6,8,24] had the reverse situation. Corneal ulcers are dendritic (Figures 25.3, 25.4). The keratitis may resemble the dendritic keratitis of herpes. The diagnosis may suggest itself to the ophthalmologist after

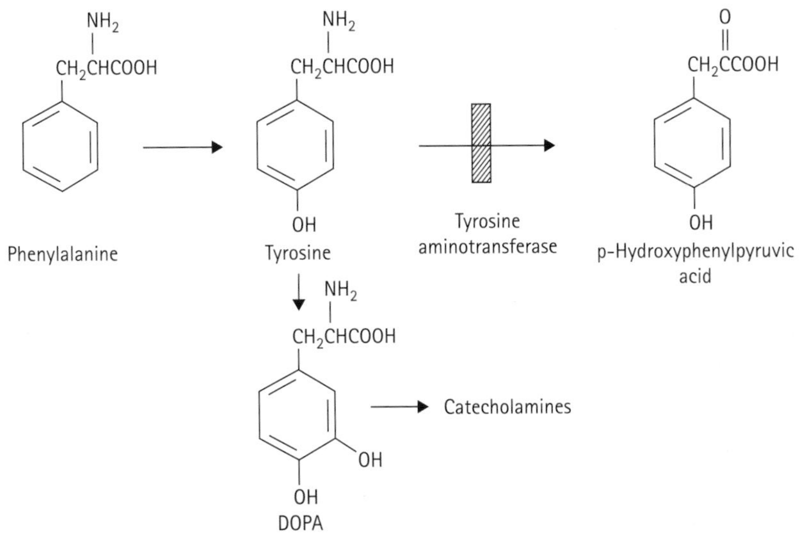

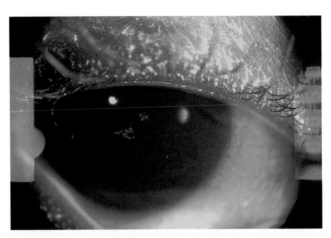

Figure 25.1   *Metabolic pathways for tyrosine and the site of the defect in oculocutaneous tyrosinemia at the tyrosine aminotransferase step.*

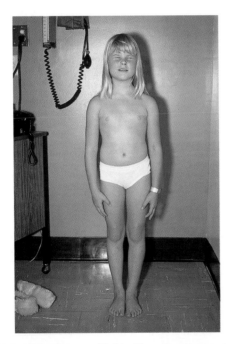

Figure 25.2   *K.P., a 9-year-old girl with oculocutaneous tyrosinemia [2]. She had recurrent photophobia and conjunctival reddening from at least 6 months-of-age. Development was mildly subnormal.*

Figure 25.3   *Corneal lesions of K.P. at 9 years-of-age. The small dendritic lesion stained weakly with fluorescein. The lesion was slightly elevated. There was no ocular inflammation at the time. (Photograph kindly provided by Dr. Perry Binder, San Diego.)*

cultures are negative or after a negative response to antiviral chemotherapy [2,7]. Corneal erosions, ulcers or plaques may be complications [25]. Ulcers may stain poorly with fluorescein. These lesions may lead to corneal clouding with central or paracentral opacities, scarring and impaired vision. There may be neovascularization of the cornea. Keratitic lesions have occurred in a transplanted cornea [26]. A white film may be visible over the cornea. Glaucoma is another reported complication [27]. The differential diagnosis of keratitis in infancy or childhood is essentially herpes or this disease. Idiopathic keratitis does not occur in childhood. Therefore, the concentration of tyrosine in the blood should be determined in any pediatric patient with keratitis.

The ocular and the cutaneous lesions in this disease are the result of the accumulation of tyrosine. Intense burning of the eyes, hands and feet have been observed within an hour of the administration of 0.7–0.8 mmol of tyrosine per kilogram [28], and erythema and pain have been observed in cutaneous lesions after a load of tyrosine [29]. Rats given a diet high in tyrosine develop keratitic ocular lesions [30]. Ocular abnormalities have been observed in other disorders in which tyrosine accumulates [31,32].

The cutaneous lesions are painful keratoses which occur particularly on the peripheral pressure-bearing areas of the palms and soles [33,34] (Figures 25.5–25.7). They may occur near the tips of the digits. Subungual lesions may be found. Typical hyperkeratotic lesions are papular, well-demarcated plaques with irregular borders. Diameters up to 2 cm are common, but lesions may be larger and may be hollow or eroded, progressing to crusted, hyperkeratotic areas. They are not pruritic. They are painful and may be associated with hyperhydrosis [35]. They may be heralded by the appearance

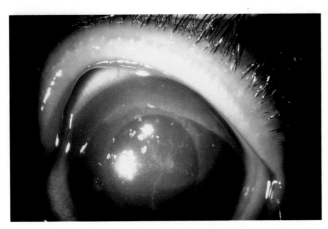

Figure 25.4   *Corneal lesions in J.F., a 3-month-old patient with oculocutaneous tyrosinemia. The appearance was dendritic, but the lesions were elevated, opaque and had mucoid material on the surface. The underlying dendritic figure stained weakly with fluorescein. (Illustration kindly provided by the US Naval Hospital, San Diego.)*

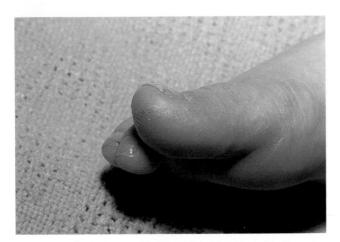

Figure 25.5   *The lesion on the left great toe of K.P. was thickened, scaly and cracked. Plasma concentration of tyrosine was 912 μmol/L (16.5 mg/dL).*

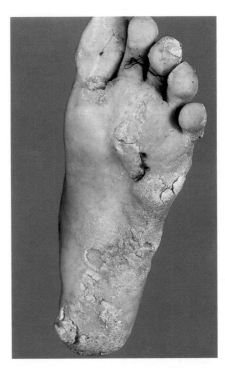

Figure 25.6   *The foot of a Saudi patient with oculocutaneous tyrosinemia (34) who presented with these painful hyperkeratotic placques.*

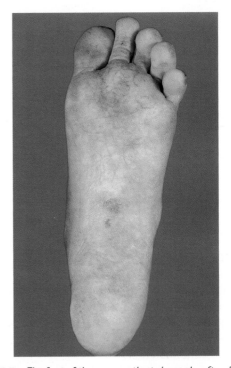

Figure 25.7   *The foot of the same patient six weeks after dietary restriction lowered blood concentrations of tyrosine.*

of blisters. Pain may be so severe that the patient will not walk. Skin lesions may be seen early in life or as late as the second decade [24]. Grayish hyperkeratotic plaques may be seen on the knees, elbows, or ankles. Hyperkeratoses have also been reported on the tongue [36]. Skin biopsy may reveal acanthosis and parakeratosis as well as hyperkeratosis [33], none of them very specific findings. Electron microscopy reveals lipid-like granules and filaments. Crystals of tyrosine were not seen, but they have been seen in the cornea.

Neurologic features of the disease are quite variable [2,24,37]. About half of the patients reported have been mentally retarded, a few severely so [11,26,38], but in most of them the level of intelligence was not very low [6,8,33,36,39]. Some have been described as having low-normal intelligence [8,27,28,40,41]. Two patients had normal intelligence, but had a learning disability [2,38]. Among the patients described there was no obvious relationship between the levels of intelligence and the levels of tyrosine in the blood [2], and it is not clear whether impairment of mental development is an integral component of the syndrome or a reflection of ascertainment bias and the frequency with which retarded individuals are studied for the possible occurrence of metabolic disease.

Hyperactivity has been observed in a number of patients, as well as abnormal language development [19]. An infant may be irritable. The first patient described [1] had self-injurious behavior, but was very severely retarded; this type of behavior has not been seen in others. Convulsions and microcephaly have been reported [42].

GENETICS AND PATHOGENESIS

Transmission of oculocutaneous tyrosinemia is autosomal recessive. Consanguinity has been documented [4,6,33,38,39], as has the occurrence of more than one involved sibling with normal parents [8,19,39]. The disease has been seen in a wide ethnic and geographic distribution, but more commonly in Italians. A registry has been developed in Italy [42]. Heterozygote detection and prenatal diagnosis have not been reported, but this should be possible in those families in which the mutation is known.

A fluorometric procedure developed permitted the initiation of programs of neonatal screening for elevated concentrations of tyrosine [43,44]. These have been supplanted by the tandem mass spectrometry (MS/MS) programs of expanded neonatal screening.

An animal model for oculocutaneous tyrosinemia is available in mink, where it produces a disorder known as pseudo-distemper in which there are exudative lesions of the eyes and volar skin [45]. The activity of tyrosine aminotransferase is reduced, and there is a reduced amount of hepatic cytosolic immunoreactive protein in these animals. There is also a canine model in German Shepherds [46].

Tyrosine aminotransferase normally converts tyrosine to p-hydroxyphenylpyruvic acid (Figure 25.1). It is the rate-limiting step in the metabolism of tyrosine. The enzyme is highly regulated. Transcription is induced by glucocorticoids and cyclic AMP [47]. It is also developmentally regulated, and human neonatal levels of activity are low [48]. The enzyme is a dimmer, that is phosphorylated and acetylated at its N terminus. Pyridoxal phosphate is bound to lysine [49]. The activity of the enzyme has been measured in liver of patients [1,15,29,50,51] and found to be low.

The gene for TAT has been sequenced in human [17], mouse [52] and rat [53]. It contains 12 exons spanning 10.9kb. The mRNA is 2.75kb. The 50.4kD protein has 454 amino acids. A rearrangement in the structural gene of one patient was demonstrated by Southern blot analysis [16]. Among a small number of point mutations reported [18,54] an R57X is frequent in Italian patients. Two missense mutations, G362V and R4331Y, converted a glycine to a valine and an arginine to an asparagine. There were two splice-site mutations and three conversions to stop codons. To date it has not been possible to correlate phenotype with genotype.

When the activity of the enzyme is deficient, tyrosine accumulates, and tyrosine is the only amino acid that accumulates. Reported levels in the blood have generally ranged

Table 25.1 *Oculocutaneous tyrosinemia*

	Plasma tyrosine concentrations μmol/L
Untreated patients on diagnosis	1100–2800
KP adlib diet – no sx	1215
KP max during 11 months with no symptoms	1099
JF asymptomatic	1073
Normal newborn	25–103
Child adult	30–90

between 1100 and 3300 μmol/L (20 and 50 mg/dL) [1,12,21,24,42,55] (Table 25.1). A level of 1000 μmol/L appears to be a threshold level below which symptoms do not occur [34]. Younger patients may have higher levels, and this is consistent with higher intakes of protein. We have observed higher levels during winter than in summer and could correlate this with a decrease in protein consumption in summer, even in San Diego, and despite no change in the diet prescribed, or in symptoms [2]. Prior to diagnosis the mother had noted that symptoms regularly improved during the summer. Some patients have avoided protein-containing foods [19].

The tyrosinemia in this disorder is generally considerably greater than in other forms of tyrosinemia. Furthermore, analysis of the amino acids of the blood permits its distinction from transient tyrosinemia of the newborn because concentrations of other amino acids, particularly phenylalanine and methionine, are not elevated. It may be distinguished from hepatorenal tyrosinemia by the absence of a generalized aminoaciduria.

In oculocutaneous tyrosinemia the excretion of tyrosine in the urine is increased to 180 and 2000 mmol/mol creatinine [4,13,26]. Acetyltyrosine is also found in the urine [13] when serum concentrations of tyrosine exceed 2500 μmol/L. Tyrosine may be converted to tyramine, and this compound may be found in the urine [13,14]. Elevated concentrations of tyrosine are also found in the cerebrospinal fluid. Levels of 190 to 450 μmol/L have been reported [27,33,36].

Analysis of the organic acids of the urine reveals large amounts of p-hydroxyphenylpyruvic acid, p-hydroxyphenyllactic acid and p-hydroxyphenylacetic acid. The excretion of large amounts of p-hydroxyphenylpyruvic acid and p-hydroxyphenyllactic acid in the urine seems at first to be inconsistent with the site of the metabolic block. It is explained (Figure 25.8) by the widespread distribution of the other transaminase, mitochondrial tyrosine aminotransferase (aspartate aminotransferase, EC 2.6.1.1), in tissues other than liver, which lack the hydroxylase that catalyzes the conversion of p-hydroxyphenylpyruvic acid to homogentisic acid [56]. Accumulated tyrosine found in the blood is converted to p-hydroxyphenylpyruvic acid in tissues such as muscle. This compound is readily reduced to p-hydroxyphenyllactic acid [57]. Both p-hydroxyl compounds are then transported in the blood to the kidney, where they are effectively cleared and excreted in the urine [56].

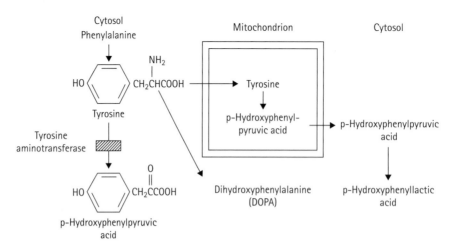

Figure 25.8   *Metabolic interrelations in deficiency of hepatic cytosolic tyrosine aminotransferase. The site of the defect is on the left. The mechanism for the excretion of p-hydroxyphenylpyruvic acid is illustrated. Accumulated tyrosine becomes a substrate for the mitochondrial tyrosine aminotransferase which leads to the formation of p-hydroxyphenylpyruvic acid (Figure 19.1, Chapter 19, p. 122). In liver this compound is readily converted to homogentisic acid and further oxidized, but this enzyme is widely distributed among other tissues of the body, and therefore p-hydroxyphenylpyruvic acid accumulates and is excreted in the urine. (Reprinted with permission from Nyhan WL:* Abnormalities in Amino Acid Metabolism in Clinical Medicine, *Appleton-Century-Crofts, Norwalk, CT; 1984.)*

Experience with maternal tyrosinemia indicates that dietary control during pregnancy should be prudent [58]. Two infants of women with untreated tyrosinemia had microophthalmia and mental retardation [42]. Two infants of a noncompliant mother were retarded [58]. Another had seizures and mental retardation [59]. On the other hand a number of normal offspring of mothers with this disease have been recorded [21,42]; so control of tyrosine levels can be rewarding.

TREATMENT

The treatment of oculocutaneous tyrosinemia consists of the institution of a diet low in tyrosine and phenylalanine. This effectively lowers concentrations of tyrosine in body fluids. Clinical symptomatology promptly resolves. Preparations (3200 AB – Mead Johnson; Tyromex – Ross) are available which are low in tyrosine and phenylalanine and simplify the preparation of formulas for the feeding of infants with tyrosinemia. Attention to compliance is important because treatment can prevent permanent ocular damage. The fact that symptoms of the disorder may be quite uncomfortable assists in the compliance of older patients. Whether early therapy prevents mental retardation is not clear, but early dietary management is prudent. There is excellent correlation between the concentration of tyrosine in the plasma and the intake of the amino acid and its precursor (Figure 25.9). Reasonable levels of control and an absence of symptoms are readily achieved using acceptable diets in childhood as well as in infancy.

Optimal blood levels have not been defined, but most patients are free of symptoms as long as the plasma concentration of tyrosine is below 550–700 μmol/L [2,60–62]. Treatment

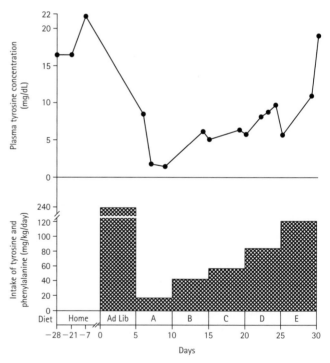

Figure 25.9   *Relation of the plasma concentration of tyrosine to the intake of tyrosine and phenylalanine. (Reprinted with permission from Nyhan WL:* Abnormalities in Amino Acid Metabolism in Clinical Medicine, *Appleton-Century-Crofts, Norwalk, CT; 1984.)*

with oral etretinate has been reported to improve skin lesions without changing levels of tyrosine [35,63], but this seems less than desirable because the skin is usually easier to control than the eye. Occasional noncompliance is not a problem as long as control is maintained most of the time.

References

1   Campbell RA, Buist NRM, Jacinto EY, *et al.* Supertyrosinemia (tyrosine transaminase deficiency) congenital anomalies and mental retardation. *Proc Soc Pediatr Res* 1967;**37**:80.

2   Ney D, Bay C, Schneider JA, *et al.* Dietary management of oculocutaneous tyrosinemia in an eleven-year-old. *Am J Dis Child* 1983;**137**:995.

3   Bardelli AM, Borgogni P, Farnetani MA, *et al.* Familial tyrosinaemia with eye and skin lesions. *Ophthalmology* (Basel) 1977;**175**:5.

4   Goldsmith LA, Reed J. Tyrosine-induced eye and skin lesions. *JAMA* 1976;**236**:382.

5   Sandberg HD. Bilateral keratopathy and tyrosinosis. *Act Ophthal* 1975; **53**:760.

6   Garibaldi LR, Siliato F, De Martini I, *et al.* Oculocutaneous tyrosinosis. Report of two cases in the same family *Helv Paediatr Acta* 1977;**32**:173.

7   Charlton KH, Binder PS, Wozniak L, Digby DJ. Pseudodendritic keratitis and systemic tyrosinemia. *Ophthalmology* 1981;**88**:355.

8   Hunziker N. Richner-Hanhart syndrome and tyrosinemia type II. *Dermatologica* 1980;**160**:180.

9   Richner H. Hornautaffektion bei Keratoma palmare et plantare heriditarium. *Klin Monatsbl Augenheilkd* 1938;**100**:580.

10 Hanhart E. Neue Sonderformen von Keratosis palmoplantaris ua eine regelmaessigdominante mit systematisieren Lipomen ferner 2 einfach-rezessive mit Schwachsinn zt mit Hornhautveraenderungen des Auges. *Dermatologica* 1947;**94**:286.

11 Kennaway NG, Buist NMR. Metabolic studies in a patient with hepatic cytosol tyrosine aminotransferase deficiency. *Pediatr Res* 1971;**5**:287.

12 Fellman JH, Buist NR, Kennaway NG, Swanson RE. The source of aromatic ketoacids in tyrosinemia and phenylketonuria. *Clin Chim Acta* 1972; **39**:243.

13 Kennaway NG, Buist NR. Metabolic studies in a patient with hepatic cytosol tyrosine aminotransferase deficiency. *Pediatr Res* 1971;**5**:287.

14 Hill A, Zaleski WA. Tyrosinosis: biochemical studies of an unusual case. *Clin Biochem* 1971;**4**:263.

15 Fellman JH, Vanbellinghen PJ, Jones RT, Koler IRD. Soluble and mitochondrial forms of tyrosine aminotransferase. Relationship to human tyrosinemia. *Biochemistry* 1969;**8**:615.

16 Natt E, Westphal EM, Toth-Fejel SE, *et al.* Inherited and *de novo* deletion of the tyrosine aminotransferase gene locus at 16q221q223 in a patient with tyrosinemia type II. *Hum Genet* 1987;**77**:352.

17 Rettenmeier R, Natt E, Hanswalter Z, Scherer G. Isolation and characterization of the human tyrosine aminotransferase gene. *Nucleic Acids Res* 1990;**18**:3853.

18 Natt E, Kida K, Odievre M, *et al.* Point mutations in the tyrosine amino-transferase gene in tyrosinemia type II. *Proc Natl Acad Sci USA* 1992; **89**:9297.

19 Rabinowitz LG, Williams LR, Anderson CE, *et al.* Painful keratoderma and photophobia: hallmarks of tyrosinemia type II. *J Pediatr* 1995;**126**:266.

20 Gounod N, Ogier H, Dufier J-L, *et al.* Tyrosinose oculo-cutanée de type II. *Ann Dermatol Venereol* 1984;**111**:697.

21 Chitayat D, Balbul A, Hani V, *et al.* Hereditary tyrosinaemia type II in a consanguineous Ashkenazi Jewish family: intrafamilial variation in phenotype; absence of parental phenotype effects on the fetus. *J Inherit Metab Dis* 1992;**15**:198.

22 Zammarchi E, La Cauza C, Calzolari C. Un caso di ipertiirosinemia con tirosiluria. *Minerva Pediatar* 1974;**26**:203.

23 Heidemann DG, Dunn SP, Bawle EV, *et al.* Early diagnosis of tyrosinemia type II. *Am J Ophthalmol* 1989;**107**:559.

24 Colditz PB, Yu JS, Billson FA, *et al.* Tyrosinaemia II. *Med J Aust* 1984; **141**:244.

25 Bienfang DC, Kuwabara T, Pueschel SM. The Richner-Hanhart syndrome. Report of a case with associated tyrosinemia. *Arch Ophthal* 1976;**94**:1133.

26 Patton TH, Hosty TS. Tyrosinosis: a patient without liver or renal disease. *Pediatrics* 1971;**48**:393.

27 Pelet B, Antener I, Faggioni R, *et al.* Tyrosinemia without liver or renal damage with plantar and palmar keratosis and keratitis (Hypertyrosinemia Type II). *Helv Paediatr Acta* 1979;**34**:177.

28 Faull KF, Gan I, Halpern B, *et al.* Metabolic studies on two patients with nonhepatic tyrosinemia using deuterated tyrosine loads. *Pediatr Res* 1977;**11**:631.

29 Billson FA, Danks DM. Corneal and skin changes in tyrosinaemia. *Aust J Ophthal* 1975;**3**:112.

30 Boctor AM, Harper AE. Tyrosine toxicity in the rat: effect of high intake of p-hydroxyphenylpyruvic acid and of force-feeding high tyrosine diet. *J Nutr* 1968;**95**:535.

31 Goldsmith LA. Tyrosinemia II: lessons in molecular pathophysiology. *Pediatr Dermatol* 1983;**1**:25.

32 Driscoll DJ, Jabs EW, Alcorn D, *et al.* Corneal tyrosine crystals in transient neonatal tyrosinemia. *J Pediatr* 1988;**113**:91.

33 Goldsmith LA, Kng E, Bienfang DC, *et al.* Tyrosinemia with plantar and palmar keratosis and keratitis. *J Pediatr* 1973;**83**:798.

34 Al-Essa M, Rashed M, Ozand PT. Tyrosinemia type II: Report of the first four cases in Saudi Arabia. *Ann Saudi Med* 1998;**18**:466.

35 Fraser NG, MacDonald J, Griffiths WA, *et al.* Tyrosinemia type II (Richner-Hanhart syndrome): report of two cases treated with etritinate. *Clin Exp Dermatol* 1987;**12**:440.

36 Larreque M, Giacomoni DE, Bressieux J-M, Grilevre M. Syndrome de Richner-Hanhart ou tyrosinose oculo-cutanée. *Ann Dermatol Vernereol* (Paris) 1979;**106**:53.

37 Goulden KJ, Moss MA, Cole DE, *et al.* Pitfalls in the initial diagnosis of tyrosinemia: three case reports and a review of the literature. *Clin Biochem* 1987;**20**:207.

38 Zaleski WA, Hills A, Kushnikuk W. Skin lesions in tyrosinosis: response to dietary treatment. *Br J Dermatol* 1973;**88**:335.

39 Goldsmith LA, Thorpe JM, Roe CR. Hepatic enzymes of tyrosine metabolism in tyrosinemia II. *J Invest Dermatol* 1979;**73**:530.

40 Callan NJ. Circumscribed palmoplantar keratoderma. *Aust J Dermatol* 1970;**11**:76.

41 Westmore R, Billson FA. Pseudoherpetic keratitis. *Br J Ophthal* 1973; **57**:654.

42 Fois A, Borgogni P, Cioni M, *et al.* Presentation of the data of the Italian registry for oculocutaneous tyrosinaemia. *J Inherit Metab Dis* 1986;**9**:262.

43 Grenier A, Laberge C. A modified automated fluorometric method for tyrosine determination in blood spotted in paper: a mass screening procedure for tyrosinemia. *Clin Chem Acta* 1974;**55**:41.

44 Halvorsen S. Screening for disorders of tyrosine metabolism: in *Neonatal Screening for Inborn Errors of Metabolism* (eds H Bickel, R Guthrie, G Hammersen) Springer-Verlag Inc, New York; 1980:**45**.

45 Goldsmith LA, Thorpe JM, Marsh RF. Tyrosine aminotransferase deficiency in mink (Mustela vison): a model for human tyrosinemia II. *Biochem Genet* 1981;**19**:687.

46 Kunkle GA, Jezyk PF, West CS, *et al.* Tyrosinemia in a dog. *J Am Anim Hosp Assoc* 1984;**20**:615.

47 Granner DK, Hargrove JL. Regulation of the synthesis of tyrosine aminotransferase: the relationship to mRNATAT. *Mol Cell Biochem* 1983;**53**:113.

48 Hargrove JL, Mackin RB. Organ specificity of glucocorticoid-sensitive tyrosine aminotransferase isoenzymes. *J Biol Chem* 1984;**259**:386.

49   Hargrove JL, Scoble HA, Matthews WR, *et al.* The structure of tyrosine aminotransferase: evidence for domains involved in catalysis and enzyme turnover. *J Biol Chem* 1989;**264**:45.

50   Lemmonier F, Charpentier C, Odievre M, *et al.* Tyrosine aminotransferase isoenzyme deficiency. *J Pediatr* 1979;**94**:931.

51   Kida A, Takahashi M, Fujisawa Y, Matsuda H. Hepatic tyrosine amino-transferase in tyrosinaemia type II. *J Inherit Metab Dis* 1982; **5**:229.

52   Muller G, Scherer G, Zentgraf H, *et al.* Isolation characterization and chromosomal mapping of the mouse tyrosine aminotransferase gene. *J Mol Biol* 1985;**184**:367.

53   Shinomoya T, Scherer G, Schmid W, *et al.* Isolation and characterization of the rat tyrosine aminotransferase gene. *Proc Natl Acad Sci USA* 1984;**81**:1346.

54   Huhn R, Stoermer H, Klingele B, *et al.* Novel and recurrent tyrosine aminotransferase gene mutations in tyrosinemia type II. *Hum Genet* 1998;**102**:305.

55   Armstrong MD, Stave U. A study of plasma free amino acid levels: II Normal values for children and adults. *Metab Clin Exp* 1973;**22**:561.

56   Kennaway NG, Buist NRM, Fellman JH. The origin of urinary p-hydroxy-phenylpyruvate in a patient with hepatic cytosol tyrosine aminotransferase deficiency. *Clin Chim Acta* 1972;**41**:157.

57   Weber WW, Zannoni VG. Reduction of phenylpyruvic acids to phenyllactic acids in mammalian tissues. *J Biol Chem* 1969;**241**:615.

58   Cerone R, Fantasia AR, Castellano E, *et al.* Pregnancy and tyrosinaemia type II. *J Inherit Metab Dis* 2002;**25**:317.

59   Garibaldi LR, Durand P. Soluble tyrosine-aminotransferase (STAT) deficiency tyrosinemia: Four cases (abstract). *Pediatr Res* 1980;**14**:1428.

60   Buist NRM, Kennaway NG, Fellman JH. Disorders of tyrosine metabolism: in *Heritable Disorders of Amino Acid Metabolism* (ed. WL Nyhan) Wiley and Sons Inc, New York;1974:**160**.

61   Herve F, Moreno JL, Ogier H, *et al.* Keratite inguerissable et hyperkeratose palmo-plantaire chronique avec hypertyrosinemia. *Arch Fr Pediatr* 1986;**43**:19.

62   Machino H, Miki Y, Kawatsu T, *et al.* Successful dietary control of tyrosinemia II. *J Am Acad Dermatol* 1983;**9**:533.

63   Saijo S, Kudoh K, Kuramoto Y, *et al.* Tyrosinemia II: report of an incomplete case and studies on the hyperkeratotic stratum corneum. *Dermatologica* 1991;**182**:168.

26

Hepatorenal tyrosinemia/fumarylacetoacetate hydrolase deficiency

MAJOR PHENOTYPIC EXPRESSION

Hepatocellular degeneration leading to acute hepatic failure, or chronic cirrhosis and hepatocellular carcinoma; renal Fanconi syndrome; peripheral neuropathy; hypertyrosinemia; succinylacetonuria; and deficiency of fumarylacetoacetate hydrolase.

INTRODUCTION

Hepatorenal tyrosinemia, which has been referred to as tyrosinemia type 1, tyrosinosis, or hereditary tyrosinemia, was first reported by Sakai and Kitagawa in 1957 [1–3]. The patient reported was the product of a consanguineous mating, who developed progressive liver disease which led to death with hematemesis and hepatic coma at 3 years-of-age. In addition, the patient had rickets, which was resistant to vitamin D. The major metabolic products in the urine were p-hydroxyphenyllactic acid, p-hydroxyphenylpyruvic acid and p-hydroxyphenylacetic acid, as well as tyrosine. Gentz, Jagenburg and Zetterstrom, in a report of seven patients with the disease, first characterized the renal component as a Fanconi syndrome [4]. It was noted that patients had neurologic crises reminiscent of porphyria [5,6], and this led to the recognition that δ-aminolevulinic acid was excreted in large amounts [6–9]. Lindblad, Lindstedt and Steen [10] reported that succinylacetone, which they found in the urine of these patients, is an inhibitor of the synthesis of porphobilinogen from δ-aminolevulinic acid. They reasoned that the fundamental defect was in the activity of fumarylacetoacetate hydrolase (Figure 26.1). This was confirmed enzymatically by these investigators [11] and others [12–14].

The gene has been cloned [15,16] and mapped to chromosome 15q23-25. Mutations have been identified [17] including founder mutations in French-Canadian Quebec and in Finland, where the disease is prevalent. The Quebec mutation is a splice mutation IVS 12 + 5 G → A [18], and that in Finland is W262X [19]. The discovery of a therapeutic agent 2-(2-nitro-4-trifluoromethylbenzoyl)-1,3-cyclohexanedione (NTBC) represents a major advance in the management of this disease [20,21].

CLINICAL ABNORMALITIES

The clinical course of hepatorenal tyrosinemia has generally followed one of two patterns: an acute or a chronic form. The former has sometimes been referred to as the French-Canadian type and the latter the Scandinavian type, but of course there is considerable overlap [4,5,14,22]. Most patients have had acute presentations. Symptoms develop in early infancy, and they are those of acute hepatic decompensation. Hepatic failure and death occurs usually under 1 year-of-age. However, some infants with an acute onset of hepatic disease survive to go on to display a chronic disease just like those patients with the chronic form. The differential diagnosis of hepatic failure

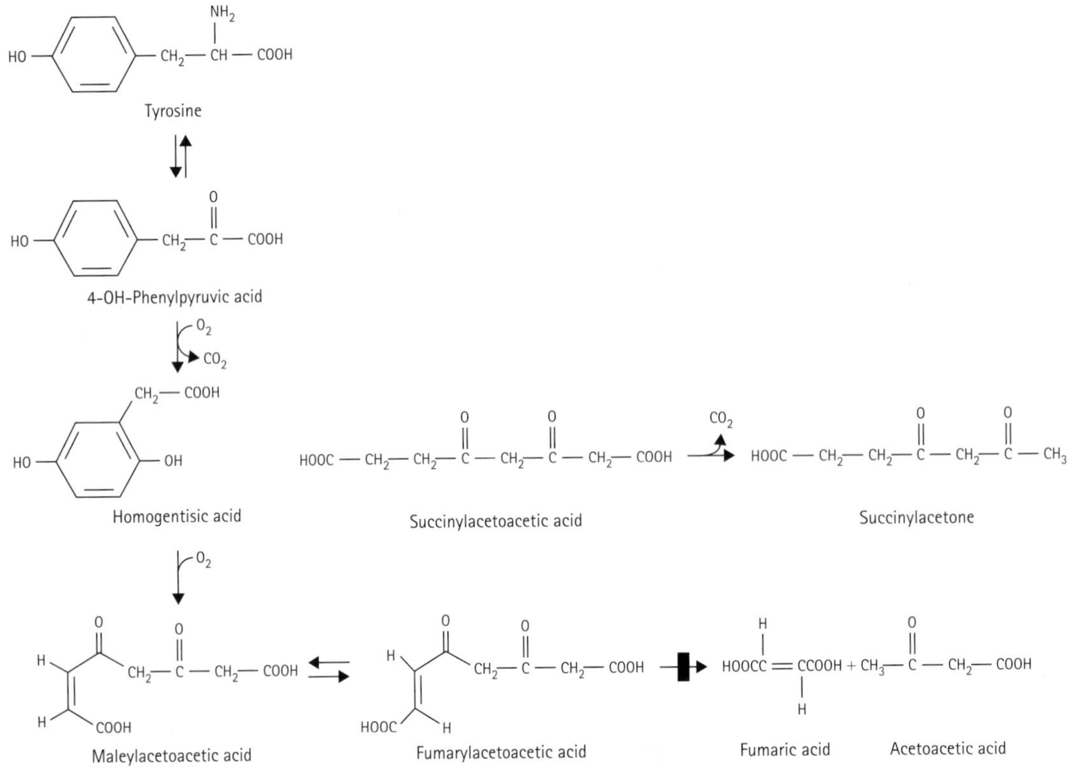

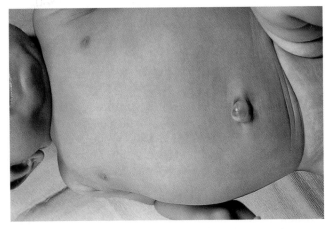

Figure 26.1   *Metabolism of tyrosine and phenylalanine. The site of defect hepatorenal tyrosinemia is in fumarylacetoacetate hydrolase.*

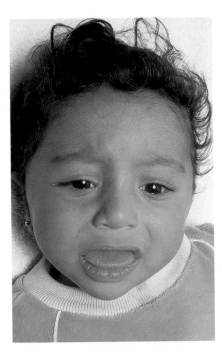

Figure 26.2   *A.Y., a 7-year-old girl with hepatorenal tyrosinemia.*

Figure 26.3   *A.M.Q., a boy with hepatorenal tyrosinemia. The abdominal enlargement resulted from the liver which was palpable 4 cm below the costal margin.*

is given in the Appendix. Until recently, most of these children died at younger than 10 years-of-age. Only one patient of those described early survived to the age of 20 years [22]. The year 1 mortality for those presenting with symptoms by 2 months was 60 percent; of those presenting between 2 and 6 months it was 20 percent and of those presenting after 6 months it was 4 percent [23]. Prognosis has changed dramatically with currently available therapy.

The earliest and the major effect of the disease is on the liver. Abdominal distension and failure to thrive are prominent, and may be associated with vomiting and/or diarrhea. (Figures 26.2–26.4). The acute hepatic crisis is the most common early presentation. The infant may appear acutely

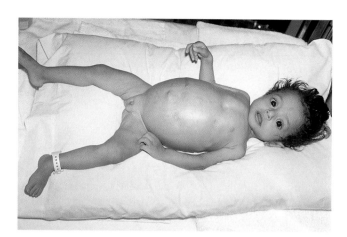

Figure 26.4   *J.Q., a girl with hepatorenal tyrosinemia. She had cirrhosis with abdominal enlargement and ascites.*

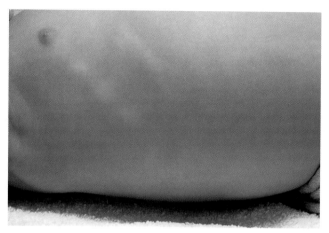

Figure 26.5   *A.Y., illustrating the rachitic rosary.*

or desperately ill and have jaundice and ascites along with hepatomegaly [24–26]. There may be gastrointestinal bleeding. Hypoglycemia may be a presenting symptom. Hepatic crises may be triggered by infection.

Several infants have been noted by the mothers to have a peculiar sweet odor. A boiled cabbage-like odor in some patients has been related to a metabolite of methionine [27–30].

Transaminase levels in the blood may be normal or slightly elevated. The rare elevation over 1000 IU/L indicates substantial damage to hepatic cells. α-Fetoprotein may be markedly elevated, ranging from 100 000 to 400 000 ng/mL. Coagulation factors may be abnormal, and there may be bleeding. Prothrombin times and partial prothrombin times may be markedly elevated. Coagulopathy is characteristically unresponsive to vitamin K. Jaundice is uncommon early in this disease.

One of our patients presented with bleeding and was investigated as a problem in coagulation before chemical evidence of hepatic disease was identified. Patients may present with epistaxis or intestinal bleeding [31]. Elevated levels of prothrombin time (PT) and partial thromboplastin time (PTT) may be found even in asymptomatic infants discovered by newborn screening. An infant presenting with liver disease and hypoglycemia may be thought to have Reye syndrome. Between acute crises the liver is enlarged. α-fetoprotein may be slightly or greatly elevated.

The chronic liver disease picture is that of hepatic cirrhosis. The differential diagnosis of hepatic cirrhosis in infancy is given in the Appendix. The pathologic picture is that of macronodular cirrhosis [32]. Splenomegaly develops. There may be acute crises of increased hepatocellular damage, often precipitated by infection, and these may lead to hepatic failure. Esophageal varices may develop, and they may be complicated by bleeding.

A more common complication is the development of hepatocellular carcinoma [33,34]. The risk of this complication has been variously reported. In a series of 42 patients reported in 1976 [35] from the United States, 37 percent of those over 2 years-of-age developed carcinoma, while information from an international series yielded an incidence of

18 percent of those over 2 years [36]. Detection of nodules by CT scan or ultrasound appears to be quite reliable, because histologic examination of 18 livers from patients subjected to liver transplantation failed to reveal focal carcinomas in patients not found to have nodules by those modalities [37]. Computed tomography (CT) should be done with and without contrast. Liver cancer has been documented as early as 33 months-of-age [38]. A 15-month-old was found to have a carcinoma following a presentation at 5 months with acute hepatic failure and a good response to NTBC with a 10-fold drop in α-fetoprotein, which then rose to 100 000 ng/mL [39]. A significant rise in the level of α-fetoprotein may herald the onset of carcinoma, but carcinoma was found in a patient whose level was only 87 ng/mL [3]. Patients should be monitored regularly by CT, magnetic resonance imaging (MRI) or ultrasound, and nodules should be biopsied.

Renal disease is another characteristic feature of this disease. Among 32 patients [40] 47 percent had enlargement of the kidneys, often palpable [31]; 47 percent had increased echogenicity of the kidneys, and 16 percent had nephrocalcinosis. In another eight patients [41] 50 percent had nephromegaly. The renal tubular disease is that of a typical renal Fanconi syndrome in which there is phosphaturia, aminoaciduria and often glycosuria. There may be proteinuria. Systemic metabolic acidosis may result from renal tubular dysfunction. The phosphate losses lead to hypophosphatemia and clinical rickets (Figures 26.5–26.7). There may also be a variable reduction in glomerular function. In the series of 32 patients [40] 48 percent had decreased glomerular filtration; 82 percent had aminoaciduria, 67 percent hypercalciuria and 59 percent renal tubular acidosis. Affected infants have been observed to have vitamin D-resistant rickets at less than 4 months-of-age [25], which is unusual.

Neurologic crises of pain and paresthesia are a result of peripheral neuropathy [42–45]. These may occur in as many as 42 percent of patients. Crises may be mistaken for porphyria [43]. There may be extensor hypotonus, or the patient may be hypertonic. Systemic, autonomic signs include hypertension, tachycardia and ileus. Pain usually begins in the legs. The patient may position the head and trunk in extreme

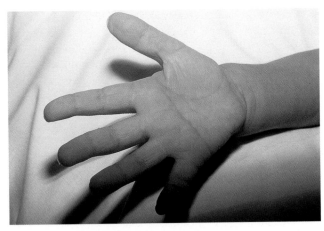

Figure 26.6   *A.Y. The wrist was enlarged because of rachitic changes at the ends of bones.*

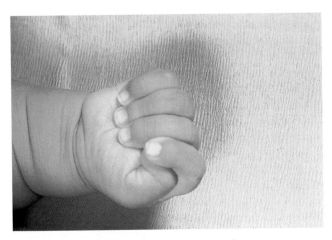

Figure 26.7   *A.M.Q. The wrist was also enlarged.*

hyperextension and may be thought to have opisthotonus or meningismus [29]. Muscular weakness may progress to paralysis requiring artificial ventilation [42]. Self-injurious behavior has been observed. Some patients have had seizures [43], some of them associated with hyponatremia [8]. Death may occur during a neurologic crisis [44,45]. During most crises consciousness is normal. These crises are not associated with hepatic relapse. Most crises subside in one to seven days and resolve slowly, but there may be residual weakness. Intelligence is usually normal.

Three infants have had obstructive hypertrophic cardiomyopathy [46,47] and this may be fatal [46]. Two patients have had macroglossia [7,36], and there may be macrosomia. Pancreatic islet hypertrophy is common, but usually asymptomatic. Hypoglycemia can usually be attributed to hepatic disease.

GENETICS AND PATHOGENESIS

Hepatorenal tyrosinemia is transmitted in an autosomal recessive fashion [26,48]. Consanguinity has been documented in

Table 26.1   *Variants of fumarylacetoacetate hydrolase in hepatorenal tyrosinemia*

Type	mRNA	CRM	Enzyme activity
A	++	0	0
B	+	+	+
C	++	++	0
D	0	0	0

a number of families [49]. A particularly high frequency of 1.46 per 1000 births has been recorded in a French-Canadian isolate in the Chicoutimi–Lac St Jean region of northeastern Quebec [49,50], where the carrier rate is 1 in 20 [47]. An overall incidence of 0.8 per 10 000 births was observed in the French-Canadian population of Quebec. The prevalence has approximated at 1 in 100 000 [51] from newborn screening programs in Scandinavia. Founder effects have been elucidated in the French-Canadian population [52,53]. The disease is frequent in French-Canada and relatively so in Scandinavia, but it may be found in any geographic or ethnic background.

The molecular defect in hepatorenal tyrosinemia is in the hepatic fumarylacetoacetic acid hydrolase (fumarylacetoacetase, EC 3.7.1.2) (Figure 26.1). This was originally proposed on the basis of the accumulation of succinylacetone [10]. Deficiency of this enzyme was then documented by assay of activity in liver [12]. The level was six percent of normal in six patients with the acute disease and 20 percent in two patients with the chronic form. The activity of maleylacetoacetic acid hydrolase was also deficient in some samples of liver. A problem with enzyme assay is that in the presence of liver disease the activity of many enzymes is reduced. The enzyme deficiency may be demonstrated in lymphocytes and fibroblasts [54]. The gold standard in the diagnosis of this disease is the demonstration of succinylacetone in the urine.

Heterozygote detection has been carried out by the assay of fumarylacetoacetate hydrolase activity in fibroblasts and lymphocytes [55]. Obligatory heterozygotes have had a mean level that is 50 percent of normal, but considerable variation and the possibility of pseudoalleles make this unreliable. Where the mutation is known or in populations like that of Quebec where a small number of mutations is responsible, molecular testing is the preferred method. Prenatal diagnosis has been accomplished by assay of the enzyme in cultured amniocytes or chorionic villus material [55–57]. It has also been accomplished by the direct assay of concentrations of succinylacetone in amniotic fluid [58,59], and this is thought to be the method of choice. However at least one affected infant has been missed in this assay [60]. In families in which the mutation is known, molecular methods are ideal.

The gene has been localized to chromosome 15q23-25 [15]. The gene contains 14 exons over a span of 30 to 34kb [61]. A number of restriction fragment length polymorphisms (RFLP) have been identified, and these RFLPs may be used for carrier detection and prenatal diagnosis [62]. A considerable number and variety of mutations have been identified (Table 26.1), and

Fumarylacetoacetate hydrolase

	Control	Patient
DNA (47)	CAA	CTA
Enzyme (16)	Asparagine	Isoleucine

Figure 26.8 *Variant fumarylacetoacetate hydrolase gene and enzyme in a French-Canadian patient with hepatorenal tyrosinemia. The numbers in parenthesis indicate nucleotide 47 in the gene and amino acid 16 in the protein.*

heterogeneity has been identified, even in the French-Canadian population [61,63]. In a French-Canadian patient an A-to-T transversion changed an asparagine to isoleucine at position 16 [17] (Figure 26.8). The IVS 12+ 5 G → A mutation is more common [18]. In a Norwegian patient, a missense mutation changed alanine at 134 to aspartic acid [61]. A splice-site mutation resulting from a G-to-A transition was found to lead to deletion of exon 12 in a French-Canadian patient [64]. A pseudo deficiency allele R341W has been found in normal individuals with low activity of the hydrolase enzyme [65]. Mutations have been shown to produce mRNA without enzyme activity or cross-reacting material (CRM); mRNA and CRM without enzyme activity; mRNA, CRM and some activity; as well as no mRNA. Patients with early onset hepatic failure tend to be CRM negative.

The deficient enzyme is on the catabolic pathway for tyrosine, and this is the cause of the hypertyrosinemia (Figure 26.1). Fumarylacetoacetate accumulates and is converted to succinylacetoacetate and to succinylacetone. In hepatorenal tyrosinemia, concentrations of tyrosine usually range from 170 to 660 μmol/L (3 to 12 mg/dL).

Increased quantities are also excreted in the urine. Of the tyrosyl compounds found in the urine, p-hydroxyphenyllactic acid is the most prominent; p-hydroxyphenylpyruvic acid and p-hydroxyphenylacetic acid are also present in appreciable quantities. Patients often have elevated concentrations of methionine in the blood. Hypoglycemia is common, especially in the acute illness. In chronic cirrhosis or after treatment, tyrosine concentrations may be normal. On the other hand, during the acute stages of hepatocellular damage many other amino acids may be found in elevated amounts in the serum, including cystathionine, proline and hydroxyproline. These patterns, along with the tyrosine, are reflected in the urinary excretion of amino acids. They are superimposed on the generalized aminoaciduria that results from the renal tubular aspects of the disease. Patients also have phosphaturia and hypophosphatemia. The presence of reducing substance completes the picture of the renal Fanconi syndrome. The sugar is usually glucose, but other sugars have been reported [4,66,67]. With progression there is systemic acidosis, increased potassium loss and hypokalemia.

The urinary excretion of δ-aminolevulinic acid is increased [8,10,68,69]. Succinylacetoacetic acid and succinylacetone are found in the serum and the urine [10,68], the direct

consequence of the defective activity of fumarylacetoacetic acid hydrolase. Accumulated fumarylacetoacetic acid is reduced to succinylacetoacetic acid and decarboxylated to form succinylacetone. Succinylacetone has immunosuppressive activity [69]. It is also a powerful inhibitor of δ-aminolevulinic acid dehydratase [70], accounting for the increased excretion of δ-aminolevulinic acid and inhibition of the synthesis of porphobilinogen from δ-aminolevulinic acid. Succinylacetone can be found in spots of blood dried on filter paper. Screening for hepatorenal tyrosinemia has been undertaken in a number of states and countries. It has recently been incorporated into expanded tandem mass spectrometry (MS/MS) programs with tyrosine as the key analyte. This has the problem that transient tyrosinemia triggers a positive screen, and the numbers are such that many programs have set the screen level so high that most patients with hepatorenal tyrosinemia would be missed. In addition, some patients with this disease have normal levels of tyrosine. Quebec now screens for succinylacetone. The development of tandem MS methodology for succinylacetone would be useful.

The pattern of laboratory findings in this disease is virtually unique. A combination of hypoglycemia, coagulopathy, tyrosinemia, succinylacetone and very high α-fetoprotein is diagnostic.

Fumarylacetocetate is an inhibitor of methionine adenosyltransferase, and this would lead to hypermethioninemia [71], but methionine levels also increase nonspecifically in hepatocellular disease. Renal tubular dysfunction is thought to result from maleylacetoacetic acid by analogy with maleic acid, which can produce an experimental Fanconi syndrome in animals [72]. Fumarylacetoacetate and maleylacetoacetate react with sulfhydryl compounds, and deficiency of glutathione has been documented in this disease [73]. Maleylacetone and succinylacetone can form glutathione adducts [74]. The accumulated products are highly reactive and could produce disease by alkylating a variety of thiols and amino groups, including those in proteins. The acute porphyria-like episodes of peripheral neuropathy in this disease are thought to result from the inhibition by succinylacetone of δ-aminolevulinic acid hydrolase and the formation of porphobilinogen.

An interesting phenomenon in this disease is the occurrence of revertant nodules in which hydrolase activity is normal [75,76]. The enzyme protein is present in these nodules in which at least one allele has mutated to the normal sequence. This of course could lead to a finding of normal activity in biopsied liver.

TREATMENT

Treatment of this disease has been revolutionized by the discovery of NTBC (Figure 26.9) [20,77]. Restriction of the dietary intake of phenylalanine and tyrosine will lower concentrations of tyrosine, and improvement in renal tubular function has been reported [35,78–81]. Coagulation problems

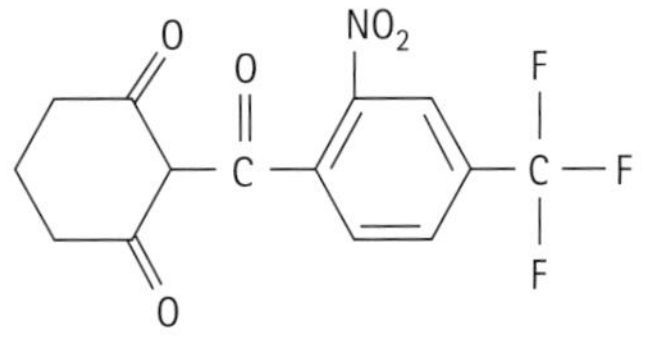

Figure 26.9 *NTBC, 2(2-nitro-4-trifluoromethylbenzyol)-1,3-cyclohexanedione.*

are also responsive. However, it is clear that hepatic disease may progress despite dietary treatment.

Acute hepatic dysfunction must be treated aggressively. Energy and nutrition may be provided parenterally, as well as the management of fluids and electrolytes. Intake of phenylalanine and tyrosine is stopped temporarily. In liver failure, transplantation of a liver is the only answer. In a neurologic crisis attention to respiration and assistance when necessary are mandatory.

Transplantation has also become the treatment choice for hepatocellular carcinoma [82,83]. In recent years, transplantation has been undertaken prior to the development of nodules in order to prevent carcinoma. [84–86]. Survival rates at 36 months following transplantation of the liver for this disease have been as high as 87 percent [86]. Tyrosyl compounds in the urine decreased to normal, while succinylacetone decreased, but as far as normal in only one patient [87]. Presumably, this succinylacetone is made in the kidney.

Excretion of δ-aminolevulinic acid also decreased but remained somewhat elevated. Renal tubular reabsorption of phosphate and bicarbonate may become normal within five days of transplantation; glycosuria and aminoaciduria correct within two weeks [88].

The advent of therapy with 2(2-nitro-4-trifluoromethylbenzoyl)-1,3-cyclohexanedione (NTBC) has changed the readiness with which hepatic transplantation is done in this disorder. The indication now is hepatic cancer. NTBC is a potent inhibitor of p-hydroxyphenylpyruvate dioxygenase [89]. Treatment with 1 mg of this compound per kilogram has led regularly to improvement in hepatic and renal function, and no side effects have been observed. Concentrations of succinylacetone and α-fetoprotein have decreased, and hepatic morphology has improved. Excretion of δ-aminolevulinic acid has decreased to near normal, and erythrocyte porphobilinogen synthesis increased. This appears to eliminate the neurologic crises of the disease in those properly treated [90]. NTBC has now been approved by the US Food and Drug Administration (FDA) for the treatment of hepatorenal tyrosinemia. As of 2003, 369 patients have been treated [91], 58 percent males, and treatment was continuing on 293. Withdrawals were 76, of which 26 had died; 21 had liver failure, of which 12 died; 25 had developed hepatocellular carcinoma, of which 7 had died, and 54 had been transplanted, of whom 8 died. Prior to NTBC survival curves in this disease indicated few long-term survivors. Now approximately 90 percent of those diagnosed before 2 years-of-age

are alive, some as long as 12 years. The figure for those diagnosed late approximates 60 percent surviving six to 12 years. There have been only three hepatic cancers in those treated before 2 years-of-age, and one of these was present at diagnosis, before treatment. Improvement has been reported when NTBC was given during a neurologic crisis [90].

References

1 Sakai K, Kitagawa T. An atypical case of tyrosinosis Part 1. Clinical and laboratory findings. *Jikeikai Med J* 1957;**4**:1.

2 Sakai K, Kitagawa T. An atypical case of tyrosinosis Part 2. A research on the metabolic block. *Jikeikai Med J* 1957;**4**:11.

3 Sakai K, Kitagawa T, Yoshioka K. An atypical case of tyrosinosis Part 3. The outcome of the patient. *Jikeikai Med J* 1959;**6**:15.

4 Gentz J, Jagenburg R, Zetterstrom R. Tyrosinemia. *J Pediatr* 1965; **66**:670.

5 Gentz J, Lindblad B, Lindstedt S, *et al*. Dietary treatment in tyrosinemia (tyrosinosis). With a note on the possible recognition of the carrier state. *Am J Dis Child* 1967;**113**:31.

6 Kang ES, Gerald PS. Hereditary tyrosinemia and abnormal pyrrole metabolism. *J Pediatr* 1970;**77**:397.

7 Gaull GE, Rassin DK, Solomon GE, *et al*. Biochemical observations on so-called hereditary tyrosinemia. *Pediatr Res* 1970;**4**:337.

8 Strife CF, Zuroweste EL, Emmett EA, *et al*. Tyrosinemia with acute intermittent porphyria: aminolevulinic acid dehydratase deficiency related to elevated urinary aminolevulinic acid levels. *J Pediatr* 1977;**90**:400.

9 Gentz J, Johansson S, Lindblad B, *et al*. Excretion of delta-aminolevulinic acid in hereditary tyrosinemia. *Clin Chim Acta* 1969;**23**:257.

10 Lindblad B, Lindstedt S, Steen G. On the enzymic defects in hereditary tyrosinemia. *Proc Natl Acad Sci USA* 1977;**74**:4641.

11 Fällström S-P, Lindblad B, Lindstedt S, Steen G. Hereditary tyrosinemia-fumarylacetoacetase deficiency. *Pediatr Res* 1979;**13**:78 (abstr).

12 Kvittingen EA, Jellum E, Stokke O. Assay of fumarylacetoacetate fumarylhydrolase in human liver-deficient activity in a case of hereditary tyrosinemia. *Clin Chim Acta* 1981;**115**:311.

13 Berger R, Smit GP, Stoker-de Vries SA, *et al*. Deficiency of fumarylacetoacetase in a patient with hereditary tyrosinemia. *Clin Chim Acta* 1981;**114**:37.

14 Gray RG, Patrick AD, Preston FE, Whitfield MF. Acute hereditary tyrosinaemia type I: clinical biochemical and haematological studies in twins. *J Inherit Metab Dis* 1981;**4**:37.

15 Phaneuf D, Labelle Y, Bérubé D, *et al*. Cloning and expression of the cDNA encoding human fumarylacetoacetate hydrolase the enzyme deficient in hereditary tyrosinemia: assignment of the gene to chromosome. *Am J Hum Genet* 1991;**48**:525.

16 Agsteribbe E, van Faassen H, Hartog MV, *et al*. Nucleotide sequence of cDNA encoding human fumarylacetoacetase. *Nucleic Acids Res* 1990;**18**:1887.

17 Phaneuf D, Lambert M, Laframboise R, *et al*. Type I hereditary tyrosinemia. Evidence for molecular heterogeneity and identification of a causal mutation in a French Canadian patient. *J Clin Invest* 1992;**90**:1185.

18 Grompe M, St-Louis M, Demers SI, *et al*. A single mutation of the fumarylacetoacetate hydrolase gene in French Canadians with hereditary tyrosinemia type I. *N Engl J Med* 1994;**331**:353.

19 Rootwelt H, Hoie K, Berger R, Kvittingen EA. Fumarylacetoacetate mutations in tyrosinaemia type I. *Hum Mutat* 1996;**7**:239.

20 Lindstedt S, Holme E, Lock EA, *et al*. Treatment of hereditary tyrosinaemia type I by inhibition of 4-hydroxylphenylpyruvate dioxygenase. *Lancet* 1992; **340**:813.

21 Holme E, Lindstedt S. Diagnosis and management of tyrosinemia Type I. *Curr Opin Pediatr* 1995;**7**:726.

22 Halvorsen S, Pande H, Loken AC, Gjessing LR. Tyrosinosis. A study of 6 cases. *Arch Dis Child* 1966;**41**:238.

23 van Spronsen FJ, Thomasse Y, Berger R, *et al.* Lifetime expectancy with dietary treatment in tyrosinemia type I: consequences for timing of liver transplantation. *Society for the Study of Inborn Errors of Metabolism;* 29th Symposium London; 1991: poster 21.

24 Scriver CR, Larochelle J, Silverberg M, Hereditary tyrosinemia and tyrosyluria in a French Canadian geographic isolate. *Am J Dis Child* 1967;**113**:41.

25 Kogut MD, Shaw KN, Donnell GN. Tyrosinosis. *Am J Dis Child* 1967;**113**:47.

26 Laberge C. Hereditary tyrosinemia in a French Canadian isolate. *Am J Hum Genet* 1969;**21**:36.

27 Cone TE Jr. Diagnosis and treatment: some diseases syndromes and conditions associated with an unusual odor. *Pediatrics* 1968;**41**:993.

28 Gahl WA, Finkelstein JD, Mullen KD, *et al.* Hepatic methionine adenosyltransferase deficiency in a 31-year-old man. *Am J Hum Genet* 1987;**40**:39.

29 Perry TL, Hardwick DF, Dixon GH, *et al.* Hypermethioninemia: a metabolic disorder associated with cirrhosis islet cell hyperplasia and renal tubular degeneration. *Pediatrics* 1965;**36**:236.

30 Perry TL. Tyrosinemia associated with hypermethioninemia and islet cell hyperplasia. *Can Med Assoc J* 1967;**97**:1067.

31 Bas AY, Kunak B, Ertan U, *et al.* Tyrosinemia type 1: a case report. *Intern Pediatr* 2003;**18**:45.

32 Fritzell S, Jagenburg OR, Schnürer L-B. Familial cirrhosis of the liver renal tubular defects with rickets and impaired tyrosine metabolism. *Acta Paediatr Scand* 1964;**53**:18.

33 Gentz J, Heinrich J, Lindblad B, *et al.* Enzymatic studies in a case of hereditary tyrosinemia with hepatoma. *Acta Pediatr Scand* 1969; **58**:393.

34 Barness L, Gilbert-Barness E. Pathological case of the month. Special feature. *Am J Dis Child* 1992;**146**:769.

35 Wehnberg AG, Mize CE, Worthen HG. The occurrence of hepatoma in the chronic form of hereditary tyrosinemia. *J Pediatr* 1976;**88**:434.

36 Mitchell GA, Lambert M, Tanguay RM. Hypertyrosinemia: in *The Metabolic and Molecular Bases of Inherited Disease* 7th edition (eds CR Scriver, AL Beaudet, WS Sly, *et al.*) McGraw Hill, New York;1995:1077.

37 Paradis K, Weber A, Seidman EG, *et al.* Liver transplantation for hereditary tyrosinemia: the Quebec experience. *Am J Hum Genet* 1990;**47**:338.

38 Mieles LA, Esquivel CO, Van Thiel DH, *et al.* Liver transplantation for tyrosinemia. A review of 10 cases from the University of Pittsburgh. *Dig Dis Sci* 1990;**35**:153.

39 Dionisi-Vici C, Boglino C, Marcellini M, *et al.* Tyrosinemia type I with early metastatic hepatocellular carcinoma: Combined treatment with NTBC chemotherapy and surgical mass removal (abstract). *J Inherit Metab Dis* 1997;**20**:(suppl 1) 3.

40 Forget S, Patriquin BH, Dubois J, *et al.* The kidney in children with tyrosinemia: sonographic CT and biochemical findings. *Pediatr Radiol* 1999;**29**:104.

41 Laine J, Salo MK, Krogerus L, *et al.* Nephropathy of tyrosinemia and its long-term outlook. *J Pediatr Gastroenterol Nutrition* 1997;**24**:113.

42 Mitchell G, Larochelle J, Lambert M, *et al.* Neurologic crises in hereditary tyrosinemia. *N Engl J Med* 1990;**322**:432.

43 Goulden KJ, Moss MA, Cole DE, *et al.* Pitfalls in the initial diagnosis of tyrosinemia: three case reports and a review of the literature. *Clin Biochem* 1987;**20**:207.

44 van Spronsen FJ, Thomasse Y, Smit GPA, *et al.* Hereditary tyrosinemia type I: A new clinical classification with difference in prognosis on dietary treatment. *Hepatology* 1994;**20**:1187.

45 Strife CF, Zuroweste EL, Emmet EA, *et al.* Tyrosinemia with acute intermittent porphyria: aminolevulinic acid dehydratase deficiency related to elevated urinary aminolevulinic acid levels. *J Pediatr* 1977;**90**:400.

46 Lindblad B, Fällström SP, Höyer S, *et al.* Cardiomyopathy in fumarylacetoacetase deficiency (hereditary tyrosinaemia): a new feature of the disease. *J Inherit Metab Dis* 1987;**10**:319.

47 Edwards MA, Green A, Colli A, Rylance G. Tyrosinaemia type I and hypertrophic obstructive cardiomyopathy. *Lancet* 1987;**1**:437 (letter).

48 De Braekeleer M, Larochelle J. Genetic epidemiology of hereditary tyrosinemia in Quebec and in Saguenay–Lac-St-Jean. *Am J Hum Genet* 1990;**47**:302.

49 Bergeron P, Laberge C, Grenier A. Hereditary tyrosinemia in the province of Quebec. Prevalence at birth and geographic distribution. *Clin Genet* 1974;**5**:157.

50 Laberge C, Dallaire L. Genetic aspects of tyrosinemia in the Chicoutimi region. *Can Med Assoc J* 1967;**97**:1099.

51 Halvorsen S. Screening for disorders of tyrosine metabolism: in *Neonatal Screening for Inborn Errors of Metabolism* (eds H Bickel, R Guthrie, G Hammersen) Springer-Verlag, New York;1980:45.

52 Laberge C. Hereditary tyrosinemia in a French Canadian isolate. *Am J Hum Genet* 1969;**21**:36.

53 Bouchard G, Laberge C, Scriver C-R. Comportements démographiques et effects fondateurs dans la population du Québec (XVIIe-Xxe siècles): in *Anonymous Societe Belege de Demographic Historiens et Populations: Liber Amicorum Etienne Hélin,* Louvain-la-Neuve Academia;1992:319.

54 Kvittingen EA, Halvorsen S, Jellum E. Deficient fumarylacetoacetate fumarylhydrolase activity in lymphocytes and fibroblasts from patients with hereditary tyrosinemia. *Pediatr Res* 1983;**17**:541.

55 Kvittingen EA, Brodtkorb E. The pre- and post-natal diagnosis of tyrosinemia type I and the detection of the carrier state by assay of fumarylacetoacetase. *Scand J Clin Lab Invest Suppl* 1986;**184**:35.

56 Kvittingen EA, Guibaud PP, Divry P, *et al.* Prenatal diagnosis of hereditary tyrosinaemia type 1 by determination of fumarylacetoacetase in chorionic villus material. *Eur J Pediatr* 1986;**144**:597 (letter).

57 Kvittingen EA, Steinmann B, Gitzelmann R, *et al.* Prenatal diagnosis of hereditary tyrosinemia by determination of fumarylacetoacetase in cultured amniotic fluid cells. *Pediatr Res* 1985;**19**:334.

58 Gagne R, Lescault A, Grenier A, *et al.* Prenatal diagnosis of hereditary tyrosinemia: measurement of succinylacetone in amniotic fluid. *Prenat Diagn* 1982;**2**:185.

59 Jakobs C, Dorland L, Wikkerink B, *et al.* Stable isotope dilution analysis of succinylacetone using electron capture negative ion mass fragmentography: an accurate approach to the pre- and neonatal diagnosis of hereditary tyrosinemia type I. *Clin Chim Acta* 1988;**171**:223.

60 Grenier A, Cederbaum S, Laberge C, *et al.* A case of tyrosinaemia type I with normal level of succinylacetone in the amniotic fluid. *Prenat Diagn* 1996;**16**:239.

61 Labelle Y, Phaneuf D, Leclerc B, Tanguay RM. Characterization of the human fumarylacetoacetate hydrolase gene and identification of a missense mutation abolishing enzymatic activity. *Hum Mol Genet* 1993;**2**:941.

62 Demers SI, Phaneuf D, Tanguay RM. Strong association of hereditary tyrosinemia type 1 with haplotype 6 in French-Canadians. Carrier detection and prenatal diagnosis by RFLP analysis. *Am J Hum Genet* 1994;**55**:327.

63 St-Louis M, Poudrier J, Phaneuf D, *et al.* Two novel mutations involved in hereditary tyrosinemia type I. *Hum Mol Genet* 1995;**4**:319.

64 Grompe M, al-Dhalimy M. Mutations of the fumarylacetoacetate hydrolase gene in four patients with tyrosinemia type I. *Hum Mut* 1993;**2**:85.

65 Kvittingen EA, Börresen AL, Stokke O, *et al.* Deficiency of fumarylacetoacetase without hereditary tyrosinemia. *Clin Genet* 1985; **27**:550.

66 Halvorsen S, Pande H, Loken AC, Gjessing LR. Tyrosinosis. A study of 6 cases. *Arch Dis Child* 1966;**41**:238.

67   Kogut MD, Shaw KN, Donnell GN. Tyrosinosis. *Am J Dis Child* 1967;**113**:47.

68   Christensen E, Jacobsen BB, Gregersen N, *et al.* Urinary excretion of succinylacetone and d-aminolevulinic acid in patients with hereditary tyrosinemia. *Clin Chim Acta* 1981;**116**:331.

69   Tschudy DP, Hess RA, Frykholm BC, Blaese RM. Immunosuppressive activity of succinylacetone. *J Lab Clin Med* 1982;**99**:526.

70   Sassa S, Kappas A. Impairment of heme synthesis by succinylacetone: a powerful inhibitor of d-aminolevulinate dehydratase activity produced in tyrosinemia. *Clin Res* 1982;**30**:551A.

71   Berger R, van Faassen H, Smith GP. Biochemical studies on the enzymatic deficiencies in hereditary tyrosinemia. *Clin Chim Acta* 1983;**134**:129.

72   Fallstrom SP, Lindblad B, Steen G. On the renal tubular damage in hereditary tyrosinemia and on the formation of succinylacetoacetate and succinylacetone. *Acta Paediatr Scand* 1981;**70**:315.

73   Stoner E, Starkman H, Wellner D, *et al.* Biochemical studies of a patient with hereditary hepatorenal tyrosinemia: evidence of glutathione deficiency. *Pediatr Res* 1984;**18**:1332.

74   Seltzer S, Lin M. Maleylacetone cis-trans-isomerase. Mechanism of the interaction of coenzyme glutathione and substrate maleylacetone in the presence and absence of enzyme. *J Am Chem Soc* 1979;**101**:3091.

75   Kvittingen EA, Rootwelt H, Brandtzaeg P. Hereditary tyrosinemia type I. *J Clin Invest* 1993;**91**:1816.

76   Kvittingen EA, Rootwelt H, Berger R, Brandtzaeg P. Self-induced correction of the genetic defect in tyrosinemia type I. *J Clin Invest* 1994;**94**:1657.

77   Holme E, Lindstedt S. Tyrosinemia type I and NTBC (2-nitro-4-trifluoromethylbenzoyl-1 3-cyclohexanedione). *J Inherit Metab Dis* 1998;**21**:507.

78   Halvorsen S. Dietary treatment of tyrosinosis. *Am J Dis Child* 1967;**113**:38.

79   Shasteen W, Zetterstrom R. Dietary treatment in tyrosinemia (tyrosinosis). *Am J Dis Child* 1967;**113**:31.

80   Halvorsen S, Gjessing LR. Studies on tyrosinosis: 1 effect of low-tyrosine and low-phenylalanine diet. *Br Med J* 1964;**2**:1171.

81   Halvorsen S, Kvittingen E-A, Flatmark A. Outcome of therapy of hereditary tyrosinemia. *Acta Paediatr Jpn* 1988;**30**:425.

82   Fisch RO, McCabe ERB, Doeden D, *et al.* Homotransplantation of the liver in a patient with hepatoma and hereditary tyrosinemia. *J Pediatr* 1978;**93**:592.

83   Starzl TE, Zitelli BJ, Shaw BW, *et al.* Changing concepts: liver replacement for hereditary tyrosinemia and hepatoma. *J Pediatr* 1985;**106**:604.

84   Paradis K, Weber A, Seidman EG, *et al.* Liver transplantation for hereditary tyrosinemia: the Quebec experience. *Am J Hum Genet* 1990;**47**:338.

85   Freese DK, Tuchman M, Schwarzenberg SJ, *et al.* Early liver transplantation is indicated for tyrosinemia type I. *J Pediatr Gastroenterol Nutrition* 1991;**13**:10.

86   Luks FI, St-Vil D, Hancock BJ, *et al.* Surgical and metabolic aspects of liver transplantation for tyrosinemia. *Transplantation* 1993;**56**:1376.

87   Tuchman M, Freese DK, Sharp HL, *et al.* Contribution of extrahepatic tissues to biochemical abnormalities in hereditary tyrosinemia type I: study of three patients after liver transplantation. *J Pediatr* 1987;**110**:399.

88   Shoemaker LR, Strife CF, Balistreri WF, Ryckman FC. Rapid improvement in the renal tubular dysfunction associated with tyrosinemia following hepatic replacement *Pediatrics* 1992;**89**:251.

89   Lindstedt S, Holme E, Lock EA, *et al.* Treatment of hereditary tyrosinemia type I by inhibition of 4-hydroxy-phenylpyruvate dioxygenase. *Lancet* 1992;**340**:813 (see comments).

90   Gibbs TC, Payan J, Brett EM, *et al.* Peripheral neuropathy as the presenting feature of tyrosinemia type I and effectively treated with an inhibitor of 4-hydroxyl-phenylpyruvate dioxygenase. *J Neurol Neurosurg Psychiatry* 1993;**56**:1129.

91   Holme E. Presentation, 3rd Swedish Orphan Conference. Karlskoga, Sweden May 15 2003.

Nonketotic hyperglycinemia

MAJOR PHENOTYPIC EXPRESSION

Potentially lethal neonatal illness, absent or poor mental development, convulsions, myoclonus, hiccups, hypotonia progressive to spasticity, abnormal electroencephalogram (EEG), hyperglycinemia, hyperglycinuria, elevated cerebrospinal fluid; plasma glycine ratio, and defective activity of the glycine cleavage system.

INTRODUCTION

Nonketotic hyperglycinemia is an inborn error of amino acid metabolism in which large amounts of glycine accumulate in body fluids, and there is no demonstrable accumulation of organic acids. A majority of patients has the classic phenotype in which life-threatening illness begins in the early days of life, and most patients die if not maintained by the use of mechanical ventilation. Survivors usually display little cognitive development and often have virtually continuous seizures. The disease was first described by Gerritsen, Kaveggia and Waisman in 1965 [1]. It was called nonketotic hyperglycinemia to distinguish it from other disorders, such as propionic acidemia (Chapter 2), in which hyperglycinemia occurs [2,3]. The high concentration of glycine in the cerebrospinal fluid (CSF) and the ratio of its concentration to that of the plasma provide the usual method of diagnosis. Analysis of organic acids of the urine is useful to exclude organic academia. Enzyme analysis is not generally available; the enzyme is fully expressed only in liver and brain.

The molecular defect is in the glycine cleavage system (EC 2.1.2.1.0) (Figure 27.1), which is a multienzyme complex with four protein components [4]. These have been labeled

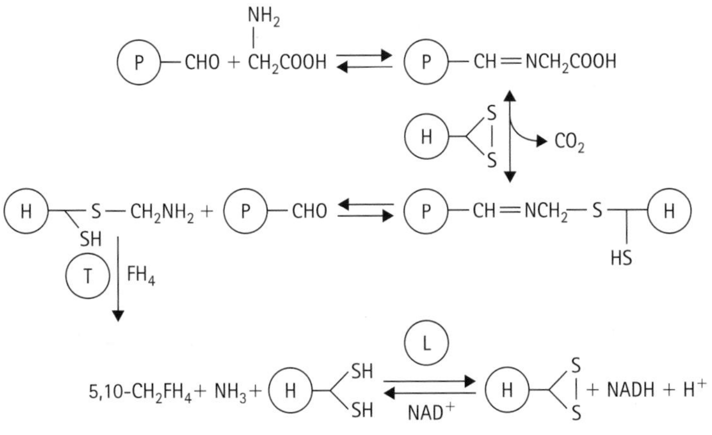

Figure 27.1 *The glycine cleavage system. The protein components, circled are labeled, P, H, T and L. (Reproduced with permission from Nyhan WL, in* The Metabolic Basis of Inherited Disease, *5th Ed. Eds Stanbury JB, Wyngaarden JB, Fredrickson DS, Goldstein JL, Brown MS. New York, McGraw Hill Book Co., 1952, p.564.)*

the P protein, H protein, T protein and L protein. In patients with nonketotic hyperglycinemia in whom the individual components have been studied, the majority has had defects in the P protein. Defective activity of the H protein and T protein have been described. The cDNA for the P protein has been cloned, and a number of mutations has been identified [5,6,7]. The genes for the T and H proteins have also been identified, and mutations have been identified [8–10].

CLINICAL ABNORMALITIES

In the classic phenotype, the infant appears normal at birth and there is a hiatus, usually up to 48 hours but ranging from a few hours to eight days, in which the patient remains well. Then, usually after the initiation of protein-containing feedings, lethargy develops, along with anorexia and failure to feed or later to suck. Feeding by nasogastric tube may be initiated. There may be some vomiting, but this is usually not a prominent feature. Lethargy is progressive to coma, and within 24 to 48 hours of the first symptom the patient is flaccid, completely unresponsive to stimuli, and apneic [1–3,11–18] (Figure 27.2). A majority of patients probably die at this point. Some are ventilated artificially using a respirator, for long enough to permit the diagnosis. Subsequent treatment with exchange transfusion, peritoneal dialysis or sodium benzoate may lead to the initiation of spontaneous respirations and the discontinuation of the respirator. However, there is seldom much evidence of cerebral development; and most patients die within the first year of life. The disorder is diagnosed in increasing fashion in neonatal intensive care units of major medical centers, but it is likely that as many or more die neonatal deaths without benefit of diagnosis.

In the infant the cry may be high-pitched. Suck, grasp and Moro responses are poor. Edema has been observed rarely [11,17]. Seizures may be myoclonic or grand mal [15]. They are prominent in almost all patients, and may be virtually continuous [1,17,19]. Hiccuping is common and often persistent [11], and we have with some frequency obtained historical evidence of recurrent prenatal hiccuping. Intermittent ophthalmoplegia or wandering eye movements have been described [20]. The electroencephalogram (EEG) is usually diffusely abnormal [21–25]. The typical pattern of burst-suppression is one of periodic or pseudoperiodic areas of large-amplitude sharp waves on a low voltage background [21–23]. The burst-suppression pattern has been observed as early as 30 minutes after birth [23]. This pattern, typical of the neonate, may change to hypsarrhythmia in later infancy. There may be multifocal epileptiform discharges [24]. Brainstem auditory evoked potentials may be abnormal [24].

Patients surviving the acute neonatal crisis develop a pattern of hypertonic spastic cerebral palsy [1,3], although they may be hypotonic throughout infancy [3,11]. Deep tendon reflexes are exaggerated, and there is ankle clonus. A position of opisthotonos is common. The patient may be completely unaware of surroundings and have few spontaneous movements. There is no head control or other evidence of psychomotor development, such as sitting or rolling over, and no adaptive or social behavior (Figures 27.3, 27.4). Eye movements may be disconjugate. Gavage or gastrostomy feeding may be required.

Nonketotic hyperglycinemia is heterogeneous, and while the majority of patients display the classic phenotype, a small number has been reported in whom a variety of milder forms have been observed. At the extreme from the classic, three affected girls [26] had only mild retardation; only one of the three was in an institution. Other families have been reported

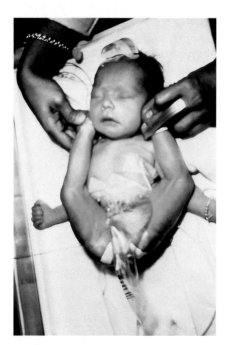

Figure 27.2 *J.S., a 4-day-old patient with nonketotic hyperglycinemia. Following exchange transfusion, assisted ventilation could be discontinued, but the patient was still in the Intensive Care Unit and unresponsive. Illustrated is the extreme hypotonicity.*

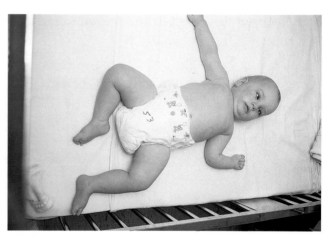

Figure 27.3 *D.G., an 8-month-old boy with nonketotic hyperglycinemia, in the tonic neck posture.*

in which there was mild developmental delay [27–32]. Acute febrile illness has been associated with involuntary movements, paresis of upward gaze, and delirium. Severe mental retardation and seizures may be found despite an atypical late onset [32]. It should be emphasized that milder variants are the exception. Of 30 patients studied by the Sendai group [5,33], 26 (87 percent) were of the classic neonatal type and the four survivors were severely retarded.

We have encountered a very different presentation [34] as a neurodegenerative disease not unlike Tay-Sachs or Krabbe disease. The patient developed relatively normally for the first months of life and then in the second half of the first year showed progressive cerebral deterioration. This led to a state of decerebrate rigidity (Figure 27.5) followed by death.

Magnetic resonance imaging (MRI) of the brain (Figure 27.6) [35–37], or computed tomography (CT), in this disease shows progressive atrophy and delayed myelination. The corpus callosum was abnormally thin in all patients and volume loss was both supra- and infratentorial. T_2-weighted images revealed decreased or absent myelination in the supratentorial white. These observations are consistent with reported neuropathology, including atrophy and corpus callosal thinning. Spongy rarefaction and vacuolation of myelin (Figure 27.7) as well as variable gliosis have been observed regularly [38,39].

Transient nonketotic hyperglycinemia represents a clinical presentation indistinguishable from the classic neonatal nonketotic hyperglycinemia [40–42]. The EEG may display the burst suppression pattern, and the concentrations of glycine in plasma and CSF, and the CSF to plasma ratios may be diagnostic. Surprisingly by two to eight weeks-of-age glycine levels have returned to normal. Five patients had normal cognitive and neurologic function at follow-up at 6 months to 13 years-of-age. One was severely retarded at report at 9 months and had MRI evidence of atrophy and abnormal signal in white matter.

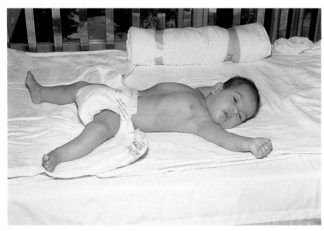

Figure 27.4   M.C., an almost 2-year-old with nonketotic hyperglycinemia. He survived a neonatal requirement for assisted ventilation following treatment with sodium benzoate but had little development or awareness of his environment. A feeding tube was required for nutrition. EEG revealed almost continuous seizure activity.

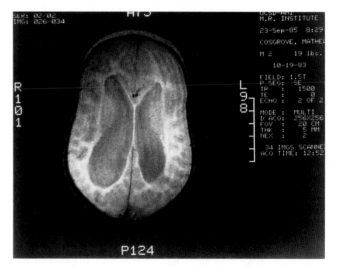

Figure 27.6   MRI of the brain of the patient in Figure 27.3. Dilated ventricles and sulci indicated a severe loss of volume of brain.

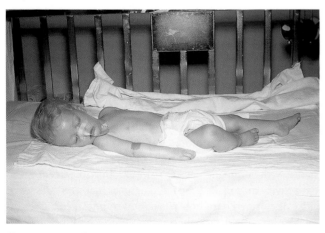

Figure 27.5   L.S. at 10 months. This patient presented with the picture of a cerebral degenerative disorder.

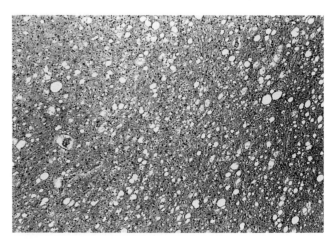

Figure 27.7   Histological section of the cortical white matter indicating the typical neuropathological finding of spongy degeneration and gliosis.

This syndrome is thought to be a consequence of immaturity of the enzyme system; support for the idea comes from studies of the development of the glycine cleavage system in the neonatal rat [43]. The existence of the syndrome has created an ethical dilemma for physicians and families of an infant in coma being artificially ventilated once a diagnosis of nonketotic hyperglycinemia has been made. Many families, once the diagnosis and its bleak prognosis have been understood have elected to discontinue life support. The alternatives seemed to be either death despite all support or, once the critical period has passed, no longer need for ventilator support, but no development either. The existence of the transient syndrome, raises the possibility of a third option. Most of us have never seen such a patient, and one wonders about the relevance of transient hyperammonemia of the newborn. Just a few years ago some of us were seeing this syndrome more frequently than permanent defects of the urea cycle and recently we do not seem to see it at all.

GENETICS AND PATHOGENESIS

Deficiency of any of the components of the glycine cleavage is transmitted in autosomal recessive fashion [33]. Defective activity of overall glycine cleavage was first described *in vivo* in studies of the metabolism of ^{14}C labeled glycine [2]. Patients displayed virtually no conversion of glycine-1-^{14}C to respiratory $^{14}CO_2$ and the conversion of glycine-2-^{14}C to the third carbon of serine was similarly defective. Assay of the enzyme in the liver homogenates was reported by Tada, Narasawa and colleagues in 1969 [44]. The enzyme system is expressed in liver, kidney and brain, and until recently could only be demonstrated in those tissues. Recently, it has been shown that the system is induced in the transformation of B lymphocytes with Epstein-Barr virus [45,46]. This has turned out to be a convenient but unreliable approach to the diagnosis.

The glycine cleavage system (Figure 27.1, p. 183) is a mitochondrial complex with four individual protein components [4,26,47]. The P protein is a pyridoxal phosphate-dependent glycine decarboxylase. The P and the H protein, a lipoic acid containing protein, are required for the formation of CO_2 from glycine. All four are required for the conversion of glycine to CO_2, NH_3 and a one-carbon tetrahydrofolate (FH_4) derivative, which can then function in one carbon transfer, as in the formation of serine from glycine. The T protein contains FH_4, and the L protein is a lipoamide dehydrogenase.

Analysis of hepatic activity of the glycine cleavage system in 30 patients in Sendai [5,33,48] revealed undetectable levels in the classic disease and some residual activity in the more indolent patients. Analysis of the components' proteins revealed that 87 percent had abnormalities in the P protein, and this included all of the classic patients. Four patients had defects in the T protein. In seven patients in whom the brain enzyme was assayed, the same component as in liver was found to be defective. Of atypical patients, two had defects in T protein

and one in H protein [33,49]. The patient with the cerebral degenerative phenotype had defective activity of both the P and H proteins [50] but the content of the P protein was normal, and it was concluded that the H protein was structurally abnormal. Immunochemical studies in patients with the classic presentation revealed virtually no P protein [51].

Molecular studies of mutation have revealed heterogeneity for the gene of the P protein, and two mutations of the T protein. None have been described for the H protein. The P protein gene [5,6] has been located on chromosome 9p13-23 [52], as first suggested by a patient with nonketotic hyperglycinemia and the 9p- syndrome [53]. It contains 25 exons over 135 kb. The gene for the H protein codes for a precursor protein of 173 amino acids and a mature protein of 125 amino acids [54]. The T protein gene maps to chromosome 3q21.1-21.3 [55]. It has 6 kb over 9 exons. In a Japanese patient a three-base deletion was found in the P protein gene, which led to deletion of a phenylalanine at position 756 [6]. Expression of the normal and mutant protein in Cos 7 cells led to abundant P protein activity in cells with the normal gene and no activity in those with the mutant gene.

Nonketotic hyperglycinemia is common in northern Finland where it occurs in 1 of 12 000 births [56]. This severe form of the disease was found to result from a point mutation of a G to T at nucleotide 1691 resulting in a change from serine to leucine at residue number 564 of the P protein [7]. The absence of this mutation in 20 non-Finnish alleles and its presence in 10 unrelated Finnish patients indicates the presence of a founder effect. Both this mutation and the Japanese deletion occurred in a region of the protein that is thought to be important for enzyme activity and for the binding of pyridoxal phosphate (Figure 27.8). In contrast a patient with late onset nonketotic hyperglycinemia had a methionine to isoleucine change at position 391 in a very different part of the molecule [5].

Mutations in the gene for the T protein have included a G to A transition coding for a glycine to aspartic acid substitution at 269 (G269D) in a patient with classic neonatal disease [8], an A to G change leading to a histidine to arginine substitution at 42 (H42R) in an Israeli-Arab family [10], a deletion (183delC) causing a frameshift, and a G to C change causing D276H [9]. An atypical patient was a compound for two G to A changes, G47R and R320H.

Conventional approaches to genetic assistance to families are difficult in disorders in which the enzyme does not express in fibroblasts or amniocytes. Prenatal diagnosis of this disease became possible with the recognition that the cleavage system did express in chorionic villus samples [7]. Thirty-one pregnancies were monitored [5], of which 23 were normal and eight affected. Similar results have been reported in experience with 50 pregnancies at risk [57], but 10 percent residual activity may make prenatal diagnosis inaccurate. Enzyme assay of cultured lymphoblasts has given intermediate results for heterozygote detection, but this approach may be inaccurate. Identification of the mutation permits prenatal diagnosis and detection of heterozygotes using molecular biology,

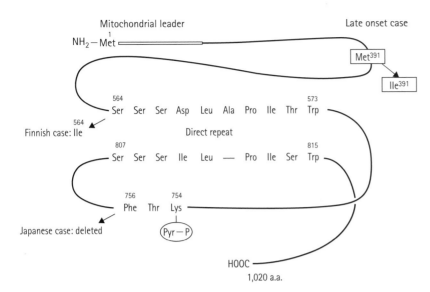

Figure 27.8 *Molecular alterations in three different forms of the P protein of the glycine cleavage enzyme. The Japanese and Finnish phenotypes were of the classic type, while the patient with the methionine to isoleucine change at 391 had a more indolent disease. (Reprinted with permission from Tada and Kure in the* Journal of Inherited Metabolic Disease *[5].)*

and a prenatal diagnosis of the Finnish mutation has been made [7].

Concentrations of glycine are elevated in the blood, urine and CSF. In spite of the large amounts of glycine found in the urine, it is possible to miss a patient with hyperglycinemia when screening the urine for amino acids by paper chromatography or electrophoresis. The normal glycine spot is very prominent. Also patients are often studied when acutely ill, not eating, and being maintained on parenterally administered fluids. Under these circumstances, the excretion of glycine in hyperglycinemic patients may be normal. In general, it is better to screen for hyperglycinemia by assaying blood rather than urine. Blood concentrations are seldom brought into the normal range.

The concentrations of glycine are uniquely elevated in the CSF. Concentrations in reported patients have varied from 130 to 360 μmol/L [11,58,59]. In a series of 12 patients summarized from the literature, the mean value was 93 μmol/L [27]. In the Finnish series of 19 patients the mean was 93 μmol/L [60]. In control subjects, the concentration has generally been less than 13 μmol/L. The ratio of the CSF concentration to that of the plasma is substantially higher in patients with nonketotic hyperglycinemia than in hyperglycinemic patients with organic acidemia. In the series of 12 patients from the literature, the mean ratio was 0.17 ± 0.09, and in the Finnish series the mean was 0.11, whereas in control individuals the ratio was 0.02 (Table 27.1). It is important to recognize that the ratio may be meaningless if concentrations are normal. A diagnosis of hyperglycinemia requires an elevated level of glycine.

We have observed patients with milder degrees of clinical expression in whom the ratios, though abnormal, were less elevated than in the classic phenotype.

Glycine has long been known to be active in the nervous system, but older information on glycine as an inhibitory neurotransmitter at strychnine receptors never fitted with the picture of intractable seizures [61]. It is now clear that glycine is an excitatory neurotransmitter (Figure 27.9) with a profound

Table 27.1 *Ratios of the concentration of glycine in the CSF to that of plasma*

Subject	Ratio
Finnish mean [60]	0.11
NKH, R.H. [11]	0.30
NKH, T.Z. [3]	0.10
Neurodegenerative variant [34]	0.07
Milder variant [29]	0.07
Control mean [58]	0.02

influence on the N-methyl-D-aspartate (NMDA) receptor, which normally responds to the excitatory amino acid glutamate [62,63]. Glycine functions as an allosteric agonist permitting glutamate to be excitatory at much smaller contractions.

TREATMENT

The management of this disease is considerably less than satisfactory. Exchange transfusion or dialysis or sodium benzoate may be life-saving in the neonatal period, and may permit weaning from the ventilator, but many families made aware of the grim prognosis prefer not to take these steps. The plasma concentrations of glycine may be lowered by dietary restriction or by the administration of sodium benzoate. It is now clear that treatment with large amounts of benzoate, which joins with glycine to form hippurate which is then excreted in the urine, can actually lower CSF concentration of glycine and that there are dose-response relationships [64]. Patients so treated had a substantial decrease in seizures. Doses employed have ranged from 250 to 700 mg/kg per day. Developmental progress has been disappointing except in one patient who was reported as developmentally normal [65].

We and others [66] have added dextromethorphan to the benzoate regimen as a noncompetitive antagonist at the

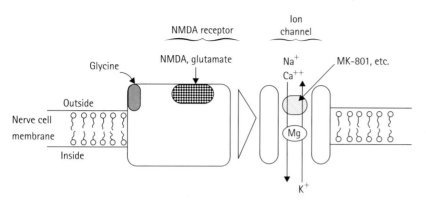

Figure 27.9 *The NMDA receptor and the role of glycine. When glutamate or NMDA binds to the receptor the channel opens and positively charged ions flow to the nerve cell. Glycine binds at a different site on the receptor and acts as a facilitator.*

NMDA receptor. Dosage employed has been in the range of 5 to 22 mg/kg per day. Among the four patients reported from Baltimore [66,67] very beneficial effects on development were observed in a patient treated from the first days of his life. This was less evident in our experience, and results were mixed in the other Baltimore patients including one who died at 12 weeks. Similarly mixed results were reported by others [68,69]. Arnold *et al.* [70] pointed out that dextromethorphan is metabolized very differently in different individuals and that measuring levels is necessary to ensure adequate dosage. Anticonvulsant effects were associated with levels of 50 to 100 ng/mL. Cimetidine, an inhibitor of P450 activity, was found to increase dextromethorphan levels in a rapid metabolizing individual.

Benzoate treatment has been observed to lead to carnitine deficiency in patients with this disease [70,71]. It would appear prudent to supplement patients under treatment with carnitine, and to measure levels. It is also prudent to avoid treatment with valproate in this disease, because it causes increase in levels of glycine [72] and inhibits the activity of the glycine cleavage system [73].

References

1　Gerritsen T, Kaveggia E, Waisman HA. A new type of idiopathic hyperglycinemia with hypo-oxaluria. *Pediatrics* 1965; **36**:882.

2　Ando T, Nyhan WL, *et al.* Metabolism of glycine in the nonketotic form of hyperglycinemia. *Pediatr Res* 1968;**2**:254.

3　Ziter FA, Bray PF, Madsen JA, Nyhan WL. The clinical findings in a patient with nonketotic hyperglycinemia. *Pediatr Res* 1968;**2**:250.

4　Kikuchi G. The glycine cleavage system: composition reaction mechanism and physiological significance. *Mol Cell Biochem* 1973;**1**:169.

5　Tada K, Kure S. Nonketotic hyperglycinaemia: molecular lesion diagnosis and pathophysiology. *J Inherit Metab Dis* 1993;**16**:691.

6　Kure S, Narisawa K, Tada K. Structural and expression analyses of normal and mutant mRNA encoding glycine decarboxylase: three base deletion in mRNA causes nonketotic hyperglycinemia. *Biochem Biophys Res Commun* 1991;**174**:1176.

7　Kure S, Takayanagi M, Narisawa K, *et al.* Identification of a common mutation in Finnish patients with nonketotic hyperglycinemia. *J Clin Invest* 1992;**90**:160.

8　Nanao K, Okamura-Ikeda K, Motokawa Y, *et al.* Identification of the mutations in the T-protein gene causing typical and atypical nonketotic hyperglycinemia. *Hum Genet* 1994;**93**:655.

9　Kure S, Shinka T, Sakata Y, *et al.* A one base deletion (183delC) and a missense mutation (D276H) in the T protein gene from a Japanese family with nonketotic hyperglycinemia. *J Hum Genet* 1998;**43**:135.

10　Kure S, Mandel H, Rolland MO, *et al.* A missense mutation (His42Arg) in the T-protein gene from a large Israeli-Arab kindred with nonketotic hyperglycinemia. *Hum Genet* 1998;**102**:430.

11　Baumgartner R, Ando T, Nyhan WL. Nonketotic hyperglycinemia. *J Pediatr* 1969;**75**:1022.

12　Simila S, Visakorpi JK. Clinical findings in three patients with nonketotic hyperglycinaemia. *Ann Clin Res* 1970;**2**:151.

13　Ferdinand W, Gordon RR, Owen G. Nonketotic hyperglycinaemia: clinical findings and amino acid analyses on the plasma of a new case. *Clin Chim Acta* 1970;**30**:745.

14　Bachmann C, Mihatsch MJ, Baumgartner RE, *et al.* Nicht-Ketotische Hyperglyzinämie: Perakuter verlauf im Neugeborenenalten. *Helv Padiatr Acta* 1971;**26**:228.

15　Von Wendt L, Simila S, Hirvasniemi A, Suvanto E. Nonketotic hyperglycinemia. A clinical analysis of 19 Finnish patients. *Monogr Hum Genet* 1978;**9**:58.

16　DeGroot CJ, Hommes FA, Touwen BCL. The altered toxicity of glycine in nonketotic hyperglycinemia. *Hum Hered* 1977;**27**:178.

17　Holmqvist P, Polberger S. Neonatal nonketotic hyperglycinemia (NKH). Diagnoses and management in two cases. *Neuropediatrics* 1985;**16**:191.

18　Dalla Bernardina B, Aicardi J, Goutieres F, Plouin P. Glycine encephalopath. *Neuropaediatrics* 1979;**10**:209.

19　Mignone F, Balbo L, Valpreda A, *et al.* Iperglicinemia non chetosica. Presentazione di un caso. *Minerva Pediatr* 1980 **32**:111.

20　Macdonald JT, Sher PK. Ophthalmoplegia as a sign of metabolic disease in the newborn. *Neurology* 1977;**27**:971.

21　Aicardi J, Goutieres F. Encephalopathie myoclonique neonatale. *Rev Electroencephalogr Neurophysiol* 1978;**8**:99.

22　Mises J, Moussalli-Salefranque F, Plouin P, *et al.* L'EEG dans les hyperglycinemies sans cetose. *Rev Electroencephalogr Neurophysiol* 1978;**8**:102.

23　Von Wendt L, Simila S, Saukkonen A-L, *et al.* Prenatal brain damage in nonketotic hyperglycinemia. *Am J Dis Child* 1981;**135**:1072.

24　Markand ON, Bhuwan PG, Brandt IK. Nonketotic hyperglycinemia: electroencephalographic and evoked potential abnormalities. *Neurology* 1982;**32**:151.

25　Bernardina BD, Dulac O, Fejerman H, *et al.* Early myoclonic epileptic encephalopathy (EMEE). *Eur J Pediatr* 1983;**140**:248.

26　Ando T, Nyhan WL, Bicknell WL, *et al.* Nonketotic hyperglycinaemia in a family with an unusual phenotype. *J Inherit Metab Dis* 1978;**1**:79.

27 Holmgren G, Blomquist HK. Nonketotic hyperglycinemia in 2 sibs with mild psycho-neurological symptoms. *Neuropaediatrie* 1977;**8**:67.

28 Flannery DB, Pellock J, Bousounis D, *et al.* Nonketotic hyperglycinemia in two retarded adults: a mild form of infantile nonketotic hyperglycinemia. *Neurology* 1983;**33**:1064.

29 Frazier DM, Summer GK, Chamberlin HR. Hyperglycinuria and hyperglycinemia in two siblings with mild developmental delays. *Am J Dis Child* 1978;**132**:777.

30 Nightingale S, Barton ME. Intermittent vertical supranuclear ophthalmoplegia and ataxia. *Mov Disord* 1991;**6**:76.

31 Steiner RD, Sweetser DA, Rohrbaugh JR, *et al.* Nonketotic hyperglycinemia: atypical clinical and biochemical manifestations. *J Pediatr* 1996;**128**:243.

32 Singer HS, Valle D, Hayasaka K, Tada K. Nonketotic hyperglycinemia: studies in an atypical variant. *Neurology* 1989;**39**:286.

33 Tada K. Nonketotic hyperglycinemia: clinical and metabolic aspects. *Enzyme* 1987;**38**:27.

34 Trauner DA, Page T, Greco C, *et al.* Progressive neurodegenerative disorder in a patient with nonketotic hyperglycinemia. *J Pediatr* 1981;**98**:272.

35 Press GA, Barshop BA, Haas RH, *et al.* Abnormalities of the brain in nonketotic hyperglycinemia: MR manifestation. *AJNR* 1989;**10**:315.

36 Dobyns WB. Agenesis of the corpus callosum and gyral malformations are frequent manifestations of nonketotic hyperglycinemia. *Neurology* 1989; **39**:817.

37 Rogers T, Al-Rayess M, O'Shea P, Ambler MW. Dysplasia of the corpus callosum in identical twins with nonketotic hyperglycinemia. *Pediatr Pathol* 1991;**11**:897.

38 Shuman RM, Leech RW, Scott CR. The neuropathology of the nonketonic and ketonic hyperglycinemias: three cases. *Neurology* 1978;**28**:139.

39 Brun A, Borjeson M, Hultberg B, *et al.* Nonketotic hyperglycinemia: a clinical biochemical and neuropathologic study including electronic microscopy findings. *Neuropaediatrie* 1979;**10**:195.

40 Luder AS, Davidson A, Goodman SI, Greene CL. Transient nonketotic hyperglycinemia in neonates. *J Pediatr* 1989;**114**:1013.

41 Eyskens FJM, Van Doorn JWD, Marlen P. Neurologic sequelae in transient nonketotic hyperglycinemia of the neonate. *J Pediatr* 1992;**121**:620.

42 Zammarchi E, Donati MA, Ciani F. Transient neonatal nonketotic hyperglycinemia: a 13-year follow-up. *Neuropediatrics* 1995;**26**:328.

43 Kalbag SS, Palekar AG. Postnatal development of the glycine cleavage system in rat liver. *Biochem Med Metab Biol* 1990;**43**:128.

44 Tada K, Narisawa K, Yoshida T, *et al.* Hyperglycinemia: a defect in glycine cleavage reaction. *Tohoku J Exp Med* 1969;**98**:289.

45 Kure S, Narisawa K, Tada K. Enzymatic diagnosis of nonketotic hyperglycinemia with lymphoblasts. *J Pediatr* 1992;**120**:95.

46 Christodoulu J, Kure S, Hayasaka K, Clarke JTR. Atypical nonketotic hyperglycinemia confirmed by assay of the glycine cleavage system in lymphoblasts. *J Pediatr* 1993;**123**:100.

47 Motokawa Y, and Kikuchi G. Glycine metabolism by rat liver mitochondria. Reconstitution of the reversible glycine cleavage system with partially purified protein components. *Arch Biochem Biophys* 1974;**164**:624.

48 Hayasaka K, Tada K, Kikuschi G, *et al.* Nonketotic hyperglycinemia: two patients with primary defects of P-protein and T-protein respectively in the glycine cleavage system. *Pediatr Res* 1983;**17**:926.

49 Tada K, Hayasaka K. Clinical and biochemical aspects. *Eur J Pediatr* 1987;**146**:221.

50 Hiraga K, Kochi H, Hayasaka K, *et al.* Defective glycine cleavage system in nonketotic hyperglycinemia. *J Clin Invest* 1981;**68**:525.

51 Hayasaka K, Tada K, Nyhan WL, *et al.* Nonketotic hyperglycinemia: analyses of the glycine cleavage system in typical and atypical cases. *J Pediatr* 1987;**110**:873.

52 Tada K, Kure S. Nonketotic hyperglycinemia: molecular lesion and pathophysiology. *Int Pediatr* 1993;**8**:52.

53 Burton BK, Pettenati MJ, Block SM, *et al.* Nonketotic hyperglycinemia in a patient with the 9p- syndrome. *Am J Med Genet* 1989;**32**:504.

54 Koyata H, Hiraga K. The glycine cleavage system: structure of a cDNA encoding human H-protein and partial characterization of its gene in patients with hyperglycinemias. *Am J Hum Genet* 1991;**48**:351.

55 Nanao K, Takada G, Takahashi E, *et al.* Structure and chromosomal localization of the gene encoding human T-protein of the glycine cleavage system. *Genomics* 1994;**19**:27.

56 Von Wendt L, Hirvasniemia A, Simila S. Nonketotic hyperglycinemia: a genetic study of 13 Finnish families. *Clin Genet* 1979;**15**:411.

57 Toone JR, Applegarth DA, Levy HL. Prenatal diagnosis of NKH: experience in 50 at-risk pregnancies. *J Inherit Metab Dis* 1994;**17**:342.

58 Perry TL, Urquhart N, Maclean J, *et al.* Nonketotic hyperglycinemia. *N Engl J Med* 1975;**292**:1269.

59 Scriver CR, White A, Sprague W, Horwood SP. Plasma–CSF glycine ratio in normal and nonketotic hyperglycinemic subjects. *N Engl J Med* 1975;**293**:778.

60 Von Wendt L, Simila S, Hirvasniemi A, Suvanto E. Altered levels of various amino acids in blood plasma and cerebrospinal fluid of patients with nonketotic hyperglycinemia. *Neuropaediatrie* 1978;**9**:360.

61 Krnjevic K. Chemical nature of synaptic neurotransmission in vertebrates. *Physiol Rev* 1974;**54**:418.

62 Newell DW, Barth A, Ricciardi TN, Malouf AT. Glycine causes receptors in the hippocampus. *Exp Neurol* 1997;**145**:235.

63 Johnson JW, Ascher P. Glycine potentiates the NMDA response in cultured mouse brain neurons. *Nature* (London) 1987;**325**:529.

64 Wolff JA, Kulovich S, Yu A, *et al.* The effectiveness of benzoate in the management of seizures in nonketotic hyperglycinemia. *Am J Dis Child* 1986;**140**:596.

65 Boneh A, Degani Y, Harari M. Prognostic clues and outcome of early treatment of nonketotic hyperglycinemia. *Pediatr Neurol* 1996;**15**:137.

66 Hamosh A, McDonald JW, Valle D, *et al.* Dextromethorphan and high-dose benzoate therapy for nonketotic hyperglycinemia in an infant. *J Pediatr* 1992;**121**:131.

67 Hamosh A, Maher JF, Bellus GA, *et al.* Long-term use of high-dose benzoate and dextromethorphan for the treatment of nonketotic hyperglycinemia. *J Pediatr* 1998;**132**:709.

68 Zammarchi E, Kure S, Hayasaka K, Clarke JTR. Failure of early dextromethorphan and sodium benzoate therapy in an infant with nonketotic hyperglycinemia. *Neuropediatrics* 1994;**25**:274.

69 Alemzadeh RMK. Efficacy of low-dose dextromethorphan in the treatment of nonketotic hyperglycinemia. *Pediatrics* 1996;**97**:924.

70 Arnold GL, Griebel ML, Valentine JL, *et al.* Dextromethorphan in nonketotic hyperglycinemia: metabolic variation confounds the dose-response relationship. *J Inherit Metab Dis* 1997;**20**:28.

71 Van Hove JL, Kishnani P, Muenzer J, *et al.* Benzoate therapy and carnitine deficiency in non-ketotic hyperglycinemia. *Am J Med Genet* 1995;**59**:444.

72 Belkinsopp WK, DuPont PA. Dipropylacetate (valproate) and glycine metabolism. *Lancet* 1977;**2**:617.

73 Kochi H, Hawasaka W, Hiraga K, Kikuchi G. Reduction of the level of glycine cleavage system in the rat liver resulting from administration of dipropylacetic acid: an experimental approach to hyperglycinemia. *Arch Biochem Biophys* 1979;**198**:589.

PART 3

Hyperammonemia and disorders of the urea cycle

28

Introduction to hyperammonemia and disorders of the urea cycle

Distinct disorders involve the enzymes of every step in the urea cycle (Figure 28.1) [1,2]. These include ornithinetranscarbamylase deficiency (Chapter 29), citrullinemia (Chapter 31), carbamyl phosphate synthetase deficiency (Chapter 30), argininosuccinic aciduria (Chapter 32) and argininemia (Chapter 33). In addition, there is a syndrome of transient hyperammonemia of the newborn [3], in which the early clinical manifestations mimic those of the severe defects of urea cycle enzymes and may be fatal, but if the patient can get through the first five days of life the problem disappears and

prognosis is good. The hyperammonemic syndrome is also characteristic of the HHH (hyperammonemia, hyperornithinemia and homocitrullinuria) syndrome (Chapter 34), which is caused by defective transport of ornithine into the mitochondria. Lysisuric protein intolerance (Chapter 35) is also associated with episodic hyperammonemia, but its major expression is as extreme failure to thrive.

Deficiencies of enzymes of the urea cycle lead to hyperammonemia, and they present classically with sudden neonatal coma and a picture of overwhelming illness. The most classic

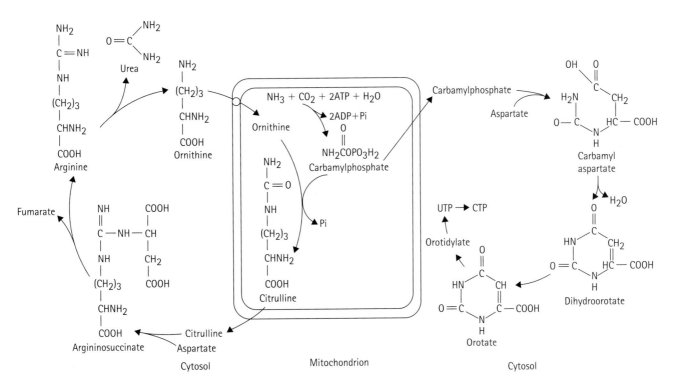

Figure 28.1   *The urea cycle.*

of these presentations is that of ornithine transcarbamylase deficiency in the male. The classic presentation of the hyperammonemic diseases is with acute neonatal life-threatening coma. Lethargy leads to a state of complete unresponsiveness reminiscent of surgical anesthesia. Breathing stops, and in the absence of intubation and artificial ventilation, death ensues. This clinical picture and concentration of ammonia from 400 to 2000 μmol/L are seen in a variety of disorders in addition to those listed above. These include the organic acidemias and the disorders of fatty acid oxidation. Effective management requires a precise diagnosis, but vigorous therapy should be initiated immediately on recognition of the hyperammonemia.

WORKUP OF THE PATIENTS WITH HYPERAMMONEMIA

A systematic approach to the workup of an infant in hyperammonemic coma is shown in Figure 28.2. The differential diagnosis is important because different disorders require very different treatments. It must proceed with dispatch in order to institute appropriate therapy. The initial studies can be carried out in any clinical laboratory and provide clear direction to the next diagnostic and therapeutic steps. Ultimately, studies must be carried out in a laboratory that specializes in biochemical genetic analysis in order to make a precise definitive diagnosis. Liver biopsy and enzymatic analysis may be required for the diagnosis of ornithine transcarbamylase deficiency, carbamyl phosphate synthetase deficiency or N-acetylglutamate synthetase deficiency. In an infant in coma the blood concentration of ammonia should be measured.

A workup for hyperammonemia should be undertaken in any newborn with an ammonia concentration greater than 150 μmol/L and in any older infant and adult at values over 100 μmol/L. The serum concentrations of bicarbonate, sodium and chloride are measured, the anion gap assessed, and the urine tested for ketones. The presence of acidosis and an anion gap, or massive ketosis, indicates that hyperammonemia is due to one of the organic acidemias. These disorders include propionic acidemia (Chapter 2), methylmalonic acidemia (Chapter 3), isovaleric acidemia (Chapter 7), glutaric aciduria Type II (Chapter 45), 3-hydroxy-3-methylglutaric aciduria (Chapter 46), and multiple carboxylase deficiency (Chapter 5). The specific diagnosis is made by organic acid analysis of the urine or of the acylcarnitine profile of the blood.

Hyperammonemia may also be seen in acute exacerbation of disorders of fatty acid oxidation. These episodes are characteristically hypoketotic. They are usually associated with hypoglycemia, raising the possibility of a diagnosis of Reye

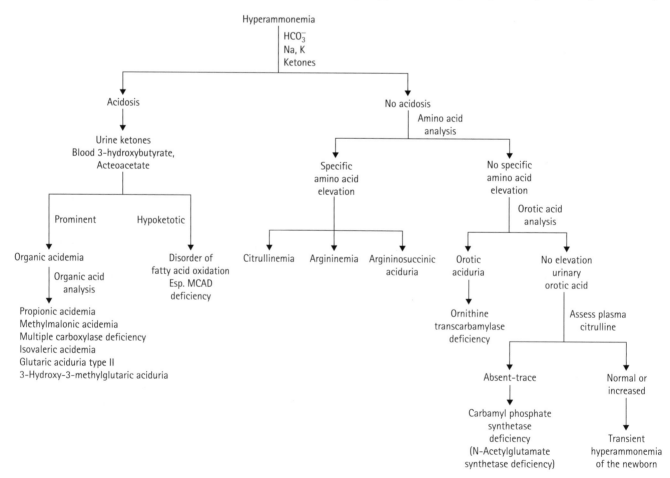

Figure 28.2 *Diagnostic workup of the hyperammonemic infant in coma. MCAD – medium chain acyl-CoA dehydrogenase deficiency (Chapter 40).*

syndrome, but we have seen an acute hyperammonemic episode in a teenage girl who turned out to have medium chain acyl CoA dehydrogenase deficiency (Chapter 40) that met all the criteria for a diagnosis of ornithine transcarbamylase (OTC) deficiency except that when the liver was biopsied its OTC activity was normal [4].

Hyperammonemic patients who do not have an organic acidemia are seldom acidotic. If there is an abnormality in acid base balance in a patient with a urea cycle defect, it is more likely to be a respiratory alkalosis, although apnea and hypoxia can lead to lactic acidosis; so adequate oxygenation and perfusion should be assured before these assessments are made once an organic acidemia is excluded. The next step toward definitive differential diagnosis is the quantitative assay of the concentrations of amino acids in blood and urine. Assessment of the plasma concentrations of amino acids will provide the diagnosis in patients with argininemia and citrullinemia. Study of the urine is required in argininosuccinic aciduria (Chapter 32).

In hyperammonemic patients found not to have diagnostic abnormality in the concentration of an amino acid, the urine should be tested for the excretion of orotic acid. Orotic aciduria is found in patients with OTC deficiency. It is also found in citrullinemia and in argininemia. In a patient without an elevation of a specific amino acid and without orotic aciduria, the expected diagnosis is carbamylphosphate synthetase (CPS) deficiency or transient hyperammonemia of the newborn [3].

The diagnosis of CPS deficiency is made by biopsy of the liver. It is preferable to make this distinction after waiting, because transient hyperammonemia of the newborn resolves within five days. Also, this gives time to bring the patient into good metabolic control. The concentration of citrulline in the blood may be helpful in making these distinctions. It is usually normal or elevated in transient hyperammonemia of the newborn, whereas it is barely detectable in neonatal carbamylphosphate synthetase or OTC deficiencies. Citrulline synthesis is coupled with the concentration of adenosine triphosphate (ATP). Hypocitrullinemia may be seen in disorders of the electron transport chain such as that resulting from the neurodegeneration, ataxia and retinitis pigmentosa (NARP) mutation (Chapter 54). In citrullinemia concentrations of citrulline in plasma usually exceed $1000\,\mu mol/L$. They are elevated to levels of $50–250\,\mu mol/L$ in argininosuccinic aciduria, and to $54 \pm 2\,\mu mol/L$ in transient hyperammonemia of the newborn [5]. The normal range is $6–20\,\mu mol/L$. Symptomatic hyperammonemia may also result from a urinary tract infection in which the infecting *Proteus mirabilis* has urease activity, which produces ammonia from urea. A patient with a prune-belly syndrome and massive dilatation of the urinary tract developed coma with a blood concentration of ammonia of $140\,\mu mol/L$ ($202\,\mu g/dL$).

Concentrations of glutamine are regularly elevated in patients with hyperammonemia, and concentrations of alanine are usually elevated as well, while concentrations of aspartic acid are elevated in some patients. These findings are nonspecific. They are not helpful in the differentiation of the different causes of hyperammonemia. They are potentially helpful in diagnosis, as sometimes an elevated level of glutamine is found in a patient that had not been expected to have hyperammonemia, and while concentrations of ammonia may vary from hour to hour, the elevated concentration of glutamine signifies a state in which there has been more chronic oversupply of ammonia. The transamination of glutamic acid and its subsequent amidation all represent detoxification mechanisms in the attempt to handle excessive quantities of ammonia.

Amino acid analysis is not specifically useful in the diagnosis of OTC deficiency and carbamyl phosphate synthetase deficiency, but in both of these conditions levels of citrulline and arginine may be low. They are distinguished by measurement of the excretion of orotic acid, which is increased in OTC deficiency, but not in carbamyl phosphate synthetase deficiency [6–8]. This is a reflection of the accumulation of carbamylphosphate, which then leaves the mitochondria and follows the cytosolic pathway of pyrimidine synthesis (Figure 28.1). There may be so much orotic acid in the urine that it forms a white crystalline precipitate. In mice with OTC deficiency calculi are found in the bladder [4].

Overproduction of pyrimidines leads to the presence of large amounts of uracil and increased amounts of uridine in the urine. In most patients with OTC deficiency orotic aciduria is always present. However, we have studied one patient [5] with a partial variant in whom orotic acid excretion was not present when he was clinically well and could not be induced by means of a protein load, but was readily evident at the time of illness induced by infection.

TREATMENT OF HYPERAMMONEMIA

The treatment of the patient with hyperammonemia has many common features that are relevant to states of elevated ammonia regardless of cause. In the acute hyperammonemic onset usually seen in infancy, all intake of protein or other sources of nitrogen is stopped. Water and electrolyte are provided intravenously and anabolism is promoted by the administration of glucose. Pharmacologic approaches to therapy include: the provision of arginine to keep the urea cycle supplied with enough ornithine to keep it running; and the provision of alternate pathways for the excretion of waste nitrogen, such as sodium benzoate and sodium phenylacetate. Extracorporeal methods such as hemodialysis are usually required in the acutely hyperammonemic newborn. The most effective treatment of the acute hyperammonemic crisis that occurs in the classic neonatal disease is hemodialysis [9–11]. Exchange transfusion is not an effective modality in such an infant, but it may reduce levels enough to buy some time while the hemodialysis is being prepared, and it has been effective in some patients with transient hyperammonemia of the newborn [3].

Peritoneal dialysis is often recommended for hyperammonemic patients, and we would agree that it is effective in an older infant, child or adult with hyperammonemia, but in our experience it has been unsatisfactory in the neonatal period [12]. Hemodialysis has been shown to be more effective than exchange transfusion, peritoneal dialysis or arteriovenous hemofiltration, but the logistics are such in most hospitals that this modality can seldom be mobilized promptly to meet the needs of a newly diagnosed newborn. This is an argument for transport of such an infant to an institution with experience in the rescue of such infants. Even so, the mechanics of hemodialysis in a tiny infant are formidable, and failure of the procedure is more common than the literature would imply. An advance in management has been the application of extracorporeal membrane oxygenation (ECMO) in the treatment of the hyperammonemic neonate [13].

The pharmacologic approach to the provision of alternate methods of waste nitrogen excretion represents a major advance in the management of hyperammonemia (Table 28.1, Figure 28.3a and b) [5,12–18]. The principle is that benzoate is effectively conjugated with glycine to form hippurate, which is efficiently excreted in the urine, and similarly phenylacetate is conjugated to form phenylacetylglutamine, and this compound is excreted in the urine; both provide pathways for getting rid of nitrogen that cannot be excreted as urea and would otherwise accumulate as ammonia. These measures have been employed along with exchange transfusion or peritoneal dialysis [3], but we have found pharmacologic therapy effective in patients in whom exchange transfusion and peritoneal dialysis were having little or no effect [12,16].

Intravenous benzoate and phenylacetate are available from Ucyclid Pharma, Phoenix, Arizona. In Europe most patients are treated with intravenous benzoate. Along with benzoate and/or phenylacetate, arginine is infused. This provides an essential amino acid in a patient with a complete block in arginine synthesis and provides ornithine substrate for any patient in whom there is not a complete block at carbamyl phosphate synthetase or ornithine transcarbamylase. It may be particularly useful as an effector of acetylglutamate synthetase and hence activator of carbamylphosphate synthetase. It is particularly useful in patients with citrullinemia or argininosuccinic aciduria (Chapters 31 and 37). It is useful to start arginine alone if benzoate and phenylacetate are not immediately available.

Supplies of benzoate, phenylacetate and arginine should ideally be kept on hand, available to the neonatal intensive care unit in anticipation of the diagnosis of such an infant. Often a patient is first recognized in a community hospital where benzoate and phenylacetate are not available but arginine is. The arginine infusion should be started and the patient then transported to the tertiary care center. We have found that many patients will respond to arginine alone. This is often

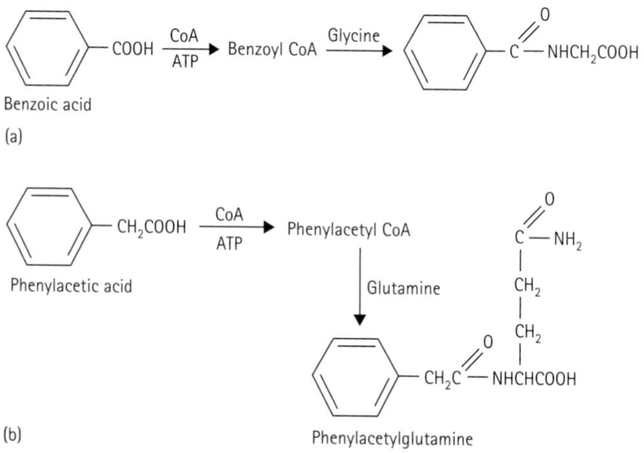

Figure 28.3 *Structures of benzoic and phenylacetic acids and the mechanism of their excretion of waste nitrogen.*

Table 28.1 *Treatment of acute hyperammonemia in neonatal period* *

Item	Action
1.	Nothing by mouth. No nitrogen intake. Start infusion of 10% glucose.
2.	Priming infusion containing 0.2–0.8 g arginine hydrochloride**/kg, 0.25 g sodium benzoate/kg and 0.25 mg sodium phenylacetate/kg in ca. 30 mL 10% glucose/kg over 1–2 hours.***
3.	Continuing infusion of 0.25 g sodium benzoate and sodium phenylacetate***/kg per 24 hours and 0.2–0.8 g arginine hydrochloride/kg in 10% glucose and maintenance electrolyte in sufficient volume to be given over 24 hours.
4.	Alert teams for hemodialysis, which must be instituted if pharmacological therapy is not successful and is often required in the initial neonatal episode, when the level of ammonia may be above 3–4 times the upper limit of normal by the time of diagnosis.
	Alert neurosurgeon, as intracranial pressure monitor will be needed if intracranial pressure is increased. Mannitol is used for increased intracranial pressure.
5.	If concentration of ammonia rises during pharmacologic therapy, start a second priming infusion while preparing to institute dialysis.
6.	Pyridoxine (5 mg) and folic acid (0.1 mg) parenterally q.d.

* Treatment of the initial episode before definitive diagnosis is established.
** Higher doses of arginine are employed in patients with citrullinemia and argininosuccinic aciduria (Chapters 31,32).
*** Both sodium benzoate and phenylacetate may be omitted in some patients with citrullinemia and most patients with argininosuccinic aciduria, especially in the treatment of an intercurrent episode that is diagnosed promptly before the serum concentration of ammonia exceeds 200 μmol/L.
Zofran may be given as an antiemetic (0.15 mg/kg intravenously) during first 15 min of the priming infusion.

true in citrullinemia or argininosuccinic aciduria, but it is also true of patients with OTC deficiency in which a variant enzyme permits activity of the urea cycle as long as the cycle does not run out of ornithine substrate. Females with OTC deficiency, with one normal X chromosome seldom completely inactivated, can respond to arginine alone. The effect of arginine as an activator of carbamyl phosphate synthetase should also be salubrious for patients with OTC deficiency, citrullinemia, and argininosuccinic aciduria. Operationally, for arginine as well as benzoate and or phenylacetate, a priming infusion is followed by a regimen of continuous infusion until the ammonia has reached the normal range (Table 28.1). The use of mannitol for cerebral edema may also provide nitrogen excretion through diuresis in patients treated with benzoate, phenylacetate and arginine.

The pharmacologic regimen is started on diagnosis in the acute neonatal hyperammonemic crisis and can be pursued while the dialysis team is being assembled. It may be effective in obviating the need for dialysis despite calculations that have been publicized [19]. It is usually effective in the management of recurrent episodes of hyperammonemia that occur in patients under therapy [17] at times of infection or other cause of catabolism, or vomiting, leading to an inability to continue oral treatment, because therapy of these episodes is generally initiated more promptly. It is also true that many patients successfully treated initially have died in later episodes of intercurrent hyperammonemia. The ideal approach to management is very early diagnosis so that hyperammonemia is prevented or treated before there is major elevation of the serum concentration of ammonia.

The drugs are supplied as concentrated solutions, which would cause hyperosmolarity if infused directly. They are diluted in 30 mL/kg of 10 percent glucose for the priming infusion and later diluted in the 24-hour maintenance fluids, which are also 10 percent with respect to glucose, providing extra calories to spare catabolism. When the sensorium clears, and there is no vomiting, further calories can be provided by nasogastric tube in the form of polycose or Mead Johnson product 80056 or Ross product Prophree usually diluted to supply 0.7 kcal/mL. Nitrogen intake is not resumed until the hyperammonemia has receded.

Long-term management of the hyperammonemic infant or child usually requires a combination of pharmacologic therapy and restriction of the intake of protein. Arginine is employed in doses of 0.4 to 0.7 g/kg. In OTC and carbamyl phosphate synthetase deficiencies sodium benzoate is given in doses of 0.25 to 0.5 g/kg/day, and citrulline, which is more palatable, is employed as a source of ornithine in a dose of 0.17 to 0.25 g/kg. Oral sodium phenylbutyrate has been employed as a source of phenylacetate in doses of 0.45 to 0.60 g/kg. It may be used as a substitute for benzoate, but many of our patients have found it unpalatable. A gastrostomy may be required. Protein is generally restricted to 0.7 g/kg and supplemented with 0.7 g/kg of a mixture of essential amino acids. We have felt that the optimal intake of whole protein should be determined in each patient and have found

supplementation with relatively small amounts of alanine to be effective [20], but in urea cycle defects, extra essential amino acids are often necessary. Treatment is continued with oral folate 0.1 mg/kg and pyridoxine 5 mg. The former is employed to enhance transamination and the latter to promote the synthesis of glycine; both have elements in the success of therapy.

Chronic management of patients with urea cycle defects has also been effective using mixtures of the keto and hydroxyacid analogs of essential amino acids [21]. These mixtures are no longer available in the US, but there may still be a place for this anabolic approach to the removal of nitrogen, and long-term therapy in which keto acids were combined with benzoate in the successful treatment of a 30-month-old infant who at report was developing normally [15]. In this patient nocturnal gavage was useful in the administration of the keto acids, arginine and benzoate.

Follow-up of 20 children treated with pharmacologic therapy who had a variety of defects of urea synthesis revealed a substantial 92 percent one-year survival, but 79 percent had significant developmental disability, and the mean IQ was 43 [22]. A significant and linear negative correlation was found between the duration of neonatal hyperammonemic coma and the IQ at 12 months. The peak level of neonatal hyperammonemia did not correlate significantly with later IQ. In this series of patients there were seven infants with ornithine transcarbamylase deficiency; two of the males died in hyperammonemic coma before 1 year-of-age. Computed tomography (CT) scans on the children in this series revealed considerable evidence of cerebral atrophy. There was a significant correlation between the presence of abnormalities seen on CT and the duration of neonatal hyperammonemic coma. The presence of abnormalities in the CT scan also correlated significantly with the ultimately determined IQ. Infants who were more than 5 days in hyperammonemic coma were invariably handicapped developmentally. In a more recent compilation of experience with 120 patients with OTC deficiency, Saudubray, Rabier and Kamoun [23] found that of 40 neonatally presenting patients, 39 male and one female, all had died, some after a few years of treatment. Of 36 late onset males, 19 died before the diagnosis was made, and 17 were alive, 11 normal and 6 with moderate sequelae. Of 37 late onset females, 26 were alive, 7 normal, of which 3 had had a liver transplantation; 14 had moderate sequelae, 5 major sequelae, and 11 had died, some after the diagnosis had been made.

References

1 Grisolia S, Baguena R, Mayor F. *The Urea Cycle.* John Wiley and Sons, New York;1976.

2 Lowenthal A, Mori A, Marescau B (eds). *Urea Cycle Diseases.* Advanced Experimental Medicine and Biology, Vol 153. Plenum Press, New York;1982.

3 Ballard RA, Vinocur B, Reynolds JW, *et al.* Transient hyperammonemia of the preterm infant. *N Engl J Med* 1978;**299**:920.

4 Marsden D, Sege-Peterson K, Nyhan WL, *et al.* An unusual presentation of medium-chain acyl coenzyme. A dehydrogenase deficiency. *Am J Dis Child* 1992;**146**:1459.

5   Nyhan WL. *Abnormalities in Amino Acid Metabolism in Clinical Medicine.* Appleton-Century-Crofts, E Norwalk Conn;1984:267.

6   Christadolu J, Qureshi IA, McInnes RR, Clarke JTR. Ornithine transcarbamylase deficiency presenting with stroke-like episodes. *J Pediatr* 1993;**122**:423.

7   Snyderman SE, Sansaricq C, Phansalkar SV, *et al.* The therapy of hyperammonemia due to ornithine transcarbamylase deficiency in a male neonate. *Pediatrics* 1975;**56**:65.

8   Oizumi J, Ng WG, Koch R, *et al.* Partial ornithine transcarbamylase deficiency associated with recurrent hyperammonemia lethargy and depressed sensorium. *Clin Genet* 1984;**25**:538.

9   Donn SM, Swartz RD, Thoene JG. Comparison of exchange transfusion peritoneal dialysis and hemodialysis for the treatment of hyperammonemia in an anuric newborn infant. *J Pediatr* 1979;**95**:67.

10 Wiegand C, Thompson T, Bock GH, *et al.* The management of life-threatening hyperammonemia: A comparison of several therapeutic modalities. *J Pediatr* 1980;**96**:142.

11 Kiley JE, Pender JC, Welsch HF, Weslch CS. Ammonia intoxication treated by hemodialysis. *N Engl J Med* 1958;**259**:1156.

12 Nyhan WL, Wolff J, Kulovich S, Schumacher A. Intestinal obstruction due to peritoneal adhesions as a complication of peritoneal dialysis for neonatal hyperammonemia. *Eur J Pediatr* 1985;**143**:211.

13 Summar M. Current strategies for the management of neonatal urea cycle disorders. *Pediatrics* 2001;**138**:S31.

14 Batshaw ML, Brusilow SW. Treatment of hyperammonemic coma caused by inborn errors of urea synthesis. *J Pediatr* 1980;**97**:893.

15 Guibaud P, Baxter P, Bourgeois J, *et al.* Severe ornithine transcarbamylase deficiency. Two and a half years' survival with normal development. *Arch Dis Child* 1984;**59**:477.

16 Nyhan WL. Urea cycle: in *Abnormalities in Amino Acid Metabolism in Clinical Medicine.* Appleton-Century-Crofts, E Norwalk Conn; 1984:267.

17 Brusilow SW, Danney M, Waber LJ, *et al.* Treatment of episodic hyperammonemia in children with inborn errors of urea synthesis. *N Engl J Med* 1983;**310**:1620.

18 Batshaw ML, Brusilow S, Waber L, *et al.* Treatment of inborn errors of urea synthesis: activation of alternative pathways of waste nitrogen synthesis and excretion. *N Engl J Med* 1982;**306**:1387.

19 Brusilow SW, Horwich AL. Urea cycle enzymes: in *The Metabolic and Molecular Bases of Inherited Disease* (eds CR Scriver, *et al.*) Mc Graw Hill Inc, New York;1976:1187.

20 Wolff J, Kelts DG, Algert S, *et al.* Alanine decreases the protein requirements of infants with inborn errors of amino acid metabolism. *J Neurogenet* 1985;**2**:41.

21 Thoene J, Batshaw M, Spector E, *et al.* Neonatal citrullinemia: Treatment with keto-analogues of essential amino acids. *Pediatrics* 1977;**90**:218.

22 Msall M, Batshaw ML, Suss R, *et al.* Neurologic outcome in children with inborn errors of urea synthesis. *N Engl J Med* 1984;**310**:1500.

23 Saudubray JM, Rabier D, Kamoun P. French experience of the long term outcome of OTC deficiencies from 120 cases diagnosed by enzymatic measurement. 1996. (Personal communication of manuscript in preparation).

Ornithine transcarbamylase deficiency

MAJOR PHENOTYPIC EXPRESSION

Potentially lethal hyperammonemic coma in the male and varying expression in the female, consistent with X-linked transmission; convulsions; elevated concentrations of glutamine and alanine; orotic aciduria; and defective activity of hepatic ornithine-transcarbamylase.

INTRODUCTION

The most classic of the infantile urea cycle presentations is that of ornithine transcarbamylase (OTC) deficiency in the male. Onset is in the neonatal period with coma and or convulsions, and in the absence of effective intervention it is rapidly fatal. A small number of males with variant enzymes has a milder and later presentation. Females who have two X chromosomes have varying phenotypes depending on the proportion of active and inactive X chromosomes.

The enzyme ornithine transcarbamylase or ornithine carbamoyl transferase (OCT) (EC 2.1.33) is found almost exclusively in liver. There is lesser activity in small intestine and a small amount in brain. The hepatic enzyme is located in the mitochondria [1]. The enzyme is a trimer in which identical subunits have a molecular weight of about 38 KD [2–4]. The OTC enzyme is synthesized in the cytosol and transported to its mitochondrial site of activity. The protein synthesized contains an N-terminal signal peptide that is specifically recognized by a receptor complex in the outer mitochondrial membrane [5]. After translocation across the membranes, proteolytic processing by two peptidases yields the mature protein [6]. Once imported into the mitochondria the OTC subunits require folding to form the active trimer, and this process is mediated by molecular chaperones.

Defective activity of the enzyme is readily demonstrable in biopsied liver [7–10]. The gene on the X-chromosome codes for the precursor protein that is imported after translation into mitochondria. The human OTC precursor cDNA has been isolated and cloned [11]. It is localized to band p2.1 in the short arm [12], just proximal to the locus for Duchenne muscular dystrophy. The genes for glycerol kinase, adrenal insufficiency, chronic granulomatous disease, Norrie disease and retinitis pigmentosa are all in this area, and a number of contiguous gene syndromes have resulted from deletions. Deletions account for about 16 percent of affected males [13]. Another 10 percent have point mutations in a TaqI recognition site in exon 5 in (TCGA) which changes the code for arginine at position 109 of the mature protein and changes it to either glutamine or a stop codon and reduces enzyme activity to one percent of normal or less [14,15]. Many other point mutations have established an enormous heterogeneity.

CLINICAL ABNORMALITIES

Ornithine transcarbamylase deficiency in its usual presentation in the neonatal male infant (Figure 29.1) provides the classic picture of a defect in the urea cycle (Figure 28.1) [16,17]. Prior to the recent development of pharmacologic approaches to the

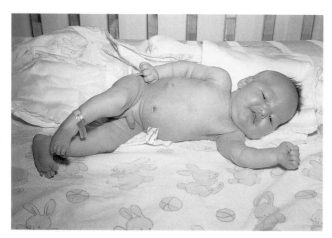

Figure 29.1   J.N., a male infant with ornithine transcarbamylase deficiency after recovery from neonatal hyperammonemia. The site of a Tenckoff catheter that had been unsuccessfully used for peritoneal dialysis is evident on the abdomen.

removal of waste nitrogen using benzoate and phenylacetate this disorder was always fatal, and usually within just a few days of birth. The mortality is still high.

Affected infants are often thought to have sepsis. Occasionally, the diagnosis of hyperammonemia is made once blood culture is found to be negative. On the other hand, we have encountered neonates with urea cycle defects who have actually had sepsis, further confusing the diagnosis. It is therefore advisable to obtain blood for ammonia in any infant in coma. A bulging fontanel may suggest intracranial hemorrhage, but it is more often the result of cerebral edema, and computed tomography (CT) scan should resolve the issue.

The infant appears normal at birth and remains so during a period of hiatus, which may be as short as a few hours and is seldom longer than 48 hours. He then begins to be lethargic and to refuse feedings. Grunting or rapid respirations may occur, and there may be a respiratory alkalosis. Convulsions may be generalized, and the electroencephalogram (EEG) is usually abnormal. The infant may be hypertonic, but there is progression to a deep coma that is indistinguishable from surgical anesthesia. Ultimately the infant stops breathing, and unless he is intubated and artificially ventilated, he dies. Despite initial improvement following dialysis or other interventions, which decrease ammonia concentrations, most of these patients have died. Those surviving because of successful pharmacologic therapy have usually had severe mental retardation, if the initial hyperammonemic coma has been profound and prolonged. Most have had recurrent hyperammonemic crises at times of catabolism induced by intercurrent illness, and each further episode appears to worsen the prognosis for mental development. If, in a family at risk, the diagnosis can be made prior to hyperammonemic coma and the patient prevented from ever having such an episode, then the development of the nervous system should be normal, but patients fitting these criteria among males with the classic form of OTC deficiency, have not yet been described. It still may be the rule rather than the exception for those patients who survive the neonatal attack to die in

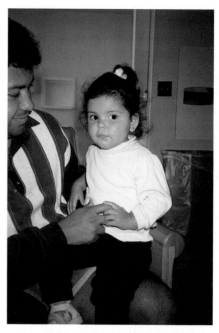

Figure 29.2   T.C., a 2-year-old girl with OTC deficiency. During infancy she had many episodes of hyperammonemia despite therapy with arginine, benzoate and phenylacetate, but each was treated promptly, and cognitive development was good. Nevertheless, she died in a subsequent hyperammonemic episode.

infancy in a subsequent hyperammonemic episode that accompanies an acute infection.

The major metabolic characteristic of patients with ornithine transcarbamylase deficiency is hyperammonemia. Levels found in the classic neonatal form of the disease are usually over 700 μmol/L (1000 μg/dL). Coma is generally present when the concentration exceeds 250 μmol/L (400 μg/dL). In infants dying of the disease, levels may range from 400 to 1700 μmol/L (600 to 2500 μg/dL). In the presence of levels over 300 μmol/L (500 μg/dL) one sees fixed dilated pupils and complete apnea. Cerebral edema occurs in some patients at these levels. Normal neonatal ammonia is <50 μmol/L. On the other hand, it is not uncommon to observe levels up to 100 μmol/L in normal infants. Problems in obtaining and handling blood samples invariably raise levels, and exercise such as squeezing a ball, can raise the level to 150 μmol/L [18]. Thus a normal level eliminates hyperammonemia, but an abnormal that does not fit with clinical findings may have to be repeated or confirmed by the presence of an elevated glutamine. Consensus has not been reached as to a specific neonatal level that should prompt intravenous therapy. Consensus was also not reached on the necessity for intravenous therapy for mild elevations of ammonia in chronically treated patients [18].

In the female the range of variation in symptomatology is very great [19–23] (Figure 29. 2). This is consistent with varying degrees of inactivation of the normal X chromosome called for by lyonization as a random process. Among these patients delay in diagnosis is common. In a series of 13 the mean interval from onset of symptoms to diagnosis was 16 months, and the range was one to 142 months. [19]. At one end of the spectrum are a small number of female infants with an overwhelming clinical picture indistinguishable from that of the male and leading to death in infancy. Others only somewhat less severe have had episodes of recurrent hyperammonemia followed by death in childhood. Others have had recurrent vomiting beginning in infancy or as late as 9 years-of-age [20]. This condition should be included in the differential diagnosis of cyclic vomiting. Attacks may be accompanied by headache, slurring of speech, or screaming. An attack may also present with ataxia. A patient with recurrent episodes of intense headache and ataxia may appear to have migraine. During the attack the patient may display muscular rigidity or opisthotonus. There may be convulsions. Any patient with ornithine transcarbamylase deficiency and symptomatic attacks of hyperammonemia may develop coma, and this may go on to death. Hepatomegaly is seen in some patients, and there may be abnormalities in liver function tests. In an older child seen for the first time with hyperammonemia these findings may be thought at first to represent primary disease of the liver. OTC deficiency has on occasion been initially diagnosed as Reye syndrome [21]. Attacks may be precipitated by a large intake of protein, infection, surgery or immunization. Mental retardation may be progressive with further episodes.

At the other end of the spectrum are women who are completely asymptomatic. They are found to be heterozygous for deficiency of ornithine transcarbamylase because a male son or other relative is found to have the classic disease. Some of these women have a dislike of protein foods and thus have not stressed the system. Others appear to have no trouble with protein. Nevertheless, a careful study of the IQ scores of heterozygotes, identified by the urinary excretion of orotic acid following a protein load, were found to be 6 to 10 points lower than in the controls, who were relatives in whom the orotic acid test was negative [23].

Some males have been reported in whom there was a much milder or late onset clinical phenotype, similar to that described in females. These patients appear to represent variants different from the classic one in that they have a defect in the enzyme that leads to partial activity [24–32]. Prominent symptoms are recurrent vomiting, lethargy, irritability and protein avoidance. A patient with one of these variants may have normal development and may progress normally in school [26,28]. The disease may present in adulthood [30]. It may present with bizarre behavior [30,31]. In fact, recurrent episodes of bizarre behavior may be the only symptoms of this type of OTC deficiency [30]. Measurement of orotic acid and orotidine even after allopurinol or a protein load failed to elucidate the diagnosis in this patient, but a high protein diet led to orotic aciduria. In the late onset male, as in the symptomatic female, the disease is nevertheless potentially lethal, and death may ultimately occur in a hyperammonemic episode even after a number of symptom-free years. In a series of 21 male patients who presented at ages ranging from 2 months to 44 years, 43 percent died [32]. The mean interval from the age at onset to that at diagnosis was 8.8 months, with a range of up to 54 months. An initial diagnosis of Reye syndrome was made in

52 percent of the patients. Among complications of OTC deficiency, sudden strokes have been reported [33]. This has also been seen in carbamylphosphate synthetase (CPS) deficiency and an enlarging group of metabolic diseases.

The diagnosis is suspected on the basis of the blood level of ammonia and suspicions are confirmed by elevations in glutamine and often alanine. An algorithmic approach to the exclusion of nonurea cycle causes of hyperammonemia and the differentiation among specific urea cycle defects (Chapter 28) identifies those disorders in which a specific amino acid, such as citrulline, is elevated. Elevated excretion of orotic acid then differentiates OTC deficiency from that of CPS in which orotic acid levels are normal. Definitive diagnosis of OTC deficiency usually requires assay of the enzyme in biopsied liver. Disorders of fatty acid oxidation may have an identical Reye-like presentation and meet all of the conditions for a diagnosis of OTC deficiency except that the enzyme activity of the liver is normal [34]. If the mutation in a family is known, analysis of the DNA will make the diagnosis.

GENETICS AND PATHOGENESIS

The gene for ornithine transcarbamylase is located on the X chromosome [11,12]. The disease is expressed as an X-linked dominant. Thus, in females in whom a major proportion of cells contain the inactivated normal X chromosome the severity of disease may be as great as in the hemizygous male. At the other end of the spectrum, even asymptomatic female heterozygotes may have lower IQs than their homozygous normal relatives [23].

The molecular defect in ornithine transcarbamylase is readily detected in the liver. This enzyme is also expressed in intestinal mucosa, and therefore the diagnosis has been made by assay of tissue obtained by rectal or duodenal biopsy [35]. However, the gold standard is the assay of biopsied liver.

In males with the lethal neonatal disease, enzyme activity is virtually absent [7–10]. In males with the partial variants, levels range from five to 25 percent of normal [26,27,36,37]. Some of these patients have been reported to have virtually zero activity [38,39], but this is not likely to reflect the level of activity that is functional in vivo. Abnormal proteins tend to be unstable and break down readily under conditions of in vitro assays. In symptomatic heterozygous females levels of activity range from four to 25 percent of normal [8]. As much as 97 percent of normal activity has been found in known heterozygous mothers of affected children. Because the female is a mosaic of hepatocytes, the level of activity found in a biopsy may not necessarily reflect the in vivo activity of their conglomerate, but the diagnosis should nevertheless be clear. In some males with partial variants the kinetic properties of the enzyme have been studied [40–42]. These variant enzymes have been found to have alterations in the K_m for ornithine or carbamyl phosphate or the optimal pH. The use of antibody prepared against the normal human enzyme has shown no cross-reacting material (CRM) in most hemizygous males, but a few were CRM positive [42].

The cloning of the gene for OTC [11] and the elucidation of its structure [43] has permitted the identification of more than 150 different mutations more [44–46]. The incidence of new mutation in the genesis of girls with OTC deficiency has been much greater than in boys [47] suggesting that mutation is more common in sperm than in ova. Among males only two of 28 had sporadic mutations, while some 95 percent inherited their mutations from their mothers. Among females only 20 percent inherited their mutations from their mothers. A mother found not to carry the mutant allele in a child could have gonadal mosaicism. This was found in a somatically normal woman who produced multiple affected males [48]. Fortunately this is very rare.

A very great amount of heterogeneity has been identified. Most families have had unique mutations. Large deletions of an exon or more were found in seven percent of families, and small deletions or insertions in 15 percent [13]. Most families have had point mutations; of families with nucleotide substitutions, less than half had mutations seen in at least one other family. All but two of these recurrent mutations occurred in CpG dinucleotides, and the mutations were spread over many of the CpG dinucleotides. The most frequent mutation was the R129H mutation in which a G to A change at the end of exon 4 replaces an arginine with a histidine. This relatively neutral substitution causes abnormal splicing and very low activity [49]. The identical mutation occurs in the *spf-ash* mouse [50]. Some correlation of phenotype and genotype are emerging. For instance, a Tyr 167 stop [51] led to truncation with loss of the ornithine binding residues, a complete loss of activity of OTC and hyperammonemic death at four days of life. A mutation reported [52] in the leader peptide region, which would lead to failure to enter the mitochondria, led to a severe neonatal phenotype and an absence of OTC activity in liver.

Defective activity of the hepatic enzyme has been documented in heterozygotes; and histochemical assay of the enzyme demonstrated the presence of two populations of hepatic cells, one normal and one deficient in the activity of ornithine transcarbamylase deficiency [53], consistent with the Lyon hypothesis. Heterozygosity has also been documented by assay of the enzyme in duodenal mucosa [54]. This method has failed to detect some known heterozygotes.

Heterozygosity has been detected by assay of the urine for orotic acid following a load of 1 g/kg of protein [23,54,55]. Urine is usually collected in three four-hour aliquots following the load. More reproducible results may be obtained using an alanine load [56]. However, it is clear that the 0.7 g/kg dose that was initially employed was too large. Such a dose can lead to alarming symptoms in a heterozygote. It also may overwhelm the system in a normal and lead to a false positive diagnosis of heterozygosity. We used [56] 0.4 g/kg along with a very sensitive method for orotic acid using stable isotope dilution, and selected ion monitoring gas chromatography-mass spectrometry [57]. Both protein and alanine loading have largely been supplanted now by the allopurinol test [58]. Allopurinol inhibits the decarboxylation of orotidine monophosphate

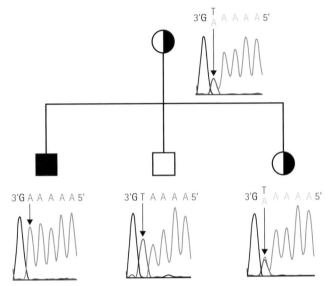

Figure 29.3   *Kindred in which an A to T mutation in exon 9 of the OTC gene specified a leucine 301 phenylalanine replacement in the enzyme was identified in three individuals in two generations. The proband had a variant late onset phenotype [60]. In each of the heterozygotes, testing for orotic acid and/or orotidine after allopurinol failed to detect heterozygosity.*

(orotidylate) (OMP) (Figure 28.1) via reaction of its phosphorylated oxidation product on the decarboxylase. When OMP accumulates it is reflected in the urine in the excretion of orotidine and orotic acid. The specificity of the test was reported to be greater when orotidine was measured than when orotic acid was measured [58]. If the mutation is known it can be effectively employed in heterozygote detection, but the enormous amount of variation in OTC deficiency often tends to make this impractical.

The ability to determine carrier status by mutational analysis (Figure 29.3) has made it clear that the allopurinol test, which was designed in families of patients with classic neonatal OTC deficiencies, is not reliable in the families of male patients with variant phenotypes [59,60]. In a series of 18 asymptomatic carriers three genotypic heterozygotes were not identified by allopurinnol testing [61]. In some instances the nature of the mutation cannot be identified. In these families linkage analysis is sometimes useful, taking advantage of restriction fragment length polymorphism. The possibility of gonadal mosaicism should be remembered in any diagnosis that a woman is not a carrier. Heterozygote detection has also been carried out for diagnostic purposes in a symptomatic girl by the ratio of transfer of administered ^{15}N-glutamine to ^{15}N-urea (^{15}N-U/G ratio) [62].

Prenatal diagnosis has been carried out by assay of the enzyme in biopsied fetal liver [63]. The risk of fetal loss makes assay for the gene much more satisfactory. Prenatal diagnosis has been carried out by assay for the *Taq*I cleavage site [64], and by assay for mutations known in probands. Certainly if precise mutation analysis is available, it should always be employed in prenatal diagnosis.

Table 29.1 *Chronic management of OTC deficiency*

	(g/kg/24 hr)			
Citrulline	Na phenylbutyrate*	Na benzoate*	Whole protein	Essential amino acids
0.170–0.250	0.450–0.600	0.250–0.500	0.7	0.7

*Na benzoate or Na phenylbutyrate are given, usually not both, but some patients have been treated with both.

TREATMENT

The treatment of the acute hyperammonemic episode, long term management, and the results of treatment have been set out in detail in Chapter 28. In the neonatal hyperammonemia of OTC deficiency the most vigorous intervention is required and even then it is often impossible to avoid death or severe neurologic disability. In neonatal onset urea cycle defects best results have been achieved in females in whom prenatal diagnosis is made, but even in these patients the risk of sudden death or disability is always present.

Most hyperammonemic infants with OTC deficiency require hemodialysis [65], and extracorporeal membrane oxygenation (ECMO) is probably preferable. Pharmacologic therapy with intravenous sodium benzoate/phenylacetate and arginine are initiated promptly and pursued vigorously. The management of intercurrent episodes of hyperammonemia in a patient rescued from the initial neonatal episode is similar, but it is hoped that treatment may be initiated promptly enough to abort the episode without the need for dialysis.

In OTC deficiency the priming infusion contains sodium benzoate acid and phenylacetate 0.25 g/kg each and 0.2 g/kg of arginine · HCl (2 mL/kg of a 10 percent solution). The sustaining infusion given over the next 24 hours has the same content of each.

In chronic management of OTC deficiency (Table 29.1) citrulline is substituted for arginine, as it is more palatable. Most patients are also treated with phenylbutyrate [66] as a source of phenylacetate, which has been thought to minimize the unpleasant odor of phenylacetate. However, phenylbutyrate is, to many, so unpalatable that a gastrostomy tube is required in order to avoid poor compliance and even then patients complain of a taste. For these reasons sodium benzoate is preferred by some patients and some authorities.

The prognosis in OTC deficiency is always guarded. In the neonatal onset hyperammonemic phenotype virtually all have died [67]. Later onset patients are nearly all female. Many of these have also died or developed major neurologic disability.

These considerations have led to the use of orthotopic transplantation of the liver [62,67,68]. Experience has been that following transplantation, levels of ammonia are no longer a problem and that protein restriction and medications to handle waste nitrogen are no longer required. Balancing the risks of the transplantation becomes a factor in later onset girls, but there is little question in patients with infantile presentations, that the risk of the disease is much higher. Technical problems make it difficult to transplant liver much before 1 year-of-age. In this way most neonatal onset males would be excluded. The use of living donor transplantation and split liver or auxiliary liver transplantation should decrease the time waiting for transplantation and increase the possibility of application before the intervention of death or severe disability.

References

1 Merker HJ. Electron microscopic demonstration of ornithine carbamyl transferase in rat liver. *Histochemia* 1969;**17**:83.

2 Marshall M, Cohen PP. Ornithine transcarbamylase from *Streptococcus faecalis* and bovine liver: I Isolation and subunit structure. *J Biol Chem* 1972;**247**:1961.

3 Clarke S. The polypeptides of rat liver mitochondria: identification of a 36 000 dalton polypeptide as the subunit of ornithine transcarbamylase. *Biochem Biophys Res Commun* 1976;**71**:1118.

4 Marshall M. Ornithine transcarbamylase from bovine liver: in *The Urea Cycle* (eds Grisolia S, Baguena R, Mayor F) John Wiley and Sons, New York;1976:169.

5 Horwich AL, Kalousek F, Fenton WA, *et al.* Targeting of pre-ornithine transcarbamylase to mitochondria: definition of critical regions and residues in the leader peptide. *Cell* 1986;**44**:451.

6 Kalousek F, Hendrick JP, Rosenberg LE. Two mitochondrial matrix proteases act sequentially in the processing of mammalian matrix enzymes. *Proc Natl Acad Sci USA* 1988;**85**:7536.

7 Campbell AGM, Rosenberg LE, Snodgrass PJ, Nuzum CT. Ornithine transcarbamylase deficiency. A cause of lethal neonatal hyperammonemia in males. *N Engl J Med* 1973;**288**:1.

8 Short EM, Conn HO, Snodgrass PJ, *et al.* Evidence for X-linked dominant inheritance of ornithine transcarbamylase deficiency. *N Engl J Med* 1973;**288**:7.

9 Kang ES, Snodgrass PJ, Gerald PS. Ornithine transcarbamylase deficiency in the newborn. *J Pediatr* 1973;**82**:642.

10 Goldstein AS, Hoogenraad HJ, Johnson JD, *et al.* Metabolic and genetic studies of a family with ornithine transcarbamylase (OTC) deficiency. *Pediatr Res* 1974;**8**:5.

11 Horwich AL, Fenton WA, Williams KR, *et al.* Structure and expression of a complementary DNA for the nuclear coded precursor of human mitochondrial ornithine transcarbamylase. *Science* 1984;**224**:1068.

12 Lindgren V, De Martinville B, Horwich AL, *et al.* Human ornithine transcarbamylase locus mapped to band Xp211 near the Duchenne muscular dystrophy locus. *Science* 1984;**226**:698.

13 Tuchman M, Morizono H, Rajagopal BS, *et al.* The biochemical and molecular spectrum of ornithine transcarbamylase deficiency. *J Inherit Metab Dis* 1998;**21**:(Suppl) 40.

14 Maddalena A, Edward SJ, O'Brien WE, Nussbaum RL. Characterization of point mutations in the same arginine codon in three unrelated patients with ornithine transcarbamylase deficiency. *J Clin Invest* 1988;**82**:1353.

15 Grompe M, Caskey CT, Fenwick RG. Improved molecular diagnostics for ornithine transcarbamylase deficiency. *Am J Hum Genet* 1991;**48**:212.

16 Leviin B, Oberholzer VG, Sinclair L. Biochemical investigations of hyperammonaemia. *Lancet* 1969;**2**:170.

17 Brusilow SW, Batshaw ML, Waber L. Neonatal hyperammonemic coma. *Adv In Pediatr* 1982;**29**:69.

18 The urea cycle disorders. Conference proceedings of a consensus conference for the management of patients with urea cycle disorders. *J Pediatr* 2001;**138**:S1–S80.

19 Rowe PC, Newman SL, Brusilow SW. Natural history of symptomatic partial ornithine transcarbamylase deficiency. *N Engl J Med* 1986;**314**:541.

20 Russell A, Levin B, Oberholzer VG, Sinclair L. Hyperammonaemia. A new instance of an inborn enzymatic defect of the biosynthesis of urea. *Lancet* 1962;**2**:699.

21 Rowe PC, Valle D, Brusilow SW. Inborn errors of metabolism in children referred with Reye's syndrome. *JAMA* 1988;**260**:3167.

22 Arn PH, Hauser ER, Thomas GH, *et al.* Hyperammonemia in women with a mutation at the ornithine carbamoyl transferase locus: a cause of post-partum coma. *N Engl J Med* 1990;**322**:1652.

23 Batshaw ML, Roan Y, Jung AL, *et al.* Cerebral dysfunction in asymptomatic carriers of ornithine transcarbamylase deficiency. *N Engl J Med* 1980;**302**:482.

24 Cathelineau L, Briand P, Petit F, *et al.* Kinetic analysis of a new ornithine transcarbamylase variant. *Biochim Biophys Acta* 1980;**614**:40.

25 Haan EA, Banks DM, Hoogenraad NJ, Roger JG. Hereditary hyperammonemic syndromes – a six year experience. *Aust Pediatr J* 1979;**15**:142.

26 Oizumi J, Ng WG, Koch R, *et al.* Partial ornithine transcarbamylase deficiency associated with recurrent hyperammonemia lethargy and depressed sensorium. *Clin Genet* 1984;**25**:538.

27 MacLeod P, Mackenzie S, Scriver CR. Partial ornithine carbamyl transferase deficiency: an inborn error of the urea cycle presenting as orotic aciduria in a male infant. *Can Med Assoc J* 1972;**107**:405.

28 Yudkoff M, Yang W, Snodgrass PJ, Segal S. Ornithine transcarbamylase deficiency in a boy with normal development. *J Pediatr* 1980;**96**:441.

29 Tallan HH, Shaffner F, Taffet SL, *et al.* Ornithine carbamoyl transferase deficiency in an adult male: significance of hepatic ultrastrucutre in clinical diagnosis. *Pediatrics* 1983;**71**:224.

30 Dimagno EP, Lowe JE, Snodgrass PJ, Jones JD. Ornithine transcarbamylase deficiency – a cause of bizarre behavior in man. *N Engl J Med* 1986;**315**:744.

31 Spada M, Guardamagna O, Rabier D, *et al.* Recurrrent episodes of bizarre behavior in a boy with ornithine transcarbamylase deficiency: diagnostic failure of protein loading and allopurinol challenge tests. *J Pediatr* 1994;**125**:249.

32 Finkelstein JE, Hauser ER, Leonard CO, Brusilow SW. Late-onset ornithine transcarbamylase deficiency in male patients. *J Pediatr* 1990;**117**:897.

33 Christadolu J, Qureshi IA, McInnes RR, Clarke JTR. Ornithine trans-carbamylase deficiency presenting with stroke-like episodes. *J Pediatr* 1993;**122**:423.

34 Marsden D, Sege-Peterson J, Nyhan WL, *et al.* An unusual presentation of medium-chain acyl coenzyme A dehydrogenase deficiency. *Am J Dis Child* 1992;**146**:1459.

35 Matsushima A, Orii T. The activity of carbamylphosphate synthetase I (CPS I) and ornithine transcarbamylase (OTC) in the intestine and the screening of OTC deficiency in the rectal mucosa. *J Inherit Metab Dis* 1981;**4**:83.

36 Cathelineau L, Saudubray JM, Navarro J, Polonovski C. Transmission par le chromosome X du gene de structure 1-ornithine carbamyl transferase. Etude de trois familles. *Ann Genet* 1973;**16**:173.

37 Levin B, Dobbs RH, Burgess EA, Palmer T. Hyperammonaemia. A variant of deficiency of liver ornithine transcarbamylase. *Arch Dis Child* 1969;**44**:162.

38 Krieger I, Snodgrass PJ, Roskamo J. Atypical clinical course of ornithine transcarbamylase deficiency due to a new mutant (comparison with Reye's disease). *J Clin Endocrinol Metab* 1979;**48**:338.

39 Matsuda I, Arashima S, Nambu H, *et al.* Hyperammonemia due to a mutant enzyme of ornithine transcarbamylase. *Pediatrics* 1971;**48**:595.

40 Cathelineau L, Saudubray JM, Polonovski C. Ornithine carbamyl transferase: the effects of pH on the kinetics of a mutant human enzyme. *Clin Chim Acta* 1972;**41**:305.

41 Cathelineau L, Saudubray JM, Polonovski C. Heterogeneous mutations of the structural gene of human ornithine carbamyl transferase as observed in five personal cases. *Enzyme* 1974;**18**:103.

42 Briand P, Francois B, Rabier D, Cathelineau L. Ornithine transcarbamylase deficiencies in human males. Kinetic and immunochemical classification. *Biochim Biophys Acta* 1981;**704**:100.

43 Hata A, Tsuzuki T, Shimada K, *et al.* Structure of the human ornithine transcarbamylase gene. *J Biochem* 1988;**103**:302.

44 Tuchman M, Plante RJ, Garcia-Perez MG, Rubio V. Relative frequency of mutations causing ornithine transcarbamylase deficiency in 78 families. *Hum Genet* 1996;**96**:274.

45 Tuchman M. Mutations and polymorphisms in the human ornithine transcarbamylase gene. *Hum Mut* 1993;**2**:174.

46 Tuchman M, Plante RJ. Mutations and polymorphisms in the human ornithine transcarbamylase gene: Update addendum. (Review) *Hum Mut* 1995;**5**:293.

47 Tuchman M, Matsuda I, Munnich A, *et al.* Proportions of spontaneous mutations in males and females with ornithine transcarbamylase deficiency. *Am J Med Genet* 1995;**55**:67.

48 Bowling F, McGown I, Mcgill S, *et al.* Maternal gonadal mosaicism causing ornithine transcarbamylase deficiency. *Am Med Genet* 1999;**85**:452.

49 Garcia-Perez MA, Sanjuro P, Rubio V. Demonstration of the *spf-ash* mutation in Spanish patients with ornithine transcarbamylase deficiency of moderate severity. *Hum Gent* 1995;**95**:183.

50 Hodges PE, Rosenberg LE. The *spf-ash* mouse: a missense mutation in the ornithine transcarbamylase gene also causes aberrant mRNA splicing. *Proc Natl Acad Sci USA* 1989;**86**:4142.

51 Garcia-Perez MA, Sanjurjo P, Briones P, *et al.* A splicing mutation a nonsense mutation (Y167X) and two missense mutations (I159T and A209V) in Spanish patients with ornithine transcarbamylase deficiency. *Hum Genet* 1995;**96**:549.

52 Grompe M, Muzny DM, Caskey CT. Scanning detection of mutations in human ornithine transcarbamylase by chemical mismatch cleavage. *Proc Natl Acad Sci USA* 1989;**86**:5888.

53 Riciutti FC, Gelehrter TD, Rosenber LE. X-chromosome inactivation in human liver: confirmation of X-linkage of ornithine transcarbamylase. *Am J Hum Genet* 1976;**28**:332.

54 Haan EA, Danks DM, Grimes A, Hoogenraad NJ. Carrier detection in ornithine transcarbamylase deficiency. *J Inherit Metab Dis* 1982;**5**:37.

55 Hokanson JT, O'Brien WE, Idemoto J, Schafer IA. Carrier detection in ornithine transcarbamylase deficiency. *J Inherit Metab Dis* 1978;**93**:75.

56 Winter S, Sweetman L, Batshaw ML. Carrier detection in ornithine transcarbamylase deficiency using L-alanine loading test. *Clin Res* 1983;**31**:112A (abstract).

57 Jakobs C, Sweetman L, Nyhan WL, *et al.* Stable isotope dilution analysis of orotic acid and uracil in amniotic fluid. *Clin Chim Acta* 1984;**143**:1231.

58 Hauser ER, Finkelstein JE, Valle D, Brusilow SW. Allopurinol-induced orotidinuria: a test for mutations at the ornithine carbamoyl transferase locus in women. *N Engl J Med* 1990;**322**:1641.

59 Barshop BA, Nyhan WL, Climent C, Rubio V. Pitfalls in the detection of heterozygosity by allopurinol in a variant form of ornithine transcarbamylase deficiency. *J Inherit Metab Dis* 2001;**24**:513.

60 Capistrano-Estrada S, Nyhan WL, Marsden DJ, *et al.* Histopathological findings in a male with late-onset ornithine transcarbamylase deficiency. *Pediatr Pathol* 1994;**14**:235.

61 Maestri NE, Lord C, Glynn M, *et al*. The phenotype of ostensibly healthy women who are carriers for ornithine transcarbamylase deficiency. *Medicine* 1998;**77**:389.

62 Scaglia F, Zheng Q, O'Brien WE, *et al*. An integrated approach to the diagnosis and prospective management of partial ornithine transcarbamylase deficiency. *Pediatrics* 2002;**109**:150.

63 Rodeck CH, Patrick AD, Pembrey ME, *et al*. Fetal liver biopsy for prenatal diagnosis of ornithine carbamyl transferase deficiency. *Lancet* 1982;**2**:297.

64 Nussbaum RL, Boggs BA, Beaudet AL, *et al*. New mutation and prenatal diagnosis in ornithine transcarbamylase deficiency. *Am J Hum Genet* 1986;**38**:149.

65 Donn SM, Swartz RD, Thoene JG. Comparison of exchange transfusion peritoneal dialysis and hemodialysis for the treatment of hyperamonemia in an anuric newborn infant. *J Pediatr* 1979;**95**:67.

66 Batshaw M, MacArthur R, Tuchman M. Alternative pathway therapy for urea cycle disorders: twenty years later. *J Pediatrics* 2001;**138**:S46.

67 Saudubray JM, Rabier D, Kamoun P. French experience of the long term outcome of OTC deficiencies from 120 cases diagnosed by enzymatic measurement (Personal communication 1996).

68 Lee B, Goss J. Long-term correction of urea cycle disorders. *J Pediatrics* 2001;**138**:S63.

Carbamyl phosphate synthetase deficiency

MAJOR PHENOTYPIC EXPRESSION

Typical neonatal hyperammonemic crisis, hypocitrullinemia and absence of activity of hepatic carbamylphosphate synthetase.

INTRODUCTION

Carbamyl phosphate synthetase (CPS) (EC 6.3.4.16) (Figure 30.1) is a mitochondrial enzyme catalyzing the formation of carbamylphosphate from ammonia in what is generally considered to be the first step in the urea cycle. Its deficiency is quite rare, compared with ornithine transcarbamylase deficiency, and usually presents with potentially lethal neonatal hyperammonia [1]. There are even rarer mutations, which lead to partial residual activity and a later onset, even adult-onset pattern of disease [2].

Transcription of the gene takes place in the nucleus. The CPS mRNA is found essentially only in the liver, but enzyme activity has been demonstrated in intestinal mucosa. Translation in the cytoplasmic ribosome yields a precursor protein, which then undergoes a complex set of molecular events that eventuate in the appearance of CPS activity in the mitochondrial matrix. The enzyme is a very large dimer with subunits of 160 kDa. The fusion of the two domains joins subunits of striking homology in various species, even including *Escherichia coli* and yeast [3]. An amino terminal leader sequence targets the protein to the mitochondria and is highly basic because of its content of lysine and arginine residues. Following transport to the mitochondria, this sequence is cleaved to yield the mature protein [4–6]. The CPS enzyme constitutes 15 to 30 percent of the hepatic mitochondrial protein. A defect at any stage of the sequence from transcription and translocation to transport, uptake and processing could lead to loss of enzyme activity and clinical disease.

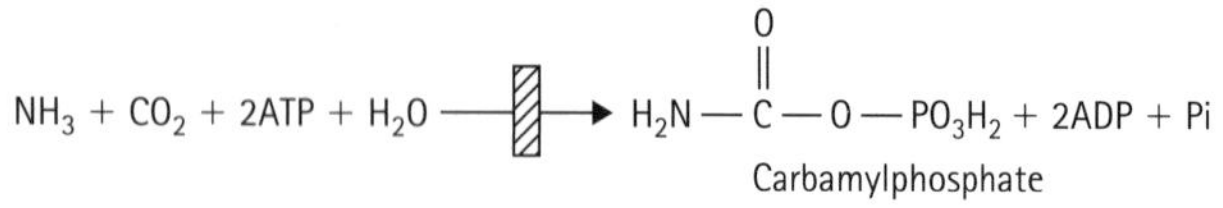

The human cDNA has been cloned and mapped to chromosome 2q35 [7,8]. To date only a few mutations have been reported, among them T1370G, and A2429G, which led to V457G and Q810R amino acid substitutions [8,9]. Molecular analysis revealed no immunoreactive enzyme and no translatable mRNA in some patients with lethal neonatal disease [10]. Gross alteration in the gene was not found in the six unrelated families studied [11]. A frequent restriction fragment length polymorphism (RFLP) is a useful genetic marker for linkage analysis in prenatal diagnosis and heterozygote detection [11].

CLINICAL ABNORMALITIES

The clinical abnormalities of CPS deficiency are indistinguishable from those of OTC deficiency (Chapter 29). In the usual situation, the infant is normal at birth and may do well for a period, usually until feedings begin. Then failure to feed well and lethargy develop. There may be grunting or rapid

$$NH_3 + CO_2 + 2ATP + H_2O \longrightarrow H_2N - \overset{\overset{\displaystyle O}{\|}}{C} - O - PO_3H_2 + 2ADP + Pi$$

Carbamylphosphate

Figure 30.1 *The carbamyl phosphate synthetase reaction. Acetylglutamate is an obligate activator of the enzyme.*

respiration, hypotonia or hypertonia, convulsions and hypothermia. This is rapidly progressive to deep coma, in which there is a complete unresponsiveness to stimuli. We have compared this state to surgical anesthesia. Apnea supervenes and the infant survives only with assisted ventilation. The history often reveals that siblings died very early in life.

A typical history was that of an infant who began to feed poorly, became lethargic, and had convulsions and an abnormal electroencephalogram [12]. She was admitted to hospital at 20 days. Two of her siblings had died with similar symptom at 4 weeks of age. Despite treatment with a low protein diet, she died at 7 months [12,13]. In similar fashion, a 2-month-old Japanese girl [2] had persistent vomiting from 7 days of life, was hypotonic and had an abnormal electroencephalogram and generalized cerebral cortical atrophy. Another full-term infant appeared normal at birth and was nursed at 10 hours; at 24 hours he developed profuse sweating and nursed poorly [1]. He had irritability, hypothermia and hypertonia, along with opisthotonus and ankle clonus. He developed coma and died at 75 hours of age. Of 20 patients reported with this neonatal presentation (outcome was known in 17), all but six died in the neonatal period, and the exceptions died at 5 to 15 months [1]. An infant with this type of disease is shown in Figure 30.2. Her brother, now mentally retarded, preceded her so she was spared the initial neonatal episode, but she had nearly monthly admissions to hospital for hyperammonemia. This clinical picture is seen in the other urea cycle disorder, which present in the neonatal period. It can be distinguished from the hyperammonemia that occurs in organic acidemias because the serum concentrations of electrolytes do not reveal an acidosis. Blood gases more often indicate a respiratory alkalosis.

A very different type of disorder, the partial deficiency of carbamylphosphate synthetase, was exemplified by a 13-year-old girl [14]. She had episodes of vomiting and lethargy at 3 weeks and 13 months of age, and she had a transient hemiparesis at 2 years. She had spastic quadriparesis and severe mental retardation. A similar patient [15] presented at 9 years of age with hyperammonemic coma and was thought to have Reye syndrome. She recovered, but with extensive damage to the brain. She had seizures at 7 days and slow psychomotor development, but was a below average student in a regular school before the episode at 9 years. From 6 years, she had episodic vomiting, abdominal pain and muscle weakness, lasting 2–3 days. Other patients have had intermittent vomiting and screaming episodes or intermittent lethargy. Mental retardation has been the rule in those with childhood onset. Seizures and cerebral atrophy on computed tomography (CT) scan are common. We have seen an adult with CPS deficiency who developed his first episode of hyperammonemic coma at the age of 36 years (Figure 30.3). This followed a fugue-like episode for which he had no memory. He gave a history of two previous episodes in which he had periods of a few days for which he had no memory and unexplained scrapes and bruises.

Metabolic stroke has been reported in CPS deficiency[16]. An 18-month old girl was admitted with somnolence and a left hemiparesis. Magnetic resonance imaging (MRI) revealed infarction of the area supplied by the right middle cerebral artery, but carotid angiography revealed no obstruction of this vessel.

The clinical chemistry of CPS deficiency may be unremarkable except for the hyperammonemia, or there may be respiratory alkalosis. Amino acid analysis of the plasma at the time of hyperammonemia reveals elevation in glutamine and usually alanine, as well as sometimes aspartic acid. In addition,

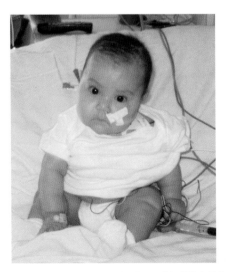

Figure 30.2 *A. O., an 8-month-old infant with CPS deficiency. The picture was taken just after recovering from hyperammonemic coma and just prior to a successful liver transplantation.*

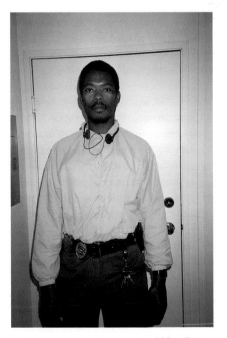

Figure 30.3 *C.B., a 38-year old man with CPS deficiency.*

the concentration of lysine maybe elevated. The concentration of citrulline is typically low. Organic acid analysis of the urine is remarkable for the absence of elevations of either orotic acid or uracil. The excretion of 3-methylglutaconic acid maybe quite high. Carnitine deficiency has been reported in CPS deficiency [17].

GENETICS AND PATHOGENESIS

CPS deficiency is determined by mutation in an autosomal recessive gene. It occurs in approximately 1 in 60 000 births in the US.

The molecular defect is in the mitochondrial carbamylphosphate synthetase (EC 6.3.4.16)[Figure 30.1]. There are two distinct carbamyl phosphate synthetases (18,19). The one found exclusively in the cytosol, which has been designated CPS II, is involved in pyrimidine biosynthesis. This enzyme is particularly active in rapidly growing tissues and preferentially utilizes glutamine rather than $NH4^+$, and it is not acetylglutamate dependent. The ammonia-dependent mitochondrial carbamylphosphate synthetase has been designated CPS I. The two-CPS enzymes are immunologically distinct [20]. In the mitochondria, CPS I catalyzes the formation of carbamyl-phosphate from $NH4^+$, $HCO3^-$ and 2 ATP. Glutamine is not an effective substrate, and acetylglutamate and Mg^{++} are required. The two CPS enzymes are located in distinct cellular compartments, but carbamylphosphate, which accumulates in mitochondria when there is a defect in OTC or more distal enzymes, readily makes its way to the cytosol and becomes a substrate for the synthesis of pyrimidines [21], and orotic acid is found in the urine. This is, of course, absent in CPS deficiency. The concentration of urea may be low. Concentrations of citrulline and arginine may be quite low.

In addition to acetylglutamate, carbamylglutamate is an activator of CPS I; glutamate and 2 oxoglutarate are inhibitors [22], as is carbamylphosphate, the product [23]. Deficiency of CPS is readily demonstrable by assay of the enzyme in biopsied liver [1,24,25]. It is possible to make the diagnosis of CPS deficiency by assay of the enzyme in biopsied rectal [25] or duodenal [26] tissue. In patients with CPS deficiency, levels of 0 to 50 percent of normal have been reported [12–14, 24, 26]. The correlation of residual activity with clinical presentation has in general been good.

Heterozygosity has been documented in a family in which intermediate levels of CPS activity were documented in biopsied liver of parents [27]. Antenatal diagnosis is possible by assay of the enzyme in biopsied fetal liver or by mutational analysis. The frequent RFLP at the CPS locus found after incubating with Bg1I is useful in heterozygote detection and prenatal diagnosis. Linkage dysequilibrium among four restriction patterns as been found; the A pattern was found in a frequency of 0.83 in affected individuals and 0.20 in controls [28].

Mutations identified to date have all been missense [8,9,29,30], which led to markedly reduced enzyme activity.

TREATMENT

The treatment of the acute hyperammonemic crisis of CPS deficiency is as outlined in Chapter 28 [31,32]. The acute and chronic management of this condition does not differ from that of OTC deficiency. Doses of Na benzoate and Na phenylacetate as well as agininine begin with 250 mL/kg of each. Maintenance in doses of 500 mg/kg of each have been given safely. An antiemetic such as Zofran (0.15–0.5 mg/kg) is sometimes useful. For chronic oral treatment Na phenylbutyrate has been employed in doses of 250–600 mg/kg/day. Citrulline is used in doses of 150–600 mg/kg. The dietary intake of protein is restricted and supplementation with a mixture of essential amino acids (Cyclinex, EAMI, UCD) is usually helpful in maintaining reasonable concentrations of amino acids in plasma while minimizing nitrogen load.

N-Carbamylglutamate is an analog of N-acetylglutamate which activates carbamyl phosphate synthetase [33]. The advantage is that it enters mitochondria and is not hydrolyzed by cytosolic deacylases, as is acetylglutamate. The compound, at 100–300 mg/kg has been reported to be effective in the management of acetylglutamate synthetase (AGS) deficiency [34,35]. Doses of 300 to 1800 mg/day have been well tolerated, and long-term management has been reported. The compound had been suggested [35] as a test for AGS deficiency, which might distinguish it from carbamylphosphate synthetase deficiency. However the compound has now been reported to be quite effective in the management of a patient with CPS deficiency [36].

References

1   Gelehrter TD, Snodgrass, PJ. Lethal neonatal deficiency of carbamyl phosphate synthetase. *N Engl J Med* 1974;**290**:430.

2   Arashima S, Matsuda I. A case of carbamyl phosphate synthetase deficiency. *Tohuku J Exp Med* 1972;**107**:143.

3   Nyunoya H, Broglie KE, Widgren EE, Lusty CJ. Characterization and derivation of the gene coding for mitochondrial carbamylphosphate synthetase I of rat. *J Biol Chem* 1985;**75**:5071.

4   Mori M, Miura S, Tatibana M, Cohen PP. Cell-free synthesis and processing of a putative precursor for mitochondrial carbamylphosphate synthetase I of rat liver. *J Biol Chem* 1979;**76**:5071.

5   Shore GL, Carignan P, Raymond Y. *In vitro* synthesis of a putative precursor to the mitochondrial enzyme carbamylphosphate synthetase. *J Biol Chem* 1979;**254**:3141.

6   Raymond Y, Shore GL. The precursor for carbamylphosphate synthetase is transported to mitochondria via a cytosolic route. *J Biol Chem* 1979;**254**:9335.

7   Adcock MW, O'Brien WE. Molecular cloning of cDNA for rat and human carbamyl phosphate synthetase I. *J Biol Chem* 1984;**259**:13471.

8   Funghini S, Donati MA, Pasquini E, *et al*. Molecular studies of CPS1 gene: determination of genomic organization and mutation detection. *Am J Hum Genet* 2000;**66**:418.

9   S. Funghini, Donati MA, Pasquini E, *et al*. Genomic organization of human CPSI gene and identification of two new mutations in a CPSD patient. *J Inherit Metab Dis* 2002;**25** (suppl. 1): 052P.

10 Graf L, McIntyre P, Hoogenraad N. A carbamylphosphate synthetase deficiency with no detectable immunoreactive enzyme and no translatable mRNA. *J Inherit Metab Dis* 1984;**7**:104.

11 Fearon ER, Mallonee RL, Phillipps JA III *et al.* Genetic analysis of carbamylphosphate synthetase 1 deficiency. *Hum Genet* 1985;**70**:207.

12 Hommes FA, DeGroot CJ, Wilmink CW, Jonxis JHP. Carbamylphosphate synthetase deficiency in an infant with severe cerebral damage. *Arch Dis Child* 1969;**44**:688.

13 Ebels EJ. Neuropathological observations in a patient with carbamylphosphate synthetase deficiency and in two sibs. *Arch Dis Child* 1972;**47**:47.

14 Batshaw M, Brusilow S, Walser M. Treatment of carbamyl phosphate synthetase deficiency with keto analogues of essential amino acids. *N Engl J Med* 1985;**292**:1085.

15 Granot E, Matoth I, Lotan C, *et al.* Partial carbamylphosphate synthetase deficiency, simulating Reye's syndrome, in a 9-year-old girl. *Isr J Med Sci* 1986;**22**:463.

16 Sperl W, Felber S, Skladal D, Wemuth B. Metabolic stroke as a novel observation in carbamylphosphate synthetase deficiency. *Proc. SSIEM,* 1995;P 036.

17 Mori T, Tsuchiyama A, Nagai K, *et al.* A case of carbamylphosphate synthetase-I deficiency associated with secondary carnitine deficiency-L carnitine treatment of CPS-I deficiency. *Euro J Pediatr* 1990;**149**:272.

18 Hager SE, Jones ME. A glutamine-dependent enzyme for the synthesis of carbamylphosphate for pyrimidine biosynthesis in fetal rat liver. *J Biol Chem* 1967;**242**:5674.

19 Tatibana M, Ito K. Control of pyrimidine biosynthesis in mammalian tissues. I. Partial purification characterization of glutamine-utilizing carbamylphosphate synthetase of mouse spleen and its tissue distribution. *J Biol Chem* 1969;**244**:5403.

20 Nakanishi S, Ito K, Tatibana M. Two types of carbamylphosphate synthetase in rat liver: chromatographic resolution and immunological distinction. *Biochem Biophys Res Commun* 1968;**33**:774.

21 Natale PJ, Tremblay GC. On the availability of intramitochondrial carbamylphosphate for the extramitochondrial biosynthesis of pyrimidines. *Biochem Biophys Res Commun* 1969;**37**:512.

22 Marshall M, Metzenberg RL, Cohen PP. Physical and kinetic properties of carbamylphosphate synthetase from frog liver. *J Biol Chem* 1961;**236**:2229.

23 Elliot KRF. Kinetic studies on mammalian liver carbamylphosphate synthetase: in *The Urea Cycle*, (eds S Grisolia, R Baguena, F Mayor), John Wiley and Sons, New York;1976:123.

24 Odievre C, Charpentier C, Cathelineau L, *et al.* Hyperammoniemie constitutionnelle avec deficit en carbamyl-phosphate-synthetase. Evolution sous regime dietetique. *Arch Fr Pediatr* 1973;**30**:5.

25 Hoogenraad NJ, Mitchell JD, Don NA, *et. al.* Detection of carbamyl phosphate synthetase I deficiency using duodenal biopsy samples. *Arch Dis Child* 1980;**55**:292.

26 Matsushima A, Orii T. The activity of carbamylphosphate synthetase I (CPS I) and ornithine transcarbamylase (OTC) in the intestine and the screening of OTC deficiency in the rectal mucosa. *J Inherit Metab Dis* 1981;**4**:83.

27 McReynolds JW, Crowley B, Mahoney MJ, Rosenberg LE. Autosomal recessive inheritance of human mitochondrial carbamyl phosphate synthetase deficiency. *Am J Hum Genet* 1981;**33**:345.

28 Malonee R, Fearon E, Philipps J III, *et al.* Genetic analysis of carbamyl-phosphate synthesis I deficiency. *Hum Genet* 1985;**70**:207.

29 Guillou F, Liao M, Garcia-Espana A, Lusty CJ. Mutational analysis of carbamylphosphate synthetase. Substitution of Glu841 leads to loss of functional coupling between the two catalytic domains of the synthetase subunit. *Biochemistry* 1992;**31**:1656.

30 Hoshide R, Matsuura T, Haraguchi Y, *et al.* Carbamylphosphate synthetase I deficiency; one base substitution in an exon of the CPS I gene causes a 9-base pair deletion due to aberrant splicing. *J Clin Invest* 1993;**91**:1884.

31 Batshaw ML, Brusilow S, Waber L, *et al.* Treatment of inborn errors of urea synthesis; activation of alternative pathways of waste nitrogen synthesis and excretion. *N Engl J Med* 1982;**306**:1387.

32 Brusilow WS, Danney M, Waber LJ, *et al.* Treatment of episodic hyper-ammonemia in children with inborn errors of urea synthesis. *N Engl J Med* 1984;**310**:1630.

33 Grisolia S, Cohen PP. The catalytic role of carbamylglutamate in citrulline biosynthesis. *J Biol Chem* 1952;**198**:561.

34 Bachmann C, Colombo JP, Jaggi K. N-Acetylglutamate synthetase (NAGS) deficiency: diagnosis, clinical observations and treatment: in *Urea Cycle Diseases* (eds Lowenthal A, *et al*). Advances in Experimental Medicine and Biology. Vol. 153. Plenum Press, New York;1982:39.

35 Rubio V, Grisolia S. Treating urea cycle defects. *Nature* 1981;**292**:496.

36 Kuchler G, Rabier D, Poggi-Travert F, *et al.* Therapeutic use of carbamylglutamate in the case of carbamylphosphate synthetase deficiency. *Proc SSIEM* 1995;P037.

Citrullinemia

MAJOR PHENOTYPIC EXPRESSION

Potentially lethal coma; convulsions; hyperammonemia; hypercitrullinemia; orotic aciduria; and defective activity of argininosuccinate synthetase.

INTRODUCTION

Citrullinemia was first reported in 1963 [1] in a patient with mental retardation. Soon after, it became apparent that the classic presentation is as a typical neonatal hyperammonemia that was, until the development of modern methods of pharmacologic therapy, uniformly lethal [2–8]. The picture is indistinguishable from that of the male neonate with ornithine transcarbamylase deficiency (Chapter 29). The activity of argininosuccinate synthetase (EC 6.3.4.5) is widely expressed in tissues (Figure 31.1). Its deficiency is readily demonstrated in cultured fibroblasts [9]. The gene has been cloned [10] and mapped to chromosome 9 at q34 [11]. A number of mutations have been described [12–15].

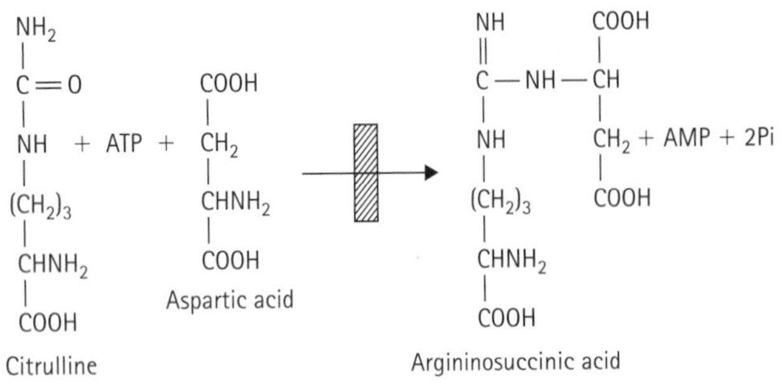

Figure 31.1 *The argininosuccinic acid synthetase reaction, site of the defect in citrullinemia.*

CLINICAL ABNORMALITIES

Citrullinemia usually presents as an overwhelming neonatal illness. Following a brief hiatus in which the newborn appears normal, anorexia, vomiting and lethargy develop, and these symptoms are followed rapidly by progression to deep coma (Figures 31.2–31.7). Apnea ensues, and death is inevitable unless the infant is intubated and provided with mechanical ventilation. Seizures often occur, and there are abnormalities of the electroencephalogram (EEG). The infant may be hypertonic, and there may be decerebrate posturing. The neurologic abnormality is progressive to flaccidity and dilated, fixed pupils. The infant is unresponsive even to deep pain. The liver may be enlarged, and serum levels of transminases are often elevated.

Citrullinemia is genetically heterogeneous, and there have been a variety of different clinical pictures in patients with partial residual activity of the defective enzyme. All of these variants are encountered less frequently than the classic infantile one. Some of these patients have had a more gradual onset of difficulty with feedings and recurrent or cyclic vomiting in infancy. Some have had hepatomegaly and elevation of the serum glutamate-oxaloacetate transaminase (SGOT) or glutamate pyruvate transaminase (SGPT), which may cause confusion by suggesting a diagnosis of hepatocellular disease [6]. This is true also of the classic acute infantile disease [16]. The prothrombin and partial thromboplastin time may be

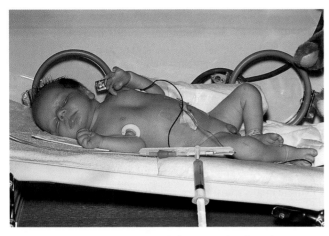

Figure 31.2 *J.P.N., a 12-day-old infant with citrullinemia, illustrating deep coma requiring assisted ventilation. The concentration of ammonia in plasma was 770 µmol/L. He was flaccid and completely unresponsive. He had required assisted ventilation, but this was discontinued after a series of exchange transfusions that temporarily lowered the ammonia to 236 µmol/L. Concentrations of ammonia were over 1000 µg/dL at 4 hours.*

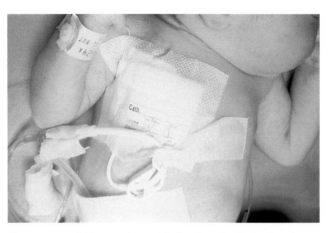

Figure 31.4 *R.M., a newborn with citrullinemia. He developed hyperammonemic coma at 3 days of age. He was treated with exchange transfusion, arginine and Na benzoate/phenylacetate. The hyperammonemia resolved, but the level of citrulline in plasma was more than 1000 µmol/L.*

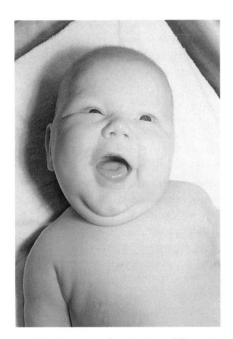

Figure 31.3 *J.P.N., 2 months after the time of Figure 31.2. Treated with keto acid analogues of amino acids, he had recovered nicely and was alert and appeared to be developing normally. He was a bit chubby. He died before his first birthday of acute hyperammonemic coma.*

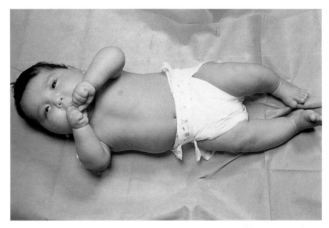

Figure 31.5 *R.M., 4 months later. He was a bit obese and had frequent diaper rashes consistent with protein inadequacy. In follow-up he was moderately retarded despite having had only two subsequent slightly hyperammonemic attacks.*

prolonged. Episodic hyperammonemia may occur with vomiting, lethargy, headaches, tremors, seizures or ataxia [17–19]. Some degree of retardation of mental development is usually present [1], and computed tomography (CT) or magnetic resonance imaging (MRI) scan usually reveals evidence of cerebral atrophy.

A late onset form of citrullinemia is especially common in Japan [20]. The first episode may begin as late as 20 years [21] with symptoms such as slurred speech, irritability, insomnia or delirium. In such a patient the intelligence may be normal. Some patients have had bizarre behavior, manic episodes or frank psychosis. Special cravings have been reported for foods such as beans, peas and peanuts, which are rich in arginine [22]. One patient in whom citrullinemia was found on routine screening had had no clinical evidence of disease at the time of report [3,23]. Even the patient with a variant form of citrullinemia, in whom symptomatology has been mild, or even absent for long periods, may become neurologically incapacitated in childhood or adulthood. Spastic paraparesis, like that seen in patients with hyperargininemia or portocaval shunts, has been reported [21].

Urinary excretion of citrulline may range from several hundred milligrams per day in an infant to several grams per day in an older patient. Some patients may also excrete homocitrulline, homoarginine or N-acetylcitrulline [1,2,6,18,19,25]. Concentrations of citrulline are also elevated in the cerebrospinal fluid, but levels are lower than in the blood.

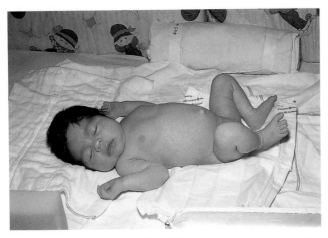

Figure 31.6   *N.F. at 4 days of age. She appeared to be normal and had a normal level of ammonia, EEG and CT scan. Treatment was initiated at birth. Her sister had died of citrulliniemia in the neonatal period. A prenatal diagnosis permitted treatment of N.F. from birth, which prevented neonatal hyperammonemia. The concentration of citrulline in the amniotic fluid at mid-gestation was 80 μmol/L (1.4 g/dL) normal range 0–23 μmol/L and the activity of the enzyme was 8 percent of the control mean.*

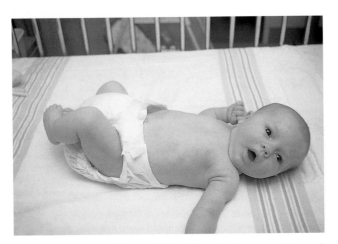

Figure 31.7   *V.T., an infant with citrullinemia who appeared normal at 2 months. A previous sibling had died of overwhelming neonatal citrullinemia.*

The most prominent metabolic characteristic of citrullinemia is the hyperammonemia, which is usually massive in the neonatal form, but deep coma mimicking anesthesia has been seen with concentrations of 400 μmol/L [16]. Concentrations in the blood of glutamine and usually of alanine are also elevated, and often that of aspartic acid as well. The concentration of arginine is usually decreased. Excretion of orotic acid is increased [24], although usually not to the degree seen in ornithine transcarbamylase deficiency.

Concentrations of citrulline in body fluids of these patients are very high. Plasma concentrations usually approximate 40 times normal; levels of 850–4600 μmol/L are commonly encountered. The lowest level reported of 290 μmol/L was found in a patient who had no clinical evidence of disease [3].

GENETICS AND PATHOGENESIS

Citrullinemia is transmitted as an autosomal recessive disease. Intermediate levels of activity of argininosuccinate synthetase have been found in fibroblasts of parents [7,8,9,16]. Prenatal diagnosis has been made by assay of the concentration of citrulline in amniotic fluid or by assay of the enzyme in cultured amniocytes [4,16] (Figure 31.6). Prenatal diagnosis may also be accomplished by assay of the enzyme in chorionic villus material [26,27], but very low levels of enzyme in heterozygotes may be a real problem. For this reason, a sensitive radiochemical assay was developed [26]. The most reliable approach is to assess the enzyme in cultured amniocytes. Restriction fragment length polymorphism (RFLP) may permit detection of heterozygotes and prenatal diagnosis, and the existence of three distinct RFLPs [28], as well as a highly polymorphic variable number tandem report (VNTR) [29], increases the likelihood that linkage analysis may be useful in an individual family.

The molecular defect in citrullinemia is in the enzyme argininosuccinic acid synthetase. This is a cytosolic enzyme in contrast to ornithine trans-carbamylase and carbamyl phosphate synthetase (Chapters 29 and 30). Argininosuccinic acid synthetase catalyzes the conversion of citrulline and aspartic acid to argininosuccinic acid (Figure 31.1). The enzyme is widely distributed in tissues. The defect has usually been demonstrated in cultured fibroblasts [8,9] and it has also been demonstrated in liver [1,4,19]. Activity in the neonatal form of the disease is usually virtually zero.

In a patient with a variant form of citrullinemia, five percent of normal activity was found in liver [30]. In the adult Japanese phenotype, levels as high as 50 percent of control have been reported [20]. Kinetic studies have revealed Km values for citrulline as high as 200 times normal in variants with alterations in the structure of the enzyme protein [9,31]. In one patient the activity of the enzyme in brain was lower than that found in the liver [32]. In the adult onset Japanese phenotype the deficiency is specific to the liver [33] and not found in other tissues. These patients have normal levels of hepatic mRNA, but a decreased amount of enzyme linked immunosorbent assay (ELISA) detectable enzyme protein [34].

Cloning of the cDNA for argininosuccinic acid synthetase was facilitated by the use of a cultured human cell line in which very high levels of mRNA for this enzyme were produced when the cells were cultivated in medium containing canavanine, an analogue of arginine [10]. The gene was sequenced and found to contain 63 kb in 16 exons [11]. It codes for a monomeric protein of 46 kDa that forms a tetramer [35]. Expression of the gene is highly regulated, increasing with fasting, dexamethasone or dibutyryl-cAMP, and the substitution of citrulline for arginine in medium, and decreasing in response to arginine.

Analysis of the DNA of 11 patients by Southern blot failed to reveal major rearrangements of the gene [36]. Analysis of the mRNA and protein of these lines revealed considerable heterogeneity. Nine of 11 were devoid of cross-reacting material (CRM), while they had all mRNA. Levels of CRM and enzyme activity below 50 percent were found in some parents. Among patients with classic citrullinemia at least 20 mutations have been reported [37], indicating a considerable heterogeneity. Most patients are compound heterozygotes.

An interesting homozygous mutation found [12] in the child of consanguineous parents was a G-to-C substitution in the splice acceptor site of the terminal intron, which abolished normal splicing and led to three abnormal splice products, the most common of which was translated to a protein 25 amino acids longer, but so unstable that CRM was not detectable. Most of the other alterations found have been missense mutations [13,37] (Table 31.1). A number have involved CpG dinucleotides. Deletions of entire exons have resulted from deletion of genomic sequences [14]. Nonsense mutations have not been reported, although a nonsense mutation in codon 86 (arginine) was found in citrullinemic cattle [15]. The missense mutations found in classic neonatal citrullinemia have all altered an amino acid that was highly conserved, most of them across eight species ranging from humans to *Saccharomyces* and *E. coli* [37].

Table 31.1   *Mutations defined in classic citrullinemia*

Mutation	Deletions, insertions	Exon
G14S		3
S18L		
		4
R86C	Δ Exon 5	5
A118T		
	Δ Exon 6	6
	IVS6-2	
R157H	Δ Exon 7	7
S180N		8
A192V		9
		10
		11
R272P		12
R279Q		
G280R		
R304W	Δ Exon 13	13
G324S		
R363W		14
R363L	IVS15-1	
G390R	Insertion 37 b, exons 15, 16	15
	Δ 76 Exon 16	16

The abbreviation b is for bases. The amino acids coded for are: A, alanine; C, cysteine; G, glycine; H, histidine; L, leucine; N, asparagine; R, arginine; S, serine; T, threonine; V, valine; and W, tryptophan.

TREATMENT

The acute management of the initial neonatal hyperammonemia and subsequent intercurrent attacks is set out in Chapter 28, along with general principles of long-term management of hyperammonemic infants using sodium benzoate and/or phenylacetate and arginine. The infant with citrullinemia differs in that even an acute crisis of hyperammonemia can be managed with intravenous arginine alone, as long as the episode is treated promptly and the level of ammonia is not too high. It would not be recommended to treat the initial infantile crisis with anything less than a full-scale attack on the hyperammonemia. In this disease, whether benzoate and/or phenylacetate is employed it is well to employ doses of arginine in both the priming and sustaining infusion of at least 0.66 g/kg.

Long-term steady state management can usually be provided with arginine and a diet modestly restricted in protein [16,38] (Figure 31.8). The principle is that if ornithine molecules can be provided through supplemental arginine, in order to keep the urea cycle operating, waste nitrogen can be adequately eliminated in the form of citrulline. Citrulline contains only one more nitrogen atom than the two provided as ornithine. Thus it is probably half as efficient as urea in eliminating nitrogen, but this is sufficient except at times of catabolism. If the patient is vomiting or for some other reason cannot take oral arginine, hospital admission for intravenous arginine therapy is mandatory. Oral doses of arginine employed have ranged from 0.25 to 0.8 g/kg per day. Normal development has been reported with such a regimen [38]. We have observed low levels of essential amino acids, especially of branched amino acids, in patients treated with benzoate, phenylacetate or phenylbutyrate. This has also been reported [39]. There may be clinical signs of protein inadequacy (Figures 31.5 and 31.9). Supplementation with mixtures of essential amino acids is preferable to increasing whole protein in this instance, and nitrogen-free analogs of amino acids are useful [40], but these mixtures are no longer available. This problem of essential amino acid depletion has not been observed with arginine treatment.

Prognosis for intellectual development probably depends on the nature of the initial hyperammonemia, especially its duration [41] or those of recurrent episodes. The ability to prevent

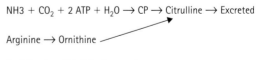

Figure 31.8   *Chronic management of citrullinemia. Of the three N atoms of citrulline, two come from ornithine administered as arginine. Hence, a net of one N is lost for every molecule of citrulline excreted. As long as ornithine is supplied, this minicycle continues to operate. CP, carbamylphosphate.*

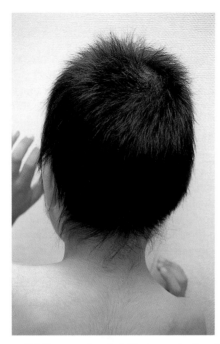

Figure 31.9 *N.F. Her very short hair illustrates the fact that among patients with urea cycle defects the loss of hair has been our most sensitive index of protein inadequacy.*

hyperammonemia by early treatment in patients diagnosed prenatally [42] should be consistent with a better prognosis, but only if recurrent attacks of hyperammonemia are prevented or treated early and effectively. In the most recent assessment of the collaborative study managed by Brusilow and colleagues [39], 24 patients had a five-year survival of 87.5 percent and 10-year survival of 72 percent, indicating the always dangerous nature of this disease. Of 15 survivors, 11 were severely or profoundly mentally retarded, and in four IQ values were in the borderline range. Growth in many was retarded, but most had height-for-weight scores within 2 SD of the mean.

References

1 McMurray WC, Rathbun JC, Mohyuddin F, *et al.* Citrullinemia. *Pediatrics* 1963;**32**:347.

2 Vander Zee SPM, Trijbels JMF, Monnens LAH, *et al.* Citrullinaemia with a rapidly fatal neonatal course. *Arch Dis Child* 1971;**48**:847.

3 Ghisolfi J, Augier D, Martinez J, *et al.* Forme neonatale de citrullinemia a l'evolution mortelle rapide. *Pediatrie* 1972;**27**:55.

4 Wick H, Bachmann C, Baumgartner R, *et al.* Variants of citrullinaemia. *Arch Dis Child* 1973;**48**:636.

5 Roerdink FH, Gouw WL, Okken A, *et al.* Citrullinemia. Report of a case with studies on antenatal diagnosis. *Pediatr Res* 1973;**7**:863.

6 Danks DM, Tipett P, Zenter G. Severe neonatal citrullinemia. *Arch Dis Child* 1974;**49**:579.

7 Buist NRM, Kennaway NG, Hepburn CA, *et al.* Citrullinemia: investigation and treatment over a four-year period. *J Pediatr* 1974;**85**:208.

8 Leibowitz J, Thoene J, Spector E, Nyhan WL. Citrullinemia. *Virchows Arch A Pathol Anat Histol* 1978;**377**:249.

9 Kennaway NG, Harwood PJ, Ramberg DA, *et al.* Citrullinemia: enzymatic evidence for genetic heterogeneity. *Pediatr Res* 1975;**9**:554.

10 Su TS, Bock HGO, O'Brien WE, Beaudet AL. Cloning of cDNA for argininosuccinate synthetase mRNA and study of enzyme over-production in a human cell line. *J Biol Chem.* 1981;**256**:11826.

11 Su TS, Nussbaum RL, Airpart S, *et al.* Human chromosomal assignments for 14 argininosuccinate synthetase pseudogenes: cloned DNAs as reagents for cytogenetic analysis. *Am J Hum Genet.* 1984;**36**:954.

12 Su TS, Lin LH. Analysis of splice acceptor site mutation which produces multiple splicing abnormalities in the human argininosuccinate synthetase locus. *J Biol Chem* 1990;**265**:19716.

13 Kobayashi K, Jackson M, Tick DB, O'Brien WE. Heterogeneity of mutations in argininosuccinate synthetase causing human citrullinemia. *J Biol Chem.* 1990;**265**:11361.

14 Jackson MJ, Allen SJ, Beaudet AL, O'Brien WE. Metabolite regulation of argininosuccinate synthetase in cultured human cells. *J Biol Chem.* 1988;**263**:16388.

15 Dennis JA, Healy PJ, Beaudet AL, O'Brien WE. Molecular definition of bovine argininosuccinate synthetase deficiency. *Proc Natl Acad Sci USA.* 1989;**86**:7947.

16 Nyhan WL, Sakati NA. Citrullinemia: in *Diagnostic Recognition of Genetic Disease* (WL Nyhan, NA Sakati). Lea and Febiger, Philadelphia;1987:159.

17 Morrow G III, Barness LA, Efron ML. Citrullinemia with defective urea production. *Pediatrics.* 1967;**40**:565.

18 Vidailhet M, Levin B, Dautrevaux M, *et al.* Citrullinemie. *Arch Franc Pediatr.* 1971;**28**:521.

19 Scott-Emuakpor A, Higgins JV, Kohrman AF. Citrullinemia: a new case with implications concerning adaptation to defective urea synthesis. *Pediatr Res* 1972;**6**:626.

20 Kooka T, Higashi Y, Uebayashi Y, Kobayashi R. A special form of hepatocerebral degeneration with citrullinemia. *Neurol Med* 1977;**6**:47.

21 Miyazaki M, Fukuda S, Aki M, *et al.* A case of hepatic encephalomyelopathy associated with citrullinemia. *Brain and Nerve* (Tokyo) 1971;**23**:19.

22 Paul AA, Southgate DAT. McCance and Widdowson's *The Composition of Foods.* 4th revised and extended edn. Elsevier/North-Holland Inc, Biomedical Press, New York;1978.

23 Wick H, Brechbühler T, Girard J. Citrullinemia: elevated serum citrulline levels in healthy siblings. *Experientia* 1970;**26**:823.

24 Bachmann C. Urea cycle: in *Heritable Disorders of Amino Acid Metabolism.* (ed. WL Nyhan) John Wiley and Sons Inc, New York;1974:361.

25 Strandholm JJ, Buist NRM, Kennaway NG, Curtis HT. Excretion of N-acetyl-citrulline in citrullinemia. *Biochim Biophys Acta* 1971;**244**:214.

26 Beaudet AL, O'Brien WE, Bock HGO, *et al.* The human arginino-succinate synthetase locus and citrullinemia: in *Advances in Human Genetics* (eds H Harris, K Hirschhorn) Plenum Press, New York;1986:161.

27 Fleisher L, Mitchell D, Koppitch F, *et al.* Chorionic villus samples (CVS) for the prenatal diagnosis of aminoacidopathies. *Am J Hum Genet* 1984;**36**:188S.

28 Northrup H, Lathrop M, Lu SY, *et al.* Multilocus linkage analysis with the human argininosuccinate synthetase gene. *Genomics* 1989;**5**:442.

29 Kwiatowski DJ, Nygaard TG, Schuback DE, *et al.* Identification of a highly polymorphic microsatellite VNTR within the argininosuccinate locus: exclusion of the dystonia gene on 9q32-34 as the cause of dopa-responsive dystonia in a large kindred. *Am J Hum Genet* 1991;**48**:121.

30 McMurray WC, Mohyuddin F, Bayer SM, Rathbun JD. Citrullinuria: a disorder of amino acid metabolism associated with mental retardation: in *Proceedings of International Copenhagen Congress on the Scientific Study of Mental Retardation.* (eds J Oster, HV Sletved) Det Berlincske Bogtrykkeri, Copenhagen;1965:117.

31 Tedesco TA, Mellman WJ. Argininosuccinate synthetase activity and citrulline metabolism in cells cultured from a citrullinemic subject. *Proc Natl Acad Sci USA* 1967;**57**:169.

32 Christensen E, Brandt NJ, Philip J, *et al.* Citrullinaemia: the possibility of prenatal diagnosis. *J Inherit Metab Dis* 1980;**3**:73.

33 Saheki T, Kobayashi K, Inoue I. Hereditary disorders of the urea cycle in man: biochemical and molecular approaches. *Rev Physiol Biochem Pharmacol* 1987;**108**:21.

34 Saheki T, Kobayashi K, Ichiki H, *et al.* Molecular basis of enzyme abnormalities in urea cycle disorders: in *Recent Advances in Inborn Errors of Metabolism* Proceedings of 4th International Congress. *Enzyme* 1987;**38**:227.

35 Bock HGO, Su TS, O'Brien WE, Beaudet AL. Sequences for human argininosuccinate synthetase cDNA. *Nucleic Acids Res* 1983;**11**:6505.

36 Su TS, Bock HO, Beaudet AL, O'Brien WE. Molecular analysis of argininosuccinate synthetase deficiency in human fibroblasts. *J Clin Invest* 1982;**70**:1334.

37 Kobayashi K, Shaheen N, Terazono H, Saheki T. Mutations in argininosuccinate synthetase mRNA of Japanese patients causing classic citrullinemia. *Am J Hum Genet* 1994;**55**:1103.

38 Melnyk AR, Matalon R, Henry BW, *et al.* Prospective management of a child with neonatal citrullinemia. *J Pediatr* 1993;**122**:96.

39 Maestri NE, Clissold DB, Brusilow SW. Long-term survival of patients with argininosuccinate synthetase deficiency. *J Pediatr* 1995;**127**:929.

40 Thoene J, Batshaw M, Spector E, *et al.* Neonatal citrullinemia: treatment with ketoanalogues of essential amino acids. *J Pediatr* 1977;**90**:218.

41 Msall M, Batshaw ML, Suss R, *et al.* Neurologic outcome in children with inborn errors of urea synthesis. *N Engl J Med* 1984;**301**:1500.

42 Donn SM, Wilson GN, Thoene JG. Prevention of neonatal hyperammonemia in citrullinemia. *Clin Res* 1984;**32**:806A.

Argininosuccinic aciduria

MAJOR PHENOTYPIC EXPRESSION

Hyperammonemia leading to lethargy and coma; convulsions; hyperglutaminemia and hyperalaninemia; argininosuccinic aciduria and defective activity of argininosuccinate lyase.

INTRODUCTION

Argininosuccinic aciduria was first recognized in patients with chronic more indolent disease where the major manifestations were nonspecific, sometimes mild or moderate mental retardation [1–4]. This may reflect the unique features of the hair in this disorder, which brought many of the early patients to attention with apparent alopecia. The disorder presents also, and probably more frequently, in the classic neonatal hyperammonemic pattern of a typical urea cycle disease [5–10]. Sometimes these infants may be suspected clinically to be different from those with other urea cycle disorders because of the magnitude of the hepatomegaly.

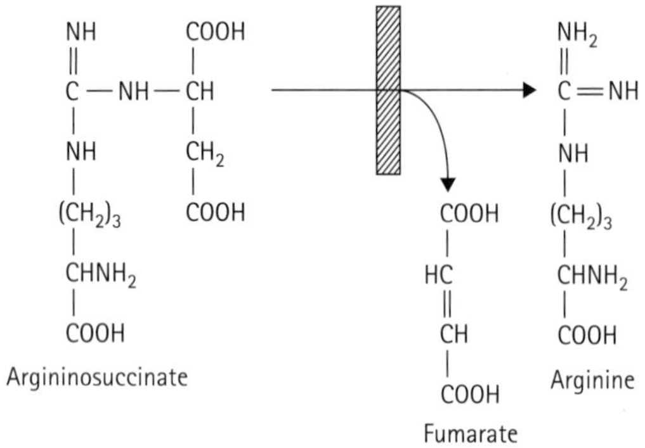

Figure 32.1 *The reaction catalyzed by argininosuccinase.*

The enzyme argininosuccinate lyase, or argininosuccinase (EC 4.3.2.1) (Figure 32.1), catalyzes the conversion of the argininosuccinate formed from citrulline and aspartate, to fumarate and arginine, the last compound of the urea cycle prior to the splitting off of urea. The cDNA for the human gene has been cloned [11], and the gene has been localized to chromosome 7 [12]. A small number of mutations has been defined [13,14], some of which have led to alternative splicing.

CLINICAL ABNORMALITIES

The classic presentation of argininosuccinic aciduria is as overwhelming illness in the newborn period. Prior to the development of modern methods of pharmacologic therapy, the end result of this presentation was uniformly fatal. The picture is indistinguishable from that of the male infant with ornithine transcarbamylase deficiency (Chapters 28 and 29). Following a brief hiatus in which the newborn appears normal, anorexia or vomiting and lethargy develop, and these symptoms are rapidly progressive to deep coma, apnea and death, unless the baby is intubated and maintained via mechanical ventilation. Seizures often occur, along with abnormalities of the electroencephalogram (EEG). The infant may be hypertonic or hypotonic or there may be decerebrate posturing. This condition is progressive to flaccidity and dilated fixed pupils. The infant is unresponsive even to deep pain. There may

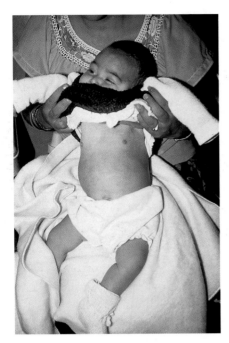

Figure 32.2   *C.G.G., a Mexican infant with argininosuccinic aciduria. The dermatitis on the abdomen and chest was unrelated.*

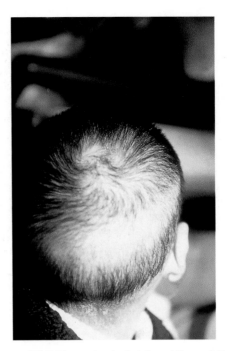

Figure 32.4   *C.G.G. More extensive hair loss at the occipital area of pressure.*

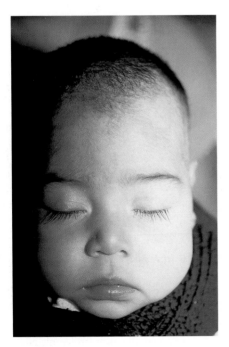

Figure 32.3   *C.G.G. Her hair was short and brittle.*

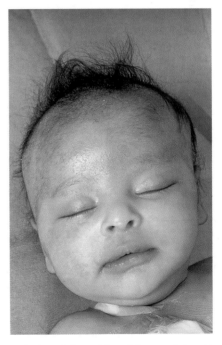

Figure 32.5   *H.H., an infant with arginino-succinic aciduria, had brittle hair and alopecia.*

be hypothermia. Patients may have tachypnea and respiratory alkalosis, which are general consequences of hyperammonemia[15]. A bulging fontanel usually indicates the presence of cerebral edema, but cerebral hemorrhages have been seen in hyperammonemic infants, as have fatal pulmonary hemorrhages.

As in the case of other disorders of the urea cycle (ornithine transcarbamylase deficiency, Chapter 29; carbamyl phosphate synthetase deficiency (CPS), Chapter 30; citrullinemia,

Chapter 31) argininosuccinic aciduria is genetically heterogeneous and patients with variant forms of the enzyme in which there is partial residual activity may have more indolent forms of the disease. Such patients may present simply with mental retardation [2,4] or a convulsive disorder. Commonly, there is episodic disease such as cyclic vomiting or recurrent headache, ataxia, tremulousness or lethargy. Abnormalities of the EEG are common. Cerebral atrophy maybe evident on

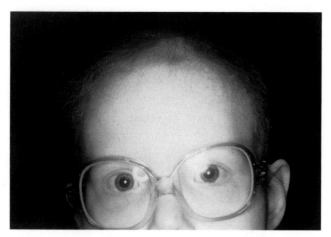

Figure 32.6   *R.W., a girl with argininosuccinase deficiency [20] who had considerable hair loss during a period of metabolic imbalance. (Kindly provided by Dr. E.V. Bawle of the Children's Hospital of Michigan.)*

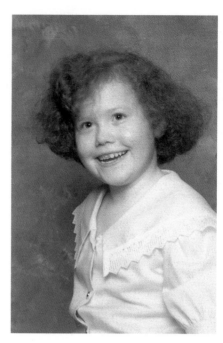

Figure 32.7   *R.W. When the hair was plentiful. (Kindly provided by Dr. E.V. Bawle of the Children's Hospital of Michigan.)*

computed tomography (CT) or magnetic resonance imaging (MRI) scan. Others may have episodes of hyperammonemic encephalopathy and coma thought to be Reye syndrome, or encephalitis. Hyperammonemia is often precipitated by infection, and such an episode may be fatal.

A unique finding in patients with variants forms of argininosuccinic aciduria is trichorrhexis nodosa (Figures 32.2–32.7) [1,2,16–18]. These patients may appear hairless at a distance, but there is always at least a fuzz of short hair. More often, they have short dry hair, but never need a haircut. The hair is very friable and breaks off easily. There may be a history of hair on the pillow. Under the microscope the hair sheaths contain tiny nodules (Figure 32.8). Break points may be seen at the nodules.

In addition, these patients have hepatomegaly [19]. Serum values of the transaminases are elevated at least at times of hyperammonemia [19,20]. Patients have been thought to have hepatic fibrosis, and there may be ultrastructural abnormalities in hepatocytes, but most synthetic functions are normal. Chronic coagulopathy was reported in an 8-year-old (Figures 32.6,32.7) with prolongation of prothrombin time and increase of the partial thromboplastin time (PTT); the only clinical consequence in the patient reported was prolonged bleeding at venipuncture sites [20].

There may be retardation of physical as well as mental development. Patients surviving episodes of coma at any age are likely to be left with mental retardation. Some have had spasticity ataxia or a seizure disorder.

Argininosuccinic aciduria has been reported in patients, detected by routine neonatal screening and treated with protein restriction and or/arginine supplementation, in whom no clinical abnormalities have been observed [21–23].

The diagnostic metabolic characteristics of this disease are hyperammonemia and argininosuccinic aciduria. Hyperammonemia may be massive in the neonatal form. In patients

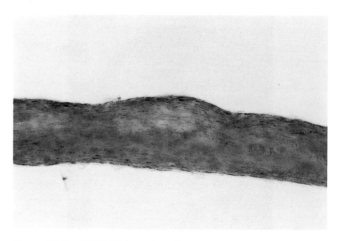

Figure 32.8   *C.G.G. Trichorexis nodosa.*

with variant forms of the disease, it is usually episodic and less dramatically elevated. Plasma concentrations of glutamine and alanine are usually elevated. Argininosuccinic acid is regularly found in the urine, but this compound is so efficiently excreted that it is not found in the blood [24]. High levels are found in the cerebrospinal fluid. In the urine, argininosuccinic acid is excreted in gram quantities. Still it may sometimes be missed on routine assays of the urine for amino acids because the compound is unstable, the peaks occur in a place unfamiliar to the operator, or they may overlap those of other amino acids. The best way to assay for argininosuccinic acid is to boil the urine; this quantitatively converts the compound to its anhydrides, which are then readily seen on the amino acid analyzer [25].

GENETICS AND PATHOGENESIS

Argininosuccinic aciduria is transmitted as an autosomal recessive disease. Its incidence approximates 1 in 70 000. The molecular defect is in argininosuccinate lyase (Figure 32.1). This enzyme is widely distributed in tissues and can be assayed in erythrocytes, as well as cultured fibroblasts. Deficient activity of the enzyme has been documented in erythrocytes, liver and fibroblasts[10,26–32]. The erythrocyte assay may be misleading; in some patients there may be substantial, even normal, activity even though there is severely defective hepatic activity. The normal enzyme in fibroblasts is immunologically indistinguishable from that of the liver. However, there have been patients reported in whom the activity in fibroblasts was less deficient than that of liver, and others in whom the activity in liver was less deficient than that of fibroblasts [32,33]. Assay conditions for the enzyme have been improved by the use of a higher concentration of citrulline. In a group of variant patients this reduced the relationship to normal from 18–75 percent to 6–28 percent [34].

Heterogeneity in the mutations responsible for deficient enzyme activity in argininosuccinic aciduria was demonstrated in complementation studies of fibroblasts of 28 patients [35], in which there was a single major complementation group, but there were 12 interallelic complementation subgroups consistent with 12 allelic mutations. The enzyme is a homotetramer in which the monomeric subunit has a molecular weight of 49.5 Kd [36,37]. Immunochemical studies of the enzyme after electrophoresis on sodium dodecylsulfate polyacrylamide gel electrophoresis revealed two bands of approximately 49 and 51 kDa in normal cells [38]. Each of 28 variants had some 49 kDa cross-reacting material (CRM). The 51 kDa band was found in only six variants in which CRM or residual enzyme activity was very high.

These data were consistent with the existence of a number of unique mutations. Definition of the nature of mutation has supported these conclusions. In four independent cell lines, six mutations were found; three missense mutations, one nonsense mutation and two deletions [13]. The missense mutations were R111W (arginine 111 to tryptophan), Q286R (glutamine 286 to arginine) and R193Q (arginine 193 to glutamine). In addition, an R95C (arginine 45 cysteine) change was found in a product of consanguinity [14], which when expressed in COS cells exhibited a normal amount of mRNA and only one percent of normal enzyme activity. The nonsense mutation changed glycine 454 to X or termination. Two deletions were found that led to skipping of exon 13 [39]. A 13 bp deletion within exon 13 is the most common mutation identified to date, occurring in eight percent of mutant alleles. The other, a 25-bp deletion, begins at exactly the same spot, which appears to be a hot spot for deletions. The deletions begin with a restriction endonuclease Topo II recognition sequence and start at the Topo II cut site, a site very similar to the ΔF508 deletion in cystic fibrosis and somewhat similar sites in hypoxanthine phosphoribosyl-transferase (HPRT)

and βglobin. In a series of five variant patients [34] three novel mutations, R385C in two patients V178M and R379C were detected in homozygous condition. One patient was a compound of R193Q and Q286R.

Parents of infants with the disease have been found to have reduced activity of argininosuccinate lyase in erythrocytes and fibroblasts [40]. Prenatal diagnosis may be carried out by analysis of the activity of the enzyme in cultured amniocytes [41–43]. Contamination with mycoplasma could cause a false negative result [14]. Prenatal diagnosis in variant families has been accomplished by ^{14}C-citrulline incorporation in amniocytes and chorionic villus cells [34]. The disease may also be detected prenatally by direct assay of the amniotic fluid for argininosuccinic acid [30,31,42–45]. It would seem reasonable always to undertake the direct assay in pregnancies at risk. In a family in which the mutation is known, prenatal diagnosis and carrier detection may be carried out by analysis for the mutation. Neonatal screening was proposed which made use of a *Bacillus subtilis* auxotroph in a Guthrie analysis of blood spots on paper [46], but experience has not been reported. In the Massachusetts program, which depended on paper chromatography of urine at 3–4 weeks of age, eight patients were found in some 600 000 samples indicating the prevalence of 1 in 70 000 [47]. Of course, some infants may have died earlier. These approaches to neonatal screening have been replaced by programs of expanded screening by tandem mass spectrometry [48].

The argininosuccinase protein has a structural function first evident from homology with the D-crystallins of avian lens [49,50]. Duck lens proteins turned out to have enormous argininosuccinate lyase activity. In birds, urea synthesis does not take place; the enzyme is required for the biosynthesis of arginine. In some birds, like chickens, evolutionary divergence has occurred, and the major crystallin does not have lyase activity.

TREATMENT

The acute management of the initial hyperammonemic episode and subsequent episodic attacks is set out in Chapter 28 along with principles of the long-term management of hyperammonemic infants. In the acute management of argininosuccinic aciduria the intravenous sustaining dose of arginine is increased to 700 mg/kg. The priming dose is given in 25 mL glucose solution/kg over 24 hours, and the sustaining dose is given in maintenance fluid over 24 hours. Because arginine is supplied as the hydrochloride for intravenous use, blood levels of chloride and bicarbonate are monitored, and hyperchloremic acidosis is treated with sodium bicarbonate. The use of sodium benzoate and phenylacetate usually may be omitted. The infant with argininosuccinic aciduria can be managed, except at times of crisis, using arginine alone and a diet modestly restricted in protein (Figure 32.9).

The principle is that if ornithine molecules can be provided through supplemental arginine in order to keep the

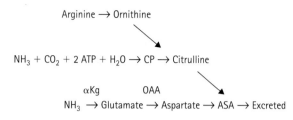

Arginine dose: 0.25–0.8 g/kg per day

Figure 32.9 *Chronic management of argininosuccinic acidemia. Of the four N atoms of arginiosuccinic acid, two came from ornithine supplied as arginine. Thus there is a net loss of two N for every molecule of argininosuccinic acid excreted, which is as efficient as urea. Continued supply of ornithine permits this minicycle to continue to operate. CP, carbamyl phosphate; αKg, α-ketoglutarate; OAA, oxaloacetate; ASA, argininosuccinate.*

urea cycle operating, waste nitrogen can be adequately eliminated in the form of argininosuccinic acid. Argininosuccinic acid contains two more N atoms than the two provided as ornithine, and it is very efficiently excreted, so that it should be as effective as urea in getting rid of unwanted nitrogen as long as there is a supply of ornithine to keep the cycle moving. As in other urea cycle disorders, an objective of therapy is to keep the levels of glutamine in normal range. Arginine therapy should be sufficient except at times of catabolism, such as during intercurrent infection. If the patient is vomiting or cannot take oral arginine, admission to hospital for parenteral arginine is mandatory. Doses of arginine employed have ranged from 0.25 to 0.89 g/kg per day.

Prognosis for intellectual development probably depends on the nature of the initial hyperammonemia, especially its duration [51] or the nature of recurrent episodes. One should expect patients rescued from neonatal hyperammonemia to be retarded. The mean IQ reported was approximately 50 [51]. The ability to prevent hyperammonemia by early treatment in patients diagnosed prenatally or during neonatal screening should be consistent with a better prognosis.

References

1 Levin B, Mackay HMM, Oberholzer VG. Argininosuccinic aciduria, an inborn error of amino acid metabolism. *Arch Dis Child* 1961;**36**:622.

2 Carson NAJ, Neill DW. Metabolic abnormalities detected in a survey of mentally backward individuals in Northern Ireland. *Arch Dis Child* 1962;**37**:505.

3 Schreir K, Leuchte G. Argininbernsteinsaure-Krankheit. Deutsch. *Med Wschr* 1965;**90**:864.

4 Blackmore RJ, Lyon ICT, Veale AMO. Argininosuccinic aciduria. *Proc U Otago Med Sch* 1972;**50**:4.

5 Carton D, DeShrijver F, Kint J, *et al.* Argininosuccinic aciduria. Neonatal variant with rapid fatal course. *Acta Paediat Scand* 1969;**58**:528.

6 Levin B, Dobbs RH. Hereditary metabolic disorders involving urea cycle. *Proc R Soc Med* 1968;**61**:773.

7 Levin B. Hereditary metabolic disorders of the urea cycle. *Adv Clin Chem* 1971;**14**:65.

8 Hambraeus L, Hardell LI, Westphal O, *et al.* Argininosuccinic aciduria: report of three cases and the effect of high and reduced protein intake on the clinical state. *Acta Paediat Scand* 1974;**63**:525.

9 Farriaux J, Pieraert C, Fontaine G. Survival of infant with argininosuccinic aciduria to 3 months of age. *J Pediatr* 1975;**86**:639.

10 Glick NNR, Snodgrass PJ, and Schaer IA. Neonatal argininosuccinic aciduria with normal brain and kidney, but absent liver argininosuccinate lyase activity. *Am J Hum Genet* 1976;**28**:22.

11 O'Brien WE, McInnes R, Kalumuck K, Adcock M. Cloning and sequence analysis of cDNA for human argininosuccinate lyase. *Proc Natl Acad Sci USA* 1986;**83**:7211.

12 Lambert MA, Simard LR, Ray PN, McInnes RR. Molecular cloning of cDNA for rat hepatoma cell lines. *Mol Cell Biol* 1986;**6**:1722.

13 Barbosa P, Cialkowski M, O'Brien WE. Analysis of naturally occurring and site-directed mutations in the argininosuccinate lyase gene. *J Biol Chem* 1991;**266**:5286.

14 Walker DC, McCloskey DA, Simard LR, McInnes RR. Molecular analysis of human argininosuccinate lyase: mutant characterization and alternative splicing of the coding region. *Proc Natl Acad Sci USA* 1990;**87**:9625.

15 Shannon DC, Wichser J, Kazemi H. Hyperventilation and hyperammonemia. *Pediatr Res* 1973;**7**:423.

16 Solitare GB, Shih VE, Nelligan DJ, Dolan TF Jr. Argininosuccinic aciduria: clinical, biochemical, anatomic and neuropathological observations. *J Ment Def Res* 1969;**13**:153.

17 Maagøe H. Argininosuccinic aciduria. *Dan Med Bull* 1969;**16**:308.

18 Farrel G, Rauschkolb EW, Moure J, *et al.* Argininosuccinic aciduria. *Tex Med* 1969;**65**:90.

19 Flick JA, Latham PS, Perman JA, Brusilow SW. Hepatic involvement in argininosuccinase deficiency. *Pediatr Res* 1986;**20**:239A.

20 Bawle EV, Warrier I. Chronic coagulopathy in a patient with argininosuccinase deficiency. *J Inherit Metab Dis* 1991;**14**:109.

21 Shih VE. Early dietary management in an infant with argininosuccinase deficiency: Preliminary report. *J Pediatr* 1972;**80**:645.

22 Applegarth DA, Davidson AGF, Perry TL, *et al.* Argininosuccinic acidemia in a healthy infant detected by urine screening program. *Clin Chem* 1975;**21**:950.

23 Shih VE, Coulombe JT, Carney MM, *et al.* Argininosuccinic aciduria detected by routine screening. *Pediatr Res* 1976;**10**:371.

24 Tomlinson S, Westall RG. Argininosuccinic aciduria. Argininosuccinase and arginase in human blood cells. *Clin Sci* 1964;**26**:261.

25 Nyhan WL, Sakati NO. Argininosuccinic aciduria: in *Diagnostic Recognition of Genetic Disease* (WL Nyhan, NO Sakati). Lea and Febiger, Philadelphia;1987:165.

26 Colombo JP, Baumgartner R. Argininosuccinate cleavage enzyme of the kidney in argininosuccinic aciduria, in *Proceedings of the 6th Annual Symposium, Society for the Study of Inborn Errors of Metabolism*, Zurich 1968. Churchill-Livingstone, London;1969:19.

27 Batshaw ML, Painter MJ, Sproul GT, *et al.* Therapy of urea cycle enzymopathies: three case studies. *Johns Hopkins Med J* 1981;**146**:34.

28 Shih VE, Littlefield JW, Moser HW. Argininosuccinase deficiency in fibroblasts cultured from patients with argininosuccinase aciduria. *Biochem Genet* 1969;**3**:181.

29 Hill HZ, Goodman SI. Detection of inborn errors of metabolism. III. Defects in urea cycle metabolism. *Clin Genet* 1974;**6**:79.

30 Goodman SI, Mace JW, Turner B, Garrett WJ. Antenatal diagnosis of argininosuccinic aciduria. *Clin Genet* 1973;**4**:236.

31 Jacoby LB, Littlefield JWR, Milunsky A, *et al.* A microassay for argininosuccinase in cultured cells. *Am J Hum Genet* 1972;**24**:321.

32 Pollitt RJ. Argininosuccinate lyase levels in blood, liver and cultured fibroblasts of a patient with argininosuccinic aciduria. *Clin Chim Acta* 1973;**46**:33.

33 VanderHeiden C, Gerards, LJ VanBiervliet JPGM, *et al.* Lethal neonatal argininosuccinate lyase deficiency in four children from same sibship. *Helv Paediat Acta* 1976;**31**:407.

34 Kleijer WJ, Garritsen VH, Linnebank M, *et al.* Clinical, enzymatic, and molecular genetic characterization of a biochemical variant type of argininosuccinic aciduria: prenatal and postnatal diagnosis in five unrelated families. *J Inherit Metab Dis* 2002;**25**:399.

35 McInness RR, Shih V, Chilton S. Interallelic complementation in an inborn error of metabolism: genetic heterogeneity in argininosuccinic acid lyase deficiency. *Proc Natl Acad Sci USA* 1984;**81**:4480.

36 O'Brien WE, Barr BH. Argininosuccinate lyase: purification and characterization from human liver. *Biochemistry* 1981;**20**:2056.

37 Palekar AG, Mantagos S. Human liver argininosuccinase purification and partial characterization. *J Biol Chem* 1981;**256**:9192.

38 Simard L, O'Brien WE, McInnes RR. Argininosuccinate lyase deficiency: evidence for heterogeneous structural gene mutations by immunoblotting. *Am J Hum Genet* 1986;**39**:38.

39 McInnes RR, Christodoulou J, Craig HJ, Walker DC. A deletion "hotspot" in the argininosuccinate lyase (ASAL) gene has both a TOPO II recognition site and a DNA polymerase a (POL a) mutation site. *Pediatr Res* 1993;**33** Abstr. 769,131A.

40 Farriaux JP, Cartigny B, Dhondt JT, *et al.* A propos d'une observation d'arginino succinylurie neonatale: essai de traitement dietetique. *Acta Paediatr Belg* 1974;**28**:193.

41 Fleisher LD, Rassin DK, Desnick RH, *et al.* Argininosuccinic aciduria: prenatal studies in a family at risk. *Am J Hum Genet* 1979;**31**:439.

42 Fensom AH, Benson PF, Baker JE, Mutton DE. Prenatal diagnosis of argininosuccinic aciduria: effect of mycoplasma contamination on the indirect assay for argininosuccinic lyase. *Am J Hum Genet* 1980;**32**:761.

43 Shih VE, Littlefield JW. Argininosuccinase activity in amniotic fluid cells. *Lancet* 1970;**2**:45.

44 Dhondt JL, Farriaux JP, Pollitt RJ, *et al.* Attempt at antenatal diagnosis of argininosuccinic aciduria. *Ann Genet* (Paris) 1973;**19**:23.

45 Hartlage PL, Coryell ME, Hall WK, Hahn DA. Argininosuccinic aciduria: prenatal diagnosis and early dietary management. *J Pediatr* 1974;**85**:86.

46 Talbot HW, Sumlin AB, Naylor EW, Guthrie R. A neonatal screening test for argininosuccinic acid lyase deficiency and other urea cycle disorders. *Pediatrics* 1982;**70**:526.

47 Levy HL, Coulombe JT, Shih VE. Newborn urine screening: in *Neonatal Screening for Inborn Errors of Metabolism.* (eds H Bickel, R Gunthrie, G Hammersen) Springer-Verlag, Berlin;1980:89.

48 Rashed MS, Rahbeeni Z, Ozand PT. Screening blood spots for argininosuccinase deficiency by electrospray tandem mass spectrometry. *Southeast As J Trop Med Publ Health* 1999;**30**:(suppl. 2):170.

49 Wistow G, Piatigorsky J. Recruitment of enzymes as lens structural proteins. *Science* 1987;**236**:154.

50 Lee HJ, Chiou SH, Chang GG. Biochemical characterization and kinetic analysis of duck delta-crystallin with endogenous argininosuccinate lyase activity. *Biochem J* 1992;**283**:597.

51 Msall M, Batshaw ML, Suss R, *et al.* Neurologic outcome in children with inborn errors of urea synthesis. *N Engl J Med* 1984;**301**:1500.

33

Argininemia

MAJOR PHENOTYPIC EXPRESSION

Spastic quadriplegia, opisthotonus, convulsions, microcephaly, psychomotor retardation, hyperargininemia, argininuria and secondary cystinuria, lysinuria and ornithinuria, orotic aciduria, and deficiency of arginase.

INTRODUCTION

Argininemia is a disorder in which the clinical picture is quite different from any of the other disorders of the urea cycle. The picture is that of a spastic diplegia or quadriplegia [1–3]. It was reported in 1965 by Serrano [1] and in 1969 by Terheggen and Colombo and their colleagues [2]. The disease is caused by a virtually complete absence [4,5] of the activity of arginase (EC 3.5.3.1) (Figure 33.1). The human and rat genes have been cloned [6,7]. The human gene is located on chromosome 6 at band q23 [7]. A small number of heterogeneous mutations have so far been identified [8,9].

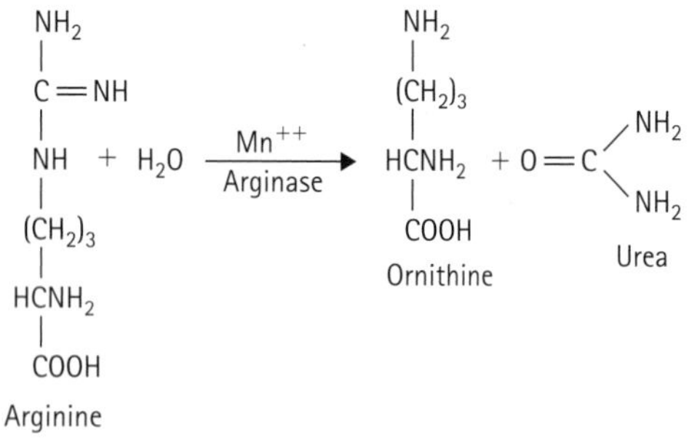

Figure 33.1 *The reaction catalyzed by arginase.*

CLINICAL ABNORMALITIES

Patients with argininemia are often recognized as abnormal because of failure to pass developmental milestones. With the advent of spasticity or opisthotonus they may be first thought to have cerebral palsy [3,10–20]. Onset may be with convulsions in the neonatal period [1–3]. Some patients may have recurrent cyclic vomiting from the early days of life [21]. Others may display anorexia, irritability or inconsolable crying; some patients have failure to thrive. Alternatively, there may be no signs in early infancy until it is apparent that development is delayed. The mother of one infant remarked on her drowsiness after feeding [3].

In the established phenotype the patient is very spastic and frequently opisthotonic (Figures 33.2, 33.3). If walking is possible, the gait is a spastic toe-walk. Scissoring of the lower extremities is common. Muscle tone is hypertonic, and the deep tendon reflexes are accentuated, both usually more so in the legs than in the arms. Patients may be hyperactive or irritable. They may be ataxic or appear clumsy. Involuntary movements may be choreic or athetoid, or there may be tremors. Drooling and dysphagia are common. Convulsions are regularly observed, and abnormalities of the electroencephalogram are the rule [22]. The pattern of the electroencephalogram (EEG) may be that of a spike and wave. Patients often become microcephalic (Figure 33.4), and cerebral atrophy is visible

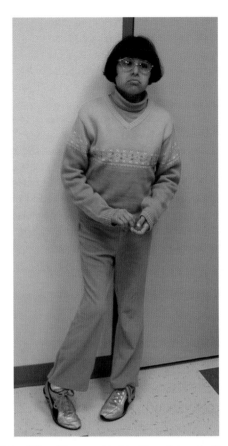

Figure 33.2   *T.G., a 19-year-old girl with argininemia. She walked with a distinct spastic gait and had equinovarus posturing of the feet. Deep tendon reflexes were brisk and there was clonus at both ankles.*

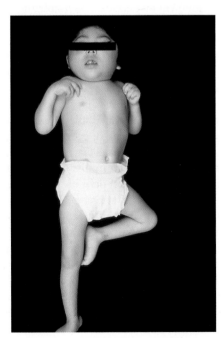

Figure 33.3   *A patient with argininemia was spastic, often opisthotonic, microcephalic and severely retarded. Convulsions began at 23 days-of-age. By 4 years-of-age she had no head control. (This illustration and Figure 33.4, were kindly provided by Dr. Makato Yoshino of Kurume University School of Medicine, Kurume, Japan.)*

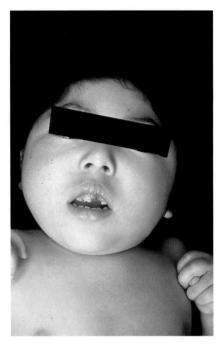

Figure 33.4   *The microcephaly of the patient. Neuroimaging revealed cerebral atrophy. Concentrations of arginine ranged from 3.1 to 19.4 mg/dL. Orotic aciduria was 6900 μg/mg creatinine.*

on computed tomography (CT) or magnetic resonance imaging (MRI) scan. Psychomotor retardation is usually severe, but it may be minimal in patients diagnosed and treated early (Figure 33.2).

Patients with argininemia may have episodic vomiting and hyperammonemia. Some have symptomatic hyperammonemia progressive to coma, and death in infancy has been reported [19,23]. In one patient hypertonicity, tachypnea, lip smacking and right-sided bicycling movements at 30 hours heralded fatal cerebral edema [23]. Also following an acute hyperammonemic episode, neurologic function may further deteriorate. However, abnormal concentrations of ammonia are less commonly encountered than in other disorders of the enzymes of the urea cycle.

Concentrations of ammonia may be elevated only intermittently, and hyperammonemia when it occurs, tend to be moderate [24]. In some patients the levels of ammonia were elevated in both the fed and fasting states [2]. In an occasional patient the concentration of ammonia may be surprisingly high in the absence of obvious symptoms of hyperammonemia [3]. On the other hand, in the patient with neonatal cerebral edema the peak ammonia was only 114 μmol/L, and it fell to 18 μmol/L with only supportive therapy [23]. There may be hepatomegaly. Serum activities of the transaminases may be elevated, and the prothrombin time may be prolonged. Unusual zones of different coloration and fragility of the hair have been reported in one patient [1]. Biopsied liver has been reported [4] to reveal multifocal hydropic changes.

Patients are generally recognized by the assessment of the concentration of amino acids in the blood or urine, the latter of which may be mistaken to be that of cystinuria (Chapter

70). All such abnormal findings should be pursued by the quantitative analysis of amino acids of the plasma. In patients with argininemia, the plasma concentration of arginine is usually four to 20 times that of the normal individuals, often up to 1500 μmol/L [14]. However, in one patient with very severe deficiency and lethal clinical disease the value was only 170 μmol/L [19].

Concentrations of arginine in cerebrospinal fluid (CSF) are also markedly elevated [3]. The concentration of the glutamine may be also increased, especially in the acute hyperammonemic crisis. In the neonate with cerebral edema [23] the plasma glutamine was 909 μmol/L and that of the CSF was 9587 μmol/L. Concentrations of other amino acids may also be elevated in the CSF [4,20]. These include ornithine, aspartate, threonine, glycine and methionine. A mechanism for their increase is not clear. The excretion of arginine in the urine is substantial. The urine also contains increased quantities of lysine, cystine and ornithine; this is the result of competition for their renal tubular reabsorption by the large amounts of arginine being processed by the kidney [22]. The amounts of cystine and ornithine are usually relatively less than observed in cystinuria. Lowering of plasma concentrations of arginine, by restriction of intake of protein, effectively reverses this pattern of urinary amino acid excretion.

GENETICS AND PATHOGENESIS

Argininemia is an autosomal recessive disease [16]. It has been reported about equally in males and females, and parents are unaffected. Incidence is approximately 1 in 363 000. The molecular defect is in the enzyme arginase. It catalyses the conversion of arginine to urea and ornithine (Figure 33.1). The activity of the enzyme is readily measured in erythrocytes, and it is through assay in this tissue that the diagnosis is usually made [3,4,10). The defect has also been demonstrated in liver [5]. The enzyme is not expressed in cultured fibroblasts [24]. The enzyme in red cells appears to be identical to that in liver. The enzyme from rat liver has been crystallized. It is a trimer of three 35 kDa monomers [25]. Negligible amounts of mRNA are found in normal tissues other than liver and erythrocytes.

Immunochemical studies using antibody to normal human hepatic arginase have shown cross-reacting material (CRM) in liver and erythrocytes of patients with argininemia in amounts equivalent to those normal individuals, indicating that a catalytically inactive structural arginase protein is made [26]. On the other hand, Western blot analyses of 15 patients were reported to reveal detectable arginase protein in only two patients [18]. Biopsy of the kidney of two patients with argininemia revealed arginase activity that was considerably greater than that of controls. Kidney contains a distinct mitochondrial arginase whose gene does not hybridize with that of the hepatic gene that is affected in argininemia [27]. The activity of the renal arginase provides the mechanism for the relatively normal production of urea in these patients.

The renal enzyme is 58 percent identical to the hepatic enzyme and 70 percent identical to *Xenopus* arginase.

The human gene at chromosome 6q 23 is 11.5 kb in size and contains 18 exons [28]. The crystal structure of the enzyme has been elucidated [29]. A dimagnesium cluster is essential for enzymatic activity and stability of the protein [30]. Mutation analysis revealed no gross deletions by Southern blot analysis in 15 patients [8]. In three, a Taq I restriction enzyme cleavage site was missing. In two of these, mutations were identified. One was homozygous for R291Y (an arginine-to-tyrosine change), and the other heterozygous for T290S (a threonine-to-serine change). Another patient, a Japanese was found to be a compound in which on one allele there was a four-base deletion in exon 3, which caused a frame shift at position 87 and a premature termination 45 residues later, while on the other allele a single base deletion in exon 2 led to a frame shift at 26 and premature termination on five residues later [31]. In another study of Japanese patients [32], the mutations found were in W122X, 6235R and L282 frame shift. The enzyme assay in expression studies in *E.coli* were zero, consistent with enzyme assays in the erythrocytes of patients. Additional mutations identified include D128G and H141L [33].

Detection of heterozygotes has been accomplished by finding arginase levels in erythrocytes or leukocytes that were appreciably less than the control levels [12,16,24,34]. The leukocyte concentration of arginine has been used to distinguish heterozygotes when arginase levels were not useful [34]. Mutation analysis is preferred for this purpose when the mutation is known. Prenatal diagnosis has been difficult because the enzyme is not expressed in fibroblasts [24]. Direct measurement by gas chromatography/mass spectrometry (GCMS) of orotic acid in amniotic fluid [35] was not useful in ornithine transcarbamylase deficiency, but it could be more reliable in argininemia. Fetal blood sampling can be employed but with risk of fetal loss. If the mutation is known this is the method of choice in prenatal diagnosis, extensive heterogeneity may make this impractical in an individual family. Fortunately, linkage analysis is available which takes advantage of restriction length polymorphism (RFLP) to PvuII should be useful in prenatal diagnosis [36] and so should a dinucleotide repeat polymorphism [33,37]. A screening method was developed that permits routine screening of newborns for deficiency of arginase [38,39]. The advent of tandem mass spectrometry and its applications to newborn screening has supplanted this approach.

In the presence of defective activity of arginase there is in addition to the accumulation of arginine, an impressive orotic aciduria [4,40]. The amounts of orotic acid found in the urine are considerably greater than those of patients with argininosuccinic aciduria and occur in the absence of hyperammonemia. So, this is not a consequence of accumulation of carbamyl phosphate behind the block, as occurs in ornithine transcarbamylase deficiency. Rather, it appears to be the direct result of the stimulation by accumulated arginine of N-acetylglutamate synthetase (NAGS), which leads to increased synthesis of carbamyl phosphate (Figure 33.5)[40]. Arginine

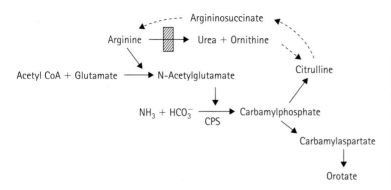

Figure 33.5 *Pathogenesis of the orotic aciduria of argininemia. Accumulation of arginine provides an effector function on N-acetylglutamate synthetase, and the product of this reaction stimulates carbamylphosphate synthetase (CPS). The carbamyl-phosphate generated does not accumulate, and since in the absence of arginase, ornithine is limiting, it flows along the pathway of pyrimidine synthesis to orotic acid.*

is a normal activator of NAGS since quantities of ornithine are limiting; this accumulation of carbamylphosphate when arginase is deficient leads preferentially to the biosynthesis of pyrimidines. Consistent with this were the low levels of ornithine reported by Yoshino [3], and the fact that, as ornithine levels were increased by treatment, the excretion of orotic acid decreased to normal levels, even though the concentration of arginine rose considerably. The orotic aciduria in this condition is also associated with increased excretion of uridine and uracil [41].

N-Acetylarginine, α-keto-guanidinovaleric acid and argininic acid, direct derivatives of arginine, are also found in the urine in this disorder, as well as guanidinoacetic acid and guanidinobutyric acid, compounds in which the amino group is donated via transamidination reaction [12,13,42,43]. Guanidinosuccinic acid excretion is not increased, whereas it does increase in individuals given an arginine load, suggesting a role for arginase in the generation of this compound [44,45]. The serum concentration of urea is usually normal in these patients.

The pathogenesis of the neurologic disability in argininemia is not clear, but doubtless it is the result of the chemical milieu in which the patient's brain develops. Intermittent or chronic elevation of ammonia could be sufficient, but the phenotype is so different from that of the other defects of the urea cycle that something about arginine or its products must have effects on the central nervous system. Neurotransmitter metabolism has been reported to be impaired in argininemia [46]. The production of nitric oxide from arginine could be another factor.

The occurrence of high levels of glutamine, especially in the CSF in the neonate with cerebral edema and only modest hyperammonemia [23] is consistent with a role for glutamine in this complication.

An arginase-deficient mouse displayed growth deficiency and hyperammonemia that led to death by 12 days of life [47].

neurologic development [4,16,17,48–53]. The methods employed have included protein restriction [13] and the use of mixtures of amino acids excluding arginine [16,51]. The latter approach has been effective in controlling levels of arginine in a patient treated from birth, as well as in older individuals [16]. Supplementation with lysine raised low levels of lysine in serum, but concentrations of arginine in plasma and CSF increased, and concentrations of ornithine in the CSF fell [50]. Supplementation with ornithine improved levels of ornithine and had a pronounced effect in lowering the amounts of orotic acid in the urine [3,50]. During combined supplementation with lysine and ornithine a patient gained weight well, and epileptiform activity on the EEG improved [50]. In one report [49], nitrogen-free analogs of some essential amino acids were employed to minimize further the nitrogenous sources of arginine in a low arginine diet.

Sodium benzoate therapy was employed in a 15-year-old patient with progressive spastic diplegia and borderline intelligence who had numerous hyperammonemic episodes, and required nasogastric tube feeding to maintain nutrition [52]. The doses employed were 250 to 375 mg/kg. This approach controlled levels of ammonia and reduced plasma concentrations of arginine. Restriction of the dietary intake of arginine reduced levels further. The excretion of orotic acid decreased to normal levels. Urinary hippurate excreted amounted to 60–80 percent of the administered benzoate and this constituted 35 to 43 percent of the urinary nitrogen. Progression of the diplegia was thought to have stopped. Phenylbutyrate or phenylacetate should have similar effects, but the resulting odor is less acceptable socially.

Phenylbutyrate increases expression of some genes, and it has been reported [54] to increase the activity of arginase in mice and in cultured cells. It was not tested in cells of patients with argininemia, but might be useful in patients with residual activity.

TREATMENT

Nutritional therapy has been designed to keep levels of arginine within normal limits, and success has been reported not only in meeting this objective, but also in promoting normal

References

1 Serrano AP. Argininuria, convulsions y oligofrenia: un nuevo error innato del metabolismo? *Rev Clin Esp* 1965;**97**:176.

2 Terheggen HG, Schwenk A, Lowenthal A, *et al.* Argininaemia with arginase deficiency. *Lancet* 1969;**2**:748.

3 Yoshino M, Kobota K, Yoshida I, *et al.* Argininemia: report of new mechanisms of orotic aciduria and hyperammonemia: in *Urea Cycle Diseases*, (eds A Lowenthal, A Mori, B Marescau), Advances in Experimental Medicine and Biology, Vol. 153. Plenum Press, New York;1982:121.

4 Cederbaum SD, Shaw KNF, Spector EB, *et al.* Hyperargininemia with arginase deficiency. *Pediatr Res* 1979;**13**:827.

5 Michels VV, Beaudet AL. Arginase deficiency in multiple tissues in argininemia. *Clin Genet* 1978;**13**:61.

6 Dizikes GJ, Grody WW, Kern RM, Cederbaum SD. Isolation of human arginase cDNA and absence of homology between two arginase genes. *Biochem Biophys Res Commun* 1986;**141**:53.

7 Sparkes RS, Dizikes GJ, Klisak I, *et al.* The gene for human liver arginase (ARGI) is assigned to chromosome band 6q23. *Am J Hum Genet* 1986;**39**:186.

8 Grody WW, Klein D, Dodson AE, *et al.* Molecular genetic study of human arginase deficiency. *Am J Hum Genet* 1992;**50**:1281.

9 Haraguchi Y, Aparicio, JM, Takiguchi M, *et al.* Molecular basis of argininemia. Identification of two discrete frame-shift deletions in the liver-type arginase gene. *J Clin Invest* 1990;**86**:347.

10 Terheggen HG, Schwenk A, Lowenthal A, *et al.* Hyperargininamie mit arginasedefekt eine neue familiare Stoffwechselstorung. *I Klin Bef Z Kinderheilk* 1970;**107**: 298.

11 Iyer R, Jenkinson CP, Vockley JC, *et al.* The human arginases and arginase deficiency. *J Inherit Metab Dis* 1998;**21**:86.

12 Terheggen HG, Lavinha F, Colombo JP, *et al.* Familial hyperargininemia. *J Hum Genet* 1972;**20**:69.

13 Terheggen HG, Lowenthal A, Lavinha F, Colombo JP. Familial hyperargininaemia. *Arch Dis Child* 1975;**50**:57.

14 Terheggen HG, Schwenk A, Lowenthal A, *et al.* Hyperargininamia mit arginasedefekt eine neue familiare stoffwechselstorung. II Biochemische Untersuchungen *Z. Kinderheilk* 1970;**107**:313.

15 Van Sande M, Terheggen HG, Clara R, *et al.* Lysine-cystine pattern associated with neurological disorders: in *Inherited Disorders of Sulfur Metabolism.* (eds Carson NAJ, Raine DN) Churchill Livingston, Edinburgh;1971:85.

16 Synderman SE, Sansaricq CC, Cheu WJ, *et al.* Argininemia. *J Pediatr* 1977;**90**:563.

17 Cederbaum SD, Shaw KNF, Valente M. Hyperargininemia. *J Pediatr* 1977;**90**:569.

18 Qureshi IA, Letarte J, Ouellet R, *et al.* Ammonia metabolism in a family affected by hyperargininemia. *Diabéte et Metabolisme* 1981;**7**:5.

19 Jorda A, Rubio V, Portoles M, *et al.* A new case of arginase deficiency in a Spanish male. *J Inherit Metab Dis* 1986;**9**:393.

20 Bernar J, Hanson RA, Kern R, *et al.* Arginase deficiency in a 12-year old boy with mild impairment of intellectual function. *J Pediatr* 1986;**108**:432.

21 Nyhan WL, Sakati SA. Argininemia: in *Diagnostic Recognition of Genetic Disease,* (eds WL Nyhan, SA Sakati), Lea and Febiger, Philadelphia;1987:169.

22 Terheggen HG, Lowenthal A, Colombo JP. Clinical and biochemical findings in argininemia: in *Urea Cycle Diseases*, (eds A Lowenthal, A Mori, B Marescalu), Advances in Medicine and Biology, Vol. 153. Plenum Press, New York;1982:111.

23 Picker JD, Puga AC, Levy HL, *et al.* Arginase deficiency with lethal neonatal expression: evidence for the glutamine hypothesis of cerebral edema. *J Pediatr* 1200;**342**:349.

24 Van Elsen A, Leroy JG. Human hyperargininemia: a mutation not expressed in skin fibroblasts. *Am J Hum Genet* 1977;**29**:350.

25 Kanyo ZF, Chen CY, Daghigh DF, *et al.* Crystallization and oligomeric structure of rat liver arginase. *J Mol Biol* 1992;**224**:1175.

26 Spector EB, Rice SCH, Cederbaum SD. Immunologic studies of arginase in tissues of normal human adult and arginase-deficient patients. *Pediatr Res* 1983;**17**:941.

27 Grody WW, Argyle C, Kern RM, *et al.* Differential expression of two human arginase genes in hyperargininemia. Enzymatic, pathologic and molecular analysis. *J Clin Invest* 1989;**83**:602.

28 Takioguchi M, Mori M. *In-vitro* analysis of the rat liver type arginase promoter. *J Biol Chem* 1991;**266**:9186.

29 Kanyo ZF, Scolnick LR, Ash DE, Christianson DW. Structure of a unique binuclear manganese cluster in arginase. *Nature* 1996;**383**:554.

30 Scolnick LR, Kanyo ZF, Cavalli RC, *et al.* Altering the binuclear manganese cluster of arginase diminishes thermostability and catalytic function. *Biochemistry* 1994;**36**:10652.

31 Haraguchi Y, Aparicio JM, Akaboshi I, *et al.* Molecular basis of argininemia. Identification of two discrete frame-shift deletions in the liver arginase gene. *J Clin Invest* 1990;**86**:347.

32 Uchino T, Haraguchi Y, Aparicia JM, *et al.* Three novel mutations in the liver-type arginase gene in three unrelated Japanese patients with Argininemia. *Am J Hum Genet* 1992;**51**:1406.

33 Vockley JG, Tabor DE, Kern RM, *et al.* Identification of mutations (D128G, HI41L) in the liver arginase gene of patients with hyperargininemia. *Hum Mutat* 1994;**4**:150.

34 Marescau B, Pintens J, Lowenthal A, *et al.* Arginase and free amino acids in hyperargininemia: leuckocyte arginine as a diagnosis parameter for heterozygotes. *J Clin Chem Clin Biochem* 1979;**17**:211.

35 Jakobs C, Sweetman L, Nyhan WL, *et al.* Stable isotope dilution analysis of orotic acid and uracil in amniotic fluid. *Clin Chim Acta* 1984;**143**:123.

36 Kidd JR, Dizikes GJ, Grody WW, *et al.* A Pvu11 RFLP for the human liver arginase (ARG1) gene. *Nucleic Acids Res* 1984;**14**:9544.

37 Meloni R, Fougerousse F, Roudaut C, Beckmann JS. Dinucleotide repeat polymorphism at the human liver arginase gene (ARG 1). *Nucleic Acids Res* 1992;**20**:1166.

38 Orfanos AP, Naylor EW, Guthrie R. Fluorometric micromethod for determination of arginase activity in dried blood spots on filter paper. *Clin Chem* 1980;**26**:1198.

39 Naylor EW, Orfanos AP, Guthrie R. A simple screening test for arginase deficiency (hyperargininemia). *J Lab Clin Me.d* 1977;**89**:876.

40 Bachmann C, Colombo JP. Diagnostic value of orotic acid excretion in heritable disorders of the urea cycle and in hyperammonemia due to organic acidurias. *Eur J Pediatr* 1980;**134**:109.

41 Naylor EW, Cederbaum SD. Urinary pyrimidine excretion in arginase deficiency. *J Inherit Metab Dis* 1981;**4**:207.

42 Marescau B, Pintens J, Lowenthal A, Terheggen HG. Excretion of alpha-keto-gamma-guanidinovaleric acid and its cyclic form in patients with hyperargininemia patients. *J Hum Genet* 1976;**24**:61.

43 Wiechert P, Mortelman J, Lavinha F, *et al.* Excretion of guanidine-derivatives in urine of hyperargininemic patients. *J Hum Genet* 1976;**24**:62.

44 Mori A, Matsumoto M, Hiramatsu C. Alpha-guanidinoglutaric acid in urine of arginine loaded rabbits. *IRCS Med Sci Biochem* 1980;**8**:75.

45 Stein IM, Cohen BD, Kornhauser RS. Guanidino-succinic acid in renal failure experimental azotemia and inborn errors of the urea cycle. *N Engl J Med* 1969;**280**:926.

47 Hyland K, Smith I, Clayton PT. Leonard JV. Impaired neurotransmitter amine metabolic deficiency. *J Neurosurg Psychiatry* 1985;**48**:1189.

48 Iyer, RK, Yu H, Kern RM, *et al.* Further studies on the arginase-1 deficient mouse. *Am J Human Genet* 2002;**71**:413.

49 Cederbaum SD, Shaw KNF, Valente M, Cotton ME. Argininosuccinic aciduria. *Am J Ment Defic* 1973;**77**:395.

50 Cederbaum SD, Moedijono SJ, Shaw KNF, *et al.* Treatment of hyperargininemia due to arginase deficiency with a chemically defined diet. *J Inher Metab Dis* 1982;**5**:95.

51   Kang SS, Wong PWK, Melyn MA. Hyperargininemia: effect of ornithine and lysine supplementation. *J Pediatr* 1983;**103**:763.

52   Synderman SW, Sansaricq C, Norton PM, Goldstein F. Argininemia treated from birth. *J Pediatr* 1979;**94**:61.

53   Qureshi IA, Letarte J, Quellet R. Treatment of hyperargininemia with sodium benzoate and arginine-restricted diet. *J Pediatr* 1984;**104**:473.

54   Kern RM, Yang Z, Grody WW, *et al.* Arginase induction by sodium phenylbutyrate in mouse tissues and human cell lines. *Am J Human Genet* 2002;**71**:425.

34

Hyperornithinemia, hyperammonemia, homocitrullinuria (HHH) syndrome

MAJOR PHENOTYPIC EXPRESSION

Episodic hyperammonemia, ataxia, vomiting, lethargy, or coma; failure to thrive; mental retardation; seizures; hyperornithinemia; homocitrullinuria; and defective transport of ornithine into mitochondria.

INTRODUCTION

The disorder was first described by Shih, Efron and Moser [1] in a patient with mental retardation, irritability and myoclonic spasms who had intermittent attacks of hyperammonemia and ataxia. He was described by the parents as having attacks in infancy of sudden jumping, as though he had been stuck by a pin. Dropping of the head was a concomitant of these myoclonic spells. A small number of patients has since been reported, six from a single consanguineous kindred [2–4]. The fundamental defect is an inability to transport ornithine into mitochondria [5–8] (Figure 34.1). The gene was cloned

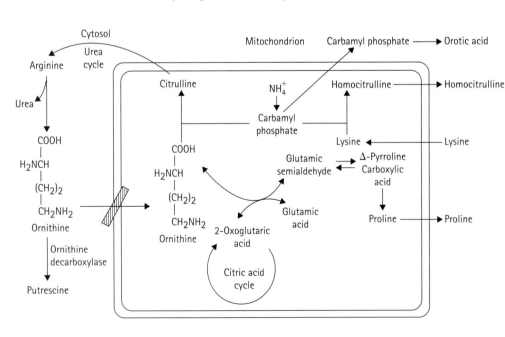

Figure 34.1 *Metabolic interrelations involving ornithine. The defect in the HHH syndrome is in the transport catalyzing the movement of ornithine into mitochondria.*

by Camacho and colleagues [9] and localized to chromosome 13q14. Three mutations were found to account for 21 of 22 possible mutant alleles including F188Δ which is common in French-Canadian patients. An additional mutation has been found in two families of Mexican descent with a mild phenotype [10].

CLINICAL ABNORMALITIES

Intermittent episodes of hyperammonemia are characteristic features of this disorder. This may be manifested in episodic vomiting, lethargy, coma, or ataxia. It was evident in the experience with the initial and subsequent patients that these symptoms vary directly with the dietary intake of protein, and the degree of hyperammonemia. This disease may first present as a Reye-like syndrome. Our patient was diagnosed as an example of Reye syndrome prior to referral despite the fact that coma developed following feeding of 8 g protein/kg following a thermal burn (Figures 34.2 and 34.3).

In infancy failure to thrive and developmental delay have been observed, although the initial patient grew along the 10th percentile [1], except when fed his lowest intake of protein, and others have grown normally while receiving diets moderately restricted in protein [6]. In our patient, failure to thrive was associated with very low levels of lysine in plasma [7]. Prior to supplementation with lysine orotate, growth in length had virtually ceased. Growth was rewarding following supplementation, which returned concentrations of lysine in plasma to normal.

Ultimate intelligence has ranged from low normal to severely retarded [1–4,10–13]. In two families IQ levels ranged from 76–80; in one, diagnosis was made as part of an evaluation for poor school performance in otherwise asymptomatic brothers; in the other family the diagnosis was made at three years-of-age on the basis of mild hyperammonemia following gastroententis, while the 13-year-old sister was asymptomatic; IQ was 79 in both siblings who were doing well in mainstream classes.

Hyperammonemic attacks may be less frequent in older patients, who may select a diet low in protein. On the other hand a 21-year-old severely retarded patient continued to have stuporous episodes, at least one a month, which lasted up to two hours. Seizures have been observed with onset from 10 months to 18 years. They may be generalized, tonic-clonic, as well as myoclonic [6]. One patient presented with attacks of headache progressive to unconsciousness beginning at 39 years-of-age [8]. Our patient has been left with a chronic seizure disorder despite an absence of symptomatic hyperammonemia since the initial episode of coma.

Ocular findings, in contrast to gyrate atrophy of the retina, have been normal except for a patient who developed papilledema during an attack of acute symptomatic hyperammonemia [3].

Progressive spastic paraparesis was emphasized as a clinical characteristic in three patients in one family [9]. This was clearly evident in the oldest patient, who began to have progressive disturbance of gait at 14 years, and at 21 had increased deep tendon reflexes, sustained ankle clonus and bilateral Babinski responses. His IQ was 67. He stuttered and had an aggressive personality that led to psychiatric consultation. His 18-year-old sister had an IQ of 60 and could not run or jump;

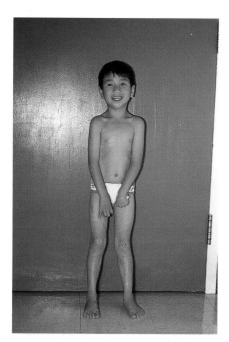

Figure 34.2 *A 5-year-old Vietnamese boy with the HHH-syndrome. Scars on his legs signify the thermal burns and its attendant treatment with large amounts of protein that led to his only episode of coma and an initial diagnosis of Reye syndrome.*

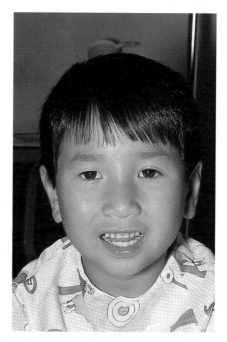

Figure 34.3 *Close-up reveals no unusual physical features. He was developmentally delayed.*

deep tendon reflexes were increased, and there were ankle clonus and Babinski responses. The 13-year-old brother had brisk deep tendon reflexes and an IQ of 51.

Cortical atrophy has been described on computed tomography (CT) scan [8]. Liver biopsy of a patient with hepatomegaly [3] revealed abnormal mitochondria containing crystalloid structures. In another patient [12] there was diffuse microvesicular fat and there were large lipid-containing vacuoles, as well as large, irregular mitochondria with paracrystalline inclusions. Our patient [7] had hepatic microvesicular fat, which had appeared to confirm the diagnosis of Reye syndrome.

Metabolic abnormality is usually first evident in hyperammonemia. The levels encountered in an acute attack, even in a patient in coma, are usually considerably less elevated than those we are accustomed to in neonatal infants with disorders of the urea cycle. The concentration of ammonia may be chronically elevated in a patient ingesting a diet high in protein. More often, the level is normal in fasting, but elevated postprandially. The concentrations of glutamine and alanine in plasma may be increased as concomitants of hyperammonemia. Orotic acid excretion has been reported to be elevated in only about half of the patients [3], but it may be induced by loading with protein or alanine. Our patient (Figures 34.2 and 34.3) had little, and often no, measurable urinary orotic acid at baseline, but loading with alanine led to a pronounced orotic aciduria (Table 34.1). He was a refugee from Vietnam, accustomed to a low protein diet. As he gradually became Americanized his protein intake increased and the amounts of orotic acid in the urine increased progressively (Table 34.2). The diagnosis may be made difficult by the increases in aspartate aminotransferase (AST) and alanine aminotransferase (ALT) that may occur acutely with the hyperammonemia [1,10].

Table 34.1 *Excretion of orotic acid following alanine**

Hours	mg/g creatine
0–2.5	18
2.5–5	236
5–6	229
6–24	242

* The dose of alanine was 400 mg/kg.

Table 34.2 *Relationship between the excretion of orotic acid and the intake of protein*

Protein intake g/kg/day	Urinary orotic acid mg/g creatine
2	–
3.7	12
4.7	19
5.4	272

GENETICS AND PATHOGENESIS

Hyperornithinemia is a hallmark feature of the metabolic abnormality. Concentrations in plasma have usually ranged from 270 to 780 μmol/L [1–4, 7]. Concentrations as high as 915 and 1439 μmol/L have been recorded [1,11]. Ornithinuria has ranged from 73 to 8160 μmol/g creatinine. The highest levels of ornithine in body fluids have been those encountered during acute episodes of hyperammonemia. Confronted with an elevated concentration of ornithine and hyperammonemia, especially in a patient with orotic aciduria, one thinks about ornithine transcarbamylase deficiency, but ornithine concentrations are never elevated in ornithine transcarbamylase deficiency, even in those with unusual kinetic properties [14,15] (Chapter 29).

There are two other types of hyperornithinemia: one with gyrate atrophy of the choroid and retina, in which the activity of ornithine-5-aminotransferase is deficient [16], and a disorder reported [17] in two siblings with mental retardation and renal tubular dysfunction, which may represent a partial deficiency of the same enzyme, because its activity in liver was reported to be 60–80 percent reduced but kinetically normal [18]. In any case, neither of these hyperornithinemic situations is ever hyperammonemic. Levels of ornithine in the two siblings were about three times normal, but later reported as normal [18], suggesting that the abnormality might be secondary to something such as acute hepatic disease; in gyrate atrophy they tend to be higher than in the HHH syndrome, on average about 1 mmol/L [19]. Oral loading with ornithine in HHH syndrome leads to higher peak levels than in normal individuals and a slower return to baseline [1,11].

The homocitrullinuria is the third major feature of the disease. In the presence of accumulated carbamylphosphate, lysine is carboxylated to form homocitrulline (Figure 34.1), which is efficiently excreted in the urine. Reported levels of excretion have ranged from 93 to 8160 μmol/g creatinine. As in the case of the orotic aciduria homocitrullinuria may be absent or not prominent in patients receiving little protein in their diets. Its levels of excretion can be correlated with protein intake [13] or the administration of lysine, and good correlation was observed between the urinary homocitrulline: creatinine ratio and the plasma lysine:ornithine ratio [13]. Homocitrulline is commonly found in the urine of infants and children, a consequence of its formation by the heat treatment of milk products, and its subsequent ingestion and excretion by the young individual [20,21]. It is often found in patients with generalized aminoaciduria and regularly follows lysine loading in normal children and adults [22,23].

Concentrations of lysine in the blood may be elevated during the acute attack of hyperammonemia as a nonspecific concomitant of hyperammonemia. During steady-state conditions, levels of lysine in blood and urine are usually low [11]. We have observed that lysine may become limiting for growth in this disease [7].

Other unusual compounds may be found in the urine of the patient. Among those identified is 3-aminopiperid-2-one, a cyclic d-lactam or methylester of ornithine [24,25]. Amounts as high as 450 μmol/g creatine have been reported [11].

The molecular defect is in the transport system responsible for the movement of ornithine into mitochondria [5,13] (Figure 34.1). This makes ornithine limiting for the synthesis of citrulline and impairs the operation of the urea cycle. This enzyme was reported by Gamble and Lehninger [26] to be uni-directional and highly stereospecific for l-ornithine. It requires respiratory energy. The driving force for entry of ornithine is a negative internal transmembrane potential produced by the entry of proton-conducting anions. The system was characterized in rat liver mitochondria; it was not operative in heart. Citrulline passes through the membrane in both directions without requiring respiratory energy.

Evidence for a defect in the ornithine transport system was obtained [6] by the study of ^{14}C-ornithine incubation in intact fibroblasts; the compartments were then separated by a digitonin method; there was significantly less incorporation into the pellet fraction in the patient than in controls. This was not confirmed in another study [27], although the methodology was somewhat different. Less direct evidence was the fact that cultured fibroblasts and phytohemagglutinin-stimulated lymphocytes produced much less labeled proline, glutamate, aspartate and CO_2 from ^{14}C-ornithine than did control cells [28]. Similar results in a simpler system were obtained in which fibroblasts of patients were defective in the incorporation of the isotope of ^{14}C-ornithine into protein [29]. The apparent Km for this process in a patient's fibroblasts was 10 times that of controls. The incorporation of the isotope of ornithine into protein requires prior conversion to proline and/or glutamate. The enzymes involved in these conversions, including pyrroline-5-carboxylate reductase, are normal [30]. Direct measurement of amino acid concentrations in hepatic mitochondria of a patient revealed the concentration of ornithine to be low [8]. Direct evidence of defective transport of ornithine was obtained in studies of mitochondria isolated from fresh liver tissue of three patients [5].

Inheritance appears to be autosomal recessive. This is consistent with the occurrence of six patients representing both sexes in one family [3]. Heterozygote detection has not been possible with current methodology [6] but would be possible in families in which the mutation is known. Fibroblasts of patients with this disorder were effectively complemented by those of a patient with gyrate atrophy, while the cells of two patients with the HHH syndrome fell into the same complementation group [29].

The ornithine transporter gene designated ORNT 1 was identified by the use of sequences from the ARG 11 and ARG 13 genes of Neurospora and Saccharomyces which encode the mitochondrial carrier family proteins that are involved in the transport of ornithine across the mitochondrial inner membrane [9]. The expression of ORNT 1 is high in liver. Expression of ORNT 1 in transformed fibroblasts of patients with HHH syndrome restored ornithine transport function. The gene contains 8 exons over 26 Kb [31].

Among mutations observed [9,10], F188Δ, a 3 bp inframe deletion in a sequence of four consecutive TTC phenylalanine codons encodes an unstable protein. This mutation was found in nine of 10 French-Canadian homozygotes and one heterozygote. E180K encodes a stable properly targeted protein and results from a G to A transition at bp 538. This mutation was found in the patient's Irish-American father, but not in his Japanese mother, who had a terminal microdeletion 13q14. Our patient [7] had a nonsense mutation R179ter [32].

A second gene, ORNT 2, has been discovered [33] which contains no introns and has a structure 88 percent identical to ORNT 1. It is located on chromosome 5q31. Overexpression of protein product ORNT 2 in fibroblasts of patients with HHH syndrome restored the metabolism of ornithine, much as did ORNT 1. The existence of this redundancy in ornithine transport was considered consistent with the generally milder phenotype in this disease than in other urea cycle abnormalities, as well as the level of residual ornithine transport observed in cultured F188Δ and E180K cells. This conceptualization has been strengthened and amplified by the finding that the Mexican families with mild phenotype had a T32R mutation in both in ORNT 1, but they also were heterozygous for the glycine 181 polymorphion in ORNT 2 which is a gain of function variant.

TREATMENT

Restriction of the dietary intake of protein to 1.5 g/kg permitted maintenance of the blood ammonia at 90–100 μg/dL and the avoidance of acute attacks of hyperammonemia, whereas 2 g/kg led to symptomatic hyperammonemia [1]. In this patient an acute load of 100 mg lysine/kg did not increase homocitrulline excretion. Supplementation of the diet with 1 g lysine hydrochloride increased its blood concentration to a low normal level but did not appreciably change the plasma ornithine or ammonia in this 19-month-old patient. Supplementation with 1 g ornithine hydrochloride per day increased the plasma concentration of ornithine but had no effect on the postprandial ammonia or the plasma lysine. On the other hand, supplementation with 6 g per day of ornithine hydrochloride or 7.5 g of arginine hydrochloride in a 32–45 kg woman were reported to lower postprandial ammonia and urinary homocitrulline [12]. In this patient, supplementation with 6 g per day of lysine hydrochloride increased the excretion of homocitrulline. Ornithine supplementation reduced plasma concentrations of lysine. In another patient [34] supplementation with ornithine reduced the concentration of ammonia following a breakfast containing 0.5 g protein/kg from 273 to 107 μg/dL.

References

1 Shih VE, Effron ML, Moser HW. Hyperornithinemia hyperammonemia and homocitrullinemia. A new disorder of amino acid metabolism associated with myoclonic seizures and mental retardation. *Am J Dis Child* 1969;**117**:83.

2 Wright T, Pollitt R. Psychomotor retardation epileptic and stuporous attacks irritability and ataxia associated with ammonia intoxication high blood ornithine levels and increased homocitrulline in the urine. *Proc Royal Soc Med* 1973;**66**:221.

3 Gatfield PD, Taller E, Wolfe DM, Haust MD. Hyperornithinemia hyperammonemia and homocitrullinuria associated with decreased carbamyl phosphate synthetase I activity. *Pediatr Res* 1975;**9**:488.

4 Valle D, Simell O. The hyperornithinemias: in *The Metabolic Basis of Inherited Disease* 5th edn (eds JB Stanbury, JB Wyngaarden, DS Fredrickson, *et al.*) McGraw-Hill Book Co Inc, New York;1983:382.

5 Inoue I, Shaheki T, Kayanuma K, *et al.* Direct evidence of decreased ornithine transport activity in the liver mitochondria from patients with hyperornithinemia hyperammonemia and homocitrullinuria: in *4th International Congress of Inborn Errors of Metabolism* May 26–30 1987, Sendai, Japan. (abstr FP-60).

6 Hommes FA, Ho CK, Roesel RA, Coryell ME. Decreased transport of ornithine across the inner mitochondrial membrane as a cause of hyperornithinaemia. *J Inherit Metab Dis* 1982;**5**:41.

7 Nyhan WL, Rice-Asaro M, Acosta P. Advances in the treatment of amino acid and organic acid disorders: in *Treatment of Genetic Diseases* (ed. Desnick RJ) Churchill Livingstone, New York;1991:45.

8 Oyanagi K, Tsuchiyama A, Itakura Y, *et al.* The mechanism of hyperammonaemia and hyperornithinaemia in the syndrome of hyperornithinaemia hyperammonaemia and homocitrullinuria. *J Inher Metab Dis* 1983;**6**:133.

9 Camacho JA, Obie C, Biery B, *et al.* Hyperornithinaemia-hyperammonaemia-homocitrullinuria syndrome is caused by mutations in a gene encoding a mitochondrial ornithine transporter. *Nature Genetics* 1999;**22**:151.

10 Camacho J, Mardach R, Rioseco-Camacho N, *et al.* Phenotypic characterization and functional consequences of a mutation in the human mitochondrial ornithine transporter (ORNT1-T32R). *J Am Hum Genet* 2002;**71**:(suppl) 418.

11 Rodes M, Ribes A, Pineda M, *et al.* A new family affected by the syndrome of hyperornithinaemia hyperammonaemia and homocitrullinuria. *J Inherit Metab Dis* 1987;**10**:73.

12 Winter HS, Perez-Atavde AR, Levy HL, Shih VE. Unique hepatic ultrastructural changes in a patient with hyperammonemia (HAM) hyperornithinemia (HOR) and homocitrulluria (HC). *Pediatr Res* 1980;**14**:583.

13 Fell V, Pollitt R, Sampson GA, Trevor W. Ornithinemia hyperammonemia and homocitrullinuria. A disease associated with mental retardation and possibly caused by defective mitochondrial transport. *Am J Dis Child* 1974;**127**:752.

14 Levin B, Oberholzer VG, Sinclair L. Biochemical investigations of hyperammonemia. *Lancet* 1969;**2**:170.

15 Oizumi J, Nf WG, Koch R, *et al.* Partial ornithine transcarbamylase deficiency associated with recurrent hyperammonemia lethargy and depressed sensorium. *Clin Genet* 1984;**25**:538.

16 O'Donnell JJ, Sandman RP, Martin SR. Gyrate atrophy of the retina: inborn error of l-ornithine: 2-oxoacid aminotransferase. *Science* 1978;**200**:200.

17 Bickel H, Feist D, Muller H, Quadbeck G. ornithinamie eine weiter aminosaurenstoff-Wechsel-sturung mit hirnschadijgung. *Dtsch Med Wochenschr* 1968;**93**:2247.

18 Kekomaki MP, Raiha Niels CR, Bickel H. Ornithine-ketoacid aminotransferase in human liver with reference to patients with hyperornithinaemia and familial protein intolerance. *Clin Chem* 1969;**23**:203.

19 Simell O, Takki K. Raised plasma ornithine and gyrate atrophy of the choroid and retina. *Lancet* 1973;**2**:1031.

20 Gerritsen T, Waisman HA, Lipton SH, Strong FM. Natural occurrence of homocitrulline: I Excretion in the urine. *Arch Biochem Biophys* 1962;**97**:34.

21 Gerritsen T, Vaughn JG, Waisman HA. Origin of homocitrulline in the urine of infants. *Arch Biochem Biophys* 1963;**100**:298.

22 Ryan WL, Wells IC. Homocitrulline and homoarginine synthesis from lysine. *Science* 1964;**144**:1122.

23 Buergi W, Colombo JP, Richterich R. Thin-layer chromatography of the acid and ether soluble DNP-amino acids in urine. *Klin Wochenschr* 1965;**43**:1202.

24 Oberholzer VG, Briddon A. 3-Amino-2-piperidone in the urine of patients with hyperornithinemia. *Clin Chim Acta* 1978;**87**:411.

25 Fell V, Pollitt RJ. 3-Aminopiperid-2-one an unusual metabolite in the urine of a patient with hyperammonaemia hyperornithinaemia and homocitrullinuria. *Clin Chim Acta* 1978;**87**:405.

26 Gamble JG, Lehninger AL. Transport or ornithine and citrulline across the mitochondrial membrane. *J Biol Chem* 1973;**248**:610.

27 Gray RGF, Hill SE, Pollitt RJ. Studies on the pathway from ornithine to proline in cultured skin fibroblasts with reference to the defect in hyperornithinaemia with hyperammonaemia and homocitrullinuria. *J Inherit Metab Dis* 1983;**6**:143.

28 Gray RGF, Hill SE, Pollitt RJ. Reduced ornithine catabolism in cultured fibroblasts and phytohaemagglutinin-stimulated lymphocytes from a patient with hyperornithinaemia hyperammonaemia and homocitrullinuria. *Clin Chim Acta* 1982;**118**:141.

29 Shih VE, Mandell R, Herzfeld A. Defective ornithine metabolism in cultured skin fibroblasts from patients with the syndrome of hyperornithinemia hyperammonemia and homocitrullinuria. *Clin Chim Acta* 1982;**118**:149.

30 Shih VE, Mandell R, Herzfeld A. Defective ornithine metabolism in the syndrome of hyperornithinaemia hyperammonaemia and homocitrullinuria. *J Inherit Metab Dis* 1981;**4**:95.

31 Camacho JA, Rioseco-Camacho N, Andrade D. Characterization of the genomic structure of the human mitochondrial ornithine transporter (HsORNT1) and annotation of its non-processed pseudogenes on chromosomes 3 10 13 22 and Y. *Personal Communication* 2002.

32 Camacho JA. *Personal Communication* 2002.

33 Camacho JA, Rioseco-Camacho N, Obie C, *et al.* Cloning and characterization of ORNT2 a second mitochondrial ornithine transporter that can rescue a defective ORNT1 in patients with the hyperornithinemia-hyperammonemia-homocitrullinemia syndrome. A urea cycle disorder. *Mol Genet Metab* 2003;**79**:257.

34 Gordon BA, Gatfield PD, Wolfe DM. Studies on the metabolic defect in patients with hyperammonemia hyperornithinemia and homocitrullinuria. *Clin Res* 1976;**24**:688A.

Lysinuric protein intolerance

MAJOR PHENOTYPIC EXPRESSION

Failure to thrive; episodic hyperammonemia; vomiting; diarrhea; pulmonary fibrosis and respiratory insufficiency; nephritis; low concentrations of lysine and other dibasic amino acids in plasma; and massive excretion of lysine in the urine along with increased excretion of ornithine and arginine; and decreased cellular transport of cationic amino acids.

INTRODUCTION

Lysinuric protein intolerance was first described by Perheentupa and Visakorpi [1] from Finland in 1965 in a report of three patients with familial intolerance to protein and abnormal transport of the basic amino acids. The disease is prevalent in Finland, where it has been estimated to occur in one in 60 000 [2], and Finns or Finnish Lapps have comprised nearly half of the patients reported [1–6]. However, the disease may be found in any ethnic population. The fundamental defect is an abnormality in the transport of basic amino acids in the basilateral or antiluminal membrane of epithelial cells [7–9] (Figure 35.1). The abnormality is in the efflux of these amino acids and can be demonstrated in cultured fibroblasts [10,11].

CLINICAL ABNORMALITIES

Most infants present with failure to thrive (Figures 35.2–35.4) [4]. There may be alopecia. Subcutaneous fat is diminished or absent, and the skin folds loose. Associated diarrhea may suggest a malabsorption syndrome. Skin lesions may resemble those of kwashiorkor or acrodermatitis and zinc deficiency (Figures 35.2, 35.3). A dry scaly rash is sometimes seen and sores on the sides of the mouth [12]. Dystrophic nails may

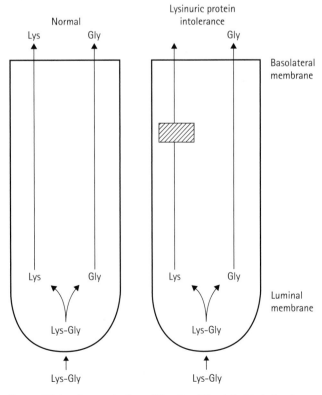

Figure 35.1 *Demonstration of the site of the defect in lysinuric protein intolerance at the antiluminal border of the epithelial cell of the jejeunal mucosa by the administration of a lysylpeptide [6].*

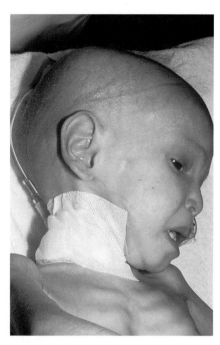

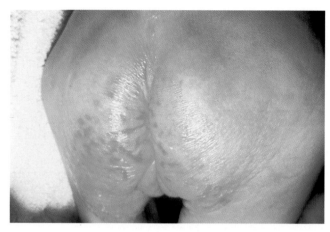

Figure 35.3 *R.Q. The perianal dermatitis was classic for a diagnosis of acrodermatitis enteropathica. Treatment of the failure-to-thrive with parenteral alimentation led to hyperammonemic coma. Levels of alanine and glutamine were elevated.*

Figure 35.2 *R.Q., a patient with lysinuric protein intolerance who presented at 5 years-of-age with failure-to-thrive, alopecia, and skin lesions reminiscent of kwashiorkor or zinc deficiency. Treatment with citrulline reversed the findings in the skin and hair.*

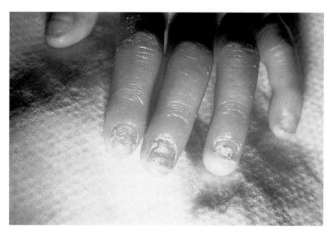

Figure 35.4 *R.Q. The fingers and nails were also reminiscent of acrodermatitis enteropathica. The day after initiating citrulline this bedridden patient was sitting up. She ultimately developed nails and hair.*

contribute to the picture of acrodermatitis enteropathica (Figure 35.4). A 5-year-old boy with chronic diarrhea and pitting edema of the lower extremities was thought to have celiac disease because villous atrophy was found on intestinal biopsy [12]. There was no improvement with a gluten free diet. There is usually some hepatomegaly. The spleen may be palpable. Body weight is reduced, and linear growth falls off. Of 20 Finnish patients [6], 16 had heights that were 2 to 6 SDs below the mean. Head circumference is normal. Skeletal maturation is usually delayed. Anemia is the rule, and leukopenia is common.

Osteoporosis develops in a majority of patients [13–15]. Two-thirds have had fractures, often after minimal trauma [3,14–16]. Compression fractures of the vertebrae may lead to deformity. Fractures may occur before the age of 5. Metabolism of calcium and phosphate is normal, but hydroxyproline excretion in the urine is elevated.

Hyperammonemia is usually manifest as episodic attacks of vomiting. These may begin in neonatal infancy or be delayed even until adult life in patients with well developed aversion to protein [6,17]. Refusal to eat meat or dairy products has also been observed in patients who have not experienced hyperammonemia [12]. The avoidance of protein-containing foods is an early characteristic, which may begin as early as a year of age. Vomiting may be associated with dizziness or headaches. There may be loss of consciousness [18] or even deep coma and an isolelectric electroencephalograph (EEG), especially in patients administered large amounts of protein by gastric tube [6,17,19–20]. Episodic psychiatric symptoms

have been observed. Some patients have been mentally retarded but most are not. Nonprogressive, asymptomatic opacities have been observed in the lens of the eye [21].

A group of patients with unusual complications has recently been described [22] from southern Italy in which consanguinity has been high. Manifestations in the patients included abnormalities of the bone marrow, in five of the six examined, in which large cells resembling sea-blue histiocytes suggested a diagnosis of Niemann-Pick disease, but sphingomyelinase was negative, and also there was prominent erythrophagocytosis. Erythrophagocytosis and immunologic abnormalities were also described in another patient with this disease [23]. This hematologic picture has been seen along with the pancytopenia of propionic acidemia [24]. It has also been observed in carnitine palmitoyl transferase I deficiency [25] and in hemochromatosis [26]. Two patients had clinical pancreatitis [22]; in one who required surgery, pancreatic fibrosis was found, indicating chronic pancreatitis, as well as acute liponecrosis.

A number of late complications have been described. Some of these patients have presented first in adult life with interstitial disease of the lung or with renal disease.

Pulmonary disease has emerged as a major complication [22,27,28]. It has ranged from mild roentgenographic changes of fibrosis to severe interstitial infiltration, alveolar proteinosis and death from respiratory failure. Respiratory insufficiency or clubbing may be the presenting complaint [28]. Cough, dyspnea and hemoptysis may occur, and there may be intermittent fever or pulmonary infection. Roentgenograms show reticulonodular interstitial densities. Biopsy of the lung may show cholesterol crystals or granulomas [28] or alveolar proteinosis. Elevated concentrations of cationic amino acids in bronchoalveolar lavage fluid suggest that transport may also be abnormal in pulmonary epithelium [29]. In a number of patients with no pulmonary symptoms there was roentgenographic evidence of pulmonary fibrosis [27].

Some patients have had chronic renal failure [22,30] with proteinuria and progressive glomerular and tubular insufficiency. A full Fanconi syndrome with clinical rickets and deformities may occur [22]. This may obscure the diagnosis because of a massive generalized aminoaciduria. Oral loading with lysine or arginine to test intestinal absorption may be required for diagnosis in such a patient.

Some children and some adults have developed terminal hepatic insufficiency. Pathology was that of extensive fatty degeneration and micronodular cirrhosis [31,32]. In other patients biopsy of the liver has been normal [4,11] or there have been fat droplets in hepatocyte cytoplasm. At autopsy in the adult, changes were noted in the glomerular basement membrane, and immunofluorescence positive for IgA indicated an active glomerular lesion [32]. Autopsy in a 21-year-old female patient who had had a typical infantile course of failure to thrive revealed terminal micronodular cirrhosis and pulmonary alveolar proteinosis [33]. Immune complex disease like that of lupus erythematosus was observed in a 3-year-old boy, and related to the pulmonary problems [34].

GENETICS AND PATHOGENESIS

The disorder is inherited in an autosomal recessive pattern [2]. Many examples have been found of multiple affected individuals in a family [17,18,30,35–37].

The defect in amino acid transport is often first evident in the analysis of amino acids in the blood. Plasma concentrations of lysine, ornithine and arginine are low. The mean concentration of lysine in 20 patients [38] was 70 μmol/L; those of ornithine and arginine were 21 and 27 μmol/L, respectively. The diagnosis may not be clear from these levels, because the normal ranges are that low. However, the plasma concentration of citrulline is impressively elevated. The mean was 232 μmol/L [38], which is about four times the upper limit of normal.

Concentrations of glutamine and alanine are also elevated, consistent with chronic excess of ammonia. Concentrations of glycine, serine and proline may also be elevated.

The urinary excretion of lysine is massively increased, and there is increased excretion of arginine and ornithine. The mean excretion of lysine per 1.73 m^2 body surface in 20 patients [38] was 4.13 mmol/24 h; those of ornithine and arginine were 0.11 and 0.36 mmol, respectively. The renal clearance of lysine was 25.7 mL/min per 1.73 m^2; those of ornithine and arginine were 3.3 and 11.5 mL/min per 1.73 m^2. Citrulline and glutamine are excreted in large amounts, but their clearance is normal. Defective renal tubular reabsorption has been demonstrated and is most marked in the case of lysine, less so for arginine, and least for ornithine [39]. The abnormal pattern of urinary amino acids may be elusive, especially when quantification is not employed, at times of very low plasma levels of the basic amino acids and rigid restriction of the dietary intake of protein. Increasing the plasma concentration of lysine clarifies the diagnosis.

Absorption of basic amino acids is defective in the small intestine [6,40–42], as well as in the renal tubule. In an interesting assessment of mechanism, the oral administration of lysylglycine to patients led to an increase in plasma concentrations of glycine, but not of lysine, while in controls both increased [6]. Thus, the lysine dipeptide was normally absorbed by patients across the luminal membrane and hydrolyzed intracellularly, but efflux of the lysine, though not of the glycine, was blocked at the antiluminal membrane. In vitro studies of biopsied jejunum confirmed this position of the defect [8]. This is very different from cystinuria, where the defect is in the luminal membrane.

The defective transport in lysinuric protein intolerance is expressed in cultured fibroblasts [9]. Labeled lysine and the nonmetabolizable analog, homoarginine [43], were found not to display the trans-stimulated efflux that occurs in the presence of a cationic amino acid on the other side of the membrane [9,44]. Heterozygotes were found to display approximately 50 percent of control activity [9].

The mechanisms by which hyperammonemia occurs are not completely understood. Concentrations of ammonia are normal in the fasting state, but increase up to 500 μmolar postprandially [4,11]. Persistent hyperammonemia may result from a large protein intake, prolonged fasting, or infection. The urinary excretion of orotic acid is usually elevated in patients [45,46] even when they are receiving diets restricted in protein, and there is a major increase after the administration of a protein or alanine load [46]. The concentration of urea in these patients is usually low.

Abnormal function of the urea cycle is thought to result from intramitochondrial shortage of ornithine, as in the HHH syndrome (Chapter 34). In lysinuric protein intolerance, intravenous infusion of ornithine or arginine (an ornithine source) prevents the hyperammonemia of protein or alanine loading [1,4,11]. Infusion of citrulline also accomplishes this effect and, furthermore, it is effective orally [41]. Oral arginine and ornithine are less effective because they are so poorly absorbed in this condition that supplementation leads to diarrhea [8,42]. Citrulline is a neutral amino acid and is absorbed via a different transport system, but once in the cell it is converted via arginine to ornithine. The nature of the defect in efflux would make for high intracellular concentration of ornithine, but the trans-stimulated system has not been found in hepatocytes [47,48], so hepatic cells would be expected to reflect the depletion of dibasic amino acids evident in the plasma. Some clinical manifestations, such as failure to thrive, anemia, hepatomegaly and osteoporosis, could be a function of a shortage of lysine.

The molecular locus for lysinuric protein intolerance was assigned to chromosome 14q11.2 in a study of 20 Finnish families [49]. This is true also of non-Finnish families. The gene for a carrier protein, SLC7A7 (solute carrier family 7, member 7) maps to this site, and a search for mutations in the Finnish families yielded a mutant allele (1181-2A→T) in which an A to T transversion at −2 of the acceptor splice site in intron 6, leading to altered splicing deleting 10 base pairs and a frame shift [50]. A common haplotype was consistent with a single founder mutation. This mutation was found independently by Italian investigators [51] who also found a frame shift mutation in Italian patients resulting from homozygosity for a 4 bp insertion (1625 ins ATAC). A 543 bp deletion was found in another Italian proband. A number of other mutations have been identified [52,53]. Expression studies of mutations have revealed proteins that failed to localize to the plasma membrane as well as proteins that localized but failed to function. Quite different clinical phenotypes have been observed in individuals with the same genotype.

TREATMENT

The effects of citrulline in this condition have formed the basis for effective therapy [5,11]. Citrulline is provided in doses of 2.5 to 8.5 g daily, usually divided into three to five doses, especially with meals. Citrulline supplementation produces an adequate quantity of urea cycle intermediates, and in this way prevents hyperammonemia. Protein intake is moderately restricted, a process most patients have begun spontaneously. Intakes of 1 to 1.5 g/kg per day in children and 0.5 to 0.7 g/kg in adults have been employed.

In an acute crisis of hyperammonemia, protein intake is stopped, and energy is supplied as intravenous glucose. Infusion of arginine, ornithine or citrulline should be effective. Dosage recommended has been 1 mmol/kg as a primary dose followed by 0.5–1 mmol/kg per hour until symptoms are eliminated. Intravenous sodium benzoate or phenylacetate, or both, may be employed as adjunctive therapy [54].

Lysine depletion may be improved with supplemental lysine [55], but this is limited by malabsorption and intestinal tolerance. ε-N-Acetyllysine has been shown to increase plasma concentrations of lysine [56]. Increase may also be accomplished by the intravenous administration of lysine [57].

Pulmonary disease may be effectively treated with high-dose regimens of prednisolone [38], but some patients have not responded. Successful treatment of renal complications has not been reported.

References

1 Perheentupa J, Visakorpi JK. Protein intolerance with deficient transport of basic amino acids. *Lancet* 1965;**2**:813.
2 Norio R, Perheentupa J, Kekomäki M, Visakorpi JK. Lysinuric protein intolerance an autosomal recessive disease. *Clin Genet* 1971;**2**:214.
3 Simell O, Rajantie J, Perheentupa J. Lysinuric protein intolerance: in *Population Structure and Genetic Disorders* (eds AW Eriksson, H Forsius, HR Nevanlinna, *et al.*), Academic Press, London;1980:633.
4 Kekomäki M, Visakorpi JK, Perheentupa J, Saxen L. Familial protein intolerance with deficient transport of basic amino acids. An analysis of 10 patients. *Acta Paediatr Scand* 1967;**56**L:617.
5 Awrich AE, Stackhouse J, Cantrell JE, *et al.* Hyperdibasicaminoaciduria hyperammonemia and growth retardation: treatment with arginine lysine and citrulline. *J Pediatr* 1975;**8**:731.
6 Simell O, Perheentupa J, Rapola J, *et al.* Lysinuric protein intolerance. *Am J Med* 1975;**59**:229.
7 Rajantie J, Simell O, Perheentupa J. Basolateral-membrane transport defect for lysine in lysinuric protein intolerance. *Lancet* 1980;**1**:1219.
8 Rajantie J, Simell O, Perheentupa J. Lysinuric protein intolerance. Basolateral transport defect in renal tubuli. *J Clin Invest* 1981;**67**:1078.
9 Desjeux JF, Rajantie J, Simell O, *et al.* Lysine fluxes across the jejunal epithelium in lysinuric protein intolerance. *J Clin Invest* 1980;**65**:1382.
10 Smith DW, Scriver CR, Tenenhouse HS, Simell O. Lysinuric protein intolerance mutation is expressed in the plasma membrane of cultured skin fibroblasts. *Proc Natl Acad Sci USA* 1987;**84**:7711.
11 Botschner J, Smith DW, Simell O, Scriver CR. Comparison of ornithine metabolism in hyperornithinemia-hyperammonemia-homocitrullinuria syndrome lysinuric protein intolerance and gyrate atrophy fibroblasts. *J Inherit Metab Dis* 1989;**12**:33.
12 Reinoso MA, Whitley C, Jessurun J, Schwarzenberg SJ. Lysinuric protein intolerance masquerading as celiac disease: a case report. *J Pediatr* 1998;**132**:153.
13 Svedström E, Parto K, Marttinen M, *et al.* Skeletal manifestations of lysinuric protein intolerance. *Skeletal Radiol* 1993;**22**:11.
14 Parto K, Penttinen R, Paronen I, *et al.* Osteoporosis in lysinuric protein intolerance. *J Inherit Metab Dis* 1993;**16**:441.
15 Carpenter TO, Levy HL, Holtrop ME, *et al.* Lysinuric protein intolerance presenting as childhood osteoporosis. Clinical and skeletal response to citrulline therapy. *N Engl J Med* 1985;**312**:290.
16 Mori H, Kimura M, Fukuda S. A case of lysinuric protein intolerance with mental-physical retardation intermittent stupor and hemiparesis. *Rinsho Shinkeigaku* 1982;**22**:42.
17 Shaw PJ, Dale G, Bates D. Familial lysinuric protein intolerance presenting as coma in two adult siblings. *J Neurol Neurosurg Psychiatry* 1989;**52**:648.
18 Yoshimura T, Kato M, Goto I, Kuroiwa Y. Lysinuric protein intolerance – two patients in a family with loss of consciousness and growth retardation. *Rinsho Shinkeigaku* 1983;**23**:140.
19 Chan H, Billmeier GJ Jr, Molinary SV, *et al.* Prolonged coma and isoelectric electroencephalogram in a child with lysinuric protein intolerance. *J Pediatr* 1977;**91**:79.
20 Coude FX, Ogier H, Charpentier C, *et al.* Lysinuric protein intolerance: a severe hyperammonemia secondary to l-arginine deficiency. *Arch Fr Pediatr* 1981;**38**:(suppl 1) 829.

21   Moschos M, Andreanos D. Lysinuria and changes in the crystalline lens. *Bull Mem Soc Fr Ophthalmol* 1985;**96**:322.

22   Parenti G, Sebastio G, Strisciuglio P, *et al*. Lysinuric protein intolerance characterized by bone marrow abnormalities and severe clinical course. *J Pediatr* 1995;**126**:246.

23   Gursel T, Kocak U, Tumer L, Hasanoglu A. Bone marrow hemophagocytosis and immunological abnormalities in a patient with lysinuric protein intolerance. *Acta Hematologica* 1997;**98**:160.

24   Stork LC, Ambruso DR, Wallner SF, *et al*. Pancytopenia in propionic acidemia: hematologic evaluation and studies of hematopoiesis *in vitro*. *Pediatr Res* 1986;**20**:783.

25   Al Aqeel AI, Rashed MS, Ijist L, Ruiter JPN, *et al*. Phenotypic variability of carnitine palmityl transferase I deficiency (CPT I) with novel molecular defect in Saudi Arabia. *Am J Hum Genet* 2002;**71**:412.

26   Parizhskaya M, Reyes J, Jaffe R. Hemophagocytic syndrome presenting as acute hepatic failure in two infants: clinical overlap with neonatal hemochromatosis. *Pediatr Dev Pathol* 1999;**2**:360.

27   Parto K, Svedstrom E, Majurin ML, *et al*. Pulmonary manifestations in lysinuric protein intolerance. *Chest* 1993;**104**:1176.

28   Kerem E, Elpeg ON, Shalev RS, *et al*. Lysinuric protein intolerance with chronic interstitial lung disease and pulmonary cholesterol granulomas at onset. *J Pediatr* 1993;**123**:275.

29   Hallman M, Maasilta P, Sipilä I, Tahvanainen J. Composition and function of pulmonary surfactant in adult respiratory distress syndrome. *Eur Respir J* 1989;**2**:(Suppl 3) 104.

30   DiRocco M, Garibotto G, Rossi GA, *et al*. Role of haematological pulmonary and renal complications in the long-term prognosis of patients with lysinuric protein intolerance *Eur J Pediatr* 1993;**152**:437.

31   Sidransky H, Verney E. Chemical pathology of diamino acid deficiency: considerations in relation to lysinuric protein intolerance. *J Exp Pathol* 1985;**2**:47.

32   Moore R, McManus DT, Rodgers C, *et al*. Lysinuric protein intolerance. *Proc SSIEM* 1995;**33**:62 (Abstr P050).

33   McManus DT, Moore R, Hill CM, *et al*. Necropsy findings in lysinuric protein intolerance. *J Clin Path* 1996;**49**:345.

34   Parsons H, Snyder F, Bowen T, *et al*. Immune complex disease consistent with systemic lupus erythematosus in a patient with lysinuric protein intolerance. *J Inherit Metab Dis* 1996;**19**:627.

35   Carson NAJ, Redmond OAB. Lysinuric protein intolerance. *Ann Clin Biochem* 1977;**14**:135.

36   Oyanagi K, Miuyra R, Yamanouchi T. Congenital lysinuria: a new inherited transport disorder of dibasic amino acids. *J Pediatr* 1970;**77**:259.

37   Kato T, Mizutani N, Ban M. Hyperammonemia in lysinuric protein intolerance. *Pediatrics* 1984;**73**:489.

38   Simell O. Lysinuric protein intolerance and other cationic aminoacidurias: in *The Metabolic and Molecular Basis of Inherited Disease* (eds CR Scriver, AL Beaudet, WS Sly, D Valle), McGraw Hill, New York;1995:4933.

39   Simell O, Perheentupa J. Renal handling of diamino acids in lysinuric protein intolerance. *J Clin Invest* 1974;**54**:9.

40   Kekamäki M. Intestinal absorption of l-arginine and l-lysine in familial protein intolerance. *Ann Paediatr Fenn* 1968;**14**:18.

41   Rajantie J, Simell O, Perheentupa J. Oral administration of urea cycle intermediates in lysinuric protein intolerance: effect on plasma and urine arginine and ornithine. *Metabolism* 1983;**32**:49.

42   Rajantie J, Simell O, Perheentupa J. Intestinal absorption in lysinuric protein intolerance: impaired for diamino acids normal for citrulline. *Gut* 1980;**21**:519.

43   Christensen HN, Cullen AM. Synthesis of metabolism-resistant substrates for the transport system for cationic amino acids; their stimulation of the release of insulin and glucagon and of the urinary loss of amino acids related to cystinuria. *Biochim Biophys Acta* 1973;**298**:932.

44   Rajantie J, Simell O, Perheentupa J. 'Basolateral' and mitochondrial membrane transport defect in the hepatocytes in lysinuric protein intolerance. *Acta Paediatr Scand* 1983;**72**:65.

45   Sanjurjo Crespo P, Vallo Boado A, Prats-Viñas JM, *et al*. Intolerancia proteica con lisinuria (aciduria dibásica). A propósito de un caso. *An Esp Pediatr* 1995;**42**:219.

46   Rajantie J. Orotic aciduria in lysinuric protein intolerance: dependence on the urea cycle intermediates. *Pediatr Res* 1981;**15**:115.

47   White MF, Christensen HN. Cationic amino acid transport into cultured animal cells. II Transport system barely perceptible in ordinary hepatocytes but active in hepatoma cell lines. *J Biol Chem* 1982;**257**:4450.

48   Christensen HN. Role of amino acid transport and countertransport in nutrition and metabolism. *Physiol Rev* 1990;**70**:43.

49   Lauteala T, Sistonen P, Savontaus M-L, *et al*. Lysinuric protein intolerance (LPI) gene maps to the long arm of chromosome 14. *Am J Hum Genet* 1997;**60**:1479.

50   Torrents D, Mykkänen J, Pineda M, *et al*. Identification of SLC7A7 encoding y$^+$LAT-1 as the lysinuric protein intolerance gene. *Nat Genet* 1999;**21**:293.

51   Borsani G, Bassi MT, Sperandeo MP, *et al*. SLC7A7 encoding a putative permease-related protein is mutated in patients with lysinuric protein intolerance. *Nat Genet* 1999;**21**:297.

52   Mykkänen J, Torrents D, Pineda M, *et al*. Functional analysis of novel mutations in y$^+$LAT-1 amino acid transporter gene causing lysinuric protein intolerance (LPI). *Hum Mol Genet* 2000;**9**:431.

53   Sperandeo MP, Bassi MT, Riboni M, *et al*. Structure of the SLC7A7 gene and mutational analysis of patients affected by lysinuric protein intolerance. *Am J Hum Genet* 2000;**66**:92.

54   Simell O, Sipilä I, Rajantie J, *et al*. Waste nitrogen excretion via amino acid acylation: benzoate and phenyl-acetate in lysinuric protein intolerance. *Pediatr Res* 1986;**20**:1117.

55   Rajantie J, Sinell O, Rapola J, Perheentupa J. Lysinuric protein I intolerance: a two-year trial of dietary supplementation therapy with citrulline and lysine. *J Pediatr* 1980;**97**:927.

56   Rajantie J, Simell O, Perheentupa J. Oral administration of ε-N-acetyllysine and homocitrulline for lysinuric protein intolerance. *J Pediatr* 1983;**102**:388.

57   Lukkarinen MJ, Nanto-Salonen KM, Pulkki KJ, *et al*. Lysine loading test in LPI-patients. *Proc SSIEM* 1995;**33**:62 (Abstr P051).

PART 4

Disorders of fatty acid oxidation

Introduction to disorders of fatty acid oxidation

The genetically determined disorders of fatty acid oxidation represent a recent rapidly growing group of inborn errors of metabolism. The field, as we know it today, really dates from the discovery in 1982 of medium-chain acyl CoA dehydrogenase (MCAD) deficiency (Chapter 40) [1,2]. Myopathic carnitine palmitoyl transferase deficiency was known for some time earlier, but considered among myopathies not a forerunner of expansive growth of knowledge, and HMG CoA lyase deficiency (Chapter 46) had been described but considered to be an organic acidemia. The fact that MCAD deficiency turned out to be common, and largely the consequence of a single mutation has contributed to the current recognition of the importance of this group of disorders. In recent years the rates of discovery of previously unrecognized disorders of fatty acid oxidation have been exponential, and the number of individual diseases is well over a dozen. The advent of diagnosis by tandem mass spectrometry and its application to programs of expanded screening of newborns [3] have opened up this entire population to the prevention of death and disability.

A summation of the various pathways involved in fatty acid oxidation and their interrelations is shown in Figure 36.1. Abnormality in those pathways has often first been suggested chemically by the excretion of dicarboxylic acids in the urine. Dicarboxylic aciduria may also be dietary, especially in infants receiving formulas containing medium-chain triglycerides. When β-oxidation is defective ω-oxidation and hydroxylation take place in the microsomal P450 system. This takes place efficiently in the case of long-chain fatty acyl CoA compounds, but the affinity of the system for medium-chain chain compounds is so low that they are thought to result from β-oxidation in peroxisomes of longer chain dicarboxylic or hydroxy acids [4].

Disorders of fatty acid oxidation may present with myopathy or cardiomyopathy. They may also present with sudden infant death syndrome (SIDS), but often the initial presentation is with a Reye-like episode of hypoketotic hypoglycemia, often with elevated blood concentrations of creatine kinase (CK), and uric acid, as well as transaminases [5]. Thus, in a hypoglycemic infant or child, evaluation of uric acid and CK (neither of which are routinely included in metabolic clinical chemistry panels in children's hospitals), serves as an alerting signal to the presence of a disorder of fatty acid oxidation. We

have developed a systematic algorithmic approach to the work-up of such a patient (Figure 36.2). The patient is often referred after the initial episode has been treated with glucose and fluids, and examination of the urine is negative except in the case of 3-hydroxy-3-methylgluraryl (HMG) CoA lyase deficiency. Modern workup begins with the assay of the DNA for the A985G mutation in the MCAD gene or tandem mass spectrometry for acylcarnitines, or both. Study of blood and urine concentrations of carnitine and its ester fraction may point to the answer. In some patients a controlled but prolonged fast is necessary to elucidate the nature of the defect, but this is less true since the availability of acylcarnitine profiles and mutational analysis for the common MCAD mutation.

The normal response to fasting and the oxidation of fat begins with lipolysis, which releases free fatty acids. In patients with disorders of fatty acid oxidation, concentrations of free fatty acids are usually higher than those of 3-hydroxybutyrate in blood at times of illness and metabolic stress. Thus, assessment of the concentrations of free fatty acids and 3-hyodroxybutyrate in the blood is essential to the diagnosis of hypoketosis. Because fatty acids that accumulate in the presence of defective oxidation undergo ω-oxidation to dicarboxylic acids, a disproportionate ratio of dicarboxylic acids to 3-hydroxybutyrate in the organic acid analysis of the urine also indicates disordered fatty acid oxidation. Transport of long-chain fatty acids into the mitochondria, where β-oxidation takes place, requires carnitine, and the entry of carnitine into cells such as muscle requires a specific transporter, which may be deficient in an inborn error of metabolism [6] (Chapter 37). Esterification of carnitine with fatty acyl CoA ester is catalyzed by acyltransferases, such as carnitine palmitoyl transferase (CPT) I (Chapter 39). The transport of the acylcarnitine across the mitochondrial membrane is catalyzed by carnitine translocase (Chapter 38); and then hydrolysis, releasing carnitine and the fatty acylCoA, is catalyzed by a second acyltransferase, CPT II. Inborn errors are known for each of these three enzymatic steps. In β-oxidation the fatty acid is successively shortened by two carbons, releasing acetyl CoA.

Specific dehydrogenases with overlapping specificities for chain length include: short-chain acyl CoA dehydrogenase (SCAD) (Chapter 43), medium-chain acyl CoA dehydrogenase (MCAD) (Chapter 40), and very long-chain acyl CoA

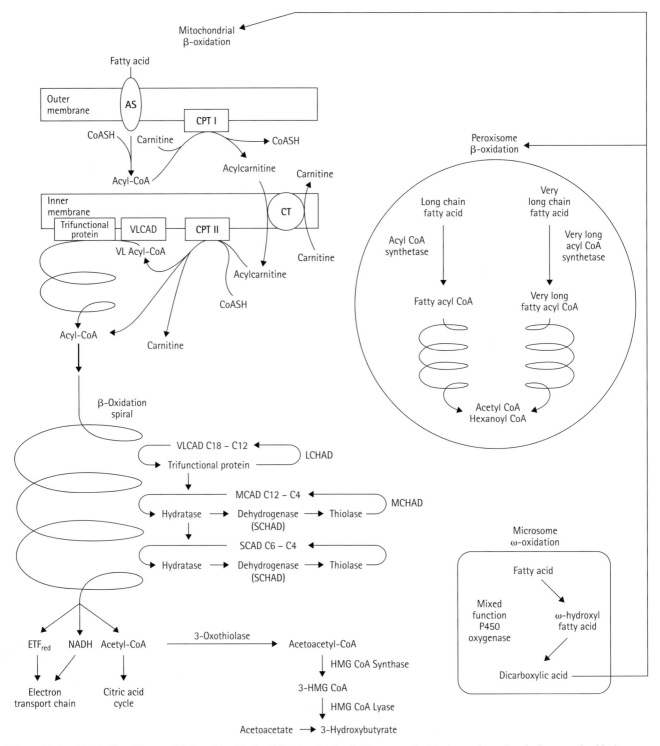

Figure 36.1 *Metabolic pathways of fatty acid oxidation. Mitochondrial activities are central, but peroxisomal and microsomal oxidation also plays a role.*

dehydrogenase (VLCAD) (Chapter 41). In addition, a trifunctional enzyme catalyzes 3-hydroxyacyl dehydrogenation, 2-enoyl-CoA hydration, and 3-oxoacyl CoA thiolysis [7]. Long chain hydroxyacyl CoA dehydrogenase (LCHAD) is now known to be one of these three enzymatic steps of the trifunctional protein (Chapter 42).

Diseases involving defects in each of these steps have also been defined. Among these diseases, and in five others that have been identified, only MCAD deficiency is easy to diagnose definitively. This is because most MCAD-deficient patients have the same mutation, an A→G change at nucleotide 985, which is readily assessed after amplification

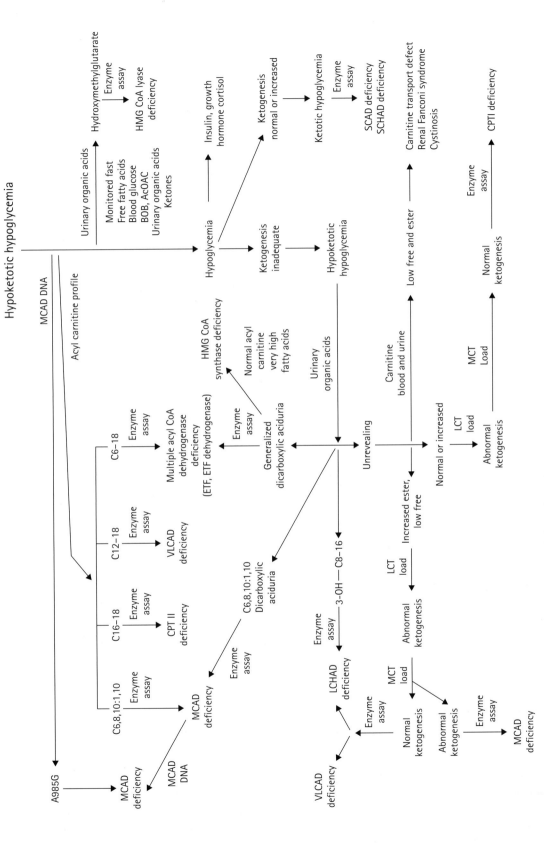

Figure 36.2   *Algorithmic approach to the elucidation of hypoketotic hypoglycemia.*

Table 36.1 *Acyl carnitine profiles of plasma in the diagnosis of disorders of fatty acid oxidation*

Disorder	Acylcarnitine	Control reference # μmol/L	Patient range μmol/L	Organic acid analysis
MCAD	C6	0.12	0.12–2.14	Hexanoyl-, suberyl-,
	C8	0.22	1.28–12.24	phenylpropionyl-,
	C8/C8:1	2.32	6.49–46.49	glycine.
	C10:1	0.22	0.26–1.84	Dicarboxylic aciduria
LCHAD	C16/C8:1	2.89	10.8–258.96	3-OH-Dicarboxylic,
	C16OH	0.02	0.12–0.60	Dicarboxylic aciduria
	C18:1OH	0.01	0.14–0.86	
VLCAD	C14:1	0.18	0.76–13.28	Dicarboxylic aciduria
	C14:1/C8:1	1.48	8.26–427.05	
	C14:2	0.08	0.30–3.48	
SCAD/EMA	C4/C3	0.98	0.71–9.0	Ethylmalonic, methyl-
	C4	0.32	0.62–1.28	succinic aciduria,
	C5/C3	0.80	0.19–4.52	Butyrylglycine
	C5	0.22	0.16–0.64	
CPT I**	C0/C16 + 18	2–32	63–291	
CPT II	C14:1/C8:1	1.48	2.50–42.79	
	C16/C8:1	2.89	101.24–221.65	
	C16	0.24	2.06–3.94	
	C16:1	0.08	0.50–0.86	
	C18	0.10	0.64–1.411	
	C16 + C18/C2	0.011–0.095	0.08–0.56	
Multiple acylCoA-dehydrogenase	C4/C3	0.98	0.70–8.19	Isobutyryl-, isovaleryl-,
	C5/C3	0.80	1.39–2.01	2-methyl-butyryl-
	C6	0.12	0.04–3.54	glycine, Glutaric acid,
	C5DC	0.06	0.04–0.08	Dicarboxylic aciduria
Carnitine transporter	C0	–	↓	
	Cesters	–	↓	
Carnitine translocase	C16	2.06–3.94	8.85	
	C18	0.64–1.44	↑	
HMG CoA lyase	C5OH	1.06	0.08–1.42	
	Methyl glutaryl	0.02	0.08–0.62	

Adapted from Vreken *et al.* [9] and other sources
* 95th percentile of the reference range except where a range is given. Abbreviations include EMA, ethylmalonic acidemia, CPT, carnitine palmitoyl transferase; DC, dicarboxylic acid.
** Absence of long chain acyl carnitines.

of the DNA by the polymerase chain reaction. Even in this disease, however, at least five infrequent mutations are known [8], and patients are not being tested for any but the most common one. Acylcarnitine profiling should lead to the diagnosis in each of these disorders [9] (Table 36.1), but experience is not yet available to indicate how often this approach might miss the diagnosis in an established patient who has become carnitine depleted.

During the long fast patients must be monitored closely so that symptomatic hypoglycemia is avoided. Testing is best done in units where the staff has experience with the protocol. An intravenous line is placed to ensure access for therapeutic glucose, and bedside monitoring of blood concentrations of glucose is done at regular intervals. In abnormalities of fatty acid oxidation, fasting must be long enough to exhaust stores

of glycogen and require the mobilization of fat and its oxidation. This usually requires 17–24 hours.

The specific enzyme assays for specific disorders are technically demanding and not generally available. A good next step following the fast, if a specific disease is not identified, is to pursue a more general study of metabolism in cultured cells [10,11] in which CoA or carnitine esters are separated and identified by high performance liquid chromatography (HPLC) after interaction with ^{14}C or ^{13}C-labeled hexadecanoate.

Experience with the diagnosis and management of disorders of fatty acid oxidation has now been summarized for a series of 107 patients with a spectrum of disorders [12]. The severity of these diseases is indicated by the fact that only 57 of the 107 patients were alive at report. An additional 47 siblings had died in infancy for a total of 97 deaths, 30 percent in the first week of life and 69 percent before 1 year. These data symbolize the importance of newborn screening in prevention, because the avoidance of fasting would prevent many deaths. Seventy three percent were judged to have hepatic clinical presentations, which included hypoketotic hypoglycemia, hepatomegaly, Reye syndrome and microscopic hepatic steatosis. True hepatic failure was seen in 11 percent and occurred only in carnitine translocase deficiency and multiple acyl CoA dehydrogenase deficiency; a single patient with LCHAD deficiency had cholestasis. In addition, a previously unrecognized defect in the transport of long chain fatty acids has been reported to cause acute liver failure and hypoketotic hypoglycemia [13]. Oxidation of ^{14}C-18 fatty acids by fibroblasts was defective. The clue to the diagnosis was low concentrations of ^{14}C-18 fatty acids and elevated carnitine, a very unusual pattern, in biopsied liver. Cardiac presentations were seen in 51 percent of patients. There were arrhythmias as well as cardiomyopathy. Skeletal muscle involvement in 51 percent of patients included myalgia, myopathy and rhabdomyolysis with myoglobinuria.

Treatment of disorders of fatty acid oxidation can be considered under two headings:

- acute management of acute metabolic imbalance
- chronic preventive therapy.

Acute management rests on the provision of a plentiful supply of glucose. This is designed to treat hypoglycemia. It is also designed to inhibit lipolysis. So intravenous solutions of 10 percent glucose or more are the rule even in those who are normo glycemia, for instance a patient with rhabdomyolysis. Insulin along with glucose may be necessary to maintain normoglycemia, and a central line or portacath may be required. Carnitine is given preferably intravenously, in doses of 100–300 mg/kg, because of greater bioavailability and the avoidance of diarrhea resulting from large oral doses. Carnitine therapy is mandatory in carnitine transporter deficiency. It has been controversial in long chain fatty acid disorders because of a theoretical risk that accumulation of long chain acyl carnitines maybe arrhythmogenic, as found in experimental situations [14]. Clinical experience is not consistent with this danger, and most support the administration of carnitine, not only to treat the deficiency of free carnitine that develops, but also to promote the detoxifying excretion of accumulated CoA esters as carnitine esters and the restoration of supplies of CoA [12].

The mainstay of long-term management is the avoidance of fasting. Our patients are supplied with letters indicating the need for parenteral glucose whenever intercurrent illness or vomiting preclude the enteral route. Overnight fasting is minimized by the use of oral corn starch. In some situations continuous nocturnal intragastric feeding has been employed. Restriction of long chain dietary fat is generally prudent as is long term oral carnitine. Medium chain triglyceride supplementation is therapeutic in long chain fatty acid defects.

References

1 Kolvraa S, Gregersen N, Christensen E, Hobolth N. *In vitro* fibroblast studies in a patient with C6-C10-dicarboxylic aciduria: Evidence for a defect in general acyl-CoA dehydrogenase. *Clin Chim Acta* 1982;**126**:53.

2 Stanley CA, Hale DE, Coates PM, *et al.* Medium-chain acyl-CoA dehydrogenase deficiency in children with non-ketotic hypoglycemia and low carnitine levels. *Pediatr Res* 1983;**17**:877.

3 Naylov EW, Chace DH. Automated tandem mass spectrometry for mass newborn screening for disorders in fatty acid organic acid and amino acid metabolism. *J Child Neurol* 1999;**14**:(suppl 1) S4.

4 Gregersen N, Mortensen PB, Kolvraa S. On the biologic origin of C_6-C_{10}-dicarboxylic and C_6-C_{10}-ω-1-hydroxy monocarboxylic acids in human and rat with acyl-CoA dehydrogenation deficiencies: *in vitro* studies on the ω- and ω-1-oxidation of medium-chain (C_6-C_{12}) fatty acids in human and rat liver. *Pediatr Res* 1983;**17**:828.

5 Marsden D, Nyhan WL, Barshop BA. Creatine kinase and uric acid: early warning for metabolic imbalance resulting from disorders of fatty acid oxidation. *Eur J Pediatr* 2001;**160**:599.

6 Treem WR, Stanley CA, Finegold DN, *et al.* Primary carnitine deficiency due to a failure of carnitine transport in kidney muscle and fibroblasts. *N Engl J Med* 1988;**319**:1331.

7 Carpenter K, Pollitt RJ, Middleton B. Human liver long-chain 3-hydroxyacyl-coenzyme A dehydrogenase is a multifunctional membrane-bound β-oxidation enzyme of mitochondria. *Biochem Biophys Res Commun* 1992;**183**:443.

8 Yakota I, Coates PM, Hale DE, *et al.* Molecular survey of a prevalent mutation ^{985}A-to-G transition and identification of five infrequent mutations in the medium-chain acyl-CoA dehydrogenase (MCAD) gene in 55 patients with MCAD deficiency. *Am J Hum Genet* 1991;**49**:1280.

9 Vreken P, van Lint AEM, Bootsma AH, *et al.* Rapid diagnosis of organic acidemias and fatty acid oxidation defects by quantitative electrospray tandem-MS acyl-carnitine analysis in plasma: in *Current Views of Fatty Acid Oxidation and Ketogenesis: From Organelles to Point Mutations* (eds PA Quant, S Eaton) Kluwer Academic/Plenum Publishers, New York; 1999;327.

10 Pourfarzam M, Schaefer J, Turnbull DM, Bartlett K. Analysis of fatty acid oxidation intermediates in cultured fibroblasts to detect mitochondrial oxidation disorders. *Clin Chem* 1994;**40**:2267.

11 Nada M, Rhead W, Sprecher H, *et al.* Evidence for intermediate channeling of mitochondrial β-oxidation. *J Biol Chem* 1995;**270**:530.

12 Saudubray JM, Martin D, De Lonlay P, *et al.* Recognition and management of fatty acid oxidation defects: a series of 107 patients. *J Inherit Metab Dis* 1999;**22**:488.

13 Odaib AA, Shneider BL, Bennett MJ, *et al.* A defect in the transport of long-chain fatty acids associated with acute liver failure. *N Engl J Med* 1998;**339**:1752.

14 Corr PB, Creer MH, Yamada KA, *et al.* Prophylaxis of early ventricular fibrillation by inhibition of acylcarnitine accumulation. *J Clin Invest* 1989;**83**:927.

Carnitine transporter deficiency

MAJOR PHENOTYPIC EXPRESSION

Hypoketotic hypoglycemia, seizures, vomiting, lethargy progressive to coma; cardiomyopathy; chronic muscle weakness; carnitine deficiency in plasma and muscle and increased excretion of free-carnitine in urine; and defective transport of carnitine into cultured fibroblasts.

INTRODUCTION

The inborn errors of fatty acid oxidation, including carnitine transporter deficiency [1], represent a newly recognized area of human disease. The rate of discovery of distinct disorders has increased rapidly since the discovery of medium-chain acyl CoA dehydrogenase (MCAD) deficiency in 1982 (Chapter 40). Deficiency of carnitine is common in these disorders in which fatty acyl CoA compounds accumulate which then form esters with carnitine and are preferentially excreted in the urine. Carnitine deficiency may also be profound in organic acidemias such as propionic acidemia for the same reason. The transport of carnitine into fibroblasts is inhibited by long and medium chain acylcarnitines [2], and this may be an additional factor in carnitine deficiency in disorders of fatty acid oxidation. Primary carnitine deficiency resulting from an abnormality in the synthesis of carnitine from protein-bound lysine has not yet been observed. Many of the patients reported early as primary carnitine deficiency have turned out to have MCAD deficiency. Deficiency of carnitine as a result of abnormality in the transporter (Figure 37.1) that facilitates its entry into certain cells has been referred to as primary carnitine deficiency [1]. The gene for the carnitine transporter SLC22A5 has been cloned, and a small number of mutations have been defined [3].

CLINICAL ABNORMALITIES

The classic, and frequently the initial, presentation of carnitine transporter deficiency (CTD) is hypoketotic hypoglycemia, as in most disorders of fatty acid oxidation. The first patient reported [1] (Figure 37.2) presented at 3 months comatose, limp and unresponsive in the afternoon after a prolonged overnight fast. She was acidotic; the serum bicarbonate was 16 mmol/L and the arterial pH 7.17. The blood concentration of glucose was 0.39 mmol/L (7 mg/dL) and that of the cerebrospinal fluid (CSF) was 0.2 mmol/L (4 mg/dL). Resuscitation required intubation, assisted ventilation and parenteral glucose and saline. Acute episodes of hypoketotic hypoglycemia are potentially fatal (Figure 37.3) [4] and may be sudden and unexpected. An infant of a vegetarian mother died at 5 days of life [5]. Episodes usually occur before 2 years of age and follow fasting [2,6].

Modest hepatomegaly is characteristic of this condition. Biopsy of the liver shows microvesicular lipid [7], a finding, like the rest of this clinical picture, that might lead to a diagnosis of Reye syndrome.

Clinical chemistry is also consistent with Reye syndrome, with hyperammonemia and increased levels of transaminases. The initial patient had an ammonia of 338 μmol/L, slightly prolonged prothrombin time, an aspartate transaminase

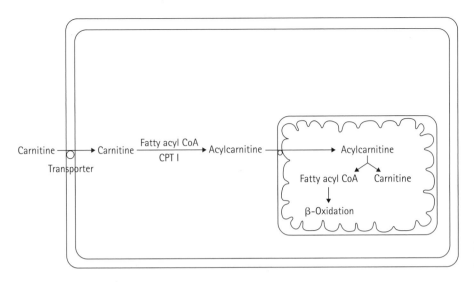

Figure 37.1   *The carnitine transporter and its role in fatty acid metabolism.*

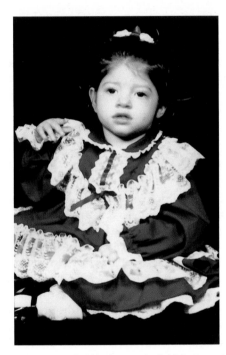

Figure 37.2   *A 17-month-old who was the initial reported patient [1] with transporter defect. She presented at 3 months with hypoglycemic coma precipitated by an intercurrent illness and prolonged fasting. This episode left her with severe brain damage reflected in her vacant expression. She died shortly after the picture was taken because of complications of a gastrostomy. (Illustration was kindly provided by Dr. Charles Stanley of the Children's Hospital of Philadelphia.)*

(AST) of 248 and alanine transaminase (ALT) of 149 IU/L [1]. Uric acid concentrations are also elevated at the time of the episode. This, along with the elevation of creatine phosphokinase (CK) [2] should strongly suggest a disorder of fatty acid oxidation.

Examination of the urine may reveal no ketonuria [1,2], and this should strongly suggest the diagnosis. However, in the height of the hypoglycemic illness, there may be misleading ketonuria in any disorder of fatty acid oxidation. Quantification of the plasma concentration of 3-hydroxybutyric acid or of acetoacetic and 3-hydroxybutyric acids at this time will provide definitive evidence of impaired ketogenesis, but this information is not usually available to the clinician. Dicarboxylic aciduria is usually notably absent [1,4].

Cardiomyopathy is the other classic way in which this disorder presents [2,7] and may be expected in any patient not given the benefit of diagnosis and treatment with carnitine [4]. It was the most common presenting complaint in 15 patients [3] and present in 100 percent of 20 reported patients. The patient of Waber and colleagues [7] reported with progressive cardiomyopathy and cardiac failure successfully treated with carnitine has been shown to have the transporter defect. The median age of onset of cardiac symptoms was 3 years [2]. Onset may be with rapidly progressive heart failure [2] or a murmur, and cardiomegaly may be found on routine physical examination or examination at the time of hypoglycemia. Roentgenograms and echocardiography reveal cardiac enlargement and increased thickness of the left ventricular wall. Electrocardiogram (EKG) reveals left ventricular hypertrophy. Nevertheless, the cardiomyopathy has been described as characteristically dilated [8], and this has repeatedly been confirmed by cardiac catheterization. This may be expected to be a lethal disease in which patients without carnitine supplementation display cardiac failure progressive to death. Death in a sibling has been recorded in 8 families [2]. A 12-year-old boy who died suddenly of cardiomyopathy following a routine surgical procedure was found to have a low concentration of carnitine in plasma and defective transport of carnitine in fibroblasts [9].

Muscle weakness or hypotonia is the third major manifestation of disease. It may be present along with other features, particularly those of the heart, but in two patients it was the only manifestation [2]. The picture may be that of a progressive proximal myopathy [8]. Biopsy of muscle reveals lipid storage myopathy [1].

Delay in diagnosis has been another characteristic of this disease. In nine patients, the delay was 1–6 years after the onset of symptoms [2], and in this time all developed cardiomyopathy, and all but one had muscle weakness. In some patients mild muscle weakness may not have been noted because of the attention devoted to the major cardiac manifestations.

GENETICS AND PATHOGENESIS

Transmission of the disorder is autosomal recessive. Affected siblings of both sexes have been observed, and consanguinity has been present in at least five families [2]. Concentrations of carnitine in plasma were low in 11 mothers studied and 10 of 11 fathers [6]. Prevalence is unknown, but there were 10 patients in the series of 107 with disorders of fatty acid oxidation in the Saudubray Paris experience [8]. Among 313 patients with an autopsy diagnosis of sudden infant death syndrome (SIDS), 3 were designated as transporter defects on the basis of hepatic steatosis and very low hepatic carnitine along with low esterified carnitine [10].

The diagnosis is usually suspected initially on the basis of a low concentration of free-carnitine in plasma. In the first patient, the total plasma carnitine ranged from 0 to 2.2 μmol/L and no free-carnitine could be detected. In 20 patients [2] total plasma carnitine ranged from 0 to 9 μmol/L, with 18 having values less than 4.2 μmol/L. In controls total carnitine was 40–60 μmol/L. The acylcarnitine profile reveals a decrease in free and esterfied carnitines.

Concentrations of carnitine in muscle are also quite low. In 13 patients studied, the range for total carnitine was from 0.05 to 17 percent of the normal mean. In liver, the total was five percent of normal. The excretion of carnitine in the urine is inappropriately high, consistent with defective renal tubular reabsorption [7]. At a time when the plasma carnitine approximated zero, the renal excretion was 121 μmol/g creatinine (normal 17–425) [1], and following a dose of 100 mg/kg of oral carnitine the plasma carnitine rose only to 21 μmol/L, but urinary excretion increased to 2911 mol/g creatinine. After four months of carnitine treatment, the plasma concentrations reached the low normal range, while urinary excretion was four to five times normal. The fractional excretion rate for free-carnitine was nearly 100 percent of the filtered load. On withdrawal of treatment the fractional excretion exceeded the filtered load.

The nature of the defect has been demonstrated by study of the uptake of carnitine *in vitro* by cultured fibroblasts [1,2] (Figure 37.3). In control cells the uptake of ^{14}C-labeled carnitine was via a high-affinity, carrier-mediated transport process with an apparent K_m of 3.24 ± 0.5 and a V_{max} of 1.67 ± 0.19 [1] consistent with previous reports [11]. Fibroblasts from patients have shown little uptake of carnitine; at a concentration of carnitine of 5 μmol/L, control uptake was 0.94 and a patient uptake was 0.1 pmol/min/mg protein [1]. High-affinity transport is best shown at lower concentrations; up to

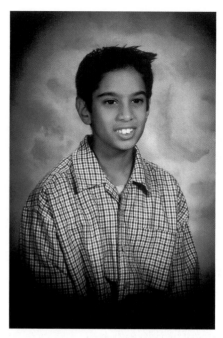

Figure 37.3   *J.S., a12-year-old boy with carnitine transporter deficiency. The disease is exquisitely responsive to carnitine. His death at 13 years highlights the dangerous nature of the disease and the importance of close follow-up of carnitine status and expert management.*

1 μmol/L uptake was negligible. Uptake in patients at high concentrations, such as 10 or 20 μmol/L reflect a second low-affinity transporter [11] or passive diffusion [12]. Transport of carnitine in control fibroblasts is sodium-dependent [1]. The uptake of carnitine by fibroblasts at 5 μmol/L showed no overlap among patients, parents and controls with the exception of one father. The velocity of carnitine uptake can be measured in lymphoblasts as well as fibroblasts [13]. Patients display rates below 10 percent of control. Heterozygosity can be demonstrated in some patients by rates below 40 percent of control. Low uptake of carnitine has also been demonstrated in cultured myocytes derived from patients [14]. Prenatal diagnosis has been accomplished by demonstration of defective uptake of carnitine from aminocytes of an affected fetus [15].

In response to the administration of carnitine, levels in liver return to normal, while those in muscle respond poorly, indicating that the transport defect includes muscle and kidney, but not liver. Consistent with this, the low K_m and preference for L-isomer that characterize the uptake of carnitine by fibroblasts is shared by heart and muscle [11,12,16], but not by liver [17].

The gene for the carnitine transporter, SLC22A5, has been mapped to chromosome 5q31, the locus for carnitine transporter deficiency in a large Japanese kindred. It codes for an organic cation transporter OCTN2 [18,19]. This is one of a family of organic cation (OCTN) sodium ion dependent transporters. The protein contains 557 amino acids and has the properties of a high affinity transporter. A number of mutations have now been identified in patients with this disease

Table 37.1 *Differential diagnosis of disorders involving carnitine*

	Plasma total μmol/L	Carnitine esterfied % of total	Urinary carnitine
Control	40–60	<30	Normal
Carnitine transporter deficiency	<5	<30	Paradoxically high free
Carnitine palmitoyl transferase (CPT) I deficiency	60–100	<20	Normal or high
Carnitine translocase deficiency	5–30	80–100	High ester
Carnitine palmitoyl transferase (CPT) II deficiency	10–40	40–80	Normal or high ester
Defects in β-oxidation	10–30	30–60	High ester
3-Hydroxy-3-methylglutaryl CoA lyase deficiency	10–30	30–60	High ester

[2,20–30]. Most individual families have had unique mutations. There have been a few instances of the same mutation in unrelated patients [22,24,25,28]. A few stop codons and frame shifts have been defined [2,20]. A lack of correlation between genotype and phenotype has been discussed [2,28]. However, decisions as to severity of phenotype often rest on whether or not hypoglycemia once occurred early in life, as in the case of one of two sibs with the R399Q missense mutation. The episode followed gastroenteritis at 2 years of age [2]. Because of her diagnosis an older sib who had proximal limb girdle weakness and mild developmental delay at 4 years-of-age was tested and found to have the mutation. Differences of this nature appear to reflect the chance occurrence of an illness that led to fasting.

Among ethnic differences an 11 bp deletion was found in unrelated patients from Switzerland and neighboring northern Italy [2], and R169W was found in two unrelated families in Italy [28]. In Japan, where the disease appears relatively frequent, most families have had a few mutations [31]. In a survey of 973 unrelated Japanese [31], 14 were found to have low levels of carnitine, and of these, six had mutations in the gene for OCTN2: W132X, S467C, W283C and M179L. These data gave a carrier frequency of one percent in Japan. Echocardiographic study indicated asymptomatic cardiac hypertrophy in these heterozygotes.

An animal model of the carnitine transporter defect, the juvenile visceral steatosis (jvs) mouse [32], has autosomal recessive fatty infiltration of the liver, hypoglycemia and hyperammonemia two weeks after birth, and very low levels of carnitine in blood and muscle, along with defective renal reabsorption of free carnitine. The hyperammonemia results from decreased expression of genes for enzymes of the urea cycle; low levels of mRNA are associated with low levels of all of the hepatic enzymes of the urea cycle [33]. Treatment with carnitine corrects the abnormal expression and urea cycle enzyme activity [34]. The jvs gene has been mapped to mouse chromosome 11, which is syntenic with the SLC22A5 locus on human chromosome 5 [35].

Analysis of the organic acids of the urine of these patients is usually normal. The absence of dicarboxylic aciduria, especially at times of acute illness and hypoglycemia, contrasts sharply with findings in patients with defects in β-oxidation such as MCAD deficiency. Patients with deficiency of carnitine palmitoyl-transferase I (Chapter 39) also develop hypoketotic hypoglycemia without dicarboxylic aciduria [36]. Comparisons of alterations of plasma carnitine in various disorders is shown in Table 37.1. Low free and total carnitine in plasma along with urinary free carnitine that is paradoxically maintained is suggestive of a transporter defect.

The response to fasting in a patient with defective carnitine transporter showed hypoketosis throughout and hypoglycemia by 12 hours (Figure 37.4) [1]. The fast was stopped when the plasma glucose reached 2.8 μmol/L (51 mg/dL) at which time the patient remained asymptomatic. Levels of free-fatty acids in plasma rose sharply to 2.22 μmol/L, but the level of 3-hydroxybutyrate remained flat at 0.27 μmol/L. Blood concentrations of ammonia rose. Treatment with carnitine corrected this patient's impaired hepatic oxidation of fatty acids; and she was able to fast for 24 hours without hypoglycemia. Levels of 3-hydroxybutyrate rose to 2 mmol/L, higher than the free-fatty acids (1.25 mmol/L).

Diet may contribute to the pathogenesis of symptoms in this disease. A 12-year old who died suddenly following surgery [9] had been exposed to an essentially vegetarian diet for some time. The 3-month-old initial patient [1] had been changed from a cow's milk protein containing formulation to a soy protein preparation that contained no carnitine, four weeks prior to the episode of hypoketotic hypoglycemia.

The pathogenesis of symptoms of hypoketotic hypoglycemia reflects the role of fat in energy metabolism. Hypoglycemia after short periods of fasting usually represent disorders of carbohydrate metabolism. The oxidation of fatty acids is not a major source of energy until relatively late in fasting. It usually takes 15 to 24 hours of fasting to induce hypoglycemia in a patient with a disorder of fatty acid oxidation. An individual who never fasted beyond 12 hours would usually be protected against this manifestation.

The metabolism of fat begins with lipolysis; those patients with defective fatty acid oxidation have high ratios of free fatty acids to 3-hydroxybutyrate in blood after fasting. Once transported into cells carnitine is esterified with acyl CoA esters including those of fatty acids resulting from lipolysis. The esterifications are catalyzed by carnitine acyl transferases such as carnitine palmitoyl transferase (CPT) I. Carnitine translocase then catalyzes the transfer of the fatty acylcarnitines across the membrane into the mitochondrion, where hydrolysis to

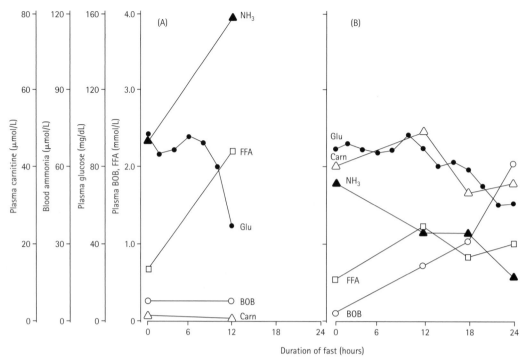

Figure 37.4 *The response to fasting in a patient with the carnitine transporter defect. (A) In the control state hypoglycemia(glu) was prominent at 12 hours, and there was no evident ketogenesis (3-hydroxybutyrate [BOB]) despite elevation of free-fatty acids (FFA). (B) Following treatment with carnitine, fasting for 24 hours was without hypoglycemia, and ketogenesis was evident in the rising BOB. (Reprinted with permission from the New England Journal of Medicine [1].)*

fatty acyl CoA and free or recycled carnitine is catalyzed by CPT II. Fatty acyl CoA compounds then undergo β-oxidation in which there is successive shortening by two carbon atoms releasing acetyl CoA. In muscle, this is largely oxidized via the citric acid cycle, while in liver ketogenesis proceeds via the successive action of 3-hydroxymethylglutaryl (HMG) CoA synthase and lyase-yielding acetoacetate, which is converted to 3-hydroxybutyrate.

TREATMENT

Treatment of this disease with carnitine has been highly successful [2,7]. Levels of free-carnitine in plasma and liver are readily restored, preventing further attacks of hypoketotic hypoglycemia. Developmental delay or seizures induced by hypoglycemic attacks prior to treatment persist, but are not progressive.

Cardiomyopathy and failure respond dramatically to treatment [6,7]. Heart size is reduced to normal within months. Doses have ranged from 50–120 mg/kg p.o. Skeletal muscle weakness improved, although mild proximal muscle weakness has occasionally persisted. However, muscle concentrations of carnitine were documented to increase only slightly to 22–80 mmol/g; control levels are 2500 to 3500 mmol/g. These observations suggested that muscle oxidation of fat and muscle

function may be unaffected until the intracellular muscle concentration of carnitine falls below 30–50 μmol/L or two to four percent of normal. Biopsied muscle revealed a decrease of stored lipid with treatment, but not a disappearance [1].

References

1 Treem WR, Stanley CA, Finegold DN, *et al*. Primary carnitine deficiency due to a failure of carnitine transport in kidney muscle and fibroblasts. *N Engl J Med* 1988;**319**:1331.

2 Stanley CA, DeLeeuw S, Coates PM, *et al*. Chronic cardiomyopathy and weakness of acute coma in children with a defect in carnitine uptake. *Ann Neurol* 1991;**30**:709.

3 Wang Y, Horman SH, Ye J, *et al*. Phenotype and genotype variation in primary carnitine deficiency. *Genet Med* 2001;**3**:387.

4 Brivet M, Boutron A, Slama A, *et al*. Defects in activation and transport of fatty acids. *J Inherit Metab Dis* 1999;**22**:428.

5 Rinaldo P, Stanley CA, Hsu B, *et al*. Sudden neonatal death in carnitine transporter deficiency. *J Pediatr* 1997;**131**:304.

6 Tein I, De Vivo DC, Bierman F, *et al*. Impaired skin fibroblast carnitine uptake in primary systemic carnitine deficiency manifested by childhood carnitine-responsive cardiomyopathy. *Pediatr Res* 1990;**28**:217.

7 Waber LJ, Valle D, Neill C, *et al*. Carnitine deficiency presenting as familial cardiomyopathy: a treatable defect in carnitine transport. *J Pediatr* 1982;**101**:700.

8 Saudubray JM, Martin D, De Lonlay P, *et al*. Recognition and management of fatty acid oxidation defects: A series of 107 patients. *Arch Neurol* 2004;**61**:570.

9   Pollitt RJ, Olpin SE, Bonham JR, *et al.* Late-presenting carnitine transport defect. *Enzyme Protein* 1993;**47**:175.

10   Boles RG, Buck EA, Blitzer MG, *et al.* Retrospective biochemical screening of fatty acid oxidation disorders in postmortem livers of 418 cases of sudden death in the first year of life. *J Pediat* 1998;**132**:924.

11   Rebouche CJ, Engel AG. Carnitine transport in cultured muscle cells and skin fibroblasts from patients with primary systemic carnitine deficiency. *In Vitro* 1982;**18**:495.

12   Vary TC, Nealy JR. Characterization of carnitine transport in isolated perfused adult rate hearts. *Am J Physiol* 1982;**242**:H585.

13   Tein I, Xie ZQ. The human plasmalemmal carnitine transporter defect is expressed in cultured lymphoblasts: A new non-invasive method for diagnosis. *Clin Chim Acta* 1996;**252**:201.

14   Pons R, Carrozzo R, Tein I, *et al.* Deficient muscle carnitine transport in primary carnitine deficiency. *Pediatr Res* 1997;**42**:583.

15   Christodoulou J, Teo SH, Hammond J, *et al.* First prenatal diagnosis of the carnitine transporter defect. *Am J Med Genet* 1996;**66**:21.

16   Rebouche CJ. Carnitine movement across muscle cell membranes: Studies in isolated rat muscle. *Biochim Biophys Acta* 1977;**471**:145.

17   Christiansen RZ, Bremer J. Active transport of butyrobetaine and carnitine into isolated liver cells. *Biochim Biophys Acta* 1976;**448**:562.

18   Wu X, Prasad PD, Leibach FH, Ganapathy V. cDNA sequence transport function and genomic organization of human OCTN2 a new member of the organic cation transporter family. *Biochem Biophys Res Commun* 1998;**246**:589.

19   Tamai I, Ohashi R, Nezu J, *et al.* Molecular and functional identification of sodium ion-dependent high affinity human carnitine transporter OCTN2. *J Biol Chem* 1998;**273**:20378.

20   Lamhonwah AH, Tein I. Carnitine uptake defect: Frameshift mutations in the human plasmalemmal carnitine transporter gene *Biochem Biophys Res Commun* 1998;**252**:396.

21   Nezu J, Tamai I, Oku A, *et al.* Primary systemic carnitine deficiency is caused by mutations in a gene encoding sodium ion-dependent carnitine transporter. *Nat Genet* 1999;**21**:91.

22   Wang Y, Ye J, Ganapathy V, Longo N. Mutations in the organic cation/carnitine transporter OCTN2 in primary carnitine deficiency. *Proc Natl Acad Sci USA* 1999;**96**:2356.

23   Tang NL, Ganapathy V, Wu X, *et al.* Mutations of OCTN2 an organic cation/carnitine transporter lead to deficient cellular carnitine uptake in primary carnitine deficiency. *Hum Mol Genet* 1999;**8**:655.

24   Burwinkel B, Kreuder J, Schweitzer S, *et al.* Carnitine transporter OCTN2 mutations in systemic primary carnitine deficiency: A novel Arg169Gln mutation and a recurrent Arg282ter mutation associated with an unconventional splicing abnormality. *Biochem Biophys Res Commun* 1999;**161**:484.

25   Vaz FM, Scholte HR, Ruiter J, *et al.* Identification of two novel mutations in OCTN2 of three patients with systemic carnitine deficiency. *Hum Genet* 1999;**105**:157.

26   Mayatepek E, Nezu J, Tamai I, *et al.* Two novel missense mutations of the OCTN2 gene (W282R and V446F) in a patient with primary systemic carnitine deficiency. *Hum Mutat* 2000;**15**:118.

27   Wang Y, Kelly MA, Cowan TM, Longo N. A missense mutation in the OCTN2 gene associated with residual carnitine transport activity. *Hum Mutat* 2000;**15**:238.

28   Wang Y, Taroni F, Garavaglia B, Longo N. Functional analysis of mutations in the OCTN2 transporter causing primary carnitine deficiency: Lack of genotype-phenotype correlation. *Hum Mutat* 2000;**16**:401.

29   Cederbaum S, Dipple K, Vilain E, *et al.* Clinical follow-up and molecular etiology of the original case of carnitine transporter deficiency. *J Inherit Metab Dis* 2000;**23**:(suppl 1) 119.

30   Christensen E, Holm J, Hansen SH, *et al.* Sudden infant death following pivampicillin treatment in a patient with carnitine transporter deficiency. *J Inherit Metab Dis* 2000;**23**:(suppl 1) 117.

31   Koizumi A, Nozaki J, Ohura T, *et al.* Genetic epidemiology of the carnitine transporter OCTN2 gene in a Japanese population and phenotypic characterization in Japanese pedigrees with primary systemic carnitine deficiency. *Hum Mol Genet* 1999;**8**:2247.

32   Horiuchi M, Hayakawa J, Yamaguchi S, Saheki T. Possible primary defect of juvenile visceral steatosis (jvs) mouse with systemic carnitine deficiency. (Abstr) *First IUBMB Conference Biochemistry of Diseases 2-a-05-p8;* 1992;Nagoya Congress Center.

33   Tomomura M, Yasushi I, Horiuchi M, *et al.* Abnormal expression of urea cycle enzyme genes in juvenile visceral steatosis (jvs) mice. *Biochim Biophys Acta* 1992;**1138**:167.

34   Horiuchi M, Kobayashi K, Tomomura M, *et al.* Carnitine administration to juvenile visceral steatosis mice corrects the suppressed expression of urea cycle enzyme by normalizing their transcription. *J Biol Chem* 1992;**267**:5032.

35   Nikaido H, Horiuchi M, Hashimoto N, *et al.* Mapping of jvs (juvenile visceral steatosis) gene which causes systemic carnitine deficiency in mice on chromosome 11. *Mamm Genome* 1995;**6**:369.

36   Bonnefont JP, Haas R, Wolff J, *et al.* Deficiency of carnitine palmitoyltransferase I. *J Child Neurol* 1989;**4**:197.

Carnitine translocase deficiency

MAJOR PHENOTYPIC EXPRESSION

Episodes of life-threatening illness with cardiac arrhythmia; coma with hypoketotic hypoglycemia, and hyperammonemia; sudden infant death; hepatomegaly; muscle weakness; deficiency of free carnitine and increased long-chain acylcarnitines; and deficiency of carnitine translocase.

INTRODUCTION

Carnitine translocase deficiency is a recently discovered disorder of fatty acid oxidation. First described in 1992 [1], the disease accounted for 10 of 107 patients in the Saudubray experience with abnormalities in the oxidation of fatty acids [2]. Many patients have developed symptoms and died in infancy [1–4].

Long chain fatty acids must be esterified with carnitine before they can be transported into the mitochondria where β-oxidation takes place. The translocase, carnitine-acylcarnitine translocase, catalyzes the transfer of the acylcarnitines across the inner mitochondrial membrane (Figure 38.1). The enzyme is one of 10 related membrane carrier proteins that shuttle proteins from the cytosol to the mitochondrial matrix.

Another is the ornithine transporter that is defective in the HHH syndrome (Chapter 34). Once inside the mitochondrion the acylcarnitine is split through the action of carnitine palmitoyltransferse II (CPTII) to free carnitine and the fatty acyl CoA ester, which is then the substrate for β-oxidation. Each step in the sequence is essential if fat is to be burned as fuel or converted to ketones and used for gluconeogenesis. The gene has been cloned, and some mutations identified.

CLINICAL ABNORMALITIES

The hallmark of disorders of fatty acid oxidation is hypoketotic hypoglycemia, and this has often occurred in the neonatal

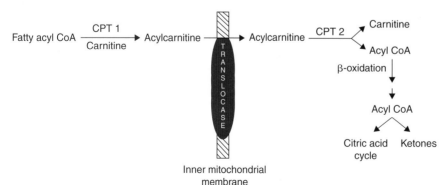

Figure 38.1 *Long chain fatty acid oxidation and the role of carnitine translocase. Abbreviations employed for carnitine palmitoyltransferase 1 and 2 were CPT I and CPT II.*

period in this disease [4]. More characteristic of this than other such disorders has been the occurrence of cardiac arrhythmias [1–4].

Episodes typically follow prolonged fasting, which is a common response of infants to intercurrent infectious disease. In one patient [3] a dextrostix reading of zero was recorded during an episode at 36 hours in which the infant was found to be pale, unresponsive, and hypothermic (34.5°C). Another patient [1] had a seizure, apnea and bradycardia at 36 hours of age. This episode, which appeared to have been provoked by fasting, led to apnea requiring mechanical ventilation and hypotension, which was treated with lidocaine and dopamine. This patient went on to have repeated episodes of vomiting, lethargy and coma following intercurrent illness and attendant fasting; each responded to the intravenous administration of glucose. Another patient [3] developed a second episode of hypoglycemia (0.7 mmol/L) on the third day of life despite receiving five percent glucose intravenously; the test for ketones in the urine was negative. The glucose was corrected by increasing the rate of infusion of glucose, but the patient deteriorated clinically and died at 8 days of age. Undetectable glucose was also the case in a patient who presented at 36 hours [5].

A previous sibling of the first patient [1] died at 4 days of age of what might be interpreted as sudden infant death syndrome. He had a sudden, unexplained cardiorespiratory arrest at 2 days and died two days later. The previous sibling of another patient [5] died of cardiorespiratory arrest at 24 hours. Two previous siblings of a patient with the disease, who died suddenly at 12 months, had died in the first 12 months [6].

Cardiomyopathy may be manifested by premature ventricular contractions, ventricular tachycardia or hypotension [1], and bradycardia due to auriculoventricular block [3]. In one patient [1] the electrocardiogram showed ventricular hypertrophy and in another [3], a left bundle branch block. Echocardiogram showed reduced ejection fraction. Intracardiac conduction defects were seen in twin siblings who died after an episode days after onset at 2 months [7].

Muscle disease may be seen very early in this disorder [4]. Weakness and hypotonia may be manifest early in poor head control, and later, inability to walk further than 15 feet [1]. The level of creatine kinase (CK) in the blood may be elevated [4,5,8,9]. Hypertonia may develop during terminal coma [1].

Hepatomegaly is a regular occurrence in this disease, and size tends to increase with time. This is among the few disorders of fatty acid oxidation in which hepatic failure has been recorded [2,9]. In one patient there was nephromegaly. Histological examination of the liver may reveal massive macrovesicular steatosis (Figures 38.2, 38.3) [2,3], as well as some fibrosis. Muscle histology has been normal. Mental development and growth has been normal [1], but most of these patients have died in infancy. One patient [5] developed microcephaly. Terminal episodes in most were cardiorespiratory failure and cardiac arrhythmia. In one there was a pulmonary hemorrhage and death at 8 days of life [3].

Clinical laboratory data have included, in addition to the hypoglycemia and deficient ketogenesis, hyperammonemia

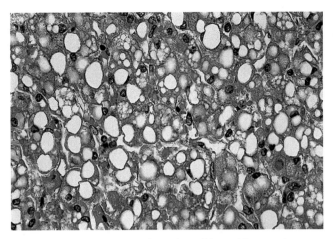

Figure 38.2 *Biopsied liver of a patient with carnitine translocase deficiency. This H and E stained section reveals extensive deposition of fat. (This illustration and Figure 38.3 were kindly provided by Dr. Jean-Marie Saudubray of l'Hopital des Enfants Malades, Paris.)*

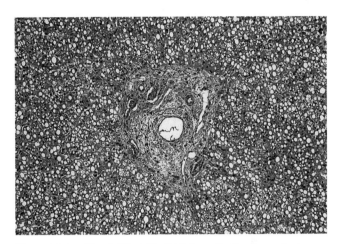

Figure 38.3 *Biopsied liver. The fat followed both microvesicular and macrovesicular patterns of steatosis.*

(491, 270, and 272 μmol/L) [1,3,9]. Patients were treated with sodium benzoate [1,9]. In some patients a urea cycle defect was considered. Some have had hyperammonemia in infancy without hypoglycemia or any of the other manifestations of a deficit in fatty acid oxidation [9]. Orotic acid excretion is however normal [9].

During the acute episode creatine phosphokinase levels in the blood as high as 4595 IU/L have been recorded, and levels remained over 500 between episodes. Acute elevations of uric acid have not been reported, but our experience with other disorders of fatty acid oxidation leads to a prediction that if measured they would be high [10]. Transaminase activities in the blood, both alanine and aspartate amino transferases have been consistently elevated. Plasma concentrations of free carnitine are low, and the esterified carnitine of blood and urine elevated. In the plasma the long chain acyl carnitine fraction was elevated. Urinary organic acid analysis may be unremarkable [1,3], or there may be mild dicarboxylic aciduria (C6, C8, C10, C12 and unsaturated C10 and C12) [4,9]. At times of acute episodes 3-hydroxydicarboxylic aciduria may also be seen [11]. In response to continued fasting, failure of ketogenesis was observed, along with a relative paucity of dicarboxylic acids [1].

The advent of acylcarnitine profiles by tandem mass spectrometry has made the diagnosis of this disease considerably easier and more reliable (Table 36.1, p. 244). The pattern is dominated by the elevation of long chain acylcarnitines, especially C16 and C18:1 and the deficiency of C0, free carnitine [4]. CPT II deficiency has an identical pattern. So enzyme assay is required for definitive diagnosis. Retrospective diagnosis of translocase deficiency has been made by the acylcarnitine profile of a neonatal blood spot [6].

A mild phenotype has been reported [11] in the seventh born of first cousin Pakistani parents. The potential lethality of even this variant is indicated by the fact that the fifth child of this union died at 3 months-of-age and the sixth had seizures, respiratory distress and an undetectable glucose at 48 hours, and he died of ventricular tachycardia later that day. Autopsy showed severe steatosis of the myocardium as well as of liver and kidneys. The patient reported was diagnosed by tandem mass spectrometry of a neonatal blood spot in which palmitoylcarnitine was 8.85 μmol/L (normal <4.82), and C2 and C0 were low. A controlled fast at 4 months revealed elevated free fatty acids without increase in 3-hydroxybutyrate and increased dicarboxylic and 3-hydroxydicarboxylic acids in the urine. Despite frequent feeding and attempted avoidance of fasting, he had a hypoglycemic seizure at 12 months. Cornstarch was added to the night-time regimen at 2 years, and he was developing normally at 3 years-of-age. Another patient with a mild phenotype was reported at 5 months of age [12].

GENETICS AND PATHOGENESIS

The fundamental defect in carnitine-acylcarnitine translocase may be demonstrated in cultured fibroblasts [1]. In the first patient, activity was barely detectable at 0.8 percent of the normal mean. Prior incubation with digitonin, to increase permeability, indicated the fibroblast assay to be linear with time and protein and that with this assay the activity in the patient studied was zero [3]. In 12 patients the activity was less than one percent of control in all but one [4]. In that patient, the one with the mild phenotype [11] activity ranged from 3 to 6.8 percent of normal [4,11]. The enzyme can be assayed in fresh lymphocytes and in amniocytes [3,4].

Intermediate levels of activity were found in fibroblasts of the mother and father of the first patient approximating 50 percent of control, consistent with an autosomal recessive mode of genetic transmission [1], as was consanguinity in other kindreds [3,11]. However, overlap between control and parent levels has been observed [4]. Better discrimination has been obtained when the results were expressed as the ratio of values of pyruvate conversion to acetylcarnitine or citric acid cycle intermediates [6].

In vitro, the oxidation of fatty acids by fibroblasts or lymphocytes reveals that oxidation of long chain fatty acids such as oleate [1] or palmitate [3] were very low while that of octanoate, which does not require carnitine-mediated transport, was normal. Oxidation of palmitate and myristate in the patient with the milder phenotype while abnormal, was somewhat better [11].

Prenatal diagnosis has been reported in six fetuses at risk [4]. Methodology included oxidation of fatty acids and enzyme assay in cultured amniocytes (n = 4) and chronic villus material (n = 3). One fetus was affected. Results were confirmed in all six. Two other prenatal diagnoses of translocase deficiency have been reported [8].

The translocase enzyme, isolated from rat liver mitochondria, is 32.5 kDa [13]. Its affinity is greatest for C12–6 acylcarnitines [14]. The human translocase cDNA has been cloned [15]. It is 1.2 Kb in length and codes for a 301 amino acid (32.9 kDa) protein. The gene is on chromosome 3p21.31 [16]. Mutations in the cDNA sequence have been defined in a few patients. A homozygous cytosine insertion causing a frameshift and elongation of the protein by 21 amino acids was found in a patient with a mild phenotype [15]. In a patient with severe disease there was compound heterozygosity for two extensive deletions [17]. In a patient with severe disease from consanguineous kindred in which seven previous siblings had had neonatal deaths, a 558 C to T transition in the cDNA led to a premature stop at amino cid 166 [4]. The transition was confirmed directly in genomic DNA of the patient and her parents [18]. In other severely affected patients missense mutations have been reported, including G81R and R133W [19,20].

Deficiency of carnitine acyl translocase leads to the accumulation of the free fatty acids outside the mitochondrial matrix; long chain acylcarnitines and short chains are also found, consistent with the fact that purified translocase catalyzes the transport of short as well as long chain acylcarnitines [21]. The long chain acyl carnitines predominate during illness following fasting induced lipolysis. Medium and short chain esters might reflect the acyl CoA products of peroxisomal oxidation that would require transfer into the mitochondria via the translocase for final oxidation. Secondary deficiency of free carnitine would be expected to result from the excretion over time of large amounts of esterified carnitine.

The hyperammonemia was associated with normal amounts of orotic acid in the urine. This would suggest an inhibition by accumulated compounds of carbamylphosphate synthetase or acetylglutamate synthetase, as has been shown for propionic academia and other organic acidemias [22]. This differs from medium chain acyl CoA dehydrogenase deficiency in which we have reported hyperammonemia and orotic aciduria [23] suggesting inhibition of the ornithine transcarbamylase step of the urea cycle.

The oxidation of long chain fatty acids is the chief source of energy during fasting for long periods and for skeletal and cardiac muscle during exercise [24]. The hepatic oxidation of long chain fats leads to ketone body production, gluconeogenesis, and maintenance of blood levels of glucose during fasting

[25]. The clinical manifestations of translocase deficiency are similar to those of the infantile form of CPT II deficiency [26] in which a similar acylcarnitine profile is observed.

TREATMENT

The ultimate courses in many of the patients described have been relentless despite treatment. However, patients with less complete defects have had milder phenotypes. Treatment should emphasize the avoidance of fasting and the use of intravenous glucose to prevent it. Supplemental carnitine and restriction of the intake of long chain fats are prudent. The acute hyperammonemia would be expected to respond to sodium benzoate, phenylacetate or phenylbutyrate. A trial of arginine might be effective. Cornstarch regimens appear to be useful in preventing hypoglycemia.

References

1   Stanley CA, Hale DE, Berry GT, et al. Brief report: A deficiency of carnitine-acylcarnitine translocase in the inner mitochondrial membrane. N Engl J Med 1992;**327**:19.

2   Saudubray JM, Martin D, De Lonlay P, et al. Recognition and management of fatty acid oxidation defects: a series of 107 patients. J Inherit Metab Dis 1999;**22**:488.

3   Pande SV, Brivet M, Slama A, et al. Carnitine-acylcarnitine translocase deficiency with severe hypoglycemia and auriculoventricular block: translocase assay in permeabilized fibroblasts. J Clin Invest 1993;**91**:1247.

4   Brivet M, Boutron A, Slama A, et al. Defects in activation and transport of fatty acids. J Inherit Metab Dis 1999;**22**:428.

5   Niezen-Koning KE, van Spronsen FJ, Ijlst L, et al. A patient with lethal cardiomyopathy and a carnitine-acylcarnitine translocase deficiency. J Inherit Metab Dis 1995;**18**:230.

6   Brivet M, Slama A, Millington DS, et al. Retrospective diagnosis of carnitine/acylcarnitine translocase deficiency by acylcarnitine analysis in the proband. Guthrie card and enzymatic studies in the parents. J Inherit Metab Dis 1996;**19**:181.

7   Brivet M, Slama A, Ogier H, et al. Diagnosis of carnitine acylcarnitine translocase deficiency by complementation analysis. J Inherit Metab Dis 1994;**17**:271.

8   Chalmers RA, Stanley CA, English N, et al. Mitochondrial carnitine acylcarnitine translocase deficiency presenting as sudden neonatal death. J Pediatr 1997;**131**:220.

9   Ogier de Baulny H, Slama A, Touati G, et al. Neonatal hyperammonemia caused by a defect of carnitine-acylcarnitine translocase. J Pediatr 1995;**127**:723.

10 Marsden D, Nyhan WL, Barshop BA. Creatine kinase and uric acid: early warning for metabolic imbalance resulting from disorders of fatty acid oxidation. Eur J Pediatr 2001;**160**:599.

11 Morris AAM, Olpin SE, Brivet M, et al. A patient with carnitine-acylcarnitine translocase deficiency with a mild phenotype. J Pediatr 1998;**132**:514.

12 Dionisi-Vici S, Garavaglia B, Bartuli A, et al. Carnitine acylcarnitine translocase deficiency: benign course without cardiac involvement [abstract]. Pediatr Res 1995;**37**:147A.

13 Indiveri C, Tonazzi A, Palmieri F. Identification and purification of the carnitine carrier from rat liver mitochondria. Biochem Biophys Acta 1990;**1020**:81.

14 Indiveri C, Tonazzi A, Prezioso G, Palmieri F. Kinetic characterization of the reconstituted carnitine carrier from rat liver mitochondria. Biochem Biophys Acta 1991;**1065**:231.

15 Huizing M, Iacobazzi V, Ijlst L, et al. Cloning of the human carnitine-acylcarnitine carrier cDNA and identification of the moelecular defect in a patient. Am J Hum Genet 1997;**61**:1239.

16 Viggiano L, Iacobazzi V, Marzella R, et al. Assignment of the carnitine-acylcarnitine translocase gene (CACT) to human chromosome band 3p2131 by in situ hybridization. Cytogenet Cell Genet 1997;**79**:62.

17 Huizing M, Wendel U, Ruitenbeek W, et al. Carnitine-acylcarnitine carrier deficiency: identification of the molecular defect in a patient. J Inherit Metab Dis 1998;**21**:262.

18 Costa C, Costa JM, Nuoffer J M, et al. Identification of the molecular defect in a severe case of carnitine acylcarnitine carrier deficiency. J Inherit Metab Dis 1999;**22**:267.
    IJlst L, Ruiter JPN, Huizing M, et al. Molecular basis of carnitine acyl-carnitine deficiency [Abstract]. J Inherit Metab Dis 1998;**21**(suppl 2) 56.

19 Invernizzi E, Garavaglia B, Parini R, et al. Identification of the molecular defect in patients with carnitine-acylcarnitine carrier deficiency. J Inherit Metab Dis 1998;**21**:(Suppl 2) 56.

20 Indiveri C, Tonazzi A, Palmieri F. Identification of the carnitine carrier from rat liver mitochondria. Biochim Biophys Acta 1990;**1020**:81.

22 Coude FX, Sweetman L, Nyhan WL. Inhibition by propionyl coenzyme A of N-acetylglutamate synthetase in rat liver mitochondria. A possible explanation for hyperammonemia in propionic and methylmalonic academia. J Clin Invest 1979;**64**:1544.

23 Marsden D, Sege-Petersen K, Nyhan WL, et al. An unusual presentation of medium-chain acyl coenzyme A dehydrogenase deficiency. Am J Dis Child 1992;**146**:1459.

24 Felig P, Wahren J. Fuel homeostasis in exercise. N Engl J Med 1975;**293**:1078.

25 McGarry JD, Foster DW. Regulation of hepatic fatty acid oxidation and ketone body production. Annu Rev Biochem 1980;**49**:395.

26 Demaugre F, Bonnefont JP, Colonna M, et al. Infantile form of carnitine palmitoyltransferase II deficiency with hepatomuscular symptoms and sudden death: physiopathological approach to carnitine palmitoyltransferase II deficiencies. J Clin Invest 1991;**87**:859.

Carnitine palmitoyl transferase I deficiency

MAJOR PHENOTYPIC EXPRESSION

Hypoketotic hypoglycemia; acute episodes leading to convulsions and coma; hepatomegaly; elevated creatine phosphokinase; and deficiency of carnitine palmitoyl transferase I.

INTRODUCTION

Deficiency of carnitine palmitoyl transferase (CPT) I was first described in 1980 by Bougneres, Saudubray, Marsac and their colleagues [1,2], in a patient who developed hypoketotic hypoglycemia and morning seizures at 8 months-of-age. They referred to the disorder as deficiency of hepatic carnitine acyl transferase, or palmitoyl transferase, to distinguish it from the deficiency of muscular CPT, in which there is a very different phenotype of muscle pain and rhabdomyolysis, usually

observed in adults after exercise [3]. They documented deficient carnitine acyl transferase activity in biopsied liver. Bonnefont, Demaugre and colleagues [4], clearly distinguished CPT I and CPT II, and demonstrated that CPT I activity was deficient in fibroblasts of the original patient and two others [4–6].

CPT I (Figure 39.1) plays an integral part in the transfer of long chain fatty acids into the mitochondria, where all the enzymes of β-oxidation are located. The enzyme is situated in the outer membrane of the mitochondrion. In the reaction

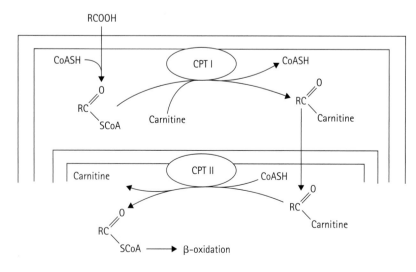

Figure 39.1 *The transport of long-chain fatty acids into the mitochondrial sites of β-oxidation involves first the formation of acylcarnitine esters, catalyzed by CPT I; once inside the membranes the liberation of fatty acyl CoA is catalyzed by CPTII. CPT I and II, carnitine palmitoyl transferase I and II; CoASH, coenzyme A; R, fatty acyl side chain.*

catalyzed, fatty acyl CoA esters are converted to carnitine esters. Medium chain and short chain fatty acids, in contrast, pass directly into mitochondria and thus, do not require esterification with carnitine [7]. CPT II is situated on the inner mitochondrial membrane, catalyzes the regeneration of carnitine and the long chain fatty acyl CoAs, which then undergo β-oxidation. Carnitine-mediated transport of fatty acids is thought to be rate-limiting in the oxidation of fats. A defect anywhere in the pathway would be expected to lead to inadequate formation of ketone bodies in response to fasting along with inadequate gluconeogenesis and hypoglycemia.

Two isoforms of CPT I have been identified [8]. Type IA or H-I, the hepatic isoform, is defective in CPT I deficiency. IB (M-I) is expressed in skeletal muscle. Human CPT IA cDNA has been cloned [9]. It codes for 773 amino acids in a mass of 88.1 Kda. Mutations have been identified [10,11].

CLINICAL ABNORMALITIES

This disorder presents usually in infancy, often in the second six months, with acute hypoketotic hypoglycemia during an episode of fasting brought in by an intercurrent, usually viral illness, or gastroenteritis [2,5,6,12,13]. Onset of symptoms may be neonatal or as late as 18 months. In the first family [2], a previous sister had had three hypoglycemic episodes and had died at 15 months after a 16 hour fast. The hypoglycemic episode may lead to convulsions and coma. Episodes tend to be recurrent until diagnosis and the institution of fast-avoidance. The disease is potentially lethal. A lethal neonatal presentation has been reported [14].

The liver is usually enlarged, but soft [2]. The acute episode has often been described as Reye-like. One patient [6], (Figures 39.2, 39.3) developed a predominantly hepatic illness at 10 months without documented hypoglycemia, in which hepatosplenomegaly and petechiae were associated with abnormal serum hepatocellular enzymes, prothrombin time, and partial thromboplastin time. She was thought to have disseminated intravascular coagulation and sepsis, consistent with an earlier *Klebsiella* sepsis at 2 days of age. At 14 months, she developed seizures and was found to have hypoglycemia with no ketonuria. An interesting hepatic effect of the disease was the occurrence of acute fatty liver of pregnancy (AFLP) in a woman pregnant with each of two siblings found to have CPT I deficiency [15]. This disease then must be added to long chain hydroxyacyl CoA dehydrogenase (LCHAD) deficiency (Chapter 42) as causative of AFLP or the hemolysis, elevated liver enzymes, low platelets (HELLP) syndrome.

Muscle biopsy may reveal lipid storage and vacuoles in electron microscopy [6], but there is no evidence of myopathy, and no cardiomyopathy. This disease has been notable for its absence of cardiac symptomatology including arrhythmias [12]. The neonatal death [14] was attributed to cardiac disease, but the only manifestations of bradycardia and arrest could reflect major systemic illness, and there were no abnormalities in cardiac or skeletal muscle at autopsy.

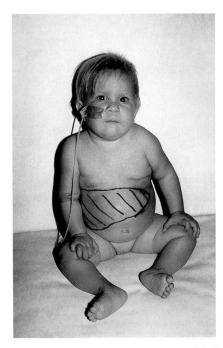

Figure 39.2 *S.V.E., an infant with CPT I deficiency [6]. She had hepatomegaly and hypoketotic hypoglycemia.*

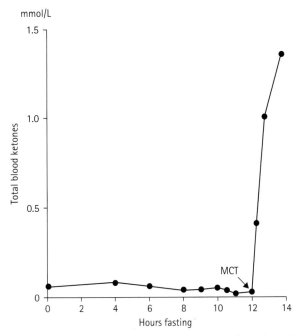

Figure 39.3 *Absence of ketogenesis with fasting to hypoglycemia in CPT I deficiency and the brisk ketogenic response to MCT. The blood sugar also rose after MCT.*

Renal tubular acidosis has been observed in three patients [6,13,16]. It may be transient. A patient displayed distal renal tubular acidosis in which there was failure to acidify the urine during spontaneous acidosis [17]. Most patients have survived, and there is a tendency to decreased frequency and severity of attacks with time and with learning to avoid fasting. In general, fasting over 15 hours is required to exhaust glycogen stores and call on fatty acid oxidation.

Cerebral deficit, or its absence, depends generally on the severity of the initial hypoglycemic episode, but many patients described have been neurologically impaired [13]. In patients with residual neurologic deficit the electroencephalograph (EEG) may show focal slowing or spike discharges, and neuroimaging may show cerebral atrophy [6]. There may be a continuing seizure disorder [17]. Linear growth and anthropometric development tend to be normal.

The creatine phosphokinase (CK) in the blood may be elevated during acute episodes [18], and this has been attributed to the MM isozyme, but the alanine transaminase (ALT) and aspartate transaminase (AST) were even more elevated; the levels of these hepatic enzymes were also elevated in other patients during acute hypoglycemic episodes [6,17]. Blood sugar levels during the acute attack have been reported at 0.3, 0.9, 1.2, 1.3 and 1.6 mmol/L [2,5,6,16,17]. In one patient there were recurrent Reye-like episodes without hypoglycemia, although there was improvement in lethargy on the administration of glucose [16].

Organic acid analysis of the urine is notable for the absence of dicarboxylic aciduria, and hydroxydicarboxylic aciduria [2,6,13], as well as the absence of elevation of 3-hydroxybutyric and acetoacetic acids in the urine at times of fasting and hypoglycemia. Plasma levels of carnitine may be normal or elevated [18,19]. Levels of both free and total carnitine may be elevated. Fractionation of the esterified carnitine of the urine revealed only acetylcarnitine. Tandem mass spectrometry of the blood reveals an absence of long chain acyl carnitines (C16, C18, C18:1) [13,20]. The ratio of C0 to C16+18 is useful in diagnosis [21]. In three patients the ratio ranged from 175 to 2000. A range of 2 to 32 was observed in control infants. Higher values were found in older infants but there was no overlap of patients and controls.

The histologic examination of the liver has revealed microvesicular and macrovesicular steatosis [6,18]. Muscle biopsy may show sarolemmal and interfibrillar accumulation of glycogen as well as the presence of lipid [6]. A hematophagocytic syndrome has been observed in a patient with otherwise clinically typical CPT I deficiency, who developed a brain abscess with candida [22]. This syndrome has also been observed in propionic acidemia and lysinuric protein intolerance.

GENETICS AND PATHOGENESIS

The disorder is transmitted in an autosomal recessive fashion. Affected children of both sexes have been observed in normal parents. Consanguinity has been documented [2,18]. In one extended inbred Hutterite kindred a brother and sister and their second cousin were affected [18]. The disorder is rare [13], but there were nine patients in the Saudubray, Paris experience of 107 patients with abnormalities of fatty acid oxidation [12].

The enzymatic defect in CPT I is most carefully documented by measuring the production of labeled palmitoylcarnitine from methyl-labeled carnitine and palmitoyl CoA in fibroblast homogenates, in which the integrity of mitochondrial membranes is preserved [5,19]. Testing with and without malonyl CoA distinguishes CPT I, which is inhibited by malonyl CoA, from CPT II, which is not. Reported activity has ranged from nine to 23 percent of control. CPT I appears to determine the overall rate of oxidation of fatty acids in the liver. Some patients have been documented to have deficiency of CPT I in liver, while activity in muscle was normal [23]. Immunochemical studies have been carried out with antibodies against CPT I and CPT II [24,25]. CPT I has been demonstrated immunochemically in rat liver and kidney. Immunochemically CPT I is absent in muscle and heart, which provided early evidence for the presence of the muscle-specific isoform. The hepatic isoform approximates 88 KD in size while that of muscle is approximately 82 KD; both variants are found in heart.

Parents of affected sibs have been found to be intermediate in levels of CPT I activity in fibroblasts, consistent with heterozygosity. Prenatal diagnosis has not been reported.

Fibroblasts from patients with CPT I deficiency incubated with labeled palmitate accumulate labeled palmitoyl CoA, but not palmitoyl carnitine [26]. The fibroblasts of CPT I-deficient patients display defective overall oxidation of long chain fatty acids, such as palmitate, whereas oxidation of octanoate and succinate is normal [5,27,28]. Similarly, the conversion of ^{3}H-palmitate to ^{3}H$_2$O in fibroblast monolayers was markedly deficient [28]. These observations are consistent with the failure of CPT I-deficient cells to transport long chain fatty acids into mitochondria, while medium chain compounds are transported normally.

The CPT IA gene on chromosome 11q13.1-13.5 [29] is expressed in liver, kidney, pancreas, ovary, leukocytes and fibroblasts [11]. The gene spans 60 Kb and contains 20 exons. The first mutation described [10], was a missense (D454G) change, which when expressed, had two percent of wild type activity. Other mutations identified [11] include Q100X, which would predict an early truncation of the protein, H414V and Y498C, which affect highly conserved sequences in the catalytic core of the enzyme. An 8 Kb deletion encompassing intron 14 to exon 17 led to loss of the mRNA [11]. The rarity of the disease and the general severity of phenotype have made genotype–phenotype correlations difficult, but the mutation leading to P479L resulted in a late onset disease in which there was proximal myopathy [30].

TREATMENT

The major element in management is the studied avoidance of fasting. In the presence of intercurrent infection or other cause of vomiting or anorexia in which the oral route is excluded, the provision of intravenous glucose is essential.

Reduction of the intake of long chain fats appears prudent. Medium chain triglycerides may be substituted (Figure 39.3).

References

1   Bougneres PF, Saudubray JM, Marsac C, *et al.* Decreased ketogenesis due to deficiency of hepatic carnitine acyl transferase. *N Engl J Med* 1980;**302**:123.

2   Bourneres PF, Saudubray JM, Marsac C, *et al.* Fasting hypoglycemia resulting from hepatic carnitine palmitoyl transferase deficiency. *J Pediatr* 1981;**98**:742.

3   Bank WJ, DiMauro S, Bonilla E, *et al.* A disorder of muscle lipid metabolism and myoglobinuria: absence of carnitine palmitoyl transferase. *N Engl J Med* 1975;**292**:443.

4   Bonnefont JP, Ogier H, Mitchell G, *et al.* Heterogeneite des deficits en palmitoyl carnitine transferase. *Arch Fr Pediatr* 1985;**42**:613.

5   Demaugre F, Bonnefont JP, Mitchell G, *et al.* Hepatic and muscular presentations of carnitine palmitoyl transferase deficiency: two distinct entities. *Pediatr Res* 1988;**24**:308.

6   Bonnefont JP, Haas R, Wolff J, *et al.* Deficiency of carnitine palmitoyl-transferase I. *J Child Neurol* 1989;**4**:198.

7   McGarry JD, Wright PH, Foster DW. Hormonal control of ketogenesis. *J Clin Invest* 1975;**55**:1202.

8   Weis BC, Esser V, Foster DW, *et al.* Rat heart expresses two forms of mitochondrial carnitine palmitoyltransferase I. *J Biol Chem* 1994;**269**:18712.

9   Britton CH, Schultz RA, Zhang B, *et al.* Human liver mitochondrial carnitine palmitoyltransferase I: characterization of its cDNA and chromosomal localization and partial analysis of the gene. *Proc Natl Acad Sci USA* 1995;**92**:1984.

10 Ijlst L, Mandel H, Oostheim W, *et al.* Molecular basis of hepatic carnitine palmitoyltransferase I deficiency. *J Clin Invest* 1998;**102**:527.

11 Gobin S, Bonnefont JP, Prip-Buus C, *et al.* Organization of the human liver carnitine palmitoyltransferase 1 gene (CPT1A) and identification of novel mutations in hypoketotic hypolgycaemia. *Hum Genet* 2002;**111**:179.

12 Saudubray J M, Martin D, De Lonlay P, *et al.* Recognition and management of fatty acid oxidation defects: A series of 107 patients. *J Inherit Metab Dis* 1999;**22**:488.

13 Brivet M, Boutron A, Slama A, *et al.* Defects in activation and transport of fatty acids. *J Inherit Metab Dis* 1999;**22**:428.

14 Invernizzi F, Burlina AB, Donadio A, *et al.* Case report: Lethal neonatal presentation of carnitine palmitoyltransferase I deficiency. *J Inherit Metab Dis* 2001;**24**:601.

15 Innes AM, Seargeant LE, Balachandra K, *et al.* Hepatic carnitine palmitoyltransferase I deficiency presenting as maternal illness in pregnancy. *Pediatr Res* 2000;**47**:43.

16 Falik-Borenstein ZC, Jordan SC, Saudubray J-M, *et al.* Renal tubular acidosis in carnitine palmitoyltransferase type 1 deficiency. *N Engl J Med* 1992;**327**:24.

17 Bergman A Donckerwolcke R, Duran M, *et al.* Rate-dependent distal renal tubular acidosis and carnitine palmitoyltransferase I deficiency. *Pediatr Res* 1994;**36**:582.

18 Haworth JC, Demaugre F, Booth FA, *et al.* Atypical features of the hepatic form of carnitine palmitoyltransferase deficiency in a Hutterite family. *J Pediatr* 1992;**121**:553.

19 Stanley CA, Sunaryo F, Hale DE, *et al.* Elevated plasma carnitine in the hepatic form of carnitine-palmitoyltransferse-1 deficiency. *J Inherit Metab Dis* 1992;**15**:785.

20 Al Aqeel A, Rashed M. Carnitine palmitoyl transferase I deficiency (CPT I) three affected siblings in one family (Abstract). *J Inherit Metab Dis* 1998;**21**:(suppl 2) 61.

21 Fingerhut R, Roschinger W, Muntau A, *et al.* Hepatic carnitine palmitoyltransferase I deficiency: Acylcarnitine profiles in blood spots are highly specific. *Clin Chem* 2001;**47**:1763.

22 Al-Aqeel AI, Rashed MS, Ijist L, *et al.* Phenotypic variability of carnitine palmityl transferase I deficiency (CPT I) with novel molecular defect in Saudi Arabia. *Am J Hum Genet* 2002;**71**: 412.

23 Tein I, Demaugre F, Bonnefont J-P, Saudubray J-M. Normal muscle CPT_1 and CPT_2 activities in hepatic presentation patients with CPT1 deficiency in fibroblasts: Tissue-specific isoforms of CPT_1. *J Neurol Sci* 1989;**92**:229.

24 Kolodziej MP, Crilly PJ, Corstorphine CG, Zammit VA. Development and characterization of polyclonal antibody against rat liver mitochondrial overt carnitine palmitoyltransferase (CPT I). Distinction of CPT I from CPT II and of isoforms of CPT I in different tissues. *Biochem J* 1992;**282**:415.

25 Demaugre F, Bonnefont J-P, Cepanec C, *et al.* Immunoquantitative analysis of human carnitine palmitoyltransferase I and II defects. *Pediatr Res* 1990;**27**:497.

26 Schaefer J, Jackson S, Taroni F, *et al.* Characterization of carnitine palmitoyltransferases in patients with a carnitine palmitoyltransferase deficiency: Implications for diagnosis and therapy. *J Neurol Neurosurg Psychiaryt* 1997;**62**:169.

27 Saudubray J M, Coude FX, Demaugre F, *et al.* Oxidation of fatty acids in cultured fibroblasts: A model system for the detection and study of defects in oxidation. *Pediatr Res* 1982;**16**:877.

28 Mitchell G, Saudubray JM, Pelet A, *et al.* The effect of D-carnitine on palmitate oxidation in cultured fibroblasts. *Clin Chim Acta* 1984;**143**:23.

29 Gellera C, Verderio E, Floridia G, *et al.* Assignment of the human carnitine palmitoyltransferase II gene to chromosome 1a32. *Genomics* 1994;**24**:195.

30 Brown NF, Mullur RS, Subramanian E, *et al.* Molecular basis of L-CPT1 deficiency in six patients: Insights into function of the native enzyme. *J Lip Res* 2001;**42**:1134.

Medium chain acyl CoA dehydrogenase deficiency

MAJOR PHENOTYPIC EXPRESSION

Hypoketotic hypoglycemia, myopathy, cardiomyopathy, sudden infant death syndrome, hyperammonemia, hyperuricemia, elevated creatine kinase, dicarboxylic aciduria, elevated levels of octanoyl and hexanoylcarnitine, deficient activity of medium chain acyl CoA dehydrogenase, and mutation in the gene, especially A → G ^{985}.

INTRODUCTION

Medium chain acyl CoA dehydrogenase (MCAD) (Figure 40.1) (Table 40.1) deficiency is the classic disorder of fatty acid oxidation, and it is the most common. Occuring in an estimated 1 in 6000 to 10 000 caucasian births, the disease was nevertheless first described in 1983, an index of the difficulties, even today, in detecting disorders of fatty acid oxidation [1].

Disorders of fatty oxidation display two general types of presentation. The first, hypoketotic hypoglycemia, is the clinical picture of Reye syndrome. In fact, it is now clear that most patients who appear to have Reye syndrome have an inborn error of metabolism, the most common being MCAD deficiency and ornithine transcarbamylase deficiency (Chapter 29) [2,3]. The other presentation reflects the chronic disruption of muscle function with symptoms relevant to myopathy or cardiomyopathy, including weakness, hypotonia, congestive heart failure, or arrhythmia. Both types of presentations may be seen in the same family or even in the same individual. Another presentation is with the sudden infant death syndrome (SIDS) [4–7]. We and others have been able to make retrospective diagnoses of MCAD in infants who had died of SIDS by retrieval of neonatal screening blood spots after making the diagnosis of MCAD deficiency in a subsequent sibling and assay for the common mutation in the DNA or for octanoylcarnitine. The introduction of the

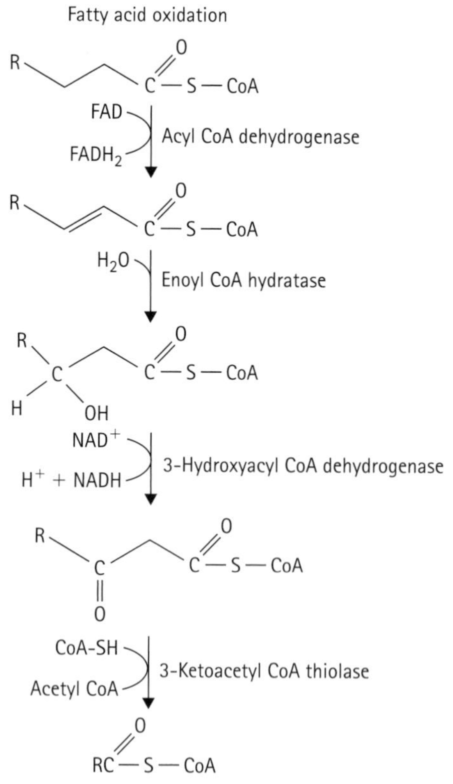

Figure 40.1 *The pathway of β-oxidation of fatty acids begins with the acyl CoA dehydrogenase step.*

Table 40.1   *Fatty acid oxidation: the acyl CoA dehydrogenases and their substrate specificities*

Enzyme	Substrate chain length	Deficiency disease
Short chain (SCAD)	C4–6	Rare
Medium-chain (MCAD)	C6–12	Common (1:10 000)
Very long-chain (VLCAD)	C12–16	Rare

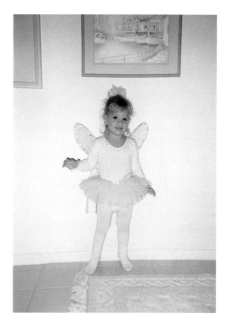

Figure 40.3   *S.E. at 26 months. These episodes were behind her; she was still receiving treatment with carnitine and cornstarch.*

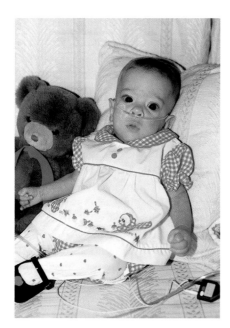

Figure 40.2   *S.E., an 8-month-old infant with MCAD deficiency, two weeks before her first episode of hypoglycemia. She had multiple episodes of hypoglycemia over the next year.*

tandem mass spectrometric analysis of acylcarnitines has greatly facilitated the diagnosis of this and other disorders of fatty acid oxidation, and its application to the screening of newborns is a major addition to preventive medicine. This should prevent further examples of SIDS due to MCAD deficiency.

CLINICAL ABNORMALITIES

Episodic illness usually occurs first between 6 months and 2 years, usually following fasting for 12 hours or more as a consequence of intercurrent infectious disease (Figures 40.2–40.4). The episode may be ushered in with vomiting or lethargy, or it may begin with a seizure. It is progressive rapidly to coma [8]. Patients are typically hypoglycemic. Hypoglycemia with a simultaneous negative urine test for ketones is very helpful in diagnosis. However, although these patients are documentably hypoketotic (Figure 40.5), the urine usually contains some ketones at times of acute illness; so this can be misleading [9]. Hepatomegaly is usually present at the time of the acute illness. Liver biopsy at the time reveals abundant deposits of lipid in

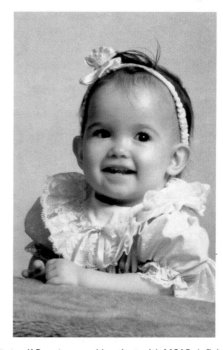

Figure 40.4   *K.B., a 1-year-old patient with MCAD deficiency. She presented at 7 months with a life-threatening episode of illness. Her sibling died in the first days of life of SIDS and was documented retrospectively to have MCAD deficiency. Since being diagnosed, this patient had not had another episode requiring admission to hospital. Nevertheless, the dangerous nature of the disease is signified by the fact that she died during sleep at home without evident prior illness.*

microvesicular pattern [10]. This and hyperammonemia have often led to a diagnosis of Reye syndrome [2,11–14]. Cerebral edema and herniation have been reported in an acute lethal episode [12]. In at least one patient [11], a documented

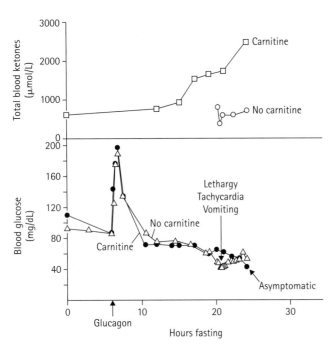

Figure 40.5 *Fasting ketogenesis in a patient with MCAD deficiency. A second fast was undertaken after initiation of treatment with carnitine, and although she again became hypoglycemic she had a better ketogenic response, did not develop symptoms of illness, did not have hypoglycemia until 24 hours and did not develop clinical evidence of illness.*

accompanying orotic aciduria permitted fulfillment of published criteria for a diagnosis of ornithine transcarbamylase deficiency, but assay of this enzyme in biopsied liver revealed normal activity. This Reye-like presentation is often the first manifestation of disease in this disorder [15].

During the intervals between episodes of illness, patients typically appear completely well. There is no muscle weakness. However, some patients are impressively hypotonic and display a reluctance to exercise or poor muscle strength. Clinical myopathy or cardiomyopathy is unusual in this condition, particularly early [15], but these problems may develop in any patient with a disorder of fatty acid oxidation. Acute cardiac arrhythmia may be seen at the time of episodic illness.

Iafolla and colleagues [16,17] have assembled data on 120 patients with MCAD deficiency referred for diagnostic testing. The mean age of onset was 12 months, and the range was 2 days to 6.5 years. Of 120 patients 23 died before the diagnosis was made; 12 siblings of patients had died previously, 11 diagnosed as SIDS and one as Reye syndrome. Emergency care or admission to hospital was required at onset in 95 percent of patients. Initial symptoms were lethargy in 84 percent, vomiting in 66 percent, encephalopathy in 49 percent and respiratory arrest in 48 percent. Cardiac arrest was the initial presentation in 36 percent and sudden death in 18 percent. Seizures were present in 43 percent and hepatomegaly in 44 percent.

The acute severity of presentation contrasts with the fact that there were no deaths in 97 surviving patients for an average of

2.6 years following diagnosis. Most of our patients have not had a second episode requiring admission to hospital. On the other hand, in follow-up data on 73 patients older than 2 years-of-age [16], there was appreciable long-term morbidity. Twenty-nine percent were judged developmentally delayed; of these, 12 had global developmental disability. Another seven had behavioral problems. Seizure disorder was present in 14 percent and attention deficit disorder in 11 percent.

Key elements of the clinical chemistry in suggesting a disorder of fatty acid oxidation are markedly elevated levels of uric acid and creatine kinase [11,18–20]. These values are elevated only during the acute episodes of illness. They are very high. Uric acid concentrations are often over 10 mg/dL and have been as high as 20 mg/dL. Creatine kinase (CK) may be over 1000 U/L. These data, along with evidence of large amounts of urate in the urine, indicate that the mechanism is cellular breakdown. Hyperuricemia and high levels of CK have been observed in patients with rabies [21]. In patients suspected of having a disorder of fatty acid oxidation it is important to order these two alerting tests specifically, as they are usually omitted from panels of clinical chemical tests in children's hospitals.

Carnitine deficiency is the rule in this disease and may be helpful in suggesting the diagnosis. Concentrations of free-carnitine are very low in plasma. Levels are also low in tissues, but muscle biopsy is not commonly available in this disorder. Levels of esterified carnitine are very high in the urine, and this is the mechanism of the secondary carnitine deficiency. In any condition in which the CoA esters of carboxylic acids accumulate, esterifications with carnitine takes place, and carnitine esters are preferentially excreted in the urine. This serves a detoxification function but it also depletes supplies of carnitine, leading to a second mechanism of impaired fatty acid oxidation. Ratios of ester to free-carnitine tend to be high in blood as well as urine, but we find this less useful than the actual levels of free-carnitine in the plasma and esterified carnitine in the urine.

Medium-chain dicarboxylic aciduria is the hallmark of the organic acid profile in the urine of the patient with this disease, and it may be diagnostic at the time of the acute episode [11]. The typical pattern is that of large amounts of the dicarboxylic acids, adipic (C6), suberic (C8), and sebacic (C10) as well as the glycine conjugates of hexanoic acid and suberic acid. The very large elevation of suberylglycine may be diagnostic [22,23]. Dicarboxylic acids as long as C12 (dodecanedoic) acid maybe elevated, and omega-1 oxidation yields the hydroxy acids, 5-hydroxy-hexanoic and 7-hydroxy octanoic acids [24]. Normal infants and children excrete large amounts of dicarboxylic acids with fasting, but the attendant ketosis is mirrored in very large excretions of 3-hydroxybutyric acid and acetoacetic acid. In contrast, in patients with disorders of fatty acid oxidation, the ratio of dicarboxylic acids to the sum of these two compounds is greater than 1 [13]. Unfortunately, these diagnostic features disappear from the urine with the disappearance of the acute episode, so that by the time the patient is referred for study, the organic acid analysis of the urine is usually completely normal.

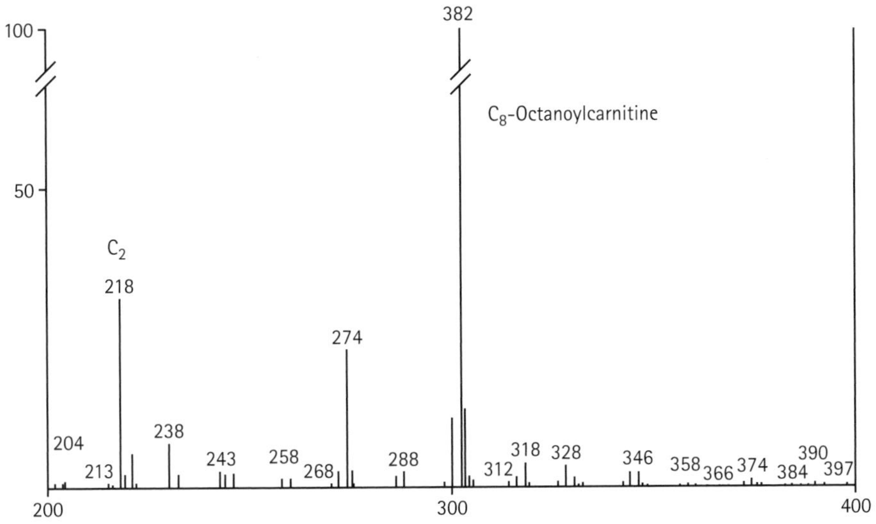

Figure 40.6 *Acylcarnitine profile of the blood plasma patient with MCAD deficiency. C8 is octanoylcarnitine. (Illustration provided by Jon Gangoiti of UCSD.)*

Fasting under controlled conditions will reproduce the typical pattern of dicarboxylic acids in the urine. We have developed a protocol for the systematic investigation of patients suspected of having disorders of fatty acid oxidation (Chapter 36). It is seldom necessary in MCAD deficiency because of the number of simple, less invasive tests that are available. Figure 40.5 illustrates its use in a patient diagnosed prior to the development of these tests. At the time that she developed hypoglycemia after 20 hours, she excreted diagnostic quantities of suberylglycine. The flat curve for the blood levels of acetoacetic and 3-hydroxy-butyric acids illustrates the impaired ketogenesis along with the development of hypoglycemia and clinical evidence of illness.

The diagnosis of MCAD deficiency in the absence of illness or fasting has been facilitated by the development of a sensitive method of gas chromatography/mass spectrometry (GCMS) using a stable isotope dilution that permits the measurement of the glycine conjugates hexanoylglycine, suberylglycine, and phenylpropionylglycine even in the normal individuals[23]. The amounts found in patients with MCAD deficiency during remission are often large enough to be diagnostic. Phenylpropionylglycine excretion depends on the conjugation of a product of intestinal microbial metabolism, and we have found that it is absent during the acute episode, when most patients are receiving antibiotic therapy.

The modern approach to the diagnosis that may be used in remission as well as during illness, is to examine the blood for specific carnitine esters by tandem mass spectrometry (MS/MS) [24,25–27]. The test is usually carried out on blood spots in programs of newborn screening. For definitive diagnosis, the analysis of plasma is preferable. Octanoylcarnitine is the compound on which reliance is usually placed (Figure 40.6) (Table 36.1, p. 244) Hexanoylcarnitine is also useful, and the ratio of C8 to C8:1 is often the best discriminator [27–29]. Normal newborns are under 0.22 μmol/L of octanoylcarnitine (C8). The mean of 16 patients with MCAD deficiency was 8.4 (range 3.1–28.3) μmol/L [28]; and of 35 patients 3.0 (0.4–21.8) μmol/L [29]. A level over 0.3 has been considered a diagnostic criteria for MCAD deficiency. With time and depletion of carnitine, levels of C8 carnitine decrease in patients with MCAD deficiency. For this test to be successful it is sometimes necessary to administer some carnitine.

The pathology of MCAD deficiency is predominantly that of the liver [10,16,30] in which microvesicular and macrovesicular deposits of fat are typical. Deposition of lipids has also been observed in the kidneys and heart [16]. Cerebral edema has been described in the neuropathology of MCAD deficiency, but this has rested on very little evidence. In the paper usually quoted [13], a 2-year-old, one of three patients reported, died and had cerebral edema and herniation on autopsy. Our teenager with MCAD deficiency [10] certainly had increased intracranial pressure, but she had hyperammonemia (235 μmol/L), a well recognized cause of cerebral edema, and her encephalopathy resolved with the level of ammonia. Cerebral edema was also reported in two patients by Duran *et al.* [31]. In the series of 120 patients with MCAD deficiency, cerebral edema was recorded in 14 of 23 studied at autopsy [16]. Cerebral edema was also recorded by Bennett *et al.* [21] in an infant with MCAD deficiency who died suddenly in her sleep.

GENETICS AND PATHOGENESIS

MCAD deficiency is autosomal recessive [8,32,33]. The gene is on chromosome 1 and the nucleotide sequence of its cDNA has been established. A single mutation in which nucleotide 985 has been changed from A to G, leading to a lysine (K) to glutamic acid (E) change in residue 329 of the protein, accounts for virtually all of the patients studied [31–33] (Figures 40.7, 40.8). Among 172 patients, 80.2 percent were homozygous for A $\rightarrow$ G ^{985}, and 17.4 percent were heterozygous for this mutation [33]. Only four percent did not have

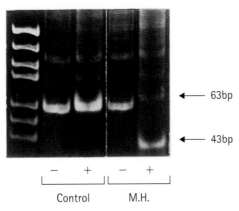

← 63bp

← 43bp

Figure 40.7 *Detection of the common mutation in MCAD deficiency; autoradiography of DNA fragments after electrophoresis on three percent agarose gel. This preparation was made by Dr. Karin Sege-Petersen with the method of Matsubara et al. [33]: Polymerase chain reaction (PCR) with a mismatched primer permitted a restriction site in the mutant but not in the normal, in which a 63 bp fragment contains the site which leads to a 43 bp fragment in the mutant when treated with NcoI. In this illustration − and + signify without and with NcoI; in normal there is no cleavage, while in the patient, M.H., the 43 bp fragment appears.*

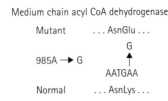

Figure 40.8 *The mutation at nucleotide 985. The A-to-G change specifies a change from the basic lysine to the acidic glutamic acid.*

this change on either allele. A second mutation was found in a patient with MCAD deficiency who was heterozygous for the A → G^{985} and a 4 bp deletion [34]. Rapid screening is available for both mutations, which account for over 93 percent of all MCAD mutations. The common mutation leads to a high frequency of missplicing of mRNA [35], which would be expected to lead to variable phenotypic expression. Heterozygote detection and prenatal diagnosis can be carried out by testing for the mutations.

Identification of newborns in the US with MCAD deficiency by MS/MS screening has yielded an incidence of 1 in 15 000 [36]. Mutation analysis revealed a lower incidence of the A985G mutation than had been observed in populations diagnosed after the onset of clinical illness. A previously unrecognized mutation, T199C, which has never been found in patients with clinical illness, appears to code for a mild phenotype. Expression of the recombinant Y42H protein coded for by T199C yielded about 80 percent of control activity and even more with chaperonin coexpression, indicating that the mutation interferes with protein folding but confers only mild interference with activity. The carrier frequency of this mutation appear to approximate 1 in 500. This mutation was

never found in a sample of more than 90 patients identified by the presence of clinical illness. In this study, a mild acylcarnitine profile, as seen in patients heterozygous for A985G and T199C, had a C8 concentration of 0.5–2.0 μmol/L and a C8/C10 ratio of 2–4, while the severe profile, found in all the A985G homozygotes, had a C8 over 2 and a ratio of over 4. These data confirm the reliability of newborn screening for clinical MCAD deficiency. Some 11 other mutations identified were rare, including IVS8+G→T, which changed a splice consensus, were associated with severe deficiency of the enzyme.

The enzyme, MCAD, is one of three mitochondrial acyl CoA dehydrogenases (Table 40.1, p. 262) that catalyze the initial steps in the β-oxidation of fatty acids (Figure 40.1, p. 261). Each is a flavin containing dehydrogenase that is specific for CoA esters of specific chain length. MCAD accepts fatty acyl CoAs in which the acid chain length is 6–12 carbons in length. The enzyme may be assayed in leukocytes, liver or cultured fibroblasts, as well as amniocytes. Immunochemical study of patients with the common mutation [37] revealed no evidence of cross reacting material (CRM), and pulse chase labeling suggests that the enzyme is unstable.

The oxidation of fatty acids is not called upon in the production of energy until fasting has proceeded for some time. Glycogen stores suffice to provide carbohydrate for energy for 12 hours in most individuals. Thus a history of hypoglycemia after a short fast implies a disorder of carbohydrate metabolism, while hypoglycemia after a prolonged fast implies a disorder of fatty acid oxidation. We have encountered exceptions to both rules, but in general when we have subjected patients in remission with disorders of fatty oxidation to fasting under controlled conditions, hypoglycemia has seldom ensued before 16–18 hours (Figure 40.5). This is consistent with the fact that the usual presentation is after 7 months (median age 13.5 months [31]), usually concomitant with a first infectious illness that leads to anorexia or prolonged vomiting and its attendant fasting. It also explains the fact that in some patients the first episode occurs in a teenager [11] or adult [38]. The recognition of asymptomatic affected adults is consistent with the fact that some people never experience a fast longer than 16 hours. We expect that the incidence of normality will be high in those infants detected through routine screening.

In our experience, the exceptional patient who developed hypoglycemia after shorter periods of fasting, was a young infant who developed multiple episodes during infancy. The occurrence of SIDS is of course another exception to the expected course [39–41], and fatal neonatal presentation has been reported [4] in an infant with hypoglycemia and normal levels of free carnitine who had severe lipid cardiomyopathy at autopsy. GCMS of the liver in patients with SIDS has yielded cis-4decenoic acid (C10:1) in each of four infants found to have had MCAD deficiency [40]. The prognosis for survival appears to be particularly bad for those with a neonatal presentation, although overall mortality in the first episode may be as high as 60 percent [39]. In patients surviving to diagnosis, the prognosis is good. Physical and intellectual development may be normal, although abnormal psychiatric tests of development were surprisingly high in the survivors reported by Iafolla et al. [16].

TREATMENT

The hallmark of treatment is the avoidance of fasting. Supplies of readily accepted and tolerated oral carbohydrate should be plentiful and accessible in the home. In a fragile infant a supply of glucose-monogel®, or even parenteral glucagon, may be useful. In the presence of vomiting or anorexia that prevents oral intake, parenteral glucose is mandatory. Admission to hospital is prudent, but sometimes remission can be accomplished in the emergency room. Rates of administration and concentrations should be adequate to reverse hypoglycemia and maintain normoglycemia. It is not sufficient to start five percent glucose and relax; we have seen patients in whom symptomatic hypoglycemia developed under those circumstances. In long-term management we have routinely employed supplemental cornstarch, at least for evening and night feedings. The initial dosage we have employed is 0.5 g/kg (1 Tbsp = 8 g), usually working up to 1.0 g/kg. In the fragile infant referred to above, 2.0 g/kg appeared to be helpful. Some reduction in the intake of fat appears prudent, but this does not need to be excessive.

Supplementation with carnitine is currently controversial, but why this is so appears difficult to understand. Patients are demonstrably deficient in free-carnitine in virtually any circumstances in which they have lived undiagnosed past early infancy [42]. The very high urinary esterified carnitine and its major increase with the specific increase in excretion of octanoylcarnitine and hexanoylcarnitine implies a detoxification function that would be well employed. During illness octanoylcarnitine excretion increases dramatically when the patient is given intravenous carnitine [43]. Figure 40.5 illustrates considerably improved ketogenesis and an absence of symptoms despite fasting hypoglycemia in a patient treated for only a few days with carnitine. An absence of effect after three months of treatment with carnitine in a 5-month-old infant was reported because of the development of symptoms and hypoglycemia after 16.5 hours of controlled fasting [41]. However, the investigators permitted this patient to fast only 12 hours prior to treatment, which did restore concentrations of carnitine in plasma to normal and markedly increased urinary carnitine excretion. Furthermore, the blood level of 3-hydroxybutyrate rose to 0.84 mmol/L, while prior to carnitine it failed to exceed 0.38 mmol/L.

In a study of five symptom-free patients [44], acylglycine excretion exceeded acylcarnitine excretion by a factor of 70 to 1, but the amounts could not be increased by supplemental oral glycine. Supplemental carnitine increased acylcarnitine excretion six-fold and caused a 60 percent reduction in acylglycine excretion. In another study of monitored fasting [45],

a patient tolerated a 12-hour fast after treatment, whereas before, 12 hours of fasting had induced a depressed sensorium and acidosis, as well as the expected accumulation of free fatty acids in the blood and dicarboxylic acids in the urine. We suspect that the failure to recognize a role for carnitine in treatment stems from the fact that, once diagnosed, these patients do so well if they avoid fasting. Most of our patients have not had a second episode requiring admission to hospital, but of course all of them have been treated with carnitine. An initial dose of 60–100 mg/kg is useful. During acute illness we use 200–300 mg/kg intravenously. Treatment with 50–150 mg riboflavin/day was reported [46] to increase the activity of MCAD in lymphocytes of five patients with MCAD deficiency. Increases were very small in four, but a major increase in one patient, who began with 19 percent of control activity, suggests that supplementation may be a useful adjunct.

References

1 Nyhan WL. Abnormalities of fatty acid oxidation. *N Engl J Med* 1988;**319**:1344.

2 Surtee R, Leonard JV. Acute metabolic encephalopathy: a review of causes, mechanisms and treatment. *J Inherit Metab Dis* 1989;**12**:(suppl) 42.

3 Rowe PC, Valle D, Brusilow SW. Inborn errors of metabolism in children referred with Reye's syndrome *JAMA* 1988;**260**:3167.

4 Leung KC, Hammond JW, Chabra S, et al. A fatal neonatal case of medium-chain acyl-coenzyme A dehydrogenase deficiency with homozygous A → G^{985} transition. *J Pediatr* 1992;**121**:965.

5 Emery JL, Variend S, Howat AJ, Vawter GF. Investigation of inborn errors of metabolism in unexpected infant deaths. *Lancet* 1988;**2**:29.

6 Harpey JP, Charpentier C, Paturneau-Jouas M. Sudden infant death syndrome and inherited disorders of fatty acid R-oxidation. *Biol Neonate* 1990;**58**:(suppl1) 70.

7 Miller ME, Brooks JG, Forbes N, Insel R. Frequency of medium-chain acyl-CoA dehydrogenase deficiency G-985 mutation in sudden infant death syndrome. *Pediatr Res* 1992;**31**:305.

8 Coates PM, Hale DE, Stanley CA, et al. Genetic deficiency of medium-chain acyl coenzyme A dehydrogenase: studies in cultured skin fibroblasts and peripheral mononuclear leukocytes. *Pediatr Res* 1985;**19**:672.

9 Patel JS, Leonard JV. Ketonuria and medium-chain acyl-CoA dehdrogenase deficiency. *J Inherit Metab Dis* 1995;**18**:98.

10 Treem WR, Witzleben CA, Piccoli DA, et al. Medium-chain and long-chain acyl-CoA dehydrogenase deficiencies: clinical pathologic and ultrastructural differentiation from Reye's syndrome. *Hepatology* 1986;**6**:1270.

11 Marsden D, Sege-Petersen K, Nyhan WL, et al. An unusual presentation of medium-chain acyl coenzyme. A dehydrogenase deficiency. *Am J Did Child* 1992;**146**:1459

12 Stanley CA, Coates PM. Inherited defects of fatty acid oxidation which resemble Reye's syndrome: IV Reye's syndrome. *J Natl Reye's Syndrome Foundation* 1985;**5**:190.

13 Stanley CA, Hale DE, Coates PM, et al. Medium chain acyl-CoA dehydrogenase deficiency in children with non-ketotic hypoglycemia and low carnitine levels. *Pediatr Res* 1983;**17**:877.

14 Green A, Hall SM. Investigation of metabolic disorders resembling Reye's syndrome. *Arch Dis Child* 1992;**67**:1313.

15 Saudubray JM, Martin D, De Lonlay P, et al. Recognition and management of fatty acid oxidation defects: A series of 107 patients. *J Inherit Metab Dis* 1999;**22**:488.

16 Iafolla AK, Thompson RJ Jr, Roe CR. Medium-chain acyl-coenzyme A dehydrogenase deficiency: Clinical course in 120 affected children. *J Pediatr* 1994;**124**:409.

17 Iafolla AK, Millington DS, Chen YT, *et al.* Natural course of medium chain acyl-CoA dehydrogenase deficiency. *Am J Hum Genet* 1991;**49**:(suppl) 99.

18 Davidson-Mundt A, Luder AS, Greene CL. Hyperuricemia in medium-chain acyl-coenzyme A dehydrogenase deficiency. *J Pediatr* 1992;**120**:444.

19 Reinehr T, Burk G, Dietz B, *et al.* Hyperuricemia as the main symptom of medium-chain acyl-CoA dehydrogenase deficiency. *Klin Padiatr* 1997;**209**:357.

20 Marsden D, Nyhan WL, Barshop BA. Creatine kinase and uric acid: early warning for metabolic imbalance resulting from disorders of fatty acid oxidation. *Arch Neurol* 2001;**160**:599.

21 Ceyhan M, Kanra G, Yilmaz Y, *et al.* Rabies (diagnosis and discussion). *Am J Dis Child* 1992;**146**:1215.

22 Bennett MJ, Rinaldo P, Millington DS, *et al.* Medium chain acyl CoA dehydrogenase deficiency: postmortem diagnosis in a case of sudden infant death and neonatal diagnosis of an affected sibling. *Pediatr Pathol* 1991;**11**:889.

23 Rinaldo P, O'Shea JJ, Coates PM, *et al.* Medium chain acyl-CoA dehydrogenase deficiency: diagnosis by stable-isotope dilution measurement of urinary N-hexanoylglycine and 3-phenylpropionylglycine. *N Engl J Med* 1988;**319**:1308.

24 Wanders RJA, Vreken P, Den Boer MEJ, *et al.* Disorders of mitochondrial fatty acyl-CoA β-oxidation. *J Inherit Metab Dis* 1999;**22**:442.

25 Roe CR, Millington DAM, Bohan TP, *et al.* Diagnostic and therapeutic implications of medium-chain acylcarnitines in the medium-chain acyl-CoA dehydrogenase deficiency. *Pediatr Res* 1985;**19**:459.

26 Roe CR, Millington DS, Maltby DA, Kinnebrew P. Recognition of medium-chain acyl-CoA dehydrogenase deficiency in asymptomatic siblings of children dying of sudden infant death or Reye-like syndromes. *J Pediatr* 1986;**108**:13.

27 Vreken P, van Lint AEM, Bootsma AH, *et al.* Rapid diagnosis of organic acidemias and fatty acid oxidation defects by quantitative electrospray tandem-MS acyl-carnitine analysis in plasma: in *Current Views of Fatty Acid Oxidation and Ketogenesis: From Organelles to Point Mutations* (eds PA Quant, S Eaton, Kluwer Academic). Plenum Publishers, New York;1999:327.

28 Chace DH, Hillman SL, Van Hover JL, Naylor EW. Rapid diagnosis of MCAD deficiency: quantitative analysis of octanoylcanitine and other acylcarnitines in newborn blood spots by tandem mass spectrometry. *Clin Chem* 1997;**43**:2106

29 Clayton PT, Doig M, Ghafari S, *et al.* Screening for medium chain acyl-CoA dehydrogenase deficiency using electrospray ionisation tandem mass spectrometry. *Arch Dis Child* 1998;**79**:109.

30 Bouve KE. Letter to the Editor. *Pediat Pathol* 1992;**12**:621.

31 Duran M, Hofkamp M, Rhead W, Sudden child death and 'healthy' affected family members with medium-chain acyl-Coenzyme A dehydrogenase deficiency. *Pediatrics* 1986;**78**:1052.

32 Workshop on Molecular Aspects of MCAD deficiency: Mutations causing medium-chain acyl-CoA dehydrogenase deficiency: A collaborative compilation of the data from 172 patients: in *New Developments in Fatty Acid Oxidation* (eds PM Coates, E Tanaka). Wiley-Liss, New York;1992:499.

33 Matsubara Y, Narisawa K, Miyabayashi S, *et al.* Identification of a common mutation in patients with medium-chain acyl-CoA dehydrogenase deficiency. *Biochem Biophys Res Comm* 1990;**171**:498.

34 Ding JH, Yang BZ, Bao Y, *et al.* Identification of a new mutation in medium-chain acyl-CoA dehydrogenase (MCAD) deficiency. *Am J Hum Genet* 1992;**50**:229.

35 Zhang Z, Zhou Y, Kelly DP, *et al.* Delineation of RFLPs and multiple ALU sequences associated with the A985G mutation in human medium chain acyl CoA dehydrogenase. *Pediatr Res* 1992;**31**:137A.

36 Andresen BS, Dobrowolski SF, O'Reilly L, *et al.* Medium-chain acyl-CoA dehydrogenase (MCAD) mutations identified by MS/MS-based prospective screening of newborns differ from those observed in patients with clinical symptoms: Identification and characterization of a new prevalent mutation that results in mild MCAD deficiency. *Am J Hum Genet* 2001;**68**:1408.

37 Coates PM, Indo Y, Young D, *et al.* Immunochemical characterization of variant medium-chain acyl-CoA dehydrogenase in fibroblasts from patients with medium-chain acyl-CoA dehydrogenase deficiency. *Pediatr Res* 1992;**31**:34.

38 Bodman M, Nyhan WL, Naviaux RK. Medium-chain acyl CoA dehydrogenase deficiency: Occurence in an infant and his mother. *Arch Neurol* 2001;**58**:811.

39 Touma EH, Charpentier C. Medium chain acylCoA dehydrogenase deficiency *Arch Dis Child* 1992;**67**:142.

40 Boles RG, Martin SK, Blitzer M, Rinaldo P. Biochemical diagnosis of fatty acid oxidation disorders by GC/MS analysis of post-mortem liver. *Pediatr Res* 1993;**33**:126A.

41 Treem WR, Stanley CA, Goodman SI. Medium-chain acyl-CoA dehydrogenase deficiency: metabolic effects and therapeutic efficacy of long term L-carnitine supplementation. *J Inherit Metab Dis* 1989;**12**:122.

42 Gillingham MB, Van Calcar SC, Ney DM, *et al.* Nutrition support of long chain 3-hydroxyacyl CoA dehydrogenase deficiency – a case report and survey. *J Inherit Metab Dis* 1999;**22**:123.

43 Roe CR, Millington DS, Kahler SG, *et al.* Carnitine homeostasis in the organic acidurias. *Prog Clin Biol Res* 1990;**2**:383.

44 Rinaldo P, Schmidt-Sommerfeld E, Posca AP, *et al.* Effect of treatment with glycine and L-carnitine in medium chain acyl-coenzyme A dehydrogenase deficiency. *J Pediatr* 1993;**122**:580.

45 Waber L, Francomano C, Brusilow S, *et al.* Medium chain acyl CoA dehydrogenase (MCD) deficiency. *Pediatr Res* 1984;**18**:302A.

46 Duran M, Cleutjens BJM, Ketting D, *et al.* Diagnosis of medium-chain acyl-CoA dehydrogenase deficiency in lymphocytes and liver by a gas chromatographic method: the effect of oral riboflavin supplementation. *Pediatr Res* 1991;**31**:39.

41

Very long-chain acyl CoA dehydrogenase (VLCAD) deficiency

MAJOR PHENOTYPIC EXPRESSION

Hypoketotic hypoglycemia, hepatomegaly, cardiomyopathy and myopathy, rhabdomyolysis, elevated creatinine kinase, lipid infiltration of liver and muscle and defective very long chain acyl CoA dehydrogenase.

INTRODUCTION

Very long-chain acyl CoA dehydrogenase (VLCAD) is a recently identified enzyme bound to the inner mitochondrial membrane. It was first reported in 1992 [1]. It catalyzes the dehydrogenation of acyl CoA esters of 14 to 20 carbon length in the first step of mitochondrial fatty acid oxidation (Figure 41.1). Within a year there were 3 reports [2–5] of patients with deficiency of VLCAD, including some that had been previously reported as having LCAD deficiency [6]. It is now recognized that most such patients have VLCAD deficiency, and the long-chain-acyl-CoA dehydrogenase (LCAD) enzyme catalyzes the specific oxidation of branched long chain acyl CoAs. The usual assay with palmitoyl CoA as substrate in the presence of electron transfer flavoprotein (ETF) would register deficiency of activity if either LCAD or VLCAD was deficient. The distinction can be made by immunochemical analysis.

VLCAD deficiency is relatively common. There were 12 patients among the series of 107 disorders of fatty acid oxidation in the Saudubray Paris experience [7]. Vianey-Saban, Divry and colleagues [8] reported 30 patients from Lyon. The VLCAD gene has been isolated [9] and found to contain 20 exons; it is situated in chromosome 17p13 [10–12]. A small number of mutations have been identified [13–16]. VLCAD deficiency is the most common disorder of fatty acid oxidation in the Saudi population.

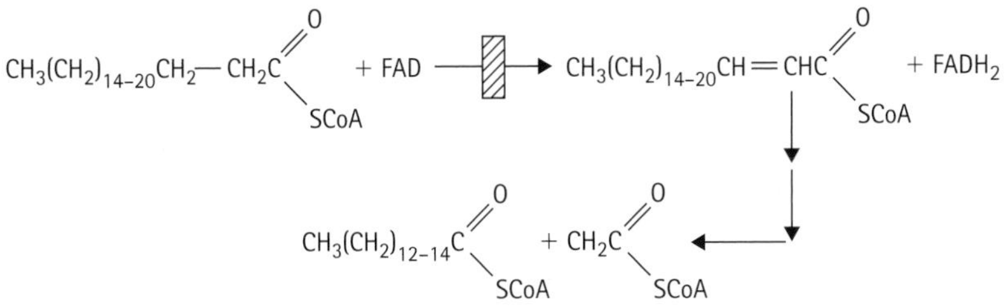

Figure 41.1 *The VLCAD reaction. Following the formation of the enol product the three successive reactions catalyzed by enoyl CoA hydratase, 3-hydroxyacyl CoA dehydrogenase and 3-ketoacyl CoA hydratase yield ultimately acetyl CoA and a fatty acyl CoA of two less carbons.*

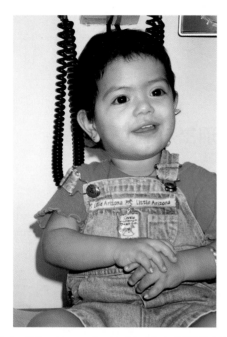

Figure 41.2   *D.S. a 16-month-old girl with the VLCAD deficiency. At 12 months-of-age she was admitted in shock with a blood sugar of 0 and a seizure. She had modest dicarboxylic aciduria. Tandem mass spectrometry revealed elevated long-chain acyl carnitine esters. She was thought to have hypopituitarism and hypothyroidism on the basis of abnormal test results at 12 months, but by 6 years these abnormalities disappeared, and she has grown well without replacement therapy since that time.*

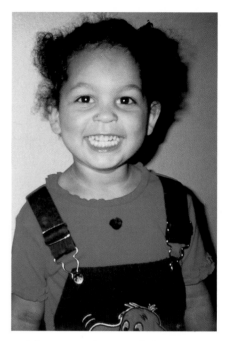

Figure 41.3   *A.G. a 2-year-old with VLCAD deficiency. Diagnosis was made at 2 days-of-age; a previous sibling had died of a disorder of fatty acid oxidation. Acylcarnitine profile revealed elevated C14:1, C16 and C18:1. She had bilateral inverted nipples.*

CLINICAL ABNORMALITIES

This disease may present in the first days of life. One patient [2] had metabolic acidosis at 2 days-of-age. The blood level of creatinine kinase (CK) was 3684, and he had impressive dicarboxylic aciduria. A sibling died suddenly without cardiac abnormalities and had massive fatty infiltration in the liver. In six families of 11 patients with VLCAD deficiency there were eight instances of sudden infant death syndrome (SIDS), or unexplained death [5]. Six of 11 patients in this series died between 3 and 14 months [5].

Hypertrophic cardiomyopathy was found in five of the six who died. This is characteristic of the severe phenotype. Nevertheless, diagnosis and treatment are consistent with survival, reversal of cardiomyopathy and relative health to at least 4 years at time of report [4,5,17]. One patient who had hypoketotic hypoglycemia and cardiomyopathy died at 8 days-of-age of a penetrating duodenal ulcer and peritonitis [18].

The disease has been divided into two forms: the early severe form with cardiac involvement [19,20], and the milder with hypoglycemia as in medium chain acyl CoA dehydrogenase (MCAD) deficiency, but both may have hypoketotic hypoglycemia (Figures 41.2, 41.3), and there really is a third phenotype characterized by episodic rhabdomyolysis and myoglobinuria. There is some merging of these clinical forms,

but distinction is useful because it tends to correlate with amounts of residual enzyme activity.

Neonatal presentations include lethargy, tachypnea, or seizures, and hypoglycemia metabolic acidosis, or arrhythmia may be found. This is followed by decompensation and evidence of hypertrophic cardiopathy. There may be pericardial effusions. Approximately 50 percent of patients have died within two months of initial symptomatology [17,21].

Some patients have had a more typical fatty acid oxidation presentation with fasting intolerance and acute hypoketotic hypoglycemia, usually presenting at the first intercurrent infection, and followed by episodic hypoglycemia. Patients or previous siblings have been diagnosed as having Reye syndrome [22]. Plasma ammonia may be elevated. Uric acid and CK are also high during attacks. An interesting variation on this theme was a patient who presented at 2 years with hypoglycemia and encephalopathy (glucose 1.7 mmol/L) and acidosis resulting from massive ketosis [23]. Because of this, a disorder of fatty acid oxidation was not considered, although the CK was 5373 U/L. The diagnosis was made when the acylcarnitine profile revealed elevated tetradecanoylcarnitine and confirmed by enzyme analysis.

A third presentation is reminiscent of that of carnitine palmitoyl transferase (CPT) II with episodic muscle pains, rhabdomyolysis and myoglobinuria [24,25]. One 28-year-old woman experienced her first symptoms, which were induced by exercise, at 19 years [25]. Levels of CK in the blood were very high.

Plasma free-carnitine may be normal or low. Urinary carnitine may be low, especially at times of acute illness, as long-chain

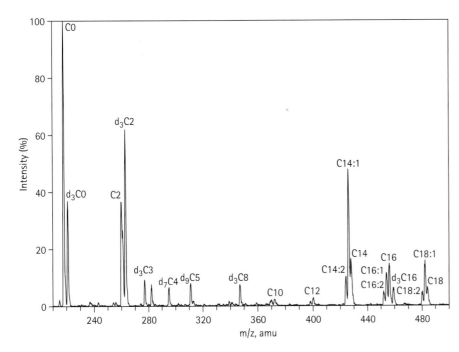

Figure 41.4 *Acylcarnitine profile of the blood plasma of a patient with VLCAD deficiency. The patient was being treated with carnitine, and the C0 was elevated. The key compound was C14:1 acylcarnitine, but all of the long chain acylcarnitine esters were elevated. (Illustration provided by Jon Gangoiti of UCSD.)*

acylcarnitine esters are not well excreted by the kidney. The accumulation in plasma of C14:1 carnitine esters is an important marker on acylcarnitine profile (Figure 41.4), and may be detected in newborn blood spots on screening cards [26]. Levels of C14, C16 and C18:1 may be elevated, and the ratios of C14:1 to C14 or C14:1 to C18:1 may be particularly useful in diagnosis [22,27]. Incubation of fibroblasts with ^{13}C-labeled palmitate revealed accumulation in C16; in this system C14:1 was not elevated [28].

Organic acid analysis of the urine reveals dicarboxylic aciduria. Unfortunately during interepisode periods of health, when many diagnostic work-ups occur, organic acid analysis is normal. During episodes there is medium chain, as well as long chain dicarboxylic aciduria indicating the functioning of peroxisomal β and ω-oxidation.

Pathologic examination reveals hepatic steatosis and deposits of lipid in cardiac and skeletal muscle. Mitochondrial appearance may be abnormal [29]. Peroxisomes may be enlarged.

GENETICS AND PATHOGENESIS

VLCAD deficiency is transmitted in an autosomal recessive fashion. The enzyme was purified from rat liver mitochondria [1]. It requires ETF as the electron receptor. Unlike the other mitochondrial acyl CoA dehydrogenases it is a heterodimer of 71 kD. It does not cross-react with antibodies against LCAD or other acyl CoA dehydrogenases. Its activity is greatest against C16, palmitoyl CoA and is 10 times that of LCAD. Deficiency of VLCAD may be demonstrated in cultured fibroblasts. Antibody against VLCAD is reduced by 66–75 percent, and this may be demonstrated by western blot analysis.

When antibody to LCAD became available, nine cell lines previously thought to be deficient in LCAD were tested and found to have normal immunoreactive LCAD protein [6], and testing via immunoblot analysis against VLCAD revealed then all to be VLCAD-deficient. Low VLCAD activity was also demonstrated by testing for enzyme activity in the presence of anti-LCAD antibody, which did not alter activity [3].

Rapid indication of the diagnosis has been reported by the study of β-oxidation and VLCAD in lymphocytes [29] and the method has been adapted for prenatal diagnosis of chorionic villus material. Prenatal diagnosis has also been made by assay of the dehydrogenation of palmitoyl CoA in amniocytes [30].

In vitro studies of the incubation of fibroblasts with deuterium labeled palmitate and carnitine followed by assay of the pattern of enrichment of acylcarnitines [31] has been reported to correlate well with the different phenotypes of severe cardiomyopathy and those without cardiomyopathy. The ratio of deuterated C16 to deuterated C12 has been discriminatory.

The gene for VLCAD has been cloned and sequenced [32]. A number of mutations have been identified in study of 32 unrelated patients [19]. In general, patients with the more severe phenotype had alleles coding for truncated proteins or proteins lacking amino acids [18,19,22,25], whereas those with the milder phenotypes had alleles with missense mutations [19]. The woman whose symptoms began at 19 years had two missense mutations (G145C/R375W) [24]. An interesting S583W mutation demonstrated that association of the mature VLCAD protein with the inner mitochondrial membrane is required for activity, because the protein is imported normally [15]. A patient who presented at 14 years with exercise induced myalgia was found to have two missense mutations (A416T and R450H), each of which expressed some temperature sensitive activity [32].

TREATMENT

Treatment aimed at the hypoglycemia emphasizes the avoidance of fasting and prompt intervention with parenteral glucose-containing solutions when fasting is unavoidable. Fasting attendant upon surgery and anesthesia, particularly for minor procedures may be particularly dangerous [33]. Cornstarch supplementation may be useful (2 g/kg at bedtime). Medium-chain triglyceride (MCT) appears to be therapeutic, and surviving patients have done well after initiation of MCT supplementation. A diet low in fat (5–10 percent of calories in long chain triglycerides) supplemented with MCT (30 percent of total calories or 85–90 percent of the calories from fat) was credited with reversal of hypertrophic cardiomyopathy [18]; the patient also received 50–100 g/kg of carnitine. Similar resolution of cardiomyopathy was reported in a boy treated with a similar regimen; he and his sister, diagnosed prenatally, had normal cardiac and developmental function at follow-up [29].

In the course of this treatment deficiency of ω-6 fatty acids, such as DHA and arachidonic acids has been reported [34], but neither patient had any symptoms of deficiency; specifically there was no pigmentary retinopathy as in LCHAD deficiency (Chapter 42), and the levels do not seem especially low to those of us monitoring very low fat diets such as those employed for lipoprotein lipase deficiency (Chapter 88). Carnitine administration, at least to restore levels of free-carnitine, appears to be indicated. Carnitine therapy has become controversial in this as well as other long-chain fatty acid oxidation disorders, largely on the basis of anecdote. Long-chain acyl carnitine esters have also been reported to promote ischemic damage or abnormal post ischemic function in experimental animals [35,36], and their prevention was reported by inhibitors of acyl carnitine formation, but another study found no effect of a CPTI inhibitor and obtained evidence that the ischemic damage resulted from the fatty acids [37]. Treatment with carnitine was reported to ameliorate recurrent myoglobinuria in an 11-year-old with VLCAD deficiency [38], but to be without effect in another patient [24].

References

1 Izai K, Uchida Y, Orii T, et al. Novel fatty acid β-oxidation enzymes in rat liver mitochondria. I Purification and properties of very-long-chain acyl-coenzyme A dehydrogenase. J Biol Chem 1992;**267**:1027.

2 Bertrand C, Largilliere C, Zabot MT, et al. Very long chain acyl-CoA dehydrogenase deficiency: identification of a new inborn error of mitochondrial fatty acid oxidation in fibroblasts. Biochem Biophys Acta 1993;**1180**:327.

3 Aoyama T, Uchida Y, Kelley RI, et al. A novel disease with deficiency of mitochondrial very-long-chain acyl-CoA dehydrogenase. Biochem Biophys Res Commun 1993;**191**:1369.

4 Yamaguchi S, Indo Y, Coates PM, et al. Identification in very-long-chain acyl-CoA dehydrogenase deficiency. Pediat Res 1993;**34**:111.

5 Vianey-Saban C, Divry P, Zabot MT, Mathieu M. Mitochondrial very long chain acyl-CoA dehydrogenase deficiency (VLCAD): identification of this new inborn error of fatty acid oxidation in 11 patients. Proceedings VI International Congress of Inborn Errors of Metabolism 1994;**88**:Wp1 (abstr).

6 Indo Y, Coates PM, Hale DE, Tanaka K. Immunochemical characterization of variant long chain acyl-CoA dehydrogenase in cultured fibroblasts from nine patients with long chain acyl CoA dehydrogenase deficiency. Pediatr Res 1991;**30**:211.

7 Saudubray JM, Martin D, De Lonlay P, et al. Recognition and management of fatty acid oxidation defects: a series of 107 patients. J Inherit Metab Dis 1999;**22**:488.

8 Vianey-Saban C, Divry P, Brivet M, et al. Mitochondrial very-long-chain acyl-coenzyme A dehydrogenase deficiency: clinical characteristics and diagnostic considerations in 30 patients. Clin Chim Acta 1998;**269**:43.

9 Aoyama T, Ueno I, Kamijo T, Hashimoto T. Rat very-long-chain acyl-CoA dehydrogenase, a novel mitochondrial acyl-CoA dehydrogenase gene product, is a rate-limiting enzyme in a long-chain fatty acid β-oxidation system. cDNA and deduced amino acid sequence and distinct specificities of the cDNA-expressed protein. J Biol Chem 1994;**269**:19088.

10 Strauss AW, Powell CK, Hale DE, et al. Molecular basis of human mitochondrial very-long-chain acyl-CoA dehydrogenase deficiency causing cardiomyopathy and sudden death in childhood. Proc Natl Acad Sci USA 1995;**92**:10496.

11 Aoyama T, Souri M, Ueno I, et al. Cloning of human very-long-chain acyl-coenzyme A dehydrogenase and molecular characterization of its deficiency in two patients. Am J Hum Genet 1995;**57**:273.

12 Orii K, Aoyama T, Souri M, et al. Genomic DNA organization of human mitochondrial very-long-chain acyl-CoA dehydrogenase and mutation analysis. Biochem Biophys Res Commun 1995;**217**:987.

13 Aoyama T, Wakui K, Fukushima Y, et al. Assignment of the human mitochondrial very-long-chain acyl-CoA dehydrogenase gene (LCACD) to 17p13 by in situ hybridization. Genomics 1996;**37**:144.

14 Souri M, Aoyama T, Orii K, et al. Mutation analysis of very-long-chain acyl-coenzyme A dehydrogenase (VLCAD) deficiency: identification and characterization of mutant VLCAD cDNAs from four patients. Am J Hum Genet 1996;**58**:97.

15 Souri M, Aoyama T, Hoganson G, Hashimoto T. Very-long-chain acyl-CoA dehydrogenase subunit assembles to the dimer form on mitochondrial inner membrane. FEBS Lett 1998;**426**:187.

16 Andresen BS, Bross P, Vianey-Saban C, et al. Cloning and characterization of human very-long-chain acyl-CoA dehydrogenase cDNA, chromosomal assignment of the gene and identification in four patients of nine different mutations within the VLCAD gene. Hum Mol Genet 1996;**5**:461.

17 Cox GF, Souri M, Aoyama T, et al. Reversal of severe hypertrophic cardiomyopathy and excellent neuropsychologic outcome in very-long-chain acyl-coenzyme. A dehydrogenase deficiency. J Pediatr 1998;**133**:247.

18 Pust B, Berger A, Hennenberger A, et al. Very-long-chain acyl-coenzyme A dehydrogenase deficiency (VLCADD) with gastrointestinal hemorrhage as a fatal complication. J Inherit Metab Dis 1996;**19**:53 P105 (abstr).

19 Andresen BS, Bross P, Lund H, et al. VLCAD deficiency – correlation between genotype and phenotype. J Inherit Metab Dis 1996;**19**:7 014 (abstr).

20 Nada MA, Vianey-Saban C, Roe CR. Very-long-chain-acyl-CoA dehydrogenase deficiency: two phenotypes with distinctive biochemical findings. J Inherit Metab Dis 1996;**19**:53 P105 (abstr).

21 Aoyama T, Souri M, Ushikubo S, et al. Purification of human very-long-chain acyl-Co A dehydrogenase and characterization of its deficiency in seven patients. J Clin Invest 1995;**95**:2465.

22 Hahn S-H, Lee E-H, Jung J-W, et al. Very long chain acyl coenzyme A dehydrogenase deficiency in a 5-month-old Korean boy: identification of a novel mutation. J Pediatr 1999;**135**:250.

23 Wraige E, Champion MP, Turner C, Dalton RN. Fat oxidation defect presenting with overwhelming ketonuria. *Arch Dis Child* 2002;**87**:428.

24 Ogilvie I, Pourfarzam M, Jackson S, *et al.* Very long chain acyl coenzyme A dehydrogenase deficiency presenting with exercise-induced myoglobinuria. *Neurology* 1994;**44**:467.

25 Pou-Serradell A, Ribes A, Briones P, *et al.* Myopathic presentation in an adult woman with a very long chain acyl-coenzyme A dehydrogenase deficiency. *J Inherit Metab Dis* 2001;**24**:(suppl 1) 70.

26 Wood JC, Magera MJ, Rinaldo P, *et al.* Diagnosis of very long chain acyl-dehydrogenase deficiency from an infant's newborn screening card. *Pediatrics* 2001;**107**:173.

27 Onkenhout W, Venizelos V, van der Poel PF, *et al.* Quantification of intermediates of unsaturated fatty acid metabolism in plasma of patients with fatty acid oxidation disorders. *Clin Chem* 1995;**41**:1467.

28 Tyni T, Pourfarzam M, Turnbull DM. Analysis of mitochondrial fatty acid oxidation intermediates by tandem mass spectrometry from intact mitochondria prepared from homogenates of cultured fibroblasts skeletal muscle cells and fresh muscle. *Pediatr Res* 2002;**52**:64.

29 Treem WR, Witzleben CA, Piccoli DA, *et al.* Medium-chain and long-chain acyl-CoA dehydrogenase deficiency. Clinical pathologic and ultrastructural differentiation from Reye's syndrome. *Hepatology* 1986;**6**:1270.

30 Sluysmans T, Tuerlinckx D, Hubinont C, *et al.* Very long chain acyl-coenzyme A dehydrogenase deficiency in two siblings: Evolution after prenatal diagnosis and prompt management. *J Pediatr* 1997;**131**:444.

31 Vianey-Saban C, Divry P, Brivet M, *et al.* Mitochondrial very-long-chain acyl-coenzyme A dehydrogenase deficiency: Clinical characteristics and diagnostic considerations in 30 patients. *Clin Chim Acta* 1998;**269**:43.

32 Fukao T, Watanabe H, Orii KE, *et al.* Myopathic form of very-long chain acyl-CoA dehydrogenase deficiency: Evidence for temperature-sensitive mild mutations in both mutant alleles in a Japanese girl. *Pediatr Res* 2001;**49**:227.

33 Roe CR, Wiltse HE, Sweetman L, Alvarado LL. Death caused by perioperative fasting and sedation in a child with unrecognized VLCAD deficiency. *J Pediatr* 2000;**136**:397.

34 Ruiz-Sanz JI. Aldamiz-Echevarria L. Arrizabalaga J. *et al.* Polyunsaturated fatty acid deficiency during dietary treatment of very-long-chain acyl-CoA dehydrogenase deficiency. Rescue with soybean oil. *J Inherit Metab Dis* 2001;**24**:493.

35 Corr PB, Creer MH, Yamada KA, *et al.* Prophylaxis of early ventricular fibrillation by inhibition of acylcarnitine accumulation. *J Clin Invest* 1989;**83**:927.

36 Yamada KA, McHowat J, Yan G-X, *et al.* Cellular uncoupling induced by accumulation of long-chain acylcarnitine during ischemia. *Circ Res* 1994;**74**:83.

37 Madden MC, Wolkowitcz PE, Pohost GM, *et al.* Acylcarnitine accumulation does not correlate with reperfusion recovery in palmitate-perfused rat hearts. *Am J Physiol* 1995;**268**:H2505.

38 Straussberg R, Harel L, Varsano I, *et al.* Recurrent myoglobinuria as a presenting manifestation of very long chain acyl coenzyme A dehydrogenase deficiency. *Pediatrics* 1997;**99**:894.

42

Long chain L-3-hydroxyacyl CoA dehydrogenase (LCHAD) deficiency – trifunctional protein deficiency

---

MAJOR PHENOTYPIC EXPRESSION

Hypoketotic hypoglycemia, episodic rhabdomyolysis, hypotonia, cardiomyopathy, hepatic disease, peripheral neuropathy, pigmentary retinopathy, 3-hydroxydicarboxylic aciduria, carnitine deficiency and defective activity of the trifunctional protein. Maternal acute fatty liver of pregnancy during carriage of a fetus with LCHAD deficiency.

INTRODUCTION

LCHAD deficiency was first reported [1,2] in 1983 in a boy who had many attacks of hypoketotic hypoglycemia starting at 9 months-of-age, had hypotonia and cardiomyopathy and went on to develop massive hepatic necrosis, and died at 19 months. There was long chain acyl carnitine accumulation in plasma and 3-hydroxydicarboxylic aciduria. The activity of LCHAD was demonstrated to be defective in an assay in which 3-ketopalmitoyl CoA was the substrate.

The enzyme is a component of the trifunctional protein (TFP) bound to the inner mitochondrial membrane [3–5]. The protein is an octamer with two distinct α and β subunits. Its three activities are long chain 2-enoyl CoA hydratase, LCHAD and long chain 3-oxoacylCoA thiolase. Its LCHAD activity against 3-hydroxyacylCoA substrates is optimal for compounds of C12–C16 chain length, in contrast to the short chain-3-hydroacylCoA dehydrogenase (SCHAD), where specificity is optimal at C6. The thiolase and enoyl hydrolase activities also have long chain specificities. The LCHAD enzyme catalyzes the reversible dehydration of the 3-hydroxy group to a 3-keto group and nicotine adenine dinucleotide (NAD) is the hydrogen acceptor (Figure 42.1). Patients with LCHAD deficiency may be deficient in LCHAD activity specifically, or may be deficient in all three activities of the TFP. The genes for the α and β subunits have been cloned [6]. The α cDNA codes for an 82,598 Da precursor of a mature 78,969 Da protein. Mutational analysis has revealed a number of distinct mutations including one that appears to be common, a G1528C point mutation in the dehydrogenase coding region that changes a glutamic acid to a glutamine [7,8,9].

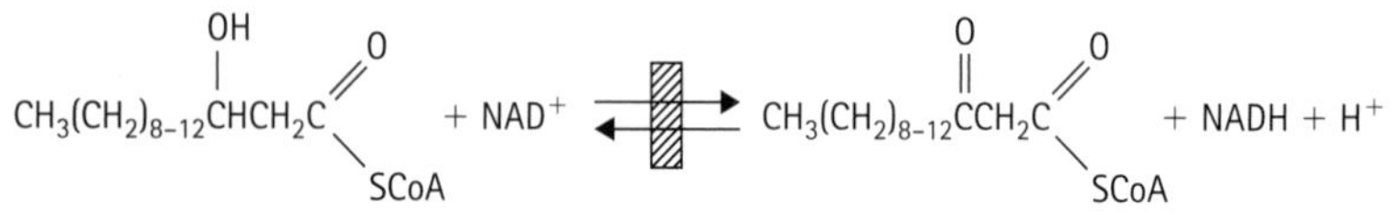

Figure 42.1 *The reaction catalyzed by LCHAD. The product is then involved in the 3-ketothiolase reaction in which the α-β bond is cleaved and acetyl CoA split off, yielding a fatty acid CoA ester of two less carbons.*

CLINICAL ABNORMALITIES

Patients with LCHAD deficiency usually present in late infancy with the typical clinical picture of a disorder of fatty acid oxidation of which the hallmark feature is acute hypoketotic hypoglycemia (Figures 42.2, 42.3). These episodes often begin late in the first year of life, with the first long fast, usually caused by an intercurrent infection illness and ushered in with vomiting [10–13]. Many have been diagnosed as having Reye syndrome. Mean age of onset in 50 patients was 5–8 months. The disease may be a cause of sudden infant death, even neonatal [14,15]. With prompt diagnosis and treatment acute neonatal cardiorespiratory arrest may yield to resuscitation and a favorable prognosis [16]. During the acute episode levels of creatine phosphokinase (CK) and uric acid are elevated [17].

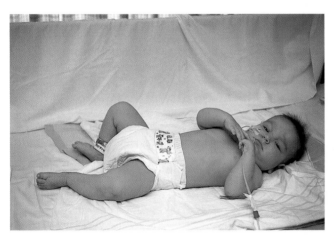

Figure 42.2   *L.J., a 9-month-old boy with LCHAD deficiency. He had a number of episodes of hypoglycemia starting at 5 months-of-age, when he was found to have hepatomegaly and hepatic steatosis. Fasting and loading with long-chain triglycerides led to hypoglycemia, while MCT loading was uneventful. Later he had an episode of myoglobinuria and massive elevation of creatinine phosphokinase.*

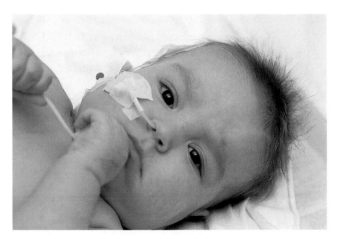

Figure 42.3   *The feeding tube reflected the need, prior to referral, for virtually continuous feeding to maintain normoglycemia.*

The acute episode may begin with a seizure; the electroencephalogram (EEG) may be abnormal. Most patients are hypotonic at least in infancy. Patients may be difficult to feed and gavage feeding may be required [14]. Some may display failure to thrive.

Later episodes are often ushered in with pains in the legs. Rhabdomyolysis leads to myoglobinuria [18]. Patients may first present as adults with exercise-induced muscle pains and rhabdomyolysis. Levels of CK may be very high (15 000–165 000 IU). Examination may reveal profound weakness, little movement and the assumption of a frog-leg position.

Some patients with myopathic presentations have had rapidly fatal cardiomyopathy in infancy [19–20]. Acute life-threatening cardiac episodes may be followed by tetraparesis [20]. Such patients may, or may not have had earlier episodes of hypoketotic hypoglycemia. Examination of the heart may reveal cardiomegaly, poor heart sounds and gallop rhythm. The electrocardiogram reveals sinus tachycardia, a long QT, ventricular tachycardia or a long left ventricular hypertrophy [20]. Echocardiography may reveal dilatation and poor contractility [19]. Pericardial effusion has been reported and tamponade [13,20]. Others have had a more indolent, myopathic presentation in which ventricular hypertrophy is found on echocardiography or electrocardiography in the absence of symptoms [14].

Hepatic dysfunction is another characteristic of the disease [1,2,13,14,18]. Most patients have hepatomegaly [12,19]. Some have had acute cholestatic jaundice as neonates, and this may be transient [12]. The other end of the scale is massive total hepatic necrosis in infancy [1]. Jaundice may develop in infancy along with elevation in the blood levels of transaminases. Ultrasound or other imaging may indicate fatty infiltration of the liver. Biopsy reveals accumulation of fat and fibrosis.

An unusual complication is the acute fatty liver of pregnancy in a mother carrying a fetus with LCHAD deficiency [21]. The heterozygous mother may have pre-eclampsia and urinary protein, or the hypertension, elevated liver enzymes and low platelets (HELLP) syndrome. As many as approximately 20 percent of pregnancies at risk may be complicated by one of these complications [12].

It has increasingly been recognized that pigmentary retinopathy is a potential complication of LCHAD deficiency [10,11,22–25]. This may occur in as many as 70 percent of patients, but as yet the true incidence is unclear, as visual problems are progressive, and few patients have been followed very long. In a series of 28 children a pattern of ophthalmologic progression emerged [22]. Of 15 patients who died at ages from 3 to 14 months vision had been normal for age. In the oldest survivors, 16 and 31 years visual loss was progressive. In 11 children granular retinal pigment was seen at 4 months to 5 years. The two long-term patients had progressive atrophy of the choroid and retina, axial myopia and scotomata. All four longer-surviving patients had lenticular opacities. The electroretinogram deteriorated during the final decade and became unrecordable in the oldest patient. Posterior staphylomas were seen in the two oldest patients.

Another clinical abnormality unusual in disorders of fatty acid oxidation that has been observed with time in LCHAD deficiency is peripheral neuropathy [18,22,23]. By adolescence neuropathy and retinopathy may be the major clinical problems [22]. Deep tendon reflexes may be absent even in infancy [24]. The patient may toe-walk and display an equinus deformity. Extensor plantar responses have been reported [24]. In one patient, mild peripheral neuropathy of adult onset was the only clinical abnormality [26]. Intelligence in these patients has usually been normal, but of course prolonged hypoglycemia always carries a risk of injury to the central nervous system, and a number of patients has been retarded and/or had a seizure disorder. Mortality has been as high as 38 percent [12]. Morbidity in surviving patients has also been high [12], especially acute muscle problems and episodic metabolic derangement [12]. On the other hand it was notable that all who died did so within three months of diagnosis. In those surviving, none had cardiomyopathy, and clinical condition was good despite recurrent muscle problems or diminished visual acuity.

The clinical chemistry in the acute illness may reveal hyperammonemia (68–400 µmol/L). This, with the hypoglycemia, hepatomegaly and elevation of transaminases is what has led to a diagnosis of Reye syndrome. The CK is elevated and so is the level of uric acid [17]. Lactic acidemia may accompany the acute episode, or there may be persistent lactic acidemia [1,14,18,24]. Fatal neonatal lactic acidemia has been reported [27] but the patient had impressive cardiomyopathy. Carnitine is low, especially free carnitine. Free fatty acids are increased, and the ratio of free fatty acids to

3-hydroxybutyrate is particularly high. With hepatic dysfunction, there is hyperbilirubinemia.

Pathologic examination has generally revealed microvesicular and macrovesicular accumulation of fat in liver, skeletal muscle and heart, but necrotic myopathy without accumulation of lipid has also been described [24] as has a predominance of type 1, slow oxidative muscle fibers. Hepatic cirrhosis has also been observed. Electron microscopy has revealed condensation of mitochondrial matrix and widening of cristal spaces [19,28].

The diagnosis is most often suggested by the findings of large amounts of 3-hydroxydicarboxylic acids in the urine, or by the determination of the acylcarnitine profile in the blood. On gas chromatography/mass spectrometry (GCMS) organic acid analysis of the urine, the key compounds are hydroxy acids of up to 14 carbons [29] but medium chain dicarboxylic and 3-hydroxydicarboxylic acids are also found [2,28]. Quantification in organic acid analysis is important in this condition as in others, for 3-hydroxydecanedioic acid and other dicarboxylic acids may be found in the urine in elevated amounts in ketosis, but in smaller quantity than in LCHAD deficiency [30]. Any of these abnormalities may become normal during an interim period of health between acute episodes. We have followed a patient in whom 3-hydroxyadipic acid is the only organic acid marker of the disease, even at times of acute rhabdomyolysis. This compound may be elevated by ketosis, but of course patients with this disease do not become ketotic. Assessment of the acylcarnitine profile of the plasma should reveal 3-hydroxyacid derivatives of the C16, C18 and C18:1 species [31] (Figure 42.4). Oral loading with 3-phenylpropionate leads to the excretion of 3-hydroxyphenylpropionate, indicating the site of the defect [15].

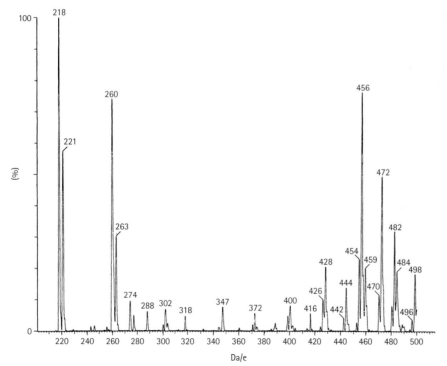

Figure 42.4 Acylcarnitine profile of the blood plasma of a patient with LCHAD deficiency. Key compounds were the 3-hydroxyl derivatives of C14, C16 and C18. (Illustration provided by Jon Gangoiti of UCSD.)

GENETICS AND PATHOGENESIS

LCHAD deficiency is transmitted as an autosomal recessive trait. The molecular defect is in the mitochondrial trifunctional protein, which contains activities of LCHAD, 2-enoyl CoA hydratase and 3-oxoacyl CoA hydratase. It differs from the trifunctional enzyme found in peroxisomes in structure and function [3], and is capable by itself of catalyzing the three sequential steps of β-oxidation. In some patients, there is defective activity of all three activities of the protein [26], but in most of the patients deficiency is isolated to LCHAD.

The diagnosis may be confirmed by study of the oxidation of ^{14}C-labeled myristic (C14:0) and palmitic (C16:0) acids by lymphocytes [32] or fibroblasts, or by mutational analysis [12]. The enzyme has usually been measured in fibroblasts in the reverse direction, with 3-oxopalmitoyl CoA as substrate and measurement of the decrease in absorbance at 340 nm of the NADH electron donor. In some patients activity is undetectable [18,33], but since the SCHAD enzyme has some activity against longer fatty acids activity is usually about 15 to 35 percent of control [2,13,18,34]. Assay in the presence of antibody against the SCHAD protein generally gives LCHAD activity values less than 10 percent of control [2,13,18]. In rare instances cross-reacting material (CRM) for trifunctional protein (TFP) is virtually undetectable and activity of the three enzymes is deficient, but in most instances immunoreactive mitochondrial TFP (MTP) is normal and activity of only LCHAD is deficient [35]. Indication of the diagnosis has also been made by incubation of fibroblasts with palmitate and analysis of the medium for free 3-hydroxyacids [36]. Levels of 3-OHC14 and 3-OHC16 were increased 11- and 14-fold.

Intermediate activity in fibroblasts has been consistent with heterozygosity. Prenatal diagnosis can be made by enzyme analysis and by mutational analysis [37].

The gene for the α protein has been cloned and localized to chromosome 2p23.3-24.1, and the common mutation has been identified [9]. This G1528C mutation changes the glutamate 510 to glutamine. A simple polymerase chain reaction (PCR), restriction fragment length polymorphism (RFLP) method of the detection of this mutation makes diagnosis and carrier detection readily performed [35]. Approximately 87 percent of chromosomes of patients with LCHAD deficiency have been found to carry the G1528C mutation [8,9,12,35]. This mutation has frequently been found in infants of mothers with acute fatty liver of pregnancy [37,38]. Expression studies indicated that the mutation induces loss of LCHAD activity [9]. Other mutations have been detected, usually in compound with G1528C. These include C1132T, which changes glutamine 342 to stop [38]. The mutation has also been designated at amino acid 474 (E474Q) [38]. Homozygosity for G1528C has been reported to lead to severe disease and death in early infancy [16,33]. An infant with neonatal hypoglycemia and death in infancy had two different splice site mutations following exon 3 [39]. An infant whose mother had acute fatty liver of pregnancy was a compound of C1678T, which converted arginine 524 to stop and TFP deficiency with the common LCHAD mutation [40]. The gene for the β subunit has been localized also to chromosome 2p23 [41]. Patients with other than the G1528C mutations are among those with complete MTP deficiency and cardiomyopathy or neuropathy. A knock out mouse lacking the α and β subunits of MTP has neonatal hypoglycemia and sudden death [42].

The lactic academia observed so regularly in this disease may result from inhibition by accumulated long chain acyl CoA esters of the pyruvate dehydrogenase complex [43], mitochondrial carriers, changing NADH/NAD ratios, or oxidative phosphorylation.

TREATMENT

The avoidance of fasting is important in the management of all patients with disorders of fatty acid oxidation, including LCHAD deficiency. The use of uncooked starch is an important adjunct to therapy. The addition of medium chain triglyceride (MCT) to the regimen has been reported to be therapeutic [1,13,14,21]. Dosage has been 1.5 g/kg. Treatment with MCT was followed by improvement almost to normal in dicarboxylic aciduria, as well as a return to normal of the plasma level of long chain acyl carnitines [14]. Carnitine therapy restored to normal the level of free-carnitine in plasma, but increased the concentrations of long chain acyl carnitines. Although many patients have improved, not all have. Peripheral neuropathy and retinopathy do not appear to benefit from MCT and dietary treatment.

Carnitine has been employed in doses approximating 50–100 mg/kg/day. Its use has become debatable because of concern that long chain acyl carnitine esters may be toxic, and some reports have suggested that carnitine-treated patients have done worse [13,19,44]. However, in the largest study, approximately half the patients were treated with carnitine, and no ill effect could be demonstrated [12]. In our view the use of carnitine in this disease makes sense. Riboflavin has been given in doses of 75 to 100 mg a day.

Dietary restriction of long chain fats in this disorder appears prudent, but it has been followed with highly variable stringency. The development of retinal degeneration has led to the hypothesis that this might be due to a shortage of essential fatty acids such as linoleic and linolenic acids, sources of docosahexanoic acid (DHA), which is important in neural and retinal development. Monkeys deficient in DHA have had retinal degeneration [45]; and there has been evidence of retinal dysfunction in premature infants that has been related to DHA [46]. DHA levels have been found to be low in patients with LCHAD deficiency [47]. For these reasons, DHA supplementation has been initiated in patients with LCHAD deficiency [25] and this approach has increased levels of DHA in the blood. In four patients studied there was electrophysiological evidence of visual improvement. An 11-year-old boy with LCHAD peripheral neuropathy had improved nerve conduction data after 12 months of treatment with cod liver oil, which is high in DHA [48].

Treatment with creatine has been reported to be followed by decrease in muscle pains and improved levels of CK [49].

References

1   Glasgow AM, Engel AG, Bier DM, *et al.* Hypoglycemia hepatic dysfunction muscle weakness cardiomyopathy free carnitine deficiency and long-chain acylcarnitine excess responsive to medium chain triglyceride diet. *Pediatr Res* 1983;**17**:319.

2   Hale DE, Thorpe C, Braat K, *et al.* The L-3-hydroxyacyl CoA dehydrogenase deficiency: in *Fatty Acid Oxidation: Clinical Biochemical and Molecular Aspects* (eds Tanaka K, Coates PM). Alan R Liss, New York;1990:503.

3   Carpenter K, Pollitt RJ, Middleton B. Human liver long-chain 3-hydroxyacyl-coenzyme A dehydrogenase is a multifunctional membrane-bound beta-oxidation enzyme of mitochondria. *Biochem Biophys Res Commun* 1992;**183**:433.

4   Uchida Y, Izai K, Orii T, Hashimoto T. Novel fatty acid β-oxidation enzymes in rat liver mitochondria. II Purification and properties of enoyl-coenzyme A (CoA) hydratase/3-hydroxyacyl CoA dehydrogenase/3-ketoacyl-CoA thiolase trifunctional protein. *J Biol Chem* 1992;**267**:1034.

5   El-Fakhri M, Middleton B. The existence of two different L-3-hydroxyacyl-coenzyme A dehydrogenases in rat tissues. *Biochem Soc Trans* 1979;**7**:392.

6   Kamijo T, Aoyama T, Komiyama A, Hashimoto T. Structural analysis of cDNAs for subunits of human mitochondrial fatty acid beta-oxidation trifunctional protein. *Biochem Biophys Res Commun* 1994;**199**:818.

7   Wanders RJA, Ijlst L, Ushikubo S, *et al.* Molecular basis of long-chain 3-hydroxyacyl-CoA dehydrogenase deficiency: identification of the major disease-causing mutation. *Abstracts 27th Meeting of the European Metabolic Group* 1994;**27**:173.

8   Ijlst L, Wanders RJA, Ushikubo S, *et al.* Molecular basis of long-chain 3-hydroxyacyl-CoA deficiency: identification of the major disease-causing mutation in the alpha-subunit of the mitochondrial trifunctional protein. *Biochim Biophys Acta* 1994;**1215**:347.

9   Ijlst L, Ruiter JPN, Hoovers JMN, *et al.* Common missense mutation G1528C in long-chain 3-hydroxyacyl-CoA dehydrogenase deficiency: characterization and expression of the mutant protein mutation analysis on genomic DNA and chromosomal localization of the mitochondrial trifunctional protein alpha subunit gene. *J Clin Invest* 1996;**98**:1028.

10   Poll-The BT, Bonnefont JP, Ogre H, *et al.* Familial hypoketotic hypoglycemia associated with peripheral neuropathy pigmentary retinopathy and C_6-C_{14} hydroxycarboxylic aciduria. A new defect in fatty acid oxidation? *J Inherit Metab Dis* 1988;**11**:183.

11   Wanders RJA, Ijlst L, Duran M, *et al.* Long chain 3-hydroxyacyl-CoA dehydrogenase deficiency: different clinical expression in three unrelated patients. *J Inherit Metab Dis* 1991;**14**:325.

12   den Boer MEJ, Wanders RJA, Morris AAM, *et al.* Long-chain 3-hydroxyacyl-CoA dehydrogenase deficiency: clinical presentation and follow-up of 50 patients. *Pediatrics* 2002;**109**:99.

13   Jackson S, Bartlett K, Land J, *et al.* Long-chain 3-hydroxy-acyl-CoA dehydrogenase deficiency. *Pediatric Res* 1991;**19**:77.

14   Duran M, Wanders RJA, de Jaguar JP, *et al.* 3-Hydroxydicarboxylic aciduria due to long chain 3-hydroxyacyl coenzyme A dehydrogenase deficiency associated with sudden neonatal death: protective effect of medium-chain triglyceride treatment. *Eur J Pediatr* 1991;**150**:190.

15   Wanders JFA, Duran M, Ijlst L. Sudden infant death and long chain 3-hydroxyacyl CoA dehydrogenase. *Lancet* 1989;**2**:52.

16   Hintz SR, Enns GM, Schelley S, Hoyme HE. Catastrophic presentation of long-chain 3-hydroxyacyl coenzyme A dehydrogenase (LCHAD) deficiency in early infancy. *Clin Res* 2001;**49**:53A.

17   Mardsen D, Nyhan WL, Barshop BA. Creatine kinase and uric acid: early warning for metabolic imbalance resulting from disorders of fatty acid oxidation. *Eur J Pediatr* 2001;**160**:599.

18   Dionisi-Vici C, Burlina AB, Bertini E, *et al.* Progressive neuropathy and recurrent myoglobinuria in a child with long-chain 3-hydroxy-acyl-coenzyme A dehydrogenase deficiency. *J Pediatr* 1991;**118**:744.

19   Rocchiccioli F, Wanders RJA, Aubourg P, *et al.* Deficiency of long chain 3-hydroxyacyl CoA dehydrogenase: a cause of lethal myopathy and cardiomyopathy in early childhood. *Pediatr Res* 1990;**28**:657.

20   Pohorecka M, Zuk M, Gradowska W, *et al.* Cardiac abnormalities in 3-hydroxyacyl-CoA dehydrogenase (LCHAD) deficiency – report of 11 cases. *J Inherit Metab Dis* 2001;**24**:70.

21   Losty HC, Shortland G, Olpin S, Pollitt RJ. Long chain hydroxy acyl CoA dehydrogenase deficiency – two further cases with obstetric complications. *Proc SSIEM* 1995;**34**:106.

22   Tyni T, Kivela T, Lappi M, *et al.* Ophthalmologic findings in long-chain 3-hyroxyacyl-CoA dehydrogenase deficiency caused by the G1528C mutation: a new type of hereditary metabolic choriorentinopathy. *Ophthalmology* 1998;**105**:810.

23   Jackson S, Kler RS, Bartlett K, *et al.* Combined defect of long-chain 3-hydroxyacyl-CoA dehydrogenase 2-enoyl-CoA hydratase and 3-oxoacyl CoA thiolase: in *New Developments in Fatty Acid Oxidation* (eds K Tanaka, P Coates). Wiley-Liss Inc, New York;1992:327.

24   Bertini E, Dionisi-Vici C, Garavaglia B, *et al.* Peripheral sensory-motor polyneuropathy pigmentary retinopathy and fatal cardiomyopathy in long-chain 3-hydroxy-acyl-CoA dehydrogenase deficiency. *Eur J Pediatr* 1992;**151**:121.

25   Harding CO, Gillingham MB, van Calcar SC, *et al.* Docosahexaenoic acid and retinal function in children with long-chain 3-hydroxyacyl-CoA dehydrogenase deficiency. *J Inherit Metab Dis* 1999;**22**:276.

26   Schaefer J, Jackson S, Dick D, Turnbull DM. Trifunctional enzyme deficiency: adult presentation of a usually fatal β-oxidation defect. *Proc SSIEM* 1996;**34**:103.

27   De Meirleir L, Vianey-Saban C, Hasaerts D, *et al.* Neonatal lactic acidosis and LCHAD deficiency. *Proc SSIEM* 1995;**34**:126.

28   Kelley RJ, Morton DH. 3-Hydroxyoctanoic aciduria: identification of a new organic acid in the urine of a patient with non-ketotic hypoglycemia. *Clin Chim Acta* 1988;**175**:19.

29   Politt RJ, Losty H, Westwood A. 3-Hydroxydicarboxylic aciduria: a distinctive type of intermittent dicarboxylic aciduria of possible diagnostic significance. *J Inherit Metab Dis* 1987;**10**:226.

30   Greter J, Lindstedt S, Seeman H, Steen G. 3-Hydroxydecanedioic acid and related homologues. Urinary metabolites in ketoacidosis. *Clin Chem* 1980;**26**:261.

31   Millington DS, Terada N, Chace DH, *et al.* The role of tandem mass spectrometry in the diagnosis of fatty acid oxidation disorders: in *New Developments in Fatty Acid Oxidation* (eds PM Coates, K Tanaka). Wiley-Liss, New York;1992:339.

32   den Boer MEJ, Akkurt EK, Wijburg FA, *et al.* Rapid diagnostic approach in LCHAD deficiency. *J Inherit Metab Dis* 1996;**19**:(suppl 1) 110.

33   Tserng K-Y, Jin S-J, Kerr DS, Hoppel CL. Urinary 3-hydroxydicarboxylic acids in pathophysiology of metabolic disorders with dicarboxylic aciduria. *Metabolism* 1991;**40**:676.

34   Przyrembel H, Jakobs C, Ijlst L, *et al.* Long-chain 3-hydroxyacyl-CoA dehydrogenase deficiency. *J Inherit Metab Dis* 1991;**14**:674.

35   Ijlst L, Ruiter JPN, Oostveen W, Wanders RJA. Long-chain 3-hydroxy-acyl-CoA dehydrogenase deficiency: new mutations and the development of a simple PCR-RFLP method to detect the G1528C mutation in blood spots. *J Inherit Metab Dis* 1996;**19**:(suppl 1) 109.

36   Jones PM, Moffitt M, Joseph D, *et al.* Accumulation of free 3-hydroxy fatty acids in the culture media of fibroblasts from patients deficient in long-chain L-3-hydroxyacyl-CoA dehydrogenase: a useful diagnostic aid. *Clin Chem* 2001;**47**:1190.

37   Ibdah JA, Bennett MJ, Zhao Y, *et al.* Effects of fetal genotype on pregnancy outcome and validity of molecular prenatal diagnosis in families with mutations in mitochondrial trifunctional protein. *Am J Human Genet* 1999;**65**:A45.

38   Sims HF, Brackett JC, Powell CK, *et al.* The molecular basis of pediatric long chain 3-hydroxyacyl-CoA dehydrogenase deficiency associated with maternal acute fatty liver of pregnancy. *Proc Nat Acad Sci USA* 1995;**92**:841.

39   Brackett JC, Sims HF, Rinaldo P, *et al.* Two alpha subunit donor splice site mutations cause human trifunctional protein deficiency. *J Clin Invest* 1995;**95**:2076.

40   Isaacs JD, Sims HF, Powell CK, *et al.* Maternal acute fatty liver of pregnancy associated with fetal trifunctional protein deficiency: molecular characterization of a novel maternal mutant allele. *Pediat Res* 1996;**40**:393.

41   Yang BZ, Heng HH, Ding JH, Roe CR. The genes for the α and β subunits of the mitochondrial trifunctional protein are both located in the same region of human chromosome 2p23. *Genomics* 1996;**37**:141.

42   Ibdah JA, Paul H, Zhao Y, *et al.* Lack of mitochondrial trifunctional protein in mice causes neonatal hypoglycemia and sudden death. *J Clin Invest* 2001;**107**:1403.

43   Moore KH, Dandurand DM, Kiechle FL. Fasting-induced alterations in mitochondrial palmitoyl-CoA metabolism may inhibit adipocyte pyruvate dehydrogenase activity. *Int J Biochem* 1992;**24**:809.

44   Tyni T, Palotie A, Viinikka L, *et al.* Long-chain 3-hydroxyacyl coenzyme A dehydrogenase deficiency with the G1528C mutation: clinical presentation of 13 patients. *J Pediatr* 1997;**130**:67.

45   Neuringer M, Connor WE, Lin DS, *et al.* Biochemical and functional effects of prenatal and postnatal omega-3 fatty acid deficiency on retina and brain in rhesus monkeys. *Proc Natl Acad Sci* 1986;**83**:4021.

46   Uauy R, Hoffman DR, Birch EE, *et al.* Safety and efficacy of omega-3-fatty acids in nutrition of premature infants – soy oil and marine oil supplementation. *J Pediatr* 1994;**124**:612.

47   Gillingham M, Van Calcar S, Ney D, *et al.* Dietary management of long-chain 3-hydroxyacyl-CoA dehydrogenase deficiency (LCHADD). A case report and survey. *J Inherit Metab Dis* 1999;**22**:23.

48   Tein I, Vajsar J, MacMillan L, Sherwood WG. Long-chain L-3-hydroxyacyl-coenzyme A dehydrogenase deficiency neuropathy: response cod liver oil. *Neurology* 1999;**52**:640.

49   Shortland GJ, Schmidt M, Losty H, Leonard JV. LCHAD deficiency treated with creatine. *J Inherit Metab Dis* 2001;**24**:(suppl 1) 71.

43

Short-chain acyl CoA dehydrogenase (SCAD) deficiency

MAJOR PHENOTYPIC EXPRESSION

Developmental delay, seizures, failure to thrive, hypotonia or muscle weakness, neonatal metabolic acidosis, ethylmalonic aciduria, elevated C_4 carnitine and deficiency in short-chain acyl CoA dehydrogenase.

INTRODUCTION

Short-chain acyl CoA dehydrogenase (SCAD) deficiency is a rare disorder of fatty acid oxidation. Clinical manifestations have been varied, but most patients have presented in the neonatal period with failure to thrive, hypotonia and/or metabolic acidosis [1–4]. Most have had delayed development. On the other hand, one of the earliest reported patients was an adult with a myopathic presentation [5,6]. The hallmark urinary metabolite is ethylmalonic acid, but it is not found with consistency in the urine, and it is found in other conditions (Chapters 45 and 109).

The enzyme is a component of the mitochondrial matrix and catalyzes the β-oxidation of fatty acyl CoA compounds of chain length 4 to 6 carbons (Figure 43.1) [7,8]. The gene for SCAD has been cloned and sequenced [9]. It has been localized to chromosome 12q22-ter [10]. A number of mutations have been defined [11,12].

Among mutations found in patients with enzymatic SCAD deficiency were a C to T 136, which changed arginine 46 to tryptophan and C to T 319, which changed arginine 107 to cysteine found in compound heterozygosity [11]. At least three other pathogenic mutations were found in patients, while two variations, G625A and C511T, were found to be present in 14 percent of the general population but to be over represented (69 percent) in patients with ethylmalonic

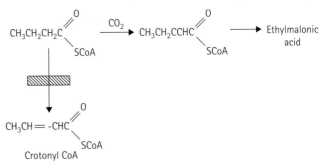

Figure 43.1 *The SCAD reaction with butyryl CoA as substrate. The conversion to ethylmalonyl CoA is catalyzed by propionyl CoA carboxylase.*

aciduria [12,13]. While enzymatic deficiency of SCAD is rare, ethylmalonic aciduria is relatively common in patients suspected of having metabolic disease. The G625A replaces a glycine at 109 with a serine. Expression of this variant in *E. coli* yielded normal SCAD enzyme activity, Km and Vmax. However, enzyme activity in the absence of a chaperonin displayed some decrease and heat stability was impaired [14]. These observations led to the hypothesis that some mutations, notably G625A and C511T represented susceptibility alleles. Individuals carrying these mutations might have asymptomatic ethylmalonic aciduria, or become ill in the presence of other environmental or genetic factors. In a study of 10 patients with ethylmalonic aciduria and SCAD deficiency in fibroblasts, sequence analysis revealed only one patient with generally accepted pathogenic mutations on both alleles; five were doubly heterozygous for such a mutation and G625A, while four had either G625A or C511T on each allele [12]. These observations imply that these are clinically relevant mutations, and that even mild ethylmalonic aciduria should lead to mutational analysis.

CLINICAL ABNORMALITIES

SCAD deficiency is unlike the classic disorders of fatty acid oxidation in that it does not present with hypoketotic hypoglycemia. Some patients have had neonatal metabolic acidosis [2,4]. In two the acidosis was profound, and in one there was hypoglycemia in the initial neonatal episode. There may be attendant lactic acidemia and hyperammonemia. The episode may be ushered in with vomiting or lethargy. The disease is potentially lethal; three of six patients died in infancy [4], one as early as 6 days of life [2].

Neuromuscular manifestations have been observed even in infancy (Figure 43.2). Most patients have been hypotonic, but hypertonicity has been observed, even in a patient also found to be hypotonic. Neonates may have compromised respiratory effort, and this may be fatal. An adult woman who developed weakness intensified by exertion had clinical and electromyographic evidence of proximal myopathy at 46 years of age [5,6]. The level of creatine phosphokinase was normal. Biopsied muscle revealed accumulation of neutral lipid in type 1 fibers. Concentrations of free-carnitine in muscle were low and those of plasma low-normal. The proportion of esterified carnitine was increased. It has been suggested [4] that this patient may have had a riboflavin-responsive multiple acyl CoA dehydrogenase deficiency because SCAD activity was deficient in muscle, but not in fibroblasts. Other patients have had low levels of free-carnitine in plasma and muscle [1].

Developmental delay has been observed in most patients with SCAD deficiency; one was stated to have delayed speech development [4]. Some have had seizures. Nystagmus has been observed [4]. One was microcephalic [1].

SCAD deficiency has been added to the list of disorders in which an affected fetus may lead to the acute fatty liver of pregnancy or the syndrome of hemolysis, elevated liver enzymes, and low platelet counts (HELLP) [15]. Two patients have been reported with SCAD deficiency and endocrine disease, one with hypopituitarism and septo-optic dysplasia and the other with hypothyroidism [16].

Organic acid analysis of the urine characteristically reveals increased excretion of ethylmalonic acid. The urine may be normal at times of relative health. Ethylmalonic acid is also found in the urine of patients with ethylmalonic aciduria (Chapter 109), in whom SCAD activity is normal, and in patients with multiple acyl CoA dehydrogenase deficiency

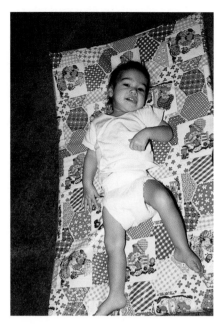

Figure 43.2   *J.G., an infant with SCAD deficiency. She was markedly hypotonic and had skeletal muscle weakness. Concentrations of free-carnitine in blood and muscle were low [1]. (Illustration was kindly provided by Dr. Susan Winter, Fresno, California.)*

(Chapter 45). Adipic acid and methylsuccinic acid may also be found in this condition and in SCAD deficiency, and there may be lactic aciduria. Multiple acyl CoA dehydrogenase deficiency can sometimes be recognized by the presence of metabolites of abnormal amino acid oxidation [17], but these are not always present. The detection of butyrylglycine in the urine may be useful in suggesting the diagnosis [2,18–20] but this may be absent from the urine in SCAD disease [21]. Butyrylcarnitine may also be found in the urine.

SCAD deficiency is now more likely to be detected by analysis of acyl carnitine profiles either in plasma or in the blood spots obtained in neonatal screening programs [21,22]. The key compound is C_4, butyrylcarnitine (Figure 43.3), but C_5 may also be elevated. The ratio of C_4 to C_3 may be particularly useful; levels as high as 9.0 μmol/L have been found, almost 10 times the control reference 95th percentile level [23].

It is important to distinguish butyrylcarnitine from isobutyrylcarnitine, which may be found in normal individuals [24], ethylmalonic aciduria [25] and in patients with a defect in branched-chain acyl CoA oxidation, isobutyryl CoA dehydrogenase deficiency [26]. These distinctions may be made by organic acid analysis, enzyme assay, mutational analysis or study of the function of labeled acylcarnitines *in vitro*.

GENETICS AND PATHOGENESIS

The disorder is transmitted in an autosomal recessive fashion. The defective enzyme, SCAD (Figure 43.1), is a homotetramer containing flavin adenine dinucleotide (FAD) moiety which is attached to the enzyme after transport into mitochondria.

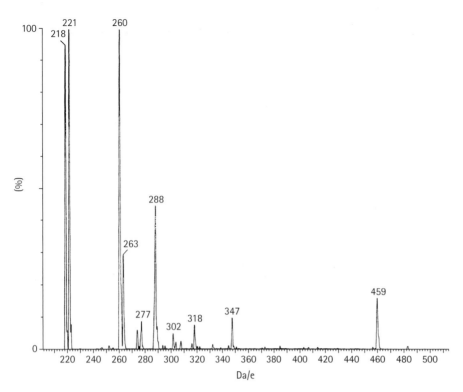

Figure 43.3 *Acylcarnitine tandem MS profile of a 3-year-old patient with SCAD deficiency. He presented with myopathy and hepatomegaly. He had episodes of hypoglycemia and lactic acidosis. He died of cardiomyopathy. The key compounds are: 288 C 4-carnitine and 302 C5-carnitine.*

The gene on chromosome 12 encodes a 412 amino acid precursor protein containing a leader peptide and a 388 amino acid mature enzyme with a molecular weight of 41 kDa.

Enzyme activity is measured with butyryl CoA as substrate. Activity found in fibroblasts of patients has approximated 50 percent of control [1,2,4], but the residual activity in most has been due to medium chain acylCoA dehydrogenase (MCAD), because when extracts were incubated with anti-MCAD antibody this activity disappeared. SCAD activity in muscle was about 25 percent of control in the adult with myopathy [6]. Immunoreactive SCAD protein was reduced in muscle in this patient and normal in fibroblasts [27]. Incubation of fibroblasts with ^{14}C-labeled butyrate and measurement of the incorporation into cellular protein has served as a screening test for this disorder [4].

There is an animal model for this disease. Defective activity and antigen of SCAD in both fibroblasts and muscle has been found in BALB/cByJ mice [28]. Affected mice have ethylmalonic and methylsuccinic aciduria, hepatic deposition of lipid and fasting hypoglycemia.

Immunochemical analysis has revealed evidence of an unstable protein of normal size [29], while in other patients the protein was stable [11]. Fibroblasts of parents have had intermediate levels of SCAD activity [1].

The G645A variant of the SCAD gene was found [19,20], in homozygous form in seven percent of the general population, and in heterozygous form in 34.8 percent [13,30,31]. At the same time, it was over-expressed in 60 percent of patients with ethylmalonic aciduria who were homozygous, and a further 30 percent who were heterozygous. It is currently recommended [12] that this and other mutations be sought in any patient

with an ethylmalonic excretion over 18 mmol per mole creatinine. Other mutations discovered include: C1147T, which converts arginine at 383 to cysteine; T529C, which converts tryptophan 177 to arginine; and G274T, which converts glycine 92 to cysteine [32].

TREATMENT

Patients have been treated with carnitine and restriction of dietary fat. Muscular symptomatology has been treated with corticosteroids. The efficacy of treatment is not clear. However treatment with carnitine would appear to be prudent. Fasting should be avoided.

References

1 Coates PM, Hale DE, Finocchiaro G, *et al*. Genetic deficiency of short chain acyl CoA dehydrogenase in fibroblasts from a patient with muscle carnitine deficiency and severe skeletal weakness. *J Clin Invest* 1988;**81**:171.

2 Amend BA, Greene C, Sweetman L, *et al*. Short chain acyl CoA dehydrogenase deficiency. *J Clin Invest* 1987;**79**:1303.

3 Sewell AC, Herwig J, Böhles H, *et al*. A new case of short-chain acyl-CoA dehydrogenase deficiency with isolated ethylmalonic aciduria. *Eur J Pediatr* 1993;**152**:922.

4 Bhala A, Willi SM, Rinaldo P, *et al*. Clinical and biochemical characterization of short-chain acyl-coenzyme A dehydrogenase deficiency. *J Pediatr* 1995;**126**:910.

5 Turnbull DM, Bartlett K, Stevens DL, *et al*. Short chain acyl-CoA dehydrogenase deficiency associated with a lipid-storage myopathy and secondary carnitine deficiency. *N Engl J Med* 1984;**311**:1232.

6 Turnbull DM, Shepard IM, Bartlett K, Sherratt HSA. Short chain-acyl CoA dehydrogenase deficiency: in *Fatty Acid Oxidation: Clinical Biochemical and Molecular Aspects* (eds K Tanaka, PM Coates) Alan R Liss Inc, New York;1990:321.

7 Davidson B, Schulz H. Separation properties and regulation of acyl coenzyme A dehydrogenases from bovine heart and liver. *Arch Biochem Biophys* 1982;**213**:155.

8 Shaw L, Engel PC. The purification and properties of ox liver short-chain acyl-CoA dehydrogenase. *Biochem J* 1984;**218**:511.

9 Naito E, Ozasa H, Ikeda Y, Tanaka K. Molecular cloning and nucleotide sequence of complementary DNAs encoding human short chain acyl-coenzyme A dehydrogenase and the study of the molecular basis of short chain acyl-coenzyme A dehydrogenase deficiency. *J Clin Invest* 1989;**83**:1605.

10 Barton DE, Yang-Feng TL, Finnocchiaro G, *et al.* Short chain acyl-CoA dehydrogenase (ACADS) maps to chromosome 12 (q22-qter) and electron transfer flavoprotein (ETFA) to 15 (q23-q25). *Cytogenet Cell Genet* 1987;**46**:577.

11 Naito E, Indo Y, Tanaka K. Identification of two variant short chain acyl-coenzyme A dehydrogenase alleles each containing a different point mutation in a patient with short chain acyl-coenzyme A dehydrogenase deficiency. *J Clin Invest* 1990;**85**:1575.

12 Corydon MJ, Vockley J, Rinaldo P, *et al.* Role of common gene variations in the molecular pathogenesis of short-chain acyl-CoA dehydrogenase deficiency. *Pediatr Res* 2001;**49**:18.

13 Gregersen N, Winter VS, Corydon MJ, *et al.* Identification of four new mutations in the short-chain acyl-CoA dehydrogenase (SCAD) gene in two patients: one of the variant alleles 511C → T is present at an unexpectedly high frequency in the general population as was the case for 625G → A together conferring susceptibility to ethylmalonic aciduria. *Hum Mol Genet* 1998;**7**:619.

14 Corydon MJ, Gregersen N, Lehnert W, *et al.* Ethylmalonic aciduria is associated with an amino acid variant of short-chain acyl-coenzyme A dehydrogenase. *Pediatr Res* 1996;**39**:1059.

15 Matern D, Hart P, Murtha AP, *et al.* Acute fatty liver of pregnancy associated with short-chain acyl-coenzyme A dehydrogenase deficiency. *J Pediatr* 2001;**138**:585.

16 Matern D, Kishnani P, Chen YT, *et al.* Hormonal imbalances in ethylmalonic aciduria. *J Inherit Metab Dis* 1999;**22**:94.

17 Gregersen N. The acyl-CoA dehydrogenation deficiencies. *Scand J Clin Lab Invest* 1985;**174**:1.

18 Costa CG, Guerand WS, Struys EA, *et al.* Quantitative analysis of urinary acylglycines for the diagnosis of betaoxidation defects using GC-NCI-MS. *J Pharm Biomed Anal* 2000;**21**:1215.

19 Kimura M, Yamaguchi S. Screening for fatty acid beta oxidation disorders. Acylglycine analysis by electron impact ionization gas chromatography-mass spectrometry. *J Chromatogr B Biomed Sci Appl* 1999;**731**:105.

20 Bonafe L, Troxler H, Kuster T, *et al.* Evaluation of urinary acylglycines by electrospray tandem mass spectrometry in mitochondrial energy metabolism defects and organic acidurias. *Mol Genet Metab* 2000;**69**:302.

21 Sim KG, Hammond J, Wilcken B. Strategies for the diagnosis of mitochondrial fatty acid β-oxidation disorders. *Clin Chim Acta* 2002;**323**:37.

22 Naylor EW, Chace DH. Automated tandem mass spectrometry for mass newborn screening for disorders in fatty acid organic acid and amino acid metabolism. *J Child Neurol* 1999;**14**:S4.

23 Vreken P, van Lint AEM, Bootsma AH, *et al.* Rapid diagnosis of organic acidemias and fatty acid oxidation defects by quantitative electrospray tandem-MS acyl-carnitine analysis in plasma: in *Current Views of Fatty Acid Oxidation and Ketogenesis: From Organelles to Point Mutations* (eds PA Quant, S Eaton; Kluwer Academic) Plenum Publishers, New York;1999:327.

24 Schmidt-Sommerfeld E, Penn D, Kerner J, Bieber LL. Analysis of acylcarnitines in normal human urine with the radioisotope exchange-high performance liquid chromatography (HPLC). *Clin Chim Acta* 1989;**181**:231.

25 Burlina AB, Dionisi-Vici C, Bennett MJ, *et al.* A new syndrome with ethylmalonic aciduria and normal fatty acid oxidation in fibroblasts. *J Pediatr* 1994;**124**:79.

26 Roe CR, Cederbaum SD, Roe DS, *et al.* Isolated isobutyryl-CoA dehydrogenase deficiency: An unrecognized defect in human valine metabolism. *Mol Genet Metab* 1998;**65**:264.

27 Farnsworth L, Shepperd IM, Johnson MA, *et al.* Absence of immunoreactive enzyme protein in short-chain acyl coenzyme A dehydrogenase deficiency. *Ann Neurol* 1990;**28**:717.

28 Amendt BA, Freneaux E, Reece C, *et al.* Short-chain acyl-coenzyme A activity antigen and biosynthesis are absent in the BALB/cByJ mouse. *Pediatr Res* 1992;**31**:552.

29 Naito E, Indo Y, Tanaka K. Short chain-acyl-coenzyme A dehydrogenase (SCAD) deficiency: immunochemical demonstration of molecular heterogeneity due to variant SCAD with differing stability. *J Clin Invest* 1989;**84**:1671.

30 Corydon MJ, Bross P, Brage Storstein A, *et al.* Structural organization of the human short-chain acyl Co A dehydrogenase gene. *J Inherit Metab Dis* 1996;**19**:114.

31 Zschocke J, Gregersen N, Lehnert W, *et al.* SCAD gene polymorphism G625A in children with neuromuscular or hepatic symptoms and ethylmalonic aciduria. *J Inherit Metab Dis* 1996;**19**:116.

32 Gregersen N, Winter VS, Corydon MJ, *et al.* Characterization of four new mutations in the short-chain acyl CoA dehydrogenase (SCAD) gene in two patients with SCAD deficiency. *J Inherit Metab Dis* 1996;**19**:115.

44

Short-chain 3-hydroxyacyl CoA dehydrogenase (SCHAD) deficiency

MAJOR PHENOTYPIC EXPRESSION

Hypoketotic hypoglycemia, recurrent myoglobinuria, encephalopathy and cardiomyopathy; or hyperketotic hypoglycemia, failure to thrive and hypotonia; elevated creatine kinase; dicarboxylic aciduria; and defective activity of SCHAD in muscle fibroblasts and leukocytes.

INTRODUCTION

Deficiency of SCHAD (EC 1.1.1.35) was first described by Tein and colleagues [1] in a 16-year-old girl with recurrent myoglobinuria and hypoketotic hypoglycemia in whom SCHAD activity was markedly diminished in muscle, but normal in fibroblasts. In contrast, we and others have seen patients in whom SCHAD activity was very low in cultured fibroblasts and freshly isolated leukocytes [2]. These patients have had what appeared to be ketotic hypoglycemia.

The enzyme, 3-hydroxyacyl CoA dehydrogenase, is a homodimer with 302 amino acids in each subunit [3–5] with activity against 3-hydroxyacyl CoA esters of C4 to C16 length, but with less activity as the chain length increases (Figure 44.1). The cDNA for the gene has been cloned and sequenced [6,7]

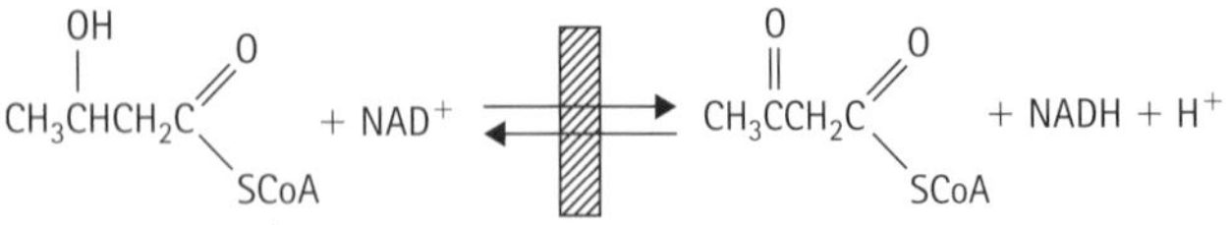

Figure 44.1 *The SCHAD reaction. Substrates 3-hydroxybutyryl CoA and the ketoacid product. The enzyme catalyzes conversion of C_4 to C_{16} esters, but activity is less as chain length increases.*

and mapped to chromosome 4q22-26 [7]. The enzyme is synthesized with a leader peptide, which is removed after import into the mitochondria. Mutations have been identified [8], but a search for mutation in patients with deficient enzyme activity is often negative, indicating a mutation in the assembly or transport of the protein resulting in decreased enzyme activity.

CLINICAL ABNORMALITIES

The initial patient [1] with deficiency of SCHAD had episodic myoglobinuria and hypoketotic hypoglycemia, as expected for a disorder of fatty acid oxidation. There was also evidence of encephalopathy and hypertrophic dilated cardiomyopathy.

Our patient [2] had a neonatal presentation of difficulty with feeding, failure to thrive and hypotonia. An elevated creatine phosphokinase (CPK) of 2000 U/L led to a muscle biopsy, which appeared normal. The CK was recorded as high as 5721 U/L. In response to fasting she developed hypoglycemia of 38 mg/dL at 23 hours, but the concentration of 3-hydroxybutyrate in the blood was 2120 μmol/L, which was a brisk ketogenic response.

Sudden infant death has also been reported [9]. This infant had brick red urine, indicative of myoglobinuria. Autopsy revealed a fatty liver. Fulminant hepatic failure has also been observed, treated by liver transplantation.

Other patients have presented with a picture of hyperketotic hypoglycaemia [10]. There may be vomiting, dehydration or lethargy; or onset may be with seizures. One patient had hyponatremia [10]. The liver may be enlarged. Another presentation may be with hyperinsulinemic hypoglycemia [8]. In one Pakistani family in which parents were doubly heterozygous documented, hyperinsulinism required treatment with diazoxide. Of four affected children two died. One was mentally retarded, and one had developed normally. An infant in another family had hyperinsulinism that was readily controlled with diazoxide and hydrochlorthiazide [11].

Laboratory evaluation has revealed hypoketosis in some patients [1,10]. Analysis of the free fatty acids of the plasma or organic acid analysis of the urine may reveal medium chain 3-hydroxy fatty acids, even when the patient is metabolically well [12,13]. However this pattern may also be seen in infants receiving medium chain triglycerides.

The concentration of free-carnitine in the plasma may be normal or low, and there may be increased quantities of carnitine esters in the urine. Medium chain dicarboxylic aciduria is characteristic, but the levels are not high and at times they may be normal. Adipic, suberic and sebacic acids are found as well as 3-hydroxydicarboxylic acids. In our patient, challenge with a load of medium-chain triglyceride led to increased excretion of dicarboxylic acids and 3-hydroxydicarboxylic acids. She always excreted elevated amounts of trans-cinnamoyl glycine.

The acylcarnitine profile reveals C_4-OH carnitine which could indicate the 3-hydroxybutyrylcarnitine of SCHAD disease, but this would not be different in the presence of 3-hydroxyisobutyryl CoA deacylase deficiency or D-3-hydroxybutyrylcarnitine in a ketone body utilization defect. In one patient [9] elevated C16 and C18 acylcarnitines were found, and no hydroxy acylcarnitines.

GENETICS AND PATHOGENESIS

The disorder is transmitted in an autosomal recessive fashion. Consanguinity has been observed, and heterozygosity has been demonstrated by enzyme assay of the liver [9]; and by mutational analysis [8].

The enzyme SCHAD is a soluble mitochondrial matrix enzyme with two identical subunits [5]. The gene encodes a 34 kDa precursor protein that, with processing, yields a mature 31 kDa subunit. Its substrate specificity is considerably broader than the name would suggest. It is most highly active against hydroxybutyryl CoA, but it is active up to C16. Deficiency of enzyme activity has been demonstrated in muscle [1], liver [9] and fibroblasts [12], as well as in mitochondria isolated from fibroblasts [11]. In some families the defective enzyme was not demonstrable in fibroblasts, but was found in muscle [1] or liver [9].

The rat and human cDNAs have been sequenced [6,7]. The human gene encodes a protein of 314 amino acids and is expressed in liver, kidney, heart and muscle. An absence of expression in fibroblasts has relevance to one of the reports [10]. The gene contains 8 exons. Compound heterozygosity for 2 mutations has been observed.

TREATMENT

Treatment with carnitine and a diet low in fat appears to be prudent. The avoidance of fasting is important, and supplemental cornstarch may be useful.

References

1   Tein I, De Vivo DC, Hale DE, *et al.* Short-chain l-3-hydroxyacyl-CoA dehydrogenase deficiency in muscle: a new cause for recurrent myoglobinuria and encephalopathy. *Ann Neurol* 1991;**30**:415.

2   Haas RH, Marsden DL. Disorders of organic acids: in *Principles of Child Neurology* (ed. BO Berg) McGraw-Hill, New York;1996:1049.

3   Uchida Y, Izai K, Orii T, Hashimoto T. Novel fatty acid b-oxidation enzymes in rat liver mitochondria. II Purification and properties of enoyl-coenzyme A (CoA) hydratase/3-hydroxyacyl-CoA dehydrogenase/3-ketoacyl-CoA thiolase trifunctional protein. *J Biol Chem* 1992;**267**:1034.

4   El-Fakhri M, Middleton B. The existence of two different l-3-hydroxyacyl-coenzyme A dehydrogenases in rat tissues. *Biochem Soc Trans* 1979;**7**:392.

5   Noyes BE, Bradshaw RA. l-3-Hydroxyacyl coenzyme A dehydrogenase from pig heart muscle. I Purification and properties. *J Biol Chem* 1973;**248**:3042.

6   Amaya Y, Takiguchi M, Hashimoto T, Mori M. Molecular cloning of cDNA for rat mitochondrial 3-hydroxyacyl-CoA dehydrogenase. *Eur J Biochem* 1986;**156**:9.

7   Vredendaal PJ, van den Berg IE, Malingre HER, *et al.* Human short-chain l-3-hydroxyacyl-CoA dehydrogenase: cloning and characterization of the coding sequence. *Biochem Biophys Res Comm* 1996;**223**:718.

8   Sovik O, Matre G, Rishaug U, *et al.* Familial hyperinsulinemic hypoglycemia with a mutation in the gene encoding short-chain 3-hydroxyacyl-CoA dehydrogenase. *J Inherit Metab Dis* 2002;**25**:63.

9   Treacy EP, Lambert DM, Barnes R, *et al.* Short-chain hydroxyacyl-coenzyme A dehydrogenase deficiency presenting as unexpected infant death: A family history. *J Pediatr* 2000;**137**:257.

10 Bennet MJ, Weinberger MJ, Kobori JA, *et al.* Mitochondrial short-chain L-3-hydroxyacyl-coenzyme A dehydrogenase deficiency: a new defect of fatty acid oxidation. *Pediatr Res* 1996;**39**:185.

11 Clayton PT, Eaton S, Aynsley-Green A, *et al.* Hyperinsulinism in short-chain L-3-hydroxyacyl-CoA dehydrogenase deficiency reveals the importance of beta-oxidation in insulin secretion. *J Clin Invest* 2001;**108**:457.

12 Jones PM, Quinn R, Fennessey PV, *et al.* Improved stable isotope dilution-gas chromatography-mass spectrometry method for serum or plasma free 3-hydroxy-fatty acids in its utility for the study of disorders of mitochondrial fatty acid beta-oxidation. *Clin Chem* 2000;**46**:149.

13 Sim KG, Hammond J, Wilcken B. Strategies for the diagnosis of mitochondrial fatty acid β-oxidation disorders. *Clin Chim Acta* 2002;**323**:37.

45

Multiple acyl CoA dehydrogenase deficiency (MADD)/Glutaric aciduria type II/Ethylmalonic-adipic aciduria

MAJOR PHENOTYPIC EXPRESSION

Overwhelming neonatal illness with metabolic acidosis, acrid odor, hypoketotic hypoglycemia and hyperammonemia; dysmorphic features; polycystic kidneys; massive urinary excretion of lactic and glutaric acids and increased concentrations of many other organic acids including ethylmalonic acid, butyric acid, methylbutyric acid, isobutyric and isovaleric acids and deficiency of electron transfer flavoprotein (ETF) or its dehydrogenase (ETF-QO).

Later onset, milder variants referred to as ethylmalonic-adipic aciduria, may first present in the neonatal period or adulthood with episodic illness characterized by vomiting, hypoglycemia and lipid storage myopathy.

INTRODUCTION

Glutaric aciduria Type II was first reported in 1976 by Przyrembel *et al.* [1] in an infant with severe hypoglycemia and profound metabolic acidosis without ketosis. Patients with this form of the disorder have overwhelming illness in the neonatal period that has been uniformly fatal. The name was employed to distinguish the disease from the glutaric aciduria due to defective activity of glutaryl CoA dehydrogenase (Chapter 8) that had been reported a year earlier by Goodman and colleagues [2]. Organic acid analysis revealed the accumulation of a wide variety of organic acids, including lactic and ethylmalonic acids, as well as glutaric acid. There is generalized defect in the activity of many acyl CoA dehydrogenases [3]. Thus, the term of multiple acyl CoA dehydrogenase deficiency is more descriptive, it has variously been abbreviated MAD deficiency and MADD; it has also been divided into severe (MAD:S) and mild (MAD:M) forms [4], but there is sufficient heterogeneity of clinical expression that these are not useful.

The fundamental molecular defect is in the mitochondrial transport of electrons from the acyl CoAs to ubiquinone (CoQ10) of the main electron transport chain [5–7]. The defect may be in any of three proteins, the alpha or beta subunits of ETF or its dehydrogenase, ETF-ubiquinone oxidoreductase (ETF-QO). (EC1.5.5.1) Both are flavoproteins. Another designation has been IIA and IIB for defects in the α and β proteins and IIC for ETF-QO defects.

The mitochondrial oxidations of glutaryl CoA and other intermediates in branched-chain amino acid metabolism, and the β-oxidation of fatty acids (Figure 45.1) are catalyzed by mitochondrial flavin adenine dinucleotide (FAD)-dependent enzymes [8–11]. Each of the dehydrogenase enzymes of fatty acid oxidation, and the amino acid catabolic enzymes catalyze the dehydrogenation of saturated acyl CoA compounds to form the 2,3-unsaturated or enoyl CoA thioesters (Figure 45.2). Both sarcosine and dimethylglycine are catabolized by specific N-methyldehydrogenases containing covalently-bound FAD and dissociable folic acid cofactors [12–14], and thus these two

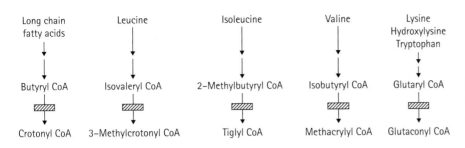

Figure 45.1   *Multiple acyl CoA dehydrogenase deficiency involves the dehydrogenation of many CoA intermediates in fatty acid and amino acid catabolism.*

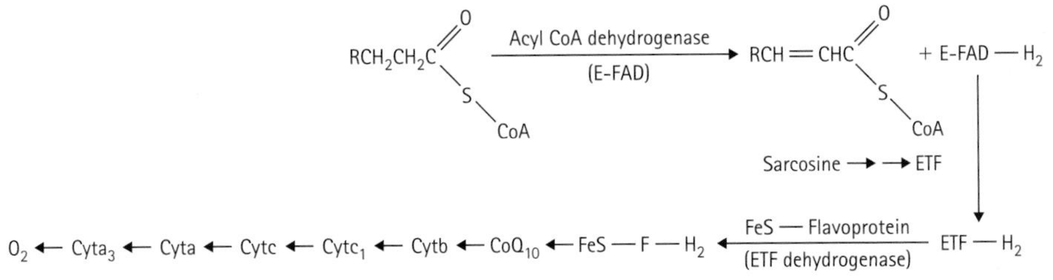

$$RCH_2CH_2C \xrightarrow[\text{(E-FAD)}]{\text{Acyl CoA dehydrogenase}} RCH = CHC + E\text{-}FAD - H_2$$

$$O_2 \leftarrow Cyta_3 \leftarrow Cyta \leftarrow Cytc \leftarrow Cytc_1 \leftarrow Cytb \leftarrow CoQ_{10} \leftarrow FeS - F - H_2 \xrightarrow[\text{(ETF dehydrogenase)}]{FeS - Flavoprotein} ETF - H_2$$

Sarcosine → → ETF

Figure 45.2   *The roles of ETF and ETF-QO oxidation and the passage of electrons along the electron transport chain.*

compounds may also accumulate in this disease. Each dehydrogenase enzyme contains a molecule of FAD. ETF is a 60 Kd heterodimer containing a single noncovalently-bound FAD which accepts hydrogens from all of the acyl CoA dehydrogenases [15–19]. ETF has an α and β subunit. ETF-QO is an iron-sulfur-containing flavoprotein (early referred to as Fe-S flavoprotein) that accepts electrons from reduced ETF and transmits them to coenzyme Q and the cytochrome chain (Figure 45.2) [7, 20–23].

The cDNAs for the α and β subunits of ETF [24,25] and ETF-QO [26] have been cloned and sequenced. α-ETF and ETF-QO have N-terminal mitochondrial import sequences, but the β subunit cDNA does not encode a leader peptide, and so does not undergo such processing. The gene for α-ETF has been localized to chromosome 15 at q23-25 [27], that of β-ETF on chromosome 19 [28] and that for ETF-QO on chromosome 4 [29] at q32-qter. Mutations have been identified in α-ETF [30,31], the most common of which appears to be a change at codon 266 from threonine to methionine. In ETF-QO a number of apparently rare mutations have been identified which lead to an absence of enzyme activity and immunoreactive proteins [32].

CLINICAL ABNORMALITIES

The infant with classic multiple acyl CoA dehydrogenase deficiency presents with life-threatening illness in the first days of life. The clinical picture is reminiscent of those of the typical organic acidemias, propionic acidemia (Chapter 2), methylmalonicacidemia, (Chapter 3) and isovaleric acidemia (Chapter 7), but the severity of illness in this disease is so great that all three of the patients we have studied died after less than 90 hours of life [33,34], and most of those reported have died within the first week [1,35–41].

These infants [1,33] develop tachypnea or dyspnea within a few hours of birth. They are found to have profound metabolic acidosis and impressive hypoglycemia. In spite of intravenous glucose and NaHCO$_3$ the concentration of glucose in the blood may decrease as does the pH, and cardiac arrest soon follows, and despite resuscitation and artificial ventilation, the course is inexorable.

The first patient was described as having a 'very disagreeable sweaty-feet odor' [1]. We described our first patient [33] as having a peculiar, acrid odor. This is the consequence of an excess of a number of short chain, volatile organic acids. A number of these patients has been described as pale [1,33,34] and one had macrocytic anemia and a hemoglobin concentration of 9.1 g/dL. Many have had convulsions consistent with the degree of depression of the blood glucose. Hyperammonemia was a consistent feature in our patients [33,34]. Fatty infiltration of the liver is found postmortem.

A number of the neonatal onset patients has had prominent dysmorphic features [33,34,42] (Figures 45.3–45.8). They include a high forehead, depressed nasal bridge and a short anteverted nose. The ears may be low-set, malrotated and abnormally formed (Figures 45.4, 45.5). Muscular defects of the abdominal wall have occurred, and genital defects such as hypospadias and chordee. Some have had macrocephaly [43]. Minor anomalies include horizontal palmar creases and rocker-bottom feet (Figure 45.6). One of our patients also had an interventricular septal defect and three umbilical vessels. Some patients [33] have been described as premature or small for gestational age.

A major malformation in these infants is the occurrence of polycystic kidneys. The kidneys may be huge and readily palpable. Abnormally small prenatal production of urine may be the cause of the semilunar folds below the eyes, as in the Potter syndrome (Figure 45.3), and typical Potter syndrome, including pulmonary hypoplasia has been observed [36]. Polycystic kidneys may be present in infants without dysmorphic features and may be found first at autopsy [37,38,42]. Ultrastructural changes have been described in the glomerular basement membrane [43]. Other pathologic abnormalities include cerebral gliosis and heterotopias giving a warty dysplastic appearance to the cortex [36]. Hepatic periportal necrosis has been reported

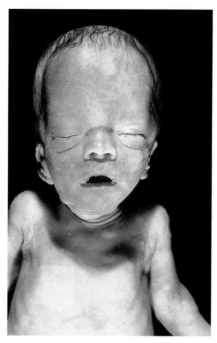

Figure 45.3   *Postmortem pictures of Baby M. [32,33] who died of glutaric aciduria type II on the first day of life. He had a low, incompletely rotated ear with a reduced anthelix, and he had three umbilical vessels. Autopsy revealed large polycystic kidneys and an interventricular septal defect.*

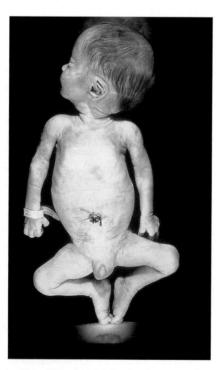

Figure 45.4   *Baby M. had a high forehead, depressed nasal bridge, short nose with anteverted nares and a long philtrum. The ears were low-set and he had semilunar folds below the eyes.*

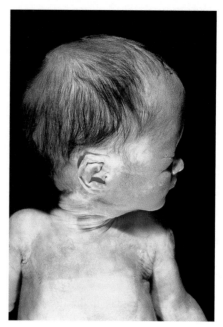

Figure 45.5   *The right ear was also abnormal in position and appearance.*

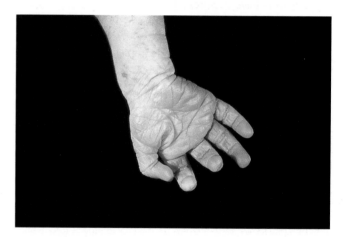

Figure 45.6   *The hand was short and broad and had a single horizontal crease.*

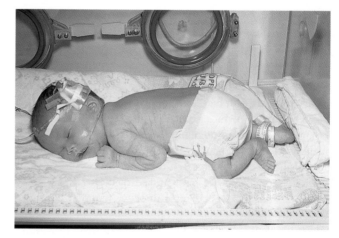

Figure 45.7   *Baby girl N. died of intractable acidosis in the first week. She had enormous polycystic kidneys.*

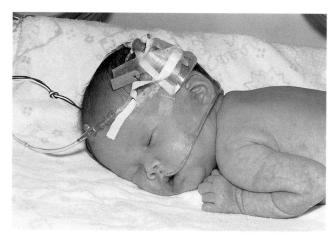

Figure 45.8 *Baby girl N. was not strikingly dysmorphic. She did have anteverted nares and a triangular-shaped mouth. The ears appeared low.*

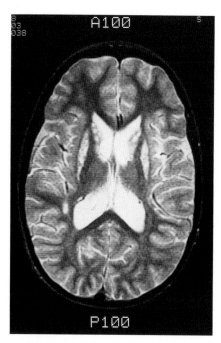

Figure 45.9 *M.H. Neuroimaging (MRI) of the brain reveals an extraordinary pattern of increased T₂ signal in the white matter.*

[43], and more commonly hepatic microvesicular lipid. Pancreatic ducts may be hypoplastic [36].

Infants without dysmorphic features and abnormal organogenesis have also presented early in life with tachypnea, acidosis, hypoglycemia and an abnormal odor. Many have had hepatomegaly. Some of these have survived the initial episode and died a few months later, often with cardiomyopathy. A small number has survived a bit longer and had episodic illness reminiscent of Reye syndrome [44–48].

The later onset multiple acyl CoA dehydrogenase deficiency, or ethylmalonic-adipic aciduria has presented with a considerable variety. The first patient reported [49] had episodic vomiting, hypoglycemia and acidosis from 7 weeks-of-age. Another [50] presented first as a 19-year-old in hypoglycemic coma and continued to have episodes of nausea, vomiting, hypoketotic hypoglycemia and hepatic dysfunction with elevated bilirubin and transaminases, but normal ammonia. Two sisters had died in childhood of the same disease. Others have had such episodes beginning in the first year of life [51–53] but one woman presented at 25 years with a history of episodic muscle weakness and vomiting [54].

The adult patient [50] had muscle weakness and low levels of carnitine in muscle. Two others had lipid storage myopathy and systemic deficiency of carnitine [55–57]. During acute episodes these patients have had hypoketotic hypoglycemia, acidosis and sometimes, especially early in life, hyperammonemia. Transaminase levels in blood may be elevated, and there may be prolongation of prothrombin or partial thromboplastin times. Lactic acidemia may be impressive.

Roentgenograms of the chest may reveal cardiomegaly, and echocardiography may be consistent with cardiomyopathy. Neuroimaging may reveal areas of increased signal on T₂ of the magnetic resonance image (MRI) in the basal ganglia [58] (Figure 45.9) or hypomyelination [59]. A macrocephalic patient was found to have symmetric hypoplasia of the temporal lobes of the brain in the first week of life [59]. He had normal psychomotor development for 11 months when he died of a sudden cardiac arrest. Autopsy showed hypomyelination and systemic hypoplasia of temporal lobes with loss of axons and focal subcortical ganglionic heterotopia, consistent with aberrant intrauterine developmental origin.

The diagnosis has usually been made on the basis of the unusual pattern of organic acid excretion in which a large number of organic acids are found in elevated amount in the urine. This is especially true in the severe neonatal onset form in which the quantities found are enormous. The most prominent of these are lactic acid and glutaric acid, but a large number of other dicarboxylic acids and hydroxy acids are found. Among the former are ethylmalonic, adipic, suberic and sebacic acids, as well as unsaturated suberic acids. Among the latter are 2-hydroxybutyric, 2-hydroxyglutaric and 5-hydroxyhexanoic acids. 3-hydroxyisovaleric and 2-hydroxyisocaproic acids are also found in the urine. Most of the same organic acids are found in increased amounts in the plasma. The concentrations of glutaric and lactic acids are prominent. p-hydroxyphenyllactic acid may be elevated in the blood and the urine, possibly an index of immaturity or of hepatic disease.

Volatile acids are demonstrable in the plasma by analysis with gas liquid chromatography. The concentrations of isovaleric, acetic, isobutyric, 2-methylbutyric, butyric and propionic acids may all be elevated to values 60 to 4800 times normal. In our first patient the concentration of isovaleric acid was 0.76 mmol/L [33]. This would account for the odor. Elevated concentrations of these compounds are also found in the urine. Isovalerylglycine is found in the urine; so is N-isovalerylglutamic acid [46]. Acylcarnitine profiles reveal multiple esters of organic acids (Figure 45.10).

The organic aciduria is not nearly so pronounced in the milder or episodic forms of the disease. Some only manifest

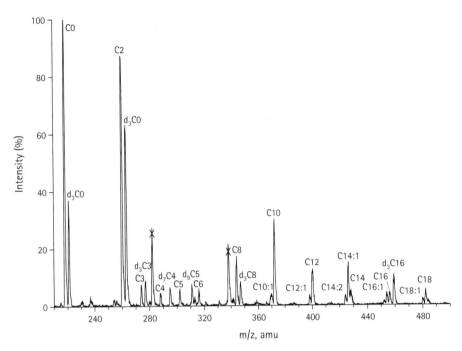

Figure 45.10 *Acylcarnitine profile of the blood plasma of a patient with multiple acyl CoA dehydrogenase deficiency. The pattern of elevation of many acylcarnitine esters follows a curve with the maximum at C10. The two peaks marked X were artifacts. The elevated C0 indicated treatment with carnitine. (Illustration provided by Jon Gangoiti of UCSD.)*

increased excretions of ethylmalonic and adipic acids [49]. In others, abnormal quantities of organic acids are found only during acute episodes of illness. The excretion of 2-hydroxyglutaric acid is a useful marker for this disease. This contrasts with glutaryl-CoA dehydrogenase deficiency (Chapter 8) in which 3-hydroxyglutaric acid is the hydroxy acid found.

In the neonatal onset disease the concentrations of the amino acids, citrulline, lysine, ornithine and proline are elevated in plasma and urine. Hydroxyproline excretion may be high, consistent with a generalized amino aciduria. The excretion of arginine may also be very high. In the later onset disease there may be elevated concentrations of sarcosine in blood and urine [36,40,44].

GENETICS AND PATHOGENESIS

The disease in each of its forms is autosomal recessive. Intermediate activities of enzymes have been documented in parents of a patient in whose fibroblasts ETF-QO was deficient [6,7], and in parents of a patient with a mild variant [49].

Prenatal diagnosis has been accomplished by the demonstration of large amounts of glutaric acid in amniotic fluid [60,61]. It has also been done by documenting impaired oxidation of substrate by cultured amniocytes [46,47,62,63].

In addition to clinical heterogeneity, heterogeneity has been observed in differing amounts of ETF and ETF-QO activity and antigen in different cell lines [64,65]. In some, this has correlated with clinical severity [6], but in others it has not. Deficiency of ETF-QO has been found in the patients with anomalies and polycystic kidneys [40]. Deficiency of ETF-QO antigen was first demonstrated [40] in liver mitochondria of

such an infant; it was also demonstrated in fibroblasts of this patient [7], and two others with renal cysts [66]. ETF-QO was nearly completely deficient in these patients, while the deficiency was less severe in patients with the later onset variants [6,57,67].

ETF deficiency was found by immunoblot analysis in fibroblasts of two neonatal patients with no congenital abnormalities [7]. In one, the α and β subunits were both deficient, and the α-subunit was of smaller size. In the other patient, the α-subunit was also small, while the β was of normal size. The biosynthesis of the α-subunit precursor in the first cell line was virtually absent; in the second an α-subunit was made that was about 1 kD smaller than usual. In another patient with severe disease and no anomalies, there were two weak bands of α-ETF, one smaller than normal [68]. ETF activity was virtually completely absent in these cells, and in another severely ill newborn; some residual activity was found in a few patients with milder disease [5,6]. In three patients, β-ETF deficiency was found by immunochemical assay [6,69]. In cell lines of some patients with multiple acyl CoA dehydrogenase deficiency with ETF and ETF-QO, activity was normal [70], raising the possibility of fundamental defects not yet discovered.

Complementation studies clearly distinguished cells of this disease from those of isovaleric acidemia [71] and provided evidence of two groups of patients with severe multiple acyl CoA dehydrogenase deficiency.

Molecular analysis of the coding sequence of six patients with neonatal onset multiple acyl CoA dehydrogenase deficiency revealed seven different mutations in the α-subunit of ETF [30,72]. The most common was a substitution of methionine for threonine at codon 266, which was found in four unrelated patients. A valine 157 to glycine change has also been reported in two patients [30,31], and a glycine 116 to arginine [30]. Three deletions were observed [30]. Mutations were not found in patients with mild disease. Mutations have not yet been reported in ETF-β, but a number have been found in the ETF-QO including a cystine 561 to alanine transition leading to a truncated protein [32].

In the presence of defective activity of ETF or ETF-QO the activities of a number of dehydrogenases are impaired. This has most commonly been demonstrated by the incubation of fibroblasts derived from the patient with ^{14}C-labeled substrates and measuring their conversion to $^{14}CO_2$. Substrates used have included labeled glutaric acid, valine, leucine, isoleucine, 2-oxoisovaleric acid and 2-oxoisocaproic acid [1], as well as labeled lysine, palmitic acid, butanoic acid and butyric acid.

The conversion of $1,5$-^{14}C-glutaryl CoA to $^{14}CO_2$ has been assessed in the absence of artificial electron acceptor as an assay for the presence of active ETF and ETF-QO [73,74]. Assay for tritium release from ^{3}H-labeled palmitic acid is also deficient in fibroblasts of patients, and this assay has been employed in complementation studies [75].

Riboflavin responsiveness has been demonstrated by the study of the oxidation of ^{14}C-labeled substrates in fibroblasts cultured in the presence and absence of riboflavin supplemented media [3]. Defective oxidation was restored to normal levels by growth in riboflavin. After growth in riboflavin depleted medium the level of the patient's ETF activity fell to 59 percent of control, as did the level of ^{14}C-FAD after growth in ^{14}C-riboflavin. This is consistent with evidence of clinical and biochemical responsiveness to riboflavin [76] in the patient whose cells were studied.

Among the consequences of multiple acyl CoA dehydrogenase deficiency is depletion of body stores of carnitine. In a later onset patient with even relatively mild disease, carnitine deficiency may be expected. An adult onset patient was reported to have low levels of free- carnitine in liver and muscle [50]. In a neonatal onset patient free-carnitine levels in the blood may be low, but they may be normal; however, carnitine esters in the urine are high [77,78]. This excretion of esters is increased after treatment with carnitine [39]. Specific carnitine esters identified include acetylcarnitine, isobutrylcarnitine, isovalerylcarnitine, hexanoylcarnitine, propionylcarnitine and butyrylcarnitine. Rapid diagnosis may be made by the analysis of acylcarnitine profiles in plasma or blood spots on filter paper [79,80], and the disease is detectable in programs of neonatal screening. In this disease there is a general accumulation of acylcarnitines from C4 to C18 [79]. It has also been documented that this approach to diagnosis may miss a patient with mild MAD deficiency [79].

TREATMENT

The treatment of the neonatal onset patient is supportive, especially the treatment of acidosis, hypoglycemia and dehydration with huge amounts of appropriate fluids. Nevertheless, most of those with polycystic kidneys die promptly.

Later onset patients, and those that survive the initial episode, should be assessed for riboflavin responsiveness, reported to be best judged by changes in the dicarboxylic aciduria. Most patients are treated with riboflavin in doses of 100 to 300 mg per 24 hours [52,53,55,76], as well as carnitine. A riboflavin-responsive boy was reported to develop progressive spasticity, ataxia and leukodystrophy without ever experiencing acute metabolic imbalance [81]. Restriction of the intake of fat and protein may be prudent, dependent on the severity of the disease. Glycine supplementation may also remove accumulated CoA esters as their glycine conjugates, as in isovaleric acidemia (Chapter 7). In a 9-year-old with milder disease glycine supplementation was as effective as carnitine supplementation in handling an MCT load [82]. Inasmuch as the major conjugated compounds excreted after glycine are different from those after carnitine, it would be prudent to treat patients with both.

References

1   Przyrembel H, Wendel U, Becker K, et al. Glutaric aciduria type II: Report of a previously underdescribed metabolic disorder. Clin Chim Acta 1976;66:22.

2   Goodman SI, Markey SP, Moe PG, et al. Glutaric aciduria: A 'new' disorder of amino acid metabolism. Biochem Med 1975;12:12.

3   Gregersen N. The acyl-CoA dehydrogenation deficiencies. Scand J Clin Invest 1985;45:1.

4   Rhead W, Roettger V, Marshall T, Amendt B. Multiple acyl-Coenzyme A dehydrogenation disorder responsive to riboflavin: Substrate oxidation flavin metabolism and flavoenzyme activities in fibroblasts. Pediatr Res 1993;33:129.

5   Amendt BA, Rhead WJ. The multiple acyl-coenzyme A dehydrogenation disorders glutaric aciduria type II and ethylmalonic-adipic aciduria: Mitochondrial fatty acid oxidation acyl-coenzyme A dehydrogenase and electron transfer flavoprotein activities in fibroblasts. J Clin Invest 1986;78:205.

6   Loehr JP, Goodman SI, Frerman FE. Glutaric acidemia type II: Heterogeneity of clinical and biochemical phenotypes. Pediatr Res 1990;27:311.

7   Frerman FE, Goodman SI. Deficiency of electron transfer flavoprotein or electron transfer flavoprotein ubiquinone oxido-reducatase in glutaric acidemia type II fibroblasts. Proc Natl Acad Sci USA 1985;82:4517.

8   Besrat A, Polan CE, Henderson LM. Mammalian metabolism of glutaric acid. J Biol Chem 1969;244:1461.

9   Hall C. Acyl CoA Dehydrogenase and electron transferring flavoprotein: in Methods in Enzymology (eds Fleisher S, Packer L) Vol 53. Academic Press, New York;1978:502.

10 Aberhart DJ, Tann CH. Substrate stereochemistry of isovaleryl CoA dehydrogenase: Elimination of the 2-pre-R hydrogen in biotin-deficient rats. Bioorg Chem 1981;10:200.

11 Ikeda Y, Tanaka K. 2-Methyl-branched chain acyl-CoA dehydrogenase from rat liver. Methods in Enzymology 1988;166:360.

12 Beinert H, Frisell WR. The functional identity of the electron-transferring flavoproteins of the fatty acyl coenzyme A and sarcosine dehydrogenase systems. J Biol Chem 1962;237:2988.

13 Frisell WR, Mackenzie CG. Separation and purification of sarcosine dehydrogenase and dimethylglycine dehydrogenase. J Biol Chem 1962;237:94.

14 Wittwer AJ, Wagner C. Identification of the folate-binding proteins of rat liver mitochondria as dimethylglycine dehydrogenase and sarcosine

dehydrogenase flavoprotein nature and enzymatic properties of the purified proteins. *J Biol Chem* 1981;**256**:4109.

15 Hoskins DD, Bjur RA. The oxidation of N-methylglycines by primate liver mitochondria. *J Biol Chem* 1964;**239**:1856.

16 Hoskins DD, Bjur RA. The electron transferring flavoprotein of primate liver mitochondria. *J Biol Chem* 1965;**240**:2201.

17 Hoskins DD. The electron transferring flavoprotein as a common intermediate in the mitochondrial oxidation of butyryl CoA and sarcosine. *J Biol Chem* 1966;**241**:4471.

18 Husain M, Steenkamp DJ. Electron transfer flavoprotein from pig liver mitochondria. A simple purification and re-evaluation of some of the molecular properties. *Biochem J* 1983;**209**:541.

19 McKean MC, Beckmann JD, Frerman FE. Subunit structure of electron transfer flavoprotein. *J Biol Chem* 1983;**258**:1866.

20 Ruzicka FJ, Beinert H. A new membrane iron-sulfur flavoprotein of the mitochondrial transfer system. The entrance point of the fatty acyl dehydrogenation pathway. *Biochem Biophys Res Commun* 1975;**66**:622.

21 Ruzicka FJ, Beinert H. A new iron-sulfur flavoprotein of the respiratory chain A component of the fatty acid β-oxidation pathway. *J Biol Chem* 1977;**252**:8440.

22 Steenkamp DJ, Ramsay RR, Husain M. Reactions of electron transfer flavoprotein and electron transfer flavoprotein: ubiquinone oxidoreductase. *Biochem J* 1987;**241**:883.

23 Frerman FE, Goodman SI. Fluorometric assay of acyl CoA dehydrogenases in normal and mutant fibroblasts lines. *Biochem Med* 1985;**33**:38.

24 Finocchiaro G, Ito M, Ikeda Y, Tanaka K. Molecular cloning and nucleotide sequence of the cDNAs encoding the α-subunit of human electron transfer flavoprotein. *J Biol Chem* 1988;**263**:15773.

25 Finocchiaro G, Colombo I, Garavaglia B, *et al*. cDNA cloning and mitochondrial import of the β-subunit of the human electron-transfer flavoprotein. *Eur J Biochem* 1993;**213**:1003.

26 Goodman SI, Bemelen KF, Frerman FE. Human cDNA encoding ETF dehydrogenase (ETF:ubiquinone oxidoreductase) and mutations in glutaric acidemia type II: in *New Developments in Fatty Acid Oxidation* (eds PM Coates, K Tanaka). John Wiley, USA;1992:567.

27 Barton DE, Yang-Feng TL, Finocchiaro G, *et al*. Short chain acyl-CoA dehydrogenase (ACADS) maps to chromosome 12 (q22-ter) and electron transfer flavoprotein (ETFα) to 15 (q23-q25). *Cytogenet Cell Genet* 1987;**46**:577.

28 Royal V, Alberts MJ, Pericak-Vance MA, *et al*. Rsal RFLP for electron transfer flavoprotein-beta (ETFB). *Nucleic Acids Res* 1991;**19**:4021.

29 Frerman FE, Goodman SI. Nuclear-encoded defects of the mitochondrial respiratory chain including glutaric acidemia type II: in *The Metabolic and Molecular Bases of Inherited Disease* (eds CR Scriver, AL Beaudet, WS Sly, D Valle) Mc-Graw Hill Inc, New York;1995:1611.

30 Freneaux E, Sheffield VC, Molin L, *et al*. Glutaric aciduria type II: Heterogeneity in the beta-oxidation flux polypeptide synthesis and complementary DNA mutations in the alpha subunit of electron transfer flavoprotein in eight patients. *J Clin Invest* 1992;**90**:1679.

31 Indo Y, Glassberg R, Yokota I, Tanaka K. Molecular characterization of variant alpha-subunit of electron transfer and identification of glycine substitution for valine-157 in the sequence of the precursor producing an unstable mature protein in a patient. *Am J Hum Genet* 1991;**49**:575.

32 Beard SE, Spector EB, Seltzer WK, *et al*. Mutations in electron transfer flavoprotein:ubiquinone oxidoreductase (ETF:QO) in glutaric academia type II (GA2). *Clin Res* 1993;**41**:271A.

33 Sweetman L, Nyhan WL, Trauner DA, *et al*. Glutaric aciduria Type II. *J Pediatr* 1980;**96**:1020.

34 Nyhan WL, Sakati NO. Glutaric aciduria type 2: in *Diagnostic Recognition of Genetic Disease*. Lea and Febiger, Philadelphia;1987:77.

35 Lehnert W, Wendel U, Lindermaier S, Bohm N. Multiple acyl-CoA dehydrogenation deficiency (glutaric aciduria type II) congenital polycystic kidneys and symmetric warty dysplasia of the cerebral cortex in two brothers. I Clinical metabolical and biochemical findings. *Eur J Pediatr* 1982;**139**:56.

36 Böhm N, Uy J, Kiessling M, Lehner W. Multiple acyl-CoA dehydrogenation deficiency (glutaric aciduria type II) congenital polycystic kidneys and symmetric warty dysplasia of the cerebral cortex in two newborn brothers. *Eur J Pediatr* 1982;**139**:60.

37 Gregersen N, Kolvraa S, Rasmussen K, *et al*. Biochemical studies in a patient with defects in the metabolism of acyl CoA and sarcosine: Another possible case of glutaric aciduria type II. *J Inherit Metab Dis* 1980;**3**:67.

38 Coude FX, Ogier H, Charpentier C, *et al*. Neonatal glutaric aciduria type II: An X-linked recessive inherited disorder. *Hum Genet* 1981;**59**:63.

39 Goodman SI, Reale M, Berlow S. Glutaric acidemia type II: A form with deleterious intrauterine effects. *J Pediatr* 1983;**102**:411.

40 Goodman SI, Frerman FE. Glutaric acidemia type II (multiple acyl-CoA dehydrogenation deficiency). *J Inherit Metab Dis* 1984;**7**:33.

41 Harkin JC, Gill WL, Shapira E. Glutaric acidemia type II: Phenotypic findings and ultrastructural studies of brain and kidney. *Arch Pathol Lab Med* 1986;**110**:399.

42 Mitchell G, Saudubray JM, Gubler MC, *et al*. Congenital anomalies in glutaric aciduria type 2. *J Pediatr* 1984;**104**:961.

43 Wilson GN, de Chadarevian J-P, Kaplan P, *et al*. Glutaric aciduria type II: review of the phenotype and report of an unusual glomerulopathy. *Am J Med Genet* 1989;**32**:395.

44 Goodman SI, McCabe ERB, Fennessey PV, Mace JW. Multiple acyl-CoA dehydrogenase deficiency (glutaric aciduria type II) with transient hypersarcosinemia and sarcosinuria: Possible inherited deficiency of an electron transfer flavoprotein. *Pediatr Res* 1980;**14**:12.

45 Goodman SI, Stene DO, McCabe ERB, *et al*. Glutaric acidemia type II. Clinical biochemical and morphologic considerations. *J Pediatr* 1982;**100**:946.

46 Niederwieser A, Seinmann B, Exner U, *et al*. Multiple acyl-CoA dehydrogenation deficiency (MADD) in a boy with nonketotic hypoglycemia hepatomegaly muscle hypotonia and cardiomyopathy. Detection of N-isovalerylglutamic acid and its monoamide. *Helv Paediatr Acta* 1983;**38**:9.

47 Bennett MJ, Curnock DA, Engel PC, *et al*. Glutaric aciduria type II. Biochemical investigation and treatment of a child diagnosed prenatally. *J Inherit Metab Dis* 1984;**7**:57.

48 Mooy PD, Przyembel H, Giesberts MAH, *et al*. Glutaric aciduria type II: Treatment with riboflavine carnitine and insulin. *Eur J Pediatr* 1984;**143**:92.

49 Mantagos S, Genel M, Tanaka K. Ethylmalonic-adipic aciduria: *In vivo* and *in vitro* studies indicating deficiency of activities of multiple acyl-CoA dehydrogenase. *J Clin Invest* 1979;**64**:1580.

50 Dusheiko G, Kew MC, Joffe BI, *et al*. Glutaric aciduria type II: A cause of recurrent hypoglycemia in an adult. *N Engl J Med* 1979;**301**:1405.

51 Vergee ZH, Sherwood WG. Multiple acyl-CoA dehydrogenase deficiency: A neonatal onset case responsive to treatment. *J Inherit Metab Dis* 1985;**8**:137.

52 Green A, Marshall TG, Bennett MJ, *et al*. Riboflavin-responsive ethylmalonic-adipic aciduria. *J Inherit Metab Dis* 1985;**8**:67.

53 Gregersen G, Wintzensen H, Kolvraa S, *et al*. C_6-C_{10} Dicarboxylic aciduria: Investigations of a patient with riboflavin responsive multiple acyl-CoA dehydrogenation defects. *Pediatr Res* 1982;**16**:861.

54 Mongini T, Doriguzzi C, Palmucci L, *et al*. Lipid storage myopathy in multiple acyl-CoA dehydrogenase deficiency: an adult case. *Europ Neurol* 1992;**32**:170.

55 De Visser M, Scholte HR, Schutgens RBH. Riboflavin-response lipid-storage myopathy and glutaric aciduria type II of early adult onset. *Neurology* 1986;**36**:367.

56 Cornelio F, DiDonato S, Peluchetti D, *et al.* Fatal cases of lipid storage myopathy with carnitine deficiency. *J Neurol Neurosurg Psychiatry* 1977;**40**:170.

57 DiDonato S, Frerman FE, Rimondi M, *et al.* Systemic carnitine deficiency due to lack of electron transfer flavoprotein:ubiquinone oxido-reductase. *Neurology* 1986;**36**:957.

58 Haas R, Nyhan WL. Disorders of organic acids: in *Neurologic Aspects of Pediatrics* (ed. Berg B) Butterworth-Heinemann, Boston;1992:47.

59 Stöckler S, Radner H, Karpf EF, *et al.* Symmetric hypoplasia of the temporal cerebral lobes in an infant with glutaric aciduria type II (multiple acyl-coenzyme A dehydrogenase deficiency). *J Pediatr* 1994;**124**:601.

60 Jacobs C, Sweetman L, Wadman SK, *et al.* Prenatal diagnosis of glutaric aciduria type II by direct chemical analysis of dicarboxylic acids in amniotic fluid. *Eur J Pediatr* 1984;**141**:153.

61 Chalmers RA, Tracy BM, King GS, *et al.* The prenatal diagnosis of glutaric aciduria type II using quantitative GC/MS. *J Inherit Metab Dis* 1985;**8**:145.

62 Mitchell G, Saudubray JM, Benoit Y, *et al.* Antenatal diagnosis of glutaric aciduria type II. *Lancet* 1983;**1**:1099.

63 Yamaguchi S, Shimizu N, Orii T, *et al.* Prenatal diagnosis and neonatal monitoring of a fetus with glutaric aciduria type II due to electron transfer flavoprotein (β-subunit) deficiency. *Pediatr Res* 1991;**30**:439.

64 Husain M, Stankovich MT, Fox BG. Measurement of the oxidation-reduction potentials for one-electron and two-electron reduction of electron transfer flavoprotein from pig liver. *Biochem J* 1984;**219**:1043.

65 Frerman FE. Reaction of electron transfer flavoprotein ubiquinone oxidoreductase with the mitochondrial respiratory chain. *Biochim Biophys Acta* 1987;**893**:161.

66 Yamaguchi S, Orii T, Suzuki Y, *et al.* Newly identified forms of electron transfer flavoprotein deficiency in two patients with glutaric aciduria type II. *Pediatr Res* 1991;**29**:60.

67 Bell RB, Brownell AKW, Roe CR, *et al.* Electron transfer flavoprotein: ubiquinone oxidoreductase (ETF:QO) deficiency in adult. *Neurology* 1990;**40**:1779.

68 Ikeda Y, Keese SM, Tanaka K. Biosynthesis of electron transfer flavoprotein in a cell-free system and in cultured human fibroblasts. Defect in the alpha subunit synthesis is a primary lesion in glutaric aciduria type II. *J Clin Invest* 1986;**78**:997.

69 Yamaguchi S, Orii T, Maeda K, *et al.* A new variant of glutaric aciduria type II deficiency of β-subunit of electron transfer flavoprotein. *J Inherit Metab Dis* 1990;**13**:783.

70 Loehr J, Frerman FE, Goodman SI. A new form of glutaric acidemia type II (GA2). *Pediatr Res* 1987;**21**:291A (Abstr).

71 Dubiel B, Dabrowski C, Wetts R, Tanaka K. Complementation studies of isovaleric academia and glutaric aciduria type II using cultured skin fibroblasts. *J Clin Invest* 1983;**72**:1543.

72 Rhead WJ, Freneaux E, Sheffield VC, *et al.* Glutaric academia type II (GAII): heterogeneity in beta-oxidation flux polypeptide synthesis and cDNA mutations in the alpha-subunit of electron transfer flavoprotein in 8 patients. *Am J Hum Genet* 199;**25**:A175.

73 Christensen E, Kolvraa S, Gregersen N. Glutaric aciduria type II: Evidence for a defect related to the electron transport flavoprotein or its dehydrogenase. *Pediatr Res* 1984;**18**:663.

74 Christensen E. Glutaryl CoA dehydrogenase activity determined with intact electron-transport chain: Application to glutaric aciduria type II. *J Inherit Metab Dis* 1984;**7**:103.

75 Moon A, Rhead WJ. Complementation analysis of fatty acid oxidation disorders. *J Clin Invest* 1987;**79**:59.

76 Gregersen N, Wintzensen H, Kolvraa S, *et al.* C_6-C_1-dicarboxylic aciduria: investigations of a patient with riboflavin-responsive multiple acyl-CoA dehydrogenation defects. *Pediatr Res* 1982;**16**:861.

77 Chalmers RA, Roe CR, Stacey TE, Hoppel CL. Urinary excretion of L-carnitine and acylcarnitines by patients with disorders of organic acid metabolism: Evidence for secondary insufficiency of L-carnitine. *Pediatr Res* 1984;**18**:1325.

78 Mandel H, Africk D, Blitzer M, Shapira E. The importance of recognizing secondary carnitine deficiency in organic acidaemias: Case report in glutaric acidaemia type II. *J Inherit Metab Dis* 1988;**11**:397.

79 Vreken P, van Lint AEM, Bootsma AH, *et al.* Rapid diagnosis of organic acidemias and fatty acid oxidation defects by quantitative electrospray tandem-MS acyl-carnitine analysis in plasma: in *Current Views of Fatty Acid Oxidation and Ketogenesis: From Organelles to Point Mutations* (eds Quant P, Eaton S, Kluwer Academic) Plenum Publishers, New York;1999:327.

80 Poplawski NK, Ranieri E, Harrison JR, Fletcher JM. Multiple acyl-CoA dehydrogenase deficiency: diagnosis by acyl-carnitine analysis of a 12-year-old newborn screening card. *J Pediatr* 1999;**134**:764.

81 Uziel G, Garavaglia B, Ciceri E, *et al.* Riboflavin-responsive glutaric aciduria type II presenting as a leukodystrophy. *Pediat Neurol* 1995;**13**:333.

82 Rinaldo P, Welch RD, Previs SF, *et al.* Ethylmalonic/adipic aciduria: Effects of oral medium-chain triglycerides carnitine and glycerol on urinary excretion of organic acids acylcarnitines and acylglycines. *Pediatr Res* 1991;**30**:216.

3-Hydroxy-3-methylglutaryl CoA lyase deficiency

MAJOR PHENOTYPIC EXPRESSION

Hypoketotic hypoglycemia, metabolic acidosis, hyperammonemia; hepatomegaly; a characteristic organic aciduria: 3-hydroxy-3-methylglutaric, 3-methylglutaconic, 3-methylglutaric and 3-hydroxyisovaleric; and deficiency of 3-hydroxy-3-methylglutaryl CoA lyase.

INTRODUCTION

3-Hydroxy-3-methylglutaric (HMG) aciduria is a disorder of leucine metabolism (Figure 46.1) that leads to life-threatening illness early in life. Once diagnosed, management, particularly the avoidance of fasting can be very rewarding. The first patient was reported in 1976 by Faull and colleagues [1]. This infant was well until 7 months-of-age when he developed diarrhea and vomiting, and within 24 hours he had lethargy, pallor, dehydration, cyanosis and apnea, requiring resuscitation.

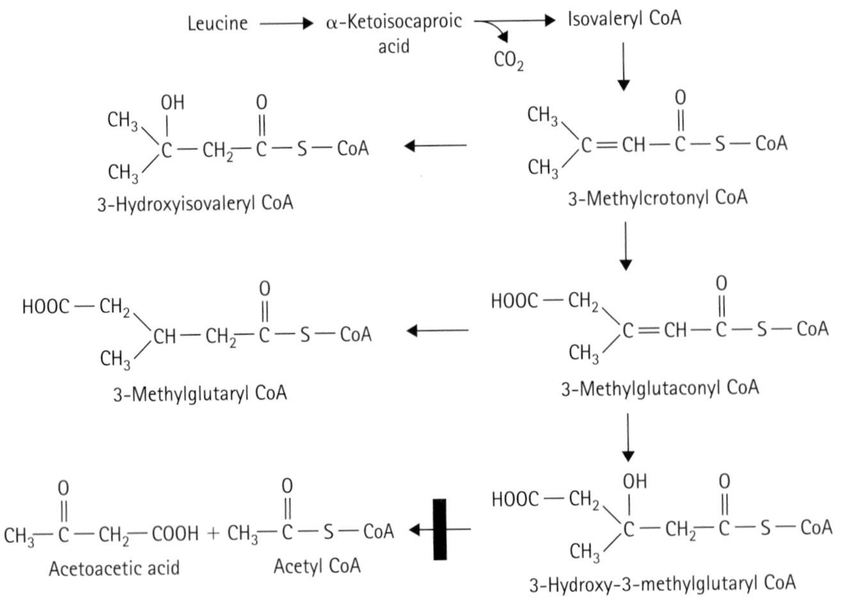

Figure 46.1   *The pathway of the catabolism of leucine and HMG CoA lyase, the site of the defect in 3-hydroxy-3-methylglutaric aciduria.*

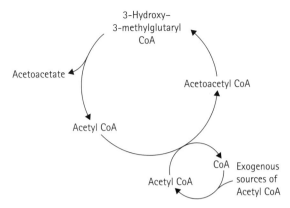

Figure 46.2   *Ketogenesis. HMG CoA and its lyase play a critical role.*

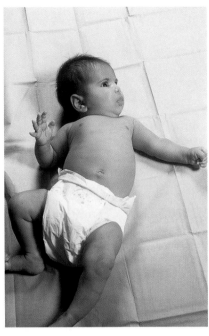

Figure 46.3   *H.H.H.A., a 1-month-old infant with HMG CoA lyase deficiency. She developed lactic acidosis and coma at 5 days-of-age and was found to have 668 mmol/creatinine of HMG in the urine. Activity of HMG CoA lyase in fibroblasts was 0.9 percent of control. The tonic neck reflex is normal at her age. Examination was unremarkable.*

At 4 years and 7 months [2] development was satisfactory. The disorder has been encountered frequently among Arab families [3].

HMG-CoA lyase deficiency may be considered an organic acidemia. It is at the same time a classic disorder of fatty acid oxidation. HMG-CoA lyase is the last step in the formation of acetoacetate (Figure 46.2) and its product, 3-hydroxybutyrate. The products of the cleavage of HMG-CoA are acetoacetate and acetyl CoA. HMG-CoA is also of course a key intermediate in the synthesis of cholesterol (Chapter 87, p. 577). Its reduction to mevalonic acid represents a feedback control point in this pathway.

CLINICAL ABNORMALITIES

The classic presentation is with a Reye-syndrome-like episode in late infancy (from 6 months to 2 years), usually following an intercurrent infection which leads to vomiting or failure to eat [1–9], some present in the neonatal period, but the majority between 3 and 11 months. Persistent vomiting may be an early symptom. There is rapid progression from lethargy and hypotonia to coma. Pallor and dehydration are commonly present. There may be seizures, including myoclonus. Hypothermia has been reported [10]. Apnea is followed by death unless the patient is artificially ventilated. Clinical chemical evaluation reveals hypoglycemia, metabolic acidosis and in some hyperammonemia. For this reason, a number of patients have initially been diagnosed as Reye syndrome [7,8]. Presentation with life-threatening acidosis is common [4,9,10]. Infants may present in the first days of life with seizures, lethargy or tachypnea. This may follow the first feeding or may precede it, an index that birth itself maybe a catabolic experience. Lactic acidemia is prominent. The initial episode may be fatal [9,10].

Recurrent episodes of acute illness have been observed particularly in those who presented in the neonatal period [9]. The patient is always at risk of acute illness, if infection or other problem leads to fasting. Some families have learned to intervene sufficiently, promptly and effectively that episodes have been prevented or aborted.

Hepatomegaly is a regular occurrence [11], and there may be elevation of levels of transaminases in the blood. However, hepatomegaly may be absent especially in the neonatal presentation. It has been absent in a 9-month old, who had elevated transaminases [12]. Histologic examination of the liver reveals infiltration of fat.

Brain injury may result from hypoglycemia, shock or both. Some patients have had a persistent seizure disorder and abnormalities of the electroencephalogram (EEG) [7,9]. Microcephaly has been observed in several patients [13,14]. One severely retarded patient was macrocephalic [15]. Hemiparesis has been reported [16] and decerebrate tetraparesis [9]. Mental retardation may be severe [9,17]. On the other hand, most patients are developmentally normal. There are no dysmorphic features (Figures 46.3–46.8).

One patient (Figure 46.5) presented at 5 years-of-age with pernicious vomiting and abdominal tenderness and was found to have acute pancreatitis [18]. She had recurrent episodes of hypoglycemia and acidosis. Pancreatitis has been described increasingly in patients with Reye syndrome [19,20] and in inborn errors of metabolism [21], suggesting further commonalties in pathogenesis of other metabolic disorders thought to be Reye syndrome.

Magnetic resonance imaging (MRI) of the brain reveals increased T2 signal indicating hypodensity of white matter [9,12,15] (Figures 46.9, 46.10). In patients in whom brain damage has occurred, the picture may be that of cerebral atrophy [9,17] (Figure 46.11).

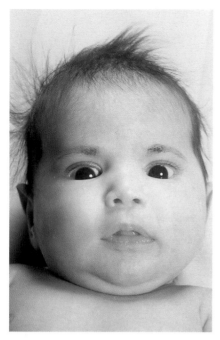

Figure 46.4 *H.H.H.A. There were no dysmorphic features. MRI showed some evidence of cerebral atrophy.*

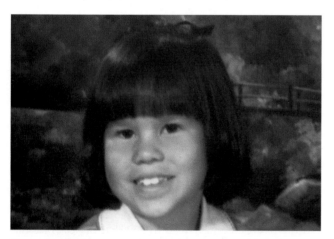

Figure 46.5 *A girl with 3-hydroxy-3-methylglutaric aciduria. She was admitted to hospital at 5 years-of-age with acute pancreatitis. The activity of 3-hydroxy-3-methylglutaryl CoA lyase in lymphocytes and fibroblasts was two percent of normal. (The illustration was kindly provided by Dr. William Wilson of the University of Virginia.)*

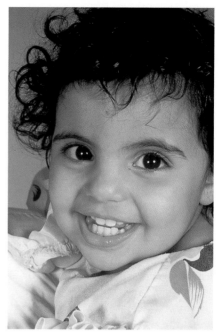

Figure 46.6 *N. A 3-year-old patient with HMG CoA lyase deficiency. She developed severe neonatal lactic acidosis, hypoglycemia and coma. Despite noncompliance with dietary treatment and multiple acidotic attacks she was developing normally. By follow-up at 7 years-of-age, she was doing better than average in school although attacks were continuing.*

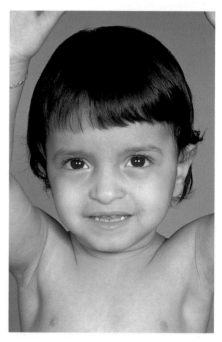

Figure 46.7 *S. A 3-year-old girl with HMG CoA lyase deficiency. She had severe lactic acidotic episodes in the neonatal period and at 5 and 14 months, in the latter of which she developed shock and convulsions along with an unmeasurable blood glucose. On follow-up at 7 years-of-age, she had no attacks for three years and was developing normally.*

The hypoglycemic acute episode is striking, often extreme and with a notable absence of ketosis. Initial concentrations of sugar in the blood have ranged from 0.2 to 1.8 mmol/L; many were below 0.4 mmol/L (8 mg/dL) and one patient died in a second episode of hypoglycemia in which the concentration recorded was less than 0.1 mmol/L. At this time the concentration of insulin was less than 1 mU/L. The episode had followed a change in diet in which the amounts of leucine ingested were increased. The infant developed cyanosis, vomiting and hypotonia. In three patients the values for the blood pH were recorded as 7.24, 7.11 and 7.29 [7,8,10]. During the acute crisis

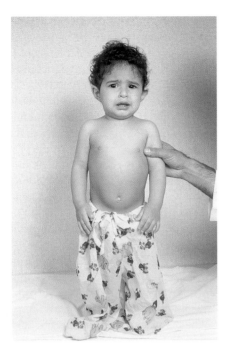

Figure 46.8   *A 21-month-old boy with HMG CoA lyase deficiency. His first acidotic episode was at 6 months-of-age following herpangina and refusal to eat. At 6 years-of-age, he had not had an attack in three years and was doing very well in school.*

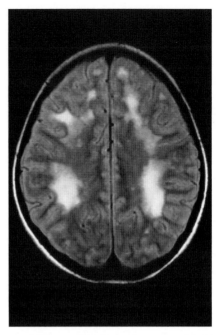

Figure 46.10   *MRI scan of the brain of a 9-year-old with HMG-CoA lyase deficiency. There was extensive increase in signal in the subcortical white matter consistent with dysmyelination. (Kindly provided by Dr. Robert Schwartz of Brown University School of Medicine.)*

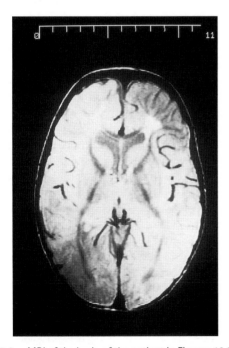

Figure 46.9   *MRI of the brain of the patient in Figures 46.3 and 46.4 at 2.5 years reveals increased signal intensity in the frontal white matter. (Reprinted with permission from the* Journal of Inherited Metabolic Disease *[9].)*

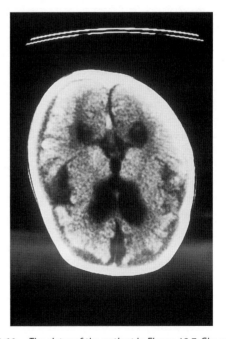

Figure 46.11   *The sister of the patient in Figure 46.7. She was diagnosed late. The CT scan at 10 months shows considerable evidence of cerebral atrophy. She was severely impaired neurologically and died at 19 months.*

a pH below 7.0 is not unusual especially in the neonatal onset patients [4,9]. The initial plasma concentrations of bicarbonate were below 16 mEq/L in five patients [4]. Lactic acidosis has been documented with levels as high as 10 and 20 mmol/L

[4]. Persistent infantile hypoglycemia in the presence of metabolic acidosis is an indication for organic acid analysis.

Hyperammonemia has been observed in about 50 percent of patients [4]. In three patients concentrations ranged from

388 μM/L to 1370 μmol/L [4] and in one patient the plasma concentration of ammonia was greater than 2000 μmol/L [3]. Abnormal liver function tests included alanine and aspartate aminotransferase [1,7]; bilirubin, gamma-glutamyl transpeptidase (γGT) [10], and prolonged prothrombin time [7,8], all of which lead to confusion with the diagnosis of Reye syndrome. In fact the provisional diagnosis was Reye syndrome in the first four patients reported. With successful treatment the abnormalities in liver function disappear. The prognosis is guarded. Death has been observed in at least five patients [9,16,17,10,22].

None of these patients had ketonuria at times of acute illness, and in some low levels of acetoacetate and 3-hydroxybutyrate have been observed in the blood [8,16,17,23]. Levels of acetoacetate and 3-hydroxybutyrate in the urine are disproportionately low. This serves to distinguish these patients from those with other organic acidurias, such as propionic acidemia (Chapter 2) or methylmalonicacidemia (Chapter 3). This is consistent with the site of the defect (Figure 46.2) in which 3-hydroxy-3-methylglutaric acid cannot be converted to acetoacetic acid and acetyl CoA. Ketone bodies decrease proteolysis in muscle and conserve muscle protein during starvation [24]; so impairment of ketogenesis could be relevant to the hyperammonemia.

GENETICS AND PATHOGENESIS

HMG-CoA lyase deficiency is transmitted as an autosomal recessive trait. Consanguinity has been observed in a number of families [7,9,10].

The molecular defect is in the enzyme HMG-CoA lyase (Figure 46.1). Defective activity of the enzyme has been demonstrated in cultured fibroblasts [25,26], leukocytes [27], and liver [10] of affected patients. Activity in 10 patients was reported to be undetectable; in 16 others it ranged from 0.7 percent to 13.7 percent of normal [4]. A variety of methods is available for enzyme analysis (28), including direct detection by high performance liquid chromatography (HPLC) of the product of the reaction [26]. In addition, the defect can be identified by measuring the incorporation of ^{14}C-isovaleric acid into trichloroacetic acid precipitable macromolecules [29] or by monitoring metabolism of ^{14}C-leucine [30].

The activity of the HMG CoA lyase in leukocyte or fibroblasts in the parents of patients is intermediate between those of the patient and controls [4,26,27]. However, in some families obligate heterozygotes have had normal values.

Prenatal diagnosis has been accomplished by the analysis of metabolites in maternal urine at 23 weeks of gestation [31]. The enzyme is active in amniocytes [32]. Prenatal diagnosis should be possible by direct measurement of HMG by stable isotope dilution gas chromatography/mass spectrometry (GC/MS) of the amniotic fluid.

The gene for HMG CoA lyase has been cloned [33]. The sequence predicts a 27 residue mitochondrial leader and a 31.6 kDa mature protein. A number of mutations have provided interesting information on the nature of the enzyme. Five mutations in the highly conserved R41 and D42 codons were found in 23 percent of the mutant alleles in 41 probands. They were R41Q, R41X, D42H, D42G and D42E [34]. R41Q is common in Saudi Arabia where six of nine probands were homozygous. This mutation has also been found in Turkish and Italian patients. Among major alterations in the gene were two large deletions [35] and three frame shift/premature terminations [33,34]. Two stop codon mutations and a two base pair deletion led to alternately spliced mRNA [36–38]. Despite these elegant studies clear relationship of genotype to phenotype has not emerged.

The pattern of organic aciduria in this disorder is characteristic [39–42] (Figure 46.12). 3-Hydroxy-3-methylglutaric acid is excreted in appreciable quantities in the urine. In acute crisis levels may reach 10 000 to 20 000 mmol/mol creatinine and between crises may be 200–4000. Normal individuals excrete in urine less than 100 mmol/mol creatinine [41]; levels are somewhat higher in young infants. Organic acid analysis by GCMS usually involves trimethylsilyl derivatives, but in the case of 3-hydroxy-3-methylglutaric acid appreciable quantities of the di-derivative are formed as well as the tri-derivative, as both must be included for quantification [43]. Large amounts of 3-methylglutaconic acid are also found in the urine. These compounds represent successive steps in the catabolism of leucine (Figure 46.1) in which isovaleryl CoA is converted to 3-methylcrotonyl CoA which is then converted to 3-methylglutaconyl CoA. The addition of H_2O across the double bond in this compound yields 3-hydroxy-3-methylglutaryl CoA which is ultimately cleaved to form acetoacetic acid and acetyl CoA. 3-Methylglutaric acid is also found; this would result from reduction of 3-methylglutaconic acid. The reaction could be catalyzed by the enzyme that catalyzes the reverse dehydrogenation of 3-methylcrotonyl CoA to isovaleryl CoA. In addition 3-hydroxyisovaleric acid is also found in the urine [42]. This compound would arise from the hydration of 3-methylcrotonyl CoA. In the acute episode a large elevation of 3-hydroxyisovaleric acid may be found, along with 3-methylcrotonylglycine [18,42–44]. Glutaric acid and adipic may also be elevated in the urine in the acute crisis [45]. Lactic acid levels may be elevated at these times [46], along with hyperammonenia. Levels of acetoacetate and 3-hydroxybutyrate in the urine, as in the blood, are disproportionately low.

3-Methylcronic (3-methyl-2-butenoic) acid may be found in the urine, along with its isomer, 3-methyl-3-butenoic acid [39], but these are artifacts of the GCMS analysis [45,47]. The abnormal metabolites in this disease may also be detected by nuclear magnetic resonance (NMR) spectroscopy [48] permitting rapid diagnosis. Rapid diagnosis is now more likely to be made by tandem mass spectrometry MS/MS. 3-Methylglutarylcarnitine has been found in the plasma and urine [49], and 3-hydroxy-isovaleryl carnitine has been found in plasma [50] (Table 1.2, p. 5.) This permits the incorporation of this disease into programs of neonatal screening.

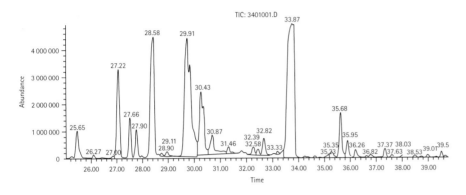

Figure 46.12 *Organic acid analysis of the urine of a patient with HMG CoA lyase deficiency. The important compounds were: 3-hydroxyisovaleric acid at 20.74; 3-methylglutaric acid at 27.90; 3-methyl glutaconic acid at 28.58 and 29.91; and 3-hydroxy-3-methyl-glutaric acid at 33.87.*

The excretion of acylcarnitine esters is elevated in this condition, and there may be a secondary deficiency of free carnitine [51].

TREATMENT

Management of the patient should be considered under two headings, long-term management and treatment of the acute crisis. The latter is an emergency, and care must be devoted first to measures of general support such as assisted ventilation and repair of deficits of fluid and electrolytes and elevation of the blood concentration of glucose. In an infant with or without hyperammonemia, exchange transfusion, or peritoneal dialysis may be necessary. Sodium benzoate or phenylacetate and arginine may be useful in management of the hyperammonemia [52]. Hypoglycemia and acidosis usually respond readily to the parenteral administration of glucose, fluid and electrolytes. Parents should be instructed to bring the patient in early, whenever the oral route is compromised by vomiting or anorexia.

Long-term management rests largely on the avoidance of hypoglycemia, and the avoidance of long fasting, especially during intercurrent illness. The importance of ketogenesis in glucose homeostasis was illustrated by the prevention of hypoglycemia with fasting in a patient with HMG CoA lyase deficiency by the infusion of 3-hydroxybutyrate [23]. Frequent feedings are advisable in infancy, with even sleeping through the night permitted only after it is documented that this does not lead to hypoglycemia. A high carbohydrate diet

is advisable; and supplementation with glucose polymers is convenient, especially during intercurrent illness. Cornstarch may be useful at bed time.

Restriction of the intake of protein has been employed, and it appears prudent to restrict the amounts of leucine ingested. Restriction of the intake of fats may reduce the levels of metabolites in the urine [11]. Carnitine supplementation has proven to be a useful adjunct to therapy [53].

References

1 Faull K, Bolton P, Halpern B, *et al*. Patient with defect in leucine metabolism. *N Engl J Med* 1976;**294**:1013.

2 Shilkin R, Wilson G, Owles E. 3-Hydroxy-3-methylglutaryl coenzyme A lyase deficiency. Follow-up of first described case. *Acta Paediatr Scand* 1981;**70**:265.

3 Ozand PT, DeVol EB, Gascon GG. Neurometabolic diseases at a national referral center: Five years experience at the King Faisal Specialist Hospital and Research Centre. *J Child Neurol* 1992;**7**:S4.

4 Gibson KM, Breuer J, Nyhan WL. 3-Hydroxy-3-methylglutaryl-coenzyme A lyase deficiency: review of 18 reported patients. *Eur J Pediatr* 1988;**148**:180.

5 Wysocki SJ, Hahnel R. 3-Hydroxy-3-methylglutaryl coenzyme A lyase deficiency: a review. *J Inherit Metab Dis* 1986;**9**:225.

6 Gibson KM, Lee CL, Kamail V, *et al*. 3-Hydroxy-3-methylglutaryl coenzyme A lyase deficiency as detected by radiochemical assay in cell extracts by thin layer chromatography and identification of two new cases. *Clin Chem* 1990;**36**:297.

7 Leonard JV, Seakins JWT, Griffin NK. β-Hydroxy-β-methylglutaric aciduria presenting as Reye syndrome. *Lancet* 1979;**1**:680.

8 Robinson BH, Oei J, Sherwood WG, *et al*. Hydroxymethylglutaryl CoA lyase deficiency: features resembling Reye syndrome. *Neurology* 1980;**30**:714.

9   Ozand PT, Al Aqeel A, Gascon GG, et al. 3-Hydroxy-3-methylglutaryl-coenzyme-A (HMG-CoA) lyase deficiency in Saudi Arabia. J Inherit Metab Dis 1991;14:174.

10   Schutgens RB, Heymans H, Ketel A, et al. Lethal hypoglycemia in a child with a deficiency of 3-hydroxy-3-methlyglutaryl-coenzyme A lyase. J Pediatr 1979;94:89.

11   Norman EJ, Denton MD, Berry HK. Gas chromatographic/mass spectrometric detection of 3-hydroxy-3-methylglutaryl-CoA lyase deficiency in double first cousins. Clin Chem 1982;28:137.

12   Gibson KM, Breuer J, Kaiser K, et al. 3-Hydroxy-3-methylglutaryl-coenzyme A lyase deficiency: report of five new patients. J Inherit Metab Dis 1988;11:76.

13   Lisson G, Leupold B, Bechinger D, Wallesch C. CT findings in a case of deficiency of 3-hydroxy-3-methylglutaryl-CoA lyase. Neuroradiology 1981;22:99.

14   Stacey TE, de Sousa C, Tracey BM, et al. Dizygotic twins with 3-hydroxy-3-methylglutaric aciduria: unusual presentation family studies and dietary management. Eur J Pediatr 1985;144:177.

15   Leupold D, Bojash M, Jakobs C. 3-Hydroxy-3-methylglutaryl-CoA lyase deficiency in an infant with macrocephaly and mild metabolic acidosis. Eur J Pediatr 1982;138:73.

16   Zoghbi HY, Spence JE, Beaudet AL, et al. Atypical presentation and neuropathological studies in 3-hydroxy-3-methylglutaryl-CoA lyase deficiency. Ann Neuro 1986;20:367.

17   Walter JH, Clayton PT, Leonard JV. 3-Hydroxy-3-methylglutaryl-CoA lyase deficiency. J Inherit Metab Dis 1986;9:287.

18   Wilson WG, Cass MB, Sovik O, et al. 3-Hydroxy-3-methylglutaryl-CoA lyase deficiency in a child with acute pancreatitis and recurrent hypoglycemia. Eur J Pediatr 1984;142:781.

19   Ellis G, Mirkin LD, Mills MC. Pancreatitis and Reye's syndrome. Am J Dis Child 1979;33:1014.

20   Morens DM, Hammar SL, Heicher DA. Idiopathic acute pancreatitis in children. Association with a clinical picture resembling Reye syndrome. Am J Dis Child 1974;128:401.

21   Kahler SG, Sherwood WG, Woolf D, et al. Pancreatitis in patients with organic acidemias. J Pediatr 1994;124:239.

22   Divry P, Rolland MO, Teyssier J, et al. 3-Hydroxy-3-methylglutaric aciduria combined with 3-methylglutaconic aciduria. A new case. J Inherit Metab Dis 1981;4:173.

23   Francois B, Bachmann C, Schutgens RBH. Glucose metabolism in a child with 3-hydroxy-3-methyl glutaryl-coenzyme A lyase deficiency. J Inherit Metab Dis 1981;4:163.

24   Felig P, Sherwin R, Palailogos G. Ketone utilization and ketone-amino acid interactions in starvation and diabetes: in Biochemical and Clinical Aspects of Ketone Body Metabolism (eds HD Soeling, CD Seufert) Thieme, Stuttgart;1978:166.

25   Wysocki SJ, Hahnel R. 3-Hydroxy-3-methylglutaric aciduria: deficiency of 3-hydroxy-3-methylglutaryl coenzyme A lyase. Clin Chim Acta 1976;71:349.

26   Gibson KM, Sweetman L, Nyhan WL, et al. 3-Hydroxy-3-methylglutaric aciduria a new assay of 3-hydroxy-3-methylglutaryl-CoA lyase using high performance liquid chromatography. Clin Chim Acta 1982;126:171.

27   Wysocki SJ, Hahnel R. 3-Hydroxy-3-methylglutaric aciduria 3-hydroxy-3-methylglutaryl-Coenzyme A lyase levels in leukocytes. Clin Chim Acta 1976;73:373.

28   Gibson KM. Assay of 3-hydroxy-3-methyl-glutaryl-coenzyme A lyase. Meth Enzymol Branched Chain Amino Acids 1988;166:219.

29   Sovik O, Sweetman L, Gibson KM, Nyhan WL. Genetic complementation analysis of 3-hydroxy-3-methylglutaryl-coenzyme A lyase deficiency in cultured fibroblasts. Am J Hum Genet 1984;26:791.

30   Yoshida I, Sovik O, Sweetman L, Nyhan WL. Metabolism of leucine in fibroblasts from patients with deficiencies in each of the major catabolic enzymes: branched-chain ketoacid dehydrogenase 3-methylcrotonyl-CoA carboxylase 3-methylglutaconyl-CoA hydratase and 3-hydroxy-3-methylglutaryl-CoA lyase. J Neurogenet 1985;2:413.

31   Duran M, Schutgens RBH, Ketel A, et al. 3-Hydroxy-3-methylglutaryl coenzyme A lyase deficiency: postnatal management following prenatal diagnosis by analysis of maternal urine. J Pediatr 1979;95:1004.

32   Hahnel R, Wysocki SJ. Potential prenatal diagnosis of 3-hydroxy-3-methylglutaryl-Coenzyme A lyase deficiency. Clin Chim Acta 1981;111:287.

33   Mitchell GA, Robert MF, Hruz PW. 3-Hydroxy-3-methylglutaryl coenzyme A lyase (HL). J Biol Chem 1993;268:4376.

34   Mitchell GA, Ozand PT, Robert M-F, et al. HMG CoA lysase deficiency: Identification of five causal point mutations in codons 41 and 42 including a frequent Saudi Arabian mutation R41Q. Am J Hum Genet 1997;62:295.

35   Wang SP, Robert M-F, Gibson KM, et al. 3-Hydroxy-3-methylglutaryl-CoA lysase (HL): mouse and human HL gene (HMGCL) cloning and detection of large gene deletions in two unrelated HL-deficient patients. Genomics 1996;33:99.

36   Buesa C, Pie J, Barcelo A, et al. Aberrantly spliced mRNAs of the 3-hydroxy-3-methylglutaryl coenzyme A lyase (HL) gene with a donor splice-site point mutation produce hereditary HL deficiency. J Lipid Res 1996;37:2420.

37   Pie J, Casals N, Casale CH, et al. A nonsense mutation in the 3-hydroxy-3-methylglutaric aciduria. Biochem J 1997;323:(Pt 2) 329.

38   Casals N, Pie J, Casale CH, et al. A two-base deletion in exon 6 of the 3-hydroxy-3-methylglutaryl coenzyme A lyase (HL) gene producing the skipping of exons 5 and 6 determines 3-hydroxy-3-methylglutaric aciduria. J Lipid Res 1997;38:2303.

39   Wysocki SJ, Wilkinson SP, Hahnel R, et al. 3-hydroxy-3-methylglutaric aciduria combined with 3-methylglutaconic aciduria. Clin Chim Acta 1976;70:399.

40   Tracey BM, Stacey TE, Chalmers RA. Urinary and plasma organic acids in dizygotic twin siblings with 3-hydroxy-3-methylglutaric aciduria studied by gas chromatography and mass spectrometry using fused silica capillary columns. J Inherit Metab Dis 1983;6:125.

41   Lippe G, Galsigna L, Rancesconi M, et al. Age-dependent excretion of 3-hydroxy-3-methylglutaric acid (HMG) and ketone bodies in the urine of full-term and pre-term newborns. Clin Chim Acta 1982;126:291.

42   Faull KF, Bolton PD, Halpern B, et al. The urinary organic acid profile associated with 3-hydroxy-3-methylglutaric aciduria. Clin Chim Acta 1976;73:558.

43   Mills GA, Hill MAW, Buchanan R, et al. 3-Hydroxy-3-methylglutaric aciduria: a possible pitfall in diagnosis. Clin Chim Acta 1991;204:131.

44   Wysocki SJ, Hahnel R. 3-Methylcrotonylglycine excretion in 3-hydroxy-3-methylglutaric aciduria. Clin Chim Acta 1978;86:101.

45   Duran M, Ketting D, Wadman SK, et al. Organic acid excretion in a patient with 3-hydroxy-3-methylglutaryl-CoA lyase deficiency. Facts and artifacts. Clin Chim Acta 1978;90:187.

46   Green CL, Cann HM, Robinson BH, et al. 3-Hydroxy-3-methylglutaric aciduria. J Neurogenet 1984;1:165.

47   Jakobs C, Bojasch M, Duran M, et al. An artefact in the urinary metabolic pattern of patients with 3-hydroxy-3-methylglutaryl-CoA lyase deficiency. Clin Chim Acta 1980;106:85.

48   Iles RA, Jago JR, Williams SR, Chalmers RA. 3-Hydroxy-3-methylglutaryl-CoA lyase deficiency studied using 2-dimensional proton nuclear magnetic resonance spectroscopy. FEBS Lett 1986;203:49.

49   Roe CR, Millington DS, Maltby DA. Identification of 3-methyl-glutarylcarnitine: a new diagnostic metabolite of 3-hydroxy-3-methylglutaryl-coenzyme A lyase deficiency. J Biol Chem 1986;77:1391.

50   van Hove JLK, Rutledge SL, Nada MA, *et al*. 3-Hydroxyisovalerylcarnitine in 3-methylcrotonyl-CoA carboxylase deficiency. *J Inherit Metab Dis* 1995;**18**:592.

51   Chalmers RA, Roe CR, Tracey BM, *et al*. Secondary carnitine insufficiency in disorders of organic acid metabolism: Modulation of acyl-CoA/CoA ratios by L-carnitine *in vivo*. *Biochem Soc Trans* 1983;**11**:724.

52   Batshaw ML, Brusilow SW. Treatment of hyperammonemia coma caused by inborn errors of urea synthesis. *J Pediatr* 1980;**97**:893.

53   Dasouki M, Buchanan D, Mercer N, *et al*. 3-Hydroxy-3-methylglutaric aciduria: response to carnitine therapy and fat and leucine restriction. *J Inherit Metab Dis* 1987;**10**:142.

PART 5

The lactic acidemias and mitochondrial disease

Introduction to the lactic acidemias

The lactic acidemias constitute a large family of distinct disorders of metabolism. There are enlarging numbers of enzymatic deficiencies, and some disorders are now characterizable on the basis of the mutation in the DNA. This is especially the case in mitochondrial DNA, but mutations are increasingly being detected in nuclear DNA. Some patients have lactic acidemia secondary to another disorder, such as propionic acidemia (Chapter 2). On the other hand, there remain a considerable number of patients with lactic acidemia in whom a molecular explanation of the abnormal metabolism cannot be found, even with the most sophisticated studies available. Elucidating the cause and the most appropriate approach to therapy in a patient with lactic acidemia requires a systematic investigation.

In considering a patient for investigation of lactic acidemia it is first necessary to establish that elevation of lactic acid in the blood is real. This may require a number of determinations even in patients with known disease. The most common reason for elevated concentration of lactic acid in blood is improper technique, the use of a tourniquet, or a real struggle in obtaining a sample. On the other hand, levels are variable even in patients with known disease. This is a function of the fact that lactic acid itself is situated some distance from most of the known defective enzymatic steps, particularly oxidative steps in the electron transport chain. The first step is the documentation of elevated levels of lactic acid, pyruvic acid and/or alanine in the blood. It is important to be rigorous about methods of sampling, to draw blood that is flowing freely without a tourniquet. Our best results are often obtained in the course of studies in the Clinical Research Center in which a catheter is placed in the vein to permit multiple sampling without the stresses of venepuncture. The concentration of lactate in the cerebrospinal fluid (CSF) may also be elevated. Increasingly, patients are encountered in whom the concentration of lactate in the CSF is elevated, whereas

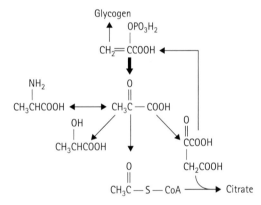

Figure 47.1 *Pyruvate plays a central role in glycolysis and in oxidative metabolism. The pyruvate does not accumulate when its metabolism is blocked; it is converted to sinks or reservoirs of lactate and alanine.*

that of plasma is normal or only slightly or intermittently elevated [1].

The lactic acidemias are disorders of pyruvate metabolism. Concentrations of pyruvate are determined, but large elevations of pyruvate are seldom seen. Accumulating pyruvate is converted to lactate and alanine (Figure 47.1). Concentrations of alanine are not raised factitiously by problems of technique, but they too are variable in patients with known enzymatic defects.

The next step is to exclude the conditions that lead to secondary elevations in concentrations of lactic acid. A major group of patients are those with hypoxia, hypoventilation, shock, or hypoperfusion. These situations are seen in patients with sepsis, cardiac and pulmonary disease, hepatic disease and severe anemia. Therefore, all of these conditions should be excluded before undertaking a metabolic workup for the elucidation of a lactic acidemia. Anaerobic exercise also these procedures are noninvasive and provide a rapid answer to the diagnosis. Most patients with disorders of gluconeogenesis in whom these two procedures do not provide the diagnosis require liver biopsy for definitive enzyme assay. Information as to the area of the defect may be obtained by loading tests, for instance with fructose, alanine or glycerol in fructose-1,6-diphosphatase deficiency [8,9] (Chapter 49). Following glycerol or fructose, phosphate should also be measured because it decreases sharply in patients with a block at this level. Concentrations of uric acid may increase. Loading with galactose should provide a positive control except in a patient with glucose-6-phosphatase deficiency. Each compound is given by mouth as a 20 percent solution 6–12 hours postprandially in a dose of 1 g/kg.

Most patients who pass the fasting test have defects in oxidation of pyruvate. A small number has essentially factitious lactic acidemia with lactic aciduria in which D-lactic acid is formed by intestinal bacteria and then absorbed. L-lactic acid and L-alanine are actually dextrarotatory in the polarimeter, but the nomenclature is employed to indicate their structural similarlity to L-glyceraldehyde (Figure 47.4) D-lactic acid and D-amino acids are bacterial components. N-Acetylmuramic acid, a compound of D-lactic acid and N-acetylglucosamine is a component of the mucopeptides of bacterial cell walls. D-Lactic aciduria is usually seen in patients with malabsorption syndromes, as well as the short bowel syndrome and necrotizing enterocolitis [10,11]. This lactic acid accumulation can even lead to systemic acidosis and coma. A course of treatment with oral neomycin or metronidazole may resolve

this problem, as may testing for lactate with an enzymatic assay specific for L-lactic acid or D-lactic acid. Factitious lactic acidemia and/or lactic aciduria may also occur in the neonatal intensive care unit or elsewhere when glucose is infused in amounts in excess of the capacity of the infant to utilize it [12].

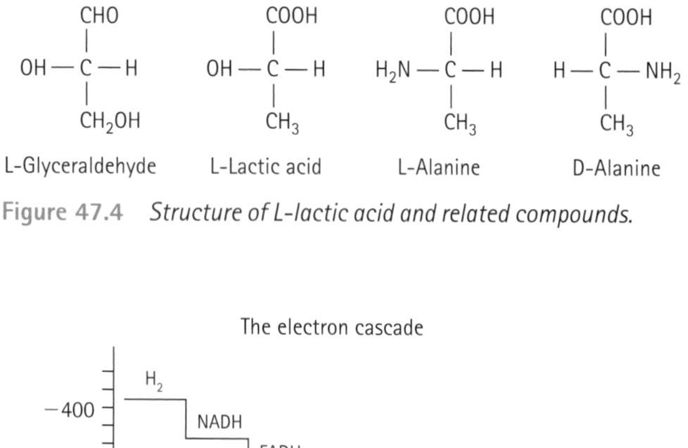

In patients who pass the test and are judged to have defective oxidation of pyruvate we carry out skin biopsies for fibroblast culture and usually initiate therapy with a diet high in fat and low in carbohydrate while the culture is being established. Once the fibroblasts are available they are assayed for defects in the pyruvate dehydrogenase complex (PDHC) and in its first enzyme, pyruvate decarboxylase (E1). E1 has an α and a β subunit. Defects in E1α can be tested for by mutational analysis (Chapter 50). The E2 transacetylase protein can be tested for by Western blot analysis, and some mutations have been defined. In patients with defects in this PDHC system it is also useful to measure the activity of α-ketoglutarate dehydrogenase and lipoamide dehydrogenase (E3) (Chapter 51).

Muscle biopsy with histology and studies of electromyography and nerve conduction are employed to elucidate patients with myopathy, or abnormalities in mitochondrial structure. Ragged red fibers are frequently seen in disorders of mitochondrial DNA. Muscle may be used as a source for analysis of mutation in the DNA. There are patients in whom analysis of muscle reveals the heteroplasmy while the blood does not. Fresh muscle obtained by open biopsy permits the best assessment of the activity of the complexes of the electron transport chain (Figure 47.5, 47.6). In some laboratories these assays are done on frozen muscle or on freshly isolated platelets. The lactate to pyruvate ratio in the blood is usually elevated in electron transport abnormalities, and this abnormality may trigger a muscle biopsy (Figure 47.3). Ragged red fibers suggest analysis of mitochondrial DNA, while their absence suggests assay for nuclear encoded defect in the respiratory chain. These complexes I to V are a mixture of mitochondrial and nuclear encoded proteins.

Figure 47.4   *Structure of L-lactic acid and related compounds.*

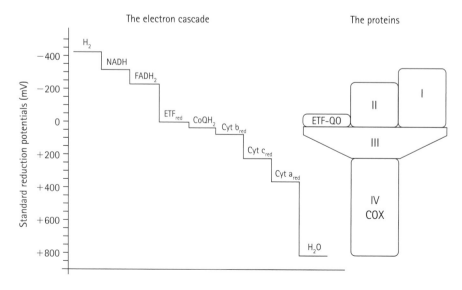

Figure 47.5   *The mitochondrial electron transport chain. Lactic acidemia and an elevated lactate: pyruvate ratio may occur with any defect that interferes with the utilization of NADH, NAD, nicotinamide adenine dinucleotide, and NADH, its flavoprotein; FeS, iron sulfur-containing flavoprotein; CoQ$_{10}$, coenzyme Q10; Cyt, cytochrome.*

Energy conversion takes place in mitochondria in which the exergonic oxidation/reduction reactions of the electron transport chain, as in chloroplasts and bacteria, are coupled to the endergonic synthesis of adenosine triphosphate (ATP) from adenosine diphosphate (ADP) and inorganic phosphate [13]. The electron flow generates a proton motive force. The ATP synthase is a large asymmetric enzyme complex of an F_0F_1 structure, in which the F_0 is a hydrophobic, membrane embedded unit that serves as a proton channel, while the F_1 contains the nucleotide binding sites and catalytic sites for ATP synthesis. When solubilized and uncoupled from its F_0 energy source, the F_1 is capable of ATP hydrolysis, and this is why it is referred to as an ATPase.

The oxidative phosphorylation system is embedded in the lipid bilayer of the mitochondrial inner membrane. In addition to the five multiprotein enzyme complexes there are two electron carriers – coenzyme Q and cytochrome C. The ATP generated by oxidative phosphorylation may be used in the mitochondrion or transported out by the adenine nucleotide transporter for other cellular purposes. Each of the complexes of the electron transport chain except complex II contains proteins encoded by the mitochondrial DNA, as well as proteins encoded by nuclear DNA (Table 47.1). Mitochondrial DNA and its mutations are maternally inherited; nuclear DNA mutations in this system are inherited autosomally.

In addition to mutations in the genes coding for proteins of the electron transport chain, there are mutations causing mitochondrial disease in proteins involved in the assembly and maintenance of mitochondrial proteins. Increasingly mutations are being found in the nuclear encoded functions of oxidative phosphorylation. A majority, so far, have been in

complex I [14–18]. Some of these mutations, which disrupt respiratory chain function, do not produce lactic academia. Knowledge of the nuclear mutation in a family permits accurate prenatal diagnosis, whereas biochemical methods have frequently been in error [19]. Among mutations in genes for proteins involved in the assembly of respiratory chain proteins SURF1, which functions in assembly of complex IV, is probably the best studied [20–22] and produces a severe clinical Leigh syndrome.

Molecular chaperones are required for the assembly of the catalytic F_1 component of the mitochondrial ATP synthase, and probably for many other proteins involved in mitochondrial function. Those for F_1 have been well studied in yeast, and mutations in *Saccharomyces* are known. The human genes

Table 47.1 *The genetic determination of the proteins of the electron transport chain*

Complex	Name	Mitochondrial genes	Nuclear genes	Total
I	NADH: ubiquinone oxidoreductase	7	>44	>51
II	Succinate: ubiquinone oxidoreductase	0	4	4
III	Cytochrome bc	1	>10	>11
IV	Cytochrome c oxidase	3	10	13
V	ATP Synthase	2	14	16
Total		13	>82	>91

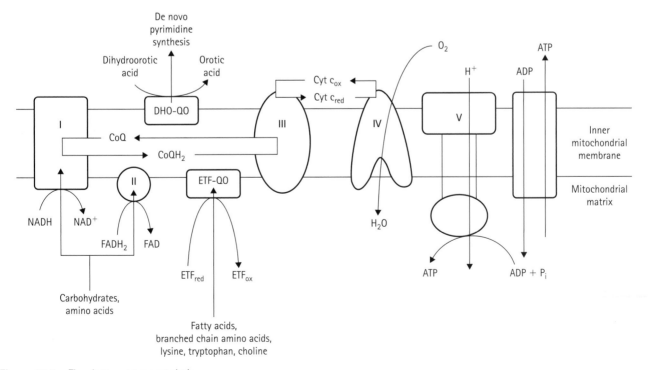

Figure 47.6 *The electron transport chain.*

for orthologs are known. Their study may reveal novel mechanisms of mitochondrial disease.

Mitochondrial proteins synthesized in the cytosol must be transported into the mitochondria. Defects in the transport proteins could provide another novel mechanism of the pathogenesis of mitochondrial disease. Two of these protein complexes, Translocation Outer Mitochondrial Membrane (TOMM) and Translocation Inner Mitochondrial Membrane (TIMM) have been extensively studied in yeast in which the genes have been characterized. The human gene encoding an ortholog of TOMM 20 has been identified [23] and the human genome project has made the genes for other orthologs available. A search for abnormalities causing human disease is under way. Among the transporters of the mitochondria is an outer membrane transporter known as Voltage-Dependent Ion Channel (VDAC) and also known as mitochondrial porin, because it forms a pore, opening the membrane for anions like phosphate, chloride and adenine nucleotides at low transmembrane voltage; at high voltage it forms a channel for cations and uncharged molecules. A deficiency in VDAC has been reported in Western blot studies [24] in a patient with developmental retardation myopathy and impaired oxidation of pyruvate in mitochondria of muscle. Lactate was elevated only mildly after 2 g/kg of glucose.

Patients with evidence of defective activity of many mitochondrial enzymes exemplify the complex nature of the pathogenesis of mitochondrial disease . For instance mitochondrial DNA depletion (Chapter 57) leads to defective activity of most of the complexes of the electron transport chain. Similarly, patients were reported [25] in whom there was defective activity of pyruvate and 2-oxoglutarate dehydrogenase complexes, the reduced form of nicotinamide-adenine dinycleotide (NADH) cytochrome C reductase, succinate dehydrogenase and succinate cytochrome reductase. This fatal disease in three siblings was shown by microcell-mediated transfer to a panel of mouse-human hybrids to be under control of a nuclear gene on chromosome 2 at 2p13-14.

Concentrations of L-lactic acid in body fluids are a function of the concentrations of pyruvate and the ratio of NAD+ to NADH. This may be expressed as:

$$K = \frac{(Lactate)\ (NAD+)}{(Pyruvate)\ (NADH)\ (H+)}$$

When NAD/NADH ratios are constant, changes in lactate concentration are a function only of the metabolism of pyruvate, but the ratio of NAD to NADH reflects the oxidative state of the cell [26]. Hypoxia increases NADH, while oxidation regenerates NAD. The normal ratio of NADH to NAD in aerobic tissues is about 10 to 1, and the ratio of lactate to pyruvate does not normally exceed 15 [27]. The ratio of 3-hydroxybutyrate to acetoacetate may more closely reflect the redox state of the mitochondria. Conditions in which there is an excess of NADH will cause an elevated lactate to pyruvate or 3-hydroxybutyrate to acetoacetate ratio. When the electron transport chain is not functioning well NADH cannot be converted to NAD and hence ATP is not produced. Compensation by conversion of pyruvate to lactate regenerates some NAD.

NADH is the fuel of the cytochrome chain (Figures 47.5, 47.6). Therefore, an abnormality in a cytochrome such as cytochrome c oxidase deficiency [28–30] will lead to abnormalities in these ratios because of diminished utilization of NADH. Defects in the respiratory chain may be demonstrated in cultured fibroblasts as well as in muscle [28,29,31–33] but a group of patients has been described [34–38] in which defects in the respiratory chain in muscle were not demonstrable in fibroblasts. In a patient with fatal neonatal lactic acidosis [39] the ratio of lactate to pyruvate was 136:1. The ratio of 3-hydroxybutyrate to acetoacetate was 42:1. In fibroblasts the conversion of 1-^{14}C-pyruvate and glutamate to $^{14}CO_2$ was defective, and when the cells were incubated with glucose an elevated lactate to pyruvate ratio of 72:1 was observed. In control cells the ratio was 20.1. The ratio of lactate to pyruvate is only useful when the level of lactate is high. The ratio in the CSF may by used, as well as that of the blood.

We regularly employ a modified oral glucose tolerance test in which the standard 1.75 g/kg is monitored by assessment of concentrations of lactate, pyruvate and alanine which may rise as much as four-fold over control levels in a patient with PDHC deficiency. This evidence of glucose intolerance may be useful in designing therapy that avoids carbohydrate and substitutes fat, as well in monitoring the efficacy of therapeutic interventions such as treatment with dichloroacetic acid (DCA).

Fructose loading has been reported [40] useful in assessing in vivo pyruvate dehydrogenase activity and its activation. After a 12 to 24 hour fast, blood samples are drawn for lactate, pyruvate, glucose and insulin before and 45 minutes after an oral load of 1 g/kg of fructose. The test is then repeated after an oral glucose load. The rise in blood pyruvate and lactate was reported to be almost twice as great in the fasted as in the postglucose state, suggesting the conversion of pyruvate dehydrogenase to its active form by glucose feeding. Studies were not reported on actual patients with problems with pyruvate dehydrogenase, and we have not found this to be especially useful. Emiprically an occasional patient has responded to fructose with a marked increase in lactic acid, but as a group the patients with mitochondrial disease have not been reliably distinguishable from control in their response to fructose.

The urinary lactate may be useful in diagnosis [2] and the lactate to creatinine ratio has been employed for this purpose. The normal range is from 0.028 to 0.22. A schematic approach to the use of the blood and urinary lactate in differential diagnosis is shown in Figure 47.7. In congenital lactic acidosis both the blood and urinary lactate should be elevated. However, each may be quite variable in any individual patient. Therefore, it is prudent in a patient suspected of having lactic acidosis to carry out a number of assays at various times.

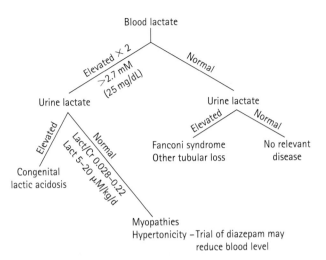

Figure 47.7   *Assessment of lactate in urine as an aid to differential diagnosis of lactic acidemia.*

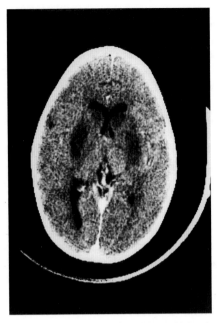

Figure 47.8   *CT scan of the head of a patient with lactic acidemia and Leigh encephalopathy, illustrating advanced degenerative changes in the brain stem as well as the basal ganglia.*

CLINICAL ABNORMALITIES

The clinical manifestations of the congenital lactic acidemias have many similarities regardless of the specific causes. There are a number of distinct clinical syndromes [41,42]. One of them is acute metabolic acidosis; usually neonatal or infantile. Congenital lactic acidosis was first described by Hartman and colleagues in 1962 [43] in patients with this clinical picture. A number of patients have been reported [44,45] in whom the picture is that of recurrent episodes of acidosis with hyperventilation, any one of which may lead to coma and death. Attacks of unexplained vomiting may herald onset. Some patients have acute symptomatic hypoglycemia. This may lead to convulsive seizures, but seizures may also occur in the absence of hypoglycemia. Any patient with chronic lactic acidosis may develop pulmonary hypertension, and this may be the cause of death.

Another presentation, especially in patients in later infancy or childhood, is with ataxia. This may be episodic or chronic. Episodes may be precipitated by stress, such as an intercurrent infection. Between attacks the patient may be clumsy. Often there is associated episodic neurologic degeneration.

Another type of presentation is with Leigh syndrome, or subacute necrotizing encephalomyelopathy [46–48]. This was essentially a histopathologic diagnosis, usually made at autopsy in an ultimately fatal disease. The neuropathologic picture resembles Wernicke encephalopathy in the basal ganglia, brain stem, and cerebellum, but in contradistinction to the picture in Wernicke disease, the mammillary bodies are usually spared. Spongiform degeneration is seen, as are increased vascularity and glial proliferation. Clinical features that lead to the diagnosis include ophthalmoplegia and other cranial nerve signs, respiratory irregularities, a central hypoventilation syndrome, or central apnea.

Computed tomography (CT) or magnetic resonance imaging (MRI) scans now provide the neuroimaging counterpart of the histology with hypodensity in the caudate and putamen [48,49] (Figure 47.8). Ultimately, the patient develops spasticity often with Babinski signs. Seizures occur in about a third of such patients. Blindness may supervene. There may be retinal pigment epithelium changes. Late in the course deep tendon reflexes may be absent. Tracheostomy and artificial ventilation may be required. This picture of Leigh encephalomyelopathy is clearly independent of etiology. It has been described with deficiency of the pyruvate dehydrogenase complex [50], and in a patient with defective activation of the pyruvate dehydrogenase complex because of deficiency of pyruvate dehydrogenase phosphatase [47]. It may be seen in patients with NARP mutation.

We have studied a small subgroup of patients with severe deficiency of the pyruvate dehydrogenase complex (PDHC) in whom there was a recognizable syndrome of dysmorphic features (Chapter 50, p. 325). A sibling had a similar clinical appearance. Our first patient appeared to be cortically-blind in infancy. Another patient had gross abnormalities in the morphogenesis of the brain.

Another group of patients has the picture of a metabolic myopathy or ophthalmoplegia [50–54]. In some there was associated neurodeafness or early cataracts. Two siblings had sideroblastic anemia. Many of these patients have had muscle weakness, usually of insidious onset, in a pattern of a proximal muscular dystrophy. Ptosis, facial muscle weakness and cardiomyopathy have also been seen. Electronmicroscopy may reveal large mitochondria, often with a bizarre appearance. Some patients have ragged, red fiber changes in the histology of muscle. Many of these have had abnormalities in mitochondrial DNA.

TREATMENT

Acute treatment of metabolic acidosis may require large amounts of sodium bicarbonate. Sodium citrate may be ineffective in a patient with an oxidative defect because citric acid cycle function is impaired. Chronic treatment may be undertaken in patients with lactic acidemia prior to the establishment of a definitive diagnosis, provided enough is known about the underlying pathophysiology. Thus, patients with disorders of gluconeogenesis should avoid fasting and require intravenous glucose during intercurrent illnesses in which the oral route is not available, as in the vomiting patient. A diet high in carbohydrate is therapeutic, and cornstarch supplementation may be helpful.

Patients with disorders of oxidation are, in contrast, often glucose-sensitive and respond with reduction in lactate concentrations to a diet high in fat [55]. Diets employed contain 50 percent or more of the calories from fat. They do not have to be ketogenic.

Lactate levels can be lowered in many patients by the administration of dichloroacetate (DCA) regardless of the cause. It is not generally recommended in disorders of gluconeogenesis, because DCA can itself produce hypoglycemia. Its use is being employed experimentally in a variety of other lactic acidemic conditions.

Dichloroacetate activates the PDHC by inhibiting PDH kinase. *In vivo* this compound reduces concentrations of lactate, pyruvate and alanine [56,57], and increases the percentage of the active form of PDHC in brain, liver and muscle. It has been used to treat congenital lactic acidosis [58–60], and levels of lactic acid have been improved. Neurologic improvement has been elusive in most patients reported, but there have been some successes. Peripheral neuropathy can be expected to worsen with DCA, and some patients may develop peripheral neuropathy [61].

References

1   Brown GK, Haan EA, Kirby DM, *et al.* 'Cerebral' lactic acidosis: Defects in pyruvate metabolism with profound brain damage and minimal systemic acidosis. *Eur J Pediatr* 1988;**147**:10.

2   Chalmers RA. Organic acids in urine of patients with congenital lactic acidoses: An aid to differential diagnosis. *J Inherit Metab Dis* 1984;**7**:79.

3   Hoffmann G, Aramaki S, Blum-Hoffmann E, *et al.* Quantitative analysis for organic acids in biological samples: Batch isolation followed by gas chromatographic-mass spectrometric analysis. *Clin Chem* 1989;**35**:587.

4   Thuy LP, Zielinska B, Zammarchi E, *et al.* Multiple carboxylase deficiency due to deficiency of biotinidase. *J Neurogenet* 1986;**3**:357.

5   Vreken P, van Lint AEM, Bootsma AH, *et al.* Rapid diagnosis of organic acidemias and fatty acid oxidation defects by quantitative electrospray tandem-MS acyl-carnitine analysis in plasma: in *Current Views of Fatty Acid Oxidation and Ketogenesis: From Organelles to Point Mutations* (eds PA Quant, S Eaton, Kluwer Academic) Plenum Publishers, New York; 1999:327.

6   Sim KG, Carpenter K, Hammond J, *et al.* Acylcarnitine profiles in fibroblasts from patients with respiratory chain defects can resemble those from patients with mitochondrial fatty acid β-oxidation disorders. *Metabolism* 2002;**51**:366.

7   Enns GM, Bennett MJ, Hoppel CL, *et al.* Mitochondrial respiratory chain complex I deficiency with clinical and biochemical features of long-chain 3-hydroxyacyl-coenzyme A dehydrogenase deficiency. *J Pediatr* 2000;**136**:251

8   Baker L, Winegrad AI. Fasting hypoglycaemia and metabolic acidosis associated with deficiency of hepatic fructose-16-diphosphatase activity *Lancet* 1970;**2**:13.

9   Pagliara AS, Karl IE, Keating JP, *et al.* Hepatic fructose-66-diphosphatase deficiency: a cause of lactic acidosis and hypoglycemia in infancy. *J Clin Invest* 1972;**51**:2115.

10 Perlmutter DH, Boyle JT, Campos JM, *et al.* D-lactic acidosis in children: An unusual metabolic complication of small bowel resection. *J Pediatr* 1983;**102**:234.

11 Garcia J, Smith FR, Cucinell SA. Urinary D-lactate excretion in infants with necrotizing enterocolitis. *J Pediatr* 1984;**104**:268.

12 Chalmers RA, Lawson AM. *Organic Acids in Man. The Analytical Chemistry Biochemistry and Diagnosis of the Organic Acidurias.* Chapman and Hall, London;1982.

13 Abrahams JP, Leslie AGW, Lutter R, Walker JE. Structure at 28 A resolution of F₁-ATPase from bovine heart mitochondria. *Nature* 1994;**370**:621.

14 Smeitink J, van den Heuvel L, DiMauro S. The genetics and pathology of oxidative phosphorylation. *Nature Rev Genet* 2001;**2**:342.

15 van den Huevel L, Ruitenbeek W, Smeets R, *et al.* Demonstration of a new pathogenic mutation in human complex I deficiency: A 5-bp duplication in the nuclear gene encoding the 18-kD (AQDQ) subunit. *Am J Hum Genet* 1998;**62**:262.

16 Triepels RH, van den Huevel LP, Loeffen JL, *et al.* Leigh syndrome associated with a mutation in the NDUFS7 (PSST) nuclear encoded subunit of complex I. *Ann Neurol* 1999;**45**:787.

17 Loeffen J, Smeitink J, Triepels R, *et al.* The first nuclear-encoded complex I mutation in a patient with Leigh syndrome. *Am J Hum Genet* 1998;**63**:1598.

18 Schuelke M, Smeitink J, Mariman E, *et al.* Mutant NDUFV1 subunit of mitochondrial complex I causes leukodystrophy and myoclonic epilepsy. *Nat Genet* 1999;**21**:260.

19 Schuelke M, Detjen A, van den Heuvel L, *et al.* New nuclear encoded mitochondrial mutation illustrates pitfalls in prenatal diagnosis by biochemical methods. *Clin Chem* 2002;**48**:772.

20 Lee N, Morin C, Mitchell G, Robinson BH. Saguenay Lac Saint Jean cytochrome oxidase deficiency: Sequence analysis of nuclear encoded COX subunits chromosomal localization and a sequence anomaly in subunit Vic. *Biochim Biophys Acta* 1998;**1406**:1.

21 Zhu Z, Yao J, Johns T, *et al.* SURF1 encoding a factor involved in the biogenesis of cytochrome c oxidase is mutated in Leigh syndrome. *Nat Genet* 1998;**20**:337.

22 Tiranti V, Hoertnagel K, Carrozzo R, *et al.* Mutations of SURF-1 in Leigh disease associated with cytochrome c oxidase deficiency. *Am J Hum Genet* 1998;**63**:1609.

23 Hernandez JM, Giner P, Hernandez-Yago J. Gene structure of the human mitochondrial outer membrane receptor Tom20 and evolutionary study of its family of processed pseudogenes. *Gene* 1999;**239**:2283.

24 Huizing M, Ruitenbeek W, Thinnes FP, *et al.* Deficiency of the voltage-dependent anion channel: A novel cause of mitochondriopathy. *Pediatr Res* 1996;**39**:760.

25 Seyda A, Newbold RF, Hudson TJ, *et al.* A novel syndrome affecting multiple mitochondrial functions located by microcell-mediated transfer to chromosome 2p14-2p13. *Am J Hum Genet* 2001;**68**:386.

26 Huckabee WE. Relationship of pyruvate and lactate during anerobic metabolism. I Effects of infusion of pyruvate or glucose and hyperventilation. *J Clin Invest* 1958;**37**:244.

27 Cohen RD. Disorders of lactic acid metabolism. *Clin Endocrinol Metabol* 1967;**5**:613.

28 Heiman-Patterson TD, Bonilla E, DiMauro S, *et al*. Cytochrome-c-oxidase deficiency in floppy infant. *Neurology* 1982;**32**:898.

29 Willems JL, Monnens LAH, Trijbels JMF, *et al*. Leigh's encephalomyelopathy in a patient with cytochrome c oxidase deficiency in muscle tissue. *Pediatrics* 1977;**60**:850.

30 Lee N, Daly MJ, Delmonte T, *et al*. A genome-wide linkage-disequilibrium scan localizes the Saguenay-Lac-Saint-Jean cytochrome oxidase deficiency to 2p16. *Am J Hum Genet* 2001;**68**:397.

31 DiMauro S, Mendell JR, Sahenk Z, *et al*. Fatal infantile mitochondrial myopathy and renal dysfunction due to cytochrome-c oxidase deficiency. *Neurology* 1980;**32**:795.

32 VanBiervliet JPGM, Bruinvis L, Ketting D, *et al*. Hereditary mitochondrial myopathy with lactic academia, a DeToni-Fanconi-Debre syndrome and a defective respiratory chain in voluntary striated muscles. *Pediatr Res* 1977;**11**:1088.

33 Miyabayashi S, Nariswar K, Tada K, *et al*. Two siblings with cytochrome-c oxidase deficiency. *J Inherit Metab Dis* 1983;**6**:121.

34 Morgan-Hughes JA, Daveniza P, Kahn SN, *et al*. A mitochondrial myopathy characterized by a deficiency of reducible cytochrome b. *Brain* 1977;**100**:617.

35 Morgan-Hughes JA, Darveniza P, Landon DN, *et al*. A mitochondrial myopathy with deficiency of respiratory chain NADH-CoQ reductase activity. *J Neurol Sci* 1979;**43**:27.

36 Spiro AJ, Moore CE, Pimeas JW, *et al*. A cytochrome related inherited disorder of the nervous system and muscle. *Arch Neurol* 1970;**23**:103.

37 Moreadith RW, Batshaw ML, Ohnishi T, *et al*. Deficiencies of the iron-sulfur clusters of mitochondrial reduced nicotinamide-adenosine dinucleotide-ubiquinone oxidoreductase (complex I) in an infant with congenital lactic acidosis. *J Clin Invest* 1984;**74**:685.

38 Clark JB, Heyes DJ, Buyrne E, Morgan-Hughes JA. Mitochondrial myopathies defects in mitochondrial metabolism in human skeletal muscle. *Biochem Soc Trans* 1983;**11**:626.

39 Robinson BH, McKay N, Toodyer P, Lancaster G. Defective intramitochondrial NADH oxidation in skin fibroblasts from an infant with fatal neonatal lactic academia. *Am J Hum Genet* 1985;**37**:938.

40 Stansbie D, Sherrif RJ, Denton RM. Fructose load test – an *in vitro* screening test designed to assess pyruvate dehydrogenase activity and interconversion. *J Inherit Metab Dis* 1978;**1**:163.

41 Robinson BH, Taylor J, Sherwood WG. The genetic heterogeneity of lactic acidosis: Occurrence of recognizable inborn errors of metabolism in a pediatric population with lactic acidosis. *Pediatr Res* 1980;**14**:956.

42 Munnich A, Rotig A, Cormier-Daire V, Rustin P. Clinical presentation of respiratory chain deficiency: in *The Metabolic and Molecular Bases of Inherited Disease* (eds CR Scriver, AL Beaudet, WS Sly, D Valle). McGraw Hill, New York;2001:2261.

43 Hartman Sr AF, Wohltmann HJ, Puckerson ML, Wesley ME. Lactic acidosis: Studies of a child with a serious congenital deviation. *J Pediatr* 1962;**61**:165.

44 Israel S, Haworth JC, Gourley B, Ford JD. Chronic acidosis due to an error in lactate and pyruvate metabolism. *Pediatrics* 1964;**34**:346.

45 Skrede S, Stromme JH, Stokke O, *et al*. Fatal congenital lactic acidosis in two siblings. II Biochemical studies *in vivo* and *in vitro*. *Acta Paediatr Scand* 1971;**60**:138.

46 Pincus JH. Subacute necrotizing encephalymyelopathy (Leigh's Disease): a consideration of clinical features and etiology. *Develop Med Child Neurol* 1972;**14**:87.

47 DeVivo DC, Haymond MW, Obert KA, *et al*. Defective activation of the pyruvate dehydrogenase complex in subacute necrotizing encephalomyelopathy (Leigh disease). *Ann Neurol* 1979;**6**:483.

48 Schwarz WJ, Hutchinson HT, Berg BO. Computerized tomography in subacute necrotizing encephalomyelopathy (Leigh disease). *Ann Neurol* 1981;**10**:268.

49 Chi JeG, Yoo HW, Chang KY, *et al*. Leigh's subacute necrotizing encephalomyelopathy: Possible diagnosis by CT scan. *Neuroradiology* 1981;**22**:141.

50 Evans OB. Episodic weakness in pyruvate decarboxylase deficiency. *J Pediatr* 1984;**105**:961.

51 Johnston K, Newth CJL, Sheu K-FR, *et al*. Central hypoventilation syndrome in pyruvate dehydrogenase complex deficiency. *Pediatrics* 1984;**74**:1034.

52 Hackett TN Jr, Bray PR, Ziter FA, *et al*. A metabolic myopathy associated with chronic lactic acidemia growth failure and nerve deafness. *J Pediatr* 1973;**83**:426.

53 VanWijngaarden GK, Bethlem J, Meijer AEFH, *et al*. Skeletal muscle disease with abnormal mitochondria. *Brain* 1967;**90**:577.

54 Shapira Y, Cederbaum SD, Cancilla PA, *et al*. Familial poliodystrophy mitochondrial myopathy and lactate academia. *Neurology* 1975;**25**:614.

55 Falk RE, Cederbaum SD, Blass JP, *et al*. Ketogenic diet in the management of pyruvate dehydrogenase deficiency. *Pediatrics* 1976;**58**:713.

56 Kuroda Y, Toshim K, Watanabe T, *et al*. Effects of dichloroacetate on pyruvate metabolism on rat brain *in vivo*. *Pediatr Res* 1984;**18**:936.

57 Stacpoole PW, Moore GW, Kornhauser DM. Metabolic effects of dichloroacetate in patients with diabetes mellitus and hyperlipoproteinemia. *N Eng J Med* 1978;**298**:526.

58 Robinson BH, Taylor J, Francois B, *et al*. Lactic acidosis neurological deterioration and compromised cellular pyruvate oxidation due to a defect in the reoxidation of cytoplasmically generated NADH. *Eur J Pediatr* 1983;**140**:98.

59 Coude FX, Saudubray JM, Demangre F, *et al*. Dichloroacetate as treatment for congenital lactic acidosis. *N Eng J Med* 1978;**299**:1365.

60 McKhann G, Francois B, Evrard P. Long term use of low doses of dichloroacetate in a child with congenital lactic acidosis. *Pediatr Res* 1980;**14**:167.

61 Sprujit L, Naviaux RX, McGowan KA, *et al*. Nerve conduction changes in patients with mitochondrial diseases treated with dichloracetate. *Muscle Nerve* 2001;**24**:916.

Pyruvate carboxylase deficiency

48

MAJOR PHENOTYPIC EXPRESSION

There are three phenotypes in each of which concentrations of lactic acid and alanine are elevated and activity of pyruvate carboxylase is deficient.

- In the simple type common in American Indians: delayed development and infantile episodes of metabolic acidosis with lactic acidemia.
- In the complex type first described from France: severe lactic acidemia, usually fatal in the early months of life, hyperammonemia, citrullinemia and hyperlysinemia.
- In a more benign presentation, episodic acidosis only.

INTRODUCTION

Pyruvate carboxylase (EC 6.4.1.1) is a biotin containing mitochondrial enzyme, which catalyzes the conversion of pyruvate to oxalacetate by CO_2 fixation (Figure 48.1) [1,2]. As in the case of other carboxylases the reaction mechanism is a two-step process in which biotin is first carboxylated and then the carboxyl group is transferred to the acceptor, pyruvate [3,4]. There is a separate catalytic site for each of the two steps. The enzyme is a tetramer of 500 kD whose individual equal-sized protomers have a different structure from other biotin-containing carboxylases [5], but the highly conserved amino acid sequence at the biotin site of biotin-containing carboxylases, Ala-Met-Lys-Met is present in pyruvate carboxylase [6]. The biotin is linked to the ε amino group of the lysine.

Pyruvate carboxylase is an important regulatory enzyme with highly tissue-specific roles. In liver and kidney, where its activity is highest, it catalyzes the first step in gluconeogenesis from pyruvate in which the oxaloacetate formed is converted via phosphoenolpyruvate carboxykinase (PEPCK) to phosphoenolpyruvate and ultimately to glucose and glycogen. It is regulated via acetylCoA, an allosteric activator, and the stimulant ratio of adenosine triphosphate/adenosine diphosphate (ATP/ADP). Conditions under which acetyl groups are generated stimulate gluconeogenesis at this step [7]. In lipogeneic tissues, such as adipose and adrenal, the enzyme participates in the synthesis of acetyl groups and reducing groups for transport into the cytosol. In other tissues such as brain, muscle and fibroblasts it has an anapleurotic role in the formation of oxaloacetate and the maintenance of four carbon intermediates for the citric acid cycle [8]. Anapleurotic is from the Greek verb to fill up. Experience with liver transplantation in this disease [9] (Figure 48.2) indicates that the liver can take over this citric acid cycle-related function for the entire body. In brain the enzyme is active not in neurons, but in astrocytes where it is involved in the synthesis and supply for the neurons of glutamine, a major precursor of the glutamate and 4-aminobutyrate neurotransmitters [10].

Deficiency of pyruvate carboxylase was first described in patients with Leigh syndrome [11–14]. It is now thought that this was a function of instability of this enzyme, especially in material obtained at autopsy. In assays of biopsied liver in six

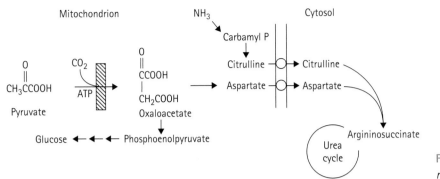

Figure 48.1   *The pyruvate carboxylase reaction.*

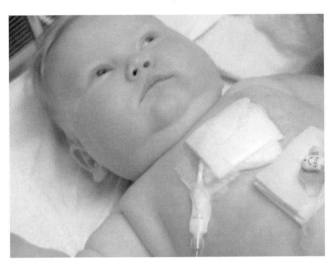

Figure 48.2   *J.M., a 5-month-old infant with pyruvate carboxylase deficiency presented first in coma. He was hypotonic to flaccid and had inverted nipples. Respirations were Kussmaul. Metabolic imbalance was judged incompatible with life, but liver transplantation reversed many features of the disease.*

patients with Leigh syndrome and of cultured fibroblasts in five, pyruvate carboxylase was not deficient [15].

The cDNA for pyruvate carboxylase has been cloned and sequenced and localized to chromosome 11 at q13.4-13.5 [6,16–19]. Absence of mRNA for the enzyme was found in four of six patients with the fatal infantile disease who also lacked pyruvate carboxylase protein [20].

CLINICAL ABNORMALITIES

Complex, French or European form

In the complex, French or European form severe neonatal lactic acidosis is the presenting picture [21,22]. The initial acidosis may be fatal, and many patients have died by 3 months-of-age. Most have hepatomegaly. Metabolic acidosis may lead to dehydration, coma, shock and apnea. This disorder has now been observed in North American, Egyptian and Saudi Arabian patients [9,20,23–25].

The term complex refers to the biochemical findings in this group of patients in whom the occurrence of hyperammonemia and citrullinemia is characteristic [22,24,26]. Hyperlysinemia is also seen, as it is in other hyperammonemic conditions. Hypoglycemia may occur, but it is usually not a major problem. Serum glutamic oxaloacetic transaminase (SGOT) and serum glutamic pyruvic transaminase (SGPT) may be elevated. Concentrations of alanine and proline are high, and there are elevated amounts of 2-oxoglutarate in the urine. Levels of lactate may be very high, and levels of pyruvate are elevated. Abnormal redox balance in which the cytosol is more reducing is indicated by a high ratio of lactate to pyruvate in the blood, while a more oxidizing mitochondrial environment is indicated by a high acetoacetate to 3-hydroxybutyrate ratio [9]. The major metabolic abnormality, significant of citric acid cycle aberration, is the massive ketoacidosis. Ketonuria is prominent.

Simple or American Indian form

In the simple or American Indian form there may be episodes of acute metabolic acidosis with lactic acidemia in the first six months of life, or the first evidence of abnormality may be slowness of development [27–29]. By the first year most are clearly retarded, and many have failure to thrive, vomiting or irritability. This clinical picture has been seen frequently in Saudi Arabia (Figures 48.3–48.8), as well as among American Indians [28]. It has been encountered in North American Caucasians and in Japanese [30]. Macrocephaly has been observed, and subdural effusions (Figures 48.4, 48.5). These effusions have also been encountered in the complex phenotype [9]. Retardation may be severe [27] (Figures 48.5–48.8). Hypoglycemia occurred on fasting for 24 hours at which time the concentration of glucose was 1.8 mMolar and lactate was 6.2 mmol/L, while the 3-hydroxybutyrate was greater than 2 mmol/L. A number of these patients have been ketotic at times of acute acidosis. There was no increase in blood glucose after an alanine load.

Seizures are frequently seen (Figure 48.5). One patient [27] presented at 3 months with fever and mild generalized seizures. Between the ages of 5 and 9 months he was admitted to hospital three times for failure to thrive and developmental delay; on each occasion mild metabolic acidosis was noted,

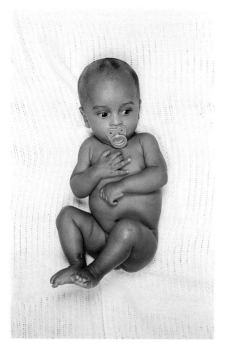

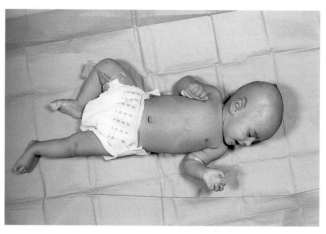

Figure 48.5   O.H., a 6-month-old female infant with pyruvate carboxylase deficiency. She presented at 2 days-of-age with grand mal seizures. The tonic neck posture is normal at this age, but she also had choreoathetosis. She had lactic acidosis and undetectable activity of pyruvate carboxylase.

Figure 48.3   T.Y.A.A.H., a 6-month-old Saudi male infant with pyruvate carboxylase deficiency. He had recurrent episodes of lactic acidosis. Plasma ammonia was normal. Levels of alanine were elevated and proline was moderately elevated. Pyruvate carboxylase in fibroblasts was 11 percent of control.

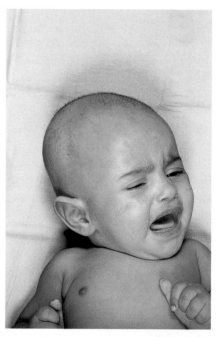

Figure 48.6   O.H. A previous sibling had died of intractable lactic acidosis.

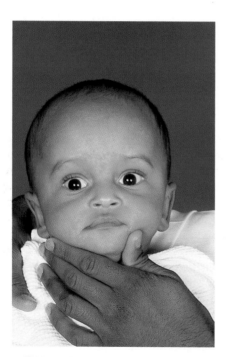

Figure 48.4   T.Y.A.A.H. The head was relatively large, just above 2SD above the mean, while length and weight were below the 50th percentile. An EEG showed diffuse slowing consistent with metabolic encephalopathy, and later he developed seizures. CT scans revealed a subdural effusion. By 2 years-of-age he was spastic and appreciably developmentally delayed.

but not evaluated further. At 9 months he had a severe metabolic acidosis and was diagnosed as having lactic acidemia. The level was 6.5 mmol/L. By 46 months he was microencephalic and severely retarded, unable to sit or feed himself and not interested in his surroundings. He had numerous sudden episodes of lactic acidosis with tachypnea and a blotchy cyanosis of the extremities. He died at that age of pneumonia and severe acidosis. This patient and others in this group had proximal renal tubular acidosis. Renal tubular acidosis has also been encountered in the complex phenotype [9].

Electroencephalography (EEG) may show prominent theta waves and abnormal slow wave activity. Histologic examination

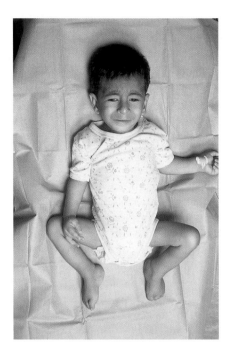

Figure 48.7 *M.S.G., a 16-month-old Saudi male with pyruvate carboxylase deficiency. Tachypnea and acidosis were noted soon after birth. Initial pH was 7.00 and the serum bicarbonate was 5 mEq/L. Lactate was 6.2 mmol/L and alanine 1074 μmol/L; proline was 775 μmol/L. The activity of pyruvate carboxylase in fibroblasts was four percent of the control mean.*

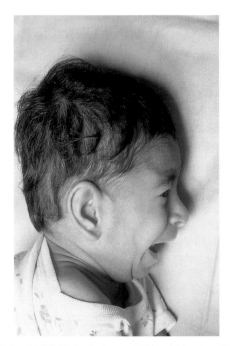

Figure 48.8 *M.S.G. He had microagnathia and hypospadias. By 16 weeks he could not sit unassisted or roll over. At 12 months his head circumference was at the 50th percentile for 4 months; but length was at the same level and weight even further behind. CT scan revealed hypodense periventricular white matter.*

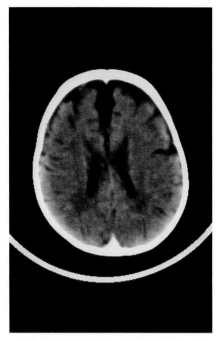

Figure 48.9 *CT scan of the brain of the 5-month-old patient shown in Figures 48.5 and 48.6. There was already marked atrophy of the brain, particularly evident over the frontal lobes. She died shortly after discharge.*

of the brain has shown depletion of neurons and poor myelin formation, as well as increased ventricular size. These changes are evident in neuroimaging (Figure 48.9). Similar findings are seen in the complex form, in which also there may be cavitated infarcts or cortical cysts [21,25]. Histologic examination of the liver in the simple and complex forms reveals steatosis.

Third form of pyruvate carboxylase deficiency

The third form of pyruvate carboxylase deficiency has to date been described in a single patient [31], who had frequent episodic lactic acidosis in infancy. She was otherwise well and developed normally. By 7 years-of-age she had slight dysarthria and learning problems in mathematics. There was no failure to thrive; she was over the 95th percentile for height and weight. Molecular evidence of mutational heterogeneity may ultimately recognize the three phenotypic distinctions as impractical. The metabolic abnormalities found in the complex phenotype are distinctive.

GENETICS AND PATHOGENESIS

All of the forms of pyruvate carboxylase deficiency appear to be inherited in an autosomal recessive fashion. A founder effect has been postulated for the abnormal gene in the Canadian Indians all of whom speak the Algonquin language [32].

Enzyme activity can be measured in lymphocytes and cultured fibroblasts [20,29], as well as tissues. Levels of enyzme activity have been very low, less than five percent of control regardless of phenotype, but some activity is usually measurable even in the most severely affected patients [9]. Assessment of the presence of pyruvate carboxylase enzyme protein has revealed differences. The enzyme can be labeled with ^{3}H-biotin or ^{35}S-streptavidin prior to SDS gel electrophoresis, which reveals a normal 125 kd band in the two milder groups of patients, while no band was detected in the fatal severe neonatal form [20,30]. Immunoprecipitation of ^{35}S-methionine- labeled protein with antibody to normal enzyme indicated absence of the protein in a number, but not all of the patients with this form of the disease. Absence of mRNA for the enzyme was found in four of six patients with this form of the disease when tested by Northern blot assay with a cloned cDNA probe [20].

The cDNA for pyruvate carboxylase codes for 19 exons over 16 kb [33]. In studies of the rat gene, alternative tissue specific transcripts led to greater expression in liver and kidney than in other tissues [34]. Among the Amerindian patients homozygosity for G1828A which changed alanine 610 to threonine, was found in the Ojibwa or Cree, consistent with a founder effect. Carrier rates were as high as 1 in 10. In another group of Amerindians there was a C2229T change, converting methionine 743 to isoleucine.

Heterozygote detection is sometimes possible in a family, but the range of normal is so great that a normal result may be inaccurate [34,35]. At the other extreme an apparent homozygote for the third type of disease with severe chronic lactic acidosis and no other abnormalities displayed 50 percent of control activity [36,37].

Prenatal diagnosis has been accomplished in families at risk [38–40]. In one family in which a sibling had died of severe neonatal disease biotin-labeled enzyme protein was absent in amniocytes.

The pathogenesis of lactic acidemia appears intuitively to be a direct consequence of the failure to metabolize pyruvate by this pathway. Pyruvate does not accumulate, but is rather converted to alanine and lactate. Hypoglycemia has been observed [34] in each of the forms of the disease, and appears likely to be a consequence of a failure of gluconeogenesis.

The complex biochemical picture reminiscent of a defect in the urea cycle appears to result from depletion of intracellular oxaloacetate and aspartate [21,22,26]. Aspartate is a source of the second nitrogen of urea (Figure 48.1); its deficiency would lead to citrullinemia and hyperammonemia. Aspartate also is involved in the shuttle of reducing equivalents from cytosol to mitochondria [41] by which the NAD$^+$/NADH ratio (nicotinamide adenine dinucleotide/reduced nicotinamide adenine dinucleotide) is very oxidized in the cytosol and reduced in mitochondria; its lack would make the cytosol more reduced and the mitochondria more oxidized, as occurs in this phenotype.

Abnormality in the anapleurotic formation of glutamine in astrocytes is consistent with diminished concentrations of glutamine found in autopsied brain of a 3-year-old patient [42]. Glutamine concentrations were low in the plasma and cerebrospinal fluid (CSF) of five living patients. Lactic acid itself may be directly toxic to brain. Depletion of oxaloacetate and interruption of the citric acid cycle would be expected to affect adversely the energy metabolism of the brain.

Experience with liver transplantation [9] has permitted a dissection of pathogenetic features of the disease. Ketoacidosis could be ameliorated by large amounts of intravenous glucose, but enteral glucose was much less effective and large amounts of enteral glucose markedly worsened the lactic acidosis. Orthotopic transplantation of the liver completely abolished life-threatening ketoacidosis, and with it the systemic metabolic acidosis. Thus, it was clear that the acidosis and its enormous requirement for sodium bicarbonate to maintain neutrality is caused by the ketoacidosis, not by the lactic academia, because lactic academia, cerebral lactic acid elevation and lactic aciduria persisted.

The provision of enzyme in the transplanted liver also abolished the abnormal redox state of this disease in which the cytosol is reducing with a high lactate to pyruvate ratio, while the mitochondrial environment is more oxidizing as indicated by a high ratio of acetoacetate to 3-hydroxybutyrate.

Glutamine levels were low and did not improve with liver transplantation. This could reflect a role for glutamine depletion in the cerebral manifestations of this disease. Cerebral depletion of glutamine could affect the replenishment of glutamate and 4-aminobutyrate (GABA) neurotransmitter pools. Liver transplantation ameliorated the lactic academia, but lactic acid concentration in the cerebrospinal fluid remained elevated post-transplantation, and the lactate to pyruvate ratio was unchanged. The central nervous system effects of the disease were not reversed, but there was surprising improvement of function during the first year of follow-up evaluation.

TREATMENT

Metabolic acidosis, and renal tubular acidosis has been treated in most patients with sodium bicarbonate. In acute episodes parenteral fluids are required. A trial of biotin would appear prudent in any patient, but to date no responses have been reported.

Supplementation with aspartic acid appears to be a rational approach to a shortage of oxalacetate [9,27,43]. Treatment appeared to reduce levels of lactate and alanine and the number of acidotic attacks [27], but in our patient, much larger amounts of Na aspartate, along with Na citrate and Na succinate failed to alter the life-threatening ketoacidosis. Glutamine 400 to 800 mg q 4 hr was thought to have diminished the number of acidotic episodes in a patient [27], but the disease proved relentless. Treatment with dichloracetic acid is effective in ameliorating the lactic academia [9].

Hepatic transplantation abolished the renal tubular acidosis, as well as the ketoacidosis. None of the treatments reported have had a major effect on the cerebral features of the disease.

References

1   Utter MF, Barden RE, Taylor BL. Pyruvate carboxylase: An evaluation of the relationships between structure and mechanism and between structure and catalytic activity. *Adv Enzymol* 1975;**42**:1.

2   Scrutton MC, Young MR. Pyruvate carboxylase: in: *The Enzymes* Vol 6 (ed. PD Boyer). Academic Press, New York;1972:1.

3   McClure WR, Lardy HA, Wagner M, Cleland WW. Rat liver pyruvate carboxylase. II Kinetic studies of the forward reaction. *J Biol Chem* 1971;**246**:3579.

4   McClure WR, Lardy HA, Cleland WW. Rat liver pyruvate carboxylase. III Isotopic exchange studies of the first partial reaction. *J Biol Chem* 1971;**246**:3584.

5   Barden RE, Taylor BL, Isohashi F, *et al.* Structural properties of pyruvate carboxylases from chicken liver and other sources. *Proc Nat Acad Sci USA* 1975;**72**:4308.

6   Freytag SW, Collier KJ. Molecular cloning of a cDNA for human pyruvate carboxylase. *J Biol Chem* 1984;**259**:12831.

7   Barrit GJ. Resolution of gluconeogenic flux by pyruvate carboxylase: in *Pyruvate Carboxylase* (eds DB Keech, JC Wallace). CRC Press, Boca Raton FL;1985:141.

8   Lee SH, Davis JE. Carboxylase and decarboxylation reactions anapleurotic flux and removal of citric acid cycle intermediates in skeletal muscle. *J Biol Chem* 1979;**254**:420.

9   Nyhan WL, Khanna A, Barshop BA, *et al.* Pyruvate carboxylase deficiency: insights from liver transplantation. *Mol Genet and Metab* 2002;**77**:143.

10   Shank RP, Bennett GS, Freytag SO, Campbell GL. Pyruvate carboxylase: an astrocyte-specific enzyme implicated in the replenishment of amino acid neurotransmitter pools. *Brain Res* 1985;**329**:364.

11   Hommes FA, Polman HA, Reerink JD. Leigh's encephalomyelopathy: an inborn error of gluconeogenesis. *Arch Dis Child* 1968;**43**:423.

12   Moosa A, Hughes EA. Proceedings: L-glutamine therapy in Leigh's encephalomyelopathy. *Arch Dis Child* 1974;**49**:246.

13   Van Biervliet JP, Duran M, Wadman SK, *et al.* Leigh's disease with decreased activities of pyruvate carboxylase and pyruvate decarboxylase. *J Inherit Metab Dis* 1980;**2**:15.

14   Gilbert EF, Arya S, Chun R. Leigh's necrotizing encephalopathy with pyruvate carboxylase deficiency. *Arch Pathol Lab Med* 1983;**107**:126.

15   Murphy JV, Isohashi F, Weinberg MB, Utter MF. Pyruvate carboxylase deficiency: an alleged biochemical cause of Leigh's disease. *Pediatrics* 1981;**68**:401.

16   Lamhonwah A, Quan F, Gravel RA. Sequence homology around biotin-binding site of human propionyl-CoA carboxylase and pyruvate carboxylase. *Arch Biochem Biophys* 1987;**254**:631.

17   Lim F, Morris CP, Occhiodoro F, Wallace JC. Sequence and domain structure of yeast pyruvate carboxylase. *J Biol Chem* 1988;**263**:11493.

18   Zhang J, Xia W-L, Brew K, Ahmand F. Adipose pyruvate carboxylase: amino acid sequence and domain structure deduced from cDNA sequencing. *Proc Natl Acad Sci USA* 1993;**90**:1766.

19   Walker ME, Baker E, Wallace JC, Sutherland GR. Assignment of the human pyruvate carboxylase gene (PC) to 11q134 by fluorescence *in situ* hybridization. *Cytogenet Cell Genet* 1995;**69**:187.

20   Robinson BH, Oei J, Saudubray JM, *et al.* The French and North American phenotypes of pyruvate carboxylase deficiency. Correlation with biotin containing protein by ^{3}H-biotin incorporation ^{35}S-streptavidin labeling and Northern blotting with a cloned cDNA probe. *Am J Hum Genet* 1987;**40**:50.

21   Saudubray JM, Marsac C, Charpentier C, *et al.* Neonatal congenital lactic acidosis with pyruvate carboxylase deficiency in two siblings. *Acta Paediatr Scand* 1976;**65**:717.

22   Coude FX, Ogier H, Marsac C, *et al.* Secondary citrullinemia with hyperammonemia in four neonatal cases of pyruvate carboxylase deficiency. *Pediatrics* 1981;**68**:914.

23   Bartlett K, Ghneim HK, Stirk JH, *et al.* Pyruvate carboxylase deficiency. *J Inherit Metab Dis* 1984;**7**:74.

24   Greter J, Gustafsson J, Holme E. Pyruvate carboxylase deficiency with urea cycle impairment. *Acta Paediatr Scand* 1985;**74**:982.

25   Wong LTK, Davidson GF, Applegarth DA, *et al.* Biochemical and histologic pathology in an infant with cross-reacting material (negative) pyruvate carboxylase deficiency. *Pediatr Res* 1986;**20**:274.

26   Charpentier C, Tetau JM, Ogier H, *et al.* Amino acid profile in pyruvate carboxylase deficiency: Comparison with some other metabolic disorders. *J Inherit Metab Dis* 1982;**5**:(suppl 1) 11.

27   Atkin BM, Buist NR, Utter MF, *et al.* Pyruvate carboxylase deficiency and lactic acidosis in a retarded child without Leigh's disease. *Pediatr Res* 1979;**13**:109.

28   Haworth JC, Robinson BH, Perry TL. Lactic acidosis due to pyruvate carboxylase deficiency. *J Inherit Metab Dis* 1981;**4**:57.

29   DeVivo DC, Haymond MW, Leckie MP, *et al.* The clinical and biochemical implications of pyruvate carboxylase deficiency. *J Clin Endocrinol Metab* 1977;**45**:1281.

30   Robinson BH, Oei J, Sherwood WG, *et al.* The molecular basis for the two different clinical presentations of classical pyruvate carboxylase deficiency. *Am J Hum Genet* 1984;**36**:283.

31   Van Coster RN, Fernhoff PM, DeVivo DC. Pyruvate carboxylase deficiency: A benign variant with normal development. *Pediatr Res* 1991;**30**:1.

32   Robinson BH. Lactic acidemia: biochemical clinical and genetic considerations: in *Advances in Human Genetics* (eds H Harris, K Hirschborn). Plenum Press, New York;1989:151.

33   Carbone MA, MacKay N, Ling M, *et al.* Amerindian pyruvate carboxylase deficiency is associated with two distinct missense mutations. *Am J Hum Genet* 1998;**62**:1312.

34   Jitrapakdee S, Booker GW, Cassady AI, Wallace JC. The rat pyruvate carboxylase gene structure. Alternate promoters generate multiple transcripts with the 5-end heterogeneity. *J Biol Chem* 1997;**272**:20522.

35   Gravel RA, Robinson BH. Biotin-dependent carboxylase deficiencies (propionyl-CoA and pyruvate carboxylase). *Ann NY Acad Sci* 1985;**447**:225.

36   Hansen TL, Christensen E, Willems JL, Trijbels JMF. A mutation of pyruvate carboxylase in fibroblasts from a patient with severe chronic lactic academia. *Clin Chim Acta* 1983;**131**:39.

37   Brunette MG, Delvin E, Hazel B, Scriver CR. Thiamine-responsive lactic acidosis in a patient with deficient low K_m pyruvate carboxylase activity in liver. *Pediatrics* 1972;**50**:702.

38   Marsac C, Augerau GL, Feldman G, *et al.* Prenatal diagnosis of pyruvate carboxylase deficiency. *Clin Chim Acta* 1982;**119**:121.

39   Robinson BH, Toon JR, Petrova-Benedict R, *et al.* Prenatal diagnosis of pyruvate carboxylase deficiency. *Prenat Diagn* 1985;**5**:67.

40   Tsuchiyama A, Oyanagi K, Hirano S, *et al.* A case of pyruvate carboxylase deficiency with later prenatal diagnosis of an unaffected sibling. *J Inherit Metab Dis* 1983;**6**:85.

41   Robinson BH, Halperin ML. Transport of reduced nicotinamide adenine dinucleotide into mitochondria of white adipose tissue. *Biochem J* 1985;**116**:229.

42   Perry TL, Haworth JC, Robinson BH. Brain amino acid abnormalities in pyruvate carboxylase deficiency. *J Inherit Metab Dis* 1985;**8**:63.

43   Ahmad A, Kahler SG, Kishnani PS, *et al.* Treatment of pyruvate carboxylase deficiency with high doses of citrate and aspartate. *Am J Med Genet* 1999;**87**:331.

Fructose-1,6-diphosphatase deficiency

MAJOR PHENOTYPIC EXPRESSION

Hypoglycemia, lactic acidosis and deficiency of hepatic fructose-1,6-diphosphatase.

INTRODUCTION

Deficiency of fructose-1,6-diphosphatase (FDP) (fructose-1,6-bisphosphatase) was first recognized in 1970 by Baker and Winegrad [1], in a girl with hypoglycemia and metabolic acidosis. A sibling had died of a similar illness. In subsequent reports in 1971 by Baerlocher, Gitzelmann and colleagues [2]

and by Hulsmann and Fernandez [3], there were multiple affected siblings of consanguineous matings.

The enzyme FDP (EC 3.1.3.11) provides an essential step in the pathway of gluconeogenesis (Figure 49.1). The enzyme catalyzes the irreversible conversion of fructose-1,6-diphosphate to fructose-6-phosphate. Another enzyme, phosphofructokinase, and adenosine triphosphate (ATP) are required to take this reaction in the reverse direction. The enzyme is most

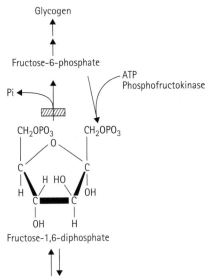

Figure 49.1 *The fructose-1,6-disphosphatase reaction and its role in gluconeogenesis. The conversion of fructose-6-phosphate to fructose-1,6-diphosphate in glycolysis is catalyzed by another enzyme, 6-phosphofructose-1-kinase.*

active in liver and kidney; and the liver enzyme is highly regulated [4]. Deficiency has most often been documented in biopsied liver. The cDNA of the rat enzyme has been cloned [5]. The common mutation in Japanese people is an insertion, 960–961insG [6], which was also the most frequent mutation in a non-Japanese population [7,8]. This mutation causes a frameshift and premature chain termination, as does 966del, and expression studies have shown both to be pathogenic. The disease is clearly genetically heterogeneous, and a variety of other mutations have been found.

CLINICAL ABNORMALITIES

FDP deficiency is a cause of life-threatening metabolic acidosis in the neonatal period. A history of a previous sibling who died in acidosis has often been the alerting episode that led to early diagnosis and survival in the subsequent affected infant [1, 2]. Onset in about 50 percent of patients is between 1 and 4 days-of-age. Most of the patients present before 6 months. An exception first developed symptoms at 4 years-of-age [9].

The first symptom in the neonatal presentation is usually hyperventilation. There may be irritability, but progression is usually rapid to somnolence, coma, apnea and cardiac arrest [2]. Physical examination may reveal tachycardia and hepatomegaly. Laboratory evaluation reveals hypoglycemia, severe acidosis and lactic acidemia [10]. The episode usually responds well to vigorous therapy with parenteral fluids containing glucose and sodium bicarbonate (Figures 49.2, 49.3).

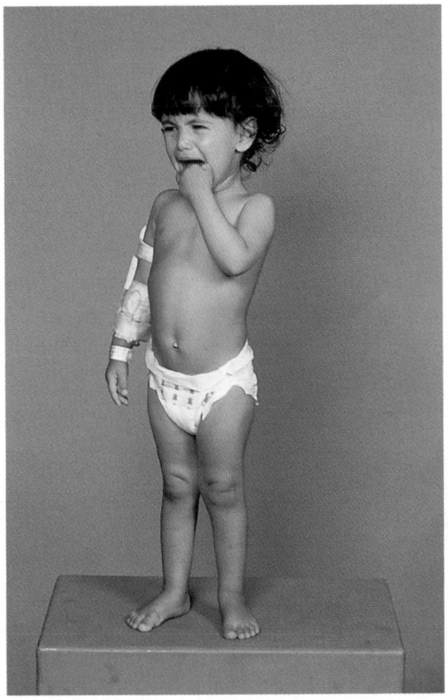

Subsequent episodes usually follow fasting, usually precipitated by intercurrent infections. Onset may be with vomiting and anorexia; attendant fasting leads to hypoglycemia and metabolic acidosis. In one patient, episodes of hyperventilation began when the infant was weaned and baby foods were begun at 6 months-of-age [10]; on admission she was hypoglycemic, and the lactic acid concentration was 20 mmol/L. Patients have been described as ketotic, and the urinary test for ketones is often 1+ to 2+ positive during the acute episode, but the disease has been classified among hypoketotic causes of metabolic acidosis and coma [11]. In the absence of gluconeogenesis, ketones would be expected to accumulate as soon as hepatic glycogen is depleted, and the usual crisis is associated with ketosis. Vomiting is not a common response to fructose, and patients do not have the aversion to fruit and its products, seen regularly in hereditary fructose intolerance. Nor do they develop proximal renal tubular dysfunction after fructose, as do the former patients.

Hepatomegaly develops regularly in infancy, but there are usually no signs of liver disease [11,12]. Neonatal hyperbilirubinemia of a severity requiring exchange transfusion was reported in three infants [13]. Failure to thrive may be seen rarely.

There may be convulsions or other manifestations of hypoglycemia. There may be flushing [2], or pallor and sweating. Vomiting may be complicated by hematemesis [14,15]. Hypotonia and muscle weakness have been observed. The electroencephalograph (EEG) may be abnormal during the acute attack and normal later. Fast spindle-shaped bursts on a slow amplitude pattern have been described [2], as well as a slow wave pattern [16]. Intellectual development is usually normal (Figures 49.2, 49.3). Of course, retardation, as well as death may

Figure 49.2   *N.M., an infant with fructose-1,6-diphosphatase deficiency. She did not have neonatal hypoglycemia. Her first episodes occurred following exposure to fruit juices in the infant's diet.*

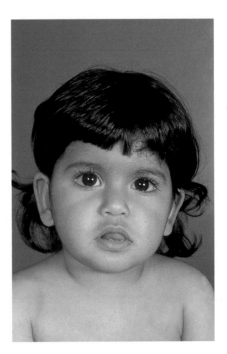

Figure 49.3   *N.M. Close-up of the face, an appearance consistent with her normal intelligence.*

accompany neonatal or early infantile hypoglycemic crises, but fasting tolerance improves with age, and patients normal by childhood usually develop normally. Analysis of the blood reveals, in addition to the lactic acidemia, increased concentrations of alanine and uric acid [17]. In some attacks there may be acidosis without hypoglycemia. Glycerol and glycerol-3-phosphate have been found in the urine [18,19].

GENETICS AND PATHOGENESIS

The disease is transmitted in an autosomal recessive fashion. There is no ethnic predominance. Consanguinity was observed early [2,3]. Most reports have been of Europeans, but there have been reports from the United States, Japan and Lebanon [10,20–25], and among the European families in one series a majority were Turkish [25]. Among nine patients from six families in Israel, two families were Jewish, three Arabic and one Druze [26]. The disease is common in Saudi Arabia, where 14 patients were reported [27]. Parents of patients have been documented to have intermediate levels of FDP activity in liver [14,28]. Testing for heterozygosity by assay of the enzyme in leukocytes may be unreliable. Prenatal diagnosis and heterozygote detection can be accomplished if the mutation is known.

The defective enzyme in patients has usually been identified in the assay of biopsied liver [1–3,29]; a majority of patients have little or no activity. Others have 20 percent or less of control activity. The enzyme is also active in kidney [3,15] and jejunum [30], and the defect has been identified in both these tissues. Assay of leukocytes is controversial, and the activity in normal individuals is quite low. The enzyme is not expressed in fibroblasts or amniocytes. The defect has been documented in tissues obtained at autopsy, but the results must be interpreted with caution because of rapid inactivation of the enzyme with autolysis [31]. The documentation of FDP enzyme activity in muscle in patients in whom activity was deficient in liver and kidney indicates that the enzyme in muscle is coded by a different gene [10,15]. Diagnosis has generally required the assay of the enzyme in biopsied liver, but mutational analysis may permit its avoidance. The enzyme in blood is expressed only in monocytes. Culture of monocytes in media rich in calcitriol has been reported [32] to permit the diagnosis by enzyme assay.

The gene FBP1 on chromosome 9 has 7 exons over 31 kb. The insG960-961 accounted for 46 percent of 22 mutant alleles in Japanese and 14 of 28 mutant alleles in non-Japanese [7]. Its frequency in diverse populations suggests a propensity for mutation. Frameshift was also observed with 807delG and 704–705insC [7]. Point mutations included A177D, N213K and G294V [7,32]. In a small number of patients a concerted search for mutation has failed to reveal any [6]; the possibility of mutation in a promoter region has been suggested.

Deficient activity of FDP interferes with gluconeogenesis, making the patient dependent on exogenous sources of glucose. The fasting that normal infants often undergo in the first days of life makes for a neonatal presentation in patients with little residual enzyme activity [33]. If tested with a provocative fast, patients become hypoglycemic when stored glycogen is exhausted. This may occur in a few hours in an infant [15], or after 14 to 20 hours in an older patient [1,2,15,34]. Depletion of glycogen previously synthesized from glucose by injection of glucagon early in the fast ensures that gluconeogenesis is being tested adequately (Chapter 47, pp. 304 and 305) [10]. The fed state response to glucagon may be normal. Administration of glucagon after the development of hypoglycemia leads to no glycemic response. In FDP deficiency, hypoglycemia induced by fasting is accompanied by increases in levels of lactate, pyruvate and alanine [2,15,34], along with acetoacetate and 3-hydroxybutyrate. Hypoglycemia may also be generated by a diet low in carbohydrate and high in protein and fat [10].

Fructose loading yields evidence of fructose intolerance. This test has been employed in patients judged on the basis of the response to fasting to have lactic acidemia, due to a defect in gluconeogenesis (Chapter 47), in order to suggest that the enzyme be assayed on biopsied liver. It should, nevertheless, be undertaken with caution, as there is risk of severe reaction. An intravenous test is preferred unless hereditary fructose intolerance can be excluded, although patients with FDP deficiency do not develop intestinal symptoms after an oral load [1,2]. The preferred intravenous dose is 200 mg/kg [31,35]. The response is dose-related. A patient became comatose after 500 mg/kg IV [16]. Following fructose, the blood sugar drops to hypoglycemic levels within 15 minutes; lactic acidemia and increased levels of alanine and uric acid accompany systemic acidosis. Fructose administration may induce hyperuricemia and uricosuria even in normal individuals, and the accumulated uric acid results from degradation of adenine nucleotides, following the utilization of ATP in the fructokinase reaction; phosphorus depletion results from the rephosphorylation of adenosine diphosphate (ADP).

These patients are also intolerant of glycerol and sorbitol. Glycerol loading leads to a response similar to that with fructose [1,7,30,36]. Concentrations of phosphate also fall. Sorbitol has been infused to treat cerebral edema; in a child not realized to have FDP deficiency and thought to have cerebral edema, repeated infusions of sorbitol were lethal [28]. Patients with FDP deficiency have normal tolerance of galactose.

TREATMENT

Treatment of the acute episode of hypoglycemia and lactic acidosis is the prompt administration of generous amounts of fluid, sodium bicarbonate and glucose. The episode usually responds readily. Avoidance of fasting is an important element of subsequent management, and if the oral route is temporarily compromised by vomiting, or intercurrent illness, an intravenous supply of glucose is mandatory.

Table 49.1 *Carbohydrate content of common medications (modified from Bosso et al. [37])*

Medication	Presentation	Sugar form	Manufacturer
ADC	Drops	Sucrose	Parke-Davis
Actifed	Syrup	Sucrose	Burroughs-Wellcome
Amcill 250	Suspension	Sucrose	Parke-Davis
Benadryl	Elixir	Sucrose	Parke-Davis
Betapen-VK	Solution	Glucose	Bristol
Cascara Sagrada Aromatic Fluid-extract	Liquid (FE 536)	Sucrose	Parke-Davis
Chlor-Trimeton	Syrup	Sucrose	Schering
Compazine	Syrup	Sucrose	Smith, Kline & French
Compocillin-VK	Drops	Sucrose	Abbott
Dilantin-30	Suspension	Sucrose	Smith, Kline & French
Erythrocin	Drops	Sucrose	Mead Johnson
Fer-in-sol	Syrup	Sucrose	Abbott
Gantrisin	Syrup	Sucrose	Roche
Ilosone 125	Liquid	Sucrose	Lilly
Keflex	Suspension	Sucrose	Lilly
Lomotil	Liquid	Sucrose	Searle
Phenobarbital	Elixir	Sucrose	Lilly
Polycillin	Suspension	Sucrose	Philips Roxane
Robicillin VK 125	Solution	Sucrose	Robins
Robitussin	Syrup	Glucose and sucrose	Robins
Sudafed	Syrup	Sucrose	Burroughs-Wellcome
Tylenol	Elixir	Sucrose	McNeil

Dietary fructose and sucrose are avoided. In most patients they do not have to be absolutely eliminated. Rather, the individual tolerance of the patient can be explored cautiously [14], while soft drinks that provide a sucrose or fructose load should be avoided. Lists are available [37] that provide the sugar content and its nature of medicinal liquids. An abbreviated list is shown in Table 49.1. Patients, families and physicians should particularly be warned about antibiotic elixirs or tylenol syrup which tend to be prescribed when the patient is already metabolically compromised with infection and vomiting-related fasting.

With treatment, hepatomegaly recedes. Subsequent episodes can largely be avoided or aborted. Tolerance to fasting improves with age [1].

References

1 Baker L, Winegrad AI. Fasting hypoglycemia and metabolic acidosis associated with deficiency of hepatic fructose-1,6-diphosphatase activity. *Lancet* 1970;**2**:13.

2 Baerlocher K, Gitzelmann R, Nussli R, Dumermuth G. Infantile lactic acidosis due to hereditary fructose-1,6-diphosphatse deficiency. *Helv Paediatr Acta* 1971;**26**:489.

3 Hulsmann WC, Fernandez J. A child with lactic acidemia and fructose-1,6-diphosphatase deficiency in the liver. *Pediatr Res* 1971;**5**:633.

4 Benkovic SJ, Demaine MM. Mechanism of action of fructose-1,6-bisphosphatase. *Adv Enzymol* 1982;**53**:45.

5 El-Maghrabi MR, Pilkis J, Marker AJ, *et al*. cDNA sequence of rat liver fructose-1,6-bisphosphatase and evidence for down-regulation of its mRNA by insulin. *Proc Natl Acad Sci USA* 1988;**85**:8430.

6 Kikawa Y, Inuzuka M, Jin BY, *et al*. Identification of genetic mutations in Japanese patients with fructose-1,6-bisphosphatase deficiency. *Am J Hum Genet* 1997;**61**:852.

7 Herzog B, Morris AAM, Saunders C, Eschrich K. Mutation spectrum in patients with fructose-1,6-bisphosphatase deficiency. *J Inherit Metab Dis* 2001;**24**:87.

8 Herzog B, Wendel U, Morris AAM, Eschrich K. Novel mutations in patients with fructose-1,6-bisphosphatase deficiency. *J Inherit Metab Dis* 1999;**22**:132.

9 De PráM, Laudanna E. La malattia di Baker-Winegard. *Minerva Pediatr* 1978;**30**:1973.

10 Pagliara AS, Karl IE, Keating JP, *et al*. Hepatic fructose-1,6-diphosphatase deficiency. A cause of lactic acidosis and hypoglycemia in infancy. *J Clin Invest* 1972;**51**:2115.

11 Saudubray JM, Charpentier C. Clinical phenotypes: diagnosis/algorithms: in *The Metabolic and Molecular Bases of Inherited Disease* (eds CR Scriver, AL Beaudet, WS Sly, D Valle) McGraw Hill, New York;1995:327.

12 Eagle RB, MacNab AJ, Ryman BE, Strang LB. Liver biopsy data on a child with fructose-1,6-diphosphatase deficiency that closely resembled many aspects of glucose-6-phosphatase deficiency (Von Gierke's type 1 glycogen-storage disease). *Biochem Soc Trans* 1974;**2**:1118.

13 Buhrdel P, Bohme H-J, Didt L. Biochemical and clinical observations in four patients with fructose-1,6-diphosphatase deficiency. *Eur J Pediatr* 1990;**149**:574.

14 Saudubray J-M, Dreyfus J-C, Cepanec C, *et al*. Acidose lactique hypoglycémie et hépatomégalie par deficit héréditaire en fructose-1,6-diphosphatase hépatique. *Arch Fr Pédiatr* 1973;**30**:609.

15 Melancon SB, Khacadurian AK, Nadler HL, Brown BI. Metabolic and biochemical studies in fructose-1,6-diphosphatase deficiency. *J Pediatr* 1973;**82**:650.

16 Corbeel L, Eggermont E, Eeckels R, *et al*. Recurrent attacks of ketotic acidosis associated with fructo-1,6-diphosphatase deficiency. *Acta Paediatr Belg* 1976;**29**:29.

17 Hopwood NJ, Holzman I, Drash AL. Fructose-1,6-diphosphatase deficiency. *Am J Dis Child* 1977;**131**:418.

18 Dremsek PA, Sacher M, Stögmann W, *et al*. Fructose-1,6-diphosphatase deficiency: glycerol excretion during fasting test. *Eur J Pediatr* 1985;**144**:203.

19 Krywawych S, Katz G, Lawson AM, *et al*. Glycerol-3-phosphate excretion in fructose-1,6-diphosphatase deficiency. *J Inherit Metab Dis* 1986;**9**:388.

20 Kinugasa A, Kusunoki T, Iwashima A. Deficiency of glucose-6-phosphate dehydrogenase found in a case of hepatic fructose-1,6-diphosphatase deficiency. *Pediatr Res* 1979;**13**:1361.

21 Ito M, Kuroda Y, Kobashi H, *et al*. Detection of heterozygotes for fructose-1,6-diphosphatase deficiency by measuring frucstose-1,6-diphosphatase activity in their cultured peripheral lymphocytes. *Clin Chim Acta* 1984;**141**:27.

22 Nakai A, Shigematsu Y, Liu YY, *et al*. Urinary sugar phosphates and related organic acids in fructose-1,6-diphosphatase deficiency. *J Inherit Metab Dis* 1993;**16**:408.

23 Nagai T, Yokoyama T, Hasegawa T, *et al*. Fructose and glucagon loading in siblings with fructose-1,6-diphosphatase deficiency in fed state. *J Inherit Metab Dis* 1992;**15**:720.

24   Alexander D, Assaf M, Khudr A, *et al.* Fructose-1,6-diphosphatase deficiency: diagnosis using leukocytes and detection of heterozygotes with radiochemical and spectrophotometric method. *J Inherit Metab Dis* 1985;**8**:147.

25   Gitzelmann R, Baerlocher K, Prader A. Hereditäre Störungen im Fructose- und Galaktosestoffwechsel. *Monatsschr Kinderheilkd* 1973;**121**:174.

26   Moses SW, Bashan N, Flasterstein BF, *et al.* Fructose-1,6- diphosphatase deficiency in Israel. *Isr Med J* 1991;**27**:1.

27   Rashed M, Ozand PT, Al Aqeel A, Gascon GG. Experience of King Faisal Specialist Hospital and Research Center with Saudi organic acid disorders. *Brain Dev* 1994;**16**:(suppl) 1.

28   Baerlocher K, Gitzelmann R, Steinmann B. Clinical and genetic studies of disorders in fructose metabolism: in: *Inherited Disorders of Carbohydrate Metabolism* (eds D Burman, JB Holton, CA Pennock). Lancaster, MTP;1980:163.

29   Gitzelmann R. Enzymes of fructose and galactose metabolism: galactose-1-phosphate: in *Clinical Biochemistry: Principles and Methods* (eds H-C Curtius, M Roth) Gruyter, Berlin;1974:1236.

30   Greene HL, Stifel FB, Herman RH. 'Ketotic hypoglycemia' due to hepatic fructose-1,6- diphosphatase deficiency. *Am J Dis Child* 1972;**124**:415.

31   Steinmann B, Gitzelmann R. The diagnosis of hereditary fructose intolerance. *Helv Paediatr Acta* 1981;**36**:297.

32   Kikawa Y, Shin YS, Inuzuka M, *et al.* Diagnosis of fructose-1,6-bisphosphatase deficiency using cultured lymphocyte fraction: A secure and noninvasive alternative to liver biopsy. *J Inherit Metab Dis* 2002;**25**:41.

33   Pagliara AS, Karl IE, Hammond M, Kipnis DM. Hypoglycemia in infancy and childhood. Parts I and II. *J Pediatr* 1973;**82**:365, 558.

34   Rallison ML, Meikle AW, Zigrang WD. Hypoglycemia and lactic acidosis associated with fructose-1,6-diphosphatase deficiency. *J Pediatr* 1979;**94**:933.

35   Steinmann B, Gitzelmann R. Fruktose und sorbitol in infusionsflüssigkeiten sind nicht immer harmlos. *Int J Vitam Nutr Res Suppl* 1976;**15**:289.

36   Odièvre M, Brivet M, Moatti N, *et al.* Déficit en fructose-1,6-diphosphatase chez deux soeurs. *Arch Fr Pédiatr* 1975;**32**:113.

37   Bosso JA, Pearson RE. Sugar content of selected liquid medicinals. *Diabetes* 1973;**22**:776.

50

Deficiency of the pyruvate dehydrogenase complex (PDHC)

MAJOR PHENOTYPIC EXPRESSION

Acute, potentially lethal metabolic acidosis, hyperventilation, Leigh syndrome, hypotonia, ataxia, failure to thrive or developmental retardation, elevated concentrations of lactic and pyruvic acids and alanine in blood, urine and cerebrospinal fluid; and defective activity of the pyruvate dehydrogenase complex.

INTRODUCTION

PDHC is a mitochondrial multienzyme system that catalyzes the oxidation of pyruvate to CO_2 and acetyl CoA and concomitantly generates reduced nicotinamide adenine dinucleotide (NADH) (Figure 50.1) [1]. Cofactors include thiaminepyrophosphate (TPP), lipoic acid, coenzyme A (CoA), flavine adenine dinucleotide (FAD) and nicotinamide adenine dinucleotide (NAD+); Mg2+ is required. There are six different protein components, in five of which human deficiency disease has been documented. The three basic components (E1, E2 and E3) are functional catalytic proteins, of types that are shared by all oxoacid dehydrogenases.

The reaction catalyzed by E1, the first enzyme in the complex (EC 1.2.4.1), which has been referred to as pyruvate decarboxylase (PDC) and even pyruvate dehydrogenase (PDH) and contains TPP, is the oxidative decarboxylation of pyruvate to CO_2 and the linkage of the remaining two-carbon unit to TPP to form a hydroxyethylthiamine pyrophosphate attached to the enzyme (TTP-E1).

The second enzyme, E2 (EC 2.3.1.12), dihydrolipoyl transacetylase, is an acyl transferase; it catalyzes the transfer of the hydroxyethyl group and its oxidation to acetyl CoA (Figure 50.1). Concomitantly, the disulfide bridge of the lipoic acid moiety attached to E2 is reduced to the SH form.

This attached dihydrolipoic acid is reoxidized in the reaction catalyzed by the E3 enzyme, dihydrolipoyl dehydrogenase or lipoamide dehydrogenase (EC 1.6.4.3). The same E3 component is shared by 2-oxoglutarate dehydrogenase and the branched-chain ketoacid decarboxylase, providing a mechanism for patients who have defective activity in all three systems [2] (Chapter 51). In PDHC a lipoyl-containing catalytic protein has been referred to as protein X, which also functions in acyl transfer [3,4]. Lipoic acid is attached to the E2 or X protein covalently to lysine moieties. Protein X may also serve in binding E3 to the rest of the complex [5].

Regulation of PDHC involves covalent modification of the protein to produce active and inactive forms. The active form is the dephosphorylated one, and this reaction is catalyzed by a specific phosphatase (PDH phosphatase). A few patients, including an infant with fatal infantile lactic acidemia, have been described in whom the inactive enzyme could not be dephosphorylated because PDH phosphatase activity was deficient [6]. Phosphorylation is catalyzed by a specific kinase, PDH kinase. Additional regulation of PDHC is via end-product inhibition by NADH and acetyl CoA [1,7]. Insulin also activates the enzyme, by fostering the prevalence of the dephosphorylated form. Dichloroacetic acid (DCA) inhibits the kinase, thus keeping the gate to the citric acid cycle locked in the open position [8].

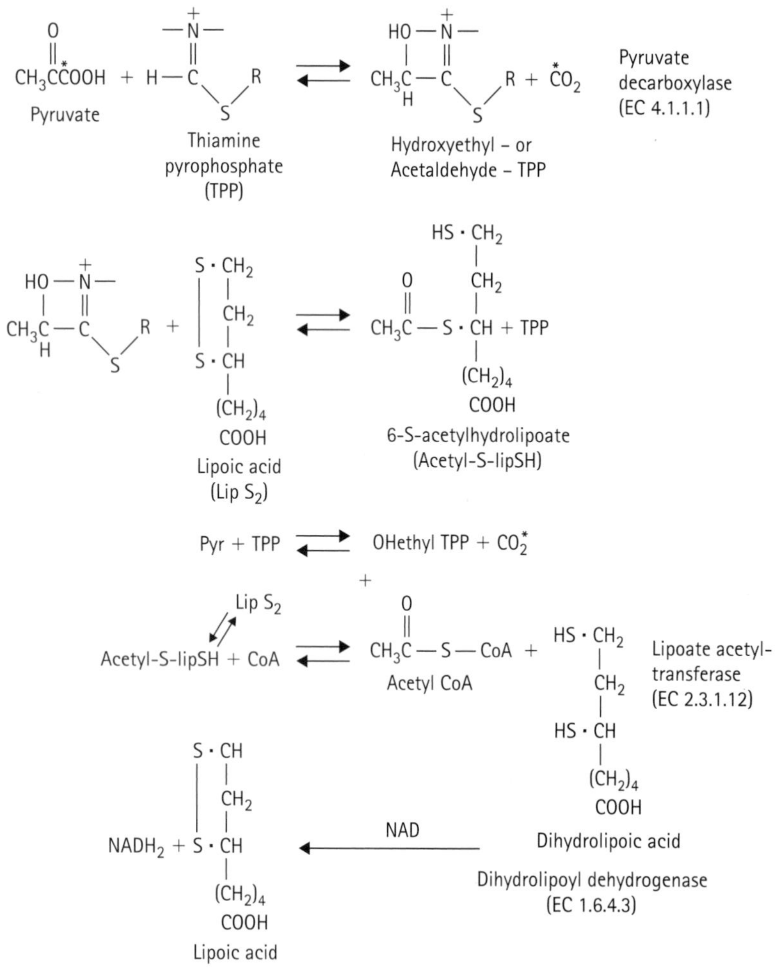

CH_3CCOOH (Pyruvate) $+$ Thiamine pyrophosphate (TPP) $\rightleftharpoons$ Hydroxyethyl – or Acetaldehyde – TPP $+ CO_2$ Pyruvate decarboxylase (EC 4.1.1.1)

Hydroxyethyl-TPP $+$ Lipoic acid (Lip S_2) $\rightleftharpoons$ 6-S-acetylhydrolipoate (Acetyl-S-lipSH) $+$ TPP

$Pyr + TPP \rightleftharpoons$ OHethyl TPP $+ CO_2^*$

Acetyl-S-lipSH $+$ CoA $\rightleftharpoons$ Acetyl CoA $+$ Lip S_2 Lipoate acetyl-transferase (EC 2.3.1.12)

$NADH_2 +$ Lipoic acid $\xleftarrow{NAD}$ Dihydrolipoic acid   Dihydrolipoyl dehydrogenase (EC 1.6.4.3)

Figure 50.1   *The pyruvate dehydrogenase complex (PDHC).*

The E1 enzyme is a tetramer of α and β subunits in an $\alpha_2\beta_2$ form. The α protein is 41 kDa and the β is 36 kDa. It is the E1α subunit that is phosphorylated and dephosphorylated by the kinase and phosphatase at serine residues [9].

Lactic acid is the major end-product of anaerobic glycolysis. It accumulates whenever production of pyruvic acid exceeds utilization. This occurs temporarily during exercise in which there is an oxygen debt, as well as in conditions in which oxygen supplies decrease because of cardiac or respiratory insufficiency or vascular perfusion problems such as shock. There is also cyclic interconversion of lactate in the Cori cycle in which glucose is converted to lactate in peripheral tissues such as brain and muscle, which oxidize carbohydrates largely to CO_2 and water, and the lactate formed circulates to the liver, where it is converted to glucose [10]. Because of gluconeogenesis, the amount of carbohydrate supplied to peripheral tissues from the liver exceeds the amount ingested. The brain is a major site of its oxidation, and this percentage is greater in infancy and childhood because of the greater proportion of the brain size to body size. The dependency of the brain on oxidative metabolism makes it particularly susceptible to damage in diseases of oxidation that lead to lactic acidosis. The activity of the pyruvate dehydrogenase complex is the rate-limiting step in the oxidation of glucose in the brain, and is central to the normal function of this organ. It has been calculated [11] that the fully activated PDHC could oxidize 180 g of glucose each day; the brain normally oxidizes 125 g a day, leaving little room for error caused by decreased activity of PDHC.

Among genetic deficiencies in PDHC, the most common result from mutations in the E1α gene on the X chromosome. The disease is expressed as an X-linked dominant. Abnormalities in E2, protein X, E3 and PDH phosphatase are rare. The gene for E1α is at Xp22.1-22.2 [12–14]. The E1$\beta\beta$gene is on chromosome 3p13-q23 [13]. The E3 gene is on chromosome 7 at q31-32 [13,15]. These three genes have been cloned and sequenced [16–18]. The gene for the X protein is on chromosome 11p [19]. A considerable number of mutations has been defined in the E1α gene [20]. Most of those in males have been missense mutations, while in females there have been major disruptions in the single affected X chromosome [21,22].

CLINICAL ABNORMALITIES

Among the defined oxidative abnormalities that lead to lactic acidemia, deficiency of PDHC has been reported to be the most common [23,24], although this certainly has not been our experience. We have seen many more mitochondrial DNA defects and electron transport chain abnormalities. In a series of 54 patients with deficiency of E1 the spectrum of clinical presentation was as broad as those of the lactic acidemias in general (Chapter 47).

The most severe presentation is of neonatal or infantile metabolic acidosis with lactic acidemia. The acute neonatal presentation may be complicated by hyperammonemia. A majority of these infants die prior to 6 months of age, many of them in the neonatal period [25–28].

There is a somewhat more indolent presentation in patients with chronic, more modest lactic acidemia who first come to attention because of delayed psychomotor development [29–36]. Some may present with failure to thrive or poor linear growth. Many of these patients have the clinical and neuropathological features of Leigh syndrome [37]. As many as 25 percent of patients with Leigh syndrome have been reported to have defects of PDHC [24,36]. Many of these patients die between 10 months and 3 years-of-age. They may experience rapid deterioration or episodic deterioration following infections. Patients may have dystonia, and ultimately they develop spastic quadriparesis. A variety of seizures includes grand mal, myoclonic, absence or akinetic convulsions. With progression, brainstem abnormalities become prominent. There may be ocular movement abnormalities and central respiratory failure. Death may be from apnea or pneumonia.

Neuroimaging may reveal attenuated signal in the basal ganglia, particularly in putamen and globus pallidus [38,39], and ultimately generalized cerebral atrophy. Histopathological examination reveals spongiform degeneration and gliosis especially in the basal ganglia. Among the neonatal acidosis group some have had cortical cysts at autopsy [24,39]. A number of these patients has also had agenesis of corpus callosum. Cerebral atrophy may be generalized.

The least severe presentations tend to be females with a slowly progressive Leigh syndrome, or males with ataxia resembling a slowly progressive spinocerebellar degeneration [40]. Among the group with psychomotor retardation surviving at report females outnumbered males 2:1 [36]. Among those with the ataxia presentation, some ataxia may be episodic, and some may be induced by carbohydrate and ameliorated by a high lipid diet [41,42]. A rare presentation is with peripheral neuropathy of infantile origin associated with hypotonia and absent deep tendon reflexes [43]. Episodic weakness has been described in a patient with ataxia and impaired reflexes [11]. Some patients have elevated concentrations of lactic acid in cerebrospinal fluid (CSF) with little or no elevation in the blood [44,45]: this has been referred to as cerebral lactic acidosis [45].

A group of patients has been described in which dysmorphic features signified prenatal onset of effects of deficiency of PDHC (Figures 50.2–50.4) [24,46–48]. Our two patients [46], who were siblings, displayed virtually complete absence of psychomotor development. Their phenotype was quite similar to the patient of Farrell and colleagues [48].

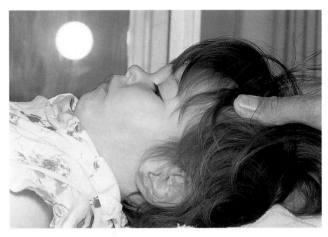

Figure 50.2   *L.R., an infant with lactic acidemia and deficiency of PDHC. In addition, she had frontal bossing, a depressed nasal bridge, and an anteverted nasal tip. The ear was large and unusual in shape.*

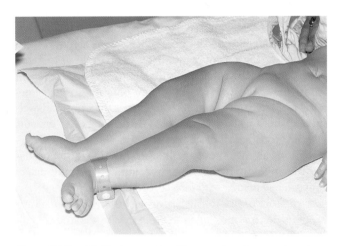

Figure 50.3   *L.R. The lower extremities were in extreme external rotation.*

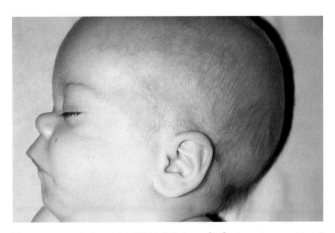

Figure 50.4   *Infant with PDHC deficiency [49] whose face and head had a similar appearance to the infant in Figure 50.2. (Illustration was kindly provided by Dr. Richard Wennberg of the University of California, Davis.)*

Characteristics were wide separation of the eyebrows, epicanthal folds, depressed nasal bridge, a small nose with anteverted flared nostrils (Figures 50.2, 50.4), and a long philtrum. There was limited extension of the elbows and ulnar deviation of the hands. Both hips appeared to be dislocated. The position of the legs was in external rotation so that the feet pointed out like those of a ballerina (Figure 50.3), and abduction was very limited. There was a ventricular septal defect. Visual evoked potentials revealed only a very small degree of cortical response. The facial features have been considered to resemble those of the fetal alcohol syndrome [49]. A common mechanism suggested would be low fetal activity of PDHC, a result in the latter condition of inhibition by acetaldehyde.

GENETICS AND PATHOGENESIS

Deficiency of E1α, the only common form of abnormality in PDHC, behaves as an X-linked dominant character in which, depending on the mutations, there may be quite severe disease in the female. All of the other defects are autosomal recessive. Reduced conversion of 1-^{14}C-pyruvate to CO_2 has been demonstrated in the fibroblasts of parents consistent with heterozygosity [50], but in four obligate heterozygotes assay of PDHC revealed somewhat lower than normal levels in two, and normal levels in two. The variability of enzyme assay makes prenatal diagnosis, as well as heterozygote detection, unreliable. In those families in which the mutation has been identified, prenatal diagnosis and heterozygote detection can be pursued with molecular methodology.

Deficiency of PDHC can be documented by assay of a variety of tissues; it is most often accomplished by the study of cultured fibroblasts [23,24]. The simplest procedure is to measure the conversion of 1-^{14}C-pyruvate to $^{14}CO_2$. Considerable variability has been the rule in the assay, and it has not been possible to correlate the amount of residual activity with the severity of the clinical phenotype. The substrate itself is unstable [51], and activity is also influenced by the methodology employed for disrupting the cell [52]. Assays generally take advantage of the use of dichloroacetate to inhibit PDH kinase and maximize the proportion of the active PDH enzyme [52–54]. Localization of the defect to the E1 component has generally been done [55] by incorporating ferricyanide into the reaction mixture as an artificial electron acceptor to oxidize the hydroxyethylthiamine and regenerate active E1 enzyme. Deficiency of activity of PDHC has been reported to range from three to 40 percent of the control level [23,24].

There is a tendency for those with severe neonatal disease and dysmorphic features to have virtually no enzymatic activity [48], and for most patients with indolent disease to have considerably more residual enzyme activity [23], but overall the correlation between survival and measured activity has not been good. In general the severity of disease also correlates with the height of the lactic acidemia; in the fatal neonatal patients it is very high. Studies of the kinetic characteristics of the enzyme in patients have been few. In one, the PDHC of autopsied liver was difficult to activate [56]. In another [11], the deficient enzyme in muscle biopsied during an acute attack was completely deactivated, although it could be activated *in vitro*.

Antisera have been prepared against purified E1, E2 and E3 [34]. In 19 of 22 patients with deficiency of PDHC in whom the defect was localized to E1, and cellular proteins were labeled with ^{35}S-methionine and immunoprecipitated by antibodies to E1, the deficiency of E1 activity was correlated with a deficient α-subunit [34]. Other patients with deficient E1 activity were immunochemically normal; consistent with simple amino acid substitution resulting in loss of activity. Visualization of PDH proteins by electrophoresis and immuno-blotting or immuno-precipitation have revealed decreased or absent E1α protein [36,57–59], as well as altered migration and an increased phosphorylated form [27,60]. Whenever E1α is decreased, there is proportional decrease in E1β. Complete absence of E1α and E1β may be associated with fatal neonatal acidosis [27,36], or with retardation and ataxia [34]. Females with deficient activity and clinical disease have been documented to have two E1α bands [58,59].

Cloning of the E1α gene has permitted extensive documentation of the nature of mutation in this disease. The E1α gene has 11 exons spanning 17 kb [16]. It is of interest that a majority of the mutations identified have been in exons 5 to 11; they include the region in which pyruvate is bound to the enzyme (amino acids 130 to 150), the TPP binding site (170–226) and the serine phosphorylation sites (231–291) [9,20,21,60]. Females with E1 deficiency have two genes, one normal E1α gene and one with the mutated gene.

Missense mutation in the pyruvate binding region, a substitution of methionine at position 138 for valine was found in two sisters with 0.6–7 percent enzyme activity and clinical mental retardation who died at 10 and 11 years [20]. Among mutations in the TPP binding area, an alanine-to-threonine 170 change led to a slowly progressive Leigh picture, while a phenylalanine 176-to-leucine change led to death in infancy with severe lactic acidosis [20,21]. An alanine-to-threonine change at 231, just before the serine phosphorylation site at 232, led to 1.7 percent activity and death from lactic acidosis at 7 days [20]. Similarly, a histidine-to-leucine 263 change just before the serine 264 phosphorylation site gave only 2.5 percent residual activity in a female. An arginine 349-to-histidine mutation very close to the N terminus of the gene occurred in a male with brain atrophy and death at 13 weeks [61]. On the other hand, milder disease was observed in 13 unrelated patients with an arginine 234-to-glycine mutation [20,62,63] and 50 percent residual activity was found in two females with an arginine 273-to-cysteine mutation [62]. A recently discovered tyrosine 243 to serine change in a patient with neonatal lactic acidemia and bilateral globus pallidus lesions was correlated in fibroblasts *in vitro* with an absence of the normal increase in activity on addition of TPP [64].

Deletions and insertions have been reported in exons 10 and 11. Many of these patients had severe lactic acidosis and died early in life [61,63,65]. An exception was a CAGT deletion at 1167 that produced a protein with 33 extra amino acids and a clinical picture of only exercise intolerance [66]. An unusual mutation in E1α [66], in a family with Leigh encephalomyelopathy presentations, led to alternate splicing in which all of exon 6 containing the TPP binding sites was lost in some transcripts. The mutation, an A-to-G substitution at position 660, did not change the glycine at this position, but led to the loss of exon 6. The mother exhibited normal activity and had 90 percent of normal alleles. A similar mutation in exon 8 of the HPRT gene led to classic Lesch-Nyhan disease (Chapter 65). In one of our patients whose mutation led to loss of the last three amino acids, onset was at 16 years, and at 35 years he displayed ataxia and dysarthria. He was also psychotic. A mutation (R20P) in a patient with Leigh syndrome has been identified in the mitochondrial targeting sequence, altering import of the precursor protein into the mitochondria [67]. Mutations in the E1β gene have not yet been defined.

Abnormalities in E2 or protein X have been reported in fewer than ten patients [68–70]. A clinical picture of severe neonatal lactic acidosis and hyperammonemia was associated with 24 percent residual activity of PDHC, and 32 percent transacetylase activity [68]. The E2 protein was absent, and protein X was reduced. Absent protein X was found in a patient with severe psychomotor retardation, with lactic acidosis and 12 percent activity of PDHC [67]. A boy with an extra band below protein X on immuno-blotting with antibody to PDH which was found to be a variant of E2 had an initial presentation of ataxia without retardation, but developed of a neuroimaging picture of Leigh disease; fibroblasts displayed 55 percent of control activity of PDHC [68]. Severe lactic acidosis and absence of the corpus callosum occurred in an infant [69] with an absence of the X component. Two patients with a Leigh syndrome presentation [70] had specific absence of the X protein.

Defects in E3 (Chapter 51) result in deficiency of 2-oxoglutarate dehydrogenase and the branched-chain oxoacid decarboxylase, as well as PDHC. In these patients lactic acidemia and systemic acidosis developed some months after birth. Elevated levels may be found of the branched-chain amino acids and of 2-oxoglutarate, as well as of pyruvate and lactate. In one patient 2-oxoisocaproic acid was found in elevated amounts. Activity of lipoamide dehydrogenase ranged from 0 to 20 percent of the control level.

Among mutations reported in the E3 gene: lysine 37 to glutamic acid, and proline 453 to leucine were found on the two alleles in a patient with no detectable activity of E3 [71].

Deficiency of pyruvate dehydrogenase phosphatase has been found in a few patients gene [6,72,73] on chromosome 8q22-23 at nucleotide 716 leading to D239V in a patient who had congenital lactic acidemia and defective activation of pyruvate decarboxylase by removing phosphate from serine residues in E1α[74]. Among other patients with deficiency of pyruvate dehydrogenase phosphatase one died at 6 months of

severe metabolic acidosis and lactic acidemia [6] and four had Leigh disease phenotypes [72,73].

TREATMENT

Patients with deficiency of PDHC are sensitive to carbohydrate [41] and may develop life-threatening acidosis when given a diet high in carbohydrates. They respond to the administration of glucose with elevation in concentrations of pyruvate and lactate [41]. The provision of a diet low in carbohydrate and high in fat may lead to reduction in the concentration of lactate and some improvement in the general condition of the patient [26,41,75]. In one patent a diet with 58 to 66 percent fat was followed by reversal of elevated concentrations of lactic acid and MRI evidence of improvement in the brain [32]. Levels of lactate in the blood may be brought within the normal range using diets in which 50 percent or more of the calories are in fat and 20 percent in carbohydrate. These diets may lead to ketonemia or ketonuria, but not to acidosis or hypoglycemia.

Despite clinical improvement attendant on amelioration of acidotic symptoms, patients with neurologic abnormalities do not improve neurologically. These diets bypass the defect by providing the product of the PDHC reaction directly as acetylCoA from the metabolism of fat. In addition, the lesser load of carbohydrate provides smaller amounts of pyruvate to accumulate behind the block and cause lactic acidosis. Caveats raised concerning the use of these diets [76] included the possibility that they could be high in protein and could cause hypercalciuria or kidney stones, as have been observed in patients with convulsions treated with ketogenic diets [77,78], but the only potentially adverse effect observed in the patients with deficiency of PDHC reviewed was hyperuricemia.

Since thiamine pyrophosphate is an integral component of the E1 enzyme, high doses of thiamine (100–600 mg/day) have been employed in the hope that a decreased affinity for the cofactor could be overcome by increasing its concentration. Improvement has been reported in a patient described as thiamine-dependent [25]. In other patients a trial of thiamine is worthwhile in the hope of stimulating residual activity of pyruvate decarboxylase.

Dichloroacetate (Chapter 47, p. 310) effectively reduces levels of lactate in most patients, consistent with the presence of residual activity in PDH in most of them. Intuitively one might not expect to achieve much in the way of clinical improvement in neurological features of this disease by treatment with DCA, but we have encountered some dramatic improvements in some patients with PDH deficiency. Responsiveness to DCA in cultured fibroblasts has been correlated with genotype in severe E1α deficiency [79]. Appreciable increase in PDHC activity in the presence of DCA was found in cell lines with R378C and R88C mutations consistent with reduced degradation of polypeptides with reduced stability. Carnitine and coenzyme Q are employed in many centers in the treatment of patients with deficiency of PDHC. The usual dose of coenzyme Q is 4 mg/kg, although we are now measuring levels of coenzyme Q, and in deficient patients, often those with electron transport defects we have employed 10–20 mg/kg.

In the management of the acute episode of lactic acidosis (Chapter 47, p. 310) the usual approach is to provide large quantities of intravenous water and electrolytes in the form of NaHCO₃. Stacpoole [80] has argued a case against the use of bicarbonate in lactic acidosis, at least in those adult patients with secondary lactic acidemia in intensive care units (ICUs). He cited evidence that infused bicarbonate forms carbon dioxide, which may diffuse across the blood–brain barrier, lowering the pH of cerebrospinal fluid; as well as evidence, in experimental lactic acidosis in animals of decreased cardiac output and increased intestinal formation of lactic acid with bicarbonate infusion as opposed to saline infusion. However, these experiments studied the hyperosmolar 1 molar NaHCO₃ solution used in ICUs compared with isotonic solutions of NaCl. They may provide an argument for the use of isotonic NaHCO₃ in the management of acidosis.

References

1 Reed LJ, Pettit FH, Yeaman SJ, et al. Structure function and regulation of the mammalian pyruvate dehydrogenase complex. *Proc Eur J Biochem Soc* 1980;**60**:47.

2 Matuda S, Kitano A, Sakaguchi Y, et al. Pyruvate dehydrogenase complex with lipoamide dehydrogenase deficiency in a patient with lactic acidosis and branched chain ketoaciduria. *Clin Chim Acta* 1984;**140**:59.

3 De Marcucci GL, Hodgson JA, Lindsay G. The Mr 50 000 polypeptide of mammalian pyruvate dehydrogenase complex participates in acetylation reactions. *Eur J Biochem* 1986;**158**:587.

4 Powers-Greenwood SL, Rahmatullah M, Radke GA, Roche TE. Separation of protein X from the dihydrolipoyl transacetylase component of the mammalian pyruvate dehydrogenase complex and function of protein X. *J Biol Chem* 1989;**264**:3655.

5 Neagle JC, Lindsay JG. Selective proteolysis of the protein X subunit of the bovine heart pyruvate dehydrogenase complex. *Biochem J* 1991;**278**:423.

6 Robinson BH, Sherwood WG. Pyruvate dehydrogenase phosphatase deficiency: a cause of congenital chronic lactic acidosis in infancy. *Pediatr Res* 1975;**9**:935.

7 Randle PJ, Sugden PH, Kerbey AL, et al. Regulation of pyruvate oxidation and the conservation of glucose. *Biochem Soc Symp* 1979;**43**:67.

8 Whitehouse S, Cooper RH, Randle PJ. Mechanism of activation of pyruvate dehydrogenase by dichloroacetate and other halogenated carboxylic acids. *Biochem J* 1974;**141**:671.

9 Randle PJ. Mitochondrial 2-oxoacid dehydrogenase complexes of animal tissues. *Philos Trans* 1987;**302**:47 (abstr).

10 Ahlborg O, Felig P. Lactate and glucose exchange across the forearm legs and splanchnic bed during and after prolonged leg exercise. *J Clin Invest* 1982;**68**:45.

11 Robinson BH, Sherwood WG. Lactic acidemia the prevalence of pyruvate decarboxylase deficiency. *J Inherit Metab Dis* 1984;**7**:69.

12 Brown RM, Dahl H-HM, Brown GK. X chromosome localization of the functional gene for E1α subunit of the human pyruvate dehydrogenase complex. *Genomics* 1989;**7**:215.

13 Olson S, Song BJ, Hueh TL, et al. Three genes for enzymes of the pyruvate dehydrogenase complex map to human chromosomes 3, 7 and X. *Am J Hum Genet* 1990;**46**:340.

14 Szabo P, Sheu KFR, Robinson RM, et al. The gene for alpha polypeptide of pyruvate dehydrogenase is X-linked in humans. *Am J Hum Genet* 1990;**46**:874.

15 Sherer SW, Otulakowski G, Robinson BH, Tsui L-C. Localization of the human dihydrolipoamide dehydrogenase gene (DLD) to 7q31-q32. *Cytogenet Cell Genet* 1991;**56**:176.

16 Maragos C, Hutchison W, Haysaka K, et al. Structural organization of the gene for the E1α subunit of the human pyruvate dehydrogenase complex. *J Biol Chem* 1989;**26**:12294.

17 Koike K, Urata Y, Koike M. Molecular cloning and characterization of human pyruvate dehydrogenase b subunit gene. *Proc Natl Acad Sci USA* 1990;**87**:5594.

18 Feigenbaum A, Robinson BH. Structural organization of the human lipoamide dehydrogenase gene. *Genomics* 1993;**17**:376.

19 Aral B, Benelli C, Ait-Ghezala G, et al. Mutations in PDX1 the human lipoyl-containing component X of the pyruvate dehydrogenase-complex gene on chromosome 11p1 in congenital lactic acidosis. *Am J Hum Genet* 1997;**61**:1318.

20 Chun K, MacKay N, Petrova-Benedict R, Robinson BH. Mutations in the X-linked E1α subunit of pyruvate dehydrogenase leading to deficiency of the pyruvate dehydrogenase complex. *Hum Mol Genet* 1993;**2**:449.

21 Dahl H-HM, Brown GK, Brown RM, et al. Mutations and polymorphisms in the pyruvate dehydrogenase E1α gene. *Hum Mutat* 1992;**1**:97.

22 Dahl H-HM, Maragos C, Brown RM, et al. Pyruvate dehydrogenase deficiency caused by deletion of a 7bp repeat sequence in the E1α gene. *Am J Hum Genet* 1990;**47**:286.

23 Robinson BH, Taylor J, Sherwood WG. The genetic heterogeneity of lactic acidosis: occurrence of recognizable inborn errors of metabolism in a pediatric population with lactic acidosis. *Pediatr Res* 1980;**14**:956.

24 Robinson BH, MacMillan H, Petrova-Benedict R, Sherwood WG. Variable clinical presentation in patients with defective E1 component of pyruvate dehydrogenase complex. A review of 30 cases with a defect in the E1 component of the complex. *J Pediatr* 1987;**111**:525.

25 Wick H, Schweizerk K, Baumgartner R. Thiamine dependency in a patient with congenital lactic acidemia due to pyruvate dehydrogenase deficiency. *Agents Actions* 1977;**7**:405.

26 Strömme JH, Borud O, Moe PJ. Fatal lactic acidosis in a newborn attributable to a congenital defect of pyruvate dehydrogenase. *Pediatr Res* 1976;**10**:60.

27 Wicking CA, Scholem RD, Hunt DS, Brown GK. Immunochemical analysis of normal and mutant forms of human pyruvate dehydrogenase. *Biochem J* 1986;**239**:89.

28 Matsuo M, Ookita K, Takemine H, et al. Fatal case of pyruvate dehydrogenase deficiency. *Acta Paediatr Scand* 1985;**74**:140.

29 Evans OB. Pyruvate decarboxylase deficiency in subacute necrotizing encephalomyelopathy. *Arch Neurol* 1981;**38**:515.

30 Papanastasiou D, Lehnert W, Schuchmann L, Hommes FA. Chronic lactic acidosis in an infant. *Helv Paediatr Acta* 1980;**35**:253.

31 Hansen TL, Christensen E, Brandt NJ. Studies on pyruvate carboxylase pyruvate decarboxylase and lipoamide dehydrogenase in subacute necrotizing encephalomyelopathy. *Acta Paediatr Scand* 1982;**71**:263.

32 Toshima K, Kuroda Y, Hashimoto T, et al. Enzymologic studies and therapy of Leigh's disease associated with pyruvate decarboxylase deficiency. *Pediatr Res* 1982;**16**:430.

33 Miyabayashi S, Ito T, Narisawa K, *et al.* Biochemical studies in 28 children with lactic acidosis in relation to Leigh's encephalomyelopathy. *Eur J Pediatr* 1985;**143**:278.

34 Ho L, Hu CWC, Packman S, *et al.* Deficiency of the pyruvate dehydrogenase component in pyruvate dehydrogenase complex-deficient human fibroblasts. Immunological identification. *J Clin Invest* 1986;**78**:844.

35 Ohtake M, Takada G, Miyabayashi S, *et al.* Pyruvate decarboxylase deficiency in a patient with Leigh's encephalomyelopathy. *Tohoku J Exp Med* 1982;**137**:379.

36 Robinson BH, Chun K, MacKay N, *et al.* Isolated and combined deficiencies of the a-keto acid dehydrogenase complexes. *Ann NY Acad Sci* 1989;**573**:337.

37 Leigh D. Subacute necrotizing encephalomyelopathy in an infant. *J Neurol Neurosurg Psychiatry* 1972;**14**:87.

38 Hall K, Gardner-Medwin D. CT scan appearances in Leigh's disease (subacute necrotizing encephalomyelopathy). *Neuroradiology* 1978;**16**:48.

39 Medina L, Chi TL, DeVivo DC, Hilal SK. MR findings in patients with subacute necrotizing encephalomyelopathy (Leigh syndrome): correlation with biochemical defect. *Am J Roentgenol* 1990;**154**:1269.

40 Blass JP, Lonsdale D, Uhlendorf BW, Hom E. Intermittent ataxia with pyruvate decarboxylase deficiency. *Lancet* 1971;**1**:1302.

41 Cederbaum SD, Blass JP, Minkoff N, *et al.* Sensitivity to carbohydrate in a patient with familial intermittent lactic acidosis and pyruvate dehydrogenase deficiency. *Pediatr Res* 1976;**10**:713.

42 Blass JP, Schulman JD, Young DS, Hom E. An inherited defect affecting the tricarboxylic acid cycle in a patient with congenital lactic acidosis. *J Clin Invest* 1972;**51**:1845.

43 Chabrol B, Mancini J, Benelli C. Leigh syndrome: pyruvate dehydrogenase defect. A case with peripheral neuropathy. *J Child Neurol* 1994;**9**:52.

44 Brown GK, Brown RM, Scholem RD, *et al.* The clinical and biochemical spectrum of human pyruvate dehydrogenase complex deficiency. *Ann NY Acad Sci* 1989;**573**:360.

45 Brown GK, Haan EA, Kirby DM, *et al.* 'Cerebral' lactic acidosis: defects in pyruvate metabolism with profound brain damage and minimal systemic acidosis. *Eur J Pediatr* 1988;**147**:10.

46 Nyhan WL, Sakati NA. Pyruvate dehydrogenase deficiency: in *Diagnostic Recognition of Metabolic Disease.* Lea and Febiger, Philadelphia;1987:228.

47 Sherwood WG, Robinson BH. Dysmorphism in congenital lactic acidosis syndrome. *Pediatr Res* 1984;**18**:300A.

48 Farrell DF, Clark AF, Scott CR, Wennberg RP. Absence of pyruvate decarboxylase activity in man: a cause of congenital lactic acidosis. *Science* 1975;**187**:1082.

49 Jones KL, Smith DW, Ulleland CW, Streissguth AP. Pattern of malformation in offspring of chronic alcoholic mothers. *Lancet* 1973;**1**:1267.

50 Robinson BH, Inborn errors of pyruvate metabolism. *Biochem Soc Trans* 1983;**11**:623.

51 Silverstein E, Boyer PD. Instability of pyruvate ^{14}C in aqueous solutions as detected by enzymic assay. *Anal Biochem* 1964;**8**:470.

52 Haas RH, Thompson J, Morris B, *et al.* Pyruvate dehydrogenase activity in osmotically-shocked rat brain mitochondria: stimulation by oxaloacetate. *J Neurochem* 1988;**50**:673.

53 Sheu KF, Hu CC, Utter MF. Pyruvate dehydrogenase complex activity in normal and deficient fibroblasts. *J Clin Invest* 1981;**67**:1463.

54 Johnston K, Newth CJL, Sheu K-FR, *et al.* Central hypoventilation syndrome in pyruvate dehydrogenase complex deficiency. *Pediatrics* 1984;**74**:1034.

55 Reed LJ, Willms CR. Purification and resolution of the pyruvate dehydrogenase complex (*Escherichia coli*). *Meth Enzymol* 1966; **9**:247.

56 MacKay N, Petrova-Benedict R, Thoene J, *et al.* Three cases of lactic acidemia due to pyruvate decarboxylase (E1) deficiency with evidence of

57 Old SE, DeVivo DC. Pyruvate dehydrogenase complex deficiency: biochemical and immunoblot analysis of cultured skin fibroblasts. *Ann Neurol* 1989;**26**:746.

58 Endo H, Miyabashi S, Toda K, Narisawa K. A four-nucleotide insertion at the E1α gene in a patient with pyruvate dehydrogenase deficiency. *J Inherit Metab Dis* 1991;**14**:793.

59 Kitano A, Endo F, Matsuda I. Immunochemical analysis of pyruvate dehydrogenase complex in two boys with primary lactic academia. *Neurology* 1990;**40**:1312.

60 Hawkins CF, Borges A, Perham RN. A common structural motif in thiamine pyrophosphate-binding enzymes. *FEBS Lett* 1989;**255**:77.

61 Hansen LL, Brown GK, Kirby DM, Dahl H-HM. Characterization of the mutations in three patients with pyruvate dehydrogenase E1α deficiency. *J Inherit Metab Dis* 1991;**14**:140.

62 Wexler ID, Hemalatha SG, Patel MS. Sequence conservation in the a and b subunits of pyruvate dehydrogenase and its similarity to branched-chain a-keto acid dehydrogenase. *FEBS Lett* 1991;**282**:209.

63 Dahl H-HM, Maragos C, Brown RM, *et al.* Pyruvate dehydrogenase deficiency caused by a 7bp repeat sequence in the E1β gene. *Am J Hum Genet* 1990;**47**:286.

64 Benelli C, Fouque F, Redonnet-Vernhet I, *et al.* A novel Y243S mutation in the pyruvate dehydrogenase E1 alpha gene subunit: Correlation with thiamine pyrophosphate interaction. *J Inherit Metab Dis* 2002;**25**:325.

65 Endo H, Hasegawa K, Narisawa K, *et al.* Defective gene in lactic acidosis: abnormal pyruvate dehydrogenase E1α-subunit caused by a frameshift. *Am J Hum Genet* 1989;**44**:358.

66 De Meirleir L, Lissens W, Benelli C, *et al.* Aberrant splicing of exon 6 in the pyruvate dehydrogenase-E1α mRNA linked to a silent mutation in a large family with Leigh's encephalomyelopathy. *Pediatr Res* 1994;**36**:707.

67 Takakudo F, Cartwright P, Hoogenraad N, *et al.* An amino acid substitution in the pyruvate dehydrogenase E1α gene affecting mitochondrial import of the precursor protein. *Am J Hum Genet*1995;**57**:772.

68 Robinson BH, MacKay N, Petrova-Benedict R, *et al.* Defects in the E2 lipoyl transacetylase and the X-lipoyl containing component of the pyruvate dehydrogenase complex in patients with lactic academia. *J Clin Invest* 1990;**85**:1821.

69 Geoffroy V, Fouque F, Benelli C, *et al.* Defect in the X-lipoyl-containing component of the pyruvate dehydrogenase complex in a patient with a neonatal lactic academia. *Pediatrics* 1996;**97**:267.

70 Marsac C, Stansbie D, Bonne G, *et al.* Defect in the lipoyl-bearing protein X subunit of the pyruvate dehydrogenase complex in two patients with encephalomyelopathy. *J Pediatr* 1993;**123**:915.

71 Liu T-C, Kim H, Arijmendi C, *et al.* Identification of two missense mutations in a dihydrolipoamide dehydrogenase deficient patient. *Proc Natl Acad Sci USA* 1993;**90**:5186.

72 DeVivo DC, Haymond MW, Obert KA, *et al.* Defective activation of the pyruvate dehydrogenase complex in subacute necrotizing encephalomyelopathy (Leigh disease). *Ann Neurol* 1979;**6**:483.

73 Sorbi S, Blass JP. Abnormal activatin of pyruvate dehydrogenase in Leigh disease fibroblasts. *Neurology* 1982;**32**:555.

74 Shinahara K, Ohigashi I, Ito M. Cloning of a cDNA for human pyruvate dehydrogenase phosphatase and detection of a mutation in a patient with congenital lactic academia. *Am J Genet* 2000;**67**:294.

75 Falk RE, Cederbaum SD, Blass JP, *et al.* Ketogenic diet in the management of pyruvate dehydrogenase deficiency. *Pediatrics* 1976;**58**:713.

76 Weber TA, Antognetti R, Stacpoole PW. Caveats when considering ketogenic diets for the treatment of pyruvate dehydrogenase complex deficiency. *J Pediatr* 2001;**138**:390.

protein polymorphism in the a subunit of the enzyme. *Eur J Pediatr* 1986;**144**:445.

77 Kinsman SL, Vining EPG, Quaskey SA, *et al.* Efficacy of the ketogenic diet for intractable seizure disorders: review of 58 cases. *Epilepsia* 1992;**33**:1132.

78 Chesney DC, Brouhard BH, Wyllie E, Powaski K. Biochemical abnormalities of the ketogenic diet in children. *Clin Pediatr* 1999;**38**:107.

79 Fouque F, Brivet M, Boutron A, *et al.* Differential effect of DCA treatment on the pyruvate dehydrogenase complex in patients with severe PDHC deficiency. *Pediatr Res* 2003;**53**:793.

80 Stacpoole PW. Lactic acidosis: The case against bicarbonate therapy. *Ann Intern Med* 1986;**105**:276.

51

Lactic acidemia and defective activity of pyruvate, 2-oxoglutarate and branched chain oxoacid dehydrogenases

MAJOR PHENOTYPIC EXPRESSION

Potentially lethal disorder of infancy, failure to thrive, hypotonia, metabolic acidosis, ketonuria, lactic acidosis, 2-oxoaciduria, and deficient activity of the three dehydrogenases for pyruvate, 2-oxoglutarate and branched-chain oxoacids.

INTRODUCTION

A small number of infants have been reported with a disorder in which severe lactic acidosis has been associated with excretion of large quantities of citric acid cycle intermediates and there is defective activity of the pyruvate dehydrogenase complex (PDHC) (Figures 51.1–51.3) and the other dehydrogenases involved in oxidative decarboxylations [1–8]. All but one [2] have died in infancy. In most, defective activity of lipoamide dehydrogenase (E_3) was reported or presumed [4–7]. In one [8] the activity of E_3 was normal, but improved catabolism of branched-chain amino acids after the growth of fibroblasts in medium supplemented with lipoic acid suggested a defect in an enzyme catalyzing the attachment of lipoic acid to a component of the enzyme complexes.

CLINICAL ABNORMALITIES

Despite the overwhelming nature of the illness, most patients have had an initial period of relative health that may have lasted as long as 5 months [8]. The first patient characterized by Robinson and colleagues in 1977 [1] was well until he became acutely ill at 8 weeks of age. He appeared pale and mottled and had labored respirations. He was lethargic and hypotonic. Failure to follow a light was consistent with bilateral optic atrophy. He had metabolic acidosis with a pH of 7.22 and a bicarbonate of 13 mEq/L. Hypoglycemia was observed on one occasion. Neurologic dysfunction was described as progressive and unremitting. He died following an aspiration at 7 months.

Among the earliest reports was that of an Indian family from Canada in which three infants had lactic acidosis, mental retardation and seizures, and two excreted large amounts of pyruvic and 2-ketoglutaric acids in the urine [2]. Cultured fibroblasts derived from one sib were found to be defective in pyruvate dehydrogenase and 2-oxoglutarate dehydrogenase. Two died at 3 and 4 months-of-age, while the third was alive at report at 23 months-of-age. These patients developed acidosis very early in infancy. We also studied a 2-year-old girl with lactic acidosis and severe retardation of growth and mental development in whom the activities of PDHC and the 2-oxoglutarate dehydrogenase complex were deficient [3]. A previous sibling had died of what appeared to be the same syndrome.

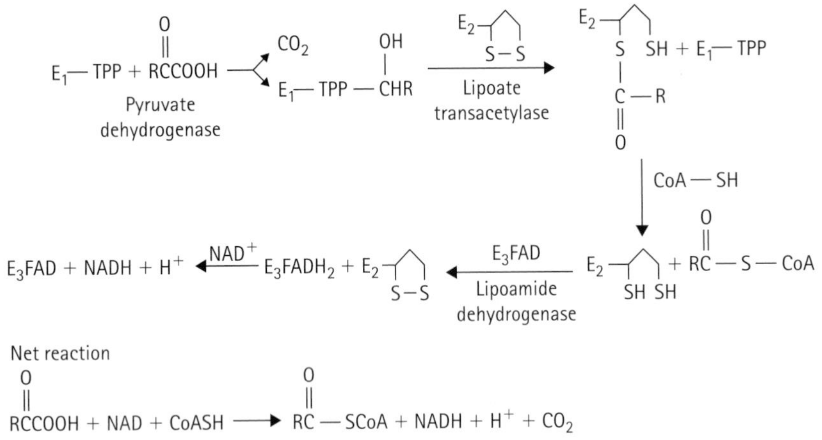

Figure 51.1   *The pyruvate dehydrogenase complex. E_1 refers to pyruvate decarboxylase; E_2 to dihydrolipoyltransacetylase; and E_3 to lipoamide dehydrogenase. Lipoic acid (Figure 51.2) is shown already attached to E_2 (Figure 51.3).*

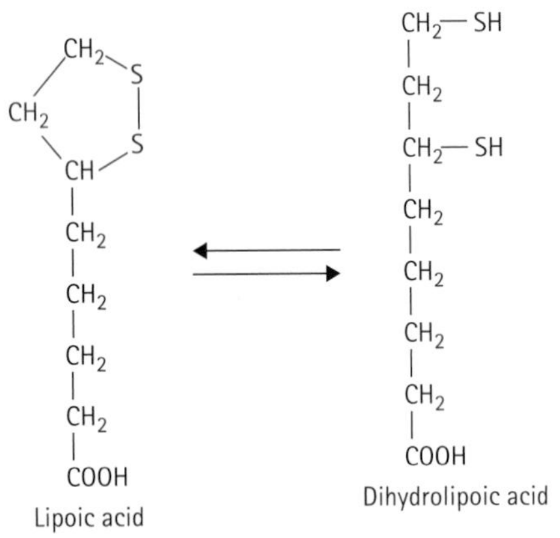

Figure 51.2   *Lipoic acid in its oxidized and reduced forms. The interaction is catalyzed by E_3.*

In another patient [4] hypotonia, a poor Moro response, left esotropia and an 'odd' cry were noted as early as 1 hour of life. At 10 weeks she developed vomiting and diarrhea and 12 hours later had a respiratory arrest. She was found to have slight hepatomegaly and a serum bicarbonate of 8 mEq/L. The blood glucose was 18 mg/dL and the lactate 8.8 mol/L. She had repeated episodes of ketoacidosis and dehydration that required admission to hospital and parenteral fluid therapy. After a second respiratory arrest at 17 months she underwent considerable neurologic deterioration, but neurologic worsening had appeared to be a consequence of each of her episodes of acute illness; by 10 months her suck was so poor a gastrostomy was placed. After 17 months she no longer responded to verbal stimuli. Seizures occurred during the second year of life.

A Japanese infant failed to thrive and fed poorly for the first four months of life [5]. This was true of our patient too [8]. The Japanese infant developed pallor and tachypnea at 6 months-of-age and was found to have a blood pH of 7.17 and a bicarbonate of 7.4 mEq/L; the blood sugar was 38 mg/dL. Neurologic features at that time were hypotonia, poor head control and dystonic movements. The developmental quotient was 78. By 17 months he had spastic quadriplegia and nystagmus. Computed tomography (CT) scan revealed lucent lesions in the basal ganglia. He died during a ketoacidotic attack at 21 months. A Tunisian infant in France [6] also fed poorly and failed to thrive from the first week, and by 6 months had hypotonia and severe developmental delay, but she did not become acutely ill until 8 months, when she had an attack of acidosis in which the pH was 7.1, the bicarbonate was 5.51 mEq/L, and there was pronounced ketonuria and lactic acidemia (10 mmol/L). She died at 18 months in an episode of severe acidosis that was precipitated by an open biopsy of the liver. Another patient failed to gain weight from the neonatal period and had recurrent episodes of vomiting and metabolic acidosis [7]. At 8 months-of-age he weighed only 4.1 kg. He had hypotonia, poor muscle mass and a pronounced head lag. CT scan revealed moderate cortical atrophy. The pH ranged from 7.0 to 7.2.

Our patient [8] (Figure 51.4) was admitted at 8 months-of-age for evaluation of lactic acidosis. He had not developed acute symptomatic acidosis until two weeks prior to admission, although he had appeared weak, sucked poorly and gained weight slowly from birth. After this long relatively benign early period, it was thereafter difficult to keep him out of the intensive care unit. The parents were first cousins. He was found to have a low serum bicarbonate and large amounts of lactic acid in blood and urine, and he was transferred to San Diego receiving 12 mEq/kg NaHCO$_3$ daily. The serum concentration of bicarbonate was 14 mEq/L. The blood concentration of lactate was 8.3 mmol/L and the pyruvate 0.34 mmol/L. Withdrawal of supplemental NaHCO$_3$ was followed by a decrease of the serum concentration of bicarbonate to 5 mEq/L. Analysis of the amino acid concentrations of the plasma revealed an elevated alanine ranging from 685 to 1000 mmol/L. Analysis of the amino acids of the urine revealed a generalized aminoaciduria. Further evidence of proximal renal tubular acidosis was a persistent urinary pH approximating 8.5 and 1–3+ glycosuria. Proteinuria of 1–3+ was also present. On admission his urine tested strongly positive for

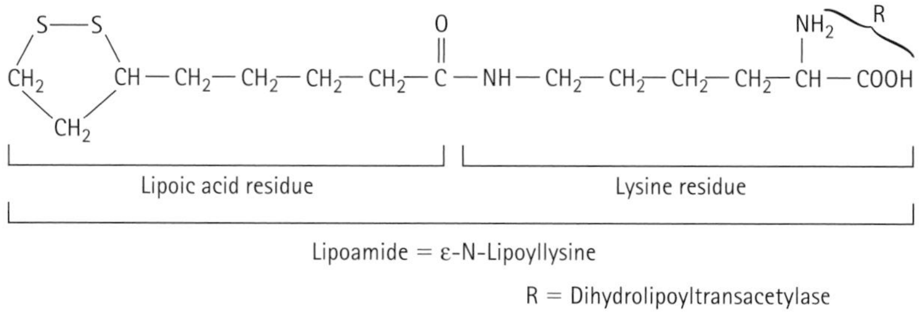

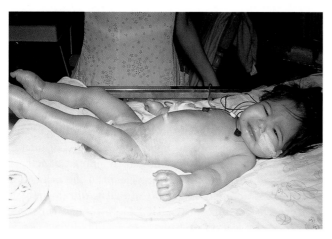

Lipoamide = ε-N-Lipoyllysine

R = Dihydrolipoyltransacetylase

Figure 51.3 *The structural attachment of lipoic acid to a lysine residue to E₂. This is reminiscent of the molecular attachment of biotin to the carboxylase apoenzymes.*

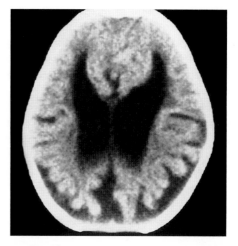

Figure 51.4 *E.B. at 10 months-of-age, two months after admission. He was symmetrically small, and at the time had hypoproteinemia and edema.*

Figure 51.5 *E.B. CT scan at 10 months. There was appreciable cerebral atrophy.*

ketones. Analysis of the organic acids of the urine revealed large amounts of lactate, acetoacetate, and 3-hydroxybutyrate. Electroencephalograph (EEG) revealed focal dysrhythmia in the left temporal region. CT scan (Figure 51.5) revealed evidence of cerebral atrophy.

Treatment was initiated with supplemental NaHCO₃ but his condition worsened progressively and his bicarbonate requirement increased. Ultimately it proved to be impossible to raise his serum concentration of bicarbonate without parenteral bicarbonate. Urinary obligatory water losses were such that he required 200 to 300 mL/kg/day, and 60 mEq/kg NaHCO₃ were required to achieve a normal serum level of bicarbonate. It was impossible to provide sufficient protein and calories to permit adequate growth without ketonuria and increasing acidosis or diarrhea. He died 7 months after admission.

Two patients [7,8] had renal tubular acidosis. We have observed renal tubular acidosis in a number of patients with organic academia [9,10]. Early death has been almost the rule, but some patients have had progressive neurologic deterioration. In some the picture has been that of Leigh encephalopathy [11]. Neuropathology was that of myelin loss and cavitation in the basal ganglia [4].

Two patients have been reported [12,13] with a milder phenotype (Figure 51.6) and normal cognitive function. One [12] had some motor problems, and one had hepatocellular disease [13].

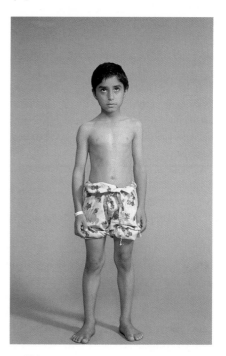

Figure 51.6 *F.M., a 7-year-old boy with a diagnosis of E₃ deficiency. At this time he looked normal, but he had episodic attacks of vomiting progressive to lethargy and lactic acidosis. Each responded to fluid and electrolyte therapy. Tandem mass spectrometry of the blood was normal between attacks, but during the attack there was mild elevation of the branched-chain amino acids.*

The acute acidotic episode in these patients differed from those of other patients with lactic acidemia because of the presence of pronounced ketonuria. This is reminiscent of the pattern in patients with pyruvate carboxylase deficiency (Chapter 48). Some patients have had hypoglycemia [1,4,5]. They have all had elevated concentrations of lactic acid and pyruvate in the blood. The characteristic urinary organic acid pattern was that of elevated excretion of lactate pyruvate and 2-oxoglutarate [5,6,8]. Elevated concentrations of 2-oxoglutarate have also been documented in the blood [1]. Other citric acid cycle intermediates, such as citrate, fumarate and malate, may be found in increased amounts in urine. Excretion of 3-hydroxybutyrate may be massive [8], and there may be secondary elevation of 2-hydroxyisovalerate, as in any patient with ketosis. Elevated amounts of 2-hydroxyglutarate and 2-oxoisocaproate have also been reported in urine [14]. The plasma and/or urinary levels of alanine are often elevated [4,6,8]. In some patients somewhat elevated concentrations of the branched-chain amino acids isoleucine, leucine and valine have been recorded [1,5,13], and alloisoleucine may be found. In one patient [5] a neonatal screen for leucine revealed an elevated concentration in the blood.

GENETICS AND PATHOGENESIS

Defective enzyme activity has regularly been observed in the case of the pyruvate dehydrogenase complex and 2-oxoglutarate dehydrogenase [1,4–8]. The assay has usually been carried out in cultured fibroblasts, but deficiency has also been demonstrated in a number of tissues, including liver [1,5]. Levels of activity for the two enzymes ranged from 10 percent and 1 percent, respectively, of control to 38 and 39 percent of control [1,4–8]. The activity of 2-oxocaproate dehydrogenase, 2-oxo-3-methylvalerate dehydrogenase and 2-oxoisovalerate dehydrogenase have also been documented to be deficient, as have the oxidation of leucine and valine to CO_2 [8]. Thus there is a generalized defect in these patients in the enzymes involved in oxidative decarboxylation.

Oxidative decarboxylation is typified by the pyruvate dehydrogenase complex (Fig. 51.1), but it is also the function of 2-oxoglutarate dehydrogenase and branched-chain amino acid dehydrogenase. The only enzyme known to be shared by the 3 enzyme complexes is lipoamide dehydrogenase (dihydrolipoyl dehydrogenase) (E_3) (EC 1.6.4.3) (Fig. 51.2). The pyruvate dehydrogenase complex consists of five known enzymatic components. Those that catalyze the actual decarboxylation include pyruvate decarboxylase (E_1) (EC 4.1.1.1) and dihydrolipoyl transacetylase (E_2) as well as E_3. E_1 exists in inactive and active forms, or phosphorylated and dephosphorylated proteins, respectively, and the activation is catalyzed by a phosphatase and the inactivation by a kinase.

An enzymatic process catalyzing the attachment of lipoic acid to the E_2 enzyme (Figure 51.3) is not known. However, it would be surprising if one did not exist. The covalent bond formed between the carboxyl group of lipoic acid and the amino group of a lysine residue of the E_2 protein would require energy. The structure suggests by analogy the attachment of biotin to the apocarboxylases propionyl CoA carboxylase, 3-methylcrotonyl CoA carboxylase and pyruvate carboxylase, which is catalyzed by holocarboxylase synthetase, the enzyme that is deficient in the neonatal form of multiple carboxylase deficiency.

Deficiency of lipoamide dehydrogenase (E_3) has been documented in a number of patients [1,4–7,14]. In the first patient activity of five to 10 percent of control was observed in a variety of tissues obtained post mortem [1]. In another, activity in cultured fibroblasts was five percent [4], while no activity could be found in biopsied liver or muscle. In another [5,13], activity was undetectable in either fibroblasts or liver. In one patient [7] with E_3 deficiency, the residual activity of the enzyme in fibroblasts was 20 percent of the control mean and the kinetics of the enzyme in both forward and reverse directions were normal. This was a patient who was reported to respond to lipoic acid, and it is of interest that he was the one with the substantial amount of activity. However, *in vitro* addition of lipoic acid to the incubation mixtures did not increase activity of PDHC or ketoglutarate dehydrogenase complex (KGDHC). One of the patients with normal cognitive function had 12 percent of residual E_3 activity [11]. Immunochemical studies with antibody to porcine E_3 enzyme revealed normal amounts of enzyme protein in fibroblasts of each of three patients studied [15].

E_3 deficiency and the other forms of combined or multiple oxoacid dehydrogenase deficiency appear to be transmitted by rare autosomal recessive genes. Consanguinity has been reported [1,8]. In another family of Canadian Indians, there were three affected siblings, a girl and two boys, and the parents were thought to be consanguineous [2].

The E_3 enzyme, as isolated from porcine heart is a homodimer with a molecular weight of 160 kDa [16]. The gene has been assigned to chromosome 7q31–32 [17]. The human cDNA codes for an enzyme with homology with glutathione reductase [18]. A number of mutations have been identified. They include K37E and P453L, found in compound heterozygous Japanese patients [19] and G229C, a frequent allele in Ashkenazi Jews [20]. A patient with A1173G/ del455–457 had delayed development and microcephaly and died at 5 years of age [20]. Two patients with a milder phenotype had an InsA105 mutation [11].

TREATMENT

Treatment has not generally been satisfactory in these patients. Most of them have died in infancy. It is important to recognize the problem because the high fat diet that is usually useful in isolated PDHC deficiency may make these patients severely acidotic [4,8]. Restriction of protein intake may result in a decrease in the excretion of 2-oxoglutarate. This would be consistent with inhibition of human KGDHC by branched-chain ketoacids, as has been observed in pig heart KGDHC *in vitro* [21]. Treatment by restriction of protein appeared to be clinically efficacious in one patient [5], but it did not prevent a fatal outcome in this patient or another [8].

Treatment with lipoic acid was reported in one patient to produce a dramatic clearing of the abnormal organic aciduria and a reduction in lactic and pyruvic acid concentrations in blood [7]. It appeared to prevent the occurrence of episodes of acidosis and to promote consistent gains in growth and development. Doses employed were 25 to 50 mg/kg per day. Similar doses appeared to be of some benefit in another patient [8]. Treatment with glutamine [4] and biotin [7] have not been of benefit. Nor have large doses of thiamine [4,7]. Nevertheless, it may be prudent to administer thiamine to patients being treated with lipoic acid because lipoic acid has been reported to be toxic to thiamine-deficient animals [22]. Lipoic acid has been thought to be useful in the management of Amanita mushroom poisoning and other forms of liver disease [23]. The adult human dose was 50–150 mg q6 hr. intravenously.

Renal tubular acidosis should be managed with sodium bicarbonate or sodium citrate.

References

1 Robinson BH, Taylor J, Sherwood WG. Deficiency of dihydrolipoyl dehydrogenase (a component of pyruvate and α-ketoglutarate dehydrogenase complexes): a cause of congenital lactic acidosis in infancy. *Pediatr Res* 1977;**11**:1198.

2 Haworth JC, Perry TL, Blass JP, *et al.* Lactic acidosis in three sibs due to defects in both pyruvate dehydrogenase and α-ketoglutarate dehydrogenase complexes. *Pediatrics* 1976;**58**:564.

3 Kuroda Y, Kline JJ, Sweetman L, *et al.* Abnormal pyruvate and α-ketoglutarate dehydrogenase complexes in a patient with lactic academia. *Pediatr Res* 1979;**12**:928.

4 Robinson BH, Taylor J, Kahler SG, Kirman HN. Lactic acidemia neurologic deterioration and carbohydrate dependence in a girl with dihydrolipoyl dehydrogenase deficiency. *Eur J Pediatr* 1981;**136**:35.

5 Sakaguchi Y, Yoshino M, Aramaki S, *et al.* Dihydrolipoyl dehydrogenase deficiency: a therapeutic trial with branched-chain amino acid restriction. *Eur J Pediatr* 1986;**145**:271.

6 Munnich A, Saudubray J-M, Taylor J, *et al.* Congenital lactic acidosis α-ketoglutaric aciduria and variant form of maple syrup urine disease due to a single enzyme defect dihydrolipoyl dehydrogenase deficiency. *Acta Paed Scand* 1982;**71**:167.

7 Matalon R, Stumpf DA, Mihals K, *et al.* Lipoamide dehydrogenase deficiency with primary lactic acidosis: Favorable response treatment with oral lipoic acid. *J Pediatr* 1984;**104**:65.

8 Yoshida I, Sweetman L, Kulovich S, *et al.* Effect of lipoic acid in patient with defective activity of pyruvate dehydrogenase and branched-chain keto acid dehydrogenase. *Pediatr Res* 1990;**27**:75.

9 Wolff JA, Strom C, Griswold W, *et al.* Proximal renal tubular acidosis in methylmalonic academia. *J Neurogenet* 1985;**2**:31.

10 Pintos-Morell G, Hass R, Prodanos C, *et al.* Cytochrome C oxidase deficiency in muscle with dicarboxylic aciduria and renal tubular acidosis. *J Child Neurol* 1990;**5**:127.

11 Schwartz WJ, Hutchinson HT, Berg BO. Computerized tomography in subacute necrotizing encephalomyelopathy (Leigh disease). *Ann Neurol* 1981;**10**:268.

12 Elpeleg ON, Shaag A, Glustein JZ, *et al.* Lipoamide dehydrogenase deficiency in Ashkenazi Jews: An insertion mutation in the mitochondrial leader sequence. *Hum Mutat* 1997;**10**:256.

13 Aptowitzer I, Saada A, Faber J, *et al.* Liver disease in the Ashkenazi-Jewish lipoamide dehydrogenase deficiency. *J Pediatr Gastroenterol Nutr* 1997;**24**:599.

14 Matuda S, Kitano A, Sakaguchi Y, *et al.* Pyruvate dehydrogenase subcomplex with lactic acidosis and branched-chain ketoacidiuria. *Clin Chim Acta* 1984;**14**:59.

15 Otulakowski G, Nyhan WL, Sweetman L, Robinson BH. Immunoextraction of lipoamide dehydrogenase from cultured skin fibroblasts in patients with combined α-ketoacid dehydrogenase deficiency. *Clin Chim Acta* 1985;**152**:27.

16 Sakurai Y, Fekuyoshi Y, Hamada M, *et al.* Mammalian α-keto acid dehydrogenase complexes. VI Nature of the multiple forms of pig heart lipoamide dehydrogenase. *J Biol Chem* 1970;**245**:4453.

17 Scherer SW, Otulakowski G, Robinson BH, Tsui L-C. Localization of the human dihydrolipoamide dehydrogenase gene (DLD) to 7q31–q32. *Cytogenet Cell Genet* 1991;**56**:176.

18 Otulakowski G, Robinson GH. Isolation and sequence determination of cDNA clones for porcine and human lipoamide dehydrogenase: Homology to other disulfide oxidoreductases. *J Biol Chem* 1987;**262**:17313.

19 Liu T-C, Kim H, Arizmendi C, *et al.* Identification of two missense mutations in a dihydrolipoamide dehydrogenase-deficient patient. *Proc Natl Acad Sci USA* 1993;**90**:5186.

20 Shaag A, Saada A, Berger I, *et al.* Molecular basis of lipoamide dehydrogenase deficiency in Ashkenazi Jews. *Am J Med Genet* 1999;**82**:177.

21 Kanzaki T, Hayakawa T, Hamada M, *et al.* Mammalian α-keto acid dehydrogenase complexes. IV Substrate specificities and kinetic properties of the pig heart pyruvate and 2-oxoglutarate dehydrogenase complexes. *J Biol Chem* 1969;**244**:118.

22 Gal EM, Razevska DE. Studies on the *in vivo* metabolism of lipoic acid. I The fate of DL-lipoic acid-S^{35} in normal and thiamine deficient rats. *Arch of Biochem Biophys* 1960;**8**:253.

23 Michel DH. Amanita mushroom poisoning. *Ann Rev Med* 1980;**31**:51.

52

Mitochondrial encephalomyelopathy, lactic acidosis and stroke-like episodes (MELAS)

MAJOR PHENOTYPIC EXPRESSION

Mitochondrial myopathy, shortness of stature, stroke-like episodes, seizures, encephalopathy progressive to dementia, migraine, diabetes mellitus, lactic acidemia, ragged red muscle fibers and mutations in the mitochondrial tRNA leucine gene.

INTRODUCTION

This syndrome was first defined as such by Pavlakis and colleagues [1] in 1984, although patients have doubtless been

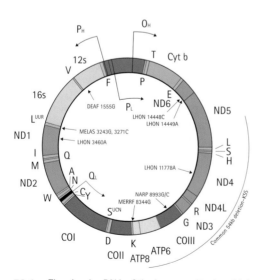

Figure 52.1 *The circular DNA of the human mitochondrial genome. Shown are the sites of the genes for the mitochondrial genes, as well as the sites for the most common mutations, including the A3243G and T3271C mutations associated with MELAS syndrome.*

reported earlier. Among the mitochondrial myopathies this is one of the more common [2].

The typical clinical presentation includes all of the features that make up the name of the syndrome, but there is enormous variability. Some affected individuals have only diabetes, or only migraine. Others have only hearing loss, or hearing loss and diabetes [3]. The disease is inherited in a maternal pattern, and the gene is on the mitochondrial genome (Figure 52.1). Most of the patients have had one of two point mutations in the mitochondrial gene for the leucine (UUR) tRNA (A3243G and T3271C) [4–7] (Figure 52.2).

CLINICAL ABNORMALITIES

There is a considerable variety of expression consistent with the varying heteroplasmy of mitochondrial inheritance. The typical picture is of normal development followed by a severe, progressive encephalomyopathy. Onset may be myopathic with exercise intolerance or weakness (Figure 52.3). Many patients have shortness of stature, and this may be the first manifestation of disease (Figure 52.4). One of our patients had been treated unsuccessfully with human growth hormone by a pediatric endocrinologist; this has also been reported by others. In many patients the onset of symptoms is with the first stroke-like episode, usually between 4 and

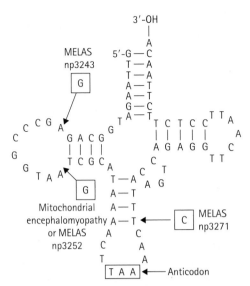

Figure 52.2   *The tRNA for leucine, the site of the defect in the MELAS syndrome. In addition to the point mutation at npA3243G, the common mutation in MELAS, and npT3271C and npA3252G the other MELAS mutations, there are a number of other known mutations in the tRNA leucine which cause mitochondrial diseases. These include: npT3250C, mitochondrial myopathy; npA3751G chronic progressive external ophthalmoplegia (CPEO) proximal weakness, sudden death; npA3260G, adult onset hypertrophic cardiomyopathy and myopathy; npA3302G, mitochondrial myopathy; and npC3303T, adult onset hypertrophic cardiomyopathy and myopathy.*

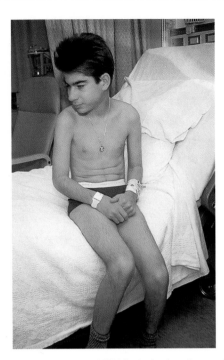

Figure 52.4   *N.F., a boy with MELAS who had strokes on three occasions and had become demented. Stature was very short. (This illustration was kindly provided by Dr. Richard Haas of UCSD.)*

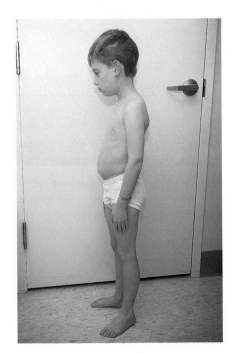

Figure 52.3   *K.S., a boy with MELAS illustrating his lordotic, myopathic posture. He presented at 4 years-of-age with weakness and exercise intolerance. He also had insulin-dependent diabetes mellitus. Blood concentration of CPK was 462 IU/L. Plasma lactate was 93.1 mg/dL. (This illustration was kindly provided by Dr. Richard Haas of UCSD.)*

15 years-of-age [1,4,8–14]. Less commonly, the onset of disease may be in infancy [8], often with delayed developmental milestones or learning disability.

The myopathy may be present before the first stroke. At one extreme is a floppy infant at 4 months-of-age [8]. More commonly, there is exercise intolerance, easy fatigability or frank weakness. Patients may have difficulty going up stairs. Myopathy may be progressive. Proximal muscles tend to be more involved than the distal [8]. Musculature is generally thin. The facial appearance may be myopathic [15]. The creatine phosphokinase activity in the blood may be elevated [13,16]. Some patients have been diagnosed as having polymyositis [11]. The electromyogram (EMG) may demonstrate a myopathic pattern.

The stroke-like episode is the hallmark feature of this syndrome. At the same time, these episodes may occur in only a few members of a pedigree, in which a much larger number has the same mutation [15,16]. In one series of four families [16] stroke-like episodes occurred only in the probands. Two of the affected mothers were clinically entirely normal. In other pedigrees no member may have had this defining manifestation. The episode may initially be manifest by vomiting and headache, convulsions or visual abnormalities [8]. Less commonly, there may be numbness, hemiplegia or aphasia. There may be recurrent episodes of headache or vomiting lasting a few hours to several days. The episode may be followed by transient hemiplegia or hemianopia lasting a few hours to several weeks. Computed tomography (CT) or magnetic resonance imaging (MRI) scan of the brain following such an episode reveals lucency consistent with infarction [17]

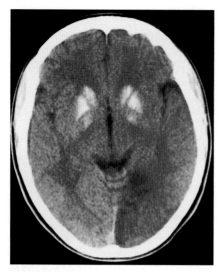

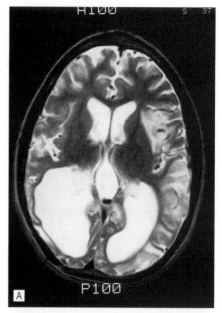

Figure 52.5   *CT of the brain of M.R., a boy with the A3243 G mutation, illustrating the posterior infarct and the extensive calcifications in the basal ganglia, including the caudate, putamen and globus pallidus. (Illustration kindly provided by Dr. Richard Haas of UCSD.)*

(Figures 52.5 and 52.6). This picture may resolve over hours or days, but later there may be cerebral atrophy and calcifications, especially in the basal ganglia [17–24] (Figure 52.6).

Infarcts are most common in the posterior temporal, parietal or occipital lobes, but histologic examination may reveal clear-cut infarcts widely scattered in the cerebrum, cerebellum or basal ganglia [18,20,25,26]. So these episodes are in fact strokes. The term 'stroke-like' may be appropriate in that no vascular changes of inflammation or atherosclerosis are found in the brain. We have tended to refer to this type of lesion as metabolic stroke in other diseases, such as propionic acidemia (Chapter 2) or methylmalonic acidemia (Chapter 3). In MELAS mitochondrial angiopathy is evident in contrast enhancement in affected areas [21,27–29], and even in the skin as purpuric lesions.

The migraine or migraine-like headaches seen in these patients may reflect the same process. Headache may be hemicranial. In pedigrees of patients with classic MELAS there are many members whose only manifestation is migraine [8,15] (Figure 52.7). Developmental delay, or learning disability [8] or attention deficit disorder [15], is mainly found in patients prior to the development of the first stroke. This was the history of the patient illustrated in Figure 52.4 who did not have his first stroke until the age of 8, but had been in a special education program for years. On the other hand, some patients with considerable myopathy and/or other symptomatology may be intellectually normal (Figure 52.3). The encephalopathy when it develops may be progressive to dementia (Figure 52.4). The patient may be apathetic and cachectic [18].

Additional neurologic features include ataxia, tremor, dystonia, visual disturbances and cortical blindness. Some have had myoclonus. Convulsive seizures may be focal or generalized

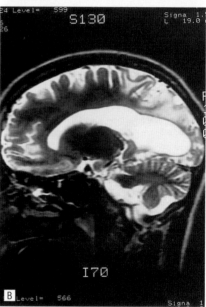

Figure 52.6   *MRI of the brain of N.F. illustrating widespread cortical atrophy, residual at a right parieto-occipital infarct with ventriculomegaly and increased T_2 signal representing preinfarction state in left temporoparieto-occipital cortex. (This illustration kindly provided by Dr. Richard Haas of UCSD.)*

tonic-clonic, but may also be myoclonic [7]. The electroencephalogram (EEG) is usually abnormal, and there are usually epileptiform spike discharges.

Some patients have had ophthalmoplegia or ptosis [11]. Others have had pigmentary degeneration of the retina [30] like those with the neurodegeneration, ataxia and retinitis pigmentosa (NARP) mutation (Chapter 54). Patients have been referred to as having the Kearns-Shy syndrome [11]. Others have presented with the picture of Leigh syndrome (Chapter 47), in which patients have recurrent attacks of

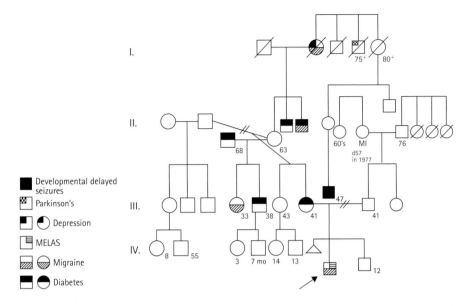

Figure 52.7   *Pedigree of the family of N.F. illustrating the occurrence of diabetes, migraine, seizures and other problems. Analysis of the blood revealed the npA3243G mutation.*

neurologic regression, pyramidal and extrapyramidal signs, brainstem abnormalities and leukodystrophy [31,32].

An interesting consequence of the MELAS mutation is the occurrence of diabetes mellitus [30] (Figure 52.7). This appears to be the most common manifestation of MELAS. It is usually type II diabetes [33], but the boy shown in Figure 52.3 had insulin-dependent diabetes mellitus.

Sensorineural hearing loss is another common manifestation, and it may be seen in individuals with or without diabetes and no other manifestations of disease [3]. It may also be seen in patients with the classic syndrome. Deafness has been reported in about 25 percent of patients [8]. The disease is a major cause of aminoglycoside-induced hearing loss [34]. This provides an argument for screening for the MELAS mutation in patients with antibiotic-induced deafness, in order to test affected relatives and avoid aminoglycosides in them.

Cardiomyopathy is a less common feature, but may be found in about 10 percent of patients. It is usually hypertrophic cardiomyopathy, but it may be dilated [35]. Patients with the MELAS mutations have been found to have MELAS and cardiomyopathy, but others have had isolated cardiomyopathy and no neurologic disease. There may be conduction abnormalities – for instance, Wolff-Parkinson-White syndrome [18] – and often an abnormal electrocardiogram [36]. Huge accumulation of mitochondria has been observed in myocardial fibers [18].

Renal involvement may take the form of renal tubular acidosis, and there may be a typical renal Fanconi syndrome [37]. One patient developed a nephrotic syndrome and had focal glomerulosclerosis [16]. A variety of other organs has been involved in individual patients. One had pancreatitis following valproate administration [15]. Others have had peripheral neuropathy with or without rhabdomyolysis [38,39]. One had ischemic colitis [40]. Pigmentary abnormalities of the skin have been reported [37].

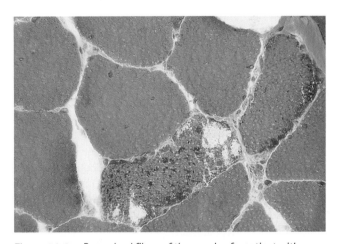

Figure 52.8   *Ragged red fibers of the muscle of a patient with MELAS. (Illustration kindly provided by Dr. Richard Haas of UCSD.)*

The histologic signature of the MELAS syndrome is the appearance of ragged red fibers in the muscle (Figure 52.8) [1,12,13,36]. These are best seen in the trichrome stain. In H and E there may be variation in fiber size and increase in connective tissue. Staining with periodic acid Schiff (PAS), NADH tetrazolium reductase or for succinic dehydrogenase may show increased subsarcolemmal activity. Electron microscopy reveals an increase in number and size of mitochondria (Figure 52.9), some with paracrystalline inclusion bodies [13,36].

The lactic acidosis is an important feature of this disorder. It does not usually lead to systemic acidosis, and it may even be absent in patients with impressive involvement of the central nervous system. The levels may be elevated in cerebrospinal fluid (CSF) and normal in blood [32]. The patient in Figure 52.4 had repeated determinations of lactate in the blood in the normal 20 mg/dL range; his CSF lactate was 56.3 mg/dL. The CSF concentration of protein may be mildly elevated.

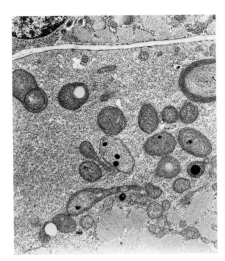

Figure 52.9   *Electronmicroscopy of the muscle of the mother of K.S. She had diabetes, but no symptoms of myopathy. Illustrated are many pleomorphic mitochondria, abnormal concentric lamellar cristae and electron-dense bodies. There is also glycogen accumulation. (Illustration kindly provided by Dr. Richard Haas of UCSD.)*

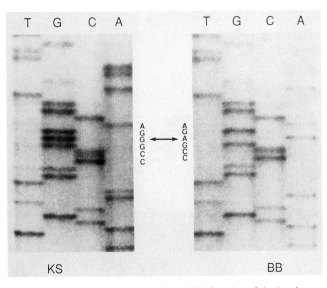

Figure 52.10   *Sequencing gel of the MELAS region of the leucine TRNA of muscle. The npA3243G mutation in K.S.; BB was a normal control. (Illustration kindly provided by Dr. Richard Haas of UCSD.)*

GENETICS AND PATHOGENESIS

The MELAS syndrome is the result of mutation in mitochondrial genes for tRNA [41]. The most common is A-to-G transition at position 3243 of the tRNALeu(UUR) [4,5] (Figure 52.1). Approximately 80 percent of affected individuals have this mutation in the dihydrouridine loop of the gene [8,16,42–44]. The other common mutation, occurring in about 8.5 percent of individuals, is also in the tRNALeu(UUR) at 3271 in the anticodon, where there is a T-to-C transversion [7]. The G-to-A transversion at 3252 of the same gene has been reported in mitochondrial encephalopathy [45]. Another mutation in the dihydrouridine loop at nucleotide 3250 is a T-to-C transition [42]. Another mutation in this gene is an A-to-T change at position 3256 [46]. A 5814G in the tRNACys gene was reported in a patient with cardiomyopathy and myopathy [35].

A quite distinct mutation, an A-to-G transition at nucleotide 11084 in the ND4 gene for the subunit of Complex I of the respiratory chain, was reported by Letrit et al. [47] in a Caucasian patient. This same mutation was later reported by Sakuta and colleagues [48] in 10–14 percent of Japanese studied, both patients with mitochondrial myopathy and normal controls, suggesting that it might be a polymorphism. On the other hand, this mutation was not found in 109 normal or patient Caucasians nor in American blacks, nor in a considerable number of patients with other mitochondrial diseases. So the issue on this transition is unresolved. A large (10.5 kg) deletion was reported in a MELAS patient with a renal Fanconi syndrome [37].

The common mutation creates a new site for Hae III leading to a 169 bp fragment in controls after electrophoresis and fragments of 97 and 72 bp in patients with MELAS [43]. Sequencing (Figure 52.10) reveals the G in MELAS where there is an A in control. Varying heteroplasmy among affected individuals appears to reflect variable segregation in the ovum. On the other hand, study of the proportion of mutant DNA in various tissues obtained from a woman and her two daughters revealed similar proportions in tissues derived from ectodermal, endodermal and mesodermal germ layers, indicating little mitotic segregation after early embryogenesis [49]. The issue of heteroplasmy, which can vary from tissue to tissue making detection difficult has been addressed in MELAS A3243G by the design of peptide nucleic acids which bond to the wild type mtDNA at 3243 preventing PCR amplification and making the mutant the dominant product [50].

Mutations in the tRNA for leucine might be expected to have an important effect on translation and hence protein synthesis in mitochondria. This has been demonstrated in studies of cybrids [25] by fusing human cell lines lacking mitochondrial DNA with exogenous mitochondria containing 0 to 100 percent of the common 3243 mutant DNA. Cybrids containing more than 95 percent mutant DNA had decreased rates of synthesis and steady state levels of mitochondrial proteins leading to respiratory chain deficiency.

Patients with the MELAS syndrome have been found to have marked deficiency in the activity of complex I of the respiratory chain [12]. In mitochondria from muscle, rotenone-sensitive NADH-cytochrome reductase activity was 0–27 percent of control value, and immunochemical study revealed a general decrease in complex I subunits. In a patient with the T-to-C 3250 mutation, complex I activity in muscle was six percent of control and that of complex IV was 47 percent of control [51]. The productions of CO_2 from labeled pyruvate, malate and 2-oxoglutarate were all reduced [36]. In a study of four patients with the 3243 mutation, the activity of complexes I and IV were reduced in muscle and other tissues, but there was no correlation between the proportion of mutant DNA in a tissue and the activity of the respiratory chain complexes [44].

TREATMENT

A variety of supportive measures is helpful in this disorder, as in other mitochondrial diseases. Riboflavin therapy has been reported to be of benefit in a patient with complex I deficiency and the T-to-C 3250 mutation [51]. A dose of 20 mg twice a day was employed in a 2-year-old patient with myopathy who could not ascend stairs and was reluctant to walk. Improvement in muscle strength occurred, and there was no further deterioration over three years of observation.

Coenzyme Q has been helpful in a number of patients [14]. Some amelioration of muscle weakness has been observed, as well as some decrease in plasma levels of lactate. CSF lactate did not improve. Doses of 30–90 mg per day were reported [14]. In MELAS, doses as high as 300 mg per day have been stated to be required for optimal effects [13,14].

Experience with dichloroacetic acid (Chapter 47) is accumulating; it is clear that levels of lactate are lowered in both plasma and CSF. MELAS may be one of the disorders that responds favorably to this agent.

References

1   Pavlakis SG, Phillips PC, DiMauro S, *et al.* Mitochondrial myopathy encephalopathy lactic acidosis and stroke-like episodes: a distinctive clinical syndrome. *Ann Neurol* 1984;**16**:481.

2   Hirano M, Ricci E, Koenigsberger MR, *et al.* MELAS: an original case and clinical criteria for diagnosis. *Neuromusc Disord* 1992;**2**:125.

3   Fischel-Ghodsian N. Mitochondrial mutations and hearing loss: Paradigm for mitochondrial genetics. *Am J Hum Genet* 1998;**62**:15.

4   Goto Y-I, Nonaka I, Horai S. A mutation in the tRNAleu(UUR) gene associated with the MELAS subgroup of mitochondrial encephalomyopathies. *Nature* 1990;**348**:651.

5   Kobayashi Y, Momoi MY, Tominaga K, *et al.* A point mutation in the mitochondrial tRNALeu(UUR) gene in MELAS (mitochondrial myopathy encephalopathy lactic acidosis and stroke-like episodes). *Biochem Biophys Res Commun* 1990;**173**:816.

6   Goto Y, Nonaka I, Horai S. An alternative mutation in the mitochondrial tRNAleu(UUR) gene associated with MELAS. *Am J Hum Genet* 1991;**49**:(suppl)190.

7   Goto Y-I, Nonaka I, Horai S. A new mutation in the tRNA-Leu(UUR) gene associated with mitochondrial myopathy lactic acidosis and stroke-like episodes. *Biochim Biophys Acta* 1991;**1097**:238.

8   Kobayashi M, Nonaka I. Mitochondrial myopathy encephalopathy lactic acidosis and stroke-like episodes (MELAS): a correlative study of the clinical features and mitochondrial DNA mutation. *Neurology* 1992;**42**:545.

9   Montagna P, Gallassi R, Medori R, *et al.* MELAS syndrome: characteristic migrainous and epileptic features and maternal transmission. *Neurology* 1988;**38**:751.

10 Ciafaloni E, Ricci E, Shanske S, *et al.* MELAS: clinical features biochemistry and molecular genetics. *Ann Neurol* 1992;**31**:391.

11 Yoda S, Terauchi A, Kitahara F, Akabane T. Neurologic deterioration with progressive CT changes in a child with Kearns-Shy syndrome. *Brain Dev* 1984;**6**:323.

12 De Quick M, Lammens M, Dom R, Carton H. MELAS: a family with paternal inheritance. *Ann Neurol* 1991;**29**:456.

13 Goda S, Hamada T, Ishimoto S, *et al.* Clinical improvement after administration of coenzyme Q10 in a patient with mitochondrial encephalomyopathy. *J Neurol* 1987;**234**:62.

14 Yamamoto M, Sato T, Anno M, *et al.* Mitochondrial myopathy encephalomyopathy lactic acidosis and stroke-like episodes with recurrent abdominal symptoms and coenzyme Q10 administration. *J Neurol Neurosurg Psychiatry* 1987;**50**:1475.

15 Dougherty FE, Ernst SG, Aprille JR. Familial recurrence of atypical symptoms in an extended pedigree with the syndrome of mitochondrial encephalomyopathy lactic acidosis and stroke-like episodes (MELAS). *J Pediatr* 1994;**125**:758.

16 Inui K, Fukushima H, Tsukamoto H, *et al.* Mitochondrial encephalomyopathies with the mutation of the mitochondrial tRNALeu(UUR) gene. *J Pediatr* 1992;**120**:62.

17 Kobayashi M, Morishita H, Sugiyama N, *et al.* Mitochondrial myopathy encephalopathy lactic acidosis and stroke-like episodes syndrome and NADH-CoQ reductase deficiency. *J Inherit Metab Dis* 1986;**9**:301.

18 Bogousslavsky J, Perentes E, Deruaz JP, Regli F. Mitochondrial myopathy and cardiomyopathy with neurodegenerative features and multiple brain infarcts. *J Neurol Sci* 1982;**55**:351.

19 Shapira Y, Cererbaum SD, Cancilla PA, *et al.* Familial poliodystrophy mitochondrial myopathy and lactate academia. *Neurology* 1975;**25**:614.

20 Kuriyama M, Umezaki H, Fukuda Y, *et al.* Mitochondrial encephalomyopathy with lactate-pyruvate elevation and brain infarctions. *Neurology* 1984;**34**:72.

21 Hasuo K, Tamura S, Yasumori K, *et al.* Computed tomography and angiography in MELAS (mitochondrial myopathy encephalopathy lactic acidosis and stroke-like episodes); report of 3 cases. *Neuroradiology* 1987;**29**:393.

22 Matthews PM, Tampieri D, Berkovic SF, *et al.* Magnetic resonance imaging shows specific abnormalities in the MELAS syndrome. *Neurology* 1991;**41**:1043.

23 Abe K, Inui T, Hirono N, *et al.* Fluctuating MR images with mitochondrial encephalopathy lactic acidosis stroke-like syndrome (MELAS). *Neuroradiology* 1990;**32**:77.

24 Rosen L, Phillips S, Enzmann D. Magnetic resonance imaging in MELAS syndrome. *Neuroradiology* 1990;**32**:168.

25 Ohama E, Ohara S, Ikuta F, *et al.* Mitochondrial angiography in cerebral blood vessels of mitochondrial encephalomyopathy. *J Dermatol* 1991;**18**:295.

26 Fujii T, Okuno T, Ito M, *et al.* CT MRI and autopsy findings in brain of a patient with MELAS. *Pediatr Neurol* 1990;**6**:253.

27 Allard JC, Tilak S, Carter AP. CT and MR of MELAS syndrome. *Am J Neuroradiol* 1988;**9**:1234.

28 Tokunaga M, Mita S, Sakuta R, *et al.* Increased mitochondrial DNA in blood vessels and ragged-red fibers in mitochondrial myopathy encephalopathy lactic acidosis and stroke-like episodes (MELAS). *Ann Neurol* 1993;**33**:275.

29 Ohama E, Ohara S, Ikuta F, *et al.* Mitochondrial angiopathy in cerebral blood vessels of mitochondrial encephalomyopathy. *Acta Neuropathol (Berl)* 1987;**74**:226.

30 King MP, Koga Y, Davidson M, Schon EA. Defects in mitochondrial protein synthesis and respiratory chain activity segregate with the tRNALeu(UUR) mutation associated with mitochondrial myopathy encephalopathy lactic acidosis and stroke-like episodes. *Molec Cell Biol* 1992;**12**:480.

31 Dahl H-H M. Getting to the nucleus of mitochondrial disorders: identification of respiratory chain-enzyme genes causing Leigh syndrome. *Am J Hum Genet* 1998;**63**:1594.

32 Rahman S, Blok R, Dahl H-H M, *et al.* Leigh syndrome: clinical features and biochemical and DNA abnormalities. *Ann Neurol* 1996;**39**:343.

33 Van den Ouweland JMW, Lemkes HHPJ, Ruitenbeek W, *et al.* Mutation in mitochondrial tRNALeu(UUR) gene in a large pedigree with maternally transmitted type II diabetes mellitus and deafness. *Nature Genet* 1992;**1**:368.

34 Prezant TR, Agapian JV, Bohlman MC, *et al.* Mitochondrial ribosomal RNA mutation associated with both antibiotic-induced and non-syndromic deafness. *Nat Genet* 1993;**4**:289.

35 Karadimas C, Tanji K, Geremek M, *et al.* A5814G mutation in mitochondrial DNA can cause mitochondrial myopathy and cardiomyopathy. *J Child Neurol* 2001;**16**:531.

36 Kobayashi M, Morishita H, Sugiyama N, *et al.* Two cases of NADH-coenzyme Q reductase deficiency: relationship to MELAS syndrome. *J Pediatr* 1987;**110**:223.

37 Campos Y, Garcia-Silva T, Barrionuevo CR, *et al.* Mitochondrial DNA deletion in a patient with mitochondrial myopathy lactic acidosis and stroke-like episodes (MELAS) and Fanconi's syndrome. *Pediatr Neurol* 1995;**13**:69.

38 Hara H, Wakayama Y, Kouno Y, *et al.* Acute peripheral neuropathy rhabadomyolysis and severe lactic acidosis associated with 3243 A to G mitochondrial DNA mutation. *J Neurol Neurosurg Psychiatry* 1994;**57**:1545 (letter).

39 Rusanen H, Majamaa K, Tolonen U, *et al.* Demyelinating polyneuropathy in a patient with the tRNALeu(UUR) mutation at base pair 3243 of the mitochondrial DNA. *Neurology* 1995;**45**:1188.

40 Hess J, Burkhard P, Morris M, *et al.* Ischaemic colitis due to mitochondrial cytopathy. *Lancet* 1995;**346**:189 (letter).

41 Enter C, Muller HJ, Zierz S, *et al.* A specific point mutation in the mitochondrial genome of Caucasians with MELAS. *Hum Genet* 1991;**88**:233.

42 Goto Y, Tojo M, Tohyama J, *et al.* A novel point mutation in the mitochondrial tRNALeu(UUR) gene in a family with mitochondrial myopathy. *Ann Neurol* 1992;**31**:672.

43 Moraes CT, Ricci E, Bonilla E, *et al.* The mitochondrial tRNALeu(UUR) mutation in mitochondrial encephalomyopathy lactic acidosis and stroke-like episodes (MELAS): genetic biochemical and morphological correlations in skeletal muscle. *Am J Hum Genet* 1992;**50**:934.

44 Obermaier-Kusser B, Paetzke-Brunner I, Enter C, *et al.* Respiratory chain activity in tissues from patients (MELAS) with a point mutation of the mitochondrial genome [tRNA(Leu(UUR))]. *FEBS Lett* 1991;**286**:67.

45 Morten KJ, Cooper JM, Brown GK, *et al.* A new point mutation associated with mitochondrial encephalomyopathy. *Hum Molec Genet* 1993;**2**:2081.

46 Sato W, Hayasaka K, Shoji Y, *et al.* A mitochondrial tRNALeu(UUR) mutation at 3256 associated with mitochondrial myopathy encephalopathy lactic acidosis and stroke-like symptoms (MELAS). *Biochem Mol Biol Int* 1994;**33**:1055.

47 Lertrit P, Noer AS, Jean-Francois MJB, *et al.* A new disease-related mutation for mitochondrial encephalopathy lactic acidosis and stroke-like episodes (MELAS) syndrome affects the ND4 subunit of the respiratory complex. *Am J Hum Genet* 1992;**51**:457.

48 Sakuta R, Goto Y, Nonaka I, Horai S. An A-to-G transition at nucleotide pair 11084 in the ND4 gene may be an mtDNA polymorphism. *Am J Hum Genet* 1993;**53**:964 (letter).

49 McMillan C, Shoubridge EA. Variable distribution of mutant mitochondrial DNAs (tRNALeu(3242)) in tissues of symptomatic relatives with MELAS: the role of mitotic segregation. *Neurology* 1993;**43**:82P (abstr).

50 Hancock DK, Schwarz FP, Song F, *et al.* Design and use of a peptide nucleic acid for detection of the heteroplasmic low-frequency mitochondrial encephalomyopathy lactic acidosis and stroke-like episodes (MELAS) mutation in human mitochondrial DNA. *Clin Chem* 2002;**48**:2155.

51 Ogle RF, Christodoulou J, Fagan E, *et al.* Mitochondrial myopathy with tRNALeu(UUR) mutation and complex I deficiency responsive to riboflavin. *J Pediatr* 1997;**130**:138.

53

Myoclonic epilepsy and ragged red fiber (MERRF) disease

MAJOR PHENOTYPIC EXPRESSION

Myoclonus, ataxia, seizures, optic atrophy, hearing loss, dementia, lipomas of neck and trunk, mitochondrial myopathy with ragged red fibers, lactic acidemia, reduced activity of oxidative phosphorylation and point mutations in the tRNA lysine gene.

INTRODUCTION

Mitochondrial disease and the abnormalities of oxidative phosphorylation were first recognized in 1962 with the description of Luft and colleagues [1] of a hypermetabolic woman with a normal thyroid, who had mitochondria that were abnormal in structure and loose coupling of oxidation and phosphorylation. The key histologic feature of mitochondrial myopathy, particularly the defects of mitochondrial DNA, was recognized first by Engel and Cunningham [2] with the modified Gomori-trichrome stain that identifies muscle with abnormal deposits of mitochondria as ragged (because of myopathic disruption) red (because of the mitochondria) muscle fibers. The ultrastructural counterpart of this appearance was first recognized by Gonatas and Shy [3], with the description of excessive proliferation of apparently normal mitochondria (pleoconial), greatly enlarged mitochondria (megaconial) or abnormalities in structure with disoriented cristae, or abnormal paracrystalline or osmiophilic inclusions.

Myoclonic epilepsy with ragged red fibers was first reported in 1973 by Tsairis and colleagues [4], but current recognition of the disease as a distinct entity was focused by the report of Fukuhara and his associates in 1980 of two patients with myoclonic epilepsy and ragged red fibers [5]. By 1988, 25 examples of the MERRF disease were reviewed by

the Columbia group [6]. In the same year Wallace and colleagues reported evidence that the disease was maternally inherited and qualified as a disease of mitochondrial DNA [7]. This group reported the point mutation in the gene for the lysine tRNA in 1990 [8] (Figure 53.1). The missense

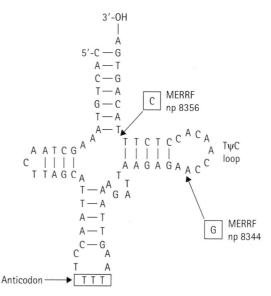

Figure 53.1 *The tRNA for lysine and the mutations that cause the MERRF disease.*

mutation A8344G has been found in approximately 80 percent of patients [8,9].

CLINICAL ABNORMALITIES

Myoclonic seizures are characteristic features of the disease [10,11,12]. They have been reported along with ataxia in the absence of ragged red fibers on muscle biopsy in patients with the documented mutation [13]. However, there is considerable phenotypic variability. In a single family with clear maternal inheritance, the clinical picture ranged all the way from an 18-year-old female who had myoclonus, ataxia, deafness, spasticity and dementia to asymptomatic status with ragged red fiber histology in two members of the family [13]. This is consistent with variable heteroplasmy. The classic picture is of a progressive myoclonic epilepsy, mitochondrial myopathy with ragged red fibers and slowly progressive dementia [7,10–23] (Figures 53.2, 53.3). Patients may also have akinetic seizures [10] or generalized grand mal seizures [24]. Myoclonic jerks may be virtually continuous and may dominate the clinical picture [10]. The onset of symptoms may be in late childhood or in adulthood [5,7,10–12,14–16,25, 26]. Truncal and limb ataxia are present, and speech may be scanning. There may be spastic paraparesis, exaggerated deep tendon reflexes in the legs and extensor plantar responses [10].

Optic atrophy is common [10]. Eye movements are visually normal, but ocular apraxia has been observed in one patient [25] and abnormal mitochondria have been observed in extraocular muscles [25] along with endomysial fibrosis [27,28]. Paracrystalline inclusions may be absent. Hearing loss is characteristic [7,12,16,17,21,29], but some patients have normal hearing [5,15,25,30]. Stature is usually short [10,11]. Peripheral neuropathy may be evident clinically; nerve conduction velocity is often reduced [10]. An absence of strokes distinguishes this disorder from mitochondrial encephalomyelopathy, lactic acidosis and stroke-like episodes (MELAS) (Chapter 52). An unusual finding seen in a few patients is the occurrence of multiple lipomas in the neck and trunk [24,31].

The electroencephalogram (EEG) is characteristically abnormal. The typical pattern is of frequent bilateral episodes of high voltage delta waves early in the disease and bilaterally synchronous bursts of slow spike and wave complexes later [10]. Visual evoked responses (VER) may be reduced [12]. Positron emission tomography of the brain and ^{31}P-nuclear magnetic resonance spectroscopy of brain and muscle have provided evidence of impairment of energy metabolism and mitochondrial capacity to generate adenosine triphosphate (ATP) [7,18,32].

Pathologic examination reveals, in addition to the characteristic myopathy with ragged red fibers (Figure 52.8), widespread neurodegeneration in the dentatorubral and pallidoluysian systems, cerebral cortex, cerebellum, pons and spinal cord [20,33–36]. Staining of the muscle for cytochrome oxidase activity may show profound deficiency [10].

Blood concentrations of lactic acid are characteristically elevated, but there are exceptions, as in the case of most features

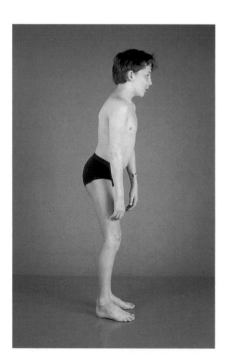

Figure 53.2 *A 12-year-old boy with the MERRF disease. He could walk, but the muscle weakness is indicated by his stooping posture. His pedigree is that of Family A of which he was the first proband in the paper of Larsson et al. [54]; other members of the family had lipomas of the neck. (This illustration and Figure 53.3 were kindly provided by Dr. Màr Tulinius of the Department of Pediatrics, Sahlgrenska University Hospital Östra, Göteberg, Sweden).*

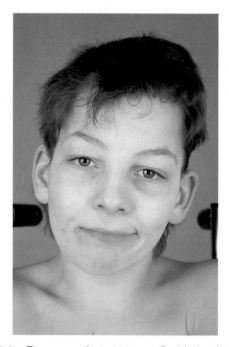

Figure 53.3 *The same patient at 16 years. By this time he was wheelchair-bound. He died at 18-years-of-age. Autopsy information was reported by Oldfors and colleagues [55]. The brain contained mutant mitochondrial DNA in 91–99 percent of tissues studied.*

of the disease, and levels are not usually very high [37]. Cerebrospinal fluid (CSF) concentrations of lactate are often higher than those of the blood. The CSF concentration of protein may be elevated, but it is usually normal [11].

GENETICS AND PATHOGENESIS

Inheritance of MERRF disease is maternal; the mutation is in the mitochondrial gene for the tRNA for lysine. The most common cause is the point mutation at nucleotide 8344 in which there is a G-to-A substitution [8,16,32]. This mutation accounts for 80–90 percent of patients [38–43]. In two families another mutation, a T-to-C change at 8356, has been identified [44,45]. A different tRNA mutation was reported [46] in a patient with manifestations called a MERRF phenotype and a mutation in the tRNA gene for leucine, a C-to-T transition at nucleotide 3256. This patient developed tonic-clonic seizures at 28 years of age. At 45 he had limb myoclonus, mild weakness of neck muscles and deltoids, mild ataxia and ragged red fibers in muscle. He did not have myoclonic seizures. In addition, he had hypothyroidism following thyroiditis, ptosis, ophthalmoparesis, hearing loss, diabetes mellitus, loss of central vision, optic atrophy and retinal pigmentary degeneration.

Abnormalities in tRNA would be expected to lead to impairment of mitochondrial translation and protein synthesis. Consistent with this hypothesis, studies of oxidative phosphorylation in muscle have revealed reduction in the activities of complexes I and IV [7,43], in which many of the protein components of the complexes are encoded by mitochondrial DNA [47,48]. Patients with MERRF have also been reported to have defects in complexes II and III [16,18,49]. Differences could suggest secondary effects or the substantial problems with methodology in assessing oxidative phosphorylation. On the other hand, phenotypic differences among patients tend to correlate with oxidative phosphorylation capacity of muscle [30].

Mitochondrial genetics differs from nuclear genetics in that the mitochondrial genome is inherited exclusively from the mother [50]. The mitochondrial DNA is transmitted via the cytoplasm of the egg. A cell may contain hundreds of mitochondria; during ovum formation the number of mitochondria increases while the number of DNAs per mitochondria decreases to one to two [51]. With growth and development, differences emerge among tissues in mitochondrial content and amounts of mitochondrial DNA. The latter is highest in brain, the organ most vulnerable to diseases of oxidative phosphorylation [52]. A cell may contain more than one sequence of mitochondrial DNA; this is referred to as heteroplasmy.

In MERRF the rule is for heteroplasmy for the mutation, and there is enormous variation within kindred in the amounts of mutated DNA and even among tissues in a patient. In oogenesis there is random segregation of mitochondria with and without mutation into daughter cells, accounting for the difference within a family. Random distribution during cytokinesis leads to different patterns in different tissues. Each tissue appears to have a threshold of production of mitochondrial ATP for adequate cellular function. As the percentage of abnormal mitochondrial DNA increases in different individuals, the threshold is exceeded and clinical disease results. A relatively high proportion of mutant DNA leads to clinical symptomatology [43]. Mitochondrial DNA also has a higher rate of mutation than does nuclear DNA [53]. One of the effects of ageing is an increase in the number of mutations in mitochondrial DNA. Thus, in a family with MERRF the severity of clinical phenotype correlates with the percentage of abnormal mutant DNA and the age of the individual. Most are phenotypically normal in infancy and childhood. As age-related decrease in oxidative phosphorylation exceeds the threshold for expression in an organ, symptoms of that organ's dysfunction appear, and they become progressively more severe with age [30]. In affected individuals the greatest percentage of mutant DNA has been found in muscle [47,54].

For this reason the work-up of a patient thought to be a candidate for this diagnosis may require muscle biopsy. The mutation may be found by analysis of the DNA of lymphocytes or platelets, but the diagnosis cannot be excluded unless the mitochondrial DNA of muscle is analyzed. Rapidly proliferating cells, such as lymphocytes, tend to have lower proportions of mutant DNA, suggesting selection against cells with high mutant content [43].

The MERRF 8344 mutation has been shown to interfere with mitochondrial protein synthesis [47,48]. When mutant mitochondrial DNA was greater than 85 percent there was impressively low synthesis of mitochondrial protein and parallel low levels of complex I and cytochrome oxidase. The effect on translation has been shown by the formation of cybrids, cells into which mitochondria were microinjected. The recipient ρ^o cells lack mitochondrial DNA and are deficient in dihydrouridine dehydrogenase required for the synthesis of uridinemonophosphate (UMP), and thus they require uridine for growth. Microinjection of human mitochondria permits growth in the absence of uridine, but cells receiving the MERRF 8344 mutation have markedly deficient synthesis of mitochondrial DNA while those receiving normal mitochondrial DNA synthesize mitochondrial protein well [48].

Family members at risk for maternal inherited MERRF may be tested for the mutation. Most often this is done on blood in those without symptoms. Examination of muscle may be required in those with any symptoms. Prenatal diagnosis is not generally reliable.

TREATMENT

Patients with this disease require supportive therapy aimed at the multiple systems involved. Seizures are managed with conventional anticonvulsant therapy.

Specific therapy is not yet available. Patients with disorders of oxidative phosphorylation, including MERRF, are generally treated with coenzyme Q, because of its place in the electron transport chain (Chapter 47). Doses of 4 mg/kg per day have usually been employed. Others have received riboflavin in doses of 100 mg/day.

Dichloroacetate is effective in lowering concentrations of lactic acid and is therefore under study. Whether or not it leads to clinical improvement in MERRF patients is not yet clear.

References

1   Luft R, Ikkos D, Palmieri G, *et al*. A case of severe hypermetabolism of nonthyroid origin with a defect in the maintenance of mitochondrial respiratory control: a correlated clinical biochemical and morphological study. *J Clin Invest* 1962;**41**:1776.

2   Engle WK, Cunningham GG. Rapid examination of muscle tissue. An improved method for fresh–frozen biopsy sections. *Neurology* 1963;**13**:919.

3   Gonatas NK, Shy GM. Childhood myopathies with abnormal mitochondria.*Excerpta Medica Int Congr Series* 1965;**100**:606.

4   Tsairis P, Engel W, Kark P. Familial myoclonic epilepsy syndrome associated with skeletal muscle mitochondrial abnormalities. *Neurology* 1973;**23**;408.

5   Fukuhara N, Tokiguchi S, Shirakawa K, Tsubaki T. Myoclonus epilepsy associated with ragged-red fibers (mitochondrial abnormalities): disease entity or a syndrome? Light- and electron-microscopic studies of two cases and review of the literature. *J Neurol Sci* 1980;**47**:117.

6   Pavlakis SG, Rowland LP, De Vivo DC, *et al*. Mitochondrial myopathies and encephalomyopathies: in *Advances in Contemporary Neurology* (ed. F Plum). FA Davis, New York;1988:37.

7   Wallace DC, Zheng XX, Lott MT, *et al*. Familial mitochondrial encephalomyopathy (MERRF): genetic pathophysiological and biochemical characterization of a mitochondrial DNA disease. *Cell* 1988;**55**:601.

8   Shoffner JM, Lott MT, Lezza AM, *et al*. Myoclonic epilepsy and ragged-red fiber disease (MERRF) is associated with a mitochondrial DNA tRNA(Lys) mutation. *Cell* 1990;**61**:931.

9   Kogelnik AM, Lott MT, Brown MD, *et al*. A human mitochondrial genome database, Atlanta Center for Molecular Medicine Emory University School of Medicine. http://www.mitomap.org (accessed December 2004).

10 Tulinius MH, Holme E, Kristiansson B, *et al*. Mitochondrial encephalomyopathies in childhood. II Clinical manifestations and syndromes. *J Pediatr* 1991;**119**:251.

11 De Vivo D. The expanding clinical spectrum of mitochondrial diseases. *Brain Dev* 1993;**15**:1.

12 Rosing HS, Hopkins LC, Wallace DC, *et al*. Maternally inherited mitochondrial myopathy and myoclonic epilepsy. *Ann Neurol* 1985;**17**:228.

13 Hammans SR, Sweeney MG, Brockington M, *et al*. Mitochondrial encephalopathies: molecular genetic diagnosis from blood samples. *Lancet* 1991;**337**:1311.

14 Fitzsimmons RB, Clifton-Bligh P, Wolfenden WH. Mitochondrial myopathy and lactic acidaemia with myoclonic epilepsy ataxia and hypothalamic infertility: a variant of Ramsay–Hunt syndrome. *J Neurol Neurosurg Psychiatry* 1981;**44**:79.

15 Feit H, Kirkpatrick J, Van Woert MH, Pandian G. Myoclonus ataxia and hypoventilation: response to l-5-hydroxytryptophan. *Neurology* 1983;**33**:109.

16 Morgan-Hughes JA, Hayes DJ, Clark JB, *et al*. Mitochondrial encephalomyopathies: biochemical studies in two cases revealing defects in the respiratory chain. *Brain* 1982;**105**:553.

17 Holliday PL, Climie AR, Gilroy J, Mahmud MZ. Mitochondrial myopathy and encephalopathy: three cases – a deficiency of NADH-CoQ dehydrogenase? *Neurology* 1983;**33**:1619.

18 Berkovic SF, Carpenter S, Evans A, *et al*. Myoclonus epilepsy and ragged-red fibres (MERRF). 1 A clinical pathological biochemical magnetic resonance spectrographic and positron emission tomographic study. *Brain* 1989;**112**:1231.

19 Lombes A, Mendell JR, Nakase H, *et al*. Myoclonic epilepsy and ragged-red fibers with cytochrome oxidase deficiency: neuropathology biochemistry and molecular genetics. *Ann Neurol* 1989;**26**:20.

20 Fukuhara N. MERRF: a clinicopathological study. Relationships between myoclonus epilepsies and mitochondrial myopathies. *Rev Neurol* (Paris) 1991;**147**:476.

21 Berkovic SF, Carpenter S, Karpati G, *et al*. Cytochrome c oxidase deficiency: a remarkable spectrum of clinical and neuropathological findings in a single family. *Neurology* 1987;**37**:223.

22 Berkovic SF, Andermann F, Karpati G, *et al*. Mitochondrial encephalomyopathies: a solution to the enigma of the Ramsay–Hunt syndrome. *Neurology* 1987;**37**:(Suppl 1) 125.

23 Ogasahara S, Engel AG, Frens D, Mack D. Muscle coenzyme Q deficiency in familial mitochondrial encephalomyopathy. *Proc Natl Acad Sci USA* 1989;**86**:2379.

24 DiMauro S, Hirano M, Bonilla E, De Vivo DC. The mitochondrial disorders; in *Principles of Child Neurology* (ed. BO Berg). McGraw Hill, New York;1996:1201.

25 Shoffner JM, Wallace DC. Oxidative phosphorylation diseases: in *The Metabolic and Molecular Bases of Inherited Disease* 7th edn (eds CR Scriver, AL Beaudet, WS Sly, D Valle) McGraw Hill, New York;1995:1535.

26 Byrne E, Dennet X, Trounce I, Burdon J. Mitochondrial myoneuropathy with respiratory failure and myoclonic epilepsy. A case report with biochemical studies. *J Neurol Sci* 1985;**71**:273.

27 Takeda S, Ohama E, Ikuta F. Involvement of extraocular muscle in mitochondrial encephalomyopathy. *Acta Neuropathol* 1990;**80**:118.

28 Takeda S, Wakabayashi K, Ohama E, Ikuta F. Neuropathology of myoclonus epilepsy associated with ragged-red fibers (Fukuhara's disease). *Acta Neuropathol (Berl)* 1988;**75**:433.

29 Berkovic SF, Andermann E, Carpenter S, *et al*. Mitochondrial encephalomyopathies: evidence for maternal transmission. *Am J Hum Genet* 1987;**41**:A47.

30 Byrne E, Trounce I, Marzuki S, *et al*. Functional respiratory chain studies in mitochondrial cytopathies. Support for mitochondrial DNA heteroplasmy in myoclonus epilepsy and ragged red fibers (MERRF) syndrome. *Acta Neuropathol (Berl)* 1991;**81**:318.

31 Berkovic SF, Shoubridge EA, Andermann F, *et al*. Clinical spectrum of mitochondrial DNA mutation at base pair 8344. *Lancet* 1991;**338**:457.

32 Eleff SM, Barker PB, Blackband SJ, *et al*. Phosphorus magnetic resonance spectroscopy of patients with mitochondrial cytopathies demonstrates decreased levels of brain phosphocreatine. *Ann Neurol* 1990;**27**:626.

33 Sasaki H, Kuzuhara S, Kanazawa I, *et al*. Myoclonus cerebellar disorder neuropathy mitochondrial myopathy and ACTH deficiency. *Neurology* 1983;**33**:1288.

34 Nakano T, Sakai H, Amano N, *et al*. An autopsy case of degenerative type myoclonus epilepsy associated with Friedreich's ataxia and mitochondrial myopathy. *Brain Nerve* 1982;**34**:321.

35 Fukuhara N. Myoclonus epilepsy and mitochondrial myopathy: in *Mitochondrial Pathology in Muscle Diseases* (eds G Scarlato, C Cerri) Pikkin Medical Books, Padua;1983:88.

36 Sengers RCA, Stadhouders AM, Trijbels JMF. Mitochondrial myopathies: clinical, morphological and biochemical aspects. *Eur J Ped* 1984;**141**:192.

37 DiMauro S, Bonilla E, Seviani M, *et al*. Mitochondrial myopathies. *Ann Neurol* 1985;**17**:521.

38 Tanno Y, Toneda M, Nonaka I, *et al.* Quantitation of mitochondrial DNA carrying tRNALys mutation in MERFF patients. *Biochem Biophys Res Commun* 1991;**179**:880.

39 Zeviani M, Amati P, Bresolin N, *et al.* Rapid detection of the A to G(8344) mutation of mtDNA in Italian families with myoclonus epilepsy and ragged-red fibers (MERRF). *Am J Hum Genet* 1991;**48**:203.

40 Seibel P, Degoul F, Bonne G, *et al.* Genetic biochemical and pathophysiological characterization of a familial mitochondrial encephalomyopathy (MERRF). *J Neurol Sci* 1991;**105**:217.

41 Noer AS, Sudoyo H, Lertrit P, *et al.* A tRNA(Lys) mutation in the mtDNA is the causal genetic lesion underlying myoclonic epilepsy and ragged-red fiber (MERRF) syndrome. *Am J Hum Genet* 1991;**49**:715.

42 Seibel P, Degoul F, Romero N, *et al.* Identification of point mutations by mispairing PCR as exemplified in MERRF disease. *Biochem Biophys Res Commun* 1990;**173**:561.

43 Chomyn A. The myoclonic epilepsy and ragged-red fiber mutation provides new insights into human mitochondrial function and genetics. *Am J Hum Genet* 1998;**62**:745.

44 Zeviani ML, Muntoni F, Savarese N, *et al.* A MERRF/MELAS overlap syndrome associated with a new point mutation of mitochondrial DNA tRNA-Lys gene. *Eur J Hum Genet* 1993;**1**:80.

45 Silvestri G, Moraes CT, Shanske S, *et al.* A new mutation in the tRNA-Lys gene associated with myoclonic epilepsy and ragged-red fibers (MERRF). *Am J Hum Genet* 1992;**51**:1213.

46 Moreas CT, Ciacci F, Bonilla E, *et al.* Two novel pathogenic mitochondrial DNA mutations affecting organelle number and protein synthesis. *J Clin Invest* 1993;**92**:2906.

47 Chomyn A, Meola G, Bresolin N, *et al. In vitro* genetic transfer of protein synthesis and respiration defects to mitochondrial DNA-less cells with myopathy-patient mitochondria. *Mol Cell Biol* 1991;**11**:2236.

48 Boulet L, Karpati G, Shoubridge E. Distribution and threshold expression of the tRNA- Lys mutation in skeletal muscle of patients with myoclonic epilepsy and ragged-red fibers (MERRF). *Am J Hum Genet* 1992;**51**:1187.

49 Riggs JE, Schochet SSJ, Fakadej AV, *et al.* Mitochondrial encephalomyopathy with decreased succinate-cytochrome c reductase activity. *Neurology* 1984;**34**:48.

50 Hutchinson CAI, Newbold JA, Potter SS, Edgell MH. Maternal inheritance of mammalian mitochondrial DNA. *Nature* 1974;**251**:536.

51 Piko L, Matsumoto L. Number of mitochondria and some properties of mitochondrial DNA in the mouse egg. *Dev Biol* 1976;**49**:1.

52 Ruiters MHJ, van Spronsen EA, Skjeldal OH, *et al.* Confocal scanning laser microscopy of mitochondria: a possible tool in the diagnosis of mitochondrial disorders. *J Inherit Metab Dis* 1991;**14**:45.

53 Wallace DC, Ye JH, Necklemann SN, *et al.* Sequence analysis of cDNAs for the human and bovine ATP synthase beta subunit: mitochondrial DNA genes sustain seventeen times more mutations. *Curr Genet* 1987;**12**:81.

54 Larsson N-G, Tulinius MH, Holme E, *et al.* Segregation and manifestations of the mtDNA tRNA-Lys A to G (8344) mutation of myoclonus epilepsy and ragged red fibers (MERRF) syndrome. *Am J Hum Genet* 1992;**51**:1201.

55 Oldfors A, Holme E, Tulinius M, Larsson N-G. Tissue distribution and disease manifestations of the tRNALys AÆG(8344) mitochondrial DNA mutation in a case of myoclonus epilepsy and ragged red fibers. *Acta Neuropathol* 1995;**90**:328.

54

Neurodegeneration, ataxia and retinitis pigmentosa (NARP)

MAJOR PHENOTYPIC EXPRESSION

Neurodegeneration, ataxia, pigmentory retinopathy, Leigh syndrome, neurogenic muscle weakness, peripheral neuropathy, and point mutation in the mitochondrial gene for subunit 6 of adenosine triphosphatase (ATPase), usually a T to G 8993, or a T to C8993 transversion.

INTRODUCTION

The 8993 mutation was first described by Holt and colleagues [1] in a family with a maternally inherited neurodegenerative disease in three generations. The major phenotype was of neurogenic muscle weakness, ataxia and retinitis pigmentosa, and this led to the acronym NARP. The 8993 T-to-G mutation is now referred to as the NARP mutation. Tatuch and colleagues in 1992 [2] reported the occurrence of this mutation in an infant who died at 7 months and at autopsy had the typical neuropathology of Leigh syndrome. It is now clear that 8933 mutation is a common cause of Leigh syndrome [3]. A second mutation at position 8993 changing T to C in the ATPase 6 gene was identified in a family with Leigh syndrome [4]. It was noted early that the percentage of mutant mitochondrial DNA varied considerably in heteroplasmic affected individuals, and this leads to considerable variability in phenotypic expression [5].

CLINICAL ABNORMALITIES

The index family was recognized as having a mitochondrial disease not previously described in which there was a variable combination of retinitis pigmentosa, neurogenic proximal muscle weakness, ataxia, sensory neuropathy, developmental delay, seizures and dementia. There were four patients in three generations. The initial patient was a 47-year-old woman who developed night blindness at 12 years-of-age and was found to have retinitis pigmentosa; she was nearly blind by 30 years. At 24 years she had a grand mal seizure and was treated with phenytoin. Unsteadiness in walking was progressive in her thirties. On examination she had marked ataxia. Ankle jerks were absent and proprioceptive and pain sensations were diminished in the distal lower extremities. Nerve conduction velocity was reduced. Her asymptomatic sister had clumps of retinal pigment and proximal muscle weakness. The daughter of this sister had reduced vision at 25 years and retinitis pigmentosa on examination along with mild proximal muscle weakness and ataxia, and extensor plantar responses. Her second daughter developed normally until she had a febrile illness at 28 months, in which she was unwell for a month, and she then stopped walking for five months. At 3 years she spoke only single words and had pigmentary retinopathy. She was ataxic and had increased tone in the limbs, exaggerated deep tendon reflexes and extensor plantar responses. The electroencephalograph (EEG) was abnormal.

Night blindness is often the first symptom of these patients [6]. This is followed by loss of peripheral vision and, in some, loss of central vision. The index patient at 47 years could just perceive light. Examination of the retina reveals evidence of retinitis pigmentosa (Figures 54.1, 54.2). The appearance of the clumps of pigment in the retina typically resembles spicules of bone [1,7]. Some retinas may have a salt-and-pepper appearance [8]. The electroretinogram may be abnormal, as

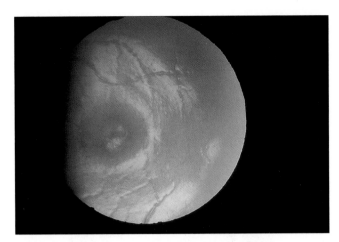

Figure 54.1 *A.A., a patient with ATP synthase deficiency had pigmentary degeneration of the retina.*

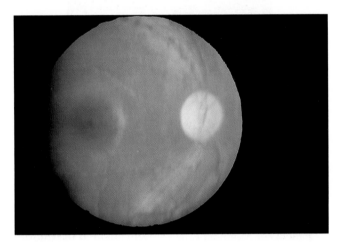

Figure 54.2 *A.A. The other fundus was also involved. His mutation was in peptide 6.*

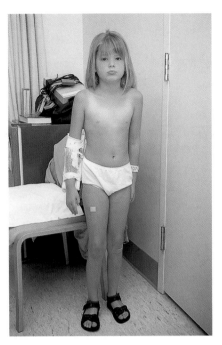

Figure 54.3 *B.F., a girl with the NARP mutation, a deletion at 8993, in mitochondrial DNA. She had been well until approximately a year before when she and her twin brother developed an acute life-threatening episode of which he died.*

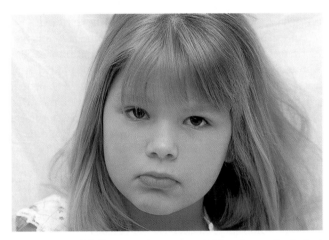

Figure 54.4 *B.F. She was quite ataxic and fell so frequently she had a raised bony area in her mid-forehead.*

may visual fields. Others have optic atrophy [9]. There may be nystagmus on horizontal or vertical gaze and esotropia [8].

Ataxia may be a prominent feature of the disease (Figures 54.3–54.5). It may lead to injuries and localized areas of traumatic hyperplasia. Cerebellar atrophy has been observed on neuroimaging [9]. Other patients have had dystonia.

Some patients have been impressively hypotonic [9]. Others have had localized proximal muscle weakness, but as recognized in the initial series the weakness is neurogenic. Muscle biopsy does not show ragged red fibers or abnormal mitochondria [1–3,9–11]. There may be evidence of denervation, lipid droplets or variation in fiber size diameter. The electromyogram (EMG) is normal.

Peripheral neuropathy may be evident on clinical examination [1]. Nerve conduction velocity is reduced in a pattern of axonal sensory neuropathy.

Seizures may be generalized and associated with spike and wave bursts on EEG [1,9]. Two patients have had infantile spasms and an EEG pattern of hypsarrhythmia [9]. Others have had myoclonic seizures. Less severely affected patients

have had migraine, some with no other manifestation of illness. Others have had depression or bulimia. Some have been developmentally delayed, some of them severely.

There have been a number of deaths in infancy [2,9] (Figure 54.3). The acute life-threatening episode may be associated with lactic acidemia [2]. The advent of dichloroacetate control of lactic acidemia has permitted us to observe episodes of acute acidemias in patients with the NARP mutation in the absence of lactic acidemia. These episodes of acute acidosis requiring admission to hospital, and parenteral fluid and electrolyte therapy have been characterized by ketoacidosis. An infant who died had lactate levels of 3–5 mmol/L [2]. Others had levels up to 5.2 mmol/L [9]. In one 50-year-old

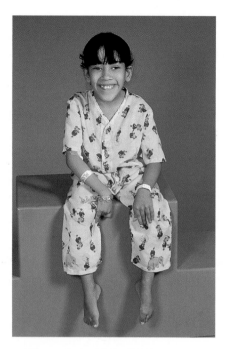

Figure 54.5   *T.S., a patient with the NARP syndrome. She had ataxia and retinitis pigmentosa.*

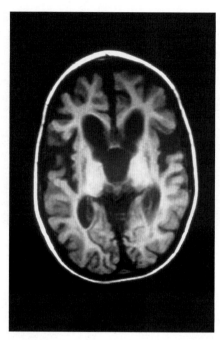

Figure 54.6   *A.A. CT scan of the brain. There was considerable atrophy.*

mildly retarded man the cerebrospinal fluid lactate was normal [9]. Cerebrospinal fluid concentrations of protein were normal [9]. Some patients have had recurrent vomiting.

An expanded spectrum of NARP syndrome [12] was recognized when the 8993G mutation was found in a patient whose diagnosis on magnetic resonance imaging (MRI) was acute demyelinating encephalomyelitis (ADEM). The patient had neurogenic muscle weakness, and ataxia, typical for NARP, but other affected family members had fewer clinical manifestations. Nevertheless, his mother died of fulminant hepatic failure following valproate administration. In four families studied none had retinitis pigmentosa. One was referred for 'cerebral palsy', attention deficit disorder, and learning disability. Later he had episodes of ataxia, headache and peripheral neuropathy following febrile illnesses.

Leigh syndrome (Chapter 47, p. 309) was first associated with the classic NARP mutation in the autopsy of an infant who died at 7 months-of-age with lactic acidemia, seizures and apnea [9]. She had been hypotonic and had head lag from early infancy. Neuropathologic examination revealed bilateral cystic lesions of the basal ganglia, thalamus, substantia nigra and tegmental brainstem. There was proliferation of astrocytes and blood vessels in these areas. A maternal aunt and uncle had died of Leigh syndrome. Another maternal uncle was normal until 12 years-of-age, when he developed a bout of weakness and ataxia from which he recovered. There were further episodes, and he developed retinitis pigmentosa. At 33 years he was ataxic, legally blind, retarded and in an institution.

Of seven patients with typical Leigh spongiform changes on neuropathology or the characteristic appearance on MRI, the classic NARP mutation was found in all [13]. In each there was heteroplasmy, but the mutation was in high proportion

in blood and muscle. It was found in four asymptomatic mothers and two asymptomatic siblings. This series was expanded to 12 patients in 10 families, all with the same mutation [3]. Consistent with the observations of Tatuch *et al.* [2] the Leigh phenotype was associated with a high percentage of abnormal mitochondrial DNA. The heterogeneity of Leigh syndrome is pointed up by the fact that the 12 patients of Santorelli *et al.* [3] were found in the study of 50 patients with typical Leigh syndrome. These authors compared 18 patients reported with the NARP mutation and Leigh syndrome with 34 and 64 in whom the underlying disease was cytochrome oxidase deficiency or pyruvate dehydrogenase complex deficiency (Chapter 48), respectively. Smaller numbers had biotinidase or complex I deficiency. Among the features of the clinical picture, only retinitis pigmentosa and positive family history seemed to distinguish the patients with NARP. An earlier-onset, more rapid course or propensity for seizures was more common among the NARP patients. Patients with the classic NARP mutation and Leigh syndrome were also reported by Ciafaloni and colleagues [10], Shoffner and colleagues [8] and Mäkelä-Bengs and colleagues [9]. Thus it is clear that the 8993 mutation in mitochondrial DNA is a common cause of Leigh syndrome.

The syndrome in these patients is characterized by developmental delay, some after a period of normal development and hypotonia, followed by psychomotor regression; some have had ataxia or dystonic posturing [8]. Spastic quadriparesis has been reported [3]. Brainstem dysfunction leads to ophthalmoplegia, apnea, ventilator dependence or death [3]. Neuroimaging reveals symmetric areas of decreased density on computed tomography (CT) or MRI in the basal ganglia, periventricular and periaqueductal areas (Figure 54.6). Blood concentrations of lactate were increased as high as 7 mmol/L with a mean concentration of 4.6 mmol/L [3]. A cerebrospinal fluid concentration of 7.12 mmol/L was reported [10]. Neuropathological examination revealed reduction in the size of the caudate, globus pallidus, putamen and cerebellum. Microscopic examination showed gliosis and demyelination of white matter and spongiform changes with relative preservation of neurons in the basal ganglia, thalamus, hypothalamus and medulla [8]. Some patients have had hypertrophic cardiomyopathy [3].

GENETICS AND PATHOGENESIS

The NARP mutation is clearly inherited in a maternal pattern [1,10–15]. Recurrence of disease in two siblings of a mother with two different mates has been reported [10]. All of the families studied have revealed degrees of heteroplasmy. In general, the correlation between the severity of phenotype and the proliferation of mutant mitochondrial DNAs has been very good [1–3,9,10]. Patients with infantile encephalopathy and Leigh syndrome have tended to have over 95 percent of mutant mitochondrial DNA. Later-onset patients have had 80–90 percent while asymptomatic patients may have had as little as 3–6 percent. Correlation has been better with the proportion of mutant DNA in the blood than in the fibroblast. For instance, an asymptomatic mother had 39 percent in blood and 71 percent in fibroblasts [2]. Prenatal diagnosis has been made in two affected pregnancies at risk by examination of chorionic villus samples [16], but, because of the random distribution of mutant DNA, neither prenatal diagnosis nor carrier detection is reliable. Calculations from 56 pedigrees relating severity of symptoms and mutant load should be useful in genetic counseling, and may be of utility in prenatal diagnosis [5].

There has been some evidence for nonrandom segregation of mutant NARP mitochondria in oocytes, such as a mother with 10 percent mutant DNAs having three offspring with 90 percent or more mutant DNAs. Examination of oocytes has revealed a predominance of mutant DNA. A bottle-neck for mitochondrial DNA in embryogenesis might lead to a reduction or enhancement of amounts of mutant mitochondrial DNA [9].

The common mutation was found originally in nucleotide 8993 of the mitochondrial genome after digestion of leukocyte mitochondrial DNA with the restriction endonuclease Ava I revealed an unusual pattern of fragments. In involved members a variable portion of the normal 14.4 kb fragment was cleaved into two, one 10.4 kb and one 4.0 kb. Further digestion with Pvu II cleaved the 10 kb fragment into two of 6 and 4 kb, respectively, which localized the gain of the Ava I site to the ATPase 6 reading frame. Both normal and mutant populations were found in muscle, as well as blood. Polymerase chain reaction (PCR) amplification with primers 8648–8665 and 9180–9199 revealed a single fragment, which was cleaved by Ava I in patients, but not in controls.

Sequencing identified the T-to-G change at 8993. This change leads to a change from the highly conserved hydrophobic leucine to the hydrophylic arginine at position 156 of subunit 6 of the mitochondrial H+ -ATPase. This would be expected to interfere with the H+ channel formed by subunits 6 and 9 and lead to failure of ATP synthesis [2]. It did not affect hydrolysis of ATP. The activity of the enzymes of the respiratory chain tend to be normal in the frozen muscle of patients [3]. However, Shoffner and colleagues [8] found deficiencies in the activities in muscle of complex I and complex III. Testing of oxidative phosphorylation revealed a reduction in the rate of generation of ATP [9]. The T-to-C mutation at 8993 replaces the leucine with proline. This would change the helical structure of the protein and would be expected to interfere with proton conduction [17]. Nevertheless, ATP production was not impaired [18]. In general the 8993C disease tends to be less severe than the 8993G [5].

TREATMENT

Supportive treatment includes the management of seizure disorder and the prompt treatment of infection. Experience with dichloroacetic acid indicates success in reducing levels of lactic acid. Effects on the neurologic features of the disease are being evaluated.

References

1 Holt IJ, Harding AE, Petty RK, Morgan-Hughes JA. A new mitochondrial disease associated with mitochondrial DNA heteroplasmy. *Am J Hum Genet* 1990;**46**:428.

2 Tatuch Y, Christodoulou J, Feigenbaum A, *et al.* Heteroplasmic mtDNA mutation (T Æ G) at 8993 can cause Leigh disease when the percentage of abnormal mtDNA is high. *Am J Hum Genet* 1992;**50**:852.

3 Santorelli FM, Shanske S, Macaya A, *et al.* The mutation at nt 8993 of mitochondrial DNA is a common cause of Leigh's syndrome. *Ann Neurol* 1993;**34**:827.

4 de Vries DD, van Engelen BGM, Gabreëls FJM, *et al.* A second missense mutation in the mitochondrial ATPase 6 gene in Leigh's syndrome. *Ann Neurol* 1993;**34**:410.

5 White SL, Collins VR, Wolfe R, *et al.* Genetic counseling and prenatal diagnosis for the mitochondrial DNA mutations at nucleotide 8993. *Am J Hum Genet* 1999;**65**:474.

6 Shoffner JM, Wallace DC. Oxidative phosphorylation diseases: in *The Metabolic and Molecular Bases of Inherited Disease* (eds CR Scriver, AL Beaudet, WS Sly, D Valle) McGraw Hill, New York;1995:1535.

7 Ortiz RG, Newman NJ, Shoffner JM, *et al.* Variable retinal and neurologic manifestations in patients harboring the mitochondrial DNA 8993 mutation. *Arch Ophthalmol* 1993;**111**:1525.

8 Shoffner JM, Fernhoff PM, Krawiecki NS, *et al.* Subacute necrotizing encephalopathy: oxidative phosphorylation defects and the ATPase 6 point mutation. *Neurology* 1993;**42**:2168.

9 Mäkelä-Bengs P, Suomalainen A, Majander A, *et al.* Correlation between the clinical symptoms and the proportion of mitochondrial DNA carrying the 8993 point mutation in the NARP syndrome. *Pediatr Res* 1995;**37**:634.

10   Ciafaloni E, Santorelli FM, Shanske S, *et al*. Maternally inherited Leigh syndrome. *J Pediatr* 1993;**122**:419.

11   Yoshinaga H, Ogino T, Ohtahara S, *et al*. A T-to-G mutation at nucleotide pair 8993 in mitochondrial DNA in a patient with Leigh's syndrome. *J Child Neurol* 1993;**8**:129.

12   McGowan KA, Naviaux RK, Barshop BA, *et al*. The expanding clinical spectrum of the NARP syndrome. *J Invest Med* 1998;**46**:86A.

13   Santorelli FM, Shanske S, Jain KD, *et al*. A new mtDNA mutation in the ATPase 6 gene in a child with Leigh syndrome. *Neurology* 1993; **43**:A171.

14   Santorelli FM, Shanske S, Sciacco M, *et al*. A new etiology for Leigh syndrome: mitochondrial DNA mutation in the ATPase 6 gene. *Ann Neurol* 1992;**32**:467 (abstr 141).

15   Puddo P, Barboni P, Mantovani V, *et al*. Retinitis pigmentosa ataxia and mental retardation associated with mitochondrial DNA mutation in an Italian family. *Br J Ophthalmol* 1993;**77**:84.

16   Harding AE, Holt IJ, Sweeney MG, *et al*. Prenatal diagnosis of mitochondrial DNA 8993 T Æ G disease. *Am J Hum Genet* 1992;**50**:629.

17   Cox GB, Fimmel AL, Gibson F, Hatch L. The mechanism of ATP synthase: a reassessment of the function of the a and b subunits. *Biochim Biophys Acta* 1986;**849**:62.

18   Anderson S, Bankier AT, Barrell BG, *et al*. Sequence and organization of the human mitochondrial genome. *Nature* 1981;**290**:457.

Kearns-Sayre syndrome

MAJOR PHENOTYPIC EXPRESSION

Onset prior to 20 years-of-age of progressive external ophthalmoplegia, ptosis, pigmentary retinopathy, block in cardiac conduction, ataxia, elevated protein in cerebral spinal fluid (CSF), and deletion in mitochondrial DNA.

INTRODUCTION

Kearns and Sayre [1] reported in 1995 a syndrome of retinitis pigmentosa, external ophthalmoplegia and complete heart block. It has for some time been recognized as an encephalomyopathy with variable neurologic manifestations, including cerebellar ataxia, muscle weakness, sensorineural deafness and mental deterioration [2]. There may be elevation of the protein in CSF to values over 100 mg/dL. Muscle biopsy reveals ragged red fibers [3]. Lestienne and Ponsot [4] and Holt and colleagues [5] in 1988 reported deletions in the DNA of mitochondria in biopsied muscle.

CLINICAL ABNORMALITIES

Patients with Kearns-Sayre syndrome usually appear normal in early childhood, developing features of the disease in later childhood or adolescence. It is probably an artificial distinction that patients developing signs of disease after the age of 20 years are referred to as having chronic progressive external ophthalmoplegia (PEO), because they have the same deletions as those presenting earlier and may develop any of the multisystem features of classic Kearns-Sayre Syndrome [2].

The earliest manifestation is often a limitation of external ocular movement or ptosis (Figures 55.1, 55.2). These manifestations are chronically progressive and the classic appearance is that of bilateral ptosis and ophthalmoplegia. There may be progression to complete ophthalmoplegia [6]. Electromyography (EMG) of the orbicularis oculi muscle may show myogenic changes.

Pigmentary degeneration of the retina may take the pattern of salt and pepper retinopathy in which there are regions of hyper- and hypopigmentation or a bone spicule appearance of retinitis pigmentosa [7,8]. There may be optic atrophy.

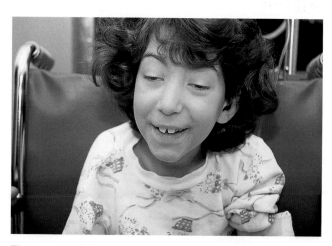

Figure 55.1   *G.F., a 10-year-old girl with Kearns-Sayre syndrome. She was very short and had pronounced ptosis bilaterally.*

Some patients have had an eventual loss of the pigment epithelium. Others have had a choroideremia pattern in which there is complete choroid atrophy [9]. Visual impairment may be the presenting complaint. Other patients with pigmentary changes on fundoscopy may have normal visual acuity. Electroretinopathy may reveal delayed A waves signifying tapeto-retinal degeneration even in patients without symptoms or abnormality visible in the fundus.

Skeletal myopathy may be evident in muscle weakness or exercise intolerance. Deep tendon reflexes may be diminished. Some patients have developed scoliosis. Cerebellar abnormality may be evident in ataxia, a broad-based gait or dysmetria. There may be an intention tremor. Sensorineural deafness is another common neurologic manifestation of the disease. Dementia may ultimately occur. Muscle biopsy classically reveals ragged red fibers [10] when the specimen is stained with Gomori trichrome. Structural abnormality may be identified by electron microscopy. There may be aggregates of mitochondria [11].

Cerebrospinal fluid concentration of protein is usually referred to as greater than 100 mg/dL, but many patients, even among those with elevated concentrations of protein, have lower levels [10]. Computed tomography (CT) or magnetic resonance imaging (MRI) scan may reveal atrophy of the cerebellum or brain stem [12], and there may be calcifications in the basal ganglia [12,13]. Some patients have had lesions in the thalamus and brainstem as seen in Leigh syndrome. Others have had diffuse white matter hypodensities [6]. The histopathology of the brain is that of spongiform degeneration [10].

Cardiac conduction (Figure 55.3) is classically abnormal and typically takes the form of a complete atrioventricular block or a right bundle branch block. The PQ interval may be prolonged on electrocardiogram (EKG), or there may be a prolonged QT [13]. Evidence of cardiomyopathy has been obtained by biopsy [11]. Clinical evidence of cardiomyopathy can range from tachycardia to frank failure. One of our

pediatric patients presented with a seizure resulting from complete heart block [14].

Other non-neurologic manifestations include shortness of stature. A variety of endocrine abnormalities have been encountered [2,15], the most common of which are diabetes mellitus and hypogonadism, including amenorrhea and delayed puberty. Hypoparathyroidism, thyroid abnormalities and hyperaldostemism are less frequent [7,16,17]. Hypomagnesemia has been observed [13]. Hypoparathyroidism has been a component of a multiple endocrine abnormality syndrome [18]. Another syndrome has been reported in four unrelated children with Kearns-Sayre syndrome who presented first with hypoparathyroidism and deafness [13]. Hypocalcemic tetany, a consequence of deficiency of parathyroid hormone, was well controlled by treatment with low doses of 1,25 dihydroxychole calciferol. Two of three patients had hypomagnesemia.

Renal tubular acidosis is another interesting manifestation [19] which is also seen in other disorders of mitochondrial electron transport function [20]. Some presentations have resembled Bartter syndrome or Lowe syndrome [21].

Lactic acidemia is not a predominant feature in many patients, but some have had lactic acidosis; some have mild elevations of levels of lactic acid in the blood. In others the CSF concentration of lactic acid is elevated in the absence of lactic acidemia.

An unusual presentation is with the Pearson-marrow syndrome (Chapter 56). Patients with the Pearson syndrome have the same area of deletion as Kearns-Sayre syndrome, and patients who have survived the early morbidity of the Pearson syndrome and whose marrow dysfunction resolved have been reported to go on to develop Kearns-Sayre syndrome [22].

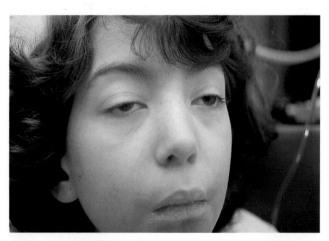

Figure 55.2   *G.F., asked to follow a light upwards, demonstrated a paresis of upward gaze.*

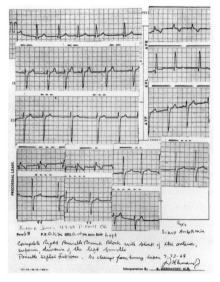

Figure 55.3   *Electrocardiogram of a patient with Kearns-Sayre syndrome illustrating a complete heart block.*

GENETICS AND PATHOGENESIS

Kearns-Sayre syndrome is virtually always sporadic [10], suggesting that the deletion in the mitochondrial genome occurred in the formation of the affected individual. Many mothers of affected individuals have been studied without finding deletions. A few pedigrees of patients with Kearns-Sayre or

chronic progressive ophthalmoplegia syndromes have displayed patterns of inheritance consistent with an autosomal dominant gene [2,23–27]. Analysis of mitochondrial DNA has revealed multiple deletions in muscle. These deletions could not be found in rapidly dividing tissues, such as leukocytes or cultured fibroblasts. It has been postulated that an abnormal mutant gene has led to the mutations in the mitochondrial genome. A similar pattern of multiple deletions in mitochondrial DNA was seen in a study in which there were two affected brothers and first cousin parents, a pattern suggesting autosomal recessive inheritance [28,29].

The vast majority of patients with Kearns-Sayre syndrome have deletions spanning approximately 5 kb and referred to as the common deletion. (Figures 55.4,55.5). Many different deletions have been observed in the O_H to O_L arc (Figure 56.1). In about half of patients this is a 4.9 kb deletion extending from the NAD dehydrogenase (ND5) to the ATPase subunit gene [30]. This is an area in which there are 13 bp direct repeats on either side, np 13,447 to 13,459 and np 8470 to 8482 [31–33]. It appears likely that this produces a situation in which hot spots promote deletion. Deletions in this area remove structural genes and some tRNA genes, which would interfere with mitochondrial protein synthesis. Overall deletions have ranged from 1.3 to 7.6 kb [16,17]. The proportion of mutated genomes ranged in these series from 27 to 85 percent of total mitochondrial DNA. In some patients the proportions in different tissues were very variable. In general the proportion of abnormal DNA increases with age, paralleling the worsening of clinical manifestations. The deletions are all large enough to be readily distinguished from control by digestion with restriction endonucleases and electrophoresis on agarose gel (Figure 55.4). Southern blots display a 16.5 kb band in normal individuals and smaller bands in those with deletions.

A 4.9 kb deletion and heteroplasmy has been observed in wild mice [34]. It has been thought that deletions in a region between two areas of direct repeats could occur through slip-replication, in which, following a break at the first direct repeat the first repeat pairs with the second direct repeat (Figure 55.6).

In some patients the abnormality in mitochondrial DNA is a duplication [35,36]. In most instances the clinical presentation is no different from those of patients with deletions.

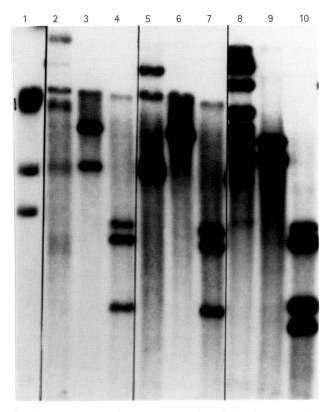

Figure 55.4   *Electrophoretic patterns of restriction fragments of mitochondrial DNA from two patients with Kearns-Sayre syndrome (lanes 2–4 and 8–10 and a control individual, lanes 5–7. Lanes 2, 5 and 8 were uncut, lanes 3, 6 and 9 cut with Bam HI, and lanes 4, 7 and 9 were cut with both Bam HI and Eco RV. Lane M represented size standards. The patient shown in lanes 8–10 had the most commonly encountered deletion. (Reprinted with permission from* Molecular Genetics and Metabolism *[14]).*

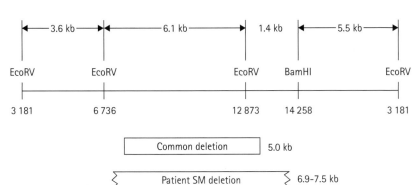

Figure 55.5   *Linear representation of the common deletion and the deletion in a patient who presented first with 2-oxoadipic aciduria [14].*

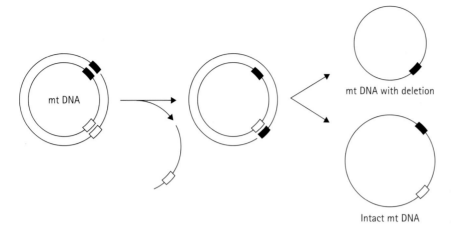

Figure 55.6 *Slip replication model for the genesis of a deletion in mitochondrial DNA. Following the development of breaks the smaller segment is removed and degraded.*

Some have had renal tubular acidosis or other renal tubular abnormality [21,19]. The children reported [13] with hypoparathyroidism and deafness in Kearns-Sayre syndrome had duplications as well as deletions. The deletions all spared four genes of complex I, including ND3 and ND6, as well as both genes of complex V, ATPase 8 and 6. The sizes of the duplications were inversely proportional to the sizes of the deletions. Homologous recombination as well as slip replication could be the mechanism of these rearrangements [37,38].

TREATMENT

Coenzyme Q10 may be of benefit. Treatment with 60–120 mg daily was reported [6] to be associated with decrease in modestly elevated levels of lactic and pyruvic acids and improvement in the prolongation of the PQ interval on the EKG as well as ocular movements. The QRS complex did not change. Concentrations of folic acid and of carnitine may be reduced in plasma or muscle, and treatment with these agents may be useful. A vitamin B complex supplement is often prescribed.

In the presence of complete A-V block a cardiac pacemaker is usually required. Corrective eyeglasses may be helpful.

References

1   Kearns T, Sayre GP. Retinitis pigmentosa, external opththalmoplegia, and complete heart block. *Arch Ophthalmol* 1958;**60**:280.

2   Berenberg RA, Pellock JM, DiMauro S, *et al.* Lumping or splitting? "Ophthalmoplegia-plus" or Kearns-Sayre syndrome? *Ann Neurol* 1977;**1**:37.

3   DiMauro S, Bonilla E, Zeviani M, *et al.* Mitochondrial myopathies. *Ann Neurol* 1985;**17**:512.

4   Lestienne P, Ponsot G. Kearns-Sayre syndrome with muscle mitochondrial DNA deletion.*Lancet* 1988; **1**:885 [Letter].

5   Holt IJ, Harding AE, Morgan-Hughes JA. Deletions of muscle mitochondrial DNA in patients with mitochondrial myopathies. *Nature* 1988;**331**:717.

6   Ogasahara S, Yorifuji S, Nishikawa Y, *et al.* Improvement of abnormal pyruvate metabolism and cardiac conduction defect with coenzyme Q10 in Kearns-Sayre syndrome. *Neurology* 1985;**35**:372.

7   Petty RK, Harding AE, Morgan HJA. The clinical features of mitochondrial myopathy. *Brain* 1986;**109**:915.

8   Mullie MA, Harding AE, Petty RK, *et al.* The retinal manifestations of mitochondrial myopathy. A study of 22 cases. *Arch Ophthalmol* 1985;**103**:1825.

9   Herzberg NH, van Schooneveld MJ, Bleeker-Wagemakers EM, *et al.* Kearns-Sayre syndrome with a phenocopy of choroideremia instead of pigmentary retinopathy. *Neurology* 1993;**43**:218.

10   Rowland LP, Blake DM, Hirano M, *et al.* Clinical syndromes associated with ragged red fibers. *Rev. Neurol.* (Paris) 1991;**147**:6, 467.

11   Bastiaensen LAK, Joosten EMG, de Rooij JAM, *et al.* Ophthalmoplegia-plus, a real nosological entity. *Acta Neurol Scand* 1978;**58**:9.

12   Robertson WC Jr., Viseskul C, Lee YE, Lloyd RV. Basal ganglia calcification in Kearns-Sayre syndrome. *Arch Neurol* 1979;**36**:711.

13   Wilichowski E, Gruters A, Kruse K, *et al.* Hypoparathyroidism and deafness associated with pleioplasmic large scale rearrangements of the mitochondrial DNA: A clinical and molecular genetic study of four children with Kearns-Sayre syndrome. *Pediatr Res* 1997;**41**:193.

14   Barshop BA, Nyhan WL, Naviaux RK, *et al.* Kearns-Sayre syndrome presenting as 2-oxoadipic aciduria. *Mol Genet Metab* 2000;**69**:64.

15   Quade A, Zierz S, Klingmuller D. Endocrine abnormalities in mitochondrial myopathy with external ophthalmoplegia. *Clin Invest* 1992;**70**:396.

16   Moraes CT, DiMauro S, Zeviani M, *et al.* Mitochondrial DNA deletions in progressive external ophthalmoplegia and Kearns-Sayre syndrome. *N Eng J Med* 1989;**320**:1293.

17   Zeviani M, Moraes CT, DiMauro S, *et al.* Deletions of mitochondrial DNA in Kearns-Sayre syndrome. *Neurology* 1988;**38**:1339.

18   Harvey JN, Barnett D. Endocrine dysfunction in Kearns-Sayre syndrome. *Clin Endocrinol* 1992;**37**:97.

19   Eviatar L, Shanske S, Gauthier B, *et al.* Kearns-Sayre syndrome presenting as renal tubular acidosis. *Neurology* 1990;**40**:1761.

20   Pintos-Morell G, Haas R, Prodanos C, *et al.* Cytochrome *c* oxidase deficiency in muscle with dicarboxylic aciduria and renal tubular acidosis. *J Child Neurol* 1990;**5**:147.

21   Moraes CT, Zeviani M, Schon EA, *et al.* Mitochondrial DNA deletion in a girl with manifestations of Kearns-Sayre and Lowe syndromes: An example of phenotypic mimicry? *Am J Med Genet* 1991;**41**:301.

22   Norby S, Lestienne P, Nelson I, *et al.* Juvenile Kearns-Sayre syndrome initially misdiagnosed as a psychosomatic disorder. *J Med Genet* 1994;**31**:45.

23   Zeviani M, Servidei S, Gellera C, *et al.* An autosomal dominant disorder with multiple deletions of mitochondrial DNA starting at the D-loop region. *Nature* 1989;**339**:309.

24 Bastiaensen LA, Jaspar HHJ, Stadhouders AM. Ophthalmoplegia-plus. *Doc Ophthalmol* 1979;**46**:365.

25 Barron SA, Heffner RRJ, Zwirecki R. A familial mitochondrial myopathy with central defect in neural transmission. *Arch Neurol* 1979;**36**:553.

26 McAuley FD. Progressive external ophthalmoplegia. *Br J Ophthalmol* 1956;**40**:686.

27 Zeviani M. Nucleus-driven mutations of human mitochondrial DNA. *J Inherit Metab Dis* 1992;**15**:456.

28 Mizusawa H, Watanabe M, Kanazawa I, *et al*. Familial mitochondrial myopathy associated with peripheral neuropathy: Partial deficiencies of complex I and complex IV. *J Neurol Sci* 1988;**86**:171.

29 Yuzaki M, Ohkoshi N, Kanazawa I, *et al*. Multiple deletions in mitochondrial DNA at direct repeats of non-D-loop regions in cases of familial mitochondrial myopathy. *Biochem Biophys Res Commun* 1989;**164**:1352.

30 Wallace DC, Lott MT, Torroni A, Brown MD. Report of the committee on human mitochondrial DNA. *Cytogenet Cell Genet* 1992;**59**:727.

31 Schon EA, Rizzuto R, Moraes CT, *et al*. A direct repeat is a hotspot for large-scale deletion of human mitochondrial DNA. *Science* 1989;**244**:346.

32 Shoffner JM, Lott MT, Voljavec AS, *et al*. Spontaneous Kearns-Sayre/chronic external ophthalmoplegia plus syndrome associated with a mitochondrial DNA deletion: A slip-replication model and metabolic therapy. *Proc Natl Acad Sci USA* 1989;**86**:7952.

33 Johns DR, Rutledge SL, Stine OC, Hurko O. Directly repeated sequences associated with pathogenic mitochondrial DNA deletions. *Proc Natl Acad Sci USA* 1989;**86**:8059.

34 Boursot P, Yonekawa H, Bonhomme F. Heteroplasmy in mice with deletion of a large coding region of mitochondrial DNA. *Mol Biol Evol* 1987;**4**:46.

35 Rotig A, Bessis JL, Romero N, *et al*. Maternally inherited duplication of the mitochondrial genome in a syndrome of proximal tubulopathy, diabetes mellitus, and cerebellar ataxia. *Am J Hum Genet* 1992;**50**:364.

36 Poulton J, Deadman ME, Gardiner RM. Duplications of mitochondrial DNA in mitochondrial myopathy. *Lancet* 1989;**1**:236.

37 Mita S, Rizzuto R, Moraes CT, *et al*. Recombination via flanking direct repeats is a major cause of large-scale deletions of human mitochondrial DNA. *Nucleic Acids Res* 1990;**18**:561.

38 Schon EA, Rizzuto R, Moraes CT, *et al*. A direct repeat is a hotspot for large-scale deletion of human mitochondrial DNA. *Science* 1989;**244**:346.

56

Pearson syndrome

MAJOR PHENOTYPIC EXPRESSION

Anemia or pancytopenia, exocrine pancreatic insufficiency, hepatic dysfunction, failure to thrive, mitochondrial myopathy, neurologic degeneration, lactic acidemia and deletions in mitochondrial DNA.

INTRODUCTION

A syndrome was first described in 1979 by Pearson and colleagues [1] from New Haven, Philadelphia, Fort Worth and Sydney, Australia, in which four unrelated patients had refractory sideroblastic anemia with variable neutropenia and thrombocytopenia and clinical and pathologic evidence

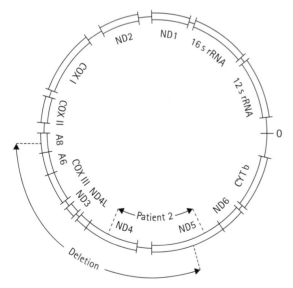

Figure 56.1 *The mitochondrial genome and the deletion of 4.9 kb most commonly found in Pearson syndrome.*

of pancreatic dysfunction. One of these patients later developed Kearns–Sayre syndrome [2]. Study of this patient by McShane and colleagues in 1991 [3] revealed a 4.9 kb deletion in mitochondrial DNA. This was the deletion most commonly observed in patients with Kearns–Sayre syndrome. The same deletion (Figure 56.1) had been reported in 1988 by Rotig and colleagues in an infant with Pearson syndrome [4]. Rotig and colleagues [5] have since studied a larger series of nine patients with Pearson syndrome, including one of Pearson's original patients; five had the previously identified 4.9 kb deletion, and four had distinctly different deletions in the same area of the genome. A consistent feature was the occurrence of direct repeats at the boundaries of the deletions [6], providing a possible mechanism for recombinations. Rotig and her colleagues [7] have since found a patient in whom there was an insertion as well as a deletion in the mitochondrial DNA. In all patients studied there was heteroplasmy of normal and deleted mitochondrial genomes.

CLINICAL ABNORMALITIES

Patients with this syndrome (Figures 56.2–56.5) have severe transfusion-dependent anemia [1]. Onset is in the early weeks of life, and pallor may be noted in the neonatal period. Anemia is macrocytic and aregenerative. Reticulocyte percentages are low. Hemoglobin F levels may be increased, and the free-erythrocyte protoporphyrin level may be increased [1].

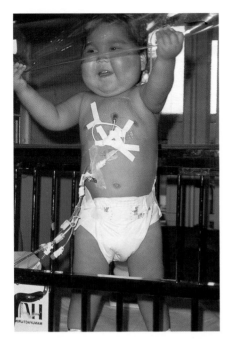

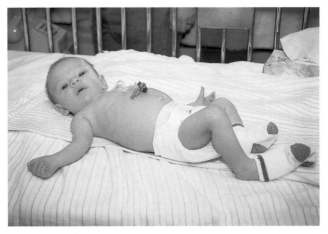

Figure 56.4 *K.K., a 4-month-old with Pearson syndrome. He had neonatal onset pancytopenia requiring transfusion. Mitochondrial DNA deletion was documented. Illustrated is the failure to thrive, a consequence of his malabsorption, and the port-a-cath for transfusion.*

Figure 56.2 *E.S., a 3-year-old boy with Pearson syndrome. He had failure to thrive, a renal Fanconi syndrome, anemia and intestinal malabsorption. Renal biopsy revealed interstitial fibrosis and mitochondrial cytopathy. A Broviac port provided venous access for alimentation as well as transfusion. He also had a gastrostomy.*

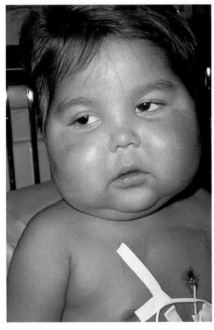

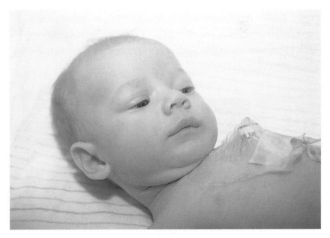

Figure 56.5 *K.K. He was pale. He had lactic acidemia and mild acidosis.*

Figure 56.3 *E.S. The face was pudgy and hyperpigmented. Despite this Cushingoid appearance there was no history of steroid treatment. He also had acanthosis nigricans.*

Neutropenia and thrombocytopenia are variable. Either or both may begin concomitantly with the anemia or shortly thereafter, or pancytopenia may become progressively worse. In some, neutropenia may be episodic. Resistance to infection is impaired and death may occur in infancy, from infection such as *E coli* sepsis. Death prior to 3 years-of-age has been reported in 62 percent of patients [7,8]. Neonatal death has been reported [9]. On the other hand, in patients surviving infancy the anemia may disappear spontaneously and the hemoglobin stabilize as early as 11 months or 2 to 3 years-of-age. In such a patient, platelet counts may remain low. On the other hand, the anemia may first be evident at 13 months-of-age [10] with spontaneous recovery 7 months later.

Bone marrow at the height of the anemia reveals increased cellularity, and there is striking vacuolization of both erythroid and myeloid precursors (Figures 56.6, 56.7). The vacuoles are not those of fat, glycogen or lysosomal material, for they were not stained by Giemsa, hematoxylin and eosin, Sudan black or periodic acid Schiff (PAS). There were increased amounts of hemosiderin in the marrow and ringed sideroblasts (Figure 56.8). Electron microscopy revealed no limiting membranes on the vacuoles. The ringed sideroblast was a nucleated red cell with hemosiderin-laden mitochondria in a perinuclear

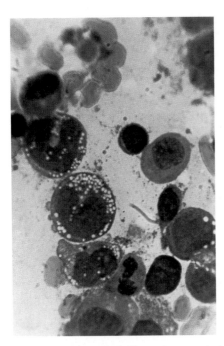

Figure 56.6   *Bone marrow aspirate illustrating vacuolation of granulocyte precursors (magnification × 1000). (Reproduced with permission from the original paper of Pearson et al. [1] in the* Journal of Pediatrics.*)*

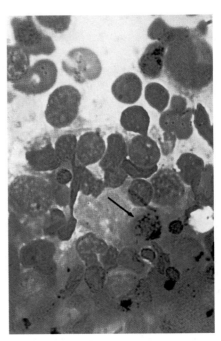

Figure 56.8   *Ringed sideroblast is indicated by the arrow. There was hemosiderin throughout the marrow (magnification × 1000, Prussian blue stain). (Reproduced with permission from the original paper of Pearson et al. [1] in the* Journal of Pediatrics.*)*

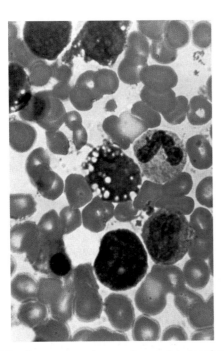

Figure 56.7   *Bone marrow also reveals vacuolated erythrocyte precursors (magnification × 1000). (Reproduced with permission from the original paper of Pearson et al. [1] in the* Journal of Pediatrics.*)*

arrangement. A variety of therapeutic modalities, such as prednisone, B$_{12}$, folate and oxymethalone, were without effect.

Patients have varying degrees of pancreatic dysfunction. Some have had steatorrhea and malabsorption, but others have not. Tests of pancreatic abnormality have included decreased response of pancreatic enzymes and bicarbonate in duodenal aspirates to secretin-pancreozymin, and absence of stool or duodenal tryptic activity. Pancreatic fibrosis was documented in two patients at autopsy [1]. Another patient had chronic diarrhea, but was not evaluated for pancreatic function. Another [11] had increased stool fat; this 2-year-old girl also had diabetes and severe renal tubular acidosis. She had polyuria, proteinuria, glycosuria, phosphaturia and generalized amino aciduria along with systemic acidosis, hypokalemia and hypophosphatemia. Renal biopsy revealed tubular dilatation, degeneration of tubular epithelium and giant mitochondria in the proximal tubules. This patient also had hypotonia and had lost the ability to walk; there was muscle wasting and failure to grow. Computed tomography (CT) scan revealed cerebral atrophy. Renal Fanconi syndrome has been observed in others [12]. Hypokalemia and hypercalciuria have been observed in other patients. One patient had renal cysts [13]. Two patients with Pearson syndrome developed insulin-dependent diabetes mellitus [14].

Similarities and differences between this syndrome and Schwachman syndrome, in which exocrine pancreatic insufficiency is associated with hematologic disease, have been highlighted [1,14]. In Schwachman syndrome, the marrow abnormality leads to leukopenia, and the histology is of pancreatic fatty replacement. There is also bony metaphyseal dysplasia. In Pearson syndrome, vacuolation of marrow cells is distinctive; there has also been autopsy evidence of splenic atrophy [1]. In a patient with severe pancytopenia early in life, fibrosis of the thyroid was found at autopsy [15].

Hepatic dysfunction is another feature of Pearson syndrome. In the initial series the first patient, who died at 26 months, had fatty infiltration of the liver; the second died of hepatic decompensation, and the liver at autopsy showed fat deposits but no cirrhosis. A number of other patients have died in infancy of hepatic insufficiency [16]. Patients recovering from the marrow dysfunction may develop evidence of hepatic disease manifested by elevated transaminases, lactic dehydrogenase and hypoprothrombinemia resistant to vitamin K. There may be jaundice.

Cataracts have been observed in Pearson syndrome [17]. Another patient had choroidal dystrophy [18].

Study of one of the original patients of Pearson *et al.* [1] at the age of 14 years revealed a very different late-childhood/adolescent phenotype [2]. His hematologic disease began to improve spontaneously at 7 months-of-age, and he had his last transfusion at 11 months, but macrocystosis and slightly decreased neutrophil and platelet counts persisted. Short stature was progressively evident; he was in the 25th percentile at 6 years and in the 5th at 8 years. Over the next 3 years growth velocity was 4 cm/year. His 24-hour integrated growth hormone level was judged to be low, and he was treated with growth hormone for 4 months. At 12 years activity and mental alertness decreased, and he developed a tremor and a stammer. Speech and handwriting deteriorated, and his tremor became increasingly debilitating. Cognitive function was normal, and his IQ was 109. Deep tendon reflexes were brisk, and there was unsustained clonus. He had a moderate lactic acidosis.

Patients with this disease may also have lactic acidemia in infancy [4,9]. Some have died in episodes of metabolic acidosis. Magnetic resonance imaging of the brain of this boy revealed diffuse increase in T2-weighted signal in the white matter of the cerebral hemispheres, with periventricular sparing, and of the globus pallidus and pons. This picture has been noted as having features of Kearns–Sayre syndrome [19]; it is more reminiscent of Leigh syndrome, at least on neuroimaging, and the dominating tremor of the clinical picture could be a different disease because of familial tremor in two generations. The fact that the affected family males were on the maternal side suggests that it is a consequence of the deletion. Other patients have had Leigh-type neuropathology [20,21].

The patient of McShane and colleagues [3], who presented in the neonatal period with Pearson-type anemia, later developed a typical Kearns-Sayre picture, with external ophthalmoplegia and pigmentary retinopathy and mitochondrial myopathy on muscle biopsy, including ragged red fibers. The patient of Nelson *et al.* [22] had Kearns–Sayre syndrome with chronic progressive ophthalmoplegia and myopathy, having had sideroblastic anemia in infancy.

GENETICS AND PATHOGENESIS

The disease is caused by alterations in the mitochondrial genome (Figure 56.1). Heteroplasmy has regularly been observed in affected individuals, and the size of the deletion may vary considerably though the location is always the same [3,5]. Deletions have been identified in every tissue tested, including leukocytes, marrow cells, fibroblasts and lymphoblasts of an original patient of Pearson [7]. The disorder is often described as sporadic, and in most families there is no evidence of disease in the mother. However, identical deletions have been reported [10] in a son with Pearson syndrome and his mother with progressive external ophthalmoplegia. A daughter was unaffected. Variability of this sort is consistent with the maternal inheritance pattern of mitochondrial mutations in which there is stochastic segregation of heteroplasmic DNA in the oocyte, and a bottle-neck effect in which few of the very many mitochondrial DNAs are selected for the oocyte and new embryo. Certainly, a mother with clinical progressive external ophthalmoplegia is at risk for production of an infant with Pearson syndrome. A clinically normal mother could also have more than one offspring with this syndrome, especially if there were germ-line mosaicism.

The most common mutation is a 4977 base pair deletion [10] (Figure 56.1) from nucleotide 8482 to 13460. This is also the most common deletion in Kearns–Sayre syndrome [23] (Chapter 55). The deletion extends from the ND5 (NADH-CoQ reductase subunit 5) gene to the adenosine triphosphatase (ATPase) subunit 8 gene. There are two origins of mitochondrial DNA replication, with two different origins O_H and O_L for heavy- and light-chains, respectively, with replication of the former in a clockwise direction and the latter in the reverse. Since deletions usually spare O_H and O_L, there are two areas in which deletions occur most often, including all of those in Pearson syndrome; that is, in the larger O_H to O_L arc. The 4977 bp deletion is bounded by a pair of 13 bp direct repeats. This is a likely hot-spot for deletion. Rotig and colleagues [5] found different types of direct repeats at the boundaries of five different deletions in the same area in nine patients. There was conservation in the 3′ repeated sequences in the deletions and a certain homology between the nucleotide composition of six direct repeats and structures normally involved in replication of mitochondrial DNA and the processing of mitochondrial RNA. These repeats were particularly rich in pyrimidine nucleotides.

The deletions span coding segments for NADH dehydrogenase, cytochrome oxidase and cytochrome b [24]. This would be expected to lead to disturbance in oxidative phosphorylation and would be consistent with the lactic acidemia observed. Abnormal redox was suggested [4] by a high lactate to pyruvate ratio of 30 (normal below 20) and 3-hydroxybutyrate to acetoacetate ratio of 4 (normal below 2). A larger 7767 bp deletion [22] led to deficient polarographic uptake of oxygen in the presence of NAD-linked substrates and enzymatic evidence of deficiency of all of the complexes of the electron transport chain.

The spontaneous improvement of the anemia with time is of considerable interest. It is consistent with a concept of critical periods in the development of individual tissues. It has been postulated that there might be selective disadvantage with time of rapidly dividing hematopoietic cells containing a high proportion of deleted DNA. The opposite appears to occur in tissues like muscle and brain, where cells turn over more slowly; mutant DNA oxidative function diminishes and mitochondrial encephalomyopathy develops. In these cells deletions and duplications appear to have selective advantage over wild type DNA, and, in contrast to mtDNA point mutations, they increase in proportion with time.

The random nature of partitioning of mitochondrial DNA during embryogenesis makes prenatal diagnosis unreliable with either amniocytes or chorionic villus cells. Rearrangements in mtDNA gradually disappear in cultured cells unless uridine is present in the culture medium.

TREATMENT

Refractory anemia requires repeated transfusion of blood. Erythropoietin is generally ineffective. Thrombocytopenia may require platelet transfusion. Pancreatic extract is useful in the management of the pancreatic insufficiency.

References

1 Pearson HA, Lobel JS, Kocoshis SA, et al. A new syndrome of refractory sideroblastic anemia with vacuolization of marrow precursors and exocrine pancreatic function. J Pediatr 1979;95:976.

2 Blaw ME, Mize CE. Juvenile Pearson syndrome. J Child Neurol 1990;5:186.

3 McShane MA, Hammans SR, Sweeney M, et al. Pearson syndrome and mitochondrial encephalopathy in a patient with a deletion of mtDNA. Am J Hum Genet 1991;48:39.

4 Rotig A, Colonna M, Blanche S, et al. Deletion of blood mitochondrial DNA in pancytopenia. Lancet 1988;2:567.

5 Rotig A, Cormier V, Koll F, et al. Site-specific deletions of the mitochondrial genome in the Pearson marrow-pancreas syndrome. Genomics 1991;10:502.

6 Kogelnik AM, Lott MT, Brown MD, et al. A human mitochondrial genome database, Atlanta Center for Molecular Medicine, Emory University School of Medicine. http://www.mitomap.org (accessed December 2004).

7 Rotig A, Cormier V, Blanche S, et al. Pearson's marrow-pancreas syndrome. A multisystem mitochondrial disorder in infancy. J Clin Invest 1990;86:1601.

8 Rötig A, Bourgeron T, Chretien D, et al. Spectrum of mitochondrial DNA rearrangements in the Pearson marrow-pancreas syndrome. Hum Mol Genet 1995;4:1327.

9 Muraki K, Goto Y, Nishinio I, et al. Severe lactic acidosis and neonatal death in Pearson syndrome. J Inherit Metab Dis 1997;20:43.

10 Bernes SM, Bacino C, Prezant TR, et al. Identical mitochondrial DNA deletion in mother with progressive external ophthalmoplegia and son with Pearson marrow–pancreas syndrome. J Pediatr 1993;123:598.

11 Majander A, Suomalainen A, Vettenranta K, et al. Congenital hypoplastic anemia diabetes and severe renal tubular dysfunction associated with a mitochondrial DNA deletion. Pediatr Res 1991;30:327.

12 Niaudet P, Heidet L, Munnich A, et al. Deletion of the mitochondrial DNA in a case of de Toni-Debre-Fanconi syndrome and Pearson syndrome. Pediatr Nephrol 1994;8:164.

13 Gurgey A, Ozalp I, Rotig A, et al. A case of Pearson syndrome associated with multiple renal cysts. Pediatr Nephrol 1996;10:637.

14 Favoreto F, Caprino D, Micalizzi C, et al. New clinical aspects of Pearson's syndrome: report of three cases. Haematologica 1989;74:591.

15 Stoddard RA, McCurnin DC, Shultenover SJ, et al. Syndrome of refractory sideroblastic anemia with vacuolization of marrow precursors and exocrine pancreatic dysfunction presenting in the neonate. J Pediatr 1981;99:259.

16 Comier V, Rotig A, Bonnefont JP, et al. Pearson's syndrome. Pancytopenia with exocrine pancreatic insufficiency: new mitochondrial disease in the first year of childhood. Arch Fr Pediatr 1991;48:171.

17 Cursiefen C, Kuckle M, Scheurlen W, Naumann GO. Bilateral zonular cataract associated with the mitochondrial cytopathy of Pearson syndrome. Am J Ophthalmol 1998;125:260.

18 Barrientos A, Casademont J, Genis D, et al. Sporadic heteroplasmic single 55 kb mitochondrial DNA deletion associated with cerebellar ataxia hypogonadotropic hypogonadism choroidal dystrophy and mitochondrial respiratory chain complex I deficiency. Hum Mutat 1997;10:212.

19 Rotig A, Colonna M, Blanche S, et al. Mitochondrial DNA deletions in Pearson's marrow/pancreas syndrome. Lancet 1989;1:902.

20 Santorelli FM, Barmada MA, Pons R, et al. Leigh-type neuropathology in Pearson syndrome associated with impaired ATP production and a novel mtDNA deletion. Neurology 1996;47:1320.

21 Yamadori I, Kurose A, Kobayashi S, et al. Brain lesions of the Leigh-type distribution associated with a mitochondriopathy of Pearson's syndrome: Light and electron microscopic study. Acta Neuropathol (Berl) 1992;84:337.

22 Nelson I, Bonne G, Degoul F, et al. Kearnes–Sayre syndrome with sideroblastic anemia: molecular investigations. Neuropediatrics 1992;23:199.

23 Wallace DC, Lott MT, Torroni A, Brown MD. Report of the committee on human mitochondrial DNA. Cytogenet Cell Genet 1992;59:727.

24 De Vivo DC, The expanding clinical spectrum of mitochondrial diseases. Brain Dev 1993;15:1.

57

The mitochondrial DNA depletion syndromes: mitochondrial DNA polymerase deficiency

MAJOR PHENOTYPIC EXPRESSION

Hepatic toddler form: episodic neurologic deterioration beginning in the second year of life, with ataxia, encephalopathy, and failure to thrive, progressive to myoclonic epilepsy, stroke-like episodes, acute fulminant hepatic failure, respiratory failure, and coma; fasting hypoglycemia, dicarboxylic aciduria, lactic acidemia, and deficient activity of intramitochondrial DNA polymerase γ.

INTRODUCTION

The first evidence for depletion of mitochondrial DNA in human disease was reported by Moraes and colleagues in 1991 [1]. Three hepatic (newborn, infantile and toddler) and two nonhepatic, myopathic (infantile and toddler) forms are now recognized (Table 57.1). The hepatic forms are more appropriately called hepatocerebral [2]. Both hepatic and myopathic phenotypes have been reported in the products of both consanguineous [3] and nonconsanguineous unions [4]. Each of the three hepatic forms is characterized by episodes of acute liver failure, fasting hypoglycemia and mitochondrial DNA depletion. The two nonhepatic forms are characterized by nonepisodic myopathy, ragged red fibers, elevated serum creatine kinase (CK) and mitochondrial DNA depletion. An enzymatic diagnosis was established for the hepatic toddler form (Alpers syndrome), in which mitochondria are deficient in the enzyme responsible for replicating mitochondrial DNA, DNA polymerase γ [5].

In the period since the initial description [1] more than 50 patients have been reported [6]. A diagnosis of mitochondrial DNA depletion may be suspected on the basis of fasting hypoglycemia and liver dysfunction characterized by elevations of gamma glutamyl transferase (GGT), often greater than alanine aminotransferase (ALT) and aspartate aminotransferase (AST), or by elevated CK and ragged red fibers. It is confirmed by quantitative analysis of mitochondrial DNA in biopsied tissue or, in the case of the hepatic toddler form, by demonstration of mitochondrial DNA polymerase deficiency. In the early infantile onset hepatocerebral disease a mutation in the deoxyguanosine kinase gene on chromosome 2p13 has been identified [7]. In addition to this single base deletion in the dGK (DGUOK) gene, missense mutations, duplications and other deletions have been described [8]. In four families with myopathic disease mutations were defined in the thymidine kinase gene (TK2) on chromosome 16q22 [9]. It is clear that there is heterogeneity, because only about 10 percent of patients with similar phenotypes that were tested were found to have mutations in these two deoxynucleoside kinases [8,10,11]. Mutations have now been found in the mitochondrial DNA polymerase γ.

CLINICAL ABNORMALITIES

In the infantile-onset hepatocerebral form of mitochondrial DNA depletion the infants were small for gestational age

Table 57.1 *Clinical and biochemical abnormalities associated with the mitochondrial DNA depletion syndromes*

Abnormality	Hepatic			Nonhepatic	
	Newborn[a]	Infantile[b]	Toddler[c]	Infantile[d]	Toddler[e]
Hypoglycemia	+	+	+	−	−
Liver failure	+	Late	Late	−	−
Gastroesophageal reflux	+	+	Late	Late	−
Anorexia, failure to thrive	+	+	Late	+	+
Setbacks with infections	+/−	+/−	Prominent	−	−
Cerebellar ataxia	?	?	+	−	−
Encephalopathy	−	+	+	Late	Late
Dicarboxylic aciduria	+	+	+	−	−
Lactic acidemia	Variable	+	Late	Variable	Variable
Cardiomyopathy	−	−	−	?	−
Skeletal myopathy	−	+	+	+	+
Elevated serum CPK	−	−	−	+	+
Ragged red fibers	−	−	−	+	+
Fibrillations on EMG	−	−	−	+	+
Hypertonia/hypotonia	+	+	+	+	+
Stroke-like episodes	−	−	Late	−	−
Renal tubulopathy	−	−	Late	−	−
Peripheral neuropathy	−	−	−	−	−
Language delay	?	?	+	−	−
Myoclonic epilepsy	+	+	+	+/−	−
Electron transport complexes	Deficient	Deficient	Deficient	Deficient	Deficient
Elevated citrate synthase	−	−	−	+	+
Abnormal brain MRI	?	?	Late	+/−	−
Mitochondrial DNA depletion	+	+	+	+	+
Mitochondrial polymerase deficiency	?	?	+	?	?

Onset: [a]birth; [b]1–3 months; [c]15–24 months; [d]12–18 months.

(1.9–2.4 kg at term) and developed severe hypoglycemia (to 18 mg/dL, 1.0 mmol/L), and signs of severe liver dysfunction (prothrombin times of 23–30 seconds) in the first day of life. Hepatic size has been increased. Lactic acidemia, metabolic acidosis and hyperbilirubinemia were inconsistent findings. Some patients had coagulopathy and increased α-fetoprotein. Mitochondrial electron transport studies showed global reductions in complexes I, II/III and IV activity in biopsied liver, normal succinate dehydrogenase, and a two-fold elevation in carnitine palmitoyl transferase II. Skeletal muscle electron transport activities were normal. Death followed progressive hepatic failure at 1–3 months of life. Neurologic abnormalities included hypotonia, failure to develop, and horizontal nystagmus [3]. Histopathology of the liver revealed micronodular cirrhosis, cholestasis, glycogen-laden hepatocytes, microvesicular steatosis and accumulation of iron. Some had giant cell formation. Electron microscopy revealed marked proliferation of pleomorphic mitochondria. In liver, the levels of mitochondrial DNA were significantly depleted (seven percent of normal). Levels of mitochondrial DNA in muscle, kidney and cultured fibroblasts were normal.

The infantile hepatocerebral form of mitochondrial DNA depletion is characterized by normal intrauterine growth, birth and delivery [12,13]. Nevertheless it may not be different from the early infantile form. The first hint of trouble may be vomiting or feeding difficulty as early as the first month of life. Death may occur as early as seven months. Hypotonia and fasting hypoglycemia often prompt admission to hospital by 2–3 months-of-age. One patient was nine weeks old upon admission [12], and was found to have hepatic dysfunction characterized by elevations in GGT (353 IU/L) greater than AST (188 IU/L) and ALT (123 IU/L); total bilirubin was 5.9 mg/dL (2.6 mg/dL conjugated, 3.3 mg/dL unconjugated). Lactate in the blood was 7.16 mmol/L, and pyruvate was 0.23 mmol/L, yielding an elevated lactate to pyruvate ratio of 31 (normal ≤20), consistent with disturbed redox resulting from a defect in mitochondrial electron transport. The serum concentration of bicarbonate was normal. Cerebrospinal fluid (CSF) concentration of lactate was 5.6 mmol/L. A monitored fast revealed hypoketotic hypoglycemia with 3-hydroxybutyric acid of 0.28 mmol/L, and acetoacetate of 0.07 mmol/L. Glucose challenge raised the fasting blood lactate from 3.1 to 6.2 mmol/L.

The patient was treated with a low fat (30 percent calories) diet, carnitine, riboflavin and thiamine, but there was no significant change in blood lactate. Hypotonia persisted and gross motor development was poor. No other neurologic abnormalities were observed. Hypoglycemia became progressively worse with age, requiring feedings every 2–3 hours. The patient died at seven months of fulminant hepatic failure and coagulopathy. Light microscopy of the liver revealed steatosis.

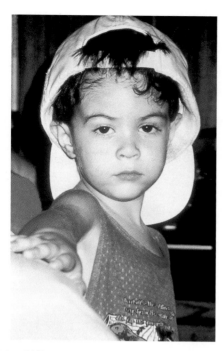

Figure 57.1   *B.W. at 2 years-of-age, with the hepatic toddler form of mitochondrial DNA depletion, 18 months before his death.*

Electromicroscopy revealed numerous mitochondria in which cristae were diminished in number or absent. Biochemical studies of liver mitochondrial electron transport complexes I, II/III, and IV revealed global reduction. Succinate dehydrogenase activity was normal. In skeletal muscle, only complex I activity was reduced. Quantitative studies of mitochondrial DNA showed normal levels in kidney, brain and heart. Skeletal muscle mitochondrial DNA was 50 percent of normal. Mitochondrial DNA in the liver was depleted to seven percent of normal.

The toddler form of hepatocerebral mitochondrial DNA depletion (Alpers syndrome) [5] is associated with an enzymatic deficiency in intramitochondrial levels of DNA polymerase γ, the enzyme responsible for replicating mitochondrial DNA. Figure 57.1 illustrates an affected child at 2 years-of-age. This child had an older brother who had died at the age of 21 months during a second acute episode of hypoglycemia, status epilepticus and acute hepatic failure associated with a 'Reye-like syndrome' that followed a febrile illness.

The toddler form of mitochondrial DNA depletion is characterized by normal intrauterine growth, birth and delivery. Growth, fine motor, gross motor, cognitive and language development were all normal in the first year of life. At 19 months-of-age, the patient depicted in Figure 57.1 had an episode of acute truncal ataxia, vomiting, hypoglycemia (34 mg/dL), associated with hypertonia and encephalopathy following a febrile diarrheal illness. The acute hypertonia gradually resolved to mild hypotonia. He recovered from almost all other deficits, leaving only mild residual truncal ataxia. After a second similar episode at 22 months and evidence of expressive language delay, he was evaluated for a

possible disorder of fatty acid oxidation. The patient developed hypoglycemia (33 mg/dL) after 15 hours of a monitored fast. Blood was 3.8 mmol/L 3-hydroxybutyrate and acetoacetate was 0.44 mmol/L at the time of hypoglycemia, reflecting intact ketogenesis for age but an elevated ratio. Urinary organic acids after the fast showed only mild elevations in adipic (70 mmol/mol creatinine), suberic (36 mmol/mol) and sebacic (18 mmol/mol) dicarboxylic acids and a trans-cinnamoyl glycine of 55 mmol/mol. Both long-chain and medium-chain triglyceride loads resulted in elevated excretion of urinary trans-cinnamoyl glycine (69 and 94 mmol/mol creatinine, respectively) and 3-hydroxydicarboxylic acids. No abnormalities in plasma amino acids were detected. Plasma free carnitine was reduced to 13.6 μmol/L. Urine carnitine was normal. ALT and AST were slightly elevated at 73 and 124 IU/L, respectively. Lactate in the blood was 2.3 mmol/L. Magnetic resonance imaging (MRI) of the brain was normal. The patient was treated with carnitine, cornstarch and a low fat diet.

The patient had six more episodes of decompensation over the following two years associated with febrile illnesses. Neurologic manifestations included truncal ataxia, erratic nystagmoid eye movements, focal myoclonic seizures, progressive failure to thrive, and stroke-like episodes. By the age of 38 months he was unable to walk. At 41 months he contracted a rotavirus infection that was associated with focal, left-sided epilepsia partialis continua (EPC), transient left hemiparesis, and cortical blindness. Liver enzymes started rising significantly at this time; the GGT was 987, AST 228 and ALT 288 IU/L. Bilirubin was normal. He died at the age of 42 months in liver failure and coma after a six-week terminal illness; lactic acid concentrations were up to 15 mmol/L.

Autopsy revealed advanced micronodular cirrhosis with regenerative nodules (Figure 57.2A). Electron microscopy of the liver revealed marked variation in mitochondrial content and morphology in neighboring hepatocytes. Some liver cells showed significant mitochondrial proliferation with a preponderance of tightly packed cristae and occasional mitochondria with concentric cristae (Figure 57.2B), while other liver cells had apparently normal mitochondria. Microvesicular fat and bile duct proliferation was noted throughout the liver. Skeletal muscle showed mild fiber size variation and mild increase in lipid staining. Electron microscopy of skeletal muscle showed mitochondrial proliferation with numerous pleomorphic forms (Figure 57.3).

In the brain, neuropathologic examination of the frontal cortex showed marked neuronal loss and astrogliosis, and the appearance of Alzheimer type II glia. Subcortical white matter was normal. The primary visual cortex showed gliosis in layers II, III and V, and perisomal and perivascular vacuolization (Figure 57.4A). Sections through the optic tracts, and chiasm, showed prominent spongiform vacuolization; however, Luxol fast-blue staining of these regions revealed normal myelination. The head of the caudate also showed gliosis. The cerebellar cortex showed a total loss of Purkinje cells, prominent Bergman gliosis and sparing of the granular layer (Figure 57.4B). The interfolial white matter displayed prominent spongy vacuolization. Sections through the vermis showed focal cerebellar sclerosis. The spinal cord also showed spongy vacuolization and gliosis affecting the anterior and posterior spinocerebellar tracts in the lateral columns. Similar but milder spongy changes were present in the cuneate and gracile fasiculi and the spinothalamic tracts of the spinal cord.

Biochemical studies of the electron transport chain from skeletal muscle showed global reduction in the activity of complexes I, II/III and IV. Mitochondrial DNA quantification revealed levels in skeletal muscle that were 30 percent of normal. Assay of purified mitochondria from skeletal muscle and liver revealed a complete absence of activity of mitochondrial DNA polymerase γ.

The nonhepatic infantile form of mitochondrial DNA depletion is characterized by normal intrauterine growth, birth and delivery [1,4]. Hypotonia, poor feeding, failure to thrive and difficulty handling oropharyngeal secretions are noted in the first month of life. Hospital admission is usually prompted by poor motor development, vomiting, dehydration, or respiratory distress by the age of 2–4 months. At this

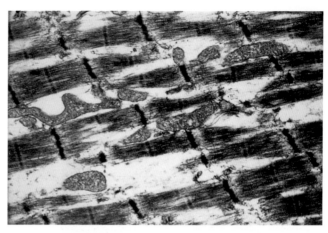

Figure 57.3   *Electron microscopy of skeletal muscle. Mitochondrial proliferation and pleomorphic appearance. There were disordered fibers and mildly increased lipid.*

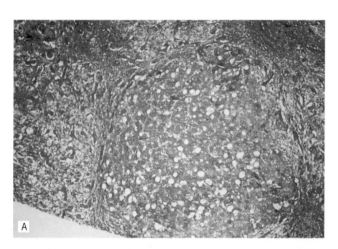

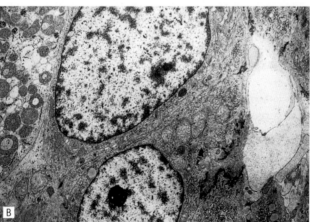

Figure 57.2   *Hepatic histology. A. Gomori-Trichrome. Micronodular cirrhosis, regenerative nodules, microvesicular fat. B. Electron microscopy. Marked cell-to-cell variation. Mitochondrial proliferation with abnormally packed lamellar and crescentic cristae in some cells, adjoining other cells with normal mitochondrial numbers and cristae.*

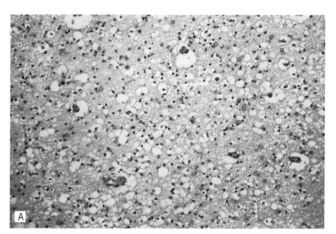

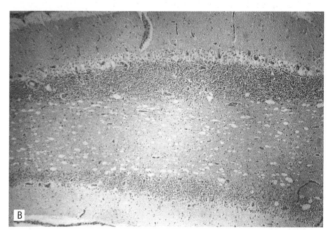

Figure 57.4   *Neuropathology. A. Occipital Visual Cortex. Fibrous gliosis in layers II, III, and V, with perisomal and perivascular vacuolization. Luxol fast-blue staining of these regions revealed normal myelination. B. Cerebellum. Total loss of Purkinje cells, prominent gliosis, and sparing of the granular layer. The interfolial white matter displayed prominent spongy vacuolization. There was also focal sclerosis in the cerebellar vermis (not shown).*

time the serum CK may exceed 1000 IU/L. Urinary organic acids are normal. Lactic acidemia may be present during periods of metabolic decompensation, but is not a consistent feature. MRI of the brain reveals delayed myelination. Focal status epilepticus is a late feature. Muscle biopsy reveals abundant ragged red fibers, increased lipid droplets by Oil Red-O staining, and increased glycogen by periodic acid Schiff PAS staining. Histochemical staining for cytochrome oxidase (COX) is absent in fibers. Biochemical studies of electron transport complexes I, II/III and IV reveal global reduction. Muscle mitochondrial DNA is 2–8 percent of normal.

A fatal neonatal outcome was reported [14] in a patient with myopathic mitochondrial DNA depletion. He developed cyanosis, a weak cry and generalized hypotonia immediately after birth. Spontaneous movements were diminished, as were reflexes. Ultrasonography of the brain showed periventricular hyperechogenicity and dilated lateral ventricles. Electroencephalograph (EEG) was abnormal. There was bilateral renal pyelectasis. There was metabolic acidosis (pH 6.99), lactic acidemia (21 mmol/L), and hyperalaninemia (1.226 mmol/L). He died at 36 hours. Activities of electron transport chain enzymes were markedly reduced in muscle while in liver there was only a mild reduction of complex I. There was a severe depletion of mitochondrial DNA in muscle while that of the liver was normal.

The nonhepatic toddler form of mitochondrial DNA depletion which may not be different from the infantile form is also characterized by normal intrauterine growth, birth and delivery [1,4]. In the first year of life, there may be frequent bouts of pneumonia, but without neurologic deficits. Cognitive and motor development are normal in the first year. Between 12 and 16 months, there may be increased stumbling or complete loss of motor milestones. Hyperlordosis and a waddling gait may be present. Serum CK is 500–2000 IU/L. Muscle biopsy reveals type I fiber predominance, abundant ragged red fibers, and a complete absence of COX activity by cytochemical staining. Patients may stop walking by the age of 2 years and be unable to sit unassisted by 2½ years. Neurodegeneration is progessive to death by respiratory failure in 2–4 years. Neuropathological examination of cerebrum, cerebellum, brainstem and spinal cord has failed to reveal abnormalities. Muscle mitochondrial DNA is 17–34 percent of normal.

Two unrelated patients with unusual clinical and biochemical phenotype were reported by Yano and colleagues [15]. Both displayed developmental delay and hypotonia. One had cerebral cortical atrophy, and she died in severe metabolic acidosis associated with pneumonia. Both had elevated plasma concentrations of glycine and methylmalonicaciduria (423 to 520 mmol/mol creatinine). Lactic acid was elevated in blood and urine. Activities of enzymes of the electron transport chain were variably reduced in muscle. The amounts of mitochondrial DNA in muscle were moderately reduced.

Mitochondrial DNA depletion has usually been documented by Southern blot analysis, but the method requires a large amount of DNA, is time-consuming and susceptible to a number of artifacts. Recent experience with real-time quantitative polymerase chain reaction (PCR) was reported to be more efficient and to have higher sensitivity [16].

GENETICS AND PATHOGENESIS

All of the forms of mitochondrial DNA depletion are transmitted as autosomal recessive disorders [1–3,12,13,16,17].

Molecular defects compatible with the clinical features of these syndromes could include abnormalities in the temporally regulated, tissue-specific expression of the mitochondrial DNA polymerase γ itself, or of one of the other essential components of the mitochondrial DNA replisome (Figure 57.5). One described defect is in the tissue-specific expression of the mitochondrial transcription factor A (mtTFA), required for the production of RNA primers [18]. The cloning of the human mitochondrial DNA polymerase [19] has facilitated molecular dissection. The patient shown in Figure 57.2 had virtually a complete absence of mitochondrial DNA polymerase γ in liver and skeletal muscle. It is likely that variants with more residual activity will soon be described.

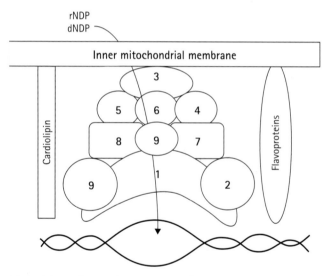

Figure 57.5 *Enzymatic components of the mitochondrial DNA replisome: nuclear contributions to mitochondrial DNA replication. All proteins involved in replication are transported to mitochondria via chaperonins (cytoplasmic transport proteins). RNA and DNA are scrolled through the membrane-fixed replisome (comprising about 20 different proteins). Diagram is a model; geometry and composition of the replisome are not yet established. Nuclear gene products known to participate in mitochondrial DNA replication and repair include: 1, DNA Pol γ ($\alpha_2\beta_2$); 2, RNAse H (removes primer RNAs); 3, ribonucleotide reductase; 4, nucleoside diphosphate kinase; 5, dihydrofolate reductase; 6, thymidylate synthetase; 7, thymidine kinase; 8, topoisomerase I; 9, DNA ligase I; 10, DNA helicase; 11, ssDNA binding protein; 12, MTFA; 13, RNAse MRP; 14, cytosine deaminase; 15, endonuclease G; 16, mTERF (mitochondrial termination (actor)); 17, T AS-A-BP (termination sequence binding protein); 18, uracil N-DNA glycosylase (UDG, UNG); 19, dUTPase; 20, mitochondrial RNA polymerase; 21, dUMP/dCMO kinase.*

Human DNA polymerase γ has been characterized as a reverse transcriptase [20,21]. Two unrelated children with Alpers syndrome were found to have a homozygous mutation in exon 17 of the POLG locus that led to a glu873 stop. In addition each was heterozygous for the G1681A mutation in exon 7 that led to an Ala467Thr substitution in the linker region of the protein [22].

The deoxynucleoside kinase defects, deoxyguanosine kinase and thymidine kinase [7,8] indicate that balanced pools of nucleotides in mitochondria are requisites for mitochondrial DNA replication. These defects provide an additional mechanism for mitochondrial DNA depletion [6]. The single base deletion in the dGK gene causes a frame shift and leads to an undetectable enzyme protein [7]. Mutations in this gene and the missense mutations in the TK2 gene accounted for only 10 percent of the patients with mitochondrial DNA depletion tested [8,10,11], and it is unlikely that all the rest had defects in mitochondrial DNA polymerase γ. So there must be other causes of this syndrome. Other kinases, such as those catalyzing the formation of di- and trinucleotides, or nucleotidases are potential candidates.

Other candidate defects lie in the tissue-specific expression of chaperonins required for accurate trafficking of nuclear gene products such as the polymerase, components of the replisome (Figure 57.5), and components of the respiratory chain into mitochondria.

The mitochondrial genome is a circular double stranded molecule containing 16 569 nucleotides and coding for 37 genes, including ribosomal RNA and 22 transfer RNAs. Each mitochondrion contains two to 10 copies of the genome.

Pathogenesis follows from mitochondrial DNA depletion. Since 13 protein subunits of complexes I, III and IV and adenosine triphosphatase (ATPase) of the electron transport chain are encoded by mitochondrial DNA, its depletion would affect the activity of oxidative phosphorylation. The prominent hepatic abnormalities may be explained by the dramatic postnatal developmental changes and mitochondrial adaptation that occur in this organ in the first few months and years of life [23]. Postnatal adaptive changes in skeletal muscle mitochondria occur only later [24]. The existence of nonhepatic (more encephalomyopathic) forms of mitochondrial DNA depletion may reflect early disturbances in the myogenic program that result in either destabilization of the muscle cell membrane, or physical muscle cell breakdown with measurable increases in CK from muscle. Liver, brain and muscle all 'learn' or undergo adaptive metabolic changes that are shaped by encounters with the postnatal environment. High ratios of NADH to NAD^+ have been found in the severe deficiencies of complexes I, III and IV in a patient with mitochondrial DNA depletion [12] and this should decrease mitochondrial β oxidation and provide a mechanism for impaired fatty acid oxidation [25,26].

Acquired mitochondrial DNA depletion syndromes have recently been described in adults as a complication of the treatment of HIV-1 and hepatitis B virus infections with the reverse transcriptase inhibitors azidothymidine (AZT) [27]

and fluoriodoarauracil (FIAU) [28]. These nucleoside analogues are potent inhibitors of the mitochondrial DNA polymerase γ. In experimental animals, the mitochondrial DNA-depleting myopathy produced by AZT is reversible upon discontinuation of the drug. The delayed liver toxicity of FIAU was apparent only after patients had received the drug for 6–8 weeks, and was not reversible upon discontinuation of the drug. Clinical trials of FIAU were suspended in 1994 when six patients died in acute liver failure. Encephalopathy and ataxia were frequent findings in patients with AZT or FIAU toxicity, but causality was difficult to establish because of coexisting disease. Secondary mitochondrial DNA depletion with near-fatal metabolic acidosis and hepatic failure has now been reported [29] in an infant with an HIV infection treated with AZT, didanosine and melfinavir. A 79 percent reduction in mitochondrial DNA of muscle reverted to normal after discontinuation of antiviral therapy.

It is interesting to note that the toxicity syndrome of FIAU more closely resembles the hepatic forms of mitochondrial DNA depletion, while the toxicity syndrome of AZT more closely resembles the nonhepatic (more encephalomyopathic) forms. The unexpected biochemical action of these reverse transcriptase inhibitors in vivo and the striking clinical overlap between the inborn and acquired forms of mitochondrial DNA depletion stand as clear reminders that our knowledge of developmentally regulated and organ-specific mitochondrial DNA metabolism and replication is far from complete.

TREATMENT

Avoidance of fasting is an important element in management of the hepatic forms of mitochondrial DNA depletion. Uncooked cornstarch at 1 g/kg three times a day, or at least at bedtime is useful in preventing hypoglycemia. Carnitine (60–100 mg/kg per day) and cofactor therapy including a multivitamin supplemented with coenzyme Q10 (4 mg/kg per day), riboflavin at 50–100 mg twice a day and niacin at 10–25 mg twice a day appear to be helpful. A diet low in fat (30 percent of calories) appears prudent.

Myoclonic seizures in the hepatic toddler form of the disease have been difficult to control. Trials of clonazepam or amantidine (5 mg/kg per day) should be considered early, if seizures are not controlled by first-line anticonvulsants or adrenocorticotropic hormone (ACTH). Valproic acid should be specifically avoided in the hepatic forms of the disease because of its mitochondrial and hepatic toxicity. Lactic acidemia is often a late complication of mitochondrial DNA depletion and may respond to treatment with dichloroacetic acid (50 mg/kg per day). Thiamine or biotin supplementation has not been successful in reducing lactic acid levels.

The multisystem abnormalities in the two later-onset hepatic forms of mitochondrial DNA depletion argue against the potential benefit of liver transplantation.

Treatment of the nonhepatic forms of mitochondrial DNA depletion also includes carnitine and cofactor therapy. Other supportive measures include good oropharyngeal secretion management, and early gastrostomy tube placement with fundoplication to avoid aspiration and provide adequate nutrition. Management of the rare bouts of metabolic acidosis is with fluids and bicarbonate. Acute lactic acidemia may be helped with dichloroacetic acid.

References

1   Moraes CT, Shanske S, Tritschler H-J, *et al*. Mitochondrial DNA depletion with variable tissue expression: A novel genetic abnormality in mitochondrial diseases. *Am J Hum Genet* 1991;**48**:492.

2   Feigenbaum A. Answers to missing mtDNA found at last. *Pediatr Res* 2002;**52**:319.

3   Bakker HD, Schotte HR, Dingemans KP, *et al*. Depletion of mitochondrial deoxyribonucleic acid in a family with fatal neonatal liver disease. *J Pediatr* 1996;**128**:683.

4   Tritschler HJ, Andreetta F, Moraes CT, *et al*. Mitochondrial myopathy of childhood associated with depletion of mitochondrial DNA. *Neurology* 1992;**42**:209.

5   Naviaux RX, Nyhan WL, Barshop BA, *et al*. Mitochondrial DNA polymerase γ deficiency and mitochondrial DNA depletion in a child with Alpers syndrome. *Ann Neurol* 1999;**45**:54.

6   Elpeleg O. Inherited mitochondrial DNA depletion. *Pediatr Res* 2003;**54**:153.

7   Mandel H, Szargel R, Labay V, *et al*. The deoxyguanosine kinase gene is mutated in individuals with depleted hepatocerebral mitochondrial DNA. *Nat Genet* 2001;**29**:337.

8   Salviati L, Sacconi S, Msancuso M, *et al*. Mitochondiral DNA depletion and dGK gene mutations. *Ann Neurol* 2002;**52**:311.

9   Saada A, Shaag A, Mandel H, *et al*. Mutant mitochondrial thymidine kinase in mitochondrial depletion myopathy. *Nat Genet* 2001;**29**:342.

10 Mancuso M, Salviati L, Sacconi S, *et al*. Mitochondrial DNA depletion: mutations in thymidine kinase gene with myopathy and SMA. *Neurology* 2002;**59**:1197.

11 Taanman JW, Kateeb I, Mantau AC, *et al*. A novel mutation in the deoxyguanosine kinase gene causing depletion of mitochondrial DNA. *Ann Neurol* 2002;**52**:237.

12 Maaswinkel-Mooij PD, Van den Bogert C, Sholte HR, *et al*. Depletion of mitochondrial DNA in the liver of a patient with lactic acidemia and hypoketotic hypoglycemia. *J Pediatr* 1996;**128**:679.

13 Mazziota MRM, Ricci E, Bertini E, *et al*. Fatal infantile liver failure associated with mitochondrial DNA depletion. *J Pediatr* 1992;**121**:896.

14 Poggi GM, Lamantea E, Ciani F, *et al*. Fatal neonatal outcome in a case of muscular mitochondrial DNA depletion. *J Inherit Metab Dis* 2000;**23**:755.

15 Yano S, Li L, Le TP, *et al*. Infantile mitochondrial DNA depletion syndrome associated with methylmalonicaciduria and 3-methylcrotonyl-CoA and proprionyl-CoA carboxylase deficiencies in two unrelated patients: A new phenotype of mtDNA depletion syndrome. *J Inherit Metab Dis* 2003;**26**:481.

16 Chabi B, Mousson de Camaret B, Duborjal H, *et al*. Quantification of mitochondrial DNA deletion depletion and overreplication: Application to diagnosis. *Clin Chem* 2003;**49**:1309.

17 Ricci E, Moraes CT, Serfidei S, *et al*. Disorders associated with mitochondrial DNA depletion. *Brain Pathol* 1992;**2**:141.

18 Poulton J, Morten K, Freeman-Emmerson C, *et al*. Deficiency of the human mitochondrial transcription factor h-mtTFA in infantile mitochondrial myopathy is associated with mtDNA depletion. *Hum Mol Genet* 1994;**3**:1763.

19 Lecrenier N, Van Der Bruggen P, Foury F. Mitochondrial DNA polymerases from yeast to man: A new family of polymerases. *Gene* 1996;**185**:147.

20 Murakami E, Feng JY, Lee H, *et al*. Characterization of a novel reverse transcriptase and other RNA-associated catalytic activities by human DNA polymerase γ: Importance in mitochondrial DNA replication *J Biol Chem* 2003;**19**:36403.

21 Naviaux RK, Markusic D, Barshop BA, *et al*. Sensitive assay for mitochondrial DNA polymerase γ. *Clin Chem* 1999;**45**:1725.

22 Naviaux RK, Nguyen KV. POLG mutations associated with Alpers syndrome and mitochondrial DNA depletion. *Ann Neurol* 2003;**55**:706.

23 Valcarce C, Nararrette RM, Encabo P, *et al*. Postnatal development of rat liver mitochondrial functions. *J Biol Chem* 1988;**263**:7767.

24 Sperl W, Sengers RCA, Trijbels JMF, *et al*. Postnatal development of pyruvate oxidation in quadriceps muscle of the rat. *Biol Neonate* 1992;**61**:188.

25 Latipää PM, Kärki TT, Hiltunen JK, Hassinen IE. Regulation of palmitoylcarnitine oxidation in isolated rat liver mitochondria: Role of the redox state of NAD(H). *Biochim Biophys Acta* 1986;**875**:293.

26 Jacobs BS, Van der Bogert C, Dacremont G, Wanders RJA. Beta-oxidation of fatty acids in cultured human skin fibroblasts devoid of the capacity for oxidative phosphorylation. *Biochim Biophys Acta* 1994;**1211**:37.

27 Arnaudo E, Dalakas M, Shanske S, *et al*. Depletion of muscle mitochondrial DNA in AIDS patients with zidovudine-induced myopathy. *Lancet* 1991;**337**:508.

28 Marwick C. NIH panel report of 'no flaws' in FIAU trial at variance with FDA report, new probe planned. *JAMA* 1994;**272**:9.

29 Church JA, Mitchell WG, Gonzalez-Gomez I, *et al*. Mitochondrial DNA depletion near-fatal metabolic acidosis and liver failure in an HIV-infected child treated with combination antiretroviral therapy. *J Pediatr* 2001;**138**:748.

Disorders of carbohydrate metabolism

Galactosemia

MAJOR PHENOTYPIC EXPRESSION

Hepatomegaly, jaundice, vomiting, failure to thrive, cataracts, mental retardation, renal Fanconi syndrome, urinary reducing substance, deficiency of galactose-1-phosphate uridyl transferase.

INTRODUCTION

Galactosemia is an inborn error of carbohydrate metabolism that results from deficiency of galactose-1-phosphate uridyl transferase (EC 2.7.7.12) (Figure 58.1). The disorder was first described in 1935 by Mason and Turner [1]. They found the reducing sugar in the urine and characterized it chemically as galactose. It is now clear that galactosuria may occur also in galactokinase deficiency, and in uridinediphosphate-4-epimerase deficiency. The enzyme deficiency was discovered by Isselbacher and colleagues [2]. The pathway of galactose metabolism had been worked out just after a few years earlier by Leloir and by Kalckar and their colleagues [3,4]. The first step in the utilization is its conversion to galactose-1-phosphate (Gal-1-P) [5], which is catalyzed by galactokinase.

$$\text{Galactose} + \text{ATP} \xrightarrow{\text{galactokinase}} \text{Gal-1-P} + \text{ADP}$$

where ATP = adenosine triphosphate; ADP = adenosine diphosphate.

Gal-1-P is then converted to glucose-1-phosphate (G-1-P) in a series of two reactions in which uridine diphosphoglucose (UDPG) functions catalytically. The first of these is the uridyl transferase reaction (Figure 58.1), which is followed by the epimerase reaction in which the uridine diphosphogalactose (UDPGal) formed is converted to UDPG [6].

$$\text{UDPGal} \leftrightarrow \text{UDPG}$$

In developed countries, galactosemia is currently detected by programs of neonatal screening in which the transferase enzyme, or galactose content, is assayed in blood. Early diagnosis and compliance with dietary treatment obviate the classic manifestations of the disease. Nevertheless, we continue to learn from experience as late complications are recognized in patients who have had early diagnosis and exemplary management. These have included abnormalities in language development [7,8] and ovarian failure [9–11].

CLINICAL ABNORMALITIES

Manifestations of galactosemia [1,12–16] appear usually within days of birth or of the initiation of milk feedings, and they increase in severity in the first months of life. Vomiting and jaundice may develop as early as a few days after milk feedings are begun. Vomiting has rarely been of sufficient severity to lead to surgery for a diagnosis of pyloric stenosis [17]. Anorexia, failure to gain weight or to increase in length, or even weight loss ensue. Hepatomegaly (Figures 58.2, 58.3) is a constant finding on examination. Parenchymal damage to the liver is progressive to typical Laennec cirrhosis. Patients may have edema, ascites (Figure 58.3), hypoprothrombinemia and bleeding. Splenomegaly may develop as portal pressure increases. If milk feedings are continued, the disease may be rapidly fatal.

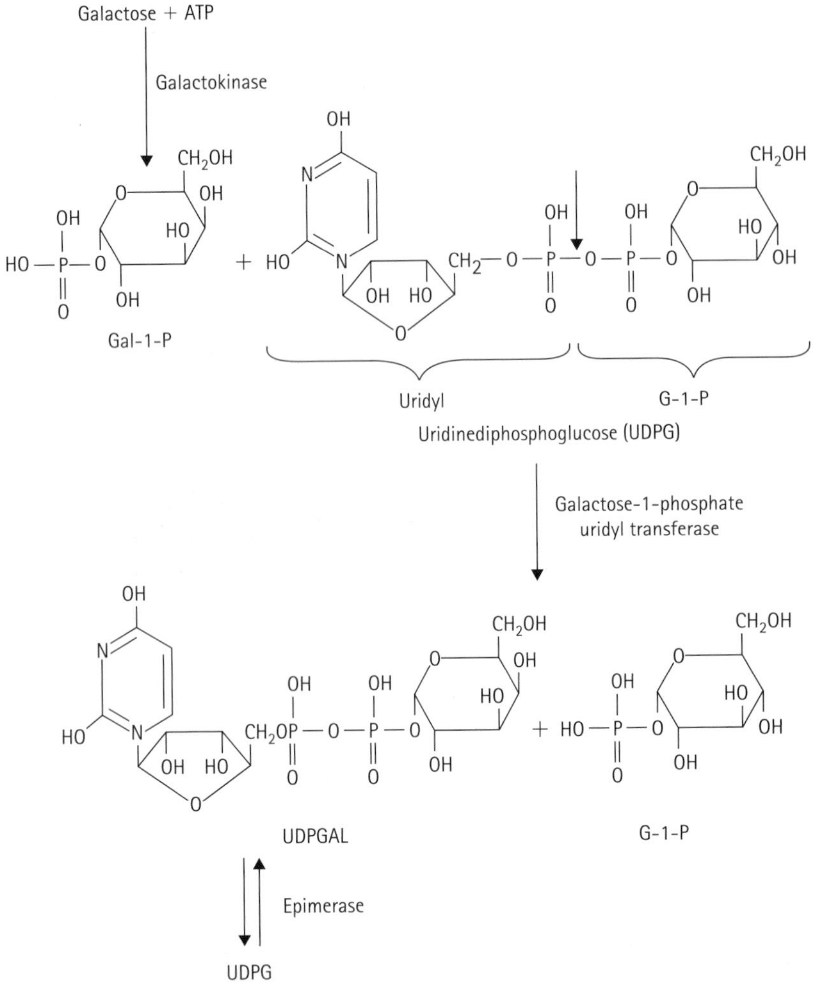

Galactose + ATP

Galactokinase

Gal-1-P

+

Uridyl   G-1-P

Uridinediphosphoglucose (UDPG)

Galactose-1-phosphate
uridyl transferase

UDPGAL   G-1-P

Epimerase

UDPG

Figure 58.1 *Galactose-1-phosphate uridyl transferase, the site of the enzyme defect in patients with galactosemia. The brackets indicate the uridyl and glucose-1-phosphate moieties of UDPG which have split at the arrow in the uridyl transferase reaction, transferring the uridyl group from G-1-P of UDPG to galactose-1-phosphate (Gal-1-P) to form uridinediphosphogalactose (UDPGal).*

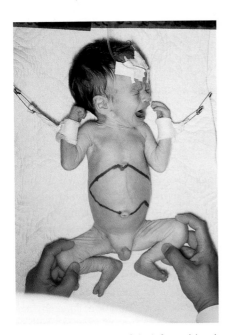

Figure 58.2 *Classic presentation of the infant with galactosemia. Hepatomegaly is outlined below the upper line of the rib cage. Failure to thrive is evident in the virtual absence of subcutaneous fat and the folds of loose skin.*

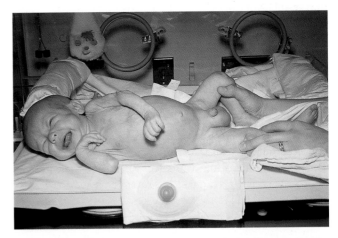

Figure 58.3 *D.S., an infant with galactosemia not diagnosed until 48 days of life. By this time, he had cataracts and failure to thrive. The abdomen was protuberant as a result of hepatomegaly and ascites. He also had edema of the legs and scrotum.*

Patients with galactosemia may present first with sepsis neonatorum. The organism is most commonly *E. coli.* In fact, prior to the advent of neonatal screening programs the recommendation for the routine testing for galactosemia in

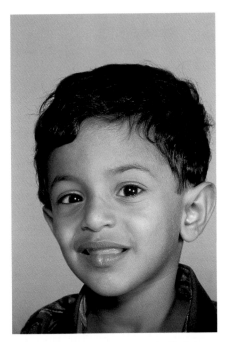

Figure 58.4   *A Saudi boy with galactosemia. Both lenses were removed because of dense cataracts. He usually wore thick glasses, but they were discarded for the photograph.*

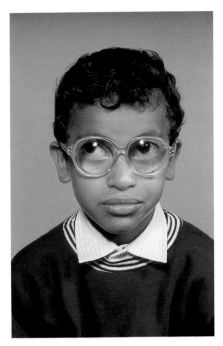

Figure 58.5   *A., another Saudi boy with galactosemia and the glasses he wore post-surgery for cataracts. His diagnosis was made at 1 year, at which time he had hepatomegaly 8 cm below the costal margin, bilateral ankle clonus and patchy white-matter abnormalities on CT, and was unable to sit or stand. Dietary treatment resolved the hepatomegaly. Developmental testing revealed borderline normal intelligence.*

all infants with sepsis led to most of the early diagnoses we encountered. A fulminant course of septicemia with early demise has been reported [18]. Complications of sepsis such as osteomyelitis and meningitis have also been observed. One patient developed gangrene of the toes bilaterally and of the dorsum of one foot [19]. Granulocyte function may be impaired [20,21].

The development of lenticular cataracts is a characteristic feature of the disease and occurs in infants who have received milk for three to four weeks (Figures 58.4, 58.5). Early cataracts maybe visible, as early as after a few days, by slit lamp examination.

Mental retardation is an important manifestation of the disease. It is most severe in patients who are not diagnosed or treated until a number of months has elapsed. Untreated or poorly compliant patients are often hyperactive. In a series of 41 patients from before the advent of neonatal screening three were severely retarded, seven had IQ levels between 70 and 84, and 29 had IQs greater than 85 [22]. This experience, of course, reflects some siblings of patients in whom treatment from birth was possible. In another series of 44 [23], eight had IQ levels below 70; 10 had levels from 71 to 89; and the rest had normal IQs, but lower than those of unaffected siblings. A relationship to compliance with diet was evident in an average IQ of 84 in 32 highly compliant patients and 77 in 22 poorly compliant patients [15].

Pseudotumor cerebri has been observed in a number of patients with galactosemia (Figure 58.6) [24]. It may be recognized by bulging of the anterior fontanel or by computed tomography (CT) [25] or magnetic resonance imaging (MRI)

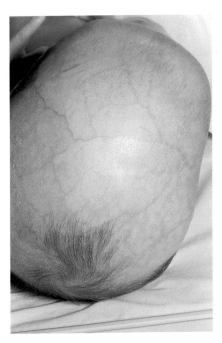

Figure 58.6   *D.S. Pseudotumor cerebri. The head circumference was increased and the fontanel bulging; the venous pattern was prominent.*

scan in which cerebral edema is evident. The occurrence of pseudotumor cerebri in patients with galactokinase deficiency [26] indicates that it is the accumulation of galactitol that causes this feature of the disease.

Renal abnormalities usually are first detected in the laboratory by the analysis of the blood and urine. Some patients have had frequency of urination. The picture is that of the renal Fanconi syndrome, in which there is renal tubular glycosuria, generalized aminoaciduria, and proteinuria, and systemically there is hyperchloremic acidosis. The glycosuria of the Fanconi syndrome may cause the galactosuria to be missed. The initial clinical suspicion of galactose has in the past come from the presence of reducing substance in a sample of urine that tests negative for glucose with a glucose oxidase, but once renal dysfunction develops both tests would be positive. In any case, most clinical laboratories now test for urinary sugar with glucose oxidase. Tests for reducing substance have become the province of the Biochemical Genetics Laboratory. At times of acute illness there may be hypoglycemia. In young infants hematological examination may reveal an erythroblastotic picture.

Long-term follow-up study on galactosemic individuals [27] showed, in general, that when diagnosis is early and compliance with therapy is good, levels of patient IQ have been normal. Experience with differing times of initiation of therapy, including sibling pairs in whom therapy could be started on the first day of life, provided a trend that indicated the earlier the diagnosis, the higher the IQ. A number of children have had problems in school, so that the performance may not be as good as the IQ would suggest, but overall results have been excellent.

While dietary therapy for galactosemia has effectively eliminated the acute toxicity syndrome of classical galactosemia, long-term complications have become evident as significant problems, even under ideal conditions of management and patient compliance.

Ovarian failure has been recognized in female patients [9–11]. It may present as either primary or secondary amenorrhea with hypergonadotrophic hypogonadism. This is seen in 75–96 percent of female patients by the age of 30. The incidence of ovarian failure is unrelated to the age at diagnosis or the degree of dietary control. The mechanism remains enigmatic. Impaired oocyte maturation and accelerated atresia have both been reported. One patient had normal ovaries at laparoscopy at 7 years-of-age and streak ovaries ten years later, suggesting a time-dependent effect. Pregnancies have occurred in female patients with classical galactosemia, although they are very rare. One patient who successfully delivered developed ovarian failure later. Many have low levels of estradiol and elevated levels of gonadotropins. Diminished or absent ovarian tissue may be revealed by ultrasonography. Evidence of hypergonadotropic hypogonadism has also been found in prepubertal girls [10]. The effect on the ovary is clearly a toxic one that takes a variable period of time to develop.

In the female patients with hypogonadism, thyroid hormone levels were normal, but low concentrations of thyroxin have been reported in two galactosemic infants in whom levels of T_4 became rapidly normal when a galactose-free diet was instituted [28]. Testing for thyroid function in such an infant would be suggested by the presence of jaundice; the finding of a low T_4 might lead away from the diagnosis of galactosemia. This problem should be less frequently encountered where there are programs of neonatal screening because now, virtually all infants are tested for galactosemia and hypothyroidism before the development of symptoms.

The second major later complication of classical galactosemia is delayed speech and language [7,8,29,30]. Onset of speech has been delayed and there have been problems of articulation and word retrieval. Most children with galactosemia have delayed language development associated with a verbal dyspraxia, but it is often overcome with time. This complication too appears to be unrelated to the time of diagnosis or the level of compliance as assessed by erythrocyte levels of galactose-1-phosphate. Some of those individuals had never received milk, and exemplary galactose-1-phosphate concentrations had been maintained.

Cognitive development is the most important long-term issue in this disease. Mental retardation is severe in patients who are diagnosed and treated late. Prior to the advent of neonatal screening 11 of 85 patients had IQ levels below 70. An average IQ of 84 was seen in 32 highly compliant patients, and 77 in 22 poorly compliant patients. Early information on the development of patients diagnosed early and complaint with therapy was optimistic [27]. By 1972 data from the largest experience in the US suggested that such patients had normal levels of IQ, and it appeared that the earlier diagnosis is, the higher the IQ.

However, more recent experience has led to a much more pessimistic prognosis. The results of a retrospective questionnaire survey of 298 patients from the US and Europe on whom IQ data were available [30] indicated that 45 percent of those at least 6 years old were developmentally delayed. This survey provided the first evidence of a definite decline in IQ with age; furthermore, the decline in females was significantly greater than in males. In a more recent retrospective study of 134 galactosemic patients in Germany there was also evidence of decline in IQ with age in that four of 34 patients less than 6 years-of-age had IQs less than 85, 10 of 18 between 7 and 12 years-of-age and 20 of 24 older than 12 years had such levels. A best fit regression line suggested a mean loss in cognitive performance of two IQ points per year; 40 points in 20 years. Of course, most of these patients, especially the older ones, antedated nationwide neonatal screening in Germany, and in the earlier international study 270 patients had clinical symptoms prior to diagnosis and treatment. Data were not specifically set out in either study for patients diagnosed presymptomatically and managed carefully. Nevertheless, decline with age in the earlier study was even shown in individuals tested at different ages. In addition, there was evidence in both studies of microcephaly and specific neurological manifestations, such as progressive ataxia and tremor.

MRI of the brain has revealed a substantial number of patients with cerebral atrophy [31]. White matter abnormalities occurred in 95 percent (52 of 55) over 1 year-of-age and persisted in follow up studies one to four years later. In addition, many patients, even with normal IQs, have had problems with behavior and school performance.

A curious syndrome of neurologic abnormality was reported [32] in siblings with galactosemia. Both had mental retardation, hypotonia, and a coarse tremor. Ataxia developed, and neurologic tests of cerebellar function were abnormal. Dietary control of galactose intake was excellent and documented by determination of levels of Gal-1-P. These manifestations are reminiscent of chicks given lethal doses of galactose [33]. On the other hand, there is a possibility that the siblings each received two rare, recessive, possibly linked genes, even in the absence of consanguinity.

GENETICS AND PATHOGENESIS

Galactosemia is inherited as an autosomal recessive trait [34]. The enzyme defect in galactosemia is in the uridyl transferase (Figure 58.1, p. 374) [2]. The abnormality can be detected in the erythrocyte. Cord blood is a useful source for early diagnosis. The defect can also be detected in cultured fibroblasts and amniotic cells, leukocytes and liver [35]. The other enzymes of galactose metabolism are normal.

The enzyme is a dimer in which each identical subunit has a molecular weight 44 kDa [36,37]. In patients with classic galactosemia, the activity of the enzyme is virtually completely absent [35,38]. In heterozygotes the levels are intermediate between patients and normals [38]. The Beutler assay [39], in which the glucose-1-phosphate product is converted to glucose-6-phosphate and the reduced form of nicotinamide-adenine dinucleotide phosphate (NADPH) formed is determined fluorimetrically, has been widely adopted for purposes of neonatal screening [40].

The demonstration of the enzyme defect in galactosemia was the first evidence for human variation at the Gal-1-P uridyl transferase locus. There has since been evidence of abundant variation [41] and the first to be discovered was the Duarte variant [42]. This enzyme has a distinct electrophoretic pattern of rapid migration [43], and its activity is about 50 percent of the normal enzyme. It produces no clinical manifestations. A number of other electrophoretic variants has been described. The Los Angeles variant, a rapidly moving enzyme with three bands, has normal or greater than normal activity [44]. The others all have less than normal activity, and in some there may be clinical manifestations. A black variant may have no erythrocytic activity but has about 10 percent of normal activity in liver and intestine [45]. These patients may have some neonatal symptoms. The Munster variant is associated with a classic galactosemic picture [46]. Gel electrophoresis [47] and isoelectric focusing [48,49] are employed to distinguish the variants.

It has become apparent that compounds in which an individual is heterozygous for two distinct variants are relatively frequent occurrences. Compounds in which one gene is the galactosemic (G) and one the Duarte (D) variant have been the most commonly encountered [50], especially in programs of neonatal screening for galactosemia [50–52]. Most individuals with this phenotype have no clinical manifestations,

but transient jaundice, lethargy, and hepatomegaly have been reported [51] in an infant whose mother had sepsis prior to the delivery; and others have displayed biochemical evidence of accumulation of galactose and Gal-1-P in the blood. Transferase levels may be very low early in life [51], and galactose tolerance tests have yielded evidence of diminished ability to metabolize ingested galactose [52].

Polymorphism complicates the determination of heterozygozity, but family study may elucidate the problem. The mean enzyme activity for heterozygotes for the galactosemia variant (GN) approximates half that of normal (N) individuals, and this is the level observed in Duarte homozygotes (DD). However, since heterozygotes for the Duarte variant have about 75 percent of normal activity, the study of parents should clarify the issue. Current practice has been to distinguish variants electrophoretically. Prenatal diagnosis has been carried out by assay of the enzyme in cultured amniocytes [53] and chorionic villus material and by the direct measurement by gas chromatography/mass spectrometry (GCMS) of galactitol in the amniotic fluid [54].

Programs of neonatal screening for galactosemia have indicated a frequency of one in 55 000 [55]. The galactosemia-Duarte (GD) compound occurs in about one in 3000 to 4000 [55]. In a recent year of experience in California, the frequency of galactosemia was one in 123 000 and that of the compound was one in 38 000, while the three-year experience with the program yielded an incidence of galactosemia of one in 86 000. In Massachusetts, screening of 6 million neonates yielded a figure of one in 62 000.

In classic galactosemia and in the Duarte variant, there are immunoreactive transferase proteins (cross-reacting material [CRM]) and the size and structure of these proteins are similar to normal [56].

The transferase gene has been localized to chromosome 9p13 [57–59] and the cDNA has been cloned from human fibroblasts [60]. The gene is small; 11 exons and 10 introns are found in 3.9 kb. A number of mutations have been identified (Table 58.1) [61–65]. In galactosemia an A to G missense mutation codes for a change from glutamine at position 188 to arginine. In the Duarte variant, an A to G mutation in exon 10 has changed an asparagine to an aspartic acid at position 314 near the carboxy terminus. The most common African mutation is S135L. The A to G mutation in the Q188R variant introduces a site of cleavage by the restriction endonuclease Hpa II, which permits family studies and population screening.

The ideal approach to diagnosis of galactosemia is through routine neonatal screening. A protocol for the screening and management of galactosemia is given in Table 58.2. The assay in the US is for the activity of galactose-1-phosphate uridyltransferase in dried blood on filter paper. In some countries the assay is for galactose, and this will also detect galactokinase deficiency. The test for galactose will also be positive in patients with congenital shunts from portal to systemic vessels [66]. A positive screening test is confirmed by quantification of activity in freshly obtained erythrocytes in the fluorimetric assay for NADPH formed along with glucose-6-phosphate from the glucose-1-phosphate product. In classic galactosemia the activity approximates zero. Variants with greater activity than this can be elucidated by electrophoresis or by mutational analysis. It is important for clinicians to recognize the early clinical manifestation of galactosemia and its infectious complications, because some developed countries have

given up neonatal screening for this disease, and even in screened infants classical disease can develop before the results of screening are known. The screening assay is followed by quantification of activity in freshly obtained erythrocytes.

In populations in which screening programs are not available, the diagnosis of infants with early symptoms is still initiated by the finding of galactose in urine. It is important to emphasize that testing of urine with glucose oxidase (Clinistix, Tes-tape) will not detect galactose; this is a strong argument for continued use of the older methods for the screening of urine for reducing substance (Benedict or Fehling test, Clinitest). We have also recognized galactosemia by finding galactose on GCMS of the urine sent for organic acid analysis. It is also true that the excretion of galactose in the urine depends on dietary intake of lactose; in an acutely ill patient admitted to hospital and treated with parenteral fluid therapy, the disease may not be recognizable by testing the urine because he or she has not received galactose for 24 to 48 hours.

Characterization of the reducing substance found in a urine sample can be done in a number of ways. It is usually done by paper chromatography [67]. Testing with paper infiltrated with galactose oxidase provides for an effective screening procedure [68]. Of course, sugar in urine of an infant that tests positive for reducing substance and negative for glucose oxidase is galactose until proved otherwise and indicates direct assay of the enzyme. In patients with normal activity of the uridyl transferase, assays are performed for galactokinase and epimerase.

The structure of galactose is identical to that of glucose except for the position of the hydroxyl on carbon 4. Lactose, the principal sugar of mammalian milks, is the predominant dietary source of galactose. It is a disaccharide in which glucose and galactose are linked in an α-1,4-glucosidic bond in which an oxygen bridge connects carbon 1 of galactose and carbon 4 of glucose.

The pathogenesis of most of the clinical manifestations of galactosemia is the accumulation of Gal-1-P in tissues [69]. Among the best evidence for this is the observation that

Table 58.1   *Protocol for galactosemia*

When newborn screening reports a low Gal-1-P uridyl transferase:
- Remove galactose/lactose from diet and prescribe a soy or other lactose/galactose-free formula. Breast feeding is stopped.
- Obtain blood for Gal-1-P and uridyl transferase electrophoresis.

Diagnosis of DD, DG, or GG.

DD diagnosis:
- Return infant to normal diet, no follow-up required.

DG diagnosis:
- Continue diet until infant is 8–12 months old
- Check Gal-1-P
- Begin full lactose/galactose diet for two weeks
- Re-check Gal-1-P
- If Gal-1-P is within normal range, continue unrestricted diet
- If Gal-1-P is elevated, then return to lactose/galactose restricted diet.

GG diagnosis:
- Continue lactose/galactose restricted diet
- Obtain blood for Gal-1-P, LFT, bilirubin, and albumin
- Refer to ophthalmologist
- Monitor monthly in metabolic clinic until four months old, checking Gal-1-P levels every two weeks
- If Gal-1-P levels indicate good control, change to monthly Gal-1-P levels and continue monthly clinic visits
- Second year of life – monitor every three months*
- 2–5 years old – monitor every six months*
- 6 years and older – monitor yearly*
- Evaluate language development at preschool age
- Evaluate ovarian function of teenage girls
- Encourage regular eye examinations
- Developmental assessment at 4, 8, 14, and 18 yr

(*may vary depending on control)

Table 58.2   *Mutations associated with galactosemia*

Codon and amino acid substitution*	Nucleotide change	Phenotype	Prevalence in classic galactosemia		
			Caucasian	Hispanic	African American
Q188R	CAG → CGG	G	62%	58%	12%
V44M	GTG → ATG	G			
S135L	TCG → TTG	G	0%		48%
M142L	ATG → AAG	G			
R148W	CGG → TGG	G			
L195P	CTG → CGG	G			
R231H	CGT → CAT	G			
H319Q	CAC → CAA	G			
R333W	CGG → TGG	G			
N314D	AAC → GAC	Duarte	5.9% of Non-galactosemia controls		

* Within galactose-1-phosphate uridyl transferase (GALT).

therapeutic measures that result in reduction of intracellular concentrations of Gal-1-P lead to prevention or disappearance of symptoms. It is clear that the manifestations of galactosemia do not occur in galactokinase deficiency. Hepatic, renal and cerebral damage is unknown. Thus, retardation is not due to galactose itself. Cataracts and pseudotumor cerebri occur in patients with galactokinase deficiency [26,70,71], and these complications are due to galactitol. This by-product of galactose accumulation occurs by its reduction at carbon-1 and is present in urine and tissues. In the lens, galactitol causes osmotic swelling and disruption of fibers. Osmotic swelling is also the mechanism of production of cerebral edema. In addition, cataracts that result from galactose treatment of rats are prevented by sorbinil, which inhibits aldose reductase, the enzyme that catalyzes the conversion of galactose to galactitol [72]. Galactitol has been demonstrated *in vivo* by proton magnetic resonance spectroscopy in the brain of an encephalopathic infant with galactosemia [73].

The pathogeneses of the later appearing dyspraxic speech and ovarian failure, as well as the potential loss of late cognitive function, are not clear. Low concentrations of UDPGal have been proposed as a mechanism [74,75]. Information on mutations has indicated that the Q188R/Q188R genotype is a significant predictor of developmental verbal dyspraxia in patients with good metabolic control as indicated by erythrocyte Gal-1-P levels less than 3.2 mg/dL [76].

TREATMENT

The treatment for galactosemia is exclusion of galactose from the diet [77]. This is accomplished by the elimination of milk and its products. The mainstay of the diet for an infant is the substitution of casein hydrolysate or a soybean preparation for milk formulas. Education of the parents, and of the child as he or she grows older, on the galactose content of foods is important. A list of foods has been published that is useful in management [78]. The determination of the Gal-1-P content of erythrocytes is employed in monitoring adherence to the diet [79], and acceptable levels have been set at 4 mg/dL (150 μmol/L). When this is not available, the serum bilirubin and the transaminase levels tend to be employed.

Experience with early treatment supports the concept that effective treatment instituted in the first weeks of life can prevent most of the classic manifestations of the disease. At the other end of the scale, mental retardation, once established, is irreversible, and if the diagnosis is delayed, some damage to the brain is inevitable. There may be abnormalities of visual perception, behavior problems or convulsions. Cataracts are reversible if treatment is started within the first three months of life. Hepatic and renal manifestations of the disease are reversible. Late manifestations of language development and ovarian failure are not prevented by otherwise effective treatment. The results of treatment on long term cognitive function are controversial but it is clear that prognosis is not as good as it was once thought.

References

1 Mason HH, Turner ME. Chronic galactosemia. *Am J Dis Child* 1935;**50**:539.

2 Isselbacher KJ, Anderson EP, Kurahashi K, Kalckar HM. Congenital galactosemia a single enzymatic block in galactose metabolism. *Science* 1956;**123**:635.

3 Leloir LF. The enzymatic transformation of uridine diphosphate glucose into a galactose derivative. *Arch Biochem Biophys* 1951;**33**:186.

4 Kalckar HM, Braganca B, Munch-Petersen A. Uridyl transferase and the formation of uridine diphosphate galactose. *Nature* 1953;**172**:1038.

5 Kosterlitz HW. The structure of the galactose-1-phosphate present in the liver during galactose assimilation. *Biochem J* 1943;**37**:318.

6 Gitzelmann R, Steinmann B. Uridine diphosphate galactose 4-epimerase deficiency. II Clinical follow-up biochemical studies and family investigation. *Helv Paediatr Acta* 1973;**28**:497.

7 Waisbren SE, Norman TR, Schnell RR, Levy HL. Speech and language deficits in early treated children with galactosemia. *J Pediatr* 1983;**102**:75.

8 Nelson CD, Waggoner DD, Donnell GN, *et al.* Verbal dyspraxia in treated galactosemia. *Pediatrics* 1991;**88**:346.

9 Kaufman FR, Kogut MD, Donnell GN, *et al.* Hypergonadotropic hypogonadism in female patients with galactosemia. *N Engl J Med* 1981;**304**:494.

10 Steinmann B, Gitzelmann R, Zachmann M. Hypergonadotropic hypogonadism found already in pre-pubertal girls but only in adult males. *Pediatr Res* 1981;**15**:1182.

11 Gibson JB. Gonadal function in galactosemics and galactose intoxicated animals. *Eur J Pediatr* 1995;**154**:S14 (suppl 2).

12 Donnell GN, Bergren WR, Cleland RS. Galactosemia. *Pediatr Clin North Am* 1960;**7**:315.

13 Holzel A, Komrower GM, Schwarz V. Galactosemia. *Am J Med* 1957;**22**:703.

14 Donnell GN, Collado M, Koch R. Growth and development of children with galactosemia. *J Pediatr* 1961;**58**:836.

15 Komrower GM, Lee DH. Long term follow-up of galactosemia. *Arch Dis Child* 1970;**45**:367.

16 Fisler K, Koch R, Donnell GN, Wenz E. Developmental aspects of galactosemia from infancy to childhood. *Clin Pediatr* 1980;**19**:38.

17 Nyhan WL. Introduction and general features: in *Abnormalities in Amino Acid Metabolism in Clinical Medicine* (ed. WL Nyhan). Appleton Century Crofts, Norwalk CT;1984:5.

18 Levy HL, Sepe SJ, Shih VE, *et al.* Sepsis due to *Escherichia coli* in neonates with galactosemia. *N Engl J Med* 1977;**297**:823.

19 Collip PJ, Donnell GN. Galactosemia presenting with gangrene. *J Pediatr* 1959;**54**:363.

20 Kobayashi R, Blum P, Gard S, *et al.* Granulocyte function in patients with galactose-1-phosphate uridyltransferase deficiency (galactosemia). *Clin Res* 1980;**28**:109A.

21 Litchfield WJ, Wells WW. Effects of galactose on free radical reactions of polymorphonuclear leukocytes. *Arch Biochem Biophys* 1978;**188**:26.

22 Donnell GN, Koch R, Bergren WR. Observations on results of management of galactosemic patients: in *Galactosemia* (ed. DYY Hsia). Charles C Thomas, Springfield IL;1969:247.

23 Nadler HL, Inouye T, Hsia DYY. Clinical galactosemia: A study of fifty-five cases. in *Galactosemia* (ed. DYY Hsia) Charles C Thomas, Springfield IL; 1969:127.

24 Huttenlocher PR, Hillman RE, Hsia YE. Pseudotumor cerebri in galactosemia. *J Pediatr* 1970;**76**:902.

25 Belman AL, Moshe SL, Zimmerman RD. Computerised tomographic demonstration of cerebral edema in a child with galactosemia. *Pediatrics* 1986;**78**:606.

26 Litman N, Kanter AI, Finberg L. Galactokinase deficiency presenting as pseudotumor cerebri. *J Pediatr* 1975;**86**:410.

27 Fishler J, Donnell GN, Bergen WR, Koch R. Intellectual and personality development in children with galactosemia. *Pediatrics* 1972;**50**:412.

28 Berger HM, Vlasveld L, Van Gelderen HH, Ruys JH. Low serum thyroxine concentrations in babies with galactosemia. *J Pediatr* 1983;**103**:930.

29 Buist NRM, Nelson D, Tuerck JM. Dyspraxia in treated galactosemic patients. *Clin Res* 1983;**34**:75.

30 Waggoner DD, Buist NRM, Donnell GN. Long-term prognosis in galactosaemia: results of a survey of 350 cases. *J Inherit Metab Dis* 1990;**13**:802.

31 Nelson MD Jr, Wolff JA, Cross CA, *et al.* Galactosemia: evaluation with MR imaging. *Radiol* 1992;**184**:255.

32 Lo W, Packman S, Nash S, *et al.* Curious neurologic sequelae in galactosemia. *Pediatrics* 1984;**73**:309.

33 Gitzelmann R, Hansen RG, Steinmann B. Biogenesis of galactose, a possible mechanism of self-intoxication in galactosemia: in *Normal and Pathological Development of Energy metabolism* (eds FA Hommes, CJ Van den Berg). Academic Press, London;1975:25.

34 Tedesco TA, Wu JW, Bioches FS, Mellman WJ. The genetic defect in galactosemia. *N Engl J Med* 1975;**292**:737.

35 Krooth R, Winberg AN. Studies on cell lines developed from the tissues of patients with galactosemia. *J Exp Med* 1961;**113**:1155.

36 Dale GL, Popjak G. Purification of normal and inactive galactosemic galactose-1-phosphate uridyl-transferase from human red cells. *J Biol Chem* 1976;**251**:1057.

37 Saito S, Ozutsumi M, Kurashashi K. Galactose-1-phosphate uridyl transferase of *E coli. J Biochem* 1967;**242**:2362.

38 Donnell GN, Bergren WR, Bretthauer MS, Hansen RG. The enzymatic expression of heterozygosity in families of children with galactosemia. *Pediatrics* 1960;**25**:572.

39 Beutler E, Baluda MC. A simple spot screening test for galactosemia. *J Lab Clin Med* 1966;**68**:137.

40 Nelson K, Hsia DYY. Screening for galactosemia and glucose-6-phosphate-dehydrogenase deficiency in newborn infants. *J Pediatr* 1967;**71**:582.

41 Harris H. Enzyme variants in human populations. *Johns Hopkins Med J* 1976;**138**:134.

42 Beutler E, Baluda MC, Sturgeon P, Day R. A new genetic abnormality resulting in galactose-1-phosphate uridyltransferase deficiency *Lancet* 1965;**1**:353.

43 Mathai CK, Beutler E. Electrophoretic variation of galactose-1-phosphate uridyltransferase. *Science* 1966;**154**:1179.

44 Ng WG, Bergren WR, Donnell GN. A new variant of galactose-1-phosphate uridyltransferase in man: the Los Angeles variant. *Ann Hum Genet* 1973;**37**:1.

45 Segal S, Blair A, Roth H. The metabolism of galactose by patients with congenital galactosemia. *Am J Med* 1965;**38**:62.

46 Matz D, Enzenauer J, Menne F. Uber einen Fall von atypischer Galactosaemie. *Humangenetik* 1975;**27**:309.

47 Ng WG, Bergren WR, Field M, Donnell GN. An improved electrophoretic procedure for galactose-1-phosphate uridyl transferase: demonstration of multiple activity bands with the Duarte variant. *Biochem Biophys Res Commun* 1969;**37**:354.

48 Shin YS, Niedermeier HP, Endres W, *et al.* Agarose gel isoelectrofocusing of UDP-galactose pyrophosphorylase and galactose-1-phosphate uridyltransferase. Developmental aspect of UDP-galactose pyrophosphorylase. *Clin Chim Acta* 1987;**166**:27.

49 Shin YS, Rieth WE, Schaub J. Prenatal diagnosis of galactosemia and properties of galactose-1-phosphate uridyltransferase in erythrocytes of galactosemic variants as well as in human fetal and adult organs. *Clin Chim Acta* 1983;**128**:271.

50 Levy HL, Sepe SJ, Walton DS, *et al.* Galactose-1-phosphate uridyltransferase deficiency due to Duarte/galactosemia combined variation: Clinical and biochemical studies. *J Pediatr* 1978;**92**:390.

51 Kelly S. Significance of the Duarte/classical galactosemia genetic compounds. *J Pediatr* 1979;**94**:937.

52 Schwarz HP, Zuppinger KA, Zimmerman A, *et al.* Galactose intolerance in individuals with double heterozygosity for Duarte variant and galactosemia. *J Pediatr* 1982;**100**:704.

53 Donnell GN, Bergeron WC, Ahi O, Golbus MS. Prenatal diagnosis of galactosemia. *Clin Chim Acta* 1977;**74**:227.

54 Jakobs C, Warner TG, Sweetman L, Nyhan WL. Stable isotope dilution analysis of galactitol in amniotic fluid: an accurate approach to the prenatal diagnosis of galactosemia. *Pediatr Res* 1984;**18**:714.

55 Levy HL. Screening for galactosemia: in *Inherited Disorders of Carbohydrate Metabolism* (eds D Burman, JB Holton, CA Penneck). MTP Press, Lancaster England;1980:133.

56 Tedesco TA. Human galactose-1-phosphate uridyl transferase. *J Biol Chem* 1972;**247**:6631.

57 Mohandas T, Sparkes RS, Sparkes MC, Schulkin JD. Assignment of the human gene for galactose-1-phosphate uridyltransferase to chromosome 9: studies with Chinese hamster-human somatic cell hybrids. *Proc Natl Acad Sci USA* 1977;**74**:5628.

58 Mohandas T, Sparkes RS, Sparkes MC, *et al.* Regional localization of human gene loci on chromosome 9: studies of somatic cell hybrids containing human translocations. *Am J Hum Genet* 1979;**31**:586.

59 Sparkes RS, Sparkes MC, Funderburk SJ, Moedjono S. Expression of GALT in 9p chromosome alterations: Assignment of GALT locus to 9cen→9p22. *Ann Hum Genet* 1980;**43**:343.

60 Reichardt KV, Berg P. Cloning and characterization of a cDNA encoding human galactose-1-phosphate uridyl transferase. *Mol Biol Med* 1988;**5**:107.

61 Elsas LJ, Langley S, Paulk EM, *et al.* A molecular approach to galactosemia. *Eur J Pediatr* 1995;**154**:(suppl 2) S21.

62 Elsas LJ, Fridovich-Keil JL, Leslie N. Galactosemia: a molecular approach to the enigma. *Int Pediatr* 1993;**8**:101.

63 Flach JE, Reichardt JKV, Elsas LJ. Sequence of a cDNA encoding human galactose-1-phosphate uridyl transferase. *Mol Biol Med* 1990;**7**:365.

64 Leslie ND, Immerman EB, Flach JE, *et al.* The human galactose-1-phosphate uridyl transferase gene. *Genomics* 1992;**14**:474.

65 Elsas LJ, Dembure PP, Langley S, *et al.* A common mutation associated with the Duarte Galactosemia allele. *Am J Hum Genet* 1994;**54**:1030.

66 Sakura N, Mizoguchi N, Ono H, *et al.* Congenital porto-systemic shunt as a major cause of galactosemia. *Int Pediatr* 2001;**16**:206.

67 Borden M. Screening for metabolic disease: in *Abnormalities in Amino Acid Metabolism in Clinical Medicine* (ed. WL Nyhan) Appleton Century Crofts, Norwalk;1984:401.

68 Dhalqvist A. Test paper for galactose in urine. *Scand J Clin Lab Invest* 1968;**22**:87.

69 Schwartz V, Golberg L, Komrower GM, Holzel A. Some disturbances of erythrocyte metabolism in galactosaemia. *Biochem J* 1956;**62**:34.

70 Van Heyningen R, Galactose cataract: a review. *Exp Eye Res* 1967;**11**:415.

71 Gitzelmann R. Hereditary galactokinase deficiency a newly recognized cause of juvenile cataracts. *Pediatr Res* 1967;**1**:14.

72 Datiles F, Fukui H, Kuwabara T, Kinoshita JH. Galactose cataract prevention with sorbinil and aldose reductase inhibitor: a light microscopic study. *Invest Ophthalmol Vis Sci* 1982;**2**:174.

73 Berry GT, Hunter JV, Wang Z, *et al. In vivo* evidence of brain galactitol accumulation in an infant with galactosemia and encephalopathy. *J Pediatr* 2001;**138**:260.

74 Kaufman FR, Xu YK, Ng WG, Donnell GN. Correlation of ovarian with galactose-1-phosphate uridyl transferase levels in galactosemia. *J Pediatr* 1988;**112**:754.

75 Kaufman FR, Ng WG, Xu YK, *et al.* Normalization of uridine disphosphate galactose (UDPGal) levels with oral uridine in patients (PTS) with classical galactosemia (G). *Clin Res* 1989;**37**:184A.

76 Robertson A, Singh RH, Guerrero NV, *et al.* Outcomes analysis of verbal dyspraxia in classic galactosemia. *Genet In Med* 2000;**2**:142.

77 Donnell GN, Bergren WR, The galactosemias: in *The Treatment of Inherited Metabolic Disease* (ed. DN Raine) MTP Press, Lancaster UK;1975:91.

78 Koch R, Acosta P, Donnell GN, Lieberman E. Nutritional therapy of galactosemia. *Clin Pediatr (Phila)* 1965;**4**:571.

79 Gitzelmann R. Alpha-D-galactose-1-phosphate determinaion as galactose after hydrolysis of phosphate: in *Methods of Enzymatic Analysis* (eds HU Bermeyer, K Gawelin) Weinheim Academic Press, New York;1974:1291.

59

Glycogen storage diseases: introduction

The glycogen storage diseases represent an enlarging group of diseases characterized by the deposition of glycogen in tissue cells. They are a heterogeneous group with different etiologies and different clinical manifestations. The classic form of glycogen storage disease was first described by von Gierke in 1929 [1]. The glycogen from this original patient was isolated by Schoenheimer [2] and was found not to differ from normal glycogen in optical rotation or in its composition of glucose residues. The resistance of this material to glycogenolysis by the patient's liver *in vitro* and its prompt degradation by normal liver led Schoenheimer to the conclusion that an enzyme essential to glycogenolysis was missing. This appears to have been the first demonstration of the concept proposed by Garrod [3] that inborn errors of metabolism result from genetically determined deficiencies of single enzymes. The demonstration by Cori and Cori [4] of the virtual absence of the activity of glucose-6-phosphatase in livers of patients with classic von Gierke disease established the deficiency of a single enzymatic step in carbohydrate metabolism as the basis of this disease.

Glycogen is a branched, polydisperse molecule that has been recognized since the time of Claude Bernard as the storage form for carbohydrates in animal tissues. This polysaccharide is composed entirely of units of α-D-glucose and the units are joined together in 1,4 and 1,6 linkages (Figure 59.1) to form molecules with molecular weights in the vicinity of 1 to 4 million. The branched, tree-like structure (Figure 59.2) was worked out through the elegant studies of Cori and Cori and their colleagues, using stepwise enzymatic degradation [5–7]. A free reducing group occurs at only one point. The strait chains of glucose residues are linked together by α-1,4 bonds; branching occurs through 1,6 linkages. In normal human glycogens, 6 to 8 percent of the glucose residues are joined to the rest of the molecule in α-1,6 linkage [8]. Glycogen contains seven tiers of branch points; the outer branches are terminated in non-reducing end groups [9].

The major pathway for the catabolism of glycogen is shown in Figure 60.1, p. 385. The splitting of the 1,4 linkages in glycogen is catalyzed in the presence of inorganic phosphate by phosphorylase to yield glucose-1-phosphate [10]. The phosphorylase is activated by phosphorylation of serine, which is stimulated by glucagon and epinephrine [11]. Phosphorylase

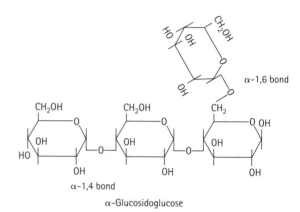

Figure 59.1   *Portion of the glycogen molecule. The predominant structure is that of straight chains of glucose molecules in α-1,4 linkage. The branch points in the structure are created by α-1,6 linkages. Cleavage of the 1,4 bonds is catalyzed by phosphorylase and cleavage of the 1,6 bonds by amylo-1,6-glucosidase, the debranching enzyme.*

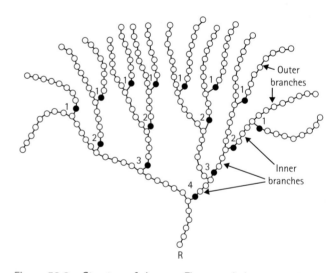

Figure 59.2   *Structure of glycogen. The open circles represent glucose moieties in α-1,4 linkage, and the black circles those in α-1,6 linkage at branch points. While four outer tiers of branch points are shown, glycogen has at least seven. R indicates the reducing end group. The outer branches terminate in nonreducing end groups. (Reproduced with permission from Cori, G.T. [7])*

Table 59.1 *Glycogen storage diseases*

Enzyme deficiency	Glycogen structure	Organs	First description	Synonyms	Type
Glucose-6-phosphatase	Normal	Liver, kidney	von Gierke	Hepatorenal glycogenosis	Ia
Glucose-6-phosphate transport protein	Normal	Liver, neutrophils	Narasawa, Lange	(Translocase) T_1 deficiency	Ib
Stabilizing protein	Normal	Liver	Burchell	Regulatory protein deficiency	Iasp
Microsomal phosphate transporter	Normal	Liver	Nordlie	T_{2B} phosphate translocase deficiency	Ic
Microsomal glucose transporter	Normal	Liver	Leonard	GLUT7 deficiency	Id
α-1,4 glucosidase	Normal	Generalized, cardiac	Pompe	Cardiac glycogenosis, generalized glycogenosis	II
Amylo-1,6-glucosidase (debrancher)	Abnormal: very short outer branches	Liver, muscle	Forbes	Limit dextrinosis	III
Amylo-(1,4→6) trans-glucosidase (brancher)	Abnormal: long, straight chains	Liver	Andersen	Amylopectinosis	IV
Muscle phosphorylase	Normal	Muscle	McArdle	Myophosphorylase	V
Liver phosphorylase	Normal	Liver	Hers	Hepatophosphorylase deficiency	VI
Muscle phosphofructokinase	Normal	Muscle, erythrocytes	Tarui	–	VII
Phosphorylase kinase	Normal	Liver	Hug, Huijing	–	VIII, IX

*Autosomal recessive and X-linked phosphorylase kinase deficiency diseases have been defined.

kinase catalyzes the phosphorylation and activation of phosphorylase [12]. Removal of phosphate from the enzyme is catalyzed by protein phosphatase, and inhibits phosphorylase activity.

The phosphorolysis of glycogen catalyzed by phosphorylase splits off glucose units until the 1,6 branch points are approached. These branches are degraded down to a limit dextrin in which three glucose residues are attached in 1,4 linkage to the 1,6-linked glucose. The transfer of this trisaccharide to the end of another glycogen chain is catalyzed by the transferase activity of the debranching enzyme. Then the exposed glucose at the branch point is cleaved by the same enzyme protein in which amylo-1,6-glucosidase activity is at a different catalytic site [13]. The product of the reaction is free glucose. The combined activity of phosphorylase and the debranching enzyme accomplish the complete degradation of glycogen.

Glycogen is stored in liver and muscle, and these are the tissues predominantly affected in the classic glycogenosis. Pompe disease, or glycogenosis II is an exception because it is a lysosomal storage disease; its major effects are cardiac; and there is no problem with this type of hepatic storage. The fact that enzymes, such as phosphorylase, have different genetically determined enzymes in liver and muscle leads to different diseases that have hepatic or myopathic clinical manifestations. Hepatic metabolism of glycogen is critical for glucose homeostasis; hepatic glycogenoses present classically with hypoglycemia. Muscle glycogen is used to make adenosine triphosphate (ATP) for contraction; glycogenoses of muscle present with cramps, weakness, stiffness or rhabdomyolysis.

Eight distinct types of glycogenosis result from specific defects in enzymes of glycogen catabolism (Table 59.1). They were given numbers in the chronological order of their description. The numbers seem less useful now that molecular defects have been identified, leading to multiple different forms of Type I, as well as the disappearance of Type VIII, which was once used for phosphorylase kinase deficiency. Nevertheless, these numbers are so commonly employed, they will be continued.

- The classic form of glycogen storage disease originally described by von Gierke [1] is caused by a deficiency of glucose-6-phosphatase (Chapter 60).
- Type II or Pompe disease (Chapter 61), is a lysosomal storage disease which usually causes death in infancy from cardiomyopathy.
- Glycogenosis Type III (Chapter 62) is the result of defective activity of the debrancher enzyme. It causes massive hepatomegaly in infancy and progressive myopathy in adults.
- Type IV, or Andersen disease, is a very different type of disorder in which defective activity of the debranching enzyme produces abnormal glycogen that appears to act as a foreign body and causes hepatic cirrhosis.
- Type V, or McArdle disease, results from defective activity of phosphorylase in muscle. Symptoms are those of muscle cramps that limit exercise tolerance, and myoglobinuria.
- Hepatic phosphorylase deficiency, type VI, leads to a mild hepatic glycogen storage disease.
- Type VII glycogenosis, or Tarui disease, is clinically identical to McArdle disease, but the enzymatic defect is in the phosphofructokinase of muscle.

- Phosphorylase kinase deficiency is now known as type IX, but this enzyme is composed of four subunits coded by different genes, and hence the inheritance of its five different clinical subtypes are variously autosomal recessive and X-linked recessive [14]. Patients with this disease and with phosphorylase deficiency often present with isolated hepatomegaly and are often first referred to the metabolic service after a liver biopsy has identified large amounts of glycogen. Most do not require treatment and as adults have normal height and modest enlargement of the liver.

References

1 Von Gierke E. Hepato-nephromegalie glykogenica. *Beitr Path Anat* 1929;**82**:497.

2 Schonheimer R. Uber eine eigenartige Storung des Kohlenhydrat-Stoffwechsels. *Zeitschr Physiol Chem* 1929;**182**:148.

3 Garrod AE. *Inborn Errors of Metabolism*. Oxford University Press, London;1923.

4 Cori GT, Cori CF. Glucose-6-phosphatase of liver in glycogen storage disease. *J Biol Chem* 1952;**199**:661.

5 Illingworth B, Cori GT. Structure of glycogens and amylopectins. III Normal and abnormal human glycogens. *J Biol Chem* 1952;**199**:653.

6 Larner J, Illingworth B, Cori GT, Cori CF. Structure of glycogens and amylopectins. II Analysis by stepwise enzyme degradation. *J Biol Chem* 1952;**199**:641.

7 Cori GT. Biochemical aspects of glycogen deposition disease. *Mod Prob Paediatr* 1957;**3**:344.

8 Cori CF. The enzymatic synthesis and molecular configuration of glycogen. in *A Symposium on the Clinical and Biochemical Aspects of Carbohydrate Utilization in Health and Disease* (ed. VA Najjar). Johns Hopkins Press, Baltimore MD;1952.

9 Cori CF. Glycogen structure and enzyme deficiencies in glycogen storage disease. *Harvey Lectures* 1952–1953;**48**:145.

10 Newgard CB, Littman DR, Van Genderen C, *et al*. Human brain glycogen phosphorylase. Cloning sequence analysis chromosomal mapping tissue expression and comparison with the human liver and muscle isozymes. *J Biol Chem* 1988;**263**:3850.

11 Cohen P, Hardie GG. The actions of cyclic AMP on biosynthetic processes are mediated indirectly by cyclic AMP dependent protein kinase. *Biochim Biophys Acta* 1991;**1094**:292.

12 Francke U, Barras BT, Zander NF, Kilimann MW. Assignment of human genes for phosphorylase kinase subunits α (PHKA) to Xq12-q13 and β (PHBK) to 16q12–q13. *Am J Hum Genet* 1989;**45**:276.

13 Liu W, Madsen NB, Braun C, Withers SG. Reassessment of the catalytic mechanism of glycogen branching enzyme. *Biochemistry* 1991;**30**:1419.

14 Van Den Berg IET, Berger R. Phosphorylase b kinase deficiency in man: A review. *J Inherit Metab Dis* 1990;**13**:442.

Glycogenosis type I – Von Gierke disease

60

MAJOR PHENOTYPIC EXPRESSION

Hypoglycemia; massive hepatomegaly from storage of glycogen in the liver; short stature; prolonged bleeding time; ketosis, hyperlipidemia, lactic acidemia and hyperuricemia; late complications of gout, hepatic adenomas, renal disease and osteoporosis; subnormal glycemic response to glucagon; and deficient hepatic glucose-6-phosphatase.

INTRODUCTION

The classic form of glycogen storage disease originally described by von Gierke [1] is caused by a deficiency of glucose-6-phosphatase (Fig 60.1). It became apparent that there were subtypes of glycogenosis I and a considerably expanded glucose-6-phosphatase system when patients were studied who appeared to have von Gierke disease in which glucose-6-phosphatase activity in frozen liver was normal. The term glycogenosis type Ib was derived to distinguish these patients from those (Ia) in whom the activity of the enzyme is deficient

[2,3]. Narisawa and colleagues in 1978 [3] found defective glucose-6-phosphatase activity in fresh liver and restored activity by adding detergents; they suggested that the defect was in glucose-6-phosphate transport. The translocase defect was reported in 1980 by Lange and colleagues [4]. Type Ic was recognized [5] on the basis of normal activity of glucose-6-phosphatase in detergent-disrupted microsomes, while activity in intact microsomes is defective for both glucose-6-phosphate and carbamylphosphate substrates. Type Id with defective microsomal transport of glucose has not yet been observed clinically [6]. A variant of type Ia is a result of the

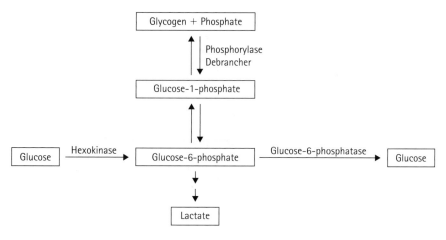

Figure 60.1 *Glucose-6-phosphatase, the site of the defect in von Gierke disease.*

deficiency of the regulatory protein, designated Iasp, for stabilizing protein which has so far been reported in a single patient [7]; it is impossible to distinguish this from deficiency of the catalytic subunit clinically, and difficult biochemically unless the entire stabilizing protein is missing.

The enzyme, glucose-6-phosphatase [8] is expressed in liver, but also in kidney, pancreatic islets and intestinal mucosa; and glycogen accumulates in all three organs. Clinical manifestations appear largely, if not entirely, consequences of the metabolic effects of the enzyme defect. Late effects, hepatic adenomas and renal disease are of uncertain pathogenesis. The enzyme is situated in the endoplasmic reticulum, and this sets the stage for transport defects.

The gene for glucose-6-phosphatase has been cloned [9] and so has that of the translocase which is deficient in type Ib [10]. Mutations have been identified in the phosphatase [9], some of which are specific for certain ethnic groups, such as R83C and Q347X in Caucasians and G727T in Japanese [11].

CLINICAL ABNORMALITIES

In classic type Ia glycogen storage disease symptoms usually occur in the first months of life and the disease may be recognized at birth. There may be neonatal hypoglycemia. Hepatomegaly is often present at birth [12] and progresses to huge enlargement of the liver without splenomegaly (Figures 60.2–60.4). The kidneys are enlarged too and may be visualized on roentgenography or may even be palpable. It is common in this condition for the liver to be palpable at the iliac crest in infancy and early childhood. The abdomen is protuberant, the posture lordotic (Figure 60.4) and the gait broad-based and rolling or swinging, all apparent consequences of the hepatomegaly. With time and growth the abdomen tends to become less prominent.

Linear growth is usually retarded (Figure 60.5). The shortness of stature is symmetrical in that there is proportionate

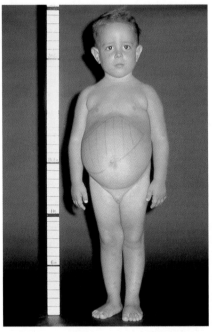

Figure 60.3 *D.A., a 5-year-old boy with glucose-6-phosphate deficiency. He had massive hepatomegaly. There was some adiposity about the face.*

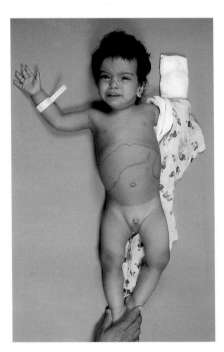

Figure 60.2 *O. H., an infant with glycogen storage disease type I. The face somewhat chubby and the liver decidedly enlarged.*

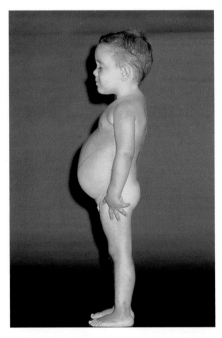

Figure 60.4 *The abdominal enlargement is more impressive in the lateral view.*

reduction in the length of the trunk and extremities [13]. Adiposity, particularly about the cheeks, is the cause of the doll-like or cherubic appearance (Figs 60.3, 60.6). Musculature tends to be flabby and poorly developed [14] and the legs appear thin.

Hypoglycemic symptoms tend to appear after 3–4 months, when the infant begins to sleep through the night. Nevertheless,

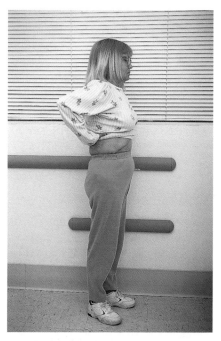

Figure 60.5   *M.S., a 60-year-old woman with glycogenosis type I. She was short. The scar represented recent surgical removal of a hepatoma. Abdominal girth was markedly reduced by the procedure.*

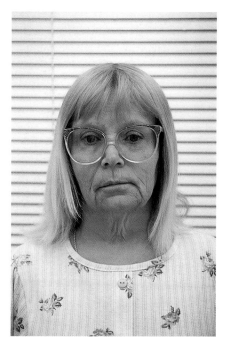

Figure 60.6   *M.S. Facial appearance was still rounded. She appeared considerably younger than her chronological age.*

symptomatic hypoglycemia may present in early infancy [15] or even in the neonatal period [16]. Manifestations of low blood sugar may include irritability, pallor, insomnia, feeding difficulties and seizures. Episodes of hypoglycemia and metabolic acidosis in the neonatal period may be refractory to treatment [15], or so easily controlled that the diagnosis is not entertained until much later [16]. Many infants present with vomiting or convulsions in the morning [17]. These symptoms are relieved by feeding or by the administration of glucose, and frequent feedings prevent their recurrence. With increase in the activity of the child at about a year of age, the frequency of hypoglycemic symptoms tends to increase. As in the case of any hypoglycemic syndrome, severe convulsions and permanent brain injury may be seen in patients with this disease.

In a series of 19 patients studied specifically for evidence of brain damage [18] abnormalities of the EE6 were found in four, only two of whom had seizures; some had abnormal evoked potentials, and all of these abnormalities correlated inversely with compliance with treatment. Abnormalities in magnetic resonance imaging (MRI) of the brain in seven correlated with neonatal hypoglycemia. None were retarded. Children with this disease have an unusual degree of tolerance to hypoglycemia, often appearing quite well at levels of blood sugar at which convulsions would ordinarily be expected [12], and the incidence of mental retardation is not high. Possibly this is a function of chronic hypoglycemia, where the rates of change of blood glucose are not very fast, but also parents and children become quite aware of the limits of tolerance for fasting. It could be relevant to utilization of lactic acid or ketones by the brain. Some patients are asymptomatic, discovered only by the presence of hepatomegaly on routine physical examination [15,19], and one of our patients came to attention at surgery for an adenoma, with evidence of glycogen storage in the adjacent liver.

Bleeding may be a major clinical manifestation in patients with this disease. It may take the form of frequent nosebleeds in which there is considerable loss of blood. Abnormal hemostasis and persistent oozing may complicate surgery. These problems are thought to represent defective platelet function. Bleeding time and platelet adhesion are abnormal, and there is defective collagen and epinephrine-induced aggregation of platelets [20]. Many small superficial vessels may be visible under the thin-looking skin.

Intermittent episodes of diarrhea have been reported [14,15,21]. This has been attributed to malabsorption of glucose [22], but in other studies no evidence was found of malabsorption of monosaccharides, disaccharides or fat [14,15,21]. Intestinal biopsy revealed no signs of inflammation and fecal α-1 antitrypsin was not increased [23]. One patient died from hemorrhagic pancreatitis [24].

Cutaneous xanthomas may develop over the buttocks, hips, elbows and knees [25,26]. Their occurrence is related to the elevated levels of triglycerides in the blood. Another consequence of hyperglycemia is the appearance of characteristic discrete, flat, yellowish retinal lesions [27] in the paramacular area; they do not adversely affect vision [18]. Patients with untreated hyperuricemia develop tophaceous gout [26,28]. Most patients have osteoporosis, and repeated spontaneous fractures have been seen in some patients [25].

In addition to the hypoglycemia a variety of abnormalities can be detected in the clinical chemistry laboratory. Lactic acidemia is a regular feature of the disease [29] and occasionally the level of pyruvate is increased. Marked hyperlipidemia and hypercholesterolemia are also features of the disease [12,30]. Concentrations of very low density lipoprotein (VLDL) and LDL are high, and the apolipoproteins apoB, C and E are high, while apoA and D are normal or low [31]. The hyperlipidemia leads not only to the formation of xanthomas, but also to large lipid-laden reticuloendothelial cells in the bone marrow. The plasma may be milky. It is important to recognize that the concentration of water in serum or plasma is markedly reduced in the presence of hyperlipidemia. Inasmuch as electrolytes and other substances are distributed only in the water phase, extremely low values are recorded for the serum sodium and other constituents. A correction must be made for the increased quantity of serum solids and decreased serum water in order to avoid a mistaken diagnosis of hyponatremia.

Ketosis and ketonuria occur promptly with minimal degrees of fasting [30]. In fact, glucose-6-phosphatase deficiency is one of the few conditions in which ketones may be observed in the urine in the neonatal period. This and the lactic acidosis concomitantly may lead to metabolic acidosis. Despite the fact that ketosis has long been considered a characteristic of the disease, patients with this disease have been reported [32,33] to be resistant to ketosis. Dicarboxylic aciduria has been observed [34], and this would be consistent with a suppression of the β-oxidation of fatty acids leading to ω-oxidation. Hyperuricemia is a regular concomitant of the disease [28]. This has been attributed to competition by lactic acid for renal tubular secretion, and decreased clearance of uric acid has been observed. However, not all patients have reduced clearance of uric acid [35], and studies of uric acid production have provided evidence of increased purine synthesis in this disease [28,36,37]. A renal Fanconi syndrome of glycosuria, aminoaciduria and phosphaturia has been reported in a number of patients with von Gierke disease [38,39]. An unusual manifestation is elevation of biotinidase activity [40]. In two patients previously not diagnosed biotinidase levels were 26 and 15 mmol/min/mL (normal mean 7); in the second it was this that led to the diagnosis.

The administration of epinephrine or glucagon fails to provoke the normal hyperglycemic response [41]. There may be some elevation of blood glucose after these agents, even in the virtual absence of glucose-6-phosphatase, for 6–8 percent of the glucose residues of glycogen are released as free-glucose as the product of the debranching enzyme. In response to glucagon or epinephrine, there is a marked increase in the concentration of lactic acid in the blood. In the absence of glucose-6-phosphatase, there is also a failure of the usual rise in blood glucose following the administration of galactose or

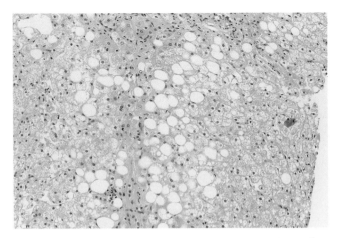

Figure 60.7 *Biopsied liver of A.K., a boy with glycogenosis type I. He clearly had storage of glycogen in distended hepatocytes, but there was also so much lipid that the initial pathologic diagnosis of Wolman disease was only discarded after the acid lipase was found to be normal, and he was referred to the metabolic service.*

fructose [15]. Similarly, following the intravenous administration of glycerol, elevation of blood glucose was less than normal and levels of lactic acid rose [42]. These abnormal responses to epinephrine, glucagon, fructose, glycerol or galactose have in the past been used to diagnose the condition. Today, the glucagon test is employed for preliminary diagnosis and decision about candidacy for liver biopsy, and the definitive finding is the assay of the enzyme and the demonstration of the accumulation of glycogen in the cells of the liver (Figure 60.4). The existence of some common mutations means it is now possible to make a definitive diagnosis by mutational analysis and avoid biopsy of the liver.

Pathologic examination [1,43] (Figure 60.7) reveals that the hepatocytes and renal tubular cells are swollen and clear as stained with hematoxylin and eosin; staining with Best's carmine reveals the stored material to be glycogen. There may also be extensive lipid storage in the liver. In fact the lipid may be so prominent that the referring pathologic diagnosis may be lipid storage disease, such as Wolman disease (Chapter 98). In the neonatal period the histology of the liver can be so normal that one is led away from the diagnosis [16].

Chemical analysis establishes that the material stored in the liver and kidneys is glycogen. Biopsy of the liver with demonstration of a glycogen content over 12 percent of the wet weight of the liver has been set out [30] as a criterion for the diagnosis of this disease. Schoenheimer [44] did not find quite that much glycogen, and most investigators would find values over 4 percent acceptable, but again, today the gold standard for diagnosis in biopsied liver is assay of the enzyme. The structure of the glycogen stored is normal [45].

A number of late complications have been observed, particularly as these patients reach adulthood. Hyperuricemia is present in infancy, but symptomatic gout occurs after adolescence. Pancreatitis [24,46] appears to be a consequence of the hypertriglyceridemia. Adult stature is low, and puberty is often delayed. Fertility is not affected, and both males and females have had children [47].

An appreciable problem in management has been the regular development of hepatic adenomas by the second or third decade [48]. These nodules are multiple, and they grow, sometimes to sizable tumors. They are usually benign, but transformations to malignant hepatocellular carcinomas have been recorded and may be fatal [48,49]. Another complication is bleeding into the adenoma [50]. Patients should therefore be investigated at intervals for these nodules, and once present their size and character should be followed. Scintigraphic scans have been recommended for this purpose [51], but ultrasonography and other forms of imaging have been useful in our hands.

A variety of renal complications has been observed. In addition to the renal Fanconi syndrome, patients have had distal renal tubular disease [52], amyloidosis [53], hypercalciuria, nephrocalcinosis and calculi. Glomerular hyperfiltration, increased renal plasma flow and microalbuminuria [54] are followed over time by proteinuria, focal segmental glomerulosclerosis and interstitial fibrosis [23,55–57]; followed in some patients by renal failure, leading to dialysis and transplantation.

Patients with glycogen storage disease type Ib [58] have the same Type I clinical phenotype, but in addition they have neutropenia and impaired neutrophil function [59] (Table 59.1, p. 383). As a consequence they have recurrent bacterial infections, inflammatory bowel disease and ulceration of oral and intestinal mucosa [59–64]. Fecal α-1 antitrypsin is increased, and biopsy of the colon reveals inflammation [23]. Among 288 patients with type I glycogenosis, 57 had type Ib [63]. Neutropenia ($<1 \times 10^9$/L) was found in 54. It is often documented in the first year of life, but may be noted first between 6 and 9 years. It may be persistent, but more commonly it is intermittent. Among 18 patients with neutropenia in whom neutrophil function was studied, it was abnormal in all. Perioral infections occurred in 37 patients, perianal infections in 27 and protracted diarrhea in 23. Inflammatory bowel disease was documented by colonoscopy or roentgenographic examination. Inflammatory bowel disease was not observed in the absence of neutropenia. Two Japanese patients were reported with no evidence of neutropenia and no recurrent bacterial infections [64]; otherwise symptoms were typical of type I glycogenosis.

GENETICS AND PATHOGENESIS

The disorder is inherited as an autosomal recessive trait. It has frequently been observed in siblings and as a concomitant of parental consanguinity [12,25,46,65]. The distribution between the sexes is about equal. Ethnic differences in the severity of disease have been observed. For example, patients from Syria and Lebanon tend to have serious disease, while those of Saudi Arabia have quite mild disease. Reduced activity of intestinal glucose-6-phosphatase has been found in

parents of patients [66]. Prenatal diagnosis has been made by biopsy of the fetal liver and enzyme assay [67].

The molecular defect in glycogenosis I is absence of activity of the catalytic subunit of the glucose-6-phosphatase enzyme complex [2]. The enzyme is expressed normally in liver, kidney and in the β cells of pancreatic islets. The diagnosis has generally been made by assay of biopsied liver. Absence or near absence of the enzyme has been required for the diagnosis [68,69] because many enzymes activities, including this one, may be reduced in liver disease or in other storage diseases. The diagnosis can be made by needle biopsy, but sufficient complexity has been recognized that open biopsy and an adequate sample of tissue are preferred. Direct vision also protects against bleeding. Samples should also be fixed for light and electron microscopy. Care should be taken to avoid destruction of hepatic cellular membrane elements, and precautions for the handling of specimens prior to assay have been set out [5].

The active site of the enzyme is within the lumen of the endoplasmic reticulum [70]. Normal activity of the enzyme requires the activity of six different proteins or subunits in the enzyme complex [71,72]. The discovery of these components and the elucidation of the function of the complex were the results of the study of patients with glycogen storage disease. The classic enzyme, or the catalytic subunit whose deficiency causes type Ia, is a 36.5kDa protein [72] that catalyzes the hydrolysis of a number of phosphate compounds, including carbamylphosphate and pyrophosphate as well as glucose-6-phosphate [73,74]. A microsomal regulatory protein has been isolated as a 21kDa stabilizing protein because it stabilizes the activity of the catalytic protein during purification [75]. It binds calcium and is essential for normal activity. Its deficiency leads to glycogenosis type Iasp [7].

The microsomal glucose-6-phosphate transport protein (T1; translocase) was recognized through the study of glycogenosis type Ib. T1 catalyzes the transport of glucose-6-phosphate into the lumens of hepatic microsomes [76,77]. In its absence, the liver is unable to release glucose from glucose-6-phosphate. The glucose-6-phosphatase catalytic protein is normal and can be assayed if membranous elements of the liver cell are disrupted by freezing or treatment with detergents, but in situ the system is nonfunctional [3,78,79]. The defect is also demonstrable in leukocytes, which have impaired uptake of glucose [80] in type Ib, and this may provide a way to test for the disorder. Activity against pyrophosphate and carbamylphosphate is not impaired.

In type Ic glycogenosis, carbamylphosphatase and pyrophosphatase activity as well as glucose-6-phosphatase activity are abnormal in microsomes. It is thought that in this disorder the microsomal phosphate transport protein, the T2 translocase, is deficient [5]. This transports phosphate, pyrophosphate and carbamylphosphate. It is a 37kDa polypeptide that has been designated T2b to distinguish it from T2a, which transports only phosphate. The glucose-6-phosphatase system also depends on the transport of glucose. A number of glucose transport proteins have been identified, and they have been designated GLUT 1–6. Deficiency of GLUT 2 causes the syndrome of hepatic glycogenosis with the renal Fanconi syndrome [81].

In glycogenosis Ia, immunochemical assay has indicated an absence of glucose-6-phosphatase catalytic enzyme protein in some patients in whom there is little or no activity, but most have had a normal amount of a protein of normal size [82]. Among patients with partial deficiencies, some have reduced levels of immunoprotein and others normal amounts [14,82,83]. In some the Km is elevated.

The cDNA for human hepatic glucose-6-phosophatase has been cloned, and a number of mutations have been identified [84]. These include an arginine-to-cysteine change at amino acid 83 (R83C) and Q347X a change from a glutamine to a stop codon, which are common in Caucasians. R83C is also common in Hispanic and Jewish patients. G727T is common in Japanese.

The cDNA for the translocase deficient in Ib has been cloned [10] and localized to chromosome 11q23 [85]. Common gene mutations in Caucasian patients are G339C and 1211delCT [86]. W118R is common in Japanese [87]. Of the two Japanese patients with type Ib without neutropenia, one had R415X, which had previously been encountered in patients with neutropenia, on one allele and G339D on the other. The other patient was homozygous for G794A, which led to a splicing error, deleting exon 3. Another patient with neutropenia, with abnormal neutrophil function and recurrent infections typical of Ib, was found to have no mutations in the translocase, but to be homozygous for G188R in the glucose-6-phosphatase gene; so she had type Ia [88].

TREATMENT

Since patients with glycogenosis type Ia are at risk of death or hypoglycemic damage to the brain in early infancy, prompt diagnosis, the avoidance of fasting and the provision of free-glucose are important in getting the patient through this critical period. Infections are particularly dangerous and the patient may require admission to hospital and treatment with parenteral fluids containing glucose and electrolytes. There is a distinct tendency for improvement with age, even by the age of 4 or 5 years [17,30]. By the time of puberty, considerable amelioration has often been observed [12]; the enlarged liver takes up considerably less of the abdomen, and hypoglycemic symptoms are much less prominent. However, little improvement in long-term prognosis as a result of treatment occurred until recently. Portacaval shunting has essentially been abandoned in the treatment of this disease, but it was noted that the parenteral alimentation attendant on the procedure led to reduction in hepatic size and reversal of metabolic abnormalities, the growth failure and the bleeding diathesis [89,90]. These observations focused attention on approaches to the more regular provision of glucose to meet tissue needs. The approaches that have been successful are continuous nocturnal nasogastric or gastrostomy feeding [90–93] and oral uncooked cornstarch [94,95].

With either regimen, frequent high carbohydrate meals in which 65–70 percent of the calories are carbohydrate are employed during the day. Dietary intake of fructose and galactose is restricted in some centers and not in others.

Uncooked cornstarch provides glucose in a slow-release fashion. Use in an infant is recommended at a dose of 1.6 g/kg every 4 hours. In older children the requirement is 1.75-2.5 g/kg every 6 hours, prepared in a 1:2 weight:volume mixture with water or diet drinks [94–98]. Argo (PC International) is prepared by suspension at room temperature. The optimal amount for each patient is determined individually; satisfactory results have been confirmed with 1 g/kg every 6 hours. Older patients may not require a feeding in the middle of the night if larger quantities (2–4 g/kg) can be taken at bedtime. This regimen has been shown to maintain euglycemia and to reverse clinical and biochemical disturbances in most patients [95,96]. Nocturnal nasogastric feeding has also been introduced in infancy at diagnosis. Glucose, polycose and elemental formulations have been employed, each providing 8–10 mg/kg per minute in an infant and 5–7 mg/kg per minute in an older child. Clinical and biochemical abnormalities can be reversed and hypoglycemia avoided. Liver size regresses and the bleeding tendency is reversed [99]. There is a tendency to the development of hypoglycemia in the morning after the nocturnal feeding is stopped; so that the first meal should be within 15 to 30 minutes of discontinuing the nocturnal feeding. Hypoglycemia and death have been reported following malfunction of the pump or dislodging the tube [100]. Some patients have required a combination of cornstarch and nocturnal nasogastric feedings. Patients with glycogenosis type Iasp and Ib should also be managed with these regimens. In type Ib, granulocyte and granulocyte-macrophage colony stimulating factors have been employed to combat the neutropenia and treat the inflammatory disease [101].

Both regimens have been employed long enough to have provided [102] encouraging long-term effects on the course of the disease [95,96,102,103]. Growth has been rewarding, and it is clear that normal adult height may be reached. Some children have remained short [102]. Surprisingly, treatment has been reported to be associated with an absence of development of hepatic adenomas [96], and regression of adenomas has been observed. Proximal renal tubular function has improved [96]. Whether treatment will prevent glomerular dysfunction and renal failure is not clear.

Allopurinol is used to lower the concentration of urate to normal levels. In patients requiring surgery, the bleeding time should be determined. If it is prolonged, it may be improved by 24–48 hours of intravenous glucose or 1-deamino-8-d-arginine vasopressin (DDAVP) [104].

Renal transplantation performed because of renal failure did not improve glucose homeostasis in this disease [105]. Transplantation of the liver provides a definitive cure of the disease [106, 107]; however, the magnitude of the procedure has tended to indicate its use in a small number of patients with refractory disease or, of course, hepatic malignancy.

References

1 Von Gierke E. Hepato-nephromegalie glykogenica. *Beitr Path Anat* 1929;**82**:497.

2 Cori GT, Cori CF. Glucose-6-phosphatase of the liver in glycogen storage disease. *J Biol Chem* 1952;**199**:661.

3 Narisawa K, Igarashi Y, Otomo H, Tada K. A new variant of glycogen storage disease type 1 probably due to a defect in the glucose-6-phosphate transport system. *Biochem Biophys Res Commun* 1978;**83**:1360.

5 Lange AJ, Arion WJ, Beaudet AL. Type 1 b glycogen storage disease is caused by a defect in the glucose-6-phosphate translocase of the microsomal glucose-6-phosphatase system. *J Biol Chem* 1980; **255**: 8381.

6 Chen Y-T. Glycogen storage diseases: in *The Metabolic and Molecular Basis of Inherited Disease* (eds FR Scriver, AL Beaudet, WS Sly, D Valle). 7th edn McGraw Hill, New York;2001:1521.

7 Burchell A, Waddell ID. Diagnosis of a novel glycogen storage disease: type 1asp. *J Inherit Metab Dis* 1990;**13**:247.

8 Nordlie R, Sukalski K. Multifunctional glucose-6-phosphatase: A critical review: in *The Enzymes of Biological Membranes* (ed. M An) Plenum Press, New York;1985: 349.

9 Lei K, Shelly L, Pan C, *et al.* Mutations in the glucose 6-phosphatase gene that cause glycogen storage disease type Ia. *Science* 1993;**262**:580.

10 Gerin I, Veiga-da-Cunha M, Achouri Y, *et al.* Sequence of a putative glucose 6-phosphate translocase mutated in glycogen storage disease type Ib. *Fed Eur Biochem Soc* 1997;**419**:235.

11 Chou J, Mansfield B. Molecular genetics of type I glycogen storage disease. *Trends Endocrinol Metab* 1999;**10**:104.

12 Van Creveld S. Glycogen storage disease. *Medicine* 1939;**18**:1.

13 Donnell GN. Growth in glycogen storage disease Type 1. Evaluation of endocrine function. *Am J Dis Child* 1969;**117**:169.

14 Howell RR, Ashton DM, Wyngaarden JB. Glucose-6-phosphatase deficiency glycogen storage disease. Studies on the interrelationships of carbohydrate lipid and purine abnormalities. *Pediatrics* 1962; **29**:553.

15 Spencer-Peet J, Norman ME, Lake BD, *et al.* Hepatic glycogen storage disease. Clinical and laboratory findings in 23 cases. *Quart J Med New Series* 1971;**40**:95.

16 Hufton BR, Wharton BA. Glycogen storage disease (type 1) presenting in the neonatal period. *Arch Dis Child* 1982;**57**:309.

17 Lowery GH, Wilson JL. Observations on the treatment of a case of glycogen storage disease. *J Pediatr* 1949;**35**:702.

18 Melis D, Parenti G, Della Casa R, *et al.* Brain damage in glycogen storage disease type I. *J Inherit Metab Dis* 2002;**25**:(Suppl 1) 248-P.

19 Keller K, Schutz M, Podskarbi T, *et al.* A new mutation of the glucose-6-phosphatase gene in a 4-year-old girl with oligosymptomatic glycogen storage disease type Ia. *J Pediatr* 1998;**132**:360.

20 Corby DG, Putnam CW, Greene HL. Impaired platelet function in glucose-6-phosphatase deficiency. *J Pediatr* 1974;**85**:71.

21 Fine RR, Kogut MB, Connell GN. Intestinal absorption in type 1 glycogen storage disease. *J Pediatr* 1969;**75**:632.

22 Milla PJ, Atherton DA, Leonard JV, *et al.* Disordered intestinal function in glycogen storage disease. *J Inherit Metab Dis* 1978;**1**:155.

23 Visser G, Rake JP, Kokke FTM, *et al.* Intestinal function in glycogen storage disease type I. *J Inherit Metab Dis* 2002;**25**:261.

24 Michels VV, Beaudet AL. Hemorrhagic pancreatitis in a patient with glycogen storage disease type 1. *Clin Genet* 1980;**17**:220.

25 Zakon SJ, Oyamada A, Rosenthal IH. Eruptive xanthoma and hyperlipemia in glycogen storage disease (von Gierke's disease). *AMA Arch Derm Syph* 1953;**67**:146.

26 Hou J-W, Wang T-R, Tunnessen WW. Picture of the month.*Arch Pediatr Adolesc Med* 1996;**150**:219.

27 Fine RN, Wilson WA, Donnell GN. Retinal changes in glycogen storage disease type 1. *Am J Dis Child* 1968;**115**:328.

28 Alepa FP, Howell RR, Klinenberg JR, Seegmiller JE. Relationships between glycogen storage disease and tophaceous gout. *Am J Med* 1967;**42**:58.

29 Mason HH, Anderson DH. Glycogen disease of the liver (von Gierke's disease) with hepatomata. Case report with metabolic studies. *Pediatrics* 1955;**16**:785.

30 Alaupovic P, Fernandes J. The serum apolipoprotein profile of patients with glucose-6-phosphatase deficiency. *Pediatr Res* 1985;**19**:380.

31 Levy E, Thibault LA, Roy CC, *et al.* Circulating lipids and lipoproteins in glycogen storage disease type 1 with nocturnal nasogastric feeding. *J Lipid Res* 1988;**29**:215.

32 Fernandes J, Pikaar NA. Ketosis in hepatic glycogenosis. *Arch Dis Child* 1972;**47**:41.

33 Binkiewicz A, Senior B. Decreased ketogenesis in von Gierke's disease (type 1 glycogenosis). *J Pediatr* 1973;**83**:973.

34 Dosman J, Crawhall JC, Klassen GA, *et al.* Urinary excretion of C6-C10 dicarboxylic acids in glycogen storage diseases types 1 and 3. *Clin Chim Acta* 1974;**51**:93.

35 Jeune M, Francois R, Jarlot B. Contribution a l'étude des polycories glycogéniques du foie. *Rev Internat Hepatol* 1959;**9**:1.

36 Jakovcic S, Sorensen LB. Studies of uric acid metabolism in glycogen storage disease associated with gouty arthritis. *Arthritis Rheum* 1967;**10**:129.

37 Kelley WN, Rosenbloom FM, Seegmiller JE, Howell RR. Excessive production of uric acid in type 1 glycogen storage disease. *J Pediatr* 1968;**72**:488.

38 Lampert F, Mayer H, Tocci PM, Nyhan WL. Fanconi syndrome in glycogen glycogen storage disease: in *Amino Acid Metabolism and Genetic Variation* (ed. WL Nyhan). McGraw Hill, New York;1967:267.

39 Garty R, Cooper M, Tabachnik E. The Fanconi syndrome associated with hepatic glycogenosis and abnormal metabolism of galactose. *J Pediatr* 1974;**85**:821.

40 Wolf B, Freehauf CL, Thomas JA, *et al.* Markedly elevated serum biotinidase activity may indicate glycogen storage disease type Ia. *J Inherit Metab Dis* 2003;**26**:805.

41 Perkoff GT, Parker JV, Hahn RF. The effects of glucagons in three forms of glycogen storage disease. *J Clin Invest* 1962;**41**:1099.

42 Senior B, Loridan L. Functional differentiation of glycogenoses of the liver with respect to the use of glycerol. *N Eng J Med* 1968;**279**:965.

43 McAdams AJ, Hug G, Bove KE. Glycogen storage disease types I to X: Criteria for morphologic diagnosis. *Hum Pathol* 1974;**5**:463.

44 Schoenheimer R. Uber eine eigenartige Storung des Kohlenhydrat-Stoffwechsels. *Zeitschr Physiol Chem* 1929;**182**:148.

45 Illingworth B, Cori GT. Structure of glycogens and amylopectins. III Normal and abnormal human glycogens. *J Biol Chem* 1952;**199**:653.

46 Kikuchi M, Hasegawa K, Handa I, *et al.* Chronic pancreatitis in a child with glycogen storage disease type 1. *Eur J Pediatr* 1991;**150**:852.

47 Van Creveld S. Clinical course of glycogen storage disease. *Chem Weekblad* 1961;**57**:445.

48 Howell RR, Stevenson RE, Ben-Menachem Y, *et al.* Hepatic adenomata in patients with type I glycogen storage disease (von Gierke's). *JAMA* 1976;**236**:1481.

49 Limmer J, Fleig WE, Leupold D, *et al.* Hepatocellular carcinoma in type I glycogen storage disease. *Hepatology* 1988;**8**:531.

50 Fink AS, Appelman HD, Thompson NW. Hemorrhage into a hepatic adenoma and type Ia glycogen storage disease: A case report and review of the literature. *Surgery* 1985;**97**:117.

51 Miller JH, Gates GF, Landing BH, *et al.* Scintigraphic abnormalities in glycogen storage diseases. *J Nucl Med* 1978;**19**:354.

52 Restiano I, Kaplan BS, Stanley C, Baker L. Nephrolithiasis hypocitraturia and a distal renal tubular acidification defect in type I glycogen storage disease. *J Pediatr* 1993;**122**:392.

53 Kikuchi M, Haginoya K, Miyabayashi S, *et al.* Secondary amyloidosis in glycogen storage disease type Ib. *Eur J Pediatr* 1990;**149**:344.

54 Baker L, Dahlem S, Goldfarb S, *et al.* Hyperfiltration and renal disease in glycogen storage disease type I. *Kidney Int* 1989;**35**:1345.

55 Chen Y-T, Coleman RA, Scheinman JI, *et al.* Renal disease in type I glycogen storage disease. *N Engl J Med* 1988;**318**:7.

56 Reitsma-Bierens WCC, Smit GPA, Troelstra JA. Renal function and kidney size in glycogen storage disease type I. *Pediatr Nephrol* 1992;**6**:236.

57 Chen Y-T. Type I glycogen storage disease kidney involvement pathogenesis and its treatment. *Pediatr Nephrol* 1991;**5**:71.

58 Lange AJ, Arion WJ, Beaudet AL. Type 1 b glycogen storage disease is caused by a defect in the glucose-6-phosphate translocase of the microsomal glucose-6-phosphatase system. *J Biol Chem* 1980;**255**:8381.

59 Beaudet AL, Anderson DC, Michels VV, *et al.* Neutropenia and impaired neutrophil migration in type IB glycogen storage disease. *J Pediatr* 1980;**97**:906.

60 Schaub J, Haas JR. Glycogenosis type Ib complicated by severe granulocytopenia resembling inherited neutropenia. *Eur J Pediatr* 1981;**137**:81.

61 Ambruso DR, McCabe ERB, Anderson D, *et al.* Infectious and bleeding complications in patients with glycogenosis Ib. *Am J Dis Child* 1985;**139**:691.

62 Roe TF, Thomas DW, Gilsanz V, *et al.* Inflammatory bowel disease in glycogen storage disease type 1b. *J Pediatr* 1986;**109**:55.

63 Visser G, Rake J-P, Fernandes J, *et al.* Neutropenia neutrophil dysfunction and inflammatory bowel disease in glycogen storage disease type Ib: Results of the European Study on Glycogen Storage Disease Type I. *J Pediatr* 2000;**137**:187.

64 Kure S, Hou D-C, Suzuki Y, *et al.* Glycogen storage disease type Ib without neutropenia. *J Pediatr* 2000;**137**:253.

65 Traisman AS, Traisman HS. Glycogen storage disease of the liver in siblings. *J Pediatr* 1953;**42**:654.

66 Field JB, Drash AL. Studies in glycogen storage disease. II Heterogeneity in the inheritance of glycogen storage disease. *Trans Assoc Am Phys* 1967;**80**:284.

67 Golbus MS, Simpson TJ, Koresawa M, *et al.* The prenatal determination of glucose-6-phosphatase activity by fetal liver biopsy. *Prenat Diagn* 1988;**8**:401.

68 Harris RC, Olmo C. Liver and kidney glucose-6-phosphatase activity in children with normal and disease organs. *J Clin Invest* 1954;**33**:1204.

69 Hers HG. Etudes enzymatiques sur fragments hepatiques; application a la classification des glycogenosis. *Rev Internat Hepatol* 1959;**9**:35.

70 Waddell ID, Burchell A. Transverse topology of glucose-6-phosphatase in rat hepatic endoplasmic reticulum. *Biochem J* 1991;**275**:133.

71 Burchell A. The molecular basis of the type I glycogen storage diseases. *Bioessays* 1992;**14**:395.

72 Countaway JL, Waddell ID, Burchell A, Arion WJ. The phosphohydrolase component of the hepatic microsomal glucose-6-phosphatase system is a 365 kilodalton polypeptide. *J Biol Chem* 1988;**263**:2673.

73 Illingworth B, Cori CF. Glucose-6-phosphatase and pyrophosphatase activities of homogenates of livers from patients with glycogen storage disease. *Biochem Biophys Res Commun* 1965;**19**:10.

74 Hefferan PM, Howell RR. Genetic evidence for the common identity of glucose-6-phosphatase pyrophosphate-glucose phosphotransferase carbamyl phosphate-glucose phosphotransferase and inorganic pyrophosphatase. *Biochim Biophys Acta* 1977; **496**:431.

75 Burchell A, Burchell B, Monaco M, *et al.* Stabilization of glucose-6-phosphatase activity by a 21000 dalton hepatic microsomal protein. *Biochem J* 1985;**230**:489.

76 Fulceri R, Bellamo G, Gamberucci A, *et al.* Permeability of the rat liver microsomal membrane to glucose-6-phosphate. *Biochem J* 1992;**286**:813.

77 Waddell ID, Hume R, Burchell A. A direct method for the diagnosis of human hepatic type Ib and Ic glycogen storage disease. *Clin Sci* 1989;**76**:573.

78 Nordlie RC. Multifunctional glucose-6-phosphatase. Characteristics and function. *Cellular Biology Life Sci* 1979;**24**:2397.

79 Sann L, Matheiu M, Bourgeois J, *et al. In vivo* evidence for defective activity of glucose-6-phosphatase in type Ib glycogenosis. *J Pediatr* 1980;**96**:691.

80 Bashan N, Hagai Y, Potashnik R, Moses SW. Impaired carbohydrate metabolism of polymorphonuclear leukocytes in glycogen storage disease type Ib. *J Clin Invest* 1988;**81**:1317.

81 Santer R, Schneppenheim R, Dombrowski A, *et al.* Mutations in GLUT2 the gene for the liver-type glucose transporter in patients with Fanconi-Bickel syndrome. *Nat Genet* 1997;**17**:324.

82 Stamm WE, Webb DI. Partial deficiency of hepatic glucose-6-phosphatase in an adult patient. *Arch Intern Med* 1975;**135**:1107.

83 Burchell A, Waddell ID. The molecular basis of the genetic deficiencies of 5 of the components of the glucose-6-phosphatase system: improved diagnosis. *Eur J Pediatr* 1993;**152**:(Suppl 1) S18.

84 Lei K-J, Pan C-J, Shelly LL, *et al.* Identification of mutations in the gene for glucose-6-phosphatase the enzyme deficient in glycogen storage disease type Ia. *J Clin Invest* 1994;**93**:1994.

85 Annabi B, Hiraiwa H, Mansfield B, *et al.* The gene for glycogen storage disease type Ib maps to chromosome 11q23. *Am J Hum Genet* 1998;**62**:400.

86 Viega-da-Cunha M, Gerin I, Chen Y-T, *et al.* A gene on chromosome 11q23 coding for a putative glucose 6-phosphatase translocase is mutated in glycogen storage disease type Ib and type Ic. *Am J Hum Genet* 1998;**63**:976.

87 Kure S, Suzuki Y, Matsubara Y, *et al.* Molecular analysis of glycogen storage disease type Ib: identification of a prevalent mutation among Japanese patients and assignment of a putative glucose-6-phosphate translocase gene to chromosome 11. *Biochem Biophy Res Commun* 1998;**248**:426.

88 Weston BW, Lin J-L, Muenzer J, *et al.* Glucose-6-phosphatase mutation G188R confers an atypical glycogen storage disease type Ib phenotype. *Pediatr Res* 2000;**48**:329.

89 Folkman J, Philippart A, Tze WJ, Cirgler J. Portacaval shunt for glycogen storage disease. Value of prolonged intravenous hyperalimentation before surgery. *Surgery* 1972;**72**:306.

90 Burr IM, O'Neill JA, Karzon DT, *et al.* Comparison of the effects of total parenteral nutrition continuous intragastric feeding and portacaval shunt on a patient with type I glycogen storage disease. *J Pediatr* 1974;**85**:792.

91 Greene HL, Slonim AE, Burr IM. Type I glycogen storage disease: a metabolic basis for advance in treatment. *Adv Pediatr* 1979;**26**:63.

92 Greene HL, Slonim AE, O'Neill JA, Burr IM. Continuous nocturnal feeding for management of type I glycogen storage disease. *N Engl J Med* 1976;**294**:423.

93 Perlman MB, Aker M, Slonim AE. Successful treatment of severe type I glycogen storage disease with neonatal presentation by nocturnal intragastric feeding. *J Pediatr* 1979;**94**:772.

94 Chen YT, Cornblath M, Sidbury JB. Cornstarch therapy in type I glycogen storage disease. *N Eng J Med* 1984;**310**:171.

95 Chen Y-T, Bazarre C, Lee MM, *et al.* Type I glycogen storage disease: nine years of management with cornstarch. *Eur J Pediatr* 1993;**152**: (Suppl 1) S56.

96 Chen Y-T, Scheinman JI, Park HK, *et al.* Amelioration of proximal renal tubular dysfunction in type I glycogen storage disease with dietary therapy. *N Eng J Med* 1990;**323**:590.

97 Leonard JV, Dunger DB. Hypoglycaemia complicating feeding regimens for glycogen-storage disease. *Lancet* 1978;**12**:1203.

98 Parker P, Burr I, Slonim A, *et al.* Regression of hepatic adenomas in GSD-Ia with dietary therapy. *Gastroenterology* 1981;**81**:534.

99 Greene HL, Slonim AE, Burr IM, Moran JR. Type I glycogen storage disease: Five years of management with nocturnal intragastric feeding. *J Pediatr* 1980;**96**:590.

100 Emmett JL, Nairns BR. Renal transplantation in Type I glycogenesis; failure to improve glucose metabolism. *JAMA* 1978;**239**:1642.

101 Schroten H, Roesler J, Breidenbach T, *et al.* Granulocyte and granulocyte-macrophage colony-stimulating factors for treatment of neutropenia in glycogen storage disease type Ib. *J Pediatr* 1991;**119**:748.

102 Fernandes J, Alaupovic P, Wit JM. Gastric drip feeding in patients with glycogen storage disease type I: its effects on growth and plasma lipids and apolipoproteins. *Pediatr Res* 1989;**25**:327.

103 Schwahn B, Rauch F, Wendel U, Schonau E. Low bone mass in glycogen storage disease type 1 is associated with reduced muscle force and poor metabolic control. *J Pediatr* 2002;**141**:350.

104 Marti GE, Rick ME, Sidbury J, Gralnick HR. DDAVP infusion in five patients with type I glycogen storage disease and associated correction of prolonged bleeding times. *Blood* 1986;**68**:180.

105 Emmett M, Narins RG. Renal transplantation in type I glycogensis: failure to improve glucose metabolism. *JAMA* 1978;**239**:1642.

106 Malatack JJ, Iwatsuki S, Gartner JC, *et al.* Liver transplantation for type I glycogen storage disease. *Lancet* 1983;**1**:1073.

107 Kirschner BS, Baker AL, Thorp FK. Growth in adulthood after liver transplantation for glycogen storage disease type 1. *Gastroenterology* 1991;**101**:238.

61

Glycogenosis type II/Pompe/lysosomal α-glucosidase deficiency

MAJOR PHENOTYPIC EXPRESSION

Cardiomegaly and congestive cardiac failure, macroglossia, weakness of skeletal muscles, accumulation of glycogen in lysosomes of cardiac and skeletal muscle, and absence of acid α-1,4-glucosidase.

INTRODUCTION

Glycogenosis type II has been referred to as generalized glycogenosis because the defect is present in all cells. Clinical expression is most prominently manifested in the heart, and therefore the disease has been considered as cardiac glycogenosis. It was first described by Pompe [1] in an infant who had died of what had been called idiopathic cardiac hypertrophy. The sections stained with Best carmine identified the material as glycogen. This material was then found in a variety of other organs. Pompe recognized the possibility that a number of other patients diagnosed as having idiopathic cardiac hypertrophy might represent examples of glycogenosis, and he called attention to the report of vacuolization in the myocardium of such a patient previously reported by Sprague and his co-workers [2]. The tissue from this patient was then re-examined and found to contain

glycogen [3]. In this family a number of patients had died of cardiac disease in early infancy. A major impact on the understanding of this disease was made by Hers [4], who identified in lysosomes an α-glucosidase that was active at acid pH and cleaved glycogen as well as maltose (Figure 61.1). He further documented that this enzyme was deficient in tissues of patients with Pompe disease.

These discoveries launched the field of lysosomal storage diseases. The gene for the enzyme has been localized to chromosome 17q25 [5]. It is now recognized that there are late onset purely myopathic forms of α-glucosidase deficiency and a spectrum of clinical phenotypes between that and the classic infantile Pompe disease [6]. Enzyme activity correlates generally with the degree of clinical severity. The gene has been cloned, and a number of mutations has been identified [7]. A few have been identified with various ethnic groups [8,9]. One mutation has accounted for a major proportion of Caucasian

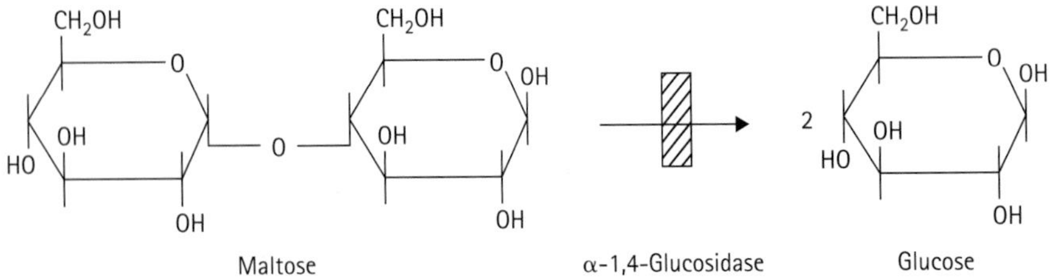

Figure 61.1   α-1,4-Glucosidase, the site of the defect in Pompe disease. This enzyme catalyzes the cleavage of other linear oligosaccharides as well as of maltose.

adult onset myopathic patients [10]. Enzyme replacement has been effective in quail [11].

CLINICAL ABNORMALITIES

The classic infantile form of glycogenosis II (Figures 61.2–61.9) is of rapidly progressive cardiomyopathy with massive cardiomegaly and death within the first year [12]. The discovery of the enzyme defect led to the recognition of a spectrum of variants. The clinical picture of those at the other end of the spectrum is that of adult-onset skeletal myopathy. Many variants have been observed between these two extremes.

In the infantile disease, manifestations begin in the first weeks or months of life [12,13]. Symptoms may even be noted at birth. Poor feeding and failure to thrive may be early complaints, but cyanosis and attacks of dyspnea begin promptly, and there is rapid progression to intractable cardiac failure [14]. Death is by congestive failure, sometimes with a complicating terminal pneumonia.

Physical examination reveals signs of cardiac failure and the hallmark feature, cardiomegaly. Massive enlargement of the heart is visible on roentgenograms (Figure 61.7). Significant cardiac murmurs are not usually present [15].

Hepatomegaly may be seen once cardiac failure begins, but it does not result from massive storage of glycogen in the liver. The electrocardiogram (Figure 61.8) may show very

large QRS complexes in all leads and a short PR interval [16]. Left axis deviation or an absence of the normal right axis deviation of this age and evidence of biventricular hypertrophy are seen, as well as T-wave changes and depression of the ST segment. Cardiac catheterization or echocardiogram show biventricular hypertrophy and obstruction of left ventricular

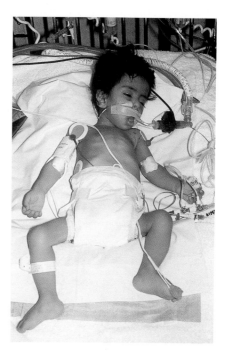

Figure 61.3   *A.M.S. An 8-month-old boy with Pompe disease. He was flaccid and intubated and had dilated cardiomyopathy.*

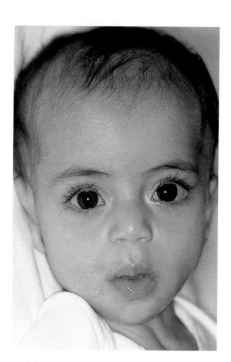

Figure 61.2   *A.A.A.D. A 6-month-old infant with Pompe disease. Dyspnea and cyanosis began at 2 months. A sibling died at 4 months. The liver was palpable 4 cm below the costal margin. There was a grade I–III systolic cardiac murmur. Electrocardiogram (EKG) and echocardiogram revealed biventricular enlargement and poor left ventricular contraction.*

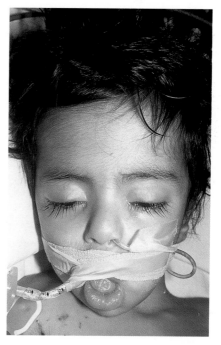

Figure 61.4   *A.M.S. The lips were thick and the tongue appeared large. The level of activity of α-glucosidase in fibroblasts was 3 percent of control. The V_{max} in muscle was markedly reduced.*

outflow [17,18]. Death within the first year of life is the usual course in this disease, but patients have been reported [19] in whom rapidly progressive cardiomegaly and cardiac failure led to death shortly after onset as late as 11 and 15 years.

Classification on the basis of age of onset appears less meaningful now that genetic variation can be expressed in terms of enzyme activity and the nature of mutation. In fact atypical or nonclassic forms of the disease have been reported with onset in infancy [20]. Most of these infants had left

ventricular hypertrophy, but they did not have left ventricular outflow obstruction. Death occurred later than the first year, often from myopathy-related pulmonary disease.

Skeletal muscle disease is prominent in all infantile patients. It is manifested by marked hypotonia and weakness associated with diminished or absent deep tendon reflexes. The clinical picture may be suggestive of amyotonia congenita [21]. Muscle mass is normal, but the muscles may feel hard. Classically the tongue is enlarged. A protuberant tongue (Figures 61.6, 61.9) with failure to thrive, hypotonia, a protuberant abdomen and possibly an umbilical hernia may suggest a diagnosis of hypothyroidism or Down syndrome. Macroglossia is caused by infiltration of the muscle fibers of

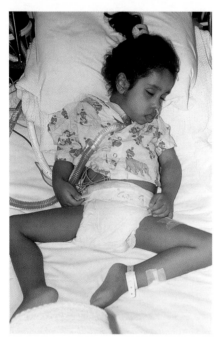

Figure 61.5   A girl with Pompe disease. The position was flaccid. She had a tracheostomy and required nasogastric feeding.

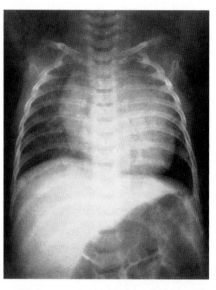

Figure 61.7   A.K. A 4-month-old infant with Pompe disease, had evidence of cardiomegaly on roentgenographic examination. (Courtesy of Dr. M.S. Ahmad, Dharan Health Centre, Dharan, Saudi Arabia.)

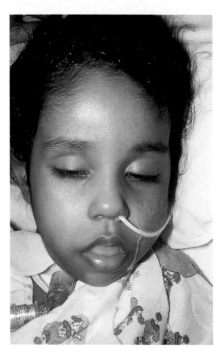

Figure 61.6   The lips were full and the tongue quite large.

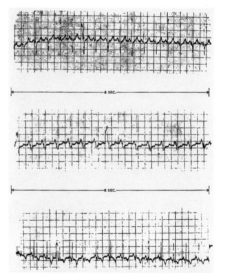

Figure 61.8   A.L. The EKG revealed biventricular hypertrophy. The leads shown, from the top, were 1, 2 and 3. (Courtesy of Dr. M.S. Ahmad, Dharan Health Centre, Dharan, Saudi Arabia.)

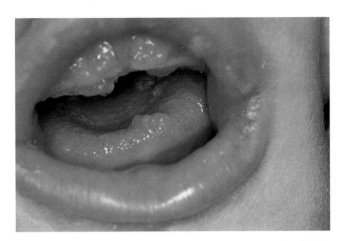

Figure 61.9   *A.A.A.D. The tongue appeared large and the lips thick. Biopsy of the right gastrocnemius revealed distention of the myocytes with stored glycogen. Activity of α-glucosidase was very low.*

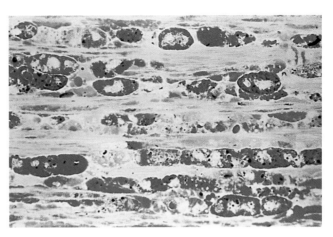

Figure 61.10   *Periodic acid Schiff (PAS)-stained longitudinal section of muscle of a patient with Pompe disease. The infant presented as very floppy and had a severe deficiency of acid maltase. The red-staining accumulations of glycogen were dramatically visible. (Courtesy of Dr. John S. Romine, Department of Neurosciences, University of California, San Diego, La Jolla, California.)*

the tongue with glycogen, but macroglossia is noted in fewer than half of patients.

A small number of patients present in infancy or early childhood with a predominantly skeletal muscle disease without cardiac disease [22–24]. They may have lordosis or scoliosis, and may require surgical treatment. There may be localized pseudohypertrophy [25]. These patients display a more slowly progressive disease and death occurs by 19 years from pneumonia or respiratory failure.

A distinct group of patients has presented in the second or third decade with muscular weakness. This is the group that has been referred to as having adult onset disease. The clinical picture in these patients is that of a slowly progressive myopathy with little or no cardiac abnormality [23,26–29]. These patients may also die of respiratory failure [26]. A patient with this form of the disease was reported to develop a Wolff-Parkinson-White syndrome and a secondary atrioventricular block [30]. The early phenotype is that of a progressive proximal muscle weakness [31]. The legs and paraspinal muscles are particularly involved. Some patients present with back pain. Deep tendon reflexes may disappear. Urinary incontinence may indicate myopathy [32]. Diaphragmatic involvement may present as sleep apnea [33], but ultimately leads to respiratory failure or pneumonia.

Electromyography (EMG) in any of the forms of type II glycogenosis reveals pseudomyotonia and high frequency discharges and fibrillations [34]. Creatine kinase (CK) is usually elevated. It may be up to tenfold in infantile patients. It may be normal, but its elevation can serve as the alerting signal for the diagnosis in a myopathic adult [35]. Transaminases may also be elevated [36]. Type II glycogenosis differs from the other glycogenoses in that no other abnormalities are detectable in the clinical chemistry laboratory. There is no hypoglycemia, and concentrations of lactic acid, uric acid and lipids are normal.

The histopathology of this disease is one of generalized deposition of increased amounts of glycogen throughout the body, but without the enormous increase in storage that tends

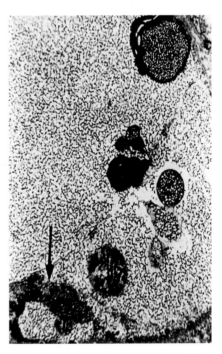

Figure 61.11   *Electron micrograph of the muscle of the same baby demonstrates the extensive accumulation of glycogen. Most of the muscle fiber was replaced by glycogen granules. The arrow in the slide points to a remnant of a muscle fiber. Also evident are membrane-bound collections of glycogen. (Courtesy of Dr. John S. Romine, Department of Neurosciences, University of California, San Diego, La Jolla, California.)*

to increase massively the size of the liver in type I and type III. The material usually stains basophilic in hematoxylin and eosin, and red with special stains for glycogen (Figure 61.10). It is digestible with amylase and contains phosphates [37]. The typical lacework appearance of sections of the myocardium results from the deposition of glycogen in cardiac fibrils. In the electron microscopic picture (Figure 61.11) it is clear that the glycogen is membrane-bound, and that the accumulation is within the lysosome in contradistinction to the appearance of other glycogenoses [38]. However, in the muscle and in the heart of type II patients there is also cytoplasmic accumulation of glycogen, and this has been correlated with destruction of contractile elements.

In addition to the accumulation in muscle and liver, deposition may be seen in motor muclei in the brainstem and in the anterior horn cells of the spinal cord [22]. There is only slight deposition in the neurons of the cerebral cortex, but it may be seen even in fetal life [39]. Histologic examination of the adult onset patient, in whom the heart is clinically normal, may reveal no accumulation of glycogen in cardiac muscle, even though the enzyme defect is no different there than in skeletal muscle [40]. The histologic appearance of skeletal muscle of infantile and adult onset patients is indistinguishable [40]. Glycogen deposition may not be seen in the heart, liver or brain of patients who have an adult onset. In classic infantile patients the diagnosis may also be made by electron microscopic examination of biopsied skin [41], in which characteristic accumulation of glycogen within a lining membrane may be demonstrated.

GENETICS AND PATHOGENESIS

Type II glycogenosis is inherited in an autosomal recessive fashion. Consanguinity has been observed. Prevalence is high in Taiwan and South China; estimated frequency was 1 in 50 000 [42]. Many patients are seen in Saudi Arabia (Figures 61.2–61.9). Elsewhere the disease is rare. The molecular defect in type II glycogenosis is in α-1,4-glucosidase (Figure 61.1, p. 394) [4]. The activity of this lysosomal enzyme in human liver at pH 4.0 is 3–10 times that at pH 7.4 [43]. It is active against maltose and other oligosaccharides, as well as glycogen. The product is free-glucose [44]. The enzyme is normally widely distributed in tissues and it is present in fibroblasts, leukocytes and amniocytes. In Pompe disease, deficiency of the enzyme has been demonstrable in all tissues measured [23,28,29] and this generalized deficiency is true of patients regardless of clinical phenotype. This explains the intralysosomal accumulation of glycogen in organs such as liver, where it would be inaccessible to other enzymes of glycogenolysis, such as phosphorylase and the debranching enzyme. In organs containing these enzymes, glycogen is not found outside the lysosomal fraction [45].

The diagnosis is best made by assay of the enzyme in muscle or fibroblasts [46]. The enzyme can be measured in transformed lymphoblasts or lymphocytes, but it may not be reliable in unfractionated leukocytes unless antibody against the enzyme is employed to prove that the activity being measured is not an unrelated glucosidase [47–49]. Among groups of patients with different clinical phenotypes there was an inverse correlation between the severity of clinical manifestation and the level of residual enzyme activity [50]. In general the classic infantile patients display virtually absent activity, while adult onset patients usually have considerable residual activity, but there is appreciable overlap among patients in between. In the infantile presentation, a catalytically inactive, immunochemically reactive enzyme has been observed. In some patients with the adult phenotype a reduction in the amount of enzyme protein has been reported [50–52]. Genetic heterogeneity is evident within both the infantile and adult forms of the disease; of nine patients with the infantile form, eight were cross-reacting material (CRM) negative and one was CRM positive [52]. In the adult phenotype CRM-negative as well as CRM-positive variants have been observed. The enzyme undergoes extensive post-translational modification: seven N-linked glycosylations and phosphorylation of mannose moieties yield the mannose-6-phosphate lysosomal recognition marker.

All of the variants of glycogenosis type II described are inherited in an autosomal recessive fashion. Analysis of affected infants in reported kindreds after subtraction of the probands yielded a figure of 21.4 percent, approximating the 25 percent expected [53]. The incidence of consanguinity was high. Reduced activity in heterozygotes of α-1,4-glucosidase has been demonstrated by assessment of fibroblasts [54]. Heterozygote detection using leukocytes from peripheral blood has been accomplished but it was unreliable [4]. An assay for heterozygosity was developed for lymphocytes stimulated by phytohemagglutinin [55]. Prenatal diagnosis has been carried out using cultivated amniocytes [56,57]. Rapid prenatal diagnosis has been accomplished by electron microscopic examination of uncultured amniotic cells [58]. Of 26 fetuses at risk, six were found to be positive. Each of these prenatal diagnoses was confirmed by enzyme assay of amniocytes, and in tissues of three fetuses terminated and in three affected infants delivered. Prenatal diagnosis has also been reported by assay of the enzyme in uncultured chorionic villus material [59].

The nature of the disease is usually quite similar in all affected members of a family. However, families have been reported in which there were examples of the typical infantile Pompe form of the disease and the late-onset adult [60,61]. This situation has been shown to reflect allelic diversity [62] in which an affected grandparent with adult onset disease had two mutant alleles, one specifying partial deficiency and one complete. This second allele was passed to a son whose spouse also turned out to have such a gene, and an infantile classic patient was produced [61]. Somatic cell hybridization studies have failed to show evidence of complementation, and so a single locus appears to exist.

The gene has been localized to chromosome 17q25 [5]. The gene has been cloned and the sequence of the cDNA determined [63]. It contains 20 exons and is approximately 20 kb. Mutations have been defined in patients with different phenotypes. Among infantile patients a majority of those studied have had undetectable mRNA [7,64,65]. A number of gross alterations in the gene have been found, such as deletion of exon 18 and stop codons [66,67]. In contrast, a number of those with adult-onset phenotypes have had missense mutations [68]. Many of the mutations reported have been genetic compounds in which different mutations were on each allele. The number and variety of mutations observed indicate that the degree of heterogeneity in this population will be very great. Expression of a G-to-A transition in exon 11 *in vitro* indicated that the mutation coded for absence of catalytic activity [69]. This is consistent with the infantile onset phenotype. The common mutation in Chinese patients [9] is an Asp645Glu. The African mutation is an Arg854X [8]. Two deletions del525T and del exon 18 are very common in Holland and in other Caucasian populations [70].

The molecular biology of this gene is complicated by the fact that considerable polymorphism has been identified in individuals with no disease or enzymatic abnormality. Eleven restriction fragment length polymorphisms (RFLPs) have been identified which result from substitution of bases within introns [64], but silent mutations in the coding regions have also been observed [63]. These RFLPs may be useful for heterozygote detection and prenatal diagnosis. Prenatal diagnosis has been carried out in a family in which the mother carried a ΔT525 deletion and whose previous child had died of glycogenosis II [71]. Mutational analysis correctly identified the absence of the mother's deletion in chorionic villus material, and enzyme analysis in the fetus was normal. However, it was concluded that enzyme analysis remains the method of choice because of the variety of mutations possible and the need to identify the mutation in each parent. If the mutation is known, this is a convenient method of prenatal diagnosis [72].

A further confounding issue is the occurrence of patients with cardiomyopathy and lysosomal storage of glycogen in whom the activity of acid α-glucosidase was normal [73,74]. Arrhythmias, especially Wolff-Parkinson-White syndrome, were common in these patients. Most of those patients have been mentally retarded.

TREATMENT

Effective treatment is not available. Supportive therapy including ventilator assistance is useful especially in advanced myopathic disease. Bone marrow transplantation has been accomplished in cattle with α-glucosidase deficiency, but there was no effect on the disease [75]. Enzyme replacement therapy has been employed, using acid maltase purified from *Aspergillus* and human placenta, without clinical evidence of improvement. Recognition of the importance of the mannose-6-phosphate receptor-mediated lysosomal uptake of enzymes and the development of recombinant human enzyme have completely changed this area of investigation. Administration intravenously to acid glucosidase-deficient quail led to increase enzyme activity in muscle and decrease in glycogen content to normal. Clinically the birds righted themselves and even flew [11]. A clinical trial of recombinant human enzyme produced in rabbit milk has been published [76] including evidence of improvement in muscle histopathology, decrease in cardiac size and improvement in function.

References

1 Pompe JC. Hypertrophie idiopathique du Coeur. *Ann Anat Pathol* 1933;**10**:23.

2 Sprague HB, Cland EF, White PD. Congenital idiopathic hypertrophy of the heart. A case with unusual family history. *Am J Dis Child* 1931;**41**:877.

3 Van Creveld S. Glycogen disease. *Medicine* 1939;**18**:1.

4 Hers HG. α-Glucosidase deficiency in generalized glycogen storage disease (Pompe's disease). *Biochem J* 1963;**86**:11.

5 Solomon E, Swallow DM, Burgess S, Evan L. Assignment of the human acid α-glucosidase gene (α-GLU) to chromosome 17 using somatic cell hybrids. *Ann Hum Genet* 1979;**42**:273.

6 Reuser AJJ, Kroos MMP, Hermans MMP, *et al*. Glycogenosis type II (acid maltase deficiency). *Muscle Nerve* 1995;**S3**:61.

7 Martiniuk F, Mehler M, Tzall S, *et al*. Extensive genetic heterogeneity in patients with acid alpha glucosidase deficiency as detected by abnormalities of DNA and mRNA. *Am J Hum Genet* 1990;**47**:73.

8 Becker JA, Vlach J, Raben N, *et al*. The African origin of the common mutation in African-American patients with glycogen storage disease type II (GSDII). *Am J Hum Genet* 1998;**62**:991.

9 Shieh J-J, Lin C-Y. Frequent mutation in Chinese patients with infantile type of GSDII in Taiwan: evidence for a founder effect. *Hum Mutat* 1998;**11**:306.

10 Kroos MA, Van Der Kraan M, Van Diggelen OP, *et al*. Glycogen storage disease type II: frequency of three common mutant alleles and their associated clinical phenotypes studied in 121 patients. *Med Genet* 1995;**32**:836.

11 Pennybacker M, Kikuchi T, Yang HW, *et al*. Clinical and metabolic correction of Pompe disease by enzyme therapy in acid maltase-deficient quail. *J Clin Invest* 1998;**101**:827.

12 di Sant' Agnese PA, Anderson DH, Mason HH, Bauman WA. Glycogen storage disease of the heart. I Report of two cases in siblings with chemical and pathological studies. *Pediatrics* 1950;**6**:402.

13 Gitzelmann R. Glukagonprobleme bei den Glykogenspeicher-krankheiten. *Helv Paediatr Acta* 1957;**21**:425.

14 Pompe JC. Over idiopatische hypertrophie van het hart. *Ned Tijdschr Geneeskd* 1932;**76**:304.

15 Cottrill CM, Johnson GL, Noonan JA. Parental genetic contribution to mode of presentation in Pompe disease. *Pediatrics* 1987;**79**:379.

16 Gillette PC, Nihill MR, Singer DB. Electrophysiological mechanisms for the short PR interval in Pompe disease. *Am J Dis Child* 1974;**128**:622.

17 Ehlers KH, Hagstrom JWC, Lukas DS, *et al*. Glycogen storage disease of the myocardium with obstruction to the left ventricular outflow. *Circulation* 1962;**25**:96.

18 Seifert BL, Snyder MS, Klein AA, *et al*. Development of obstruction to ventricular outflow and impairment of inflow in glycogen storage disease of the heart: serial echocardiographic studies from birth to death at 6 months. *Am Heart J* 1992;**123**:239.

19 Antopol W, Boas EP, Levison W, Tuchman LR. Cardiac hypertrophy caused by glycogen storage disease in a 15-year-old boy. *Am Heart J* 1940;**20**:546.

20 Slonim AE, Bulone L, Ritz S, *et al*. Identification of two subtypes of infantile acid maltase deficiency. *J Pediatr* 2000;**137**:283.

21 Clement DH, Godman GC. Glycogen disease resembling mongolism cretinism and amyotonia congenital. *J Pediatr* 1950;**36**:11.

22   Gambetti P, Di Mauro S, Baker L. Nervous system in Pompe's disease: ultrastructure and biochemistry. *J Neuropathol Exp Neurol* 1971;**30**:412.

23   Engel AG, Gomez MR, Seybold ME, Lambert EH. The spectrum and diagnosis of acid maltase deficiency. *Neurology* 1973;**23**:95.

24   Tanaka K, Shimazu S, Oya N, *et al*. Muscular form of glycogenosis type II (Pompe's disease). *Pediatrics* 1979;**63**:124.

25   Iancu TC, Lerner A, Shiloh H, *et al*. Juvenile acid maltase deficiency presenting as paravertebral pseudotumour. *Eur J Pediatr* 1988;**147**:372.

26   Rosenow EC, Engel AE. Acid maltase deficiency in adults presenting as respiratory failure. *Am J Med* 1978;**64**:485.

27   Engel AG. Acid maltase deficiency in adults: studies in four cases of a syndrome which may mimic muscular dystrophy or other myopathies. *Brain* 1970;**93**:599.

28   Martin JJ, DeBarsy T, den Tandt WR. Acid maltase deficiency in nonidentical adult twins: a morphological and biochemical study. *J Neurol* 1976;**213**:105.

29   DiMauro S, Stern LZ, Mehler M, *et al*. Adult onset acid maltase deficiency: a postmortem study. *Muscle Nerve* 1978;**1**:27.

30   Francesconi M, Auff E. Cardiac arrhythmias and the adult form of type II glycogenosis (Letter). *N Engl J Med* 1982;**306**:937.

31   Cinnamon J, Slonim AE, Black KS, *et al*. Evaluation of the lumbar spine in patients with glycogen storage disease: CT demonstrations of patterns of paraspinal muscle atrophy. *Am J Neuroradiol* 1991;**12**:1099.

32   Chancellor AM, Warlow CP, Webb JN, *et al*. Acid maltase deficiency presenting with a myopathy and exercise-induced urinary incontinence in a 68-year-old male (Letter). *J Neurol Neurosurg Psychiatry* 1991;**54**:659.

33   Margolis ML, Howlett P, Goldgerg R, *et al*. Obstructive sleep apnea syndrome in acid maltase deficiency. *Chest* 1994;**105**:947.

34   Lenard HG, Schauab J, Keutel J, Osang M. Electromyography in type II glycogenosis. *Neuropaediatrie* 1974;**5**:410.

35   Ausems MGEM, Lochman P, Van Diggelen OP, *et al*. A diagnostic protocol for adult-onset glycogen storage disease type II. *Neurology* 1999;**52**:851.

36   DiFiore MT, Manfredi R, Marri L, *et al*. Elevation of transaminases as an early sign of late-onset glycogenosis type II (Letter). *Eur J Pediatr* 1993;**152**:784.

37   Martin JJ, DeBarsy T, van Hoof F, Palladini G. Pompe's disease: an inborn lysosomal disorder with storage of glycogen: a study of brain and striated muscle. *Acta Neuropathol (Berl)* 1973;**23**:229.

38   Baudhuin P, Hers HG, Loeb H. An electron microscopic and biochemical study of type II glycogenosis. *Lab Invest* 1964;**13**:1139.

39   Hug G. Pre-and postnatal pathology enzyme treatment and unresolved issues in five lysosomal disorders. *Pharmacol Rev* 1979;**30**:565.

40   Hug G. Glycogen storage diseases. *Birth Defects: Original Article Series* 1976;**12**(6):145.

41   O'Brien JS, Bernett J, Veath L, Paa D. Lysosomal storage disorders. Diagnosis by ultrastructural examination of skin biopsy specimens. *Arch Neurol* 1975;**32**:592.

42   Lin CY, Hwang B, Hsiao KJ, Yin YR. Pompe's disease in Chinese and the prenatal diagnosis by determination of alpha-glucosidase activity. *J Inherit Metab Dis* 1987;**10**:11.

43   Hers HG, van Hoof F. Glycogen storage diseases: type II and type VI glycogenosis: in *Carbohydrate Metabolism and Its Disorders* (eds Dickens F, Randle PJ, Whelan WJ). Academic Press Inc, New York; 1968:151.

44   Hers HG. Glycogen storage disease. *Adv Metab Disord* 1964;**1**:1.

45   Garancis JC. Type II glycogenosis. Biochemical and electron microscope study. *Am J Med* 1968;**44**:289.

46   Angelini C, Engel AG, Titus JL. Adult acid maltase deficiency. Abnormalities in fibroblasts cultured from patients. *N Engl J Med* 1972;**287**:948.

47   Koster JF, Slee RG, Hulsmann WC. The use of leukocytes as an aid in the diagnosis of a variant of glycogen storage disease type II (Pompe's disease). *Eur J Clin Invest* 1972;**2**:467.

48   Broadhead DM, Butterworth J. α-Glucosidase in Pompe's disease. *J Inherit Metab Dis* 1978;**1**:153.

49   Dreyfus JC, Poënaru L. Alpha glucosidases in white blood cells with reference to the detection of acid α-14-glucosidase deficiency. *Biochem Biophys Res Commun* 1978;**85**:615.

50   Reuser AJJ, Koster JF, Hoogeveen A, Galjaard H. Biochemical immunological and cell genetic studies in glycogenosis type II. *Am J Hum Genet* 1978;**30**:132.

51   Beratis NG, LaBadie GU, Hirschhorn K. Characterization of the molecular defect in infantile and adult acid alpha-glucosidase deficiency fibroblasts. *J Clin Invest* 1978;**62**:1264.

52   Beratis NG, LaBadie GU, Hirschhorn K. Genetic heterogeneity in acid α-glucosidase deficiency. *Am J Hum Genet* 1983;**35**:21.

53   Sidbury JB Jr. The genetics of the glycogen storage diseases. *Prog Med Genet* 1965;**IV**:32.

54   Nitowsky HM, Grunfield A. Lysosomal α-glucosidase type II glycogenosis: activity in leukocytes and cell cultures in relation to genotype. *J Lab Clin Med* 1967;**69**:472.

55   Hirschhorn K, Nadler HL, Waithe WI, *et al*. Pompe's disease: detection of heterozygotes by lymphocytes stimulation. *Science* 1969;**166**:1632.

56   Butterworth J, Broadhead DM. Diagnosis of Pompe's disease in cultured skin fibroblasts and primary amniotic fluid cells using 4-methylumbelliferyl-α-glycopyranoside as substrate. *Clin Chim Acta* 1977;**78**:335.

57   Cox RP, Douglas G, Hutzler J, *et al*. In-utero detection of Pompe's disease. *Lancet* 1970;**1**:893.

58   Hug G, Soukup S, Ryan M, Chuck G. Rapid prenatal diagnosis of glycogen storage disease type II by electron microscopy of uncultured amniotic-fluid cells. *N Engl J Med* 1984;**310**:1018.

59   Minelli A, Piantanida M, Simoni G, *et al*. Prenatal diagnosis of metabolic diseases on chorionic villi obtained before the ninth week of pregnancy. *Prenat Diag* 1992;**12**:959.

60   Koster JF, Busch HFM, Slee RG, van Weerden TW. Glycogenosis type II. The infantile and late-onset acid maltase deficiency observed in one family. *Clin Chim Acta* 1978;**87**:451.

61   Loonen MCB, Busch HFM, Koster JF, *et al*. A family with different clinical forms of acid maltase deficiency (glycogenosis type II): biochemical and genetic studies. *Neurology* 1981;**31**:1209.

62   Hoefsloot LH, Van Der Ploeg AT, Kroos MA, *et al*. Adult and infantile glycogenosis type II in one family explained by allelic diversity. *Am J Hum Genet* 1990;**46**:45.

63   Martiniuk F, Mehler M, Tzall S, *et al*. Sequence of the cDNA and 5′ flanking region for human acid alpha glucosidase detection of an intron in the 5′untranslated leader sequences definition of 18 base pair polymorphisms and additional differences with previous cDNA and amino acid sequences. *DNA Cell Biol* 1990;**9**:85.

64   Martiniuk F, Mehler M, Pellicer A, *et al*. Isolation of a cDNA for human acid alpha glucosidase and detection of genetic heterogeneity for mRNA in three alpha glucosidase deficient patients. *Proc Natl Acad Sci USA* 1986;**83**:9641.

65   Van der Ploeg AT, Hoefsloot LH, Hoogeveen-Westerveld M, *et al*. Glycogenosis Type II: protein and DNA analysis in five South African families from various ethnic origins. *Am J Hum Genet* 1989;**44**:787.

66   Huie ML, Chen AS, Grix A, *et al*. A de novo 13nt deletion a newly identified C647W missense mutation and a deletion of exon 18 in infantile onset glycogen storage disease type II (GSDII). *Hum Mol Genet* 1994;**3**:1081.

67   Huie ML, Chen AS, Grix AW, Hirschhorn R. De novo mutation (13nt deletion) resulting in infantile GSDII (Pompe) in a child carrying a missense mutation on the other allele. *Am J Hum Genet* 1993;**53**:(suppl) 906.

68 Hermans MMP, Kroos MA, de Graff E, *et al*. Two mutations affecting the transport and maturation of lysosomal alpha-glucosidase in an adult case of glycogen storage type II. *Hum Mutat* 1993;**2**:268.

69 Hermans MMP, de Graaff E, Kroos MA, *et al*. Identification of a point mutation in the human lysosomal alpha glucosidase gene causing infantile glycogenosis Type II. *Biochem Biophys Res Commun* 1991;**179**:919.

70 Hirschhorn R, Huie ML. Frequency of mutations for glycogen storage disease type II in different populations: The del525T and delexon18 mutations are not generally "common" in Caucasian populations. *J Med Genet* 1999;**36**:85.

71 Kleijer WJ, van der Kraan M, Kroos MA, *et al*. Prenatal diagnosis of glycogen storage disease Type II: enzyme assay or mutation analysis? *Pediatr Res* 1995;**38**:103.

72 Kroos MA, Waitfield AE, Joosse M, *et al*. A novel acid alpha-glucosidase mutation identified in a Pakistani family with glycogen storage disease type II. *J Inherit Metab Dis* 1997;**20**:556.

73 Danon MJ, Oh SJ, Di Mauro S, *et al*. Lysosomal glycogen storage disease with normal acid maltase. *Neurology* 1981;**31**:51.

74 Byrne E, Dennett X, Crotty B, *et al*. Dominantly inherited cardioskeletal myopathy with lysosomal glycogen storage and normal acid maltase levels. *Brain* 1986;**109**:523.

75 Howell JM, Dorling PR, Shelton JN, *et al*. Natural bone marrow transplantation in cattle with Pompe's disease. *Neuromusc Disord* 1991;**6**:449.

76 Van den Hout H, Reuser AJJ, Vulto AG, *et al*. Recombinant human α-glucosidase from rabbit milk in Pompe patients. *Lancet* 2000;**356**:397.

62

Glycogenosis type III/Amylo-1,6-glucosidase (debrancher) deficiency

---

MAJOR PHENOTYPIC EXPRESSION

Hepatomegaly, hypoglycemia, late myopathy, storage of glycogen in liver and muscle, elevated transaminases and creatine phosphokinase, and deficient activity of the glycogen debranching enzyme amylo-1-6-glucosidase.

INTRODUCTION

The first patient described with glycogenosis type III was reported by Forbes in 1953 [1]. She had been noted at 1 year-of-age to have a large abdomen, and when she presented at 3.4 years-of-age, the liver was palpated at the left iliac crest. By 13 years-of-age she was described as not appearing chronically ill [2]. The liver was studied by Illingworth and the Cori [3,4], who found the glycogen content of both muscle and liver to be increased. The structure of the glycogen was very abnormal and resembled a phosphorylase limit dextrin (Figure 62.1). The outer chains were abnormally short, and the number of branch points was increased. The structure of the glycogen suggested that the defect was in the debrancher enzyme. This hypothesis was promptly confirmed by assay of the enzyme [4]. Activity of amylo-1,6-glucosidase was virtually absent in liver and muscle [4,5]. The history of the disease is impressive in that the nature of the disorder and the enzyme defect were worked out in studies on the index case within a few years of the first report. The cDNA has been cloned, and heterogeneity has been demonstrated in study of mRNAs [6]. The gene has been mapped to chromosome 1p21 [7].

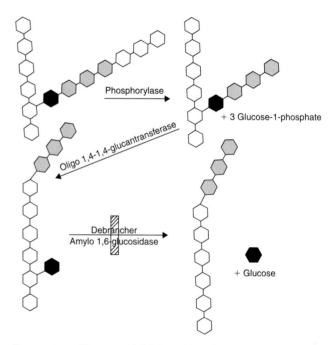

Figure 62.1 *The sequential debranching of glycogen. Phosphorylase catalyzes the cleavage of glycosyl units in α-1,4 glucose unit before the amylo-1,6-glucosidase can cleave the glucose moiety in 1,6 linkage. This debrancher is the site of the defect in glycogenosis type III.*

CLINICAL ABNORMALITIES

The clinical manifestations of glycogenosis III tend to be milder than those of type I (Chapter 60), but the diseases cannot reliably be distinguished without laboratory procedures. Death in infancy has been recorded [2]. The most consistent clinical feature is hepatomegaly, and it may be the only clinical abnormality at the time of presentation [1] (Figures 62.2–62.7). In contrast to the patient with type I, these patients may also have some enlargement of the spleen [8]. The kidneys are not enlarged in this disease; in fact, assessment of renal size by imaging of the abdomen may aid in distinguishing types I and III [9]. The enlargement of the liver may be massive; in infancy it may interfere with walking or even standing. A 2-year-old patient of ours simply toppled over if not supported in the standing position.

With time and growth, the patient's size tends to catch up with the liver which, while prominent, is less impressive. By adulthood the abdomen usually appears normal [2]. The size of the liver may be normal by puberty [10].

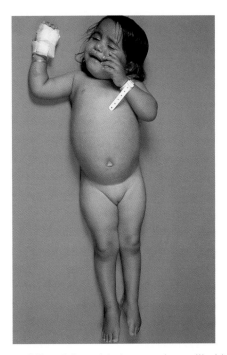

Figure 62.4   *S.H., an infant with glycogenosis type III with protruberant abdomen.*

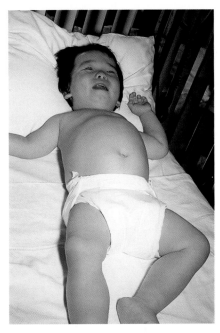

Figure 62.2   *J.L., an 18-month-old boy with glycogenosis type III [12] who presented with a history of increasing abdominal protuberance. He woke routinely at 4 a.m. for breakfast. (Kindly provided by Dr. Jon Wolff.)*

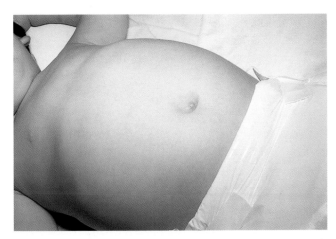

Figure 62.3   *J.L. Close-up of the abdomen highlighted the relatively enormous size of the liver. With time he grew and the liver could only be found by palpation. (Kindly provided by Dr. Jon Wolff.)*

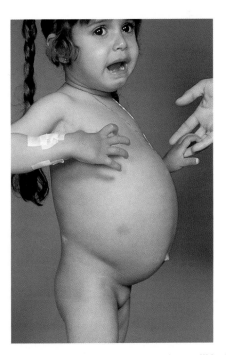

Figure 62.5   *M.S. This infant with glycogenosis type III had a highly prominent abdomen.*

Hypoglycemia is usually not a prominent feature of this disease, but fasting concentrations of glucose are usually moderately reduced, and some patients, especially in infancy, have severe hypoglycemia (Figure 62.8) and even convulsions. Some patients have developed mental retardation [11], presumably as a consequence of hypoglycemia. It is thought that hypoglycemia of infancy and early childhood may reflect

developmental inadequacy of gluconeogenesis [9], but the behavior may also modulate the problem. For instance, one of our patients ate five meals a day and woke at 4 a.m. for breakfast [12]. In any case, by the second decade fasting hypoglycemia improves and most adults with this disease tolerate fasting well [9]. Ketonuria may be observed after a moderate fast when the blood glucose approximates 40 mg/dL [13]. Hyperketonuria tends not to lead to metabolic acidosis or symptoms.

Vigorous catabolism of fatty acids and hyperactive fasting ketonuria are indicated by a 10-fold elevation in concentrations of 3-hydroxybutyric acid after a 12-hour fast. Concentrations of lipids may be elevated, but not to the degree seen in von Gierke disease [1,14]. The concentration of cholesterol may be elevated in the absence of hypertriglyceridemia, and there may be hyperbetalipoproteinemia [9]. Over the years, levels of lipids in the blood tend to decrease [1] and those of sugar to increase. Patients with type III disease do not develop xanthomas. Concentrations of uric acid are normal and levels of lactate are also usually normal. Concentrations of transaminases are usually elevated in infancy, and this may make the clinical picture confusing, suggesting hepatitis or hepatocellular insult as a cause of the hepatomegaly. On the other hand, the creatine kinase is usually elevated [12]; so some of the enzyme levels could represent myopathy. Nevertheless, the histologic appearance of the liver usually indicates at least some fibrosis in this disease [8,12]. Frank cirrhosis may be encountered, but cirrhosis does not usually progress with age [15]. Cirrhosis appeared to be more common in Japan [16–18], and progressive cirrhosis and hepatic failure have

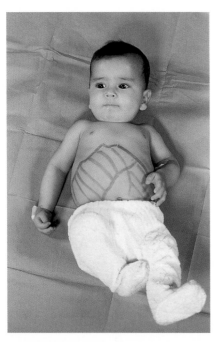

Figure 62.6   *F.M.S. The enlarged liver created a very protruberant abdomen of this infant with glycogenosis type III.*

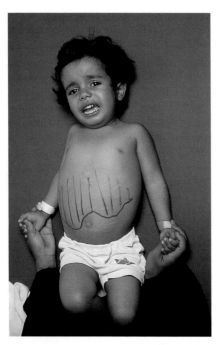

Figure 62.7   *Another girl with glycogenosis type III and marked hepatomegaly.*

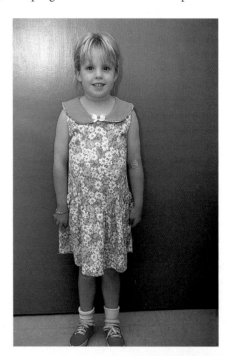

Figure 62.8   *A 5-year-old girl with glycogenosis type III. Unlike most patients with this disease, she had problems with hypoglycemia and was using an overnight glucose drip. Introduction of a cornstarch regimen at this time permitted its discontinuation.*

been observed, particularly in that country [19–21]. Hepatic adenomas have been described [22], but they have not developed malignant change. On the other hand hepatocellular carcinoma has been observed in end-stage cirrhosis [18,21]. Pallor has been described [23], but patients are usually not anemic.

Growth and development may be completely normal in this disease [1], but in some patients retardation of linear growth may be striking [12]. Many children are of normal size, although in a lower percentile for height than for weight and head circumference.

Renal tubular acidosis has been reported in two patients, along with severe failure to thrive [24]. One of the patients had a typical distal renal tubular acidosis, while the other had glycosuria and bicarbonate wasting, suggesting a Fanconi syndrome, as seen in type I glycogenosis (Chapter 60, p. 388).

It has been recognized since the first patient that glycogen accumulates in muscle as well as liver. It has only more recently been recognized that this leads to a myopathy, especially by adulthood [25–27]. In fact, the late myopathy is the major morbidity of type III glycogenosis. There may be hypotonia, but muscle atrophy occurs as well as weakness. It is often notable in the interossei and over the thumbs. Atrophy in the legs has suggested diagnosis of Charcot-Marie-Tooth disease [28]. Weakness tends to be slowly progressive. Walking rapidly or upstairs brings out the weakness. Strenuous exercise cannot be effectively performed, but there is no tenderness, cramping or myoglobinuria. Some patients have presented first in adulthood with progressive muscular weakness. Ultimately, the patient may be wheelchair-bound or bedridden. The electromyogram (EMG) may reveal a myopathic pattern [27]. Nerve conduction may be abnormal. Activity of creatine kinase (CK) in serum is elevated [25] in the presence or absence of myopathic symptoms, but a normal level of creatine kinase (CK) does not rule out deficiency of debranching enzyme in muscle [29]. Deformity of the chest and kyphoscoliosis may be progressive. Some patients have had muscular fasciculations suggestive of motor neuron disease, and peripheral nerve involvement has been documented [30] in this disease. Electron microscopic study of a 20-month-old boy [12] revealed selective massive accumulation of glycogen in the Schwann cells of unmyelinated nerve fibers.

Cardiomyopathy may also occur; in fact, abnormalities of the electrocardiogram and echocardiographic evidence of biventricular hypertrophy are frequently observed, although rarely accompanied by cardiac symptoms [31,32]. However, congestive cardiac failure has been described [26], as has exertional dyspnea and chest pain, and sudden death may occur [33].

Polycystic ovaries have been described in this disease, as in Type I, but without effect on fertility [34]. Histologic examination reveals the cells of the liver to be swollen and finely granular with an open nucleus. The material stored may be identified by Best stain as glycogen. Large vacuoles in the hepatocytes may be filled with periodic acid-Schiff (PAS)-positive material. There is evidence of an increase amount of fibrous tissue within the lobules of the liver. In addition, there may be some

proliferation of the bile ducts. Unlike the picture in glycogenosis type I, there is no infiltration with fat. Histologic examination of the muscle reveals abundant amounts of glycogen visible in subsarcolemmic areas of myofibrils [15]. The glycogen in this disease is more soluble than a normal glycogen, and therefore it tends to disappear more readily from conventional histologic preparations. Cryostat sections may be useful for biopsies. Electron microscopy reveals large pools of monoparticulate glycogen in hepatocytes [35]. Ovoid subunits measure 45–60 Å. In muscle, the glycogen accumulates beneath the sarcolemma. Glycogen is also seen between and within myofibrils. Glycogen may also be demonstrated by electron microscopy in granulocytes [35].

A variety of functional studies has been employed to document the presence of type III glycogenosis and to distinguish it from type I (Table 62.1). Among the most useful is the administration of glucagon after a 14-hour fast, following which there is little or no increase in blood glucose; and again 2–3 hours after a meal, following which there is a blood glucose response [36,37]; the rise in glucose may be normal, but it is usually reduced, though clearly present. This is consistent with the availability of glucose moieties on the elongated outer branches of glycogen to degradation of phosphorylase, even in the total absence of debranching activity. These patients also do not have lactic acidemia and, in particular contrast to patients with type I, the concentration of lactic acid does not increase after glucagon. Also in contrast to type I, there is a normal level of conversion of galactose, fructose or glycerol to glucose [38].

The absence of highly elevated concentrations of lactic acid has been cited [39] as a reason why patients with this disease have been observed to have seizures at higher concentrations of glucose than those with type I disease, in whom the brain may be able to substitute lactate for glucose. On the other hand, seizures are not common in glycogenosis type III, and

Table 62.1 *Features by which type III glycogenosis may be distinguished from type I*

Feature	Type III	Type I
Hypoglycemia	+	Severe
Bleeding diathesis	0	+
Splenomegaly	+/−	0
Enlarged kidneys	0	+
Myopathy	+	0
Elevated creatine kinase, transaminases	++	0
Fasting ketogenesis	++	+
Lactic acidemia	0	+
Alanine in plasma	Low	High
Hyperuricemia	0	+
Little or no response to glucagon after fast	+	+
Normal postprandial response to glucagon	+	0
Increase in blood glucose after galactose, fructose or glycerol	+	0

concentrations of ketones in blood are elevated in this disease [40]. Mobilization of fat is very active, as is gluconeogenesis.

Metabolism of amino acids in glycogenosis type III is distinctly different from that of normal individuals and of patients with type I disease [41]. The major difference is in the responses of the principal gluconeogenic amino acid, alanine. The concentrations of alanine in plasma were significantly lower in 11 patients than in 27 controls [41]. This would be consistent with an overactive process of gluconeogenesis. In contrast in type I, concentrations of alanine are increased, consistent with defective gluconeogenesis. In type III there were significantly lower concentrations of a number of other amino acids, notably threonine, valine, methionine, isoleucine, leucine, tyrosine, phenylalanine and lysine. This would be consistent with the operation of the alanine-glucose cycle in which branched-chain and other essential amino acids in muscle are depleted in order to serve as donors of nitrogen for the net synthesis of alanine from pyruvate in muscle [42]. Alanine is the only amino acid whose concentration in venous blood draining muscle is higher than arterial. The alanine formed is then transported through the blood to the liver, where it is converted to glucose.

Following the ingestion of glucose in a glucose tolerance test, concentrations of alanine in the blood rise dramatically in type III patients, while in type I patients they fall [41]. In controls, the level of alanine does not change after glucose. After a protein challenge with 4 g beef/kg, levels of alanine rose, but much less than in normals or than in type I patients and significantly less than the rise in alanine in type III after glucose. All of these data are compatible with an enhanced level of gluconeogenesis in type III disease.

The concentration of glycogen in the liver is markedly elevated. The amounts vary from 15 to 21 percent [10,35]. Normal liver has less than six percent glycogen. Concentrations in muscle are less, approximating six percent in patients with type III disease and less than 1.5 percent in controls. Accumulation of glycogen of abnormal structure has also been reported in erythrocytes [43].

Depressed levels of enzymes other than the debranching enzyme are sometimes found in biopsies of these patients. For instance, glucose-6-phosphatase activities are sometimes somewhat low. That these are secondary effects has been suggested by the successful induction of increase to normal activity by the administration of triamcinolone [44].

GENETICS AND PATHOGENESIS

The disorder is transmitted by an autosomal recessive gene. Heterozygote detection has been carried out by the assay of debrancher enzyme activity in leukocytes and erythrocytes; intermediate levels were obtained [11,45–47]. In families in which the patient lacks immunoprecipitable debrancher protein, carrier detection can be accomplished by Western blot [48].

The disorder has been recognized to be relatively high in frequency in Israel [11], where it makes up 73 percent of patients with glycogen storage disease. All of these are Sephardic Jews of North African origin, in whom the incidence figure was estimated at one in 5420. Gene frequency also appears to be high in the Faroe islands [49]. Prenatal diagnosis has been accomplished by the study of the enzyme activity of immunoblot in cultured amniocytes and chorionic villus cells [50–52], but the assay of the enzyme is demanding, because activity is so low in these materials, and immunoassay is only useful in families in which patients have no enzyme protein.

The molecular defect is in the activity of amlyo-1,6-glucosidase (Figure 62.1, p. 402) [4,5,53,54]. A number of different methods has been used to assay the enzyme. The overall reaction catalyzes the production of glucose from phosphorylase limit dextrin. The partial reactions, transferase and glucosidase, appear to reside on a single polypeptide chain [55]. Enzyme deficiency has been demonstrated in leukocytes [45,50,56,57], erythrocytes [58,59] and cultured fibroblasts [60], as well as liver and muscle [4,5,53,54]. In most patients there is parallel reduction in all tissues tested, regardless of the assay method employed. However, there are some discrepancies, and it is clear that a few patients with proven hepatic deficiency of the enzyme have had normal activity in muscle, leukocytes, erythrocytes or fibroblasts [6, 46,48,61–63]. This means that the diagnosis cannot be excluded without assay of the liver. It also seems likely that myopathy would only be expected in those with abnormal enzyme in muscle and this seems to be the case [29]. The most common situation in which activity is deficient in both liver and muscle is sometimes referred to as IIIa; when the deficiency is found only in liver it is referred to as IIIb; and the instances in which there is selective loss of only the glucosidase activity or only the transferase activity have been called IIIc and IIId, respectively [48,54].

Studies using antibody to the normal debranching enzyme have revealed absence or considerable reduction of cross-reacting material (CRM) [48,64]. The amounts of protein do not correlate with clinical severity [65].

The gene on chromosome 1p21 is in the area to which amylase genes have been mapped [7]. A variety of different mutations are responsible for this disease [6]. The isolation of the gene and determination of its sequence [6,66] has elucidated a structure of 85 kb with 35 exons. The protein is a large monomeric structure of approximately 170 KDa. There is a single gene in liver and muscle, and the coding sequences of the two mRNAs are the same and code for a protein of 1532 amino acids. Isoforms differing in the 51 untranslated region appear to account for tissue differences.

Determination of the nature of mutation has provided correlations between molecular abnormality and clinical phenotype. In a patient with quite severe IIIa disease, an apparently homozygous mutation was found in which a single base (A4529) was inserted, changing a tyrosine to a stop codon at amino acid 1510 [67,68]. Two mutations in exon 3 at amino acid codon 6, 17delAG and Q6X, and were found in three patients with type IIIb and not in type IIIa. Two patients had deletion of AG at nucleotides 17 and 18, leading to a truncated protein. The third had a C-to-T change at nucleotide

6, which changed glutamine to a stop. These mutations were not found in 31 patients with IIIa, two with IIId or 28 controls. This permits DNA diagnosis on a blood sample in patients suspected of having type IIIb disease. A deletion, 4455delT, was found in all of the Sephardic Jewish patients [69]. A donor splice site mutation was found in a Japanese patient [70].

TREATMENT

Frequent high carbohydrate feedings in infancy and early childhood are often all that is necessary for the management of the hypoglycemia of glycogenosis III. Cornstarch supplementation has facilitated this regimen, particularly if used at bedtime, or during infant feedings at night [71–73]. Few if any patients need nocturnal enterogastric infusion, which may be dangerous if the tube becomes disconnected in a hyperinsulinemic state in the middle of the night. Serious, permanent brain damage may ensue. There is no need to restrict fructose and galactose in this disease.

A diet high in protein has been advocated for patients with this disease, but it has been our experience that pediatric patients will seldom eat a diet high enough in protein to make an appreciable difference in any of the abnormalities we could measure. Added protein has been obtained by mixing supplemental cornstarch with yogurt and other products [73].

The enhanced gluconeogenesis in this condition makes the use of high protein feedings logical [41]. Diets in which 20–25 percent of the calories are from protein and only 40–50 percent from carbohydrate have been employed. One approach has been to give between a fourth and a third of the calories as nocturnal enteral therapy high in protein. This has been recommended for patients with myopathy or growth retardation [74,75]. Patients were reported to experience improved muscle performance, in some cases quite dramatic. In others, effects were minimal or temporary [27]. In younger patients there was improvement in growth [68,72,73]. An older patient who discontinued the regimen experienced a recurrence of weakness that did not remit when therapy was resumed.

In asymptomatic patients in childhood who nevertheless had elevated levels of CK and transaminases in the blood, we found no effects of cornstarch or a high protein diet on these abnormalities. In contrast, we reasoned that if muscle were being broken down to provide alanine for gluconeogenesis, the provision of supplemental alanine might be therapeutic. We have observed a considerable improvement in levels of CK and transaminases [76]. Doses of alanine have ranged from 0.25 to 2.0 g/kg/day. A teaspoonful of alanine weighs 3.78 g.

References

1   Forbes GB. Glycogen storage disease. Report of a case with abnormal glycogen structure in liver and skeletal muscle. *Pediatrics* 1953;**42**:645.

2   Recant L. Recent developments in the field of glycogen metabolism and in the diseases of glycogen storage. *Am J Med* 1955;**19**:610.

3   Illingworth B, Cori GT. Structure of glycogens and amylopectins. III Normal and abnormal human glycogens. *J Biol Chem* 1952;**199**:653.

4   Illingworth B, Cori GT, Cori CF. Amylo-16-glucosidase in muscle tissue in generalized glycogen storage disease. *J Biol Chem* 1956;**218**:123.

5   Hers HG. Etudes enzymatiques sur fragments hépatiques; application à la classification des glycogénoses. *Rev Internat Hepatol* 1959;**9**:35.

6   Yang B-Z, Ding J-H, Enghild JJ, *et al*. Molecular cloning and nucleotide sequence of cDNA encoding human muscle glycogen debranching enzyme. *J Biol Chem* 1992;**267**:9294.

7   Yang-Zeng TL, Zheng K, Yu J, *et al*. Assignment of the human glycogen debrancher gene to chromosome 1p21. *Genomics* 1992;**13**:931.

8   Brandt IK, De Luca VA Jr. Type III glycogenosis: a family with an unusual tissue distribution of the enzyme lesion. *Am J Med* 1966;**40**:779.

9   Moses SW. Pathophysiology and dietary treatment of the glycogen storage diseases. *J Pediatr Gastroenterol Nutr* 1990;**11**:155.

10 Brown BI, Brown DH. The glycogen storage diseases: types I III IV V VII and unclassified glycogenoses: in *Carbohydrate Metabolism and Its Disorders* (ed. WJ Whelan). Academic Press Inc, New York;1968:Vol 2,123.

11 Levin S, Moses SW, Chayoth R, *et al*. Glycogen storage disease in Israel. A clinical biochemical and genetic study. *Israel J Med Sci* 1967;**3**:297.

12 Nyhan WL, Sakati NO. Glycogenosis type III; amylo-16-glucosidase (debrancher) deficiency: in *Diagnostic Recognition of Genetic Disease* (eds WL Nyhan, NO Sakati). Lea and Febiger, Philadelphia;1987:205.

13 Von Buerhrdel P, Boehme HJ, Hubald J. Metabolische adaptation im Nahrungskarenztest bei Kinder mit Glykogenosen der Typen III und VI. *Kinderarztl Prax* 1987;**55**:543.

14 Vitek B, Srachova D, Toma M, *et al*. Hyperlipidemia in type III glycogenosis. *Acta Pediatr Scand* 1970;**59**:701.

15 Starzl TE, Putnam CW, Portern KA, *et al*. Portal diversion for the treatment of glycogen storage disease in humans. *Ann Surg* 1973;**178**:525.

16 Fellows IW, Lowe JS, Ogilvie AL, *et al*. Type III glycogenosis presenting as liver disease in adults with atypical histological features. *J Clin Pathol* 1983;**36**:431.

17 Coleman RA, Winter HS, Wolf B, Chen Y-T. Glycogen debranching enzyme deficiency: Relationship of serum enzyme activities to biochemical diagnosis and clinical features. *J Inherit Metab Dis* 1992;**15**:869.

18 Momoi T, Sano H, Yamanaka C, *et al*. Glycogen storage disease type III with muscle involvement. Reappraisal of phenotypic variability and prognosis. *Am J Med Genet* 1992;**42**:696.

19 Rosenfeld EL, Popova IA, Chibisov IV. Some cases of type III glycogen storage disease. *Clin Chim Acta* 1976;**67**:123.

20 Markowitz A, Chen Y-T, Muenzer J, *et al*. A man with type III glycogenosis associated with cirrhosis and portal hypertension. *Gastroenterology* 1993;**105**:1882.

21 Haagsma E, Smit G, Niezen-Koning K, *et al*. Type IIIb glycogen storage disease associated with end-stage cirrhosis and hepatocellular carcinoma. The Liver Transplant Group. *Hepatology* 1997;**25**:537.

22 Labrune P, Trioche P, Duvaltier I, *et al*. Hepatocellular adenomas in glycogen storage disease type I and III: A series of 43 patients and review of the literature. *J Pediatr Gastroenterol Nut* 1997;**24**:276.

23 Spencer-Peet J, Norman ME, Lake BD, *et al*. Hepatic glycogen storage disease. Clinical and laboratory findings in 23 cases. *Quart J Med New Series* 1971;**40**:95.

24 Chen J, Friedman M. Renal tubular acidosis associated with type III glycogenosis. *Acta Pediatr Scand* 1979;**68**:779.

25 Brunberg JA, McCormick WF, Schochet SS. Type III glycogenosis: An adult with diffuse weakness and muscle wasting. *Arch Neurol* 1971;**25**:171.

26 DiMauro S, Hartwig GB, Hays A, *et al*. Debrancher deficiency: Neuromuscular disorder in 5 adults. *Ann Neurol* 1976;**5**:422.

27   Moses SW, Gadoth N, Bashan N, *et al*. Neuromuscular involvement in glycogen storage disease type III. *Acta Pediatr Scand* 1986;**75**:289.

28   Cornelio F, Bresolin N, Singer PA, *et al*. Clinical varieties of neuromuscular disease in debrancher deficiency. *Arch Neurol* 1984;**41**:1027.

29   Coleman RA, Winter HS, Wolf B, *et al*. Glycogen storage disease type III (glycogen debranching enzyme deficiency: correlation of biochemical defects with myopathy and cardiomyopathy). *Ann Intern Med* 1992;**116**:896.

30   Powell HC, Haas R, Hall CL, *et al*. Peripheral nerve in type III glycogenosis: Selective involvement of unmyelinated fiber Schwann cells. *Muscle Nerve* 1985;**8**:667.

31   Moses SW, Wanderman KL, Myroz A, Friedman M. Cardiac involvement in glycogen storage disease type III. *Eur J Pediatr* 1989;**431**:1.

32   Olson LJ, Reeder GS, Noller KL, *et al*. Cardiac involvement in glycogen storage disease III: Morphologic and biochemical characterization with endomyocardial biopsy. *Am J Cardiol* 1984;**53**:980.

33   Miller CG, Alleyne GA, Brooks SEH. Gross cardiac involvement in glycogen storage disease type III. *Br Heart J* 1972;**34**:862.

34   Lee P, Patel A, Hindsmarsh P, *et al*. The prevalence of polycystic ovaries in the hepatic glycogen storage diseases: Its association with hyperinsulinism. *Clin Endocrinol* 1995;**42**:601.

35   Garancis JC, Panares RR, Good TA, Kuzman JF. Type III glycogenosis A biochemical and electron microscopic study. *Lab Invest* 1970;**22**:468.

36   Hug G, Krill CE Jr, Perrin EV, Guest GM. Cori's disease (amylo-16-glocosidase deficiency). Report of a case in a Negro child. *N Engl J Med* 1963;**268**:113.

37   Perkoff GT, Parker VJ, Hahan RE. The effects of glucagons in three forms of glycogen storage disease. *J Clin Invest* 1962;**41**:1099.

38   Senior B, Loridan L. Studies of liver glycogenosis with particular reference to the metabolism of intravenously administered glycerol. *N Engl J Med* 1968;**279**:958.

39   Huijing F. Glycogen metabolism and glycogen-storage diseases. *Physiol Rev* 1975;**55**:609.

40   Fernandes J, Pikaar NA. Ketosis in hepatic glycogenosis. *Arch Dis Child* 1972;**47**:41.

41   Slonim AE, Coleman RA, Moses S, *et al*. Amino acid disturbances in type III glycogenosis: differences from type I glycogenosis. *Metabolism* 1983;**32**:70.

42   Odessey R, Kairallath EA, Goldberg AL. Origin and possible significance of alanine production by skeletal muscle. *J Biol Chem* 1974; **249**:7623.

43   Sidbury JB Jr, Cornblath M, Fisher J, House E. Glycogen in erythrocytes of patients with glycogen storage disease. *Pediatrics* 1961;**27**:103.

44   Moses SW, Leven S, Chayoth R, Steinitz K. Enzyme induction in a case of glycogen storage disease. *Pediatrics* 1966;**38**:111.

45   Williams HE, Kendig EM, Field JB. Leukocyte debranching enzyme in glycogen-storage disease. *J Clin Invest* 1963;**42**:656.

46   Williams C, Field JB. Studies in glycogen-storage disease: limit dextrinosis a genetic study. *J Pediatr* 1968;**72**:214.

47   Shin YS, Ungar R, Rieth M, Endres W. A simple assay for amylo-16-glucosidase to detect heterozygotes for glycogenosis type III in erythrocytes. *Clin Chem* 1984;**30**:717.

48   Ding J-H, de Barsy T, Brown BI, *et al*. Immunoblot analyses of glycogen debranching enzyme in different subtypes of glycogen storage disease type III. *J Pediatr* 1990;**116**:95.

49   Cohn J, Wang P, Hauge M, *et al*. Amylo-16-glucosidase deficiency (glycogenosis type III) in the Faroe Islands. *Hum Hered* 1975;**25**:115.

50   Yang B-Z, Ding J-H, Brown BI, Chen Y-T. Definitive prenatal diagnosis for type III glycogen storage disease. *Am J Hum Genet* 1990;**47**:735.

51   Maire I, Mandon G, Mathieu M. First trimester prenatal diagnosis of glycogen storage disease type III. *J Inherit Metab Dis* 1989;**12**:(suppl 2) 292.

52   Van Diggelen OP, Janse HC, Smit GPA. Debranching enzyme in fibroblasts amniotic fluid cells and chorionic villi: pre- and postnatal diagnosis of glycogenosis type III. *Clin Chim Acta* 1985;**149**:129.

53   Hers HG, Verhue W, Van Hoof F. The determination of amylo-16-glucosidase. *Eur J Biochem* 1967;**2**:257.

54   Hoof F, Hers HG. The subgroups of type III glycogenosis. *Eur J Biochem* 1967;**2**:265.

55   Lee EYC, Smith EE, Whelan WJ. Glycogen and starch debranching enzymes. *Enzymes* 1971;**5**:191.

56   Huijing F. Amylo-16-glucosidase activity in normal leukocytes and in leukocytes of patients with glycogen storage disease. *Clin Chim Acta* 1964;**9**:269.

57   Steinitz K, Bodur H, Arman T. Amylo-16-glucosidase activity in leukocytes from patients with glycogen-storage disease. *Clin Chim Acta* 1963;**8**:807.

58   Chayoth R, Moses SW, Steinitz K. Debrancher enzyme activity in blood cells of families with type III glycogen storage disease. *Israel J Med Sci* 1967;**3**:422.

59   Van Hoof F. Amylo-16-glucosidase activity and glycogen content of the erythrocytes of normal subjects patients with glycogen-storage disease and heterozygotes. *Eur J Biochem* 1967;**2**:271.

60   Justice P, Ryan C, Hsia DY, Krmpotik E. Amylo-16-glucosidase in human fibroblasts: studies in type III glycogen-storage disease. *Biochem Biophys Res Commun* 1970;**39**:301.

61   Deckelbaum RJ, Russell A, Shapira E, *et al*. Type III glycogenosis: atypical enzyme activities in blood cells in two siblings. *J Pediatr* 1972;**81**:955.

62   Gutman A, Barash V, Schramm H, *et al*. Incorporation of (^{14}C) glucose into alpha-14-bonds of glycogen by leukocytes and fibroblasts of patients with type III glycogen storage disease. *Pediatr Res* 1985;**19**:218.

63   Brown BI. Diagnosis of glycogen storage disease: in *Congenital Metabolic Disease Diagnosis and Treatment* (ed. RA Wapnir). Dekker, Basel;1985:227.

64   Dreyfus JC, Alexandre Y. Immunological studies on glycogen-storage disease type III and V. Demonstration of the presence of an immunoreactive protein in one case of muscle phosphorylase deficiency. *Biochem Biophys Res Commun* 1971;**44**:1364.

65   Yang B-Z, Stewart C, Ding J-H, Chen Y-T. Type III glycogen storage disease: An adult case with mild disease but complete absence of debrancher protein. *Neuromusc Dis* 1991;**1**:173.

66   Liu W, de Castro ML, Takrama J, *et al*. Molecular cloning sequencing and analysis of the cDNA for rabbit muscle glycogen debranching enzyme. *Arch Biochem Biophys* 1993;**306**:1.

67   Yang B-Z, Ding J-H, Bao Y, *et al*. Molecular basis of the enzymatic variability in type III glycogen storage disease (GSD-III). *Am J Hum Genet* 1992;**51**:A28.

68   Shen J, Bao Y, Chen Y-T. A nonsense mutation due to a single base insertion in the 3′-coding region of glycogen debranching enzyme gene is associated with a severe phenotype in a patient with GSD type IIIa. *Hum Mutat* 1997;**9**:37.

69   Parvar R, Moses S, Shen J, *et al*. A single base deletion in the 3′ coding region of glycogen debranching enzyme gene is prevalent in glycogen storage disease type IIIa in a population of North African Jewish patients. *Eur J Hum Genet* 1998;**5**:266.

70   Okubo M, Aoyama Y, Murase T. A novel donor splice-site mutation in the glycogen debranching enzyme gene is associated with glycogen storage disease type III. *Biochem Biophysi Res Commun* 1996;**255**:695.

71   Borowitz SM, Green HL. Cornstarch therapy in a patient with type III glycogen storage disease. *J Pediatr Gastroenterol Nutr* 1987;**6**:631.

72   Gremse DA, Bucuvals JC, Balistreri WF. Efficacy of cornstarch therapy in type III glycogen-storage disease. *Am J Clin Nutr* 1990;**52**:671.

73   Ullrich K, Schmidt H, van Teeffelen-Heithoof A. Glycogen storage disease type I and III and pyruvate carboxylase deficiency: results of long-term treatment with uncooked cornstarch. *Acta Paediatr Scand* 1988;**77**:531.

74   Slonim AE, Weisberg C, Benke P, *et al*. Reversal of debrancher deficiency myopathy by the use of high protein nutrition. *Ann Neurol* 1982;**11**:420.

75   Slonim AE, Coleman RA, Moses WS. Myopathy and growth failure in debrancher enzyme deficiency: Improvement with high-protein nocturnal enteral therapy. *J Pediatr* 1984;**105**:906.

76   Nyhan WL, Rice-Asaro M, Acosta P. Advances in the treatment of amino acid and organic acid disorders: in *Treatment of Genetic Diseases* (ed. RJ Desnick). Churchill Livingstone, New York;1991:45.

Peroxisomal disorders

Adrenoleukodystrophy

MAJOR PHENOTYPIC EXPRESSION

X-linked cerebral demyelinating disease with onset in males in childhood, usually with behavioral abnormalities progressive to dementia, speech difficulty and loss of vision and hearing; relentless progression to decorticate spastic quadriparesis; pigmentation of the skin; adrenal insufficiency; cytoplasmic inclusions; accumulation of very long-chain fatty acids, particularly hexacosanoate (C26:0); defective activity of very long-chain acylCoA synthetase; and abnormal adenosine triphosphate- (ATP)-binding cassette (ABC) peroxisomal transmembrane transporter protein.

INTRODUCTION

Adrenoleukodystrophy is a progressive cerebral degenerative disorder with onset in childhood, in which there is increased pigmentation of the skin and laboratory evidence of degenerative disease of the adrenals [1,2]. The disease appears to have been first described by Haberfield and Spielerwere in 1910 [3], and the neuropathological findings by Schilder [4]. Siemerling and Creutzfeld were in 1923 [5] the first to put together the adrenal and cerebral disease in the definitive description; they referred to it as a bronzed disease in which there was sclerosis and encephalomyelitis, and it has been referred to as a bronzed Schilder disease, but in spite of the pigment, which may serve as the alerting sign to the diagnosis, most patients have full progression of the cerebral manifestations without the clinical symptomatology of adrenal insufficiency [2,6,7]. The lipid inclusions in the adrenal were first recognized by Schaumberg and colleagues [6,7] who found that they were composed of cholesterol esters [8]. The term adrenoleukodystrophy was first employed by Blaw [9]. This disease appears to be the cause of Schilder disease in most males [9].

Neonatal adrenoleukodystrophy (Chapter 64) is a very different disease with an entirely different phenotype and an autosomal recessive, as opposed to X-linked transmission.

The X-linked nature of the disease was first recognized by Fanconi, Prader and colleagues [10]. A more indolent, slowly progressive phenotype with onset even in adulthood was described in 1976 [11], and this has been referred to as adrenomyeloneuropathy [12]. Despite the slower course, characterized mainly by progressive spastic paraparesis, this is fundamentally the same disorder and the two phenotypes have been observed in siblings [13]. The disease expresses in a portion of heterozygotes, in whom the picture is of adrenomyeloneuropathy.

The cholesterol esters found in the adrenal glands contain large amounts of very long-chain fatty acids (VLCFA) [8]. Moser and colleagues [14,15] found that these elevated VLCFA could be demonstrated in blood and cultured fibroblasts, and this has become the method of choice for diagnosis. They can be demonstrated by gas chromatography and gas chromatography/mass spectrometry (GCMS). The oxidation of VLCFA takes place in peroxisomes. The enzyme that catalyzes the formation of the CoA esters of these very long-chain fatty acids is defective in this disorder (Figure 63.1) [16,17]. However, the defective gene is that of a peroxisomal membrane transporter protein [18]. The gene was mapped to Xq28 [19]. It was isolated and found to be a member of the ABC transporter family [18,20]. Of more than 200 mutations identified approximately 50 percent were missense and 24

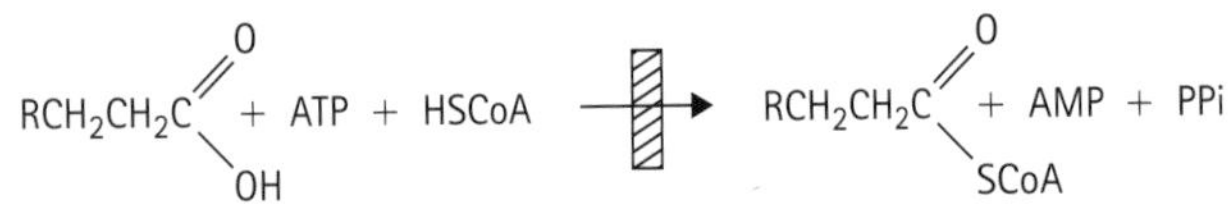

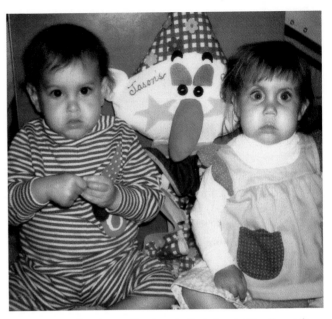

Figure 63.1 *Very-long-chain acylCoA synthetase (VLCAS), the activity is defective in adrenoleukodystrophy.*

percent frameshifts; large deletions, insertions and splicing defects are uncommon [21–23]. The gene is now referred to as ABCD1 and its product as ALDP.

CLINICAL ABNORMALITIES

The presenting findings in adrenoleukodystrophy are often behavioral [2,9,24,25] (Figures 63.2, 63.3). Some patients, who have passed early milestones normally, begin by 4 to 8-years-of age to be hyperactive and withdrawn. Others may be aggressive or belligerent, and this behavior may occur in bizarre outbursts. Initial referral is often to a psychiatrist or psychologist. Poor school performance may be another presenting problem, but often there is inattentiveness and poor concentration. Diagnosis of attention deficit disorder and treatment with stimulants such as Ritalin is a common history. There may be changes in or failing memory. Difficulty in communication or loss of acquired skills in speech is commonly encountered. In testing patients at risk the earliest manifestations may be detected by neuropsychometric testing for abnormalities in visual or auditory processing, new learning or short-term visual memory [26]. This is the classic or childhood cerebral onset phenotype that occurs in approximately 40 percent of patients. In a small number of these patients onset is in adolescence, but most begin by 3–10 years [2,8,24,25].

Visual disturbances are common in these patients and may occur early. Homonymous hemianopsia has been observed in at least two patients [2], and there may be a striking loss in visual recognition of objects. There may be a transient horizontal nystagmus in the early stages of visual loss. There may be strabismus or double vision. Ultimately, virtually all patients have a loss of vision as a prominent feature. Optic atrophy is usually a late finding, but rarely it may be seen early. The pupillary response to light remains intact until late in the illness. Hearing loss is also characteristic and may occasionally be seen as an early finding. Difficulty in understanding speech in a noisy room or over the telephone may be an early sign of impaired auditory discrimination.

Abnormalities in gait may be seen early. Characteristically, the gait is stiff-legged and unsteady. Deep tendon reflexes may be increased. Asymmetry of relatively early findings may confuse the diagnosis. A number of patients have had hemiparesis, but eventually they all develop spastic quadriparesis. Astereognosis, graphesthesia and apraxia may be seen early. Dysarthyria and dysphagia occur regularly. Once they appear, neurologic manifestations are progressive rapidly, usually over months or years, to a decorticate state in which the patient is blind and deaf. Seizures are relatively common late in the disease and may be

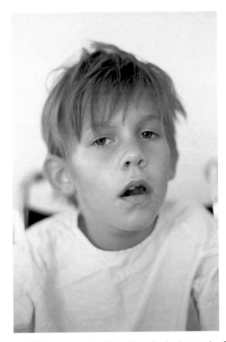

Figure 63.2 *Two boys with adrenoleukodystrophy. The diagnosis was made at 6 and 8 years-of-age, respectively. Onset was with attention deficit and hyperactivity followed by loss of verbal skills. Hyperpigmentation was particularly prominent in inguinal areas.*

Figure 63.3 *Eight-year-old with adrenoleukodystrophy. The blank open-mouthed expression was characteristic. By 9 years-of-age he was spastic and blind and had multiple contractures.*

focal or generalized. In some patients they may occur early, even as the first neurologic feature. In a series of 167 patients, the duration of disease from the onset of neurological manifestations until death was 1.9 ± 2; range was 0.5 to 10.5 years [25].

The brown pigmentation may be evident at the onset of symptoms, but it is usually found later. It occurs particularly in areas not exposed to the sun, such as skin folds, inguinal areas, areolas and the buccal mucosa. Clinical signs of adrenal insufficiency are seen in some patients and have antedated the neurologic manifestations in some patients [2]. For this reason it is worth a specific assessment for adrenoleukodystrophy in any boy who develops adrenal insufficiency during childhood. The onset of adrenal failure is usually insidious, with fatigue and intermittent vomiting. Two patients have been reported who had arterial hypotension but it is easy to see how the other manifestations of adrenal failure could be missed in a patient with advanced neurologic disease. The most useful test of adrenal function is to assess the response to adrenocorticotropin (ACTH) [25,26]. Levels of cortisol in plasma or urinary 17-hydroxy steroids may be low, but more important is a failure to respond to ACTH. Testing with metyrapone early in the illness, when the ACTH stimulation test may be normal, reveals normal pituitary function. Concentrations of electrolytes in serum have regularly been normal. Plasma levels of ACTH may be increased.

Among variant presentations patients with adrenomyeloneuropathy were so characterized because of prominent spinal cord involvement [11,12]. Initial symptoms of stiffness or clumsiness in the legs progress to spastic paraplegia. Generalized weakness, loss of weight, hyperpigmentation and attacks of vomiting are signs of adrenal insufficiency. The neurologic disease often progresses slowly over five to 15 years. The patient becomes wheelchair-bound and may develop problems with urination. Somatosensory and brainstem auditory evoked responses are abnormal. Cognitive function is abnormal in about half of the patients. Vibration sense in the lower extremities may be impaired and so may nerve conduction velocity. Impotence is common [27]. Gonadal insufficiency is ultimately common [28].

Symptoms in the female heterozygote may resemble those of adrenomyeloneuropathy. In a few, there is severe disability with paraparesis [29,30]. These women may be thought to have multiple sclerosis if there is no family history of involved males [31]. One patient had intermittent paresthesia from the age of 40 years [31]. Some asymptomatic patients have had hyperreflexia and impaired vibration sensation in the legs. Some have been diagnosed, only after they had an affected son [31]. Adrenal function is normal in most heterozygotes. Some have had dementia. Others have had an adolescent onset of the kind of progressive cerebral disease seen in the male, even with adrenal insufficiency [30,32].

Rarely, males have had an adult onset of cerebral disease without cord involvement [29]. Some have been thought to have schizophrenia, or a Kluver-Bucy syndrome [33]. Psychotic symptoms in a patient with Addison disease should trigger this diagnosis, but adrenal function may be normal.

A small number of male patients, mostly from Japan, has presented with a picture of olivopontocerebellar atrophy [34–37]. Most were adults. A Japanese 5-year-old presented with cerebellar ataxia [38]. Imaging revealed cerebellar and pontine atrophy. The disease was progressive.

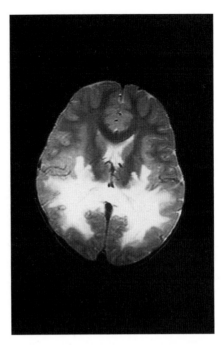

Figure 63.4   *MRI of the brain of G.Q., a 7-year-old boy with adrenoleukodystrophy. He had experienced the sudden onset of seizures after a period of disturbed behavior. He had pyramidal tract signs and spatial agnosia. Imaging revealed the typical white matter disease.*

At the other end of the spectrum three infants have been reported [39] whose phenotype was that of a peroxisomal disorder such as neonatal adrenoleukodystrophy (ALD) (Chapter 69). They had profound hypotonia (Chapter 64), failure to thrive and cholestatic hepatic disease. Two had seizures and the third episodic opisthotonus. In a single autopsy available the adrenals were small and fibrotic.

Some patients with this disease have had pure Addison disease without neurologic findings [39,40]. In areas in which adrenal tuberculosis is rare, this disorder may represent a significant proportion of patients with Addison disease. Some patients, found by testing relatives of known patients, have been asymptomatic for long periods of time, but it is expected that they will all sooner or later develop neurologic abnormalities. Some have developed prominent cerebellar signs or a picture of olivopontocerebellar degeneration [35–37,41].

Neuroimaging by computed tomography (CT) or magnetic resonance imaging (MRI) [42–44] reveals evidence of leukodystrophy in the cerebral white matter (Figures 63.4–63.6). Temporal and parieto-occipital involvement is seen most frequently, but there may be widespread involvement including the cerebellar white matter and the corticospinal tracts. Some patients have had cerebral atrophy. There are widespread symmetric, confluent, low density lesions on CT or T1-weighted MRI or increased density on T2 in the periventricular white matter of the parieto-occipital areas that enhance anteriorly in the CT on infusion of contrast material. Repeated scans over time show a caudal-rostral progression of the demyelination. The enhancement with contrast reflects breakdown of the blood–brain barrier, and this is seen also on brain

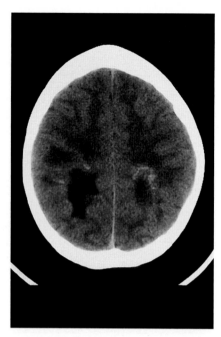

Figure 63.5   *CT scan of the brain of H.M., a boy with adrenoleukodystrophy. There was extensive leukodystrophy and calcification around the lucent area of demyelination.*

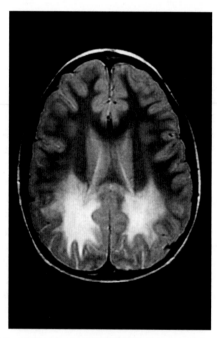

Figure 63.6   *MRI of the brain of H.M. The intense T2 signal in the white matter was indicative of the leukodystrophy.*

scintiscan, which shows increased uptake in the involved areas. In some patients the lesions found on imaging the white matter have been the first clue to the diagnosis. In a few patients atypical unilateral lesions have, along with, in one patient, symptomatology of unilateral headache, visual loss, weakness and hyperreflexia, led to a diagnosis of brain tumor [45]. Biopsy revealed leukodystrophy and led to the diagnosis.

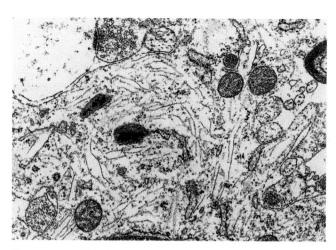

Figure 63.7   *Electron microscopic section of the brain, illustrating the characteristic fine thin spicules. These cytoplasmic inclusions may be straight or curved and contain a central electrolucent space bound by a thin electrodense membrane. (Illustration kindly provided by Henry Powell of the University of California, San Diego.)*

Brainstem auditory evoked responses in adrenoleukodystrophy may be abnormal [46] asymmetry in that wave VI on one side may be absent. There may be progressive loss so that ultimately only a prolonged wave I is recordable bilaterally [47]. Electroencephalograms (EEG) are usually abnormal, most commonly showing diffuse slow activity or large-amplitude slow waves over the posterior regions [48].

Pathological examination of the nervous system reveals extensive diffuse demyelination in the cerebral white matter, most prominent in the occipital and posterior parietal areas and spreading in a caudal-rostral direction [2,49,50]. There is secondary loss of axons and gliosis. Late findings may be cavitation or calcification. In addition there are diffuse perivascular infiltrations of lymphocytes. These inflammatory findings are not seen in adrenomyeloneuropathy, which is predominantly a distal axonopathy [50]. In the adrenal gland there are ballooned cortical cells, which have characteristic striations [7].

The nature of the disorder was originally clarified by the finding of characteristic cytoplasmic inclusions in large glial cells or macrophages of the central nervous system and in adrenal cortical cells [49,51,52]. The inclusions in the central nervous system stain positive with periodic acid-Schiff (PAS) and Oil Red O stains. Sudanophilia is common, but may be absent. The electron microscope reveals the pathognomonic ultrastructure of curvilinear spicules with central lucent spaces (Figures 63.7, 63.8) [49,51]. Similar inclusions have been seen in Schwann cells [52], making the diagnosis possible by sural nerve biopsy, but this has more often been negative [2]. Testicular tissue may show identical ultrastructural lamellar lesions [53]. Characteristic ultrastructural lesions have been seen in Schwann cells obtained by conjunctival biopsy, and vacuoles have been seen in eccrine glands of the skin [54]. Chemical methods have largely supplanted biopsy approaches to diagnosis.

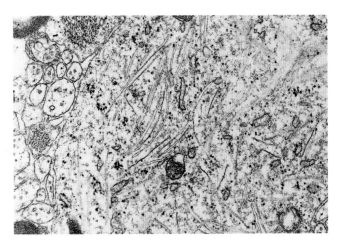

Figure 63.8 *Cytoplasm of this brain cell illustrates the characteristic scimitar-shaped inclusions. (Illustration kindly provided by Dr. Henry Powell of the University of California, San Diego.)*

GENETICS AND PATHOGENESIS

Adrenoleukodystrophy is an X-linked disorder that is not fully recessive in its expression, as there may be clinical expression in female heterozygotes.

The specific biochemical abnormality in adrenoleukodystrophy is the accumulation of very long-chain unbranched fatty acids, which are saturated or mono-unsaturated. The carbon lengths of these compounds are 24 to 30. They are found normally among the fatty acids of the cholesterol esters and gangliosides of the cerebral white matter and the adrenal cortex, and C26:0 makes up as much as five percent of the total fatty acids of cerebrosides and sulfatides of the normal brain [8,55–57]. Similarly, the VLCFA that accumulate in adrenoleukodystrophy are predominantly those with a chain length of 26. They are largely hexacosanoic acid (C26:0) (cerotic acid). Accumulation of these VLCFA has been demonstrated in cultured fibroblasts [14,57,58] and muscle cells [59,60]. In cultured fibroblasts, the ratio of C26 to C22 fatty acids has been useful in diagnosis, as well as the level of C26:0 [14]. The ratio was 0.76 in six patients with clinically typical disease and 0.78 in five patients with autopsy proven disease, while in controls it was 0.06. The concentrations of these same very long-chain saturated fatty acids in plasma are also increased [61], and this is the most convenient method for definitive diagnosis. The levels of C24 (lignoceric acid), C25 and C26 are significantly elevated, while those of C20 and C22 are normal. The C26:C22 ratios of hemizygotes are approximately five times those of controls. In general, the plasma assay is sufficient for diagnosis. In instances in which the data are equivocal, the fibroblast assay is employed. The accumulation of VLCFA in patients with adrenomyeloneuropathy is no different than in patients with classic adrenoleukodystrophy [14].

The accumulation of VLCFA in adrenoleukodystrophy is a consequence of abnormality in the oxidation of these VLCFA, which takes place in peroxisomes [62,63]. Studies of oxidation to $^{14}CO_2$ of ^{14}C-labeled fatty acids in fibroblasts revealed impaired production of CO_2 in adrenoleukodystrophy [64]. Oxidation of hexacosanoic (C26:0) acid was 14 percent of control, and that of lignoceric (tetracosanoic) (C24:0) was eight percent of control.

Heterozygotes can be detected by assay of the very long-chain fatty acids of plasma or cultured fibroblasts [64]. Levels in both plasma and fibroblasts, especially using the ratios of C26:C22, or C24:C22, were intermediate between patients and controls, and significantly different from the latter, but there was a small amount of overlap. By assaying both fibroblasts and plasma, over 90 percent of obligate heterozygotes can be identified [65]. Cloning of fibroblasts from heterozygotes yielded two populations of cells, one normal and the other identical to patients with adrenoleukodystrophy in its C26 fatty acid content [65]. These experiments proved that the gene is on the X chromosome and that it is subject to inactivation. Studies of women doubly heterozygous for glucose-6-phosphate dehydrogenase (G-6-PD) revealed close linkage between the two loci [65].

The gene for G-6-PD has been mapped to Xq28 [66], localizing the gene for adrenoleukodystrophy to this locus of the X chromosome. This has led to the exploration of DNA probes, and DXS52 was found to be closely linked to adrenoleukodystrophy [67,68]. The only instance so far tested that looked like recombination turned out to be gonadal mosaicism in a grandmother [69]. The linkage can be used in heterozygote detection [70] and effectively resolves any situations in which the assay of VLCFA is not clear. Mutation analysis is the most reliable method for detection of heterozygosity [70].

The linkage to DXS52 has also been used successfully in prenatal diagnosis [71,72]. The assay for VLCFA is usually employed as the procedure of choice for prenatal identification of the affected male fetus [73]. Cultured amniocytes and chorionic villus material have been used, but normal VLCFA have been found in cultured chorionic villus cells in pregnancies where the fetus turned out to be affected [74,75]. Oxidation of C26:0 fatty acid in cultured chorionic villus material has been employed for prenatal diagnosis [76]. In terminated pregnancies, fetal ultrastructural as well as chemical abnormalities were clearly present. When the mutation is known it provides a definitive method of prenatal diagnosis [77,78].

Defective oxidation of VLCFA in this disease is a consequence of failure to form the coenzyme A esters. The synthetase enzyme (Figure 63.1) whose activity is defective has been localized to the peroxisome [79–81].

The gene for adrenoleukodystrophy was found by positional cloning within the Xq28 region [18]. It spans approximately 20 kb in 10 exons. The deduced amino acid sequence placed it among the ATP-binding cassette superfamily of transmembrane transporter proteins [82]. The structure has extensive similarities to the 70 kDa peroxisomal membrane protein, PXMP 1 [18]. A few deletions in the gene were identified in patients by Southern blot analysis [18]. A majority of the mutations are missense, and a majority of all mutations are unique to the family in which they are found [23].

Mutations have clustered in the membrane spanning region and in the nucleotide binding region, and there is a hot spot in exon 5. Correlation between genotype and phenotype has not been possible. Polymorphism has also been identified (N13T) which caused amino acid change but does not affect function of the ALDP [21]. In the 3 patients with neonatal presentations suggestive of peroxisomal disease [39] there was no immunochemically defectable ALDP, and large deletions were found in the ABCD1 promoter region and the adjacent DXS1357E gene. Deletions in this latter gene cause creatine deficiency in brain as a result of deficiency in the X-linked creatine transporter gene (SLC6A8) [83].

It is not clear how the defect in the gene affects VLCFA synthetase activity, and ALDP does not function as a synthetase. Nevertheless, it appears likely that the disease in the central nervous system and in the adrenal results from the accumulation of VLCFA [84,85].

TREATMENT

The course of adrenoleukodystrophy has usually been relentless, and no therapeutic measures appear to be effective. Symptomatic therapy is important [86], and support groups may be helpful to families. Physiologic amounts of adrenal steroid replacement therapy are effective in the management of the adrenal disease.

Bone marrow transplantation has been carried out without improvement in neurologic status, but encouraging results have been obtained in patients treated early in their courses [87–91]. It is reported that some patients have become clinically stable after transplantation, and some have even improved. In patients studied with proton MR spectroscopy, transplanted patients fell midway between controls and untreated patients in the ratios of N-acetylaspartate (NAA) to creatinine and NAA to choline [91]. Criteria for transplantation remain unclear, but increasingly patients are transplanted for worsening MR imaging before clinical regression.

Studies using deuterium-labeled hexacosanoic acid indicated that a substantial amount of the C26 fatty acids in the brain is of dietary origin [92]. Although there is also evidence that fibroblasts of patients are able, unlike controls, to synthesize C26 fatty acid from stearic acid [93], these observations have raised the possibility of dietary therapy. Restriction of the intake of very long-chain fatty acids has been undertaken in this disease without effect on levels of VLCFA or clinical course. The observation [94] that the addition of mono-unsaturated fatty acids such as oleic acid to cultured fibroblasts of patients leads to reduction in accumulation of VLCFA, led to the use of glyceryltrioleate in therapy. Glyceryltrierucate was even more effective *in vitro* [95], and this has led to the development of Lorenzo's oil, a 4:1 mixture of trioleate and trierucate oils, named after the patient. Treatment does bring plasma levels of C26:0 to normal, but it is clear that the neurologic progression of the disease is not halted. Double blind placebo-controlled studies have not been done, but Lorenzo's oil does not appear to be useful in patients who have demonstrated neurological regression [96,97]. It may be worth exploring in patients with adrenomyeloneuropathy, but the evidence is against it [98]. Many patients develop thrombocytopenia [99] and so platelet counts must be monitored. Levels of essential fatty acids should be monitored to prevent deficiency.

By analogy with its beneficial effect in sickle cell anemia, where it increases fetal hemoglobin, butyrate and 4-phenylbutyrate have been explored in adrenoleukodystrophy. Cultured cells from patients were found to have improvement in the oxidation of VLCFA and amounts of stored VLCFA in the brain of a mouse model were decreased by exposure to phenylbutyrate [100]. Preliminary studies in man are underway.

References

1 Moser HW, Moser AB, Kawamura N, *et al.* Adrenoleukodystrophy: studies of the phenotype genetics and biochemistry. *Johns Hopkins Med J* 1980;**147**:217.

2 Schaumberg HH, Powers JM, Raine CS, *et al.* Adrenoleukodystrophy. A clinical and pathological study of 17 cases. *Arch Neurol* 1975;**32**:577.

3 Haberfeld W, Spieler F. Zur diffusen Hirn-Rueckenmarksclerose im Kindesalter. *Dtch Z Nervenh* 1910;**40**:436.

4 Schilder P. Zur frage der encephalitis periaxialis diffusa (sogenannet diffuse sklerose). *Z Neuro Psych* 1913;**15**:359.

5 Siemerling E, Creutzfeld HG. Bronzekrankheit und sklerosierende encephalomyelitis. *Arch Psychiatr Nervenkr* 1923;**68**:217.

6 Schaumberg HH, Richardson EP, Johnson PC, *et al.* Schilder's disease: sex-linked transmission with specific adrenal changes. *Arch Neurol* 1972;**27**:458.

7 Powers JM, Schaumberg HH. The adrenal cortex in adrenoleukodystrophy. *Arch Pathol* 1973;**96**:305.

8 Igarashi M, Schaumberg HH, Powers JM, *et al.* Fatty acid abnormality in adrenoleukodystrophy. *J Neurochem* 1976;**26**:851.

9 Blaw ME. Melanodermic type leukodystrophy (adrenoleukodystrophy): in *Handbook of Clinical Neurology* Vol 10 (eds PJ Vinken, GW Bruyn). American Elsevier, New York;1970:128.

10 Fanconi VA, Prader A, Isler W, *et al.* Morbus Addison mit hirnsklerose im kindesalter D. Ein hereditares syndrom mit X-chromosomaler vererbung? *Helv Paediatr Acta* 1963;**18**:480.

11 Budka H, Sluga E, Heiss WD. Spastic paraplegia associated with Addison's disease: adult variant of adrenoleukodystrophy. *J Neurol* 1976;**213**:237.

12 Griffin JW, Goren E, Schaumberg H, *et al.* Adrenomyeloneuropathy: a probable variant of adrenoleukodystrophy. *Neurology* 1977;**27**:1107.

13 Davis LE, Snyder RD, Orth DN, *et al.* Adrenoleukodystrophy and adrenoneuropathy associated with partial adrenal insufficiency in three generations of a kindred. *Am J Med* 1979;**66**:342.

14 Moser HW, Moser AB, Kawamura N, *et al.* Elevated C-26 fatty acid in cultured skin fibroblasts. *Ann Neurol.* 1980;**7**:542.

15 Moser HW, Moser AB, Frayer KK, *et al.* Adrenoleukodystrophy: increased plasma content of saturated very-long-chain fatty acids. *Neurology* 1981;**31**:1241.

16 Wanders RJA, van Roermund CWT, van Wijland MJA, *et al.* Direct evidence that the deficient oxidation of very-long-chain fatty acids in X-linked adrenoleukodystrophy is due to an impaired ability of peroxisomes to activate very-long-chain fatty acids. *Biochem Biophys Res Commun* 1988;**153**:618.

17 Lazo O, Contreras M, Hashmi M, *et al*. Peroxisomal lignoceroyl-CoA ligase deficiency in childhood adrenoleukodystrophy and adrenomyeloneuropathy. *Proc Natl Acad Sci USA* 1988;**85**:7647.

18 Mosser J, Douar AM, Sarde CO, *et al*. Putative X-linked adrenoleukodystrophy gene shares unexpected homology with ABC transporters. *Nature* 1993;**361**:726.

19 Aubourg P, Sack GH, Meyers DA, *et al*. Linkage of adrenoleukodystrophy to a polymorphic DNA probe. *Ann Neurol* 1987;**21**:349.

20 Higgins CF. ABC transporters: from microorganisms to man. *Annu Rev Cell Biol* 1992;**8**:67.

21 Dvorakova L, Storkanova G, Unterrainer G, *et al*. Eight novel ABCD1 gene mutations and three polymorphisms in patients with X-linked adrenoleukodystrophy: the first polymorphism causing an amino acid exchange. *Hum Mutat* 2001;**18**:52.

22 Electronic database http://www.x-aldnl (accessed December 2004).

23 Smith KD, Kemp S, Braiterman LT, *et al*. X-linked adrenoleukodystrophy: genes mutations and phenotypes. *Neurochem Res* 1999;**24**:521.

24 Aubourg P, Chaussain JL, Dulac O, Arthuis M. Adrenoleukodystrophy in childhood: a review of 20 cases. *Arch Fr Pediatr* 1982;**39**:663.

25 Moser HW, Naidu S, Kumar AJ, Rosenbaum AE. The adrenoleukodystrophies. *CRC Crit Rev Neurobiol* 1987;**3**:29.

26 Forsyth CC, Forbes M, Cummings JH. Adrenocortical atrophy and diffuse cerebral sclerosis. *Arch Dis Child* 1971;**46**:273.

27 Powers JM, Schaumburg HH. A fatal cause of sexual inadequacy in men: adrenoleukodystrophy. *J Urol* 1980;**124**:583.

28 Assies J, van Geel B, Barth P. Signs of testicular insufficiency in adrenomyeloneuropathy and neurologically asyptomatic X-linked adrenoleukodystrophy; a retrospective study. *Int J Androl* 1997;**20**:315.

29 Moser HW, Moser AB, Naidu S, Bergin A. Clinical aspects of adrenoleukodystrophy and adrenomyeloneuropathy. *Dev Neurosci* 1991;**13**:254.

30 Noetzel MJ, Landau WM, Moser HW. Adrenoleukodystrophy carrier state presenting as a chronic nonprogressive spinal cord disorder. *Arch Neurol* 1987;**44**:566.

31 Dooley JM, Wright BA. Adrenoleukodystrophy mimicking multiple sclerosis. *Can J Neurol Sci* 1985;**12**:73.

32 Heffungs W, Hameisier H, Ropers HH. Addison's disease and cerebral sclerosis in an apparently heterozygous girl: evidence of inactivation of the adrenoleukodystrophy locus. *Clin Genet* 1980;**18**:184.

33 Powers JM, Schaumburg HH, Gaffney CL. Kluver-Bucy syndrome caused by adrenoleukodystrophy. *Neurology* 1980;**30**:1131.

34 Tateish J, Sato Y, Suetsugu M, Takshiba T. Adrenoleukodystrophy with olivopontocerebellar atrophy-like lesions. *Clin Neuropath* 1986;**5**:34.

35 Marsden CD, Obeso JA, Lang AE. Adrenoleukomyeloneuropathy presenting as spinocerebellar degeneration. *Neurology* 1982;**32**:1031.

36 Kuroda S, Kirano A, Yuasa S. Adrenoleukodystrophy: cerebello-brainstem dominant case. *Acta Neuropath* 1983;**60**:149.

37 Ohno T, Tsuchida H, Fukuhara N, *et al*. Adrenoleukodystrophy: a clinical variant presenting as olivopontocerebellar atrophy. *J Neurol* 1984;**231**:167.

38 Kurihara M, Kumagai K, Yagishita S, *et al*. Adrenoleukomyeloneuropathy presenting as cerebellar ataxia in a young child: a probable variant of adrenoleukodystrophy. *Brain Dev* 1993;**15**:377.

39 Corzo D, Gibson W, Johnson K, *et al*. Contiguous deletion of the X-linked adrenoleukodystrophy gene (ABCD1) and DXS1357E: a novel neonatal phenotype similar to peroxisomal biogenesis disorders. *Am J Hum Genet* 2002;**70**:1520.

40 Moser HW, Bergin A, Naidu S, Ladenson PW. Adrenoleukodystrophy: new aspects of adrenal cortical disease. *Endocrinol Metab Clin N Am* 1991;**20**:297.

41 Takada K, Onoda J, Takahashi K, *et al*. An adult case of adrenoleukodystrophy with features of olivo-ponto-cerebellar atrophy. *Jpn J Exp Med* 1987;**57**:53.

42 Duda EE, Huttenlocher PR. Computed tomography in adrenoleukodystrophy: correlation of radiological and histological findings. *Radiology* 1976;**120**:349.

43 Kumar AJ, Rosenbaum AE, Naidu S, *et al*. Adrenoleukodystrophy: correlating MR imaging with CT. *Radiology* 1987;**165**:496.

44 Aubourg P, Adamsbaum C, Lavallard-Rosseau MC, *et al*. Brain MRI and electrophysiologic abnormalities in preclinical and clinical adrenomyeloneuropathy. *Neurology* 1992;**42**:85.

45 Afifi AK, Menenez X, Reed LA, Bell WA. Atypical presentation of X-linked childhood adrenoleukodystrophy with an unusual magnetic resonance imaging pattern. *J Child Neurol* 1996;**11**:497.

46 Black HA, Fariello RG, Chun RW. Brain stem auditory evoked response in adrenoleukodystrophy. *Ann Neurol* 1979;**6**:269.

47 Kaga K, Tokoro Y, Tanaka Y, Ushijima H. The progress of adrenoleukodystrophy as revealed by auditory brainstem evoked responses and brainstem histology. *Arch Otorhinolaryngol* 1980;**228**:17.

48 Mamoli B, Graf M, Toifi K. EEG pattern-evoked potentials and nerve conduction velocity in a family with adrenoleukodystrophy. *Electroencephalogr Clin Neurophysiol* 1979;**14**:411.

49 Schaumburg HH, Powers JM, Suzuki K, Paine CS. Adrenoleukodystrophy (sex-linked Schilder's disease). Ultrastructural demonstration of specific cytoplasmic inclusions in the central nervous system. *Arch Neurol* 1974;**31**:210.

50 Powers JM. Adrenoleukodystrophy (adreno-testiculo-leukomyelo-neuropathic-complex). *Clin Neuropathol* 1985;**4**:181.

51 Powell H, Tindall R, Schultz P, *et al*. Adrenoleukodystrophy: electron microscopic findings. *Arch Neurol* 1975;**32**:250.

52 Powers JM, Schaumburg HH. Adrenoleuko-dystrophy: similar ultrastructural changes in adrenal cortical cells and Schwann cells. *Arch Neurol.* 1974;**30**:406.

53 Powers JM, Schaumburg HH. The testis in adrenoleukodystrophy. *Am J Pathol* 1981;**81**:90.

54 Martin JJ, Ceuterick C, Martin L, Libert J. Skin and conjunctival biopsies in adrenoleukodystrophy. *Acta Neuropath* 1977;**38**:247.

55 Brown FR III, Chen WW, Kirschner DA, *et al*. Myelin membrane from adrenoleukodystrophy brain white matter – isolation and physical/chemical properties. *J Neurochem* 1983;**41**:341.

56 Menkes JH, Corbo LM. Adrenoleukodystrophy. Accumulation of cholesterol esters with very-long-chain fatty acids. *Neurol (Minneapolis)* 1977;**27**:928.

57 Kawamura N, Moser AB, Moser HW, *et al*. High concentration of hexacosanoate in cultured skin fibroblast from adrenoleukodystrophy patients. *Biochem Biophys Res Commun* 1978;**82**:114.

58 Tonshoff B, Lehnert W, Ropers H-H. Adrenoleukodystrophy: diagnosis and carrier. Detection by determination of long-chain fatty acids in cultured fibroblasts. *Clin Genet* 1982;**22**:25.

59 Askanas V, McLaughlin JM, Engel WK, Adornato BT. Abnormalities in cultured muscle and peripheral nerve of a patient with adrenomyeloneuropathy. *N Engl J Med* 1979;**301**:588.

60 McLaughlin J, Askanas V, Engel WK. Adrenomyeloneuropathy: increased accumulation of very long-chain fatty acid in cultured skeletal muscle. *Biochem Biophys Res Commun* 1980;**92**:1202.

61 Rezanker T. Very long chain fatty acids from the animal and plant kingdoms. *Prog Lipid Res* 1989;**28**:147.

62 Schutgens RBH, Heymans HSA, Wanders RJA, *et al*. Peroxisomal disorders: a newly recognized group of genetic diseases. *Eur J Pediatr* 1986;**144**:430.

63 Singh I, Moser HW, Moser AB, Kishimoto Y. Adrenoleukodystrophy: impaired oxidations of long chain fatty acids in cultured skin fibroblasts and adrenal cortex. *Biochem Biophys Res Commun* 1981;**102**:1223.

64 Moser HW, Moser AB, Trojak JE, Supplee SW. Identification of female carriers of adrenoleukodystrophy. *J Pediatr* 1983;**103**:54.

65 Migeon BR, Moser HW, Moser AB, *et al*. Adrenoleukodystrophy: evidence for X linkage inactivation and selection favoring the mutant allele in heterozygous cells. *Proc Natl Acad Sci USA* 1981;**78**:5066.

66 Pai GS, Sprenkle JA, Do TT, *et al.* Localization of loci for hypoxanthine phosphoribosyltransferase and glucose-6-hypoxanthine dehydrogenase and biochemical evidence of nonrandom X-chromosome expression from studies of a human X-autosome translocation. *Proc Natl Acad Sci USA* 1980;**77**:2810.

67 Oberle I, Drayna D, Camerino G, *et al.* The telomere of the human X-chromosome long arm: presence of a highly polymorphic DNA marker and analysis of recombination frequency. *Proc Natl Acad Sci USA* 1985;**82**:2824.

68 Willems PJ, Vits L, Wanders RJ, *et al.* Linkage of DNA markers at Xq28 to adrenoleukodystrophy and adrenomyeloneuropathy present within the same family. *Arch Neurol* 1990;**47**:665.

69 Graham CE, MacLeod PM, Lillicrap DP, Bridge PJ. Gonadal mosaicism in a family with adrenoleukodystrophy: molecular diagnosis of carrier status among daughters of a gonadal mosaic when direct detection of the mutation is not possible. *J Inherit Metab Dis* 1992;**15**:68.

70 Boehm CD, Cutting GR, Lachtermacher MB, *et al.* Accurate DNA-based diagnostic and carrier testing for X-linked adrenoleukodystrophy. *Mol Genet Metab* 1999;**66**:128.

71 Boue J, Oberle I, Mandel JL, *et al.* First trimester prenatal diagnosis of adrenoleukodystrophy by determination of very-long-chain fatty acid levels and by linkage analysis to a DNA probe. *Hum Genet* 1985;**69**:272.

72 Moser AB, Moser HW. The prenatal diagnosis of X-linked adrenoleuko-dystrophy. *Prenat Diag* 1999;**19**:46.

73 Moser HW, Moser AB, Powers JM, *et al.* The prenatal diagnosis of adrenoleukodystrophy. Demonstration of increased hexacosanoic acid levels in cultured amniocytes and fetal adrenal gland. *Pediat Res* 1982;**16**:172.

74 Carey WF, Poulos A, Sharp P, *et al.* Pitfalls in the prenatal diagnosis of peroxisomal beta oxidation defects by chorionic villus sampling. *Prenat Diag* 1994;**14**:813.

75 Gray RGF, Green A, Cole T, *et al.* A misdiagnosis of X-linked adrenoleukodystrophy in cultured chorionic villus cells by the measurement of very long chain fatty acids. *Prenat Diag* 1995;**15**:486.

76 Wanders RJA, van Wijland MJA, van Roermund CWT, *et al.* Prenatal diagnosis of Zellweger syndrome by measurement of very-long-chain fatty acid (C26:0) b-oxidation in cultured chorionic villus fibroblasts: implications for early diagnosis of other peroxisomal disorders. *Clin Chim Acta* 1987;**165**:303.

77 Maier EM, Roscher AA, Kammerer S, *et al.* Prenatal diagnosis of X-linked adrenoleukodystrophy combining biochemical immunocytochemical and DNA analyses. *Prenat Diag* 1999;**19**:364.

78 Imamura A, Suzuki Y, Song XQ, *et al.* Prenatal diagnosis of adrenoleuko-dystrophy by means of mutation analysis. *Prenat Diagn* 1996;**16**:259.

79 Mannaerts GP, van Veldhoven P, Van Broekhoven A, *et al.* Evidence that peroxisomal acyl-CoA synthetase is located at the cytoplasmic side of the peroxisomal membrane. *Biochem J* 1982;**204**:17.

80 Lageweg W, Tager JM, Wanders JA. Topography of very-long-chain fatty acid activating activity in peroxisomes from rat liver. *Biochem J* 1991;**276**:53.

81 Lazo O, Contreras M, Yoshida Y, *et al.* Cellular oxidation of lignoceric acid is regulated by the subcellular localization of lignoceroyl-CoA ligases. *J Lipid Res* 1990;**31**:583.

82 Sarde C-O, Mosser J, Kioschis P, *et al.* Genomic organization of the adrenoleukodystrophy gene. *Genomics* 1994;**23**:13.

83 Salomons GS, van Dooren SJ, Verhoeven NM, *et al.* X-linked creatine-transporter gene (SLC6A8) defect: a new creatine-deficiency syndrome. *Am J Hum Genet* 2001;**68**:1497.

84 Theda C, Moser AB, Powers JM, Moser HW. Phospholipids in X-linked adrenoleukodystrophy white matter – fatty acid abnormalities before the onset of demyelination. *J Neurol Sci* 1992;**110**:195.

85 Reinecke CJ, Knoll DP, Pretorius PJ, *et al.* The correlation between biochemical and histopathological findings in adrenoleukodystrophy. *J Neurol Sci* 1985;**70**:21.

86 Brown FR III, Stowens DW, Harris JC Jr, Moser HW. The leukodystrophies: in *Current Therapy in Neurologic Disease* (ed. RT Johnson) Decker, Philadelphia;1985:313.

87 Krivit W, Shapiro EG, Balthazor M, *et al.* Hurler syndrome: outcomes and planning following bone marrow transplantation: in *Correction of Genetic Diseases by Transplantation III* (eds CC Steward, JR Hobbs). Westminster, London;1995:25.

88 Aubourg P, Blanche S, Jambaque I, *et al.* Reversal of early neurologic and neuroradiologic manifestations of X-linked adrenoleukodystrophy by bone marrow transplantation. *N Engl J Med* 1990;**322**:1860.

89 Moser HW, Moser AB, Smith KD, *et al.* Adrenoleukodystrophy: phenotypic variability. Implications for therapy. *J Inherit Metab Dis* 1992;**15**:645.

90 Baumann M, Korenke GC, Weddige-Diedrichs A, *et al.* Haematopoietic stem cell transplantation in 12 patients with cerebral X-linked adrenoleukodystrophy. *Eur J Pediatr* 2003;**162**:6.

91 Rajanayagam V, Grad J, Krivit W, *et al.* Proton MR spectroscopy of childhood adrenoleukodystrophy. *Am J Neuroradiol* 1996;**17**:1013.

92 Kishimoto Y, Moser HW, Kawamura N, *et al.* Adrenoleukodystrophy: evidence that abnormal very long-chain fatty acids of brain cholesterol esters are of exogenous origin. *Biochem Biophys Res Commun* 1980;**96**:69.

93 Tsuji S, Sano T, Ariga T, Miyatake T. Increased synthesis of hexacosanoic acid (C26:0) by cultured skin fibroblasts from patients with adrenoleukodystrophy (ALD) and adrenomyeloneuropathy (AMN). *J Biochem* 1981;**90**:1233.

94 Rizzo WB, Watkins PA, Phillips MW, *et al.* Adrenoleukodystrophy: oleic acid lowers fibroblast saturated C22:C26 fatty acids. *Neurology* 1986;**36**:357.

95 Rizzo WB, Leshner RT, Odone A, *et al.* Dietary erucic acid therapy for X-linked adrenoleukodystrophy. *Neurology* 1989;**39**:1415.

96 van Geel BM, Assies J, Haverkort EB, *et al.* Progression of abnormalities in adrenomyeloneuropathy and neurologically asymptomatic X-linked adrenoleukodystrophy despite treatment with 'Lorenzo's Oil'. *J Neurol Neurosurg Psychiatry* 1999;**67**:290.

97 Moser HW. Lorenzo Oil therapy for adrenoleukodystrophy: a prematurely amplified hope. *Ann Neurol* 1993;**34**:121.

98 Aubourg P, Adamsbaum C, Lavallard-Rousseau M-C, *et al.* A two-year trial of oleic and erucic acids ('Lorenzo's Oil') as treatment for adrenomyeloneuropathy. *N Engl J Med* 1993;**329**:745.

99 Zinkham WH, Kickler T, Borel J, Moser HW. Lorenzo's oil and thrombocytopenia in patients with adrenoleukodystrophy. *N Engl J Med* 1993;**328**:1126.

100 Lu J-F, Lawler AM, Watkins PA, *et al.* A mouse model for X-linked adrenoleukodystrophy. *Proc Natl Acad Sci USA* 1997;**94**:9366.

64

Neonatal adrenoleukodystrophy/disorders of peroxisomal biogenesis

---

MAJOR PHENOTYPIC EXPRESSION

Profound hypotonia, seizure disorder, hepatic fibrosis, atrophic adrenals, accumulation of very long-chain saturated fatty acids, pipecolic aciduria and defective biogenesis of peroxisomes as a result of failure to import peroxisomal proteins.

INTRODUCTION

Neonatal adrenoleukodystrophy was first described in 1978 by Ulrich and colleagues [1]. A relatively small number of patients has since been recognized [2–12]. Accumulation of very long-chain fatty acids (VLCFA) in this condition is indicative of multiple defective peroxisomal functions. This disorder, infantile Refsum disease, hyperpipecolic aciduria and Zellweger syndrome fall into the same group of disorders of peroxisomal biogenesis, but at least 12 complementation groups have been identified, indicating fundamental defects in a number of steps in peroxisomal biogenesis [13–15]. Among them Zellweger is the most severe, but neonatal adrenoleukodystrophy is also a very severe disease. No correlation between complementation group and phenotype has emerged. Zellweger syndrome is found in at least 10 complementation groups and neonatal adrenoleukodystrophy in at least six of the same groups. Among patients with Zellweger syndrome, one has been shown to have a defect in peroxisomal assembly factor 1 (PAF 1), a 35 kDa membrane protein involved in the assembly of peroxisomes [16]. Two patients were found to have mutated alleles in the 70 kDa peroxisomal membrane protein (PMP70) [17], which is a member of the multiple drug resistance-related adenosine triphosphate-(ATP)-binding cassette transporter superfamily. Patients with defective biogenesis of peroxisomes have abnormality in virtually every peroxisomal function, notably the peroxisomal β-oxidation of fatty acids (Figure 64.1).

Another peroxisomal assembly protein, PXR1, is the site of the defect in some patients with neonatal adrenoleukodystrophy. Two mutations have been identified: a nonsense and a missense mutation [18]. Genes for peroxisomal biogenesis in yeast have been extensively studied; they are referred to as PEX genes, and this usage has been adopted for the human orthologs [19]. Proteins that mediate the import of peroxisomal matrix proteins are called peroxins, and they are encoded by PEX genes. Members of the various complementation groups have mutations in what are now known as the human PEX genes. Thus the mutations in the patient with neonatal adrenoleukodystrophy, referred to initially as PXR1 are in the PEX 5 gene on chromosome 12p13. PEX1, the first PEX gene to be identified in yeast [20] situated on human chromosome 7q21-22 is the most common cause of neonatal adrenoleukodystrophy and Zellweger syndrome [21].

CLINICAL ABNORMALITIES

The clinical picture of neonatal adrenoleukodystrophy is dominated by extreme hypotonia and a severe convulsive disorder

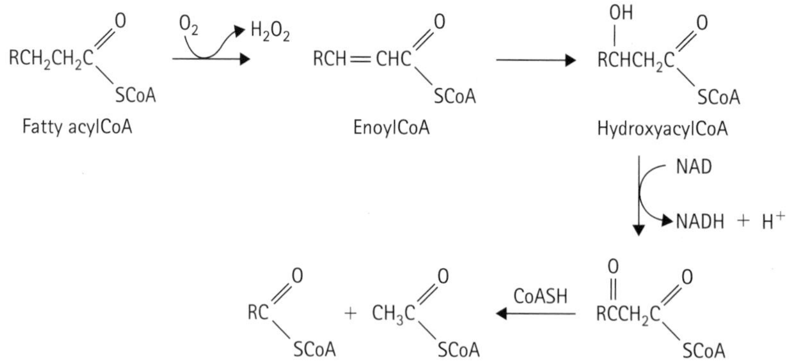

Figure 64.1   *The pathway of carnitine-independent oxidation in peroxisomes. The NAD-dependent step and the one preceding it are analogous to mitochondrial enzymes enoylCoA hydratase and 3-hydroxyacylCoA dehydrogenase and they are catalyzed by the bifunctional enzyme. This pathway catalyzes the metabolism of long- and medium-chain fatty acids, as well as the very-long-chain fatty acids. Short-chain acylCoAs and acetylCoA can then be transferred into carnitine esters via peroxisomal carnitine transferases.*

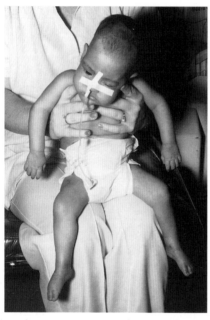

Figure 64.2   *A.A. at 3½ months-of-age, illustrating the hypotonia and the ptosis on the left. She had a peroxisome biogenesis disorder resulting from mutation T1467G in the PXR gene [18].*

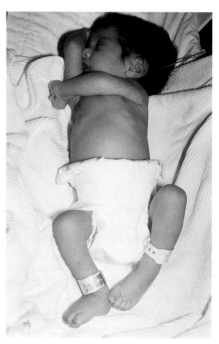

Figure 64.3   *Baby girl M., a neonate with neonatal adrenoleukodystrophy who presented with severe neonatal seizures. She was extremely hypotonic. She trembled at slight touch. There was mild hepatomegaly and absent neonatal reflexes. MRI was consistent with abnormal myelination. Analysis of VLCFA revealed a C26 of 3.25 µg/mL and a C26/C22 ratio of 1.05. She died at 3–4 months-of-age at home.*

(Figures 64.2–64.5) [1,3,9]. The hypotonia may be evident on the initial neonatal examination and is severe enough to suggest a diagnosis of myopathy [9]. Cerebral manifestations are profound. Most of these infants show little evidence of psychomotor development. Sucking reflex is poor. They feed poorly and may fail to thrive unless tube-fed. There are few or no spontaneous movements. The grasp and Moro responses are poor or absent. Tonic neck, stepping and placing reactions are absent. Deep tendon reflexes are usually diminished. Two patients were reported to be macrocephalic [3]. Ocular abnormalities reported include nystagmus, optic atrophy and pigmentary degeneration of the retina [1,7,22,23].

Seizures usually begin within the first days of life and continue as a major problem. They tend to be refractory to anticonvulsant therapy. Seizures may be myoclonic, as well as grand mal. Shivering or trembling may be stimulated by light touch and may be reminiscent of autumn leaves. Electroencephalograms (EEG) are abnormal, usually showing multifocal spike discharges [1,3]. In one patient the pattern changed at one month to that of hypsarrhythmia [1]. Decreased nerve conduction has been reported [3]. The computed tomography (CT) scan may be normal, or show a mild decrease in white

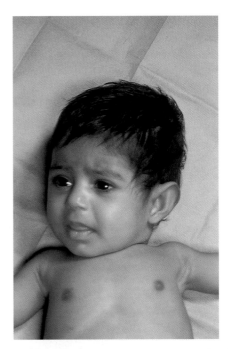

Figure 64.4 *A.H., a 6-month-old who had severe early infantile myoclonic seizures. VLCFA were elevated. He died at 1 year-of-age.*

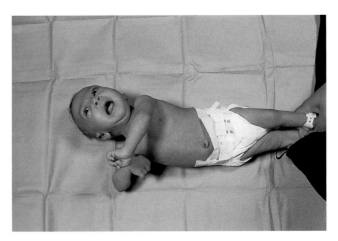

Figure 64.5 *A.H., the brother of the patient in Figure 64.4 at 4 months. He had uncontrollable early infantile seizures and elevated VLCFA. He died at 10 months-of-age.*

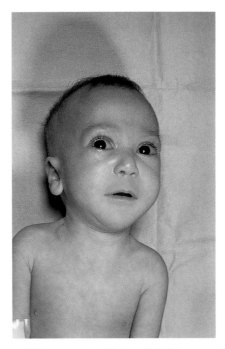

Figure 64.6 *H.S., a 1-month-old girl with Zellweger syndrome, had the typical facial appearance along with severe hypotonia, absent development and hepatomegaly. VLCFA were elevated. She died at 4-months-of-age.*

matter, or there may be many patchy lucencies on CT or magnetic resonance imaging (MRI) scan [3]. There may be enlargement of the ventricular system. Cerebrospinal fluid protein may be elevated [1,3].

Hepatomegaly may be progressive [3]. Levels of transaminase activity in the blood may be elevated [3]. With time there is little evidence of developmental progress. One patient could smile and roll from supine position at 7–9 months, but lost these functions shortly thereafter. Another developed some lateral head movement and a smile, which she lost after 12 months [3]. One patient had a cataract [3]. Most patients have died before the second birthday [1,3,9]. Mean age of death of the patients was 15 months, while in classical

Zellweger syndrome it was 5.7 months (n = 50). In neonatal adrenoleukodystrophy death has occurred as early as 4 months. A small number of patients has survived to teenage, albeit severely handicapped and dysmorphic [24,25]. Impaired hearing and retinopathy have suggested a diagnosis of Usher syndrome. The mental age of patients has seldom exceeded 12 months, and some have regressed at 3 to 5 years.

Dysmorphic features may be like those of Zellweger syndrome, but may be absent [9,10]. Renal cysts are not found, nor is chondrodysplasia punctata. The typical facial appearance of the Zellweger syndrome includes a prominent high forehead and flat occiput with large fontanels and wide cranial sutures, abnormal helices of the ears, a broad nasal bridge, epicanthal folds and hypoplastic supraorbital ridges [26,27] (Figures 64.6–64.10). In addition there are hepatorenal abnormalities and stippled calcifications in the patellae. Nipples and external genitalia may be hypoplastic.

The advent of molecular understanding of the disorders of peroxisomal biogenesis may ultimately render the earlier distinct clinical phenotypes obsolete. It is clear that there is a spectrum from the very severe Zellweger phenotype to the severe neonatal adrenoleukodystrophy to the more indolent infantile Refsum disease, and that mutations in the same gene can produce any of these phenotypes. The infantile Refsum phenotype may include some dysmorphic features such as epicanthal folds, a flat nasal bridge and low set ears [28]. Hypotonia is impressive in all of these diseases [29]. Retinitis pigmentosa and sensorineural hearing loss is characteristic [30]. These patients learn to walk but with an ataxic gait, and they are severely retarded [29].

The same phenotype can also be found in deficiencies of single peroxisomal enzymes (Figures 64.11–64.13). The enzymes include acylCoA oxidase-1 [31,32], which phenotype has been referred to as pseudoneonatal adrenoleukodystrophy, D-bifunctional protein [33,34] and peroxisomal thiolase-1 [35], which phenotype was originally referred to as pseudo-Zellweger syndrome. In these disorders VLCFA are elevated, but plasmalogen synthesis is normal. Among these disorders, deficiency of the D-bifunctional enzyme is much more common. This protein has both enoyl CoA hydratase and 3-hydroxyacylCoA dehydrogenase activity. Among these patients three subgroups have been identified [35,36], one with

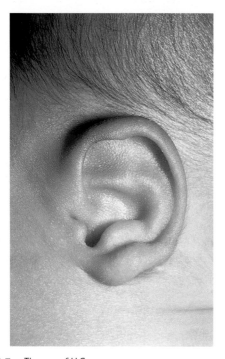

Figure 64.7   The ear of H.S.

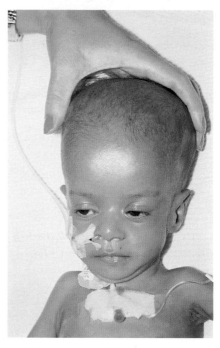

Figure 64.9   A.M., a 4-month-old infant with Zellweger syndrome and the typical facies. He had cataracts, hypotonia and retinitis. The patellae were stippled. VLCFA were elevated, and there was pipeocolic aciduria. He died at 6-months-of-age.

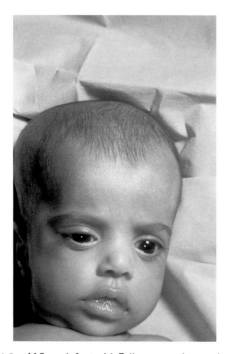

Figure 64.8   M.B., an infant with Zellweger syndrome whose clinical and chemical presentation was like that of H.S., but who was alive at 18 months when the family was lost to follow-up. The forehead was striking.

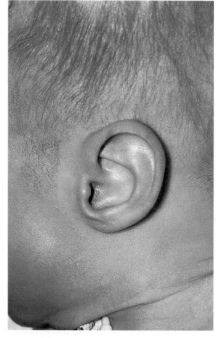

Figure 64.10   The ear of A.M.

deficient hydratase activity, one with deficient hydroxyacyl dehydrogenase activity, and one with absent protein and deficiency of both activities.

Patients with neonatal adrenoleukodystrophy usually have no clinical evidence of adrenal insufficiency. Electrolyte concentrations are normal. One patient had a low level of cortisol in the serum, but the cortisol response to adrenocorticotropin (ACTH) was normal. Most have had impaired cortisol responses to ACTH. One patient developed hypoglycemia in response to fasting [9]. Very small adrenals have been observed at autopsy [1,3]. Histological examination of adrenals has revealed extensive cortical atrophy with nodules of ballooned cells that stained for lipid with Oil Red O. Electron microscopy showed lamellar, needle-like lipid inclusions. It was this similarity to X-linked adrenoleukodystrophy that led to the naming of this disease. This adrenal pathology is also seen in Zellweger syndrome [37]. ACTH was demonstrated immunohistochemically in the pituitary, indicating the adrenal changes to be primary [1].

The neuropathology is characterized in some patients by polymicrogyria, as well as patchy demyelination throughout the cerebral white matter [1]. Some have had only mild abnormalities in neuronal migration and heterotopias [11]; in others the cortex and neurons appeared normal [6,38]. The olivary nuclei were normal in all. Cytoplasmic inclusions were seen, as in the adrenal, and were like those seen in X-linked adrenoleukodystrophy, as was perivascular accumulation of the lymphocytes. Demyelination of a widespread sudanophilic leukodystrophy tends to be more extensive than in X-linked adrenoleukodystrophy. It includes the cerebellum and brainstem. Periventricular rarefactions and microcalcifications have been observed [3]. Abnormalities of the gray matter include neuronal loss and inclusions in cortical neurons. Ocular histopathology includes ganglion cell loss and retinitis pigmentosa-like changes [22]. Retinitis pigmentosa may be seen in a variety of the peroxisomal disorders. Figure 64.12 illustrates the retina of a patient with defective activity of the bifunctional enzyme protein, which is a single enzyme defect in the pathway of peroxisomal β-oxidation (Figure 64.1) rather than a defect in peroxisome assembly.

Extensive hepatic fibrosis was reported in two patients at autopsy [3] and periportal fibrosis was observed at biopsy at 3 months-of-age [9]. Periodic acid-Schiff (PAS) positive macrophages have been reported in the liver [6] but not uniformly [3]. Hepatic peroxisomes may be absent or diminished in number [12,39,40].

Chemical analysis of the lipid of the brain revealed an increase in cholesterol esters and a diminution in constituents of myelin [1]. Hexacosanoic (C26:0) acid accounted for 25 percent of the total fatty acid [24,41]. Examination of the very long-chain fatty acids of the plasma and cultured fibroblasts also reveals accumulation of VLCFA. Levels are similar to those found in X-linked adrenoleukodystrophy [4]. The mean C26:C22 ratio in fibroblasts in two patients [3] was 0.5, while that in adrenoleukodystrophy was 0.7. The value for controls was 0.03. The accumulation tends to be less than that seen in Zellweger syndrome. In another patient the ratio was 1.8 [9]. The levels of C26:0 in postmortem liver and adrenal were higher than those reported in adrenoleukodystrophy [3]. Accumulation of very long-chain fatty acids has also been observed in retina [23]. Oxidation of lignoceric acid (C24:0) in cultured fibroblasts is impaired [3], and the level of activity is similar to that of cells derived from patients with adrenoleukodystrophy. Defective plasmalogen synthesis tends to be less than that of Zellweger syndrome [42].

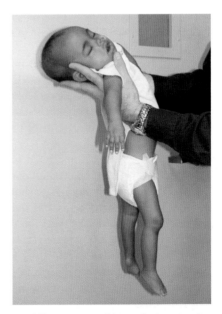

Figure 64.12   *S.E., a neonate with a typical neonatal adrenoleukodystrophy phenotype with intractable seizures and essentially no muscle tone. VLCFA were highly elevated, but plasmalogens were normal, indicating a single enzyme defect in peroxisomal fatty acid oxidation rather than a defect in peroxisomal biogenesis. A deficiency of the D-bifunctional protein was likely, but has not yet been tested. (Patient was kindly referred by Dr. Keith Vaux.)*

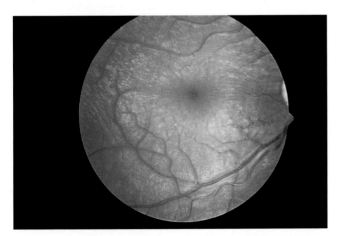

Figure 64.11   *The tigroid retinitis pigmentosa of S.M., a girl with peroxisomal bifunctional protein deficiency.*

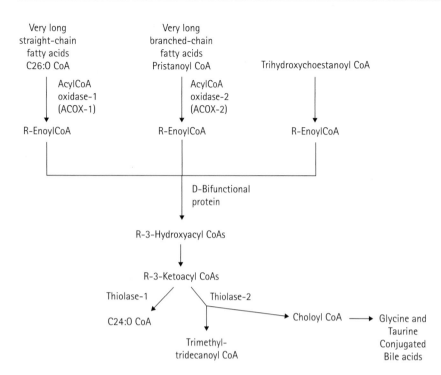

Figure 64.13   *Peroxisomal β-oxidation of very-long-chain fatty acids.*

GENETICS AND PATHOGENESIS

All of the disorders of peroxisomal biogenesis are transmitted in an autosomal recessive fashion. Patients of both sexes have been reported with identical phenotypes. In the Zellweger syndrome, consanguinity was observed in 17 of 78 patients [43]. The frequency of Zellweger syndrome was estimated to be one in 100 000 [44] and that of all disorders of peroxisome biogenesis to be one in 25 000 to 50 000 [27].

Testing of parents for levels of very long-chain fatty acids in plasma and in fibroblasts yielded normal levels [3]. This is in contrast to the findings in X-linked adrenoleukodystrophy. Normal levels of very long-chain fatty acids have also been found in plasma and fibroblasts of parents of patients with Zellweger syndrome [41].

Prenatal diagnosis has been accomplished in Zellweger syndrome [41], as it has been in X-linked adrenoleukodystrophy [45], by assay of cultured amniocytes, or chorionic villus samples, for very long-chain fatty acids and the activity of dihydroxyacetonephosphate acyltransferase [46–48], as well as by demonstration that catalase activity is present in the cytosol [49]. The same approaches should also be effective in neonatal adrenoleukodystrophy. False negatives have been observed in testing chorionic villus samples, so it has been recommended that tests be followed up by testing cultured chorionic villus cells, though this would not obviate the problem of overgrowth of maternal cells [45,50]. In patients shown to have mutations in any of the PEX genes [16,17,51], these can be the basis of prenatal diagnosis and heterozygote detection.

The fundamental defect in the disorders of peroxisomal biogenesis is a failure in the process of protein import into the peroxisomal matrix. This may lead to an absence of demonstrable peroxisomes as reported in Zellweger syndrome [52]. Actually, fibroblasts of these patients have been shown to have peroxisomal ghosts, or empty peroxisomal structures containing membrane proteins, but no catalase or other matrix proteins [53–56]. In milder examples, including some patients with neonatal adrenoleukodystrophy, there may be small amounts of catalase within the ghosts [57].

Peroxisomal biogenesis requires the synthesis of proteins on cytosolic polyribosomes and post-translational import to pre-existing peroxisomes, which enlarge until they divide and form new peroxisomes. Matrix proteins include catalase, the bifunctional hydratase-dehydrogenase enzyme, the thiolase, and acyl CoA oxidase [6]. Peroxisomal matrix proteins carrying either a carboxy terminal peroxisomal targeting sequence (PTS1) or a cleavable amino terminal sequence (PTS2) are translocated across the peroxisomal membrane [58–60]. A defect in a peroxin, caused by mutation in a PEX gene leads to failure of protein import via either the PTS1 or PTS2 import pathway and, as a consequence, to functional deficiency of the peroxisomes.

The PEX1 gene codes for a member of the AAA protein family of ATPases, which interacts with another ATPase coded for by PEX6, and this interaction is required for matrix protein import [61,62]. Defects in the PEX1 gene account for over half of patients with defects of peroxisomal biogenesis [63–65]. A variety of mutations has been identified. Two mutations, G843D [21] and 2097insT [66] are common in the general population; one or the other allele accounts for a great majority of patients with defects in peroxisomal biogenesis [63,64]. Genotype tends to correlate with phenotype in the sense that missense mutations have been found in milder presentations and nonsense mutations, deletions and insertions in severe disease [64]. Thus the type of mutation can be helpful in prognosis. The G843D mutation not only leads to milder disease in the homozygote, but also appears to ameliorate the effects of genes that usually cause severe disease.

PEX2 deficiency is defective in patients in complementation group 10 [16]. The gene is on chromosome 8q21.1 [67]. It codes for a 35 kDa peroxisomal membrane protein that restores proper assembly in a CHO cell mutant that is defective in peroxisome assembly [68]. In the initial homozygous patient a point mutation led to a premature termination of the protein, and addition of wild type protein to cultured cells of the patient restored peroxisomal assembly. Other point mutations in this protein have been identified [69], a G-to-A 737 change that led to a cysteine-to-tyrosine change in the region of the carboxyl terminus resembling the zinc finger motif of DNA binding proteins, and a C-to-T 370 change which formed a stop codon.

The identification of the molecular defect in the PEX5 gene, defective in complementation group 2 was the result of imaginative studies [18] on the patient [9] shown in Figure 64.2 (p. 420). She was found to have a T-to-G transversion of nucleotide 1467 which changed an asparagine to a lysine. The same mutation was found in another, unrelated Arabian patient with a neonatal adrenoleukodystrophy phenotype in complement group 2 [70]. Another member of complement group 2 was found to be homozygous for a nonsense mutation T 1168C that changed an arginine to a premature termination in PXR1 [18]. PEX1 codes for a receptor for proteins with PTS1 targeting signals, the targeting signal on the majority of matrix proteins. Fibroblasts of these patients were unable to import PTS1-containing proteins into peroxisomes.

Mutations in other genes involved in the import of peroxisomal matrix proteins have been identified, in the PEX6 [61], PEX7 [71], PEX12 [72] and PEX13 [73]. In addition mutations have been observed in PEX3 [74], PEX1 [75] and PEX19 [76], which code for proteins of peroxisomal membrane synthesis, all of them in patients with the Zellweger phenotype. Mutations have recently been found in PEX26, the cause of peroxisome biogenesis complementation group 8 [77]. This relatively common group contains patients with all three phenotypes. Cells of these patients have defective import of catalase and PTS2 proteins, such as 3-ketoacylCoA thiolase, but not PTS1 proteins, and the import defect is temperature sensitive [77]. The temperature-sensitive variants tend to cause less severe disease than the nonsensitive variants.

In the presence of defective processing of peroxisomal matrix proteins, these enzymes are found in the cytosol, where some, such as the oxidase and thiolase, are degraded rapidly, while catalase accumulates and is degraded more slowly than in normal cells [78]. Among the consequences of defective peroxisomal assembly is a variety of abnormalities of morphogenesis. These are most notable externally in Zellweger syndrome, but abnormal neuronal migration takes place in neonatal adrenoleukodystrophy, as well as Zellweger syndrome [78,79]. Abnormal migration is demonstrable in fetal tissue. Neurons normally found in the outer layers of the cerebral cortex are found in inner layers and in the white matter. Abnormal migration leads to microgyria and to thick pachygyria. Abnormal migration is not seen in rhizomelic

chondrodysplasia punctata, and other peroxisomal disorders in which plasmalogen synthesis is defective, so this could not be the mechanism of the abnormal migration. On the other hand, VLCFA do not accumulate in the chondrodysplasias, so this could be involved in the abnormal neuronal pathogenesis [79]. Deficiency of plasmalogens does make cells sensitive to ultraviolet irradiation [80].

The subcellular localization of catalase correlates with the status of peroxisomes in histologic studies of tissues. In Zellweger patients, catalase is essentially all cytosolic, while in normal individuals as much as 65 percent of catalase sediments with the peroxisomal particles.

Defective peroxisomal function is manifest in pathways of plasmalogen synthesis, pipecolic acid and phytanic metabolism, branched chain fatty acid oxidation and cholesterol metabolism. Plasma levels of VLCFA and bile acid intermediates are elevated. The VLCFA accumulate in this condition and in Zellweger syndrome because of failure to catabolize them [81]. All of the enzymes of peroxisomal β-oxidation are defective. These enzymes are synthesized normally, but they are degraded rapidly because they cannot target into peroxisomes. Cultured fibroblasts of a patient with neonatal adrenoleukodystrophy have been shown to make mRNA normally for an enzyme of fatty acid oxidation whose activity could not be found in autopsied liver [82].

Patients with Zellweger syndrome and neonatal adrenoleukodystrophy have dicarboxylic aciduria of predominantly medium-chain length [83], such as adipic (C6), suberic (C8) and sebacic (C10) acids. This reflects the failure of peroxisomal β-oxidation. The dicarboxylic aciduria may be modest compared with that seen in abnormalities of mitochondrial β-oxidation.

Levels of docosahexanoic acid (DHA) are low in brain, retina, liver and plasma in patients with disorders of peroxisomal biogenesis [84,85]. The mechanism is not yet clear, but may be a consequence of defective β-oxidation. DHA is important for the integrity of both brain and retina [86] and so may play a role in the pathogenesis of some clinical manifestations.

Bile acids are also metabolized to deoxycholic acid in peroxisomes, and precursors such as tri-hydroxycholestanoic acid (THCA) and dihydroxy-cholestanoic acid are present in high concentrations in patients [87]. This could relate to the pathogenesis of hepatic abnormality, and levels of transaminases and bilirubin in plasma are regularly elevated in Zellweger patients.

The accumulation of pipecolic acid and its increased excretion in urine [44] as the L-isomer. It appears to result from a failure to metabolize pipecolic acid to α-aminoadipic acid which normally takes place in peroxisomes [88].

TREATMENT

No effective treatment has been developed for the disorders of peroxisome biogenesis. The dietary regimens under exploitation in X-linked adrenoleukodystrophy are currently being explored in the milder examples of disorders of peroxisomal biogenesis. Improvement in a patient with neonatal adrenoleukodystrophy has been reported [89] following treatment with docosahexanoic acid (250 mg per day) but these observations have not generally been accepted. Clofibrate has been used without success to induce the formation of hepatic peroxisomes in Zellweger syndrome. Symptomatic therapy, such as the use of anticonvulsants may be helpful in management.

References

1 Ulrich H, Herschkowitz N, Heitz P, *et al*. Adrenoleukodystrophy. Preliminary report of a connatal case. Light and electron microscopical immunohistochemical and biochemical findings. *Acta Neuropathol* 1978;**43**:77.

2 Moser HW, Moser AB, Kawamura N, *et al*. Adrenoleukodystrophy: elevated C26 fatty acid in cultured skin fibroblasts. *Ann Neurol* 1980;**7**:542.

3 Jaffe R, Crumrine P, Hashida Y, Moser HW. Neonatal adrenoleukodystrophy. Clinical pathological and biochemical delineation of a syndrome affecting both males and females. *Am J Pathol* 1982;**108**:100.

4 Moser HW, Moser AB, Kawamura N, *et al*. Adrenoleucodystrophy: studies of the phenotype genetics and biochemistry. *Johns Hopkins Med J* 1980;**147**:217.

5 Moser HW, Moser AB, Frayer KK, *et al*. Adrenoleukodystrophy: increased plasma content of saturated very long chain fatty acids. *Neurology* 1981;**31**:1241.

6 Haas HE, Johnson ES, Farrell DL. Neonatal-onset adrenoleukodystrophy in a girl. *Ann Neurol* 1982;**12**:449.

7 Benke PJ, Reyes PF, Parker JC. New form of adrenoleukodystrophy. *Hum Genet* 1981;**58**:204.

8 Mobley WC, White CL, Tennekoon G, *et al*. Neonatal adrenoleukodystrophy. *Ann Neurol* 1982;**12**:204.

9 Wolff J, Nyhan WL, Powell H, *et al*. Myopathy in an infant with a fatal peroxisomal disorder. *Ped Neurol* 1986;**2**:141.

10 Kelley RI, Datta NS, Dobyns WB, *et al*. Neonatal adrenoleukodystrophy: new cases biochemical studies and differentiation from Zellweger and related peroxisomal polydistrophy syndromes. *Am J Med Genet* 1986;**23**:869.

11 Aubourg P, Scotto J, Rocchiccioli F, *et al*. Neonatal adrenoleukodystrophy. *J Neurol Neurosurg Psychiatry* 1986;**49**:77.

12 Vamecq J, Draye J-P, Van Hoof F, *et al*. Multiple peroxisomal enzymatic deficiency disorders. A comprehensive biochemical and morphological study of Zellweger cerebrohepatorenal syndrome and neonatal adrenoleukodystrophy. *Am J Pathol* 1986;**125**:524.

13 Brul S, Westerveld A, Strijland A, *et al*. Genetic heterogeneity in the cerebrohepatorenal (Zellweger) syndrome and other inherited disorders with a generalized impairment of peroxisomal function – a study using complementation analysis. *J Clin Invest* 1988;**81**:1710.

14 Roscher AA, Hoefler S, Hoefler G, *et al*. Genetic and phenotypic heterogeneity in disorders of peroxisome biogenesis – a complementation study involving cell lines from 19 patients. *Pediatr Res* 1989;**26**:67.

15 Yajima S, Suzuki T, Shimozawa N, *et al*. Complementation study of peroxisome-deficient disorders by immunofluorescence staining and characterization of fused cells. *Hum Genet* 1992;**88**:491.

16 Shimozawa N, Tsukamoto T, Suzuki Y, *et al*. A human gene responsible for Zellweger syndrome that affects peroxisome assembly. *Science* 1992;**255**:1132.

17 Gartner J, Moser H, Valle D. Mutations in the 70 K peroxisomal membrane protein gene in Zellweger syndrome. *Nat Genet* 1992;**1**:16.

18 Dodt G, Braverman N, Wong C, *et al*. Mutations in the PTS1 receptor gene PXR1 define complementation group 2 of the peroxisome biogenesis disorders. *Nature Genet* 1995;**9**:115.

19 Gould SJ, Valle D. The genetics and cell biology of the peroxisome biogenesis disorders. *Trends Genet* 2000;**16**:340.

20 Erdmann R, Wiebel FF, Flessau A, *et al*. PAS1 a yeast gene required for peroxisome biogenesis encodes a member of a novel family of putative ATPases. *Cell* 1991;**64**:499.

21 Reuber BE, Collins CS, Germain-Lee E, *et al*. Mutations in PEX1 are the most common cause of Zellweger syndrome neonatal adrenoleukodystrophy and infantile Refsum disease. *Nat Genet* 1997;**17**:445.

22 Cohen SMZ, Green WR, de la Cruz ZC, *et al*. Ocular histopathological studies of neonatal and childhood adrenoleukodystrophy. *Am J Opthalmol* 1983;**95**:82.

23 Cohen SM, Brown FR III, Martyn L, *et al*. Ocular histopathologic and biochemical studies of the cerebro-hepatorenal (Zellweger) syndrome and its relation to neonatal adrenoleukodystrophy. *Am J Ophthalmol* 1983;**96**:488.

24 Brown RF III, McAdams AJ, Cummins JW, *et al*. Cerebro-hepato-renal (Zellweger) syndrome and neonatal adrenoleukodystrophy: similarities in phenotype and accumulation of very long chain fatty acids. *Johns Hopkins Med J* 1982;**151**:344.

25 Noetzel MJ, Clark HB, Moser HW. Neonatal adrenoleukodystrophy with prolonged survival. *Ann Neurol* 1983;**14**:380.

26 Gootjes J, Elpeleg O, Eyskens F, *et al*. Novel mutations in the PEX2 gene of four unrelated patients with a peroxisome biogenesis disorder. *Pediatr Res* 2004;**55**:431.

27 Zellweger H. The cerebro-hepato-renal (Zellweger) syndrome and other peroxisomal disorders. *Dev Med Child Neurol* 1987;**29**:821.

28 Torvik A, Torp S, Kase BE, *et al*. Infantile Refsum's disease: a generalized peroxisomal disorder. Case report with postmortem examination. *J Neurol Sci* 1988;**85**:39.

29 Budden SS, Kennaway NG, Buist NR, *et al*. Dysmorphic syndrome with phytanic acid oxidase deficiency abnormal very long chain fatty acids and pipecolic acidemia: studies in four children. *J Pediatr* 1986;**108**:33.

30 Weleber RG, Tongue AC, Kennaway NG, *et al*. Ophthalmic manifestations of infantile phytanic acid storage disease. *Arch Ophthalmol* 1984;**102**:1317.

31 Poll-Thá; BT, Roels F, Ogier H, *et al*. A new peroxisomal disorder with enlarged peroxisomes and a specific deficiency of acyl-CoA oxidase (pseudo-neonatal adrenoleukodystrophy). *Am J Hum Genet* 1988;**42**:422.

32 Fournier B, Saudubray JM, Benichou B, *et al*. Large deletion of the peroxisomal acyl-CoA oxidase gene in pseudoneonatal adrenoleukodystrophy. *J Clin Invest* 1994;**94**:526.

33 Watkins PA, Chen WW, Harris CJ, *et al*. Peroxisomal bifunctional enzyme deficiency. *J Clin Invest* 1989;**83**:771.

34 van Grunsven EG, van Berkel E, Mooijer PAW, *et al*. Peroxisomal bifunctional protein deficiency revisited: resolution of its true enzymatic and molecular basis. *Am J Hum Genet* 1999;**64**:99.

35 Goldfischer S, Collins J, Rapin I, *et al*. Deficiencies in several peroxisomal oxidative activities. *J Pediatr* 1986;**108**:25.

36 van Grunsven EG, van Roermund CWT, Denis S, Wanders RJA. Complementation analysis of fibroblasts from peroxisomal fatty acid oxidation deficient patients shows high frequency of bifunctional enzyme deficiency plus intragenic complementation: unequivocal evidence for differential defects in the same enzyme protein. *Biochem Biophys Res Commun* 1997;**235**:176.

37 Goldfischer S, Powers JM, Johnson AB, *et al*. Striated adrenocortical cells in cerebro-hepato-renal (Zellweger) syndrome. *Virchows Arch* 1983;**401**:355.

38   Manz HJ, Schuelein M, McCullough DC, *et al*. New phenotypic variant of adrenoleukodystrophy: pathologic ultrastructural and biochemical study in two brothers. *J Neurol Sci* 1980;**45**:245.

39   Singh I, Moser AB, Goldfischer S, Moser HW. Lignoceric acid is oxidized in the peroxisome: implications for the Zellweger cerebro-hepato-renal syndrome and adrenoleukodystrophy. *Proc Natl Acad Sci USA* 1984;**81**:4203.

40   Goldfischer S, Collins J, Rapin I, *et al*. Peroxisomal defects in neonatal onset and X-linked adrenoleuko-dystrophies. *Science* 1985;**227**:67.

41   Moser AE, Singh I, Brown FR III, *et al*. The cerebro-hepato-renal (Zellweger) syndrome and neonatal adrenoleukodystrophy: increased levels and impaired degradation of very long chain fatty acids and their use in prenatal diagnosis. *N Engl J Med* 1984;**310**:1141.

42   Roscher A, Molzer B, Bernheimer H, *et al*. The cerebrohepatorenal (Zellweger) syndrome: an improved method for the biochemical diagnosis and its potential value of prenatal detection. *Pediatr Res* 1985;**19**:930.

43   Heymans HSA. Cerebro-hepato-renal (Zellweger) syndrome: clinical and biochemical consequences of peroxisomal dysfunction. Thesis, University of Amsterdam;1984.

44   Danks DM, Tippett P, Adams C, Campbell P. Cerebro-hepato-renal syndrome of Zellweger: a report of eight cases with comments upon the incidence the liver lesion and fault in pipecolic acid metabolism. *J Pediatr* 1975;**86**:382.

45   Moser HW, Moser AB, Powers JM, *et al*. The prenatal diagnosis of adrenoleukodystrophy. Demonstration of increased hexacosanoic acid levels in cultured amniocytes and fetal adrenal gland. *Pediatr Res* 1982;**16**:172.

46   Hajra AK, Datta NS, Jackson LJ, *et al*. Prenatal diagnosis of Zellweger cerebrohepatorenal syndrome. *N Engl J Med* 1985;**312**:445.

47   Wanders RJA, van Wijland MJA, van Roermund CWT, *et al*. Prenatal diagnosis of Zellweger syndrome by measurement of very long chain fatty acid (C26:0) β-oxidation in cultured chorionic villus fibroblasts: implications for early diagnosis of other peroxisomal disorders. *Clin Chim Acta* 1987;**165**:303.

48   Rocchiccioli F, Aubourg P, Choiset A. Immediate prenatal diagnosis of Zellweger syndrome by direct measurement of very long chain fatty acids in chorionic villus cells. *Prenat Diagn* 1987;**7**:349.

49   Wanders RJA, Schrakamp G, van den Bosch H, *et al*. A prenatal test for the cerebro-hepatorenal (Zellweger) syndrome by demonstration of the absence of catalase-containing particles (peroxisomes) in cultured amniotic fluid cells. *Eur J Pediatr* 1986;**145**:136.

50   Carey WF, Robertson EF, Van Crugten C, *et al*. Prenatal diagnosis of Zellweger's syndrome by chorionic villus sampling – and a caveat. *Prenat Diagn* 1986;**6**:227.

51   Shimozawa N, Suzuki Y, Orii T, *et al*. Standardization of complementation grouping of peroxisome-deficient disorders and the second Zellweger patient with peroxisomal assembly factor-1 (PAF-1) defect. *Am J Hum Genet* 1993;**52**:843 (letter to the editor).

52   Goldfischer S, Moore CL, Johnson AB, *et al*. Peroxisomal and mitochondrial defects in the cerebro-hepato-renal syndrome. *Science* 1973;**182**:62.

53   Santos MJ, Imanaka T, Shio H, *et al*. Peroxisomal membrane ghosts in Zellweger syndrome – aberrant organelle assembly. *Science* 1988;**239**:1536.

54   Santos MJ, Imanaka T, Shio H, Lazarow PB. Peroxisomal integral membrane proteins in control and Zellweger fibroblasts. *J Biol Chem* 1988;**263**:10502.

55   Aikawa J, Chen WW, Kelley RI, *et al*. Low-density particles (W-particles) containing catalase in Zellweger syndrome and normal fibroblasts. *Proc Natl Acad Sci USA* 1991;**88**:10084.

56   Santos M, Imanaka T, Shio H, *et al*. Peroxisomal membrane ghosts in Zellweger syndrome – aberrant organelle assembly. *Science* 1988;**239**:1536.

57   Santos MJ, Hoefler S, Moser AB, *et al*. Peroxisome assembly mutations in humans: structural heterogeneity in Zellweger syndrome. *J Cell Physiol* 1992;**151**:103.

58   Gould SJ, Keller GA, Subramani S. Identification of peroxisomal targeting signals located at the carboxy terminus of four peroxisomal proteins. *J Cell Biol* 1988;**107**:897.

59   Subramani S. Protein translocation into peroxisomes. *J Biol Chem* 1996;**271**:32483.

60   Terlecky SR, Legakis JE, Hueni SE, Subramani S. Quantitative analysis of peroxisomal protein import *in vitro*. *Exp Cell Res* 2001;**263**:98.

61   Geisbrecht BV, Collins CS, Reuber BE, Gould SJ. Disruption of a PEX1-PEX6 interaction is the most common cause of the neurologic disorders Zellweger syndrome neonatal adrenoleukodystrophy and infantile Refsum disease. *Proc Natl Acad Sci USA* 1998;**95**:8630.

62   Tamura S, Shimozawa N, Suzuki Y, *et al*. A cytoplasmic AA family peroxin Pex1p interacts with Pex6p. *Biochem Biophys Res Commun* 1998;**245**:883.

63   Maxwell MA, Nelson PV, China SJ, *et al*. A common PEX1 frameshift mutation in patients with disorders of peroxisome biogenesis correlates with the severe Zellweger syndrome phenotype. *Hum Genet* 1999;**105**:38.

64   Preuss N, Brosius U, Biermanns M, *et al*. PEX1 mutations in complementation group 1 of Zellweger spectrum patients correlate with severity of disease. *Pediatr Res* 2002;**51**:706.

65   Wanders RJA, Mooijer PAW, Dekker C, *et al*. Disorders of peroxisome biogenesis: complementation analysis shows genetic heterogeneity with strong overrepresentation of one group (PEX1 deficiency). *J Inherit Metab Dis* 1999;**22**:314.

66   Collins CS, Gould SJ. Identification of a common mutation in severely affected PEX1-deficient patients. *Hum Mutat* 1999;**14**:45.

67   Masuno M, Shimozawa N, Suzuki Y, *et al*. Assignment of the human peroxisome assembly factor-1 gene (PXMP3) responsible for Zellweger syndrome to chromosome 8q211 by fluorescence *in situ* hybridization. *Genomics* 1994;**20**:141.

68   Tsukamoto T, Mijura S, Fujiki Y. Restoration by a 35K membrane protein of peroxisome assembly in a peroxisome-deficient mammalian cell mutant. *Nature* 1991;**350**:77.

69   Thieringer R, Raetz CRH. Peroxisome-deficienct. Chinese hamster ovary cells with point mutations in peroxisome assembly Factor-1*. *J Biol Chem* 1993;**268**:12631.

70   Steinberg SJ, Fensom AH. Complementation analysis in patients with the clinical phenotype of a generalised peroxisomal disorder. *J Med Genet* 1996;**33**:295.

71   Braverman N, Steel G, Lin P, *et al*. PEX7 gene structure alternative transcripts and evidence for a founder haplotype for the frequent RCDP allele 1292ter. *Genomics* 2000;**63**:181.

72   Chang C-C, Warren DS, Sacksteder KA, Gould SJ. PEX12 interacts with PEX5 and PEX10 and acts downstream of receptor docking in peroxisomal matrix protein import. *J Cell Biol* 1999;**147**:761.

73   Shimozawa N, Suzuki Y, Zhang Z, *et al*. Nonsense and temperature-sensitive mutations in PEX13 are the cause of complementation group H of peroxisome biogenesis disorders. *Hum Mol Genet* 1999;**8**:1077.

74   South ST, Sacksteder KA, Li X, *et al*. Inhibitors of COPI and COPII do not block PEX3-mediated peroxisome synthesis. *J Cell Biol* 2000;**149**:1345.

75   Honsho M, Tamura S, Shimozawa N, *et al*. Mutation in PEX16 is causal in the peroxisome-deficient Zellweger syndrome of complementation group D. *Am J Hum Genet* 1998;**63**:1622.

76   Matsuzono Y, Kinoshita N, Tamura S, *et al*. Human PEX19:cDNA cloning by functional complementation mutation analysis in a patient with Zellweger syndrome and potential role in peroxisomal membrane assembly. *Proc Natl Acad Sci USA* 1999;**96**:2116.

77   Matsumoto N, Tamura S, Furuki S, *et al.* Mutations in novel peroxin gene PEX26 that cause peroxisome-biogenesis disorders of complementation group 8 provide a gentoype-phenotype correlation. *Am J Hum Genet* 2003;**73**:233.

78   Wanders RJA, Los M, Roest B, *et al.* Activity of peroxisomal enzymes and intracellular distribution of catalase in Zellweger syndrome. *Biochem Biophys Res Commun* 1984;**123**:1054.

79   Powers JM, Tummons RC, Caviness VS Jr, *et al.* Structural and chemical alterations in the cerebral maldevelopment of fetal cerebro-hepato-renal (Zellweger) syndrome. *J Neuropathol Exp Neurol* 1989;**48**:270.

80   Hoefler G, Paschke E, Hoeffler S, *et al.* Photosensitized killing of cultured fibroblasts from patients with peroxisomal disorders due to pyrene fatty acid-mediated ultraviolet damage. *J Clin Invest* 1991;**88**:1873.

81   Suzuki Y, Orii T, Mori M, *et al.* Deficient activities and proteins of peroxisomal b-oxidation enzymes in infants with Zellweger syndrome. *Clin Chim Acta* 1986;**156**:191.

82   Chen WW, Watkins PA, Osumit T, *et al.* Peroxisomal beta-oxidation enzyme proteins in adrenoleukodystrophy: distinction between X-linked adrenoleukodystrophy and neonatal adrenoleukodystrophy. *Proc Natl Acad Sci USA* 1987;**84**:1435.

83   Pampols T, Ribes A, Pineda M, *et al.* Medium chain dicarboxylic and hydroxydicarboxylic aciduria in a case of neonatal adrenoleukodystrophy. *J Inherit Metab Dis* 1987;**10**:217.

84   Martinez M. Abnormal profiles of polyunsaturated fatty acids in the brain liver kidney and retina of patients with peroxisomal disorders. *Brain Res* 1993;**583**:171.

85   Martinez M. Severe deficiency of docosahexaenoic acid in peroxisomal disorders. A defect of delta-4 desaturations? *Neurology* 1990;**40**:1292.

86   Bazan NG. Supply of n-3 polyunsaturated fatty acids and their significance in the central nervous system: in *Nutrition and the Brain* (eds Wurtman RJ, Wurtman JJ). Vol 8, Raven, New York;1990:1.

87   Hanson RF, Szczepanick-Van Leeuwen P, Williams GC, *et al.* Defects of bile acid synthesis in Zellweger's syndrome. *Science* 1979;**203**:1107.

88   Wanders RJA, Romeyn GJ, van Roermund CWT, *et al.* Identification of L-pipecolate oxidase in human liver and its deficiency in the Zellweger syndrome. *Biochem Biophys Res Commun* 1988;**154**:33.

89   Martinez M, Pineda M, Vidal R, Martin B. Docosahexaenoic acid: a new therapeutic approach to peroxisomal patients. Experience with two cases. *Neurology* 1993;**43**:1389.

Disorders of purine metabolism

65

Lesch-Nyhan disease and the non-Lesch-Nyhan variants of HPRT

LESCH-NYHAN DISEASE

MAJOR PHENOTYPIC EXPRESSION

Retardation of motor development, spasticity, involuntary movements, self-injurious behavior, hyperuricemia, uricosuria, urinary tract calculi, nephropathy, tophi, gouty arthritis, and deficient activity of hypoxanthine guanine phosphoribosyl transferase (HPRT).

Introduction

Lesch-Nyhan disease was first described in 1964 [1] as a syndrome in which disordered purine metabolism, as exemplified by hyperuricemia, uricaciduria, increased turnover of an enlarged uric acid pool and enormous overproduction of

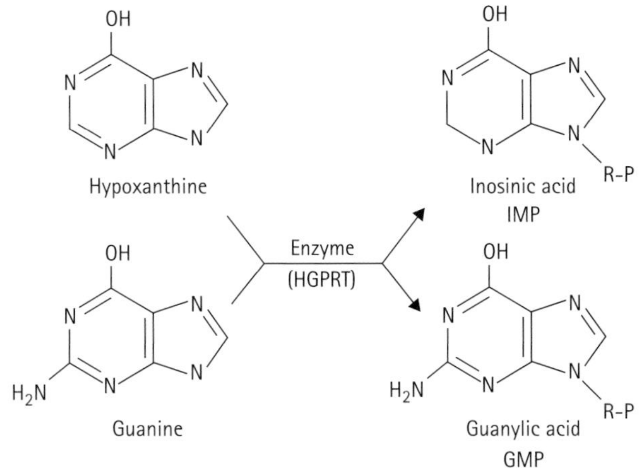

Figure 65.1 *Hypoxanthine-guanine phosphoribosyl transferase (HPRT), the site of the defect in the Lesch-Nyhan disease.*

purine *de novo*, was associated with a neurological picture resembling athetoid cerebral palsy and bizarre, compulsive, self-mutilative behavior. The overproduction of purine from an intravenous glycine precursor was 20 times the normal value [2], whereas in adults with gouty arthritis the largest rates observed were twice the normal value. The hallmark feature of the behavior was loss of tissue because of biting. The gene was recognized early from pedigree studies to be situated on the X chromosome [3], and transmission is as a fully recessive character. There have been a few affected females, most reflecting a nonrandom inactivation of the normal X chromosome. The enzyme defect in HPRT (Figure 65.1) was discovered in 1967 by Seegmiller, Rosenbloom and Kelley [4]. The gene was cloned in 1982 by Friedmann, Jolly and colleagues [5,6]. A large number of mutations have been defined [7].

Clinical abnormalities

Male infants with Lesch-Nyhan disease appear normal at birth and usually develop normally for the first 6 to 8 months. The first sign is usually the appearance of orange crystals or orange sand in the diapers [8] and this history is regularly obtained from the parents. This manifestation of crystalluria would permit early diagnosis, prior to the development of neurologic

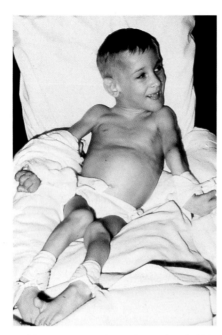

Figure 65.2   *M.J., a 7-year-old boy with the Lesch-Nyhan syndrome illustrating the motor disability as exemplified by an inability to sit without support; choreoathetoid posturing in the position of the upper extremities; spasticity; and a left spontaneous Babinski.*

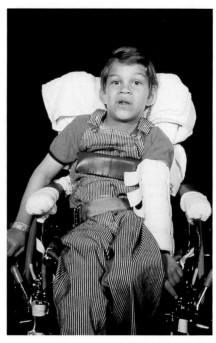

Figure 65.3   *O.K., a Lesch-Nyhan patient in the typical position. Supported properly, the patient can be part of the action, and he can get around in a wheelchair.*

or behavioral features, and I am pleased to say that we have recently encountered a patient who was detected early on this basis. Hematuria or urinary tract stones may develop as well as crystalluria during the early months of life.

Defective motor development usually becomes evident in the second six months of life. Commonly it is the failure to reach developmental milestones, or poor head control that brings the infant to attention. At this age hypotonia is commonly evident, but some patients may have hypertonic lower extremities. Patients with Lesch-Nyhan disease do not learn to walk, and must have some support even to sit unaided (Figure 65.2). No patient with this disease has learned to walk. Patients do learn to sit in a chair if they are fastened securely about the chest as well as the waist, and narrow wheelchairs are preferred (Figure 65.3). Involuntary movements have been seen in 100 percent of our patients [8]. Extrapyramidal features indicating abnormality in the function of the basal ganglia occur in all of the patients with this disease [8,9].

Varying descriptions in the literature probably reflect varying use of the language rather than variation in the neurologic phenotype. Increasingly, we have recognized dystonia as a major feature with its extensive cocontraction of agonist and antagonist muscles, dystonic posturing especially on intention, and overflow muscular contractions elsewhere. There may be flailing movements of the extremities that have been called ballismus. Choreic movements are particularly common with excitement, either emotionally positive or negative. We have also observed fine, typically athetoid movements (Figure 65.2). Opisthotonic spasms or periodic arching of the

back are characteristic. They begin in infancy but continue even into adult life, becoming in some patients a semivoluntary component of the behavior. Among pyramidal features spasticity is usually considerable. Scissoring of the lower extremities is common. The increased muscle pull leads ultimately to dislocation of both hips in most patients. Many patients develop contractures, predominantly in flexion. Deep tendon reflexes are increased, but reflexes may be difficult to obtain because excitement engendered by the examination leads to so much activity. Babinski reflexes are regularly found, but may be absent. Spontaneous dorsiflexion of the toe (Figure 65.2) may be easier to observe than one elicited by a detailed neurologic examination. Seizures occur in some patients, but are not a major feature of the disease, and the electroencephalogram (EEG) is usually normal. Oculomotor abnormalities were described [10] as an impairment in the initiation of voluntary saccades. Patients often initiated a saccade with a thrust of the head, and when this was inhibited by holding the head, the response was delayed. This would be consistent with dysfunction of oculomotor circuits in the basal ganglia.

Mental retardation is a prominent but controversial feature of the disease. In most patients the IQ as tested has approximated 50. However, adequate testing is very difficult because the behavior and a short attention span get in the way of the testing. Clearly, these patients have cognitive abilities well above the level of the motor disability. A few patients have been observed in whom there has been normal or near normal intelligence. Many parents feel that their sons are intellectually normal. Two of our patients were doing grade level work in normal high schools. These patients were toilet trained. None

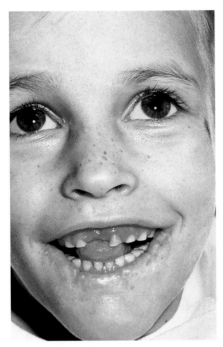

Figure 65.4   *M.J. The degree of the mutilation of the lip is relatively mild.*

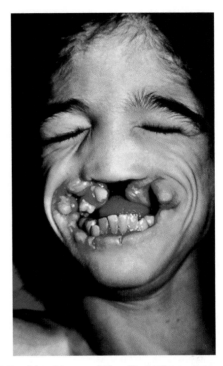

Figure 65.5   *J.J., a 14-year-old boy, illustrating an extreme degree of mutilation around the face.*

of the others we have studied was. All of them learn to speak, but dysarthria makes their speech difficult to understand. Despite the gravity of the cerebral disease there is no evidence that this is a progressive, degenerative disease. Behavioral features are integral to the disease and the behavior is compulsive and aggressive. In our experience self-injurious behavior occurs in 100 percent of patients [8]. On the other hand there are exceptions to every rule, and Puig *et al.* [11] have reported two patients, one 6 years-of-age, but the other 21 years, who have not mutilated despite having uncles, and in one case a brother, who displayed the complete phenotype including self-injurious behavior. While aggressive activity is predominantly directed against the patients themselves, they do attempt to injure others and sometimes succeed, but the motor disability largely prevents such success.

The most characteristic feature is self-destructive biting of the lips (Figures 65.4, 65.5) and fingers (Figures 65.6–65.8). Unlike many other retarded patients who engage in self-mutilative behavior, these patients bite with a ferocity that leads to significant loss of tissue. Partial amputation of fingers has been observed (Figure 65.8). The differential diagnosis of self-injury of this disease includes the De Lange syndrome and dysautonomia. It does not really include sensory neuropathy and indifference to pain. Those patients tend to look like pugilists, and the injuries are accidental. Lesch-Nyhan patients do not have sensory abnormalities; they scream in pain when they bite and cry in terror of its anticipation. As patients become older, they learn to become aggressive with speech. Four letter Anglo-Saxon expressions are common.

Apraxic discoordination of the lips and tongue make feeding difficult, and swallowing is imperfect. In addition, most

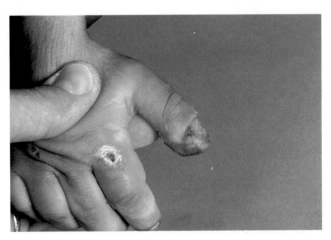

Figure 65.6   *Freshly bitten lesions of the thumb and forefinger of a 6-year-old Saudi boy with the Lesch-Nyhan syndrome.*

have lost teeth in order to protect against damage by biting. Patients with this disease feed poorly. Virtually all vomit, and this, too, seems to be incorporated into the behavior. In most patients, growth in height and weight are well below the norms for chronological age [8]. Autopsy studies have revealed no consistent abnormalities in the brain and a number of brains has been judged to be normal. So too have routine neuroimaging studies. However, quantitative magnetic resonance imaging (MRI) comparison of patients and age-matched controls has revealed a 34 percent decrease in the volume of the caudate [12], which appeared to reflect abnormal development as opposed to atrophy.

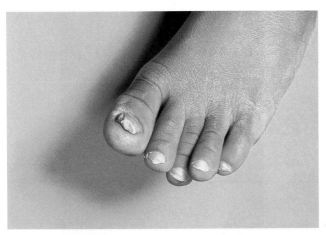

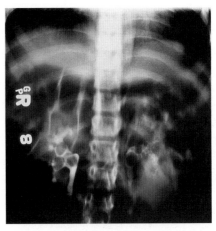

Figure 65.7   *This same boy managed to bite his great toe as well. He also had loss of tissue from biting the lower lip, banged his head and created sores on his chin by rubbing it on the floor.*

Figure 65.9   *Intravenous pyelogram of a patient with Lesch-Nyhan disease. There were numerous radiolucent calculi.*

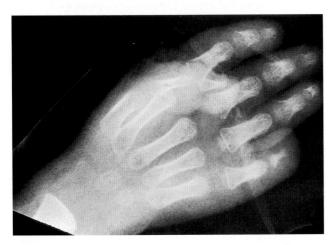

Figure 65.8   *M.J. Roentgenogram of the left hand, illustrating partial amputation of the fifth finger.*

Hyperuricemia is present in virtually all patients. The concentration of uric acid in the plasma is usually between 9 and 12 mg/dL, which is at the limit of solubility of urate in plasma. Patients with some degree of acute or chronic glomerular insufficiency may have high concentrations of uric acid, and some who are very efficient at excreting urate may have lower values, occasionally in the normal range. The clinician must be careful about accepting a conclusion that a plasma uric acid is normal from a laboratory whose norms were established on adult males in whom hyperuricemia is common. All patients excrete large amounts of uric acid in the urine. Twenty-four-hour excretions of 600 to 1000 mg are the rule in patients weighing 15 kg or more. Throughout childhood patients with this disease excrete three to four times as much uric acid as do control individuals of comparable size. In relation to body weight they excrete 40–70 mg of uric acid per kg. Another pitfall in interpreting uric acid data arises from the propensity of micro-organisms to consume purines including uric acid; conditions of collection of a 24-hour

sample at room temperature are ideal for bacterial purposes. For this reason it is best to avoid collecting 24-hour samples except for research purposes under which each sample is added to the batch in the freezer as soon as obtained. For diagnostic purposes it is more convenient to collect a fresh sample and analyze promptly for uric acid and creatinine [13]. These patients regularly excrete 3–4 mg of uric acid/mg of creatinine, while in control individuals older than 1 year-of-age the level is less than one.

The clinical consequences of the accumulation of large amounts of uric acid in body fluids are manifestations classic for gout. Episodes of hematuria and crystalluria are the rule and may cause abdominal pain. Urinary tract calculi are regularly observed (Figure 65.9) and they may occur as early as the first months of life, and they lead to urinary tract infections. In the absence of treatment, urate nephropathy develops as a result of the deposition of sodium urate in the renal parenchyma. Death from renal failure at less than 10 years-of-age was the expected outcome before the development of allopurinol. Tophi (Figure 65.10) may be seen in those unusual patients who survive without treatment beyond 10 years. Acute gouty arthritis is even more rare but has occurred uniformly in untreated patients reaching adult life.

Genetics and pathogenesis

The molecular defect in Lesch-Nyhan disease is in the activity of the enzyme hypoxanthine-guanine phosphoribosyl transferase (HPRT) (EC 2.4.2.8) (Figure 65.1, p. 431). This enzyme catalyzes the reaction of hypoxanthine or guanine with phosphoribosyl pyrophosphate (PRPP) to form their respective nucleotides, inosinic and guanylic acids. The enzyme is present in all cells of the body. It is particularly active in basal ganglia and testis. The defect is readily detectable in erythrocyte hemolysates and in cultured fibroblasts. In the erythrocyte quantitative assays reveal no activity.

HPRT is determined by a gene on the long arm of the X chromosome at Xq26-27. The disease is transmitted as an

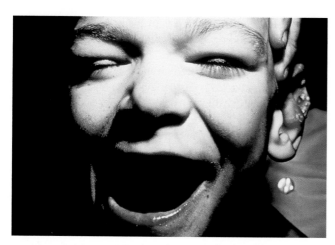

Figure 65.10 *A 17-year-old boy with prominent tophaceous deposits in the ears. The violaceous inflammatory reaction is unusual around tophi. It subsided following treatment with colchicine.*

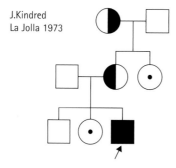

J.Kindred
La Jolla 1973

Figure 65.11 *Pedigree of M.J. Symbols employed were black box for hemizygous male, half black circle, heterozygous female, and circle with a dot, a female tested and found to be normal.*

X-linked recessive trait (Figure 65.11). It is essentially a disease of the male, occurring at a frequency of approximately 1 in 380 000 births. Six females have been observed [14,15].

The heterozygous carrier can be detected by assay of the enzyme in individual cells, such that the two populations of cells specified in the Lyon hypothesis are demonstrated. This has been accomplished by cloning or pharmacologic selection in thioguanine or azaguanine. A more convenient but still tedious method is hair root analysis [16], which takes advantage of the largely clonal nature of individual hair follicles but requires the plucking of at least 30 individual hairs and enzyme analysis of each one. Definition of the molecular defect in an individual family permits direct testing for carriers of the mutation. This is labor intensive because of the large number of mutations, but in families in which the mutation is known it is the method of choice. It can be simplified especially where a new restriction site is created or an old one eliminated by the mutation.

In informative families, linkage analysis of restriction fragment length polymorphism (RFLP) has been used for heterozygote detection [17]. Study of the carrier status of mothers has indicated that the incidence of new mutation is considerably

less than the one-third of affected patients predicted by population genetics theory for an X-linked lethal gene [18]. There is some evidence for an effect of paternal age and of mutation occurring in the genesis of the carrier mother. Simple testing of erythrocytes or leukocytes for enzyme activity is not useful for carrier detection, because the activity in heterozygotes is always normal [18], an index probably of selection against mutant cells.

Prenatal diagnosis has regularly been accomplished by assay of the enzyme in amniocytes [19,20] or chorionic villus samples, and a considerable number of affected and nonaffected fetuses has been detected. Nucleotidase activity, which is high in villus material, may lead to the breakdown of newly formed inosinic acid (IMP) and thus cause a false positive diagnosis of an affected fetus [20] so it is important to inhibit the nucleotidase during the assay. Among normal individuals a certain amount of RFLP has been identified and the linkage appears to be quite tight. This has permitted its use in informative families in which the mother carries identifiable alleles for prenatal diagnosis as well as for the detection of heterozygosity [17]. In families in which the mutation is known, determination of its presence or absence is the method of choice for prenatal diagnosis.

The gene for the HPRT enzyme has been cloned and its nucleotide sequence determined [5,6]. It spans more than 44 kb of DNA; its coding region contains 654 nucleotides in 9 exons. The mRNA is 1.6 kb, but the reading frame approximates 700 bases and the enzyme contains 217 amino acids [21], which forms a tetramer.

The introduction of the polymerase chain reaction has permitted the identification of a number of mutations in patients with HPRT deficiency [7,22–27]. In the most recent summary 236 mutations were recorded [7]. In most families studied a unique mutation has been found. The same mutation has only rarely been found in unrelated pedigrees. In most patients the gene is not grossly altered; on the other hand, in classic Lesch-Nyhan patients the results of the mutation have been major ones leading to essentially no activity of the enzyme. In eight classic Lesch-Nyhan phenotypes [22] an entire exon was deleted in two; and in three, nonsense mutations led to a stop mutation and hence a markedly truncated protein. In classic Lesch-Nyhan patients a complete spectrum of mutations has been observed including major disruptions, such as deletions, insertions, frame shift mutations leading to exon skipping and stop codons leading to truncated unstable proteins which are readily degraded [7]. Missense mutations were generally nonconservative; for instance an aspartic acid for a glycine at position 16; a leucine for a phenylalanine at position 74; and a tyrosine for an aspartic acid at position 201. A very small number of CpG mutational hot spots were identified, for instance at arginine 51 and 170 of the HPRT protein. These are thought to represent deamination of 5-methylcytosine to thymine changing the message for arginine to stop. This mutation has occurred eleven times among reported patients [7,22,28]. In Lesch-Nyhan patients some large deletions have been detectable by Southern blot analysis [29]. Deletions have involved single exons, multiple exons, and the entire gene. Single base substitutions tend to be nonconservative, such as a change from aspartic acid to a large tyrosine ring structure that would be expected to interfere with protein function. Among other mutations of the gene reported are duplications, one of which resulted from recombination of Alu sequences in introns 6 and 8 [30]. This patient, though 22 years old and severely retarded, had no self-injurious behavior; so he could represent a variant.

Prenatal diagnosis and heterozygote detection can readily be carried out in a family in which the mutation is known. In one family [31] a nonsense mutation of the CpG site for arginine 169 was identified in a fetus and five female heterozygotes, in three of whom X chromosomal mosaicism could not be demonstrated by repeated hair root analysis or by selection of fibroblasts in azaguanine and thioguanine. Presumably this represents an extreme example of selection against the mutant cell. We recommend prenatal diagnosis in pregnancies in which a mother has had an affected infant even if she is found not to be a heterozygote in order to avoid the problem of gonadal mosaicism. Also, since there have now been documented affected females we recommend prenatal diagnosis of HPRT status even when the fetus is found to have two X chromosomes.

Establishment of the diagnosis in a patient with the typical phenotype requires determination that the activity of HPRT in a hemolysate is zero. However, some patients with different variants and different clinical phenotypes pp. 437–43 may also have zero activity in the erythrocyte assay. Assay of the enzyme in intact cultured fibroblasts has permitted the distinction of these populations: patients with Lesch-Nyhan disease have activity that is less than 1.4 percent of normal [32]; the variants have all had more activity.

In the presence of defective activity of HPRT, concentrations of phosphoribosyl-pyrophosphate rise, and there may be diminished feedback inhibition of glutamine amidotransferase by purine nucleotides. The rate of synthesis of purines via the de novo pathway increases markedly as studied in vivo with labeled glycine. Concentrations of hypoxanthine have been found to be elevated; in the cerebrospinal fluid (CSF), levels were four-fold greater than those of control individuals [33]. Concentrations of uric acid are not elevated in the spinal fluid.

The pathogenesis of the cerebral and particularly behavioral features of the disease remain unclear, while those features that are shared with patients with gout are clearly consequences of the accumulation of uric acid. Substantial evidence indicates that there is an imbalance of neurotransmitters. The best evidence for altered dopaminergic function came from the postmortem study of the brains of three patients in which there was statistically significant depression specifically of dopaminergic function in the caudate, putamen, nucleus accumbens and external pallidum [34]. Levels of homovanillic acid (HVA) in the spinal fluid were found to be low [35]. Studies of positron emission tomography (PET)

with ligands specific for targets in the basal ganglia revealed reduction in binding to dopamine uptake transporters by 73 percent in the putamen and 56 percent in the caudate [36]. Another study showed over 60 percent reduction in fluorodopa uptake [37]. Further evidence for neurotransmitter imbalance was the transient cessation of self-injurious behavior following treatment with the serotonin precursor, 5-hydroxytryptophan with carbidopa [38].

Treatment

Allopurinol has been effective in reducing concentrations of uric acid and alleviating all of its direct clinical consequences. Doses of 200–400 mg/day lead promptly to normal plasma concentrations. Calculi and tophi are prevented or resorbed as concentrations of uric acid in blood and in urine fall. Nephropathy and arthritis are prevented. The total production of purine does not change; concentrations of xanthine and hypoxanthine increase. Some patients develop xanthine calculi. Determination of the levels of the oxypurines may be useful in providing the optimal dose of allopurinol. We aim to maximize the content of hypoxanthine without running the risk of oxypurinol lithiasis.

Dietary approaches to reduction of purine and uric acid output by reducing intake of purine-rich foods are ineffective. Similarly, feeding purines does not increase it. The production level appears set by the metabolism. On the other hand, these patients are virtually all thin and predominantly short. The enormous loss of nitrogen and preformed purine in the urine along with dysphagia and vomiting make keeping up nutrition difficult. A diet high in protein and calories appears prudent. The occurrence of megaloblastic anemia and the requirement for folate-containing cofactors at two steps in purine synthesis would make the provision of folate prudent as folate rich foods or a supplement.

Pharmacologic approaches to therapy based on the neurotransmitter imbalance have not yet been successful, but this is a promising direction, possibly aided by PET and the demonstration of a reduction in dopamine transporters [36]. The availability of the cloned normal gene raises the possibility of gene therapy. Transfection of Lesch-Nyhan cells in vitro has been demonstrated, along with expression of normal enzyme [39]. Long-term expression in vivo remains an objective.

The only successful approaches to the self-injurious behavior have been the removal of teeth and physical restraint. Tooth removal can be selective. In addition to physical restraint it is useful to be imaginative in finding ways to encourage purposeful activity to replace self-injurious behavior [40]. For instance, one adult patient in a community placement regularly managed on entering an automobile to leave a hand in place to be caught when the door was closed. His caretaker learned to avoid this problem by the simple expedient of asking the patient to close the door himself.

NON-LESCH-NYHAN VARIANTS OF HPRT

MAJOR PHENOTYPIC EXPRESSION

Hyperuricemia, gout or renal calculi in each variant; in a neurologic variant the neurologic phenotype is identical to that of Lesch-Nyhan disease, but self-mutilation is absent and intelligence may be normal; in another variant the expression is of spastic diplegia, and mild mental retardation; variant HPRT enzymes may have activity that is 0 or as much as 50 percent of normal in hemolysates, but over 1.4 percent of control in the intact cell assay.

Introduction

The discovery of the enzyme defect in Lesch-Nyhan disease was followed shortly by the recognition of deficiency of the enzyme in patients with gout [41] or urinary tract calculi [42]. Initial expectations that these populations might be quite large have turned out not to be true, and most patients with abnormal HPRT enzymes have classic Lesch-Nyhan disease. Nevertheless, a certain number of variants has been described – enough that assay for HPRT activity should be performed in any patient with overproduction hyperuricemia, and any hyperuricemic patient with a diagnosis of cerebral palsy. In an infant found to have HPRT deficiency distinction between the classic Lesch-Nyhan prognosis and that of the variant forms is of major importance. Molecular studies of the nature of mutation in these populations are providing information on the genetic basis of altered phenotype [7].

Clinical abnormalities

The populations of patients initially described [41,42] had hyperuricemia, with gout or renal stones and HPRT enzyme activity greater than zero. For this reason they have been referred to as partial variants. However, additional experience shows that some of these patients have zero activity in the erythrocyte lysate assay and cannot in this way be distinguished from patients with Lesch-Nyhan disease. The phenotype of the patient with the classic partial variant enzyme consists of manifestations that can be directly related to the accumulation of uric acid in body fluids. The central nervous system and behavior are normal.

These patients pass large amounts of urate crystals in the urine (Figure 65.12). The earliest presentation, as in the Lesch-Nyhan disease, should be orange sand in the diaper. Advantages of the earliest diagnosis possible should be effective therapy to prevent renal complications. Renal calculi have been observed even early in childhood [42]. Such patients may present with hematuria, colic, urinary tract infection, or passage of a stone (Figure 65.13). There may be acute obstruction of one or both ureters and hydronephrosis. Crystalluria is so massive that an intercurrent infection that leads to vomiting or dehydration may result in complete obstruction of the ureters with sludge

requiring emergency surgery and ureteral lavage. We have observed this complication in which the crystals were of uric acid, but also of oxypurinol [43], the oxidation product of allopurinol. In the initial evaluation and follow-up of a patient with overproduction hyperuricemia, renal ultrasound

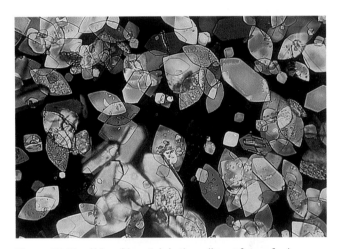

Figure 65.12 *Uric acid crystals in the sediment from a fresh, centrifuged sample of urine viewed through polarized light. (Reprinted with permission from Stapleton FB, Linshaw MA. N Eng J Med 1994;330:762.)*

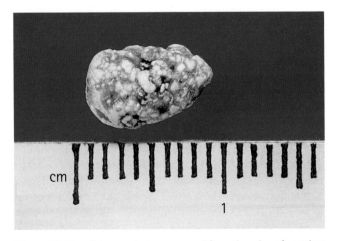

Figure 65.13 *Urinary calculus recovered from the urine of a patient with HPRT deficiency.*

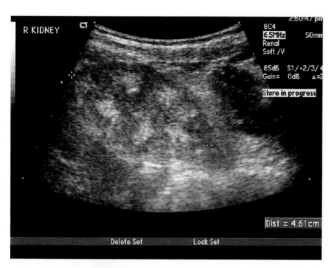

Figure 65.14   *Ultrasonograph of the kidneys of an infant with HPRT deficiency. Uric acid crystals are echogenic.*

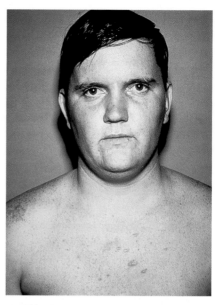

Figure 65.16   *R.L., a young man with a partial variant HPRT, was diagnosed after he passed a uric acid calculus during his second episode of renal colic. He and three male relatives displayed approximately five percent of the control level of HPRT by erythrocyte assay.*

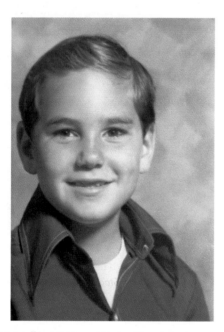

Figure 65.15   *T.L., a 7-year-old boy with a variant enzyme HPRT whose initial presentation was with painless hematuria. The initial episode was thought to be hemorrhagic cystitis but recurrent episodes suggested chronic glomerulonephritis. Biopsy was normal. HPRT activity was three percent in the erythrocyte assay at high concentration of substrates.*

or an intravenous pyelogram is essential to assess for the presence of uric acid or xanthine stones, which are radiolucent. A radiopaque stone in a patient with hyperuricemia indicates the codeposition of calcium salts. Ultasonography (Figure 65.14) may reveal echogenic crystals in the substance of the kidney. Untreated accumulation of uric acid can lead to urate nephropathy and renal failure.

Another presentation is with painless hematuria in a pattern that suggests a diagnosis of hemorrhagic cystitis or glomerulonephritis [44] (Figure 65.15). Cystourethography in this

patient led to transient hypertension, oliguria and azotemia; following anesthesia and renal biopsy oliguria/anuria recurred, and the blood urea nitrogen (BUN) rose to 80 mg/dL.

A majority of patients with partial variants have presented with gout [41,45,46]. Acute attacks of gouty arthritis and tophi usually occur first in adult life even though the hyperuricemia has been present since birth. It appears to require approximately 20 years of hyperuricemia before the conditions are appropriate for precipitation of the needle-like crystals of urate that produce the inflammatory response of the acute attack of arthritis. There are exceptions to every rule, and we have found a variant enzyme in a patient in whom acute attacks of arthritis began at one year.

Behavior is normal in these variant patients (Figure 65.16). Antisocial behavior that has rarely been described [47] may be completely unrelated to the defect in HPRT.

A quite different phenotype is what we have called the neurologic variant [48]. This picture, which has been observed in a small, but important group of patients, is characterized by a neurological examination that is identical to that of the classic Lesch-Nyhan patient. These patients are generally diagnosed as having cerebral palsy or athetoid cerebral palsy. They are confined to wheelchairs and unable to walk. The index patient was reported by Catel and Schmidt [49], as a patient with the Lesch-Nyhan syndrome in whom intelligence and behavior were normal. He has since been followed by Manzke [50], and we had the opportunity to study him just after his graduation from university (Figure 65.17). He spoke English and German. There were no abnormalities of intelligence or behavior. His variant HPRT was zero in erythrocyte lysates, but activity was readily distinguished from the

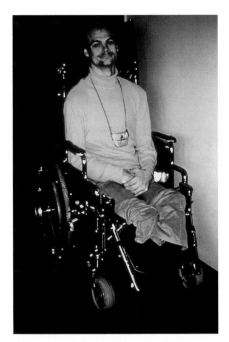

Figure 65.17 *H.C.B., a 21-year-old patient with the classic neurological variant [51]. Neurologic manifestations were identical to those of the Lesch-Nyhan disease, but intelligence and behavior were normal. A variant enzyme was documented by the intact cell assay.*

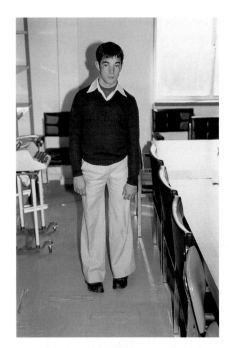

Figure 65.18 *A.A., a boy with HPRT$_{Salamanca}$. He had a pronounced spastic diplegia and a mild degree of developmental retardation.*

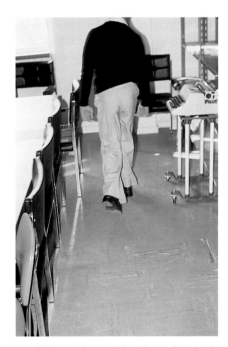

Figure 65.19 *A.A., rear view walking illustrating the dragging of his toes.*

Lesch-Nyhan disease by the intact cell assay [51]. Activity approached 10 percent of control, and there was enough activity to permit kinetic studies. A maternal uncle had had a similar syndrome. Other patients have since been studied in whom variant enzymes have produced this phenotype [52,32]. Behavior is normal, and intelligence is normal or nearly normal.

Virtually complete deficiency of HPRT in erythrocyte lysates was recently reported [53] in a 28-year-old patient with hyperuricemia and gout along with deficiency of glucose-6-phosphate dehydrogenase who had mild developmental retardation, mild dysarthria and hypotonia. Puig and colleagues [11] observed a variant patient who was intellectually normal but so dystonic and spastic that he could not walk.

Another phenotype has been observed in a family with an HPRT variant that we have called HPRT$_{Salamanca}$ [22,54]. In this pedigree four males in three generations had an identical phenotype, the most prominent feature of which was spastic diplegia. They were all able to walk, albeit with a spastic gait. The boy we studied (Figures. 65.18, 65.19) wore out the tops of the toes of his shoes because of the way he dragged his feet. Muscle tone and deep tendon reflexes were much more increased in the legs than in the arms. Babinski responses were positive bilaterally. There was a bilateral pes cavus and exaggerated lumbar lordosis. Mental retardation was mild. Involved members of the family were effectively employed as migrant grape pickers in Southern France. The proband had developed tophaceous gout by 32 years-of-age. Each of the involved members of the family had clinodactyly of the fifth fingers and proximally-placed thumbs. The abnormal enzyme displayed approximately eight percent of control activity in the whole cell assay. Other abnormalities observed in Lesch-Nyhan patients such as megaloblastic anemia or testicular dysfunction maybe seen in variants.

Genetics and pathogenesis

The gene for HPRT is on the long arm of the X chromosome and the pattern of inheritance is X-linked recessive. A kindred similar to that shown in Figure 65.20 with four involved males in two generations was recently reported [55]. In variants, in contrast to the Lesch-Nyhan disease, the heterozygote may display varying degrees of expression of the abnormal gene including hyperuricemia, uricosuria, gout, or the renal complication of uric acid excess. The presence of residual enzyme activity may make carrier detection or prenatal diagnosis unreliable with methods that depend on enzyme assay. Linkage analysis with RFLP [17] has been employed in informative families. In the case of HPRT$_{Toronto}$ a Taq 1 polymorphism was the only method that permitted the detection of heterozygosity [56]. Of course in a family in which the mutation is known, this may be effectively employed in both carrier detection and prenatal diagnosis.

Patients with variant forms of abnormal HPRT can all be characterized as different from normal by the assay [41,42,45] of the enzyme in erythrocytes, which identifies the presence of enzyme deficiency. In families in which there is a considerable amount of activity in the assays they are also distinguishable from Lesch-Nyhan variants. There may be one percent, five percent, 15 percent or more of the normal level of activity; and in a kindred in which there are a number of involved members [42,55] (Figure 65.20), each involved member has the same deficiency. All four males in one kindred (Figure 65.16, 65.20) had five percent of control activity. In other families, altered kinetics may be illustrated by different activity at saturating concentrations of substrates than at low concentrations (Figure 65.15), therefore, we routinely carry out the assay under these two conditions. In one of our patients with gout the erythrocyte activity was 60 percent of control [57].

On the other hand, the difficulty arises because a number of patients with phenotypes very different from the Lesch-Nyhan disease have been found to have no activity of HPRT as measured in erythrocyte or fibroblast lysates. This is a likely result of the fact that structurally abnormal enzymes are often unstable, and activity disappears rapidly once cell walls are broken. It is for this reason that no correlation has been found between the level of activity of the enzyme in hemolysates and clinical features in patients [58]. This is not because patients with the Lesch-Nyhan disease display any appreciable activity in these assays; it is because patients with quite mild phenotypes, including no central nervous system abnormality, also have no activity.

This problem has been solved by the development of a more physiological method in which enzyme activity is assessed in intact cells [59,60]. Cultured fibroblasts are incubated with ^{14}C-hypoxanthine, the products are separated by high performance liquid chromatography, and the total number of picomoles of isotope incorporated into purine compounds is expressed per nanomole of total purine compounds present [32]. The method permits the determination of kinetic properties of the enzyme. The K_m for hypoxanthine found in normal fibroblasts was identical to that of purified human HPRT, and a number of kinetic variants have been documented [61]. The patient illustrated in Figure 65.17 was shown with this method [51] to have a variant different from the classic Lesch-Nyhan enzyme; his HPRT converted nine percent of ^{14}C-hypoxanthine and 27 percent of ^{14}C-guanine to products that were mostly adenine and guanine nucleotides. In a series of patients with varying phenotypes a roughly inverse correlation was obtained between enzyme activity and clinical severity [32] (Figure 65.21). The activity obtained with hypoxanthine correlated better than did that obtained with guanine, and for this reason we routinely carry out the assay with hypoxanthine substrate. In this analysis Lesch-Nyhan patients

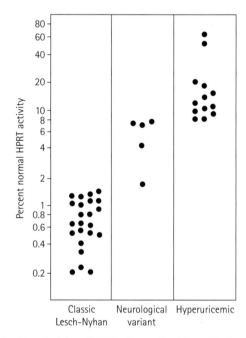

Figure 65.21 *Activity of HPRT in intact fibroblasts. The level of enzyme activity was roughly inversely proportional to the degree of clinical severity. Actually, the values fell into three groups, correlated with phenotype: the Lesch-Nyhan; the neurologic variant, and the classic partial variant.*

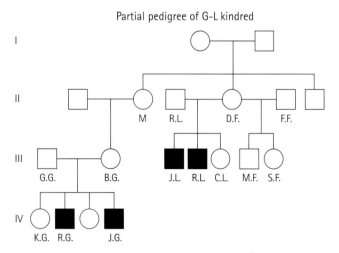

Figure 65.20 *Partial pedigree of the G.-L. kindred [42] (Figure 65.15).*

have displayed activity below 1.2 percent to 1.4 percent of normal, and the classic partial variants all had greater than 10 percent of control activity. The neurologic variants have had intermediate levels of activity.

Variant enzymes have been observed to have a variety of other properties that have aided their characterization as distinct, such as unusual sensitivity to fluoride [44], unusual kinetic properties, or altered heat stability [41,42]. Electrophoretic analysis has revealed mobilities that were both faster and slower than the normal enzyme [43,57,62]. Antibody generated against normal human HPRT has demonstrated the presence [57] and the absence [63] of cross-reacting material (CRM). In all of the variants studied the activity of adenine phosphoribosyl transferase (APRT) is increased; the level usually approximates 150 percent of control.

When the primary structure of normal human HPRT was determined [64] it became possible to determine the amino acid substitutions in variants in which a substantial amount of activity permitted purification and the preparation of peptide maps. For instance, in HPRT$_{Toronto}$ the substitution of glycine for arginine at position 50 is far removed from the binding sites for substrate, and, consistent with this, the kinetics were normal, and the phenotype was that of a classic hyperuricemic variant. In similar fashion, the transposition in HPRT$_{London}$ was far removed from substrate binding sites.

These issues are being clarified by the availability of the gene for human HPRT and of labeled probes for areas of the cDNA permitting amplification by PCR and definition by sequencing of the mutation [7,22]. In contrast to the mutations in Lesch-Nyhan disease the majority of these variants had missense mutations (Figure 65.22). Most had a single nucleotide change. Among seven variant patients reported from Spain [11] none had mutations that predicted altered protein size. Of the 271 mutations summarized by Jinnah et al. [7] there were 2 deletions in variant patients in contrast to 63 in Lesch-Nyhan patients. The one insertion observed in a variant added a single amino acid and did not alter the reading frame. Changes such as a leucine to valine at codon 78 appeared relatively conservative and led to a variant phenotype whereas

a leucine to glutamine change at 78 lead to a Lesch-Nyhan phenotype [7]. In HPRT$_{Salamanca}$ there were two mutations: a T to G change at position 128 and a G to A at 130. These led to conversions of two adjacent amino acids at position 43 and 44 in the protein: a methionine to an arginine and an aspartic acid to an asparagine. These alterations appear nonconservative. However they illustrate another issue: mutations in the variants have tended to cluster in the amino end of the molecule. In contrast, Lesch-Nyhan alterations in this area tended to be those with stop codons.

The pathogenesis of the hyperuricemia in patients with variant enzymes is no different from the typical Lesch-Nyhan situation. Overproduction of purines via the *de novo* pathway is probably largely a consequence of accumulation of phosphoribosylpyrophosphate (PRPP). Increased amounts of uric acid accumulating in body fluids lead to the clinical manifestations of gout and its renal complications. It is important to remember that normals for routine chemistry laboratories in general hospitals are established for adults. A serum concentration of 5 mg/dL in an infant or child is distinctly elevated [65]. The degree of overproduction in these variants is the same as in the Lesch-Nyhan disease. It is as if the production of purines has been reset at maximum or at a similar high plateau; they all have the same elevation in the amounts of uric acid in the urine and in the blood.

Treatment

These patients should all be treated with allopurinol. Relatively large doses may be required, with the objective of maintaining the plasma concentration less than 3 mg/dL. The encouragement of a high fluid intake and the avoidance of dehydration are prudent. Radiolucent urate stones are dissolved if the concentrations of uric acid bathing the calculus are sufficiently low as a result of treatment with allopurinol. Radiopaque stones will not, and they must be managed with lithotripsy or surgery if they are too large to pass spontaneously. This is also true of xanthine stones, which develop in the allopurinol-treated

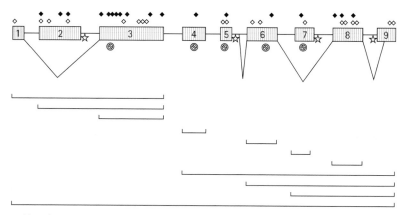

Figure 65.22   *The HPRT gene. The nine exons and sites of mutations are shown. The open diamonds represent variants. The filled diamonds represent classic Lesch-Nyhan patients. The stars indicate frame shifts and the stop signs, stop codons. Deletions of various sizes are shown below, virtually all in Lesch-Nyhan patients.*

patient. In a patient who develops xanthine stones it may be useful to measure the excretion of xanthine and hypoxanthine in the urine and adjust the dose such that amounts of the soluble hypoxanthine are maximal and the insoluble xanthine minimal.

References

1   Lesch M, Nyhan WL. A familial disorder of uric acid metabolism and central nervous system function. *Am J Med* 1964;**36**:561.

2   Nyhan WL. Introduction – clinical features: in *Seminars on the Lesch-Nyhan syndrome* (ed. JH Bland). *Fed Proc* 1968;**27**:1027.

3   Nyhan WL, Pesek J, Sweetman L, *et al.* Genetics of an X-linked disorder of uric acid metabolism and cerebral function. *Pediatr Res* 1967;**1**:5.

4   Seegmiller JE, Rosenbloom FM, Kelley WN. Enzyme defect associated with sex-linked human neurological disorder and excessive purine synthesis. *Science* 1967;**155**:1682.

5   Jolly DJ, Esty AC, Bernard HU, Friedmann T. Isolation of a genomic clone encoding human hypoxanthine guanine phosphoribosyl transferase. *Proc Natl Acad Sci USA* 1982;**79**:5038.

6   Jolly DJ, Okayama H, Berg P, *et al.* Isolation and characterization of a full length expressible cDNA for human hypoxanthine guanine phosphoribosyl transferase. *Proc Natl Acad Sci USA* 1983;**80**:477.

7   Jinnah HA, De Gregorio L, Harris JC, *et al.* The spectrum of inherited mutations causing HPRT deficiency: 75 new cases and a review of 196 previously reported cases. *Mutat Res* 2000;**463**:309.

8   Christie R, Bay C, Kaufman IA, *et al.* Lesch-Nyhan disease: clinical experience with nineteen patients. *Dev Med Child Neurol* 1982;**24**:293.

9   Jinnah HA, Harris JC, Reich SG, *et al.* The motor disorder of Lesch-Nyhan disease. *Mov Disord* 1998;**13**:98.

10 Jinnah HA, Harris JC, Rothstein JD, *et al.* Ocular motor abnormalities in Lesch-Nyhan disease. *Ann Neurol* 1998;**44**:453.

11 Puig JG, Torres RJ, Mateos FA, *et al.* The spectrum of hypoxanthine-guanine phosphoribosyltransferase (HPRT) deficiency. Clinical experience based on 22 patients from 18 Spanish families. *Medicine* 2001;**80**:102.

12 Harris JC, Lee RR, Jinnah HA, *et al.* Craniocerebral magnetic resonance imaging measurement and findings in Lesch-Nyhan syndrome. *Arch Neurol* 1998;**55**:547.

13 Kaufman JM, Greene ML, Seegmiller JE. Urine uric acid to creatinine ratio: screening test for disorders of purine metabolism. *J Pediatr* 1968;**73**:583.

14 Ogasawara N, Yamada Y, Goto H. HPRT gene mutations in a female Lesch-Nyhan patient: in *Purine and pyrimidine metabolism in man VII part B* (eds RA Harkness, *et al.*). Plenum Press, New York;1991:109.

15 De Gregorio L, Nyhan WL, Serafin E, Chamoles NA. An unexpected affected female patient in a classical Lesch-Nyhan family. *Mol Genet Metab* 2000;**69**:263.

16 Page T, Bakay B, Nyhan WL. An improved procedure for the detection of hypoxanthine-guanine phosphoribosyl transferase heterozygotes. *Clin Chem* 1982;**28**:1181.

17 Nussbaum RL, Crowder WE, Nyhan WL, Caskey CT. A three-allele restriction-fragment-length polymorphism at the hypoxanthine phosphoribosyltransferase locus in man. *Proc Natl Acad Sci USA* 1983;**80**:4035.

18 Francke U, Felsenstein J, Gartler SM, *et al.* The occurrence of new mutants in the X-linked recessive Lesch-Nyhan disease. *Am J Hum Genet* 1976;**28**:123.

19 Bakay B, Francke U, Nyhan WL, Seegmiller JE. Experience with detection of heterozygous carriers and prenatal diagnosis of Lesch-Nyhan disease: in *Purine Metabolism in Man II: Regulation of Pathways and Enzyme Defects* (eds MM Muller, E Kaiser, JU seegmiller). Plenum Press, New York;1977:351.

20 Page T, Broock RL. A pitfall in the prenatal diagnosis of Lesch-Nyhan syndrome by chorionic villus sampling. *Prenat Diagn* 1990;**10**:153.

21 Wilson JM, Tarr GE, Mahoney WC, Kelley WN. Human hypoxanthine-guanine phosphoribosyl-transferase. *J Biol Chem* 1982;**257**:10978.

22 Sege-Peterson K, Chambers J, Page T, *et al.* Characterization of mutations in phenotypic variants of hypoxanthine phosphoribosyltransferase deficiency. *Hum Molec Genet* 1992;**1**:427.

23 Gibbs RA, Nguyen P, McBride LJ, *et al.* Identification of mutations leading to the Lesch-Nyhan syndrome by automated direct DNA sequencing of *in vitro* amplified cDNA. *Proc Natl Acad Sci USA* 1990;**86**:1919.

24 Gibbs RA, Nguyen P, Edwards A, *et al.* Multiplex DNA deletion detection and exon sequencing of the hypoxanthine phosphoribosyltransferase gene in Lesch-Nyhan families. *Genomics* 1990;**7**:235.

25 Davidson BL, Tarle SA, Palella TD, Kelley WN. Molecular basis of hypoxanthine-guanine phosphoribosyltransferase deficiency in ten subjects determined by direct sequencing of amplified transcripts. *J Clin Invest* 1989;**84**:342.

26 Davidson BL, Tarle SA, van Antwerp M, *et al.* Identification of 17 independent mutations responsible for human hypoxanthine-guanine phosphoribosyltransferase (HPRT) deficiency. *Am J Hum Genet* 1991;**48**:951.

27 Tarle SA, Davidson BL, Wu VC, *et al.* Determination of the mutations responsible for the Lesch-Nyhan syndrome in 17 subjects. *Genomics* 1991;**10**:499.

28 Ehrlich M, Wang RY-H. 5-Methylcytosine in eukaryotic DNA. *Science* 1981;**212**:1350.

29 Yang TP, Patel PI, Stout JT, *et al.* Molecular evidence for new mutations in the HPRT locus in Lesch-Nyhan patients. *Nature* 1984;**310**:412.

30 Marcus S, Hellgren D, Lambert B, *et al.* Duplication in the hypoxanthine phosphoribosyl-transferase gene caused by Alu-Alu recombination in a patient with Lesch Nyhan syndrome. *Hum Genet* 1993;**90**:477.

31 Marcus S, Steen A-M, Andersson B, *et al.* Mutation analysis and prenatal diagnosis in a Lesch-Nyhan family showing non-random X-inactivation interfering with carrier detection tests. *Hum Genet* 1992;**89**:395.

32 Page T, Bakay B, Nissinen R, Nyhan WL. Hypoxanthine-guanine phosphoribosyl transferase variants: correlation of clinical phenotype with enzyme activity. *J Inherit Metab Dis* 1981;**4**:203.

33 Sweetman L. Urinary and cerebrospinal oxypurine levels and allopurinol metabolism in the Lesch-Nyhan syndrome. *Fed Proc* 1968;**27**:1055.

34 Lloyd KG, Hornykewicz O, Davidson L, *et al.* Biochemical evidence of dysfunction of brain neurotransmitters in the Lesch-Nyhan syndrome. *N Engl J Med* 1981;**305**:1106.

35 Silverstein FS, Johnston MV, Hutchinson RJ, Edwards NL. Lesch-Nyhan sydnrome: CSF neurotransmitter abnormalities. *Neurology* 1985;**35**:907.

36 Wong DF, Harris JC, Naidu S, *et al.* Dopamine transporters are markedly reduced in Lesch-Nyhan disease *in vivo*. *Proc Natl Acad Sci USA* 1996;**93**:5539.

37 Ernst M, Zametkin AJ, Matochik JA, *et al.* Presynaptic dopaminergic deficits in Lesch-Nyhan disease. *N Engl J Med* 1996;**334**:1568.

38 Nyhan WL, Johnson HG, Kaufman IA, Jones KL. Serotonergic approaches to the modification of behavior in the Lesch-Nyhan syndrome. *Appl Res in Mental Retard* 1980;**1**:25.

39 Miller AD, Jolly DJ, Friedmann T, Verma IM. A transmissable retrovirus exposing human hypoxanthine phosphoribosyl transferase (HPRT): gene transfer into cells obtained from humans deficient in HPRT. *Proc Natl Acad Sci USA* 1983;**80**:4709.

40 Barabas G, Zumoff PJ. Overview of Lesch-Nyhan disease. *Matheny Bulletin Special Edition* 1993;**III**:1.

41 Kelley WL, Greene ML, Rosenbloom FM, *et al.* Hypoxanthine-guanine phosphoribosyltransferase deficiency in gout: a review. *Ann Intern Med* 1969;**70**:155.

42 Kogut MD, Donnell GN, Nyhan WL, Sweetman L. Disorder of purine metabolism due to partial deficiency of hypoxanthine-guanine phosphoribosyltransferase. *Am J Med* 1970;**48**:148.

43 Landgrebe AR, Nyhan WL, Coleman M. Urinary-tract stones resulting from the excretion of oxypurinol. *N Engl J Med* 1975;**292**:626.

44 Sweetman L, Hoch MA, Bakay B, *et al.* A distinct human variant of hypoxanthine-guanine phosphoribosyl transferase. *J Pediatr* 1978;**92**:385.

45 Henderson JF, Kelley WN, Rosenbloom FM, Seegmiller JE. Inheritance of purine phosphoribosyltransferase in man. *Am J Hum Genet* 1969;**21**:61.

46 Wilson JM, Young AB, Kelley WN. Hypoxanthine-guanine phosphoribosyltransferase deficiency. The molecular basis of the clinical syndromes. *N Engl J Med* 1983;**309**:900.

47 Benke PJ, Herrick H. Azaguanine-resistance as a manifestation of a new form of metabolic overproduction of uric acid. *Am J Med* 1972;**52**:547.

48 Nyhan WL. Inborn errors of purine metabolism: in *Inborn Errors of Metabolism in Humans.* Monograph based upon Proceedings of the International Symposium held in Interlaken, Switzerland, September 1980. (eds F Cockburn, R Gitzelmann) MTP Press, Lancaster England;1982:13.

49 Catel VW, Schmidt J. Uber familiar gichtisch Diathese in Verbindung mit zerebralen und renalen Symptomen bei einem Kleinkind. *Dtsch Med Wochenschr* 195;**84**:2145.

50 Manzke H, Harms D, Dormer K. Zur Problematic der Behandlung der kongenitalen Hyperuyrikamie. *Monatsschr Kinderheilkd* 1971;**119**:424.

51 Bakay B, Nissinen E, Sweetman L, *et al.* Utilization of purines by an HPRT variant in an intelligent nonmutilative patient with features of the Lesch-Nyhan syndrome. *Pediatr Res* 1979;**13**:1365.

52 Gottlieb RP, Koppel MM, Nyhan WL, *et al.* Hyperuricaemia and choreoathetosis in a child without mental retardation or self-mutilation – a new HPRT variant. *J Inherit Metab Dis* 1982;**5**:183.

53 Micheli V, Jacomelli G, Notarantonio L, *et al.* Purine and pyrimidine metabolism in a patient with virtually complete HPRT deficiency but not Lesch-Nyhan syndrome. *European Society for Study of Purine and Pyrimidine Metabolism in Man* 2001:95.

54 Page T, Nyhan WL, Morena de Vega V. Syndrome of mild mental retardation spastic gait and skeletal malformations in a family with partial deficiency of hypoxanthineguanine phosphoribosyltransferase. *Pediatrics* 1987;**79**:713.

55 Augoustides-Savvopoulou P, Papachristou F, Fairbanks LD, *et al.* Partial HPRT deficiency as the cause of renal disease in a large kindred. *European Society for Study of Purine and Pyrimidine Metabolism in Man* 2001:26.

56 Wilson JM, Kobayashi R, Fox IH, Kelley WN. Human hypoxanthine-guanine phosphoribosyltransferase: molecular abnormality in the mutant of the enzyme (HPRT_Toronto). *J Biol Chem* 1983;**258**:6458.

57 Sweetman L, Borden M, Lesh P, *et al.* Diminished affinity for purine substrates as a basis for gout with mild deficiency of hypoxanthine guanine phosphoribosyl transferase: in *Purine Metabolism in Man: II Regulation of Pathways and Enzyme Defects* (eds MM Muller, E Kaiser, JE Seegmiller) Plenum Press, New York;1977:329.

58 Emmerson BT, Thompson L. The spectrum of hypoxanthine guanine phosphoribosyl transferase deficiency. *Quart J Med* 1973;**166**:423.

59 Bakay B, Nissinen E, Sweetman L. Analysis of radioactive and nonradioactive purine bases nucleosides nucleotides by high-speed chromatography on a single column. *Anal Biochem* 1978;**86**:65.

60 Bakay B, Nissinen EA, Sweetman L, Nyhan WL. Analysis of radioactive and nonradioactive purine bases purine nucleosides and purine nucleotides by high-speed chromatography on a single column. *Monogr Hum Genet* Vol 10. Karger, Basel;1978:127.

61 Page T, Bakay B, Nyhan WL. Kinetic studies of normal and variant hypoxanthine phosphoribosyltransferases in intact fibroblasts. *Anal Biochem* 1982;**122**:144.

62 Bakay B, Nyhan WL, Fawcett N, Kogut MD. Isoenzymes of hypoxanthine-guanine phosphoribosyl transferase in a family with partial deficiency of the enzyme. *Biochem Genet* 1972;**7**:73.

63 Bakay B, Becker MA, Nyhan WL. Reaction of antibody to normal human hypoxanthine phosphoribosyltransferase with products of mutant genes. *Arch Biochem Biophys* 1976;**177**:415.

64 Arnold WJ, Kelley WN. Molecular basis of hypoxanthine guanine phosphoribosyltransferase purification and subunit structure. *J Biol Chem* 1971;**246**:7398.

65 Monkus E StJ, Nyhan WL, Fogel BJ, Yankow S. Concentrations of uric acid in the serum of neonatal infants and their mothers. *Am J Obstet Gynecol* 1970;**108**:91.

66

Adenine phosphoribosyl-transferase (APRT) deficiency

MAJOR PHENOTYPIC EXPRESSION

Renal calculi and crystalluria, excretion of 2,8-dihydroxyadenine and deficiency of adenine phosphoribosyltransferase.

INTRODUCTION

Deficiency of APRT was first reported in 1976 by Simmonds and colleagues [1], and by Debray and colleagues [2], as a cause of urinary tract stones in children [1–3]. Initially, the calculi were mistaken for those of uric acid, and this is still a potential problem [4] when a routine chemical colorimetric reaction for uric acid is used to determine the compound being excreted in excessive quantity, or if lucency of the stone is considered diagnostic. The disease has most often been recognized in children, in whom urinary calculi are rare and thus more likely to trigger a search for an unusual cause, but the disease is now recognized in adults more commonly than in children [4]. This is particularly true in Japan, where the disease is more commonly encountered [5,6].

The enzyme APRT (EC 2.4.2.7.) (Figure 66.1) catalyzes the conversion of free-adenine to its mononucleotide (AMP).

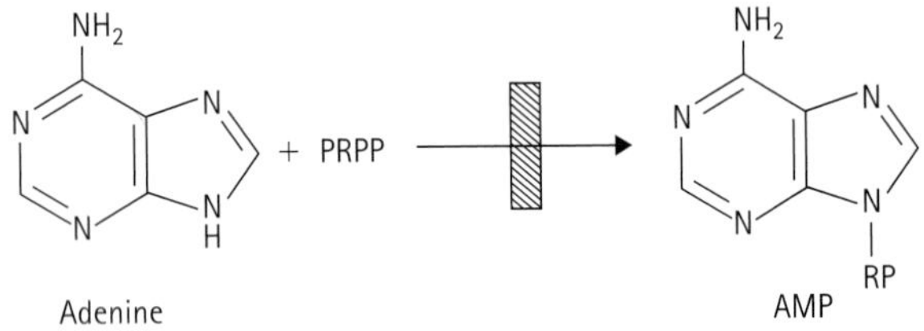

Figure 66.1 *The reaction catalyzed by APRT. Magnesium is a cofactor. Abbreviations include PRPP: phosphoribosyl pyrophosphate and AMP, adenylic acid.*

This enzyme and HPRT (Chapter 65) have been referred to as purine salvage enzymes. Deficiency is readily documented by assay of erythrocyte lysates. The gene has been localized to chromosome 16q24.3 [7–9] and has been cloned and sequenced. A number of mutations have been identified [10,11], including three mutations that account for 96 percent of the mutant alleles found in Japan [12].

CLINICAL ABNORMALITIES

The clinical picture of APRT deficiency is entirely a function of the excretion of 2,8-dihydroxyadenine and its propensity to cause nephrolithiasis and nephropathy (Figure 66.2) [13–16]. The severity of the disease is quite variable, ranging from no symptoms to life-threatening renal disease. A number of asymptomatic patients with APRT deficiency has been reported; they were found because they were screened family members of a known patient [4,13,14,17]. Onset of symptoms has ranged from birth to 74 years [5,13]. Rarely the disease may be indicated by the presence of brown spots on the diaper.

Patients may have hematuria, dysuria, crystalluria or urinary tract calculi. The presenting complaint may be fever resulting from a complicating urinary tract infection. Calculi may also lead to renal colic or urinary retention. Obstructive crystals may lead to acute renal failure even in infancy. This may be reversible, but the long-term outcome in some patients is chronic renal failure leading to dialysis or renal

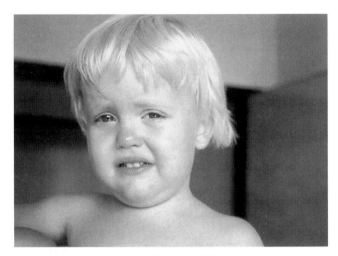

Figure 66.2 *An 18-month-old with APRT deficiency who began passing stones at birth. At last report he was a young, fit 24-year-old. (Illustration was kindly provided by Dr. H. Anne Simmonds of the United Medical and Dental Schools, University of London.)*

transplantation [4,15,16,18–22]. On the other hand some patients are asymptomatic.

Plain roentgenograms of the abdomen are usually negative in these patients since 2,8-dihydroxyadenine stones, like those of uric acid, are radiolucent; rarely, admixture of calcium will render these stones radio-opaque. Abdominal ultrasound or intravenous urography should be done if there is a suspicion of radiolucent stones. Calculi are usually thought first to be those of uric acid, and routine colorimetric analysis of the urine will not differentiate between uric acid and 2,8-dihydroxyadenine. A simple fluorescence method has been developed for the identification of 2,8-dihydroxyadenine stones. Mass spectrometry or scanning electron microscopy can be used for the correct identification of calculi [23].

It has become clear with increasing experience that there are no problems with other systems. Intelligence is normal. There is no abnormality of immune function.

GENETICS AND PATHOGENESIS

APRT deficiency is transmitted in an autosomal recessive fashion. Early reports of disease in heterozygotes have not held up. Consanguinity has been observed [3,13,24,25]. The disease has been divided into two subtypes: in type I erythrocyte lysates have no activity and in type II there is residual activity. Now that it is possible to determine the mutation these distinctions may become less useful, but homozygous type II patients have been found only in Japan; type I patients have been widely distributed, including in Japan [12,26]. The frequency of a heterozygous allele for APRT deficiency has been given as 0.4 to 1.2 percent in various Caucasian populations [27–29], but the incidence of diagnosed homozygotes is much lower than would be expected from these figures. This would be consistent with the asymptomatic nature of some patients described.

The enzyme (Figure 66.1) is a dimer with a subunit molecular weight of approximately 19 kDa and 179 amino acids [30]. 2,6-Diaminopurine (DAP) and 8-azaadenine are substrates for the enzyme, as are many adenine analogs that are toxic to cells after conversion to their nucleotides. These compounds are used in selective media [31]. Cells from either type I or type II patients will not grow in azaserine-alanosine-adenine (AAA) medium, and they are resistant to the adenine analogs 6-methylpurine and 2,6-diaminopurine. APRT is widely distributed in tissues and it is most commonly assayed in erythrocyte lysates, where normal activity is 16–32 nmol/h/mg hemoglobin.

In patients with the classic type I disease, there is less than one percent of control activity and immunoreactive protein [32–34]. Patients with residual enzyme activity of 10–25 percent of control in the type II group have displayed a variety of different properties, such as sigmoidal kinetics [26,35], reduced affinity for phosphoribosylpyrophosphate (PRPP) and altered heat stability. Decreased amounts of immunoprotein have been found [36].

Heterozygotes for type I deficiency have activity in hemolysates approximating 25 percent of control. Levels of immunoreactive protein may be 22 percent to normal [32–34]. In contrast, in lymphoblasts or fibroblasts activity is 46 percent and cross-reacting material (CRM) 41 percent of control. This raises the issue of distinguishing type II homozygotes from type I heterozygotes. Testing for resistance of cultured cells to medium containing DAP or 6-methylpurine should resolve the question [27]. Also cells of patients with type II disease will not grow in AAA medium, while those of type I heterozygotes do. Documentation of the mutation will also resolve the question. In general, anyone with APRT activity of 25 percent or more will have no clinical symptoms.

The gene at 16q24 is the most telomeric gene on chromosome 16 [37]. It contains five exons and a 540 base pair coding region [38,39]. A number of mutations have been identified, many of them single base substitutions. Many patients are compounds of two mutant alleles. A T insertion in intron 4 at the splice donor site has been found in five families from Europe and the United States; it leads to abnormal splicing and loss of exon 4 in the mRNA [11,14,40–42]. The T insertion creates an MseI restriction site that is useful in diagnosis [41]. Another intron 4 splice donor site mutation, a G-to-T transversion, would also disrupt splicing. A relatively common mutation in Britain and Iceland was an A-to-T change in exon 3, which converts aspartate 65 to valine [11]. Five Icelandic patients were homozygous for this mutation.

Among Japanese patients with the type II phenotype the most common mutation is a T-to-C mutation which changes methionine 136 to threonine (M136T) [12,43]. This has to date been found exclusively in type II patients. Actually three mutations account for 95 percent of the mutant alleles in Japanese patients [12]. The M136T accounts for 67 percent. The other two are a G-to-A substitution which changed tryptophan 98 to a stop codon in patients with the type I phenotype [44,45], and a four base, CCGA insertion in exon 3.

Restriction fragment length polymorphism in this area has been useful in family and population studies, leading, for instance, to a prediction that the M136T mutation has been in existence for between 4000 and 40 000 years [46]. A partial deficiency of APRT has also been reported in a patient with the type II mutation on one allele and a null or type I mutation on the other allele [47].

The direct consequence of deficiency of APRT is the accumulation of adenine, which is oxidized in the presence of xanthine oxidase to 2,8-dihydroxyadenine, which is very insoluble. The solubility of 2,8-dihydroxyadenine in water is less than 3 mg/L [13] but the compound may be supersaturated in urine. The excretion of adenine and 2,8-dihydroxyadenine occur in a ratio of 1:1.5. 8-Hydroxyadenine is excreted in lesser amount. Concentrations of 2,8-dihydroxyadenine up to 80 mg/L (0.5 mmol/L) have been found in patients [13].

TREATMENT

Therapy is aimed at reducing the formation of 2,8-dihydroxyadenine by the use of a low purine diet and allopurinol [3,13,15,48,49]. A dose of allopurinol of 10 mg/kg per day up to 300 mg in an adult has virtually eliminated 2,8-dihydroxyadenine from the urine [15,50]. Adenine still accumulates. A high fluid intake is prudent. Alkali therapy is not beneficial; the solubility of 2,8-dihydroxyadenine is not altered by changes of urinary pH in the range obtainable physiologically. Stones already formed may be treated with lithotripsy [51–53].

References

1 Simmonds HA, Van Acker KJ, Cameron JS, Snedden W. The identification of 28-dihydroxyadenine a new compound of urinary stones. *Biochem J* 1976;**157**:485.

2 Debray H, Cartier P, Temstet A, Cendron J. Child's urinary lithiasis revealing a complete deficit in adenine phosphoribosyltransferase. *Pediatr Res* 1976;**10**:762.

3 Barratt TM, Simmonds HA, Cameron JS, *et al.* Complete deficiency of adenine phosphoribosyltransferase. A third case presenting as renal stones in a young child. *Arch Dis Child* 1979;**54**:25.

4 Ceballos-Picot I, Perignon JL, Hamet M, *et al.* 28-Dihydroxyadenine urolithiasis an underdiagnosed disease. *Lancet* 1992;**339**:1050.

5 Kamatani N, Terai C, Kuroshima S, *et al.* Genetic and clinical studies on 19 families with adenine phosphoribosyltransferase deficiencies. *Hum Genet* 1987;**75**:163.

6 Kamatani N, Sonoda T, Nishioka K. Distribution of patients with 28-dihydroxyadenine urolithiasis and adenine phosphoribosyltransferase deficiency in Japan. *J Urol* 1988;**140**:1470.

7 Kahan B, Held KR, DeMars R. The locus for human adenine phosphoribosyltransferase on chromosome No 16. *Genetics* 1974;**78**:1143.

8 Tischfield JA, Ruddle FH. Assignment of the gene for adenine phosphoribosyltransferase to human chromosome 16 by mouse–human somatic cell hybridization. *Proc Natl Acad Sci USA* 1974;**71**:45.

9 Fratini A, Simmers RN, Callen DF, *et al.* A new location for the human adenine phosphoribosyltransferase gene (APRT) distal to the haptoglobin (HP) and fra (16)(q23)(FRA16D) loci. *Cytogenet Cell Genet* 1986;**43**:10.

10 Sahota A, Chen J, Stambrook PJ, Tischfield JA. Mutational basis of adenine phosphoribosyltransferase deficiency. *Adv Exp Med Biol* 1991;**309B**:73.

11 Sahota A, Chen J, Stambrook PJ, Tischfield JA. Genetic basis of adenine phosphoribosyltransferase deficiency: in *Molecular Genetics, Biochemistry and Clinical Aspects of Disorders of Purine and Pyrimidine Metabolism* (ed. U Gresser). Springer-Verlag, Heidelberg;1993:54.

12 Kamatani N, Hakoda M, Otsuka S, *et al.* Only three mutations account for almost all defective alleles causing adenine phosphoribosyltransferase deficiency in Japanese patients. *J Clin Invest* 1992;**90**:130.

13 Sahota AS, Tischfield K, Simmonds AH. Adenine phosphoribosyltransferase deficiency and 28-dihydroxyadenine lithiasis: in *The Metabolic and Molecular Bases of Inherited Disease* (eds CR Scriver, AL Beaudet, WS Sly, D Valle) 8th edn. McGraw Hill, New York;2001:2571.

14 Van Acker KJ, Simmonds HA, Potter CF, Cameron JS. Complete deficiency of adenine phosphoribosyltransferase: report of a family. *N Engl J Med* 1977;**297**:127.

15 Greenwood MC, Dillon MJ, Simmonds HA, *et al.* Renal failure due to 28-dihydroxyadenine urolithiasis. *Eur J Pediatr* 1982;**138**:346.

16 Fye KH, Sahota A, Hancock DC, *et al.* Adenine phosphoribosyltransferase deficiency with renal deposition of 28-dihydroxyadenine leading to nephrolithiasis and chronic renal failure. *Arch Int Med* 1993;**153**:767.

17 Laxdal T, Jonasson TA. Adenine phospho-ribosyltransferase deficiency in Iceland. *Acta Med Scand* 1988;**224**:621.

18 Schabel F, Doppler W, Hirsch-Kauffman M, *et al.* Hereditary deficiency of adenine phosphoribosyltransferase *Paëdiatr Paëdol* 1980;**15**:233.

19 Gliklich D, Gruber HE, Matas AJ, *et al.* 28-dihydroxyadenine lithiasis: report of a case first diagnosed after renal transplant. *Q J Med* 1988;**69**:785.

20 Takemoto M, Nagano S. Urolithiasis containing 28-dihydroxyadenine: report of a case. *Acta Urol Jpn* 1979;**25**:265.

21 Gagne ER, Deland E, Daudon M, *et al.* Chronic renal failure secondary to 28-dihydroxyadenine deposition: the first report of recurrence in a kidney transplant. *Am J Kid Dis* 1994;**24**:104.

22 de Jong DJ, Assmann KJ, De Abreu RA, *et al.* 28-Dihydroxyadenine stone formation in a renal transplant recipient due to adenine phosphoribosyltransferase deficiency. *J Urol* 1996;**156**:1754.

23 Winter P, Hesse A, Klocke K, Schaefer RM. Scanning electron microscopy of 28-dihydroxyadenine crystals and stones. *Scanning Microsc* 1993;**7**:1075.

24 Kuroda M, Miki T, Kiyohara H, *et al.* Urolithiasis composed of 28-dihydroxyadenine due to partial deficiency of adenine phosphoribosyl-transferase. *Jpn J Urol* 1980;**71**:283.

25 Ishidate T, Igarashi S, Kamatani N. Pseudodominant transmission of an autosomal recessive disease adenine phosphoribosyltransferase deficiency. *J Pediatr* 1991;**118**:90.

26 Fujimori S, Akaoka I, Sakamoto K, *et al.* Common characteristics of mutant adenine phosphoribosyltransferase. From four separate Japanese families with 28-dihydroxy-adenine urolithiasis associated with partial enzyme deficiencies. *Hum Genet* 1985;**7**:171.

27 Hakoda M, Yamanaka H, Kamatani N, Kamatani N. Diagnosis of heterozygote states for adenine phosphoribosyltransferase. Deficiency based on detection of *in vivo* somatic mutants in blood T cells: application to screening of heterozygotes. *Am J Hum Genet* 1991;**48**:552.

28 Simmonds HA. 28-dihydroxyadenine lithiasis. *Clin Chim Acta* 1986;**160**:103.

29 Fox IH, La Croix S, Planet G, Moore M. Partial deficiency of adenine phosphoribosyltransferase in man. *Medicine* 1977;**56**:515.

30 Wilson JM, O'Toole TE, Argos P, *et al.* Human adenine phosphoribosyltransferase: complete amino acid sequence of the erythrocyte enzyme. *J Biol Chem* 1986;**261**:13677.

31 Steglich C, DeMars R. Mutations causing deficiency of APRT in fibroblasts cultured from human heterozygous for mutant APRT alleles. *Somat Cell Genet* 1982;**8**:115.

32   Kishi T, Kidani K, Komazawa Y, *et al.* Complete deficiency of adenine phosphoribosyl-transferase: a report of three cases and immunologic and phagocytic investigations. *Pediatr Res* 1984;**18**:30.

33   Wilson JM, Daddona PE, Simmonds HA, *et al.* Human adenine phosphoribosyltransferase: immunochemical quantitation and protein blot analysis of mutant forms of the enzyme. *J Biol Chem* 1982;**257**:1508.

34   O'Toole TE, Wilson JM, Gault MH, Kelley WN. Human adenine phosphoribosyltransferase: characterization from subjects with a deficiency of enzyme activity. *Biochem Genet* 1983;**21**:1121.

35   Fujimori S, Akaoka I, Takeuchi F, *et al.* Altered kinetic properties of a mutant adenine phosphoribosyltransferase. *Metabolism* 1986;**35**:187.

36   Abe S, Hayasaka K, Narisawa K, *et al.* Partial and complete adenine phosphoribosyltransferase deficiency associated with 28-dihydroxyadenine urolithiasis: kinetic and immunochemical properties of APRT. *Enzyme* 1987;**37**:182.

37   Richards RI, Holman K, Lane S, *et al.* Chromosome 16 physical map: mapping of somatic cell hybrids using multiplex PCR deletion analysis of sequence tagged sites. *Genomics* 1991;**10**:1047.

38   Broderick TP, Schaff DA, Bertino AM, *et al.* Comparative anatomy of the human APRT gene and enzyme: nucleotide sequence divergence and conservation of a non-random CpG dinucleotide arrangement. *Proc Natl Acad Sci USA* 1987;**84**:3349.

39   Hidaka Y, Tarle SA, Kelley WN, Palella TD. Nucleotide sequence of the human APRT gene. *Nucleic Acids Res* 1987;**15**:9086.

40   Hidaka Y, Palella TD, O'Toole TE, *et al.* Human adenine phosphoribosyltransferase. Identification of allelic mutations at the nucleotide level as a cause of complete deficiency of the enzyme. *J Clin Invest* 1987;**80**:1409.

41   Gathof BS, Zollner N. The restriction enzyme MseI applied for the detection of a possibly common mutation of the APRT locus. *Clin Invest* 1992;**70**:535.

42   Chan J, Sahota A, Martin GF, *et al.* Analysis of germline and *in vivo* somatic mutations in the human adenine phosphoribosyltransferase genes: mutational hotspots at the intron 4 splice donor site and at codon 87. *Mutat Res* 1993;**287**:217.

43   Hidaka Y, Tarle SA, Fujimori S, *et al.* Human adenine phosphoribosyltransferase deficiency. Demonstration of a single mutant allele common to the Japanese. *J Clin Invest* 1988;**81**:945.

44   Sahota A, Chen J, Asako K, *et al.* Identification of a common nonsense mutation in Japanese patients with type I adenine phosphoribosyltransferase deficiency. *Nucleic Acids Res* 1990;**18**:5915.

45   Mimori A, Hidaka Y, Wu VC, *et al.* A mutant allele common to the type I adenine phosphoribosyltransferase deficiency in Japanese subjects. *Am J Hum Genet* 1991;**48**:102.

46   Kamatani N, Kuroshima S, Hakoda M, *et al.* Crossover within a short DNA sequence indicates a long evolutionary history of APRT*J mutation. *Hum Genet* 1990;**85**:600.

47   Takeuchi H, Kaneko Y, Fujita J, Yoshida O. A case of compound heterozygote for adenine phosphoribosyltransferase deficiency (APRT*J/ APRT*QO) leading to 28-dihydroxyadenine urolithiasis: review of the reported cases with 28-dihydroxyadenine stones in Japan. *J Urol* 1993;**149**:824.

48   Cartier P, Hamet M, Vincens A, Perignon JL. Complete adenine phosphoribosyl-transferase (APRT) deficiency in two siblings: report of a new case. *Adv Exp Biol Med* 1980;**122A**:343.

49   Chevet D, Le Pogamp P, Gie S, *et al.* 28-Dihydroxy-adenine (28-DHA) urolithiasis in an adult – complete adenine phosphoribosyl-transferase deficiency – family study. *Kidney Int* 1984;**26**:226.

50   Simmonds HA, Cameron JS, Barratt TM, *et al.* Purine enzyme defects as a cause of acute renal failure in childhood. *Pediatr Nephrol* 1989; **3**:433.

51   Jung P, Becht E, Ziegler M, *et al.* New diagnostic and therapeutic aspects of 28-dihydroxyadenine lithiasis. Another case of complete adenine phosphoribosyltransferase deficiency. *Eur J Urol* 1988;**14**:493.

52   Coupris L, Champion G, Duverne C, *et al.* La lithiase 28-dihydroxyadeninique 2 nouvelles observations pédiatriques d'un deficit métabolique méconnu. Apport de la lithotripsie extra-corporelle *Chir Pediatr* 1990;**31**:26.

53   Frick J, Sarica K, Kohle R, Kunit G. Long-term follow-up after extracorporeal shock wave lithotripsy in children. *Eur Urol* 1991;**19**:225.

67

Phosphoribosylpyrophosphate (PRPP) synthetase and its abnormalities

MAJOR PHENOTYPIC EXPRESSION

Hyperuricemia, uricosuria, hematuria, crystalluria, urinary tract calculi, gouty arthritis, nephropathy, sensorineural deafness and abnormal phosphoribosylpyrophosphate synthetase in which activity is greater than normal.

INTRODUCTION

A familial disorder, in which accelerated activity of PRPP synthetase was associated with overproduction of uric acid and gout, was first reported in 1972 by Sperling and colleagues [1,2]. A small number of patients has now been identified, establishing the relationship with hyperuricemia [1–10]. In some kindreds there has been sensorineural deafness [11–13].

5-Phosphoribosylpyrophosphate synthetase (EC 2.7.6.2) (Figure 67.1) catalyzes the initial step in the *de novo* synthesis of purines in which ribose-5-P reacts with adenosine triphosphate (ATP) to form PRPP. The PRPP formed provides the substrate for the first rate-limiting step in the 10-step reaction. Increased quantities of intracellular PRPP lead to overproduction of purine *de novo* and of uric acid. PRPP is coded for by two genes on the X chromosome at Xq22-24 and

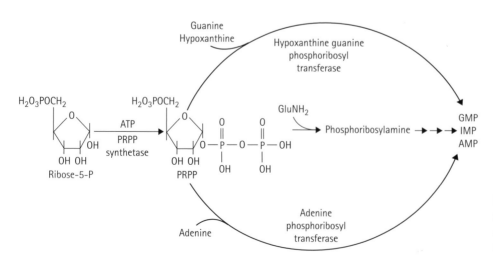

Figure 67.1 *PRPP synthetase. The role of the product PRPP is central in the interrelation of purines and their nucleotides.*

Xp22.2-22.3 [14,15]. The genes have been cloned and sequenced [16] and referred to as PRPS1 and S2 [17]. A small number of point mutations have been defined in PRPS1 in patients with overactivity and altered allosteric properties of the enzyme.

In six patients with overactivity of PRPP synthetase no mutation in the cDNA of PRPS1 or S2 were found; instead there were increased quantities of the S1 isoform whose physical and catalytic properties were normal [18].

CLINICAL ABNORMALITIES

The invariant clinical features of this disease are hyperuricemia and uricosuria. Therefore, a patient is subject to any of the clinical consequences of the accumulation of uric acid in body fluids. Gouty arthritis has been reported with onset as early as 21 years-of-age [1]. Renal colic has been observed, as well as the passage of calculi [3]. One boy developed hematuria at the age of 2 months and was found to have crystalluria, hyperuricemia and uricosuria [4]. In families with this early onset phenotype females have manifestations of hyperuricemia prior to menopause [13].

A small number of families has been reported [5,6,11,12] in which deafness has been associated with an abnormally active PRPP synthetase. In one family there were three involved males, each of whom also had severe neurodevelopmental retardation. The mother had high tone deafness. A large kindred had previously been reported in which there were X-linked deafness and hyperuricemia; an enzyme defect was not demonstrated at the time of report [19].

Another patient [5] appeared initially to be mentally retarded, and his behavior was thought to be autistic (Figure 67.2). With time it became apparent that he was deaf, and his behavior was quite appropriate (Figure 67.3). As an infant he failed to cry with tears and was found to have absent lachrymal glands. Other structural anomalies were a glandular hypospadias and hypoplastic teeth. The relationship of all of these problems to the metabolic abnormality is not clear, but the mother also had the abnormal PRPP synthetase and hearing loss, and she and her father had problems with behavior.

Patients with late teenage or young adult gout or urolithiasis have been exclusively male and have had no neurologic abnormalities [10,13]. These patients have had overabundance of the normal S1 isoform.

All of these patients have had increased amounts of uric acid in the blood and urine. In our patient prior to treatment, the concentration in serum ranged from 8.5 to 11.6 mg/dL [5]. Urinary excretion ranged from 1.84 to 3.26 mg/mg creatinine. In the initial proband [1] uric acid excretion was 2400 mg per 24 hr. Overproduction of purine *de novo* was documented [5] by measuring the *in vivo* in conversion of ^{14}C-glycine to urinary uric acid. In seven days 0.7 percent of the isotope of glycine administered was converted to uric acid – seven times the control level of 0.1 percent.

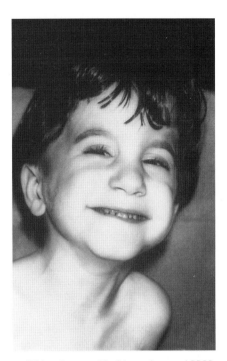

Figure 67.2   *S.M., a 3-year-old with an abnormal PRPP synthetase. The odd grimace was characteristic. (Reprinted with permission from the* Journal of Pediatrics *[5]).*

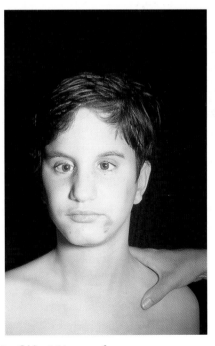

Figure 67.3   *S.M., at 14 years-of-age.*

GENETICS AND PATHOGENESIS

The S1 isoform of PRPP synthetase, while coded for by a gene on the long arm of the X chromosome [14] may be fully recessive [1] or may be expressed in the heterozygous female [3]. This could reflect different degrees of Lyonization. On the other hand, it is easier for an overactive enzyme, rather than the more common deficient one encountered in inborn errors, to function as an X-linked dominant.

The cDNAs of human S1 PRPP synthetase encodes a transcript of 2.3 kb and a protein of 317 amino acids. PRPS1 and S2 cDNAs have 80 percent nucleotide sequence identity in the translated regions. A third gene (S3) maps to chromosome 7 and is expressed only in testis [20]. In six male patients with overactivity of PRPP synthetase and resistance to purine nucleotide feedback, there was a single base transition, which led to a single amino acid change at positions 51, 89, 113, 128, 182 and 192 [16,17].

The molecular basis of the disease in the patients with superactive enzyme activity is an altered PRPP synthetase structure. Activity may be three times that of the normal enzyme [3]. In one of the families studied, increased enzyme activity was demonstrable only at low concentrations of phosphate and there was diminished responsiveness to feedback inhibition by purine nucleotides [2]. In another family an elevated level of enzyme-specific activity was demonstrable over a wide range of phosphate concentrations, and feedback inhibition was normal [3]. The amounts of immunoreactive enzyme protein were normal [21]. These observations indicate the presence in normal amounts of a protein in which structural alteration leads to increased specific activity. The data are consistent with the presence of two important sites on the enzyme: a catalytic site altered by one mutation and a regulatory site altered by the other. In one patient the altered structure affected both catalytic and regulatory sites [6]. The enzyme may have increased affinity for the substrate ribose-5-phosphate [22].

In addition to its other properties the PRPP synthetase in one patient had diminished stability to heat [6]. Distinctly diminished levels were found in old as opposed to young erythrocyte obtained by density separation. For these reasons the activity of PRPP as determined in erythrocyte lysates was not elevated, but in fact was lower than normal. This same observation was made in another family in which erythrocyte levels of PRPP were not elevated [11]. In the first patient the activity of PRPP synthetase in hemolysates was less than 10 percent of normal at concentrations of inorganic phosphate over 1 mM. In this sense a direct assay that indicates a deficiency of the erythrocytes' enzyme could be the clue to the presence of an abnormal enzyme that is superactive *in vivo*. Nevertheless, in a patient who appears clinically to be a candidate for a diagnosis of PRPP synthetase overactivity, a normal result of an erythrocyte assay should be followed up by an intact cell method.

Intact cultured fibroblasts can be shown to incorporate each of the purine bases, adenine, guanine and hypoxanthine, more rapidly into nucleotides than do controls [6]. Adenosine conversion to nucleotide is normal. Incorporation of ^{14}C-formate into formylglycinamide ribotide (FGAR) in the presence of azaserine is also accelerated. These findings indicate the presence of increased intracellular concentrations of PRPP. Concentrations can be measured in fibroblasts or lymphoblasts and found to be elevated [6].

The single amino acid substitutions in the S1 enzyme are clearly scattered over much of the protein; yet they all lead to decreased responsiveness to feedback inhibition by adenosine diphosphate (ADP) and guanosine diphosphate (GDP) [16]. Also the binding of MgATP to the active site is normal. The mechanism for the allosteric changes resulting in superactivity is unknown, but it must be structurally diffuse. Mechanisms for the increased transcription in the patients in whom no structural changes were found are even less clear, although a number of possibilities have been excluded [23].

An entirely different variation in PRPP synthetase has been described [24] in an infant with markedly decreased activity of PRPP synthetase in erythrocytes. The patient was severely retarded mentally and had a megaloblastic bone marrow. PRPP synthetase deficiency led to low levels of uric acid in blood and urine and large amounts of orotic acid in the urine; which would be consistent with a shortage of PRPP substrate for the orotate phosphoribosyltransferase (OPRT) reaction.

TREATMENT

Allopurinol is the treatment of choice in overproduction hyperuricemia. Treatment of abnormalities in PRPP synthetase is simpler than that of hypoxanthine guanine phosphoribosyl transferase (HPRT) deficiency because in the presence of normal HPRT activity there is extensive reutilization of hypoxanthine accumulating behind the block in xanthine oxidase, leading to a substantial decrease in the overall excretion of oxypurines in the urine. In contrast, in HPRT deficiency there is simple substitution of hypoxanthine or xanthine for uric acid, and the total oxypurine excretion does not change.

Hearing should be tested promptly and appropriate intervention provided.

References

1   Sperling O, Eilma G, Persky-Brosh S, DeVries A. Accelerated erythrocyte 5-phosphoribosyl-1-pyro-phosphate synthesis: a familial abnormality associated with excessive uric acid production and gout. *Biochem Med* 1972;**6**:310.

2   Sperling O, Boer P, Persky-Brosh S, *et al*. Altered kinetic property of erythrocyte phosphoribosylpyrophosphate synthetase in excessive purine production. *Eur J Clin Biol Res* 1972;**17**:73.

3   Becker MA, Meyer LJ, Seegmiller JE. Gout with purine overproduction due to increased phosphoribosylpyrophosphate synthetase activity. *Am J Med* 1973;**55**:232.

4   DeVries A, Sperling O. Familial gouty malignant uric acid lithiasis due to mutant phosphoribosyltransferase synthetase. *Urologe A* 1973;**12**:153.

5   Nyhan WL, James JA, Teberg AJ, *et al*. A new disorder of purine metabolism with behavioral manifestations. *J Pediatr* 1969;**74**:20.

6   Becker MA, Raivio KO, Bakay B, *et al*. Variant human phosphoribosylpyrophosphate synthetase altered in regulatory and catalytic functions. *J Clin Invest* 1980;**65**:109.

7   Nishida Y, Akaoka I, Horiuchi Y. Altered isoelectric property of a superactive 5-phosphoribosyl-1-pyrophosphate (PRPP) synthetase in a patient with clinical gout. *Biomed Med* 1981;**26**:387.

8 Akaoka I, Fujimori S, Kamatani N, *et al.* A gouty family with increased phosphoribosylpyrophosphate synthetase activity: case reports familial studies and kinetic studies of the abnormal enzyme. *J Rheumatol* 1981;**8**:563.

9 Sperling O, Boer P, Browsch S, *et al.* Overproduction disease in man due to enzyme feedback resistance mutation. *Enzyme* 1978;**23**:1.

10 Becker MA, Losman MH, Rosenberg AL, *et al.* Phosphoribosylpyrophosphate synthetase superactivity. A study of five patients with catalytic defects in the enzyme. *Arthritis Rheum* 1986;**29**:880.

11 Simmonds HA, Webster DR, Wilson J, *et al.* Evidence of a new syndrome involving hereditary uric acid overproduction neurological complications and deafness: in *Purine Metabolism in Man – IV* (eds CHMM DeBruyn, HA Simmonds, MM Muller) Plenum Press, New York;1984:97.

12 Simmonds HA, Webster DR, Lingam S, Wilson J. An inborn error of purine metabolism deafness and neurodevelopmental abnormality. *Neuropediatrics* 1985;**16**:106.

13 Becker MA, Puig JG, Mateos FA, *et al.* Inherited superactivity of phosphoribosylpyrophosphate synthetase: association of uric acid overproduction and sensorineural deafness. *Am J Med* 1988;**85**:383.

14 Becker MA, Yen RCK, Itkin P. Regional localization of the gene for human phosphoribosylpyrophosphate synthetase on the X chromosome. *Science* 1979;**203**:1016.

15 Becker MA, Heidler SA, Bell GI, *et al.* Cloning of cDNAs for human phosphoribosylpyrophosphate synthetases 1 and 2 and X chromosome localization of PRPS1 and PRPS2 genes. *Genomics* 1990;**8**:555.

16 Becker MA, Smith PR, Taylor W, *et al.* The genetic and functional basis of purine nucleotide feedback-resistant phosphoribosylpyrophosphate synthetase superactivity. *J Clin Invest* 1995;**96**:2133.

17 Roessler BJ, Nosal JM, Smith PR, *et al.* Human X-linked phosphoribosylpyrophosphate synthetase superactivity is associated with distinct point mutations in the PRPS1 gene. *J Biol Chem* 1993;**268**:26476.

18 Becker MA, Taylor W, Smith PR, Ahmed M. Overexpression of the normal phosphoribosylpyrophosphate synthetase isoform 1 underlies catalytic superactivity of human phosphoribosylpyrophosphate synthetase. *J Biol Chem* 1996;**271**:19894.

19 Rosenberg AL, Bergstrom L, Troost BT, Bartholomew BA. Hyperuricaemia and neurological deficits: a family study. *N Engl J Med* 1970;**282**:992.

20 Taira M, Iizasa T, Shimada H, *et al.* A human testis-specific mRNA for phosphoribosylpyrophosphate synthetase that initiates from a non-AUG codon. *J Bio Chem* 1990;**265**:16491.

21 Becker MA, Kostel PJ, Meyer LJ, Seegmiller JE. Human phosphoribosylpyrophosphate synthetase: increased enzyme specific activity in a family with gout and excessive purine synthesis. *Proc Natl Acad Sci USA* 1973;**70**:2749.

22 Becker MA, Losman MH, Simmonds HA. Inherited phosphoribosylpyrophosphate synthetase superactivity due to aberrant inhibitor and activator responsiveness: in *Purine and Pyrimidine Metabolism in Man, V Part A: Clinical Aspects Including Molecular Genetics* (eds WL Nyhan, LF Thompson, RWE Watts) Plenum Press. New York;1986:59.

23 Ahmed M, Taylor W, Smith PR, Becker MA. Accelerated transcription of PRPS1 in X-linked overactivity of normal human phosphoribosylpyrophosphate synthetase. *J Biol Chem* 1999;**274**:7482.

24 Wada Y, Nishimura Y, Tanabu M, *et al.* Hypouricemic mentally retarded infant with a defect of 5-phosphoribosyl-1-pyrophosphate synthetase of erythrocytes. *Tohoku J Exp Med* 1974;**113**:149.

Adenosine deaminase deficiency

MAJOR PHENOTYPIC EXPRESSION

Severe combined immunodeficiency disease, involving immunoglobulins and cell-mediated immunity; clinical immunodeficiency triad of persistent diarrhea, progressive pulmonary disease, and extensive moniliasis; skeletal abnormalities; and deficiency of adenosine deaminase.

INTRODUCTION

The discovery of the association between adenosine deaminase (ADA) (EC 3.5.4.4) deficiency and severe combined immunodeficiency disease in the early 1970s [1] provided exciting evidence of metabolic causation of immunodeficiency. This established a relationship between the metabolism of purines and developmental immunobiology, and this was reinforced by the discovery of purine nucleoside phosphorylase deficiency.

The discovery of this disorder was an interesting example of important observations made by a prepared mind. Giblett, a pediatric pathologist [1,2] was reviewing polymorphic markers in candidates for a bone marrow transplantation and found one deficient in ADA; a sample from a second unrelated patient studied a week later was also ADA-deficient. Within a year a number of immunodeficient patients with ADA deficiency were reported [3]. Giblett and her colleagues used the same approach to discover purine nucleoside phosphorylase (PNP) (EC 2.4.2.1) deficiency [4].

Adenosine deaminase and PNP deficiencies represent enzymatic defects in the metabolism of purines that affect primarily cells of the immune system. The mechanism appears to be the accumulation of purine nucleotides which are toxic to T and B cells [5]. Adenosine deaminase is an enzyme of purine interrelations, which converts adenosine to inosine (Figure 68.1). This is an important reaction because adenosine is not a

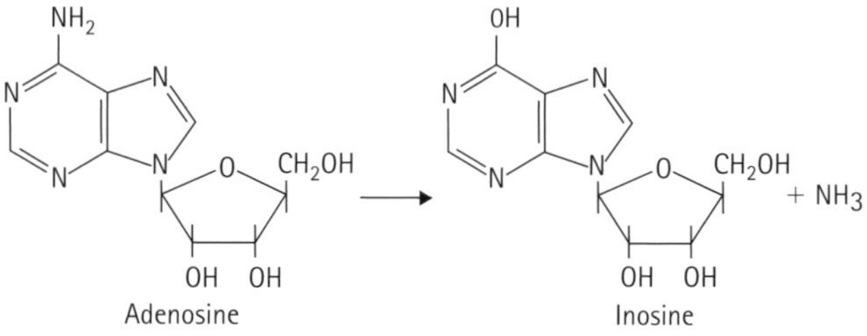

Figure 68.1 *The adenosine deaminase reaction.*

substrate for nucleoside phosphorylase, which converts inosine and guanosine to hypoxanthine and guanine. Adenosine deaminase is widely distributed in animal tissues. This enzyme is determined by a gene on chromosome 20q13.11 [6]. The gene for ADA has been cloned and sequenced [7]. A considerable number of mutations have been identified [8–10], most of them single amino acid changes.

CLINICAL ABNORMALITIES

Classic patients with ADA deficiency have a distinct syndrome of severe combined immunodeficiency disease (SCID). In common with other patients with severe combined immunodeficiency disease, they have both defective immunoglobulins or bone marrow-derived B-cell function and defective cell-mediated immunity or thymus-derived T-cell function. Patients with B cell or humoral immunodeficiency have infections caused by organisms such as the pneumococcus with capsules as well as some viruses. Patients with T cell or cell-mediated immunodeficiency have infections caused by opportunistic organisms, such as monilia, or by viruses. Patients with combined immunodeficiency have both types of infection.

Most patients with SCID present in the first months of life with failure to thrive and recurrent or persistent diarrhea [1,3,11–14]. The diagnosis is usually not made until the onset of infection that follows the disappearance of maternal antibody. Severe bacterial and viral infections occur very early in life. A majority of patients have had extensive candidiasis. Many have presented in the first weeks or months of life with thrush, diarrhea and pneumonia. Many have had bacterial infections of the skin. Recurrent otitis media is common, and pneumonia is a frequent complication. Many patients have died, often of infections with opportunistic organisms, some viral and some bacterial, that are not usually productive of severe infections in ordinary individuals.

Isolated defects of the cellular immune system, as well as severe forms of combined immunodeficiency, have been described in 10–15 percent of individuals with ADA deficiency [6,15]. These patients have had a milder course of disease, often with a later onset. A number of patients have been observed with milder forms of the disease reflecting higher levels of residual ADA activity. Adult-onset immunodeficiency was reported in two sisters with a residual ADA activity of 5–13 percent [16]. Furthermore, ADA deficiency has been described without abnormality in immune function [17]. A tandem mass spectrometry (MS/MS) method for the detection of ADA deficiency has been developed [18]; so neonatal screening is now possible, and this should lead to complete ascertainment and better definition of the clinical spectrum. In general it appears that immune function may be normal if levels of ADA are over five percent of control.

Patients with ADA deficiency, like those with other types of SCID, are at risk for the development of graft-versus-host disease if they receive blood transfusion from a donor with immunocompetent T cells. They are also at risk for disseminated diseases following immunization with live attenuated vaccines, such as poliomyelitis. Active infection has occurred following administration of oral polio vaccine. Known patients are better immunized for this disease with Salk inactivated vaccine.

The majority of patients reported with ADA deficiency have been infants with SCID and recurrent infections [19,20]. Pneumonia may be caused by *Pneumocystis carinii* or by viruses. Candidiasis may involve the skin, the mucosa of the mouth, esophagus, or vagina, and stool cultures may reveal this organism. Patients surviving infancy may have pulmonary insufficiency, a consequence of repeated infection. Among late onset presentations were pulmonary insufficiency and recurrent warts in adult sisters [21].

Autoimmune disease is also a feature of ADA deficiency. Presentations have included autoimmune thyroid insufficiency [22,23], autoimmune thrombocytopenia [24] and fatal autoimmune hemolytic anemia [25].

Neurologic abnormalities may occur in ADA deficiency; they are more common in PNP deficiency. They may be a consequence of infection or possibly of the severe failure to thrive. However, in some patients neurologic abnormality has appeared to be a metabolic consequence of the disease. Patients have had spasticity, nystagmus, tremors, dystonic posturing, athetosis, hypotonia and head lag [20,26–28]. In at least one patient, improvement was documented after successful treatment with enzyme replacement [26]. Developmental delay has been reported to be more prevalent in ADA-deficient patients with SCID than in ADA-normal patients with SCID [20]. In a similar study of patients with SCID treated with bone marrow transplantation [29] tests of cognitive function revealed no differences between the two groups, ADA-deficient and non-ADA deficient. However, among the ADA-deficient patients there was significant inverse correlation between the levels of deoxyadenosine triphosphate (dATP) at diagnosis and IQ. In behavioral assessment the ADA-SCID patients functioned in the pathologic range in all domains while the non-ADA patients scored in the normal range. Neurologic examinations were unremarkable in these patients, and none had seizures.

Hepatic dysfunction has been observed in this disease [30,31], and many patients have elevated serum transaminase levels; levels have improved with replacement therapy. Recurrent hepatitis has been followed by chronic hepatobiliary disease. B cell lymphomas have been related to infection with Epstein-Barr virus.

Physical examination may be remarkable only for evidence of infection and poor growth, failure to thrive. Absence of lymphatic tissue may be striking, and this may be evident on palpation or examination of the pharynx. It is often first recognized roentgenographically. In roentgenograms the upper mediastinum is narrow. In lateral views there may be retrosternal radiolucency and no thymus shadow can be seen. Examination of the blood reveals profound lymphopenia [31]. Total lymphocyte count may be less than 500 per μL. Most of these patients have chronic pulmonary changes such as those seen in infections with *Pneumocystis carinii*. A bony dysplasia is an impressive feature of the syndrome [32]. The sacroiliac notch may be large, as in achondroplasia, and the ilium flares outward, resembling Mickey Mouse ears. The acetabular angle is reduced, also like that of achondroplasia. The pubis is short and the ischium squared off. The ribs are flared, enlarged anteriorly, and cupped at the costochondral ends, resembling changes seen in rickets. In the spine there is platyspondyly and an appearance reminiscent of mucopolysaccharidosis. In contrast to the spine in achondroplasia, the interpedicular distance in these patients does not decrease from L1 to L5. Growth arrest lines may be unusually thick. Roentgenograms of the bones may reveal profound osteoporosis. One patient had compression fractures of two vertebral bodies.

Skin tests for delayed hypersensitivity are deficient, and skin tests for candida are negative in patients known to have had candidal infection. Skin tests for streptokinase and other antigens are negative. The response of lymphocytes *in vitro* to phytohemagglutinin and other lectins is reduced or absent, and the formation of T-cell rosettes is poor. All of the immunoglobulins in these patients are decreased in concentration, once the infant is old enough to have lost immunoglobulin transferred from the mother. These include IgG, IgM, IgA and others, but often it is to a variable degree of each. The antibody response to the injection of an immunizing antigen is faulty.

Pathologic examination of the thymus at autopsy has revealed a very small organ with little differentiation into lobules. No Hassall's corpuscles were seen. There was no central medullary area and no differentiation into cortex and medulla. Huber and Kersey [33], who analyzed tissues from four patients with adenosine deaminase deficiency and five without, all of whom had died of combined immunodeficiency disease, believed that they could distinguish between the two groups. The patients without ADA deficiency appeared to have failed to develop thymic tissue in early embryonic life, whereas the ADA-deficient patients had what they called extreme involution. The thymus in these patients appeared to have known better days.

GENETICS AND PATHOGENESIS

Adenosine deaminase deficiency is transmitted as an autosomal recessive disease. In heterozygous carriers for adenosine deaminase deficiency, levels of enzyme activity are about half the normal level [5,34–36], but detection of carriers by enzyme assay in erythrocytes or fibroblasts is not reliable. Polymorphism in the ADA cDNA has been successfully used for this purpose, and of course in a family in which the mutation is known, this is a reliable approach to carrier detection. The incidence of the disease from neonatal screening in New York approximated one in 400 000 to 500 000 births [19,37]. ADA deficiency accounts for about half of the patients with autosomal recessive SCID. Prenatal diagnosis has been accomplished by assay of the enzyme in cultured amniocytes and chorionic villus samples [34,38,39].

The molecular basis of the disease is the deficiency of the activity of ADA, a 41 kDa single polypeptide chain enzyme, the N terminal of which is post translationally removed to yield 332 amino acids [40]. The ADA gene [7] consists of 12 exons spanning about 32000 bases of DNA. Analyses of the ADA genes isolated from patients with ADA deficiency have revealed a heterogeneous pattern of mutations as causes of deficient enzyme activity [8,9,41–44]. Most patients are compounds of two mutant genes. Severe combined immunodeficiency and low levels of mRNA and protein have been seen with a 5 base pair deletion in exon 10 [41] and a glycine 20 to arginine point mutation [43], while later-onset, milder disease was found with a point mutation changing arginine 253 to proline [44] and substitution at 156 of histidine for arginine. Splicing and other missense mutations have been identified [42]. The same mutation found in more than one family has

often arisen at CpG hot spots [45,46]. A329V, a relatively common mutation has been found in a number of unrelated patients [8]; so has R211H. Most deletions are small but may introduce stop signals. Splicing site mutations, such as a G to A change in IVS10, which inserts 100 amino acids, have been observed in patients with more indolent disease, suggesting that alternate splicing may provide useful amounts of the wild type enzyme [47,48]. Prenatal diagnosis has been accomplished by the assessment of mutation in the ADA-gene [49].

ADA catalyzes the irreversible deamination of adenosine (Figure 68.1) to form inosine. Deoxyadenosine also serves as a substrate for the enzyme. Intracellular adenosine is produced in the catabolism of RNA and also by the hydrolysis of S-adenosylhomocysteine, an intermediary in transmethylation reactions [50].

Adenosine deaminase may be assayed in the erythrocyte by means of a technique that measures ammonia liberated from adenosine. The enzyme in intact erythrocytes of normal individuals had a mean activity of 0.29 nmol/min/mL packed cells. There has been no detectable ADA activity in most patients studied [5,34,35]. A screening test has been developed [51] which permits the diagnosis on spots of dried blood on filter paper and is employed in neonatal screening.

In ADA deficiency there is accumulation of adenosine and 2′-deoxyadenosine. Normal plasma concentrations of adenosine are 0.05 to 0.4 μM/L; levels of deoxyadenosine are below the level of detection. In ADA-deficient patients, plasma concentrations of adenosine and deoxyadenosine range from 0.5 to 10 μM/L. Large amounts of deoxyadenosine are excreted in the urine.

Inhibitors of ADA are toxic to cells. The pathophysiological mechanism by which ADA deficiency produces immunodeficiency appears to be the consequence of the accumulation of adenosine and deoxyadenosine, which are converted to ATP and deoxyadenosine triphosphate (dATP). ATP and, especially, dATP have been shown to be toxic to lymphoid cells of the immune system [6,52–56]. It is thought that accumulated dATP inhibits ribonucleotide reductase, which catalyzes the conversion of ribonucleotide diphosphates to deoxyribonucleotide diphosphates and in this way inhibits the synthesis of DNA [54]. Consistent with hypothesis, deoxynucleosides of cytosine, thymine and guanine are capable of reversing the toxic effects of the adenosine deaminase inhibitor, deoxycoformycin [55], but there appear to be many possible mechanisms of the deficiency of immune function. Deoxyadenosine itself also leads to chromosomal breakage through inhibition of DNA repair.

Adenosine deaminase inhibitors coformycin and deoxycoformycin produce a metabolic pattern in normal cells similar to that of ADA-deficient cells, and so does an inhibitor of nucleoside transport; neither compound had any effect on ADA-deficient cells [35]. Lymphocytes and lymphoblasts undergo apoptosis when treated with deoxyadenosine [57]. CD26, a T cell surface activation molecule also known as depeptidyl peptidase IV (DPPIV), has been found to bind to ADA [58] and has been called ADA complexing protein.

It could have a role in T cell activation. The activity of S-adenyosylhomocysteine (SAH) hydrolase is reduced in ADA deficiency, a consequence of suicide-like inactivation by deoxyadenosine [59]. Accumulation of adenosyl-homocystine could inhibit transmethylation. ADA-deficient murine cultured thymocytes could be rescued by an adenosine kinase inhibitor 5′-amino-5′deoxyadenosine indicating that dATP is responsible for the toxicity of deoxyadenosine [60] and that dATP-induced release of mitochondrial cytochrome followed by apoptosis is the mechanism of reduced T cells in ADA deficiency. SAH hydrolase remained deficient in the rescued cells.

Adenosine also serves as a regulator of blood flow and an inhibitor of platelet aggregation, lipolysis and neurotransmitter release. It modulates beta-adrenergic receptor and insulin-mediated responses; it stimulates steroidogenesis and histamine release; and it inhibits superoxide and hydrogen peroxide release from neutrophils [61,62]. Adenosine mediates these varied functions through specific membrane receptors. It is not clear that any of theses functions is altered in ADA deficiency.

TREATMENT

The current definitive treatment of ADA deficiency is bone marrow transplantation. The first survivors of SCID due to ADA deficiency were those that had been successfully treated with bone marrow transplantation [63] or with transplantation from fetal liver (Figures 68.2, 68.3). Successful treatment by bone marrow transplantation has readily been accomplished when a histocompatible donor has been available; or, in the absence of such a donor, with half-matched parental marrow after removal of most of the post-thymic T cells [64]. In the presence of histocompatibility antigens (HLA)-identical bone marrow, the engraftment rate is around 80 percent, and full immune repopulation occurs in approximately 6 months [62]. In experience with patients with SCID, four of whom were ADA deficient, all received HLA-identical bone marrow grafts and survived [65].

It has been found that transfusion of frozen irradiated red blood cells from normal individuals provided circulating levels of ADA and restored normal and cell-mediated immunity [27,66,67]. Levels of dATP were reduced [67]. The half-life of transfused ADA activity is 30 days, and so treatment must be repeated every four weeks.

These observations led to the development of enzyme replacement therapy using bovine ADA conjugated to polyethylene glycol (PEG-ADA). which has proved to be useful for many patients [24,68]. It is given initially twice a week, and later weekly as an intramuscular injection. PEG-ADA treatment restores immune competence. PEG-ADA has been employed to prepare very ill patients for transplantation.

ADA deficiency has also been treated by gene therapy [69,70]. Cells (CD 34) isolated from autologous peripheral blood of the patient's cord blood have been used as recipients

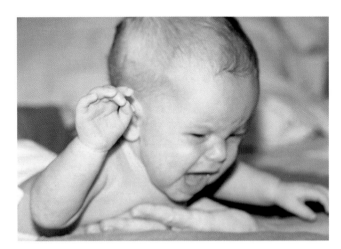

Figure 68.2   *M.R., a 3-month-old boy with combined immuno-deficiency. He had failed to thrive, had sparse facial and scalp hair, and had begun to have repeated infections. (Courtesy of Dr. R. Keightly of the University of Alabama.)*

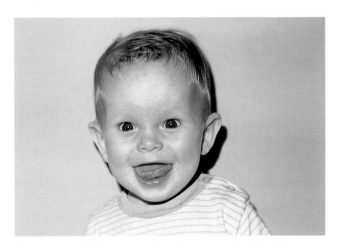

Figure 68.3   *M.R., at 10 months-of-age, 9 months following transplantation with fetal liver. He was thriving and looked well. (Courtesy of Dr. R. Keightly of the University of Alabama.)*

for transfer of a viral vector containing the human ADA gene and then infused into the patient. In others treatment was with repeated infusions of transduced peripheral mononuclear cell or stem cells from the marrow. To date, all patients have also received PEG-ADA, making the issue of expression of ADA protein difficult to assess, but long-term presence of the gene has been demonstrated. It has been concluded that it is premature to attribute benefit to gene therapy [71] but promising new trials are underway [72].

References

1   Giblett ER, Anderson JE, Cohen F, *et al.* Adenosinedeaminase deficiency in two patients with severely impaired cellular immunity. *Lancet* 1972;**2**:1067.

2   Giblett ER. ADA and PNP deficiencies: How it all began. *Ann NY Acad Sci* 1985;**451**:1.

3   Pollara B, Pickering RJ, Meuwissen HJ. Combined immunodeficiency disease associated with adenosine deaminase deficiency an inborn error of metabolism. *Pediatr Res* 1973;**7**:362.

4   Giblett ER, Ammann AJ, Wara DW, *et al.* Nucleoside-phosphorylase deficiency in a child with severely defective T-cell immunity and normal B-cell immunity. *Lancet* 1975;**1**:1010

5   Hirschhorn R. Overview of biochemical abnormalities and molecular genetics of adenosine deaminase deficiency. *Pediatr Res* 1993;**33**: (suppl 1) S35.

6   Petersen MB, Tranebjaerg L, Tommerup N, *et al.* New assignment of the adenosine deaminase gene locus to chromosome 20q1311 by study of a patient with interstitial deletion 20q. *J Med Genet* 1987;**24**:93.

7   Wiginton DA, Kaplan DJ, States JC, *et al.* Complete sequence and structure of the gene for human adenosine deaminase. *Biochemistry* 1986;**25**:8234.

8   Hirschhorn R, Ellenbogen A, Tzall S. Five missense mutations at the adenosine deaminase locus (ADA) detected by altered restriction fragments and their frequency in ADA: patients with severe combined immunodeficiency (ADA-SCID). *Am J Med Genet* 1992;**42**:201.

9   Markert ML. Molecular basis of adenosine deaminase deficiency. *Immunodeficiency* 1994;**5**:141.

10 Akeson AL, Wiginton DA, Dusing MR, *et al.* Mutant human adenosine deaminase alleles and their expression by transfection into fibroblasts. *J Biol Chem* 1988;**263**:16291

11 Meuwissen HJ, Pollara B, Pickering RJ. Combined immunodeficiency disease associated with adenosine deaminase deficiency. *J Pediatr* 1975;**86**:169.

12 Dissing J, Knudsen B. Adenosine-deaminase deficiency and combined immunodeficiency syndrome. *Lancet* 1972;**2**:1316.

13 Ochs HD, Yount JE, Giblett ER, *et al.* Adenosine-deaminase deficiency and severe combined immunodeficiency syndrome. *Lancet* 1973;**1**:1393.

14 Parkman R, Gelfand EW, Rosen FS, *et al.* Severe combined immunodeficiency and adenosine deaminase deficiency. *N Engl J Med* 1975;**292**:714.

15 Morgan G, Levinsky RJ, Hugh-Jones K, *et al.* Heterogeneity of biochemical clinical and immunological parameters in severe combined immunodeficiency due to ADA deficiency. *Clin Exp Immunol* 1987;**70**:491.

16 Shovlin CL, Simmonds HA, Fairbanks LD, *et al.* Adult onset immunodeficiency caused by inherited adenosine deaminase deficiency. *J Immunol* 1994;**153**:2331.

17 Borkowsky W, Gershon AA, Shenkman LS, Hirschhorn R. Adenosine deaminase deficiency without immunodeficiency: clinical and metabolic studies. *Pediatr Res* 1980;**14**:885.

18 van Gennip AH, van Cruchten AG, Bootsma AH, *et al.* Detection of patients with adenosine deaminase deficiency by HPLC/ESI tandem-MS analysis of blood spots. *J Inherit Metab Dis* 2002;**25**:156 (suppl 1).

19 Hirschhorn R. Incidence and prenatal detection of adenosine deaminase deficiency and purine nucleoside phosphorylase deficiency: in *Inborn Errors of Specific Immunity* (eds B Pollara, RJ Pickering, HJ Meuwissen, IH Porter). Academic Press, New York;1979:5.

20 Stephan JL, Vlekova V, Le Deist F, *et al.* A retrospective single center study of clinical presentation and outcome in 117 patients. *J Pediatr* 1993; **123**:564.

21 Shovlin CL, Hughes JMB, Simmonds HA, *et al.* Adult presentation of adenosine deaminase deficiency. *Lancet* 1993;**341**:1471.

22 Hong R, Gatti R, Rathbun JC, Good RA. Thymic hypoplasia and thyroid dysfunction. *N Engl J Med* 1970;**282**:470.

23 Geffner ME, Stiehm ER, Stephure D, Cowan MJ. Probable autoimmune thyroid disease and combined immunodeficiency disease. *Am J Dis Child* 1986;**140**:1194.

24 Hershfield MS, Chaffee S, Sorensen RU. Enzyme replacement therapy with polyethylene glycol-adenosine deaminase in adenosine deaminase deficiency: Overview and case reports of three patients including two now receiving gene therapy. *Pediatr Res* 1993;**33**:(suppl) 42.

25 Hirschhorn R. Adenosine deaminase deficiency: in *Immunodeficiency Reviews* (eds FS Rosen, M Seligmann). Harwood Academic, New York;1990:175.

26 Hirschhorn R, Papageorgiou PS, Kesariwala HH, Taft LT. Amelioration of neurologic abnormalities after 'enzyme replacement' in adenosine deaminase deficiency. *N Engl J Med* 1980;**303**:377.

27 Polmar SH, Stern RC, Schwartz AL, *et al.* Enzyme replacement therapy for adenosine deaminase deficiency and severe combined immunodeficiency. *N Engl J Med* 1976;**295**:1337.

28 Tanaka C, Hara T, Suzaki I, *et al.* Sensorineural deafness in siblings with adenosine deaminase deficiency. *Brain Dev* 1996;**18**:304.

29 Rogers MH, Lwin R, Fairbanks L, *et al.* Cognitive and behavioral abnormalities in adenosine deaminase deficient severe combined immunodeficiency. *J Pediatr* 2001;**139**:44.

30 Ozsahin H, Arredondo-Vega FX, Santisteban I, *et al.* Adenosine deaminase (ADA) deficiency in adults. *Blood* 1997;**89**:2849.

31 Buckley RH, Schiff RI, Schiff SE, *et al.* Human severe combined immunodeficiency: Genetic phenotypic and functional diversity in one hundred eight infants. *J Pediatr* 1997;**130**:378.

32 Wolfson JJ, Cross VF. The radiographic findings in 49 patients with combined immunodeficiency: in *Combined Immunodeficiency Disease and Adenosine Deaminase Deficiency A Molecular Defect* (eds HJ Meuwissen, RJ Pickering, B Pollara, IH Porter). Academic Press, New York;1975:225.

33 Huber J, Kersey J. Pathological findings: in *Combined Immunodeficiency Disease and Adenosine Deaminase Deficiency A Molecular Defect* (eds HJ Meuwissen, RJ Pickering, B Pollara, IH Porter). Academic Press, New York;1975:279.

34 Hirschhorn R, Beratis N, Rosen FS, *et al.* Adenosine deaminase deficiency in a child diagnosed prenatally. *Lancet* 1975;**1**:73.

35 Agarwal RP, Crabtree GW, Parks RE Jr, *et al.* Purine nucleoside metabolism in the erythrocytes of patients with adenosine deaminase deficiency and severe combined immunodeficiency. *J Clin Invest* 1976;**57**:1025.

36 Scott CR, Chen SH, Giblett ER. Detection of the carrier state in combined immunodeficiency disease associated with adenosine deaminase deficiency. *J Clin Invest* 1974;**53**:1194.

37 Moore EC, Meuwissen HJ. Screening for ADA deficiency. *J Pediatr* 1974;**95**:802.

38 Dooley T, Fairbanks LD, Simmonds HA, *et al.* First trimester diagnosis of adenosine deaminase deficiency. *Prenat Diag* 1987;**7**:561.

39 Ziegler JB, Van der Weyden MB, Lee CH, Daniel A. Prenatal diagnosis for adenosine deaminase deficiency. *J Med Genet* 1981;**18**:154.

40 Schrader WP, Stacy AR. Purification and subunit structure of adenosine deaminase from human kidney. *J Biol Chem* 1977;**252**:6409.

41 Gossage DL, Norby-Slycord CJ, Hershfield MS, Markert ML. A homozygous 5 base-pair deletion in exon 10 of the adenosine deaminase (ADA) gene in a child with severe combined immunodeficiency and very low levels of ADA mRNA and protein. *Hum Mol Genet* 1993;**2**:1493.

42 Santisteban I, Arrendondo-Vega FX, Kelly S. Novel splicing missense and deletion mutations in seven adenosine deaminase-deficient patients with late/delayed onset of combined immunodeficiency disease. Contribution of genotype to phenotype. *J Clin Invest* 1993;**92**:2291.

43 Yang DR, Huie ML, Hirschhorn R. Homozygosity for a missense mutation (G20R) associated with neonatal onset adenosine deaminase-deficient severe combined immunodeficiency (ADA-SCID). *Clin Immunol Immunopathol* 1994;**70**:171.

44 Hirschhorn R, Yang DR, Insel RA, Ballow M. Severe combined immunodeficiency of reduced severity due to homozygosity for an adenosine deaminase missense mutation (Arg253Pro). *Cell Immunol* 1993;**152**:383.

45 Cooper DN, Krawczak D. The mutational spectrum of single base-pair substitutions causing human genetic disease: Patterns and predictions. *Hum Genet* 1990;**85**:55.

46 Cooper DN, Youssoufian H. The CpG dinucleotide and human genetic disease. *Hum Genet* 1988;**78**:151.

47 Hirschborn R, Yang DR, Israni A, *et al.* Somatic mosaicism for a newly identified splice-site mutation in a patient with adenosine deaminase-deficient immunodeficiency and spontaneous clinical recovery. *Am J Hum Genet* 1994;**55**:59.

48 Arredondo-Vega FX, Santisteban I, Kelly S, *et al.* Correct splicing despite a G → A mutation at the invariant first nucleotide of a 5′ splice site: A possible basis for disparate clinical phenotypes in siblings with adenosine deaminase (ADA) deficiency. *Am J Hum Genet* 1994;**54**:820.

49 Brinkmann B, Brinkmann M, Martin H. A new allele in red cell adenosine deaminase polymorphism: ADA0. *Hum Hered* 1973;**23**:603.

50 De La Haba G, Cantoni GL. The enzymatic synthesis of S-adenosyl-L-homocysteine from adenosine and homocysteine. *J Biol Chem* 1959;**234**:603.

51 Naylor EW, Orfanos AP, Guthrie R. An improved screening test for adenosine deaminase deficiency. *J Pediatr* 1978;**93**:473.

52 Coleman MS, Donofrio J, Hutton JJ, *et al.* Identification and quantitation of adenine deoxynucleotides in erythrocytes of a patient with adenosine deaminase deficiency and severe combined immunodeficiency. *J Biol Chem* 1978;**253**:1619.

53 Cohen A, Hirschhorn R, Horowitz SD, *et al.* Deoxyadenosine triphosphate as a potentially toxic metabolite in adenosine deaminase deficiency. *Proc Natl Acad Sci USA* 1978;**75**:472.

54 Henderson JF, Scott FW, Lowe JK. Toxicity of naturally occurring purine deoxyribonucleotides. *Pharmacol Ther* 1980;**8**:573.

55 Matsumoto SS, Yu AL, Bleeker LC, *et al.* Biochemical correlates of the differential sensitivity of subtypes of human leukemia to deoxyadenosine and deoxycoformycin. *Blood* 1982;**60**:1096.

56 Carson DA, Kaye J, Seegmiller JE. Differential sensitivity of human leukemic T-cell lines and B-cell lines to growth inhibition by deoxyadenosine. *J Immunol* 1978;**121**:1726.

57 Seto S, Carrera CJ, Kubota M, *et al.* Mechanism of deoxyadenosine and 2-chlorodeoxyadenosine toxicity to nondividing human lymphocytes. *J Clin Invest* 1985;**75**:377.

58 Kameoka J, Tanaka T, Nojima Y, *et al.* Direct association of adenosine deaminase with a T cell activation antigen CD26. *Science* 1993;**261**:466.

59 Hershfield MS. Apparent suicide inactivation of human lymphoblast S-adenosylhomocysteine hydrolase by 2′-deoxyadenosine and adenine arabinoside. A basis for direct toxic effects of analogs of adenosine. *J Biol Chem* 1979;**254**:22.

60 Van De Wiele CJ, Vaughn JG, Blackburn MR, *et al.* Adenosine kinase inhibition promotes survival of fetal adenosine deaminase-deficient thymocytes by blocking dATP accumulation. *J Clin Invest* 2002;**110**:395.

61 Stiles GL. Adenosine receptors: structure function and regulation. *Trends Physiol Sci* 1986;**7**:486.

62 Gerlach E, Becker BF. *Topics and Perspectives in Adenosine Research.* Springer-Verlag, Berlin Heidelberg 1987.

63 Meuwissen HJ, Moore E, Pollara B. Maternal marrow transplant in a patient with combined immunodeficiency disease (CID) and adenosine deaminase (ADA) deficiency. *Pediatr Res* 1973;**7**:362.

64 Buckley RH. Breakthroughs in the understanding and therapy of primary immunodeficiency. *Pediatr Clin North Am* 1994;**41**:665.

65 Buckley RH, Schiff SE, Schiff RI, *et al.* Hematopoietic stem-cell transplantation for the treatment of severe combined immunodeficiency. *N Engl J Med* 1999;**340**:508.

66 Dyminski JW, Daoud A, Lampkin BC, *et al.* Immunological and biochemical profiles in response to transfusion therapy in an adenosine-deaminase deficient patient with severe combined immunodeficiency. *Clin Immunol Immunopathol* 1979;**14**:307.

67 Donofrio J, Colmena MS, Hutton JJ, *et al.* Overproduction of adenine deoxynucleosides and deoxynucleotides in adenosine deaminase deficiency with severe combined immunodeficiency disease. *J Clin Invest* 1978;**62**:884.

68 Hershfield MS, Buckley RH, Greenberg ML, *et al.* Treatment of adenosine deaminase deficiency with polyethylene glycol-modified adenosine deaminase. *N Engl J Med* 1987;**316**:589.

69 Parkman R, Gelfland EW. Severe combined immunodeficiency disease adenosine deaminase deficiency and gene therapy. *Curr Opinion Immunol* 1991;**3**:547.

70 Blaese RM. Development of gene therapy for immunodeficiency: Adenosine deaminase deficiency. *Pediatr Res* 1993;**33**:(suppl 1) S49.

71 Orkin S, Motulsky A. Report and recommendations of the panel to assess the NIH investment in research on gene therapy. 1995 *World Wide Web* http://wwwnihgov/news/panelrephtml (accessed November 2004).

72 Cavazzana-Calvo M, Hacein-Bey S, de Saint Basile G, *et al.* Gene therapy of human severe combined immunodeficiency (SCID)-X1 disease. *Science* 2000;**288**:669.

Adenylosuccinate lyase deficiency

MAJOR PHENOTYPIC EXPRESSION

Developmental retardation, seizures, autistic behavior, excretion of adenylosuccinate and succinylaminoimidazolecarboxamide riboside in the urine and deficient activity of adenylosuccinate lyase.

INTRODUCTION

Adenylosuccinate lyase (ASL) deficiency was first described by Jaeken and Van den Berghe [1] in 1984. This created enormous interest because autistic behavior was observed in the affected patients in this family, and it would be of considerable interest if it were possible to relate molecular changes in the gene for ASL to the genetics of autism [2]. However,

extensive survey of autistic populations has failed to turn up additional patients with lyase deficiency.

The enzyme adenylosuccinate lyase (adenylosuccinase, ASL; EC 4.3.2.2) catalyzes the eighth step in the *de novo* synthesis of purines in which succinylaminoimidazolecarboxamide ribotide (SAICAR, SAICAMP) is converted to aminoimidazolecarboxamide ribotide (AICAR, AICAMP, ZMP) [3,4] (Figure 69.1). The same enzyme catalyzes the conversion of

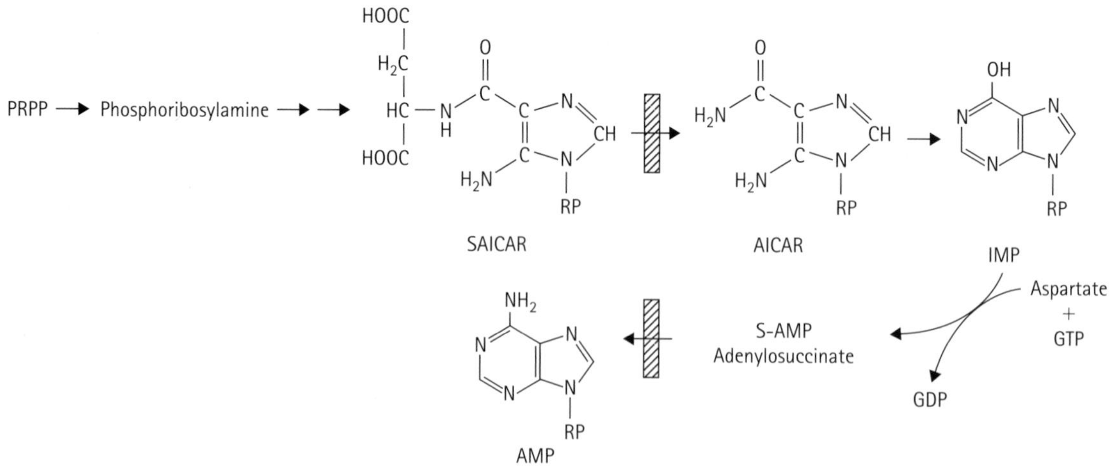

Figure 69.1 *The reaction catalyzed by adenylosuccinate lyase. In the* de novo *pathway of purine nucleotide synthesis the conversion of 5-phosphoribosyl-5-amino-4-imidazole succinyl-carboxamide (SAICAR) to 5-phosphoribosyl-5-amino-4-imidazole carboxamide (AICAR) and in the purine interrelations cycle the conversion of adenylosuccinate to adenylic acid (AMP).*

adenylosuccinate to adenosine monophosphate (AMP) in the cycle of purine nucleotide conversions that yield adenine nucleotides [5]. Deficient activity of the enzyme was documented in 1988 by Jaeken, Wadman, Duran and colleagues [3]. The human gene has been mapped to chromosome 22q1.3.1.-1.3.2 [6]. The human cDNA has been cloned and the nature of the point mutation was defined in the initial family reported [1,2]. A majority of the 30 different mutations delineated have been missense, most of them in compound heterozygotes. The most common mutation, R426H was found in 13 families from many countries [7].

CLINICAL ABNORMALITIES

Adenylosuccinate lyase deficiency has been diagnosed in more than 60 patients; the phenotype is variable, but it is clear that psychomotor retardation is a regular manifestation of the disease [1,3,5,8,9]. Many have had seizure disorders. Some of the patients with early onset seizures have died in infancy [10–14]. More have had moderate to severe mental retardation and seizures after the first year [1,3,8,15]. Autistic features in some have included absence of eye contact, repetitive behavior, temper tantrums and self-injurious behavior, none of them rare in retarded individuals. Retardation of growth and muscle wasting have also been observed [3]. One patient had only mild developmental delay [3], and she has been referred to as type II to distinguish her from all the other patients in type I, in whom mental retardation is more severe [16]. Another patient was described [8] as having an intermediate degree of symptomatology, and another had only delayed motor development and severe hypotonia [17]. Siblings shown in Figure 69.2 had less severely retarded development [10]. It seems likely that once a large number of patients is observed, a spectrum will be the case rather than discrete groups of phenotypes.

A distinctive feature of ASL deficiency that simplifies the detection of this disorder is the accumulation of the metabolites adenylosuccinate (succinyladenosine) and SAICAriboside (succinyl-AICAriboside), the dephosphorylated products of the substrates for the deficient enzyme. It is possible to screen for the latter compound, because it gives a positive Bratton-Marshall reaction [18] (Figure 69.3). Confirmation of a positive screening test is done by identification of adenylosuccinate and SAICAriboside in urine or blood [1]. Both compounds are also readily found in the cerebrospinal fluid, where concentrations are 20 to 100 fold those of plasma and are as high as 500 µmol/L [1,19]. Urinary excretions range from 25–700 mmol/mol creatinine [1,3,19]. In most patients the ratio of the two compounds adenylosuccinate/succinyl-AICAriboside approximates 1 [9]. Patients with milder phenotypes have had more adenylosuccinate, sometimes as much as four-fold higher or even 100-fold [3].

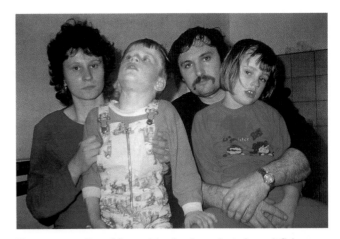

Figure 69.2   *Two siblings with adenylosuccinate lyase deficiency, shown with their parents. Their degree of mental retardation was described as less severe. (This illustration was kindly provided by Dr. Ivan Sebesta of Universita Karlova, Prague, Czech Republic.)*

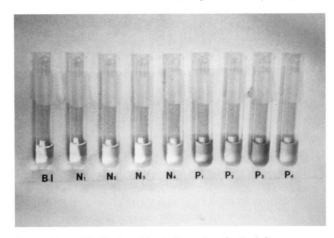

Figure 69.3   *The Bratton-Marshall reaction. On the left are negative tubes; on the right, the urine of two patients with adenylosuccinate lyase deficiency.*

GENETICS AND PATHOGENESIS

The disorder is inherited as an autosomal recessive trait. Consanguinity has been described [1]. The enzyme has been generally assayed by following the conversion of adenylosuccinate to AMP spectrophotometrically [20]. Liver fibroblasts and lymphocytes have been used to document the deficiency of enzyme activity in individuals with ASL deficiency [3,9,21,22]. The very different metabolite ratio in the type II patient suggested that the enzyme be assayed with both substrates. It was found that in classic type I ASL deficiency the activities of the enzyme toward the two substrates are decreased in parallel to about 30 percent of control [8]. In contrast, in fibroblasts derived from the patient in type II, activity against succinylAICAR was about 30 percent of control, but when adenylosuccinate was the substrate the activity was only three percent of control [9]. Certainly, these data provide an explanation for the higher concentration of adenylosuccinate in the type II patient.

Kinetic studies have indicated that in lymphoblasts [23] as well as in fibroblasts [9] the affinity for adenylosuccinate is normal even at physiological temperatures [2]. Furthermore, the variant enzyme has been shown to have decreased stability to heat [23], and this would account for the reduced residual activity. An increase in the Km for succinylAICAR in some patients [9] indicates the modification of the active site. The kinetics of the type II enzyme differed in that the Km for adenosylsuccinate was markedly increased [9]; its V_{max} was strongly inhibited by KCl and nucleoside triphosphates, neither of which affected the kinetics of type I. Mammalian ASL is a heteropolymer of about 52 kDa containing four subunits [24].

The cDNA for the gene contains 1452 nucleotides and codes for a protein of 484 amino acids [25]. Molecular analysis in the first reported Moroccan family with four affected children [1–3] indicated homozygosity for a point mutation in the ASL gene resulting in a serine to proline change originally placed at amino acid 413, but now called S438P in the 484 amino acid protein. This might be expected to increase the flexibility of the peptide backbone of the enzyme, which might account for decreased stability. Analysis of genomic polymerase chain reaction (PCR) products from the parents of the patients revealed both a normal and a mutant allele, documenting heterozygosity [2]. Another mutation identified [26] in a Gypsy patient without known consanguinity, G1279A converted a well conserved arginine at 401 to histidine. Other missense mutations identified have indicated a high degree of molecular heterogeneity [26–28]. A 39bp deletion in the cDNA was caused by a C to A change in exon 5 creating a consensus 5′ donor splice site [29]. One nonsense mutation has been observed [25].

An interesting mutation found in three unrelated patients. In them the coding sequence was normal in the allele with the mutation, which was a I49C change in 5′ untranslated region (UTR) [7]. This led to a reduction to 25 percent and 33 percent of wild type promoter function and mRNA. The mutation affected the binding of a known activator of transcription, nuclear respiratory factor 2 (NRF-2).

TREATMENT

Specific therapy has not been devised. Seizures may be treated with the usual anticonvulsant drugs. Management is designed for optimal developmental potential.

References

1 Jaeken J, Van den Berghe G. An infantile autistic syndrome characterized by the presence of succinylpurines in body fluids. *Lancet* 1984;**2**:1058.

2 Stone RL, Aimi J, Barshop BA, *et al*. A mutation in adenylosuccinate lyase associated with mental retardation and autistic features. *Nature Genet* 1992;**1**:59.

3 Jaeken J, Wadman SK, Duran M. *et al*. Adenylosuccinase deficiency: an inborn error of purine nucleotide synthesis. *Eur J Pediatr* 1988;**148**:126.

4 Lowy BA, Ben-Zion D. Adenylosuccinase activity in human and rabbit erythrocyte lysates. *J Biol Chem* 1970;**245**:3043.

5 Van den Berghe G, Bontemps F, Vincent MF, Van den Bergh F. The purine nucleotide cycle and its molecular defects. *Prog Neurobiol* 1992;**39**:547.

6 Fon EA, Demczuk S, Delattre O, *et al*. Mapping of the human adenylosuccinate lyase (ADSL) gene to chromosome 22q131-q132. *Cytogenet Cell Genet* 1993;**64**:201.

7 Marie S, Race V, Nassogne M-C, *et al*. Mutation of a nuclear respiratory factor 2 binding site in the 5′ untranslated region of the ADSL gene in three patients with adenylosuccinate lyase deficiency. *Am J Hum Genet* 2002;**71**:14.

8 Jaeken JF, Van der Bergh F, Vincent MF, *et al*. Adenylosuccinase deficiency: a newly recognized variant. *J Inherit Metab Dis* 1992;**15**:416.

9 Van den Bergh F, Vincent MF, Jaeken J, Van den Berghe G. Residual adenylosuccinase activities in fibroblasts of adenylosuccinase deficient children: parallel deficiency with adenylosuccinate and succinyl-AICAR in profoundly retarded patients and on-parallel deficiency in a mildly retarded girl. *J Inherit Metab Dis* 1993;**16**:415.

10 Sebesta I, Krijt J, Kmoch S, *et al*. Adenylosuccinase deficiency – clinical and biochemical findings in 5 Czech patients. *J Inherit Metab Dis* 1996;**19**:2 (abstr 04).

11 Van den Bergh FAJTM, Boschaart AN, Hageman G, *et al*. Adenylosuccinase deficiency with neonatal onset severe epileptic seizures and sudden death. *Neuropediatrics* 1998;**29**:51.

12 Krijt J, Sebesta I, Svehlakova A, *et al*. Adenylosuccinate lyase deficiency in a Czech girl and two siblings. *Adv Exp Med Biol* 1995;**370**:367.

13 Maaswinkel-Mooij PD, Laan LAEM, Onkenhout W, *et al*. Adenylosuccinase deficiency presenting with epilepsy in early infancy. *J Inherit Metab Dis* 1997;**20**:606.

14 Köhler M, Assmann B, Bräutigam C, *et al*. Adenylosuccinase deficiency: Possibly underdiagnosed encephalopathy with variable clinical features. *Eur J Pediatr Neurol* 1999;**3**:6.

15 Salerno C, Crifo C, Giardini O. Adenylosuccinase deficiency: A patient with impaired erythrocyte activity and anomalous response to intravenous fructose. *J Inherit Metab Dis* 1995;**18**:602.

16 Van den Berghe G, Vincent MF, Jaeken J. Inborn errors of the purine nucleotide cycle: Adenylosuccinase deficiency. *J Inherit Metab Dis* 1997;**20**:193.

17 Valik D, Miner PT, Jones JD. First US case of adenylosuccinate lyase deficiency with severe hypotonia. *Pediatr Neurol* 1997;**16**:252.

18 Laikind PK, Seegmiller JE, Gruber HE. Detection of 5′-phosphoribosyl-4-(N-succinylcarboxamide)-5-aminoimidazole in urine by use of the Bratton–Marshall reaction: identification of patients deficient in adenylosuccinate lyase activity. *Anal Biochem* 1986;**156**:81.

19 De Bree PK, Wadman SK, Duran M, Faabery de Jonge H. Diagnosis of inherited adenylosuccinase deficiency by thin-layer chromatography of urinary imidazoles and by automated cation exchange column chromatography of purines. *Clin Chim Acta* 1986;**156**:279.

20 Schultz V, Lowenstein JM. Purine nucleotide cycle. Evidence for the occurrence of the cycle in brain. *J Biol Chem* 1976;**251**:485.

21 Van der Bergh F, Vincent MF, Jaeken J, Van den Berghe G. Radiochemical assay of adenylosuccinase: demonstration of parallel loss of activity toward both adenylosuccinate and succinylaminoimidazole carboxamide ribotide in liver of patients with the enzyme defect. *Anal Biochem* 1991;**193**:287.

22 Van den Berghe G, Jaeken J. Adenylosuccinase deficiency. *Adv Exp Med Biol* 1986;**195A**:27.

23 Barshop BA, Alberts AS, Gruber HE. Kinetic studies of mutant human adenylosuccinase. *Biochim Biophys Acta* 1989;**999**:19.

24 Casey PJ, Lowenstein JM. Purification of adenylosuccinate lyase from rat skeletal muscle by a novel affinity column. Stabilization of the enzyme and effects of anions and fluoro analogues of the substrate. *Biochem J* 1987; **246**:263.

25 Kmoch S, Hartmannová H, Stiburková B, *et al*. Human adenylosuccinate lyase (ADSL) cloning and characterization of full-length cDNA and its isoform gene structure and molecular basis for ADSL deficiency in six patients. *Hum Mol Genet* 2000;**9**:1501.

26 Kmoch S, Hartmannova H, Krijt J, Sebesta I. Adenylosuccinase deficiency – identification of a new disease causing mutation. *J Inherit Metab Dis* 1996;**19**:13.

27 Kmoch S, Hartmannova H, Krijt J, *et al*. Genetic heterogeneity in adenylosuccinate lyase deficiency. *Clin Biochem* 1997;**30**:22.

28 Verginelli D, Luckow B, Crifo C, *et al*. Identification of new mutations in the adenylosuccinate lyase gene associated with impaired enzyme activity in lymphocytes and red blood cells. *Biochim Biophys Acta* 1998;**1406**:81.

29 Marie S, Cuppens H, Heuterspreute M, *et al*. Mutation analysis in adenylosuccinate lyase deficiency. Eight novel mutations in the re-evaluated full ADSL coding sequence. *Hum Mut* 1999;**13**:197.

PART 9

Disorders of transport and mineral metabolism

Cystinuria

MAJOR PHENOTYPIC EXPRESSION

Calculi in the urinary tract leading to colic or infection, urinary excretion of large amounts of cystine, lysine, ornithine and arginine, and impaired intestinal absorption of these amino acids.

INTRODUCTION

Cystine (Figure 70.1) owes its name to the fact that it was first recovered from stones obtained from the urinary bladder [1,2]. The stones of the earliest known cystinuric patients were described by Wollaston in 1810 [1]. He called the material cystic oxide to reflect the origin in the bladder, but Berzelius recognized that the compound in the stones was an amine not an oxide and named it cystine [2]. Its chemical nature was delineated in 1902 by Friedman [3]. Garrod in 1908 discussed cystinuria in the famous Croonian lectures, as being among the original inborn errors of metabolism [4]. Today we continue to consider that aberrations in transepithelial transport are among the disorders of metabolism.

The renal transport of cystine and the dibasic amino acids has been clarified to a considerable extent by studies over the years on patients with cystinuria. The facts that these patients excrete cystine, lysine, ornithine and arginine [5–8] and that the plasma concentrations are not increased indicated that they must share a common transport mechanism – one that is defective in cystinuria. That there are similarities in structure

(Figure 70.2) makes this intuitively reasonable. It is now clear from studies on rat renal tubular fragments and isolated brush-border membrane vesicles that there are two transport systems for cystine: one with a high affinity, low Km that is shared with the dibasic amino acids [9,10], and a low affinity system that is not shared. These observations are consistent with physiological studies that had been carried out *in vivo* in cystinuric patients by Dent and Rose [11] who first formulated the idea of a common transport mechanism, shared by the four amino acids, that was defective in cystinuria.

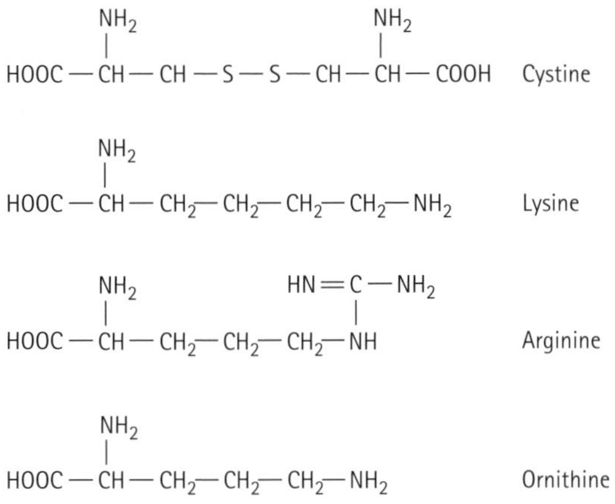

Figure 70.2 *Structures of cystine and the dibasic amino acids whose transport is defective in cystinuria.*

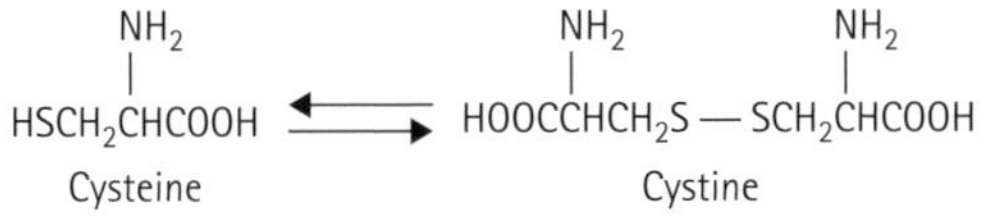

Figure 70.1 *Structure of cystine and its relationship to cysteine.*

Cystinuria has been divided into at least two types, Type I which is fully recessive and displays normal amino acid excretion in heterozygotes, and an incomplete recessive form in which heterozygotes excrete the relevant amino acids at levels between normal and homozygotes (Types II and III) [12].

The gene for cystinuria Type II has been mapped to chromosome 2p16.3-21 [13–15]. This is the locus for a gene cloned from rabbit renal cortex, and therefore called rBAT [16], whose cDNA expresses the high affinity transport of cystine and dibasic amino acids [16]. A considerable number of missense mutations have been defined in this gene (SLC3A1) [14]. A second locus has been identified in Type II and III patients at chromosome 19q13.1–13.2 [17,18]. The gene (SLCA9) appears to code for the light subunit that forms a complex with rBAT to form a holotransporter.

CLINICAL ABNORMALITIES

Cystinuria is of clinical significance because of the insolubility of cystine. The excretion of the dibasic amino acids is without clinical consequences, but cystine is so insoluble that the formation of stones in the urinary tract of cystinuric patients is the rule rather that the exception. Calculi may develop in infancy or childhood (Figures 70.3, 70.4) [19]. They are usually present before the age of 30 years and they may vary in size from tiny sands or gravel to large staghorn calculi in the renal pelvis or huge calculi in the bladder. They may induce colic or urinary tract obstruction and may require surgical removal. Repeated urinary tract infections can be expected in any patient with renal stone disease. Physical examination may reveal flank tenderness. All of these problems may ultimately lead to renal failure. Some patients have hypertension. Cystine is radio-opaque (Figure 70.4); therefore, the stones can usually be recognized roentgenographically without the use of contrast [20,21]. They can also

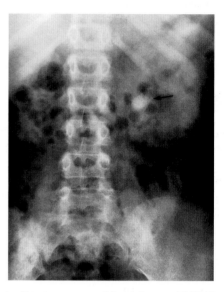

Figure 70.4   *Roentgenogram of the abdomen of C.M., illustrating radioopaque renal calculi.*

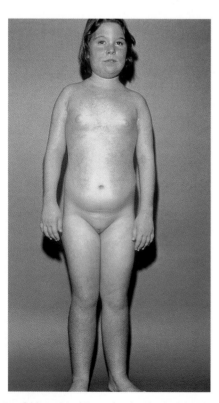

Figure 70.3   *C.M., a girl with cystinuria, also had dermatomyositis; a disease as common as cystinuria is often found in conjunction with other unrelated conditions.*

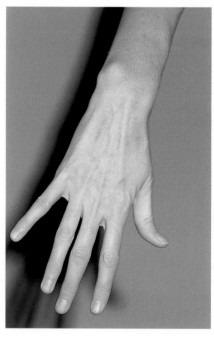

Figure 70.5   *J. Family. Illustrated is the hand of a woman who had cystinuria. She and a number of her family also had Marfan syndrome, another instance of two unrelated diseases, but in this instance they were referred because a positive cyanide-nitroprusside test had led to a diagnosis of homocystinuria.*

be demonstrated by ultrasound. Cystine stones themselves are usually yellow-brown in color and have a maple-sugar crystal appearance to the surface. They may contain secondary deposits of calcium, especially following infection.

Twenty-five to 30 percent of patients have evidence of calculi in the first 10 years of life [22], 30–35 percent in the next 10 years, and some first encounter symptomatic stone disease in adulthood. Some patients with cystinuria are asymptomatic even as adults (Figure 70.5).

Cystine stones represent 6–8 percent of urinary tract stones of childhood [23], and 1–3 percent of those found in adulthood [24].

GENETICS AND PATHOGENESIS

Cystinuria is transmitted in an autosomal recessive fashion. It is a relatively common inherited disease and neonatal screening programs have yielded prevalence figures from one in 2000 to one in 15 000 [25–27] with a consensus figure of one in 7000 [28]. Both sexes are equally affected, but there is a tendency for more severe disease in males.

The first evidence of heterogeneity in cystinuria came with approaches to carrier detection. It was found that parents of cystinuric patients could be divided into two groups: those who excreted increased amounts of cystine and lysine and those who did not [29]. Cystinuric homozygotes have been classified into three allelic [30] groups on the basis of *in vitro* studies of intestinal transport. The urine was normal in the families of type I patients, in whom *in vitro* transport of cystine and lysine was absent, while cystinuria-lysinuria was found in families of patients of types II and III. The quantities of amino acid excreted tended to be larger in type II than in type III heterozygotes [12,31], but it was evident early that there were a number of compounds [12,32], and types II and III may be heterogeneous in intestinal absorption. The excretion of arginine was found to be greater in Type II than in Type III heterozygotes [12]. Studies of the nature of mutation have begun to clarify the observed heterogeneity.

Cystine has been recognized by the visualization of the typical hexagonal crystals in microscopic examination of the urinary sediment. However, it has been our experience that uric acid crystals are often mistakenly identified as those of cystine [33]. Many cystinuric individuals are first identified using the cyanide nitroprusside test [34] (Figure 70.6). The red color obtained is also found in patients with homocystine or other sulfur-containing amino acids in the urine. Confirmation of the amino acid being excreted has been obtained using high voltage electrophoresis, or chromatography on paper or thin layer plates, but the excretion of amino acids should always be quantified. Quantitative amino acid analysis defines the nature of the multiple amino aciduria in cystinuria, and also makes possible the distinction (not always easy) of homozygote from heterozygote and provides prognostic information on the likelihood of the formation of calculi.

Normal individuals excrete cystine, lysine, arginine and ornithine in amounts less than 10, 60, 5 and 5 mmol/mol creatinine (18, 130, 16 and 22 mg/g creatinine), respectively. Cystinuric individuals have been variously defined as those who excrete more than 120–200 mmol cystine/mol of creatinine (250–400 mg/g creatinine). A patient may be expected to form calculi if the concentrations of cystine in urine regularly exceed 1250 μmol/L (300 mg/L).

In order to separate heterozygotes from homozygotes Crawhall [35,36] developed data for 24 stone-forming subjects in 12 different families on the excretion of cystine, lysine, ornithine and arginine into a canonical variant analysis that has been put into a computer program that generally distinguishes these two populations, but there is overlap between the normal and heterozygous populations. Slow rates of development of renal malabsorption may make the distinction of heterozygotes from homozygotes particularly less reliable in infancy.

The cystinuric pattern of amino aciduria is characterized also by a marked increase in the excretion of lysine and somewhat less of ornithine and arginine [8,11]. The plasma concentrations of these amino acids are normal. That they are not usually low probably reflects the fact that intestinal absorption of the amino acids of ingested proteins normally proceeds via small peptide absorption, and this is normal in cystinuria [37]. The cystinuric pattern of urinary excretion has also been observed in infants with organic acidemias such as propionic acidemia, methylmalonic acidemia and isovaleric acidemia [38], often reverting to normal with metabolic control and reduced excretion of organic acids.

The renal clearance of the dibasic amino acids is increased in cystinuria to a rate usually equal to or somewhat less than the glomerular filtration rate, but in some patients it has exceeded the clearance of inulin [32,39,40]. The clearance of lysine is usually 50–70 percent of the glomerular filtration rate, and the abnormalities in ornithine and arginine reabsorption are usually less than that of lysine [41]. The excretion of lysine exceeds that of cystine, and the excretion of arginine and ornithine may exceed it as well.

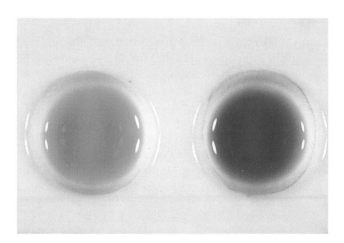

Figure 70.6 *Cyanide-nitroprusside test. The red color on the right indicates the presence of a sulfur containing amino acids.*

Increasing the filtered load of one of the four amino acids by, for instance, infusion of lysine reduces the reabsorption and increases the clearance of the others in normal individuals and in patients with cystinuria [41–43], although increased cystine excretion may sometimes not occur after a lysine load in a cystinuric patient, presumably because it is already being excreted maximally.

Some other amino acids may be excreted in large amounts in cystinuria; these include glycine [39], cystathionine [44], methionine [45]. The cysteine-homocysteine disulfide [46] is found regularly. Homoarginine [47] and citrulline [48] have also been found in the urine of cystinuric patients.

Studies *in vitro* with isolated tubules and brush border membrane vesicles clarified the nature of renal transport defect in cystinuria. There are two renal tubular transport systems for cystine [9,10,49]. A high Km system is not shared by the dibasic amino acids. It is the low Km shared system that is defective in cystinuria.

Defective intestinal transport has also been demonstrated in cystinuria [50,51]. Evidence for defective absorption of cystine and the dibasic amino acids was obtained *in vivo* [7,50–52] by oral loading tests [53]. Intestinal absorption of cysteine is not impaired in cystinuria [54].

Accumulation of basic amino acids in the intestine leads to bacterial decarboxylation to form the diamines, cadaverine, agmatine and putrescine, which are then absorbed and excreted in the urine. The heterocyclic amine piperidine is also formed from lysine, and pyrrolidine from arginine and ornithine, and these compounds may also be excreted in the urine.

Defective intestinal amino acid transport was also demonstrated in biopsied jejunal mucosa [55–58]. Evidence for heterogeneity was obtained in these studies and among the cystinuric patients three types were identified [59].

- In type I there was no accumulation of cystine or the dibasic amino acids against a gradient;
- In type II cystine accumulated, but the dibasic amino acids did not;
- In type III there was accumulation of cystine and the dibasic amino acids to a limited degree.

Family studies suggested that some patients classified as type III might be compounds of I and II. These types could also be identified by analysis of amino acid excretion in patients and parents.

The molecular biology of cystinuria has been advanced by the discovery of the gene for a renal and intestinal cystine transporter and by expression in Xenopus oocytes of mRNA derived from rat intestine [60] or renal cortex [61]. cDNA clones of rat [61] and rabbit [16] origin were obtained. The cDNA of the rabbit clone, named rBAT, expressed in Xenopus a high affinity transport for cystine and dibasic amino acids. The human cDNA, called human rBAT or D2H, has been isolated [62,63] and mapped to chromosome 2p16.3-21 [62]. The mRNA contains 2.3 kb and codes for a protein of 78.8 kDa with 663 amino acids [62,64].

Mutations identified in the human SLC3A1 gene for rBAT have largely been missense, such as R180Q, M467K, M467T, P615T, T652R and L678P but a few stop codons, deletions, frameshift mutations and splicing errors have been observed [65,66]. The missense mutations have generally involved important, highly conserved amino acids. Most mutations have occurred only on a single population, but M467T, the most common to date, has been observed in a broad distribution. Expression of M467T in Xenopus led to a protein with 20 percent of normal transport activity [14]. The mutation does not interfere with the affinity of the protein for its substrates, but rather with cellular trafficking so that a small proportion arrives at the plasma membrane where transport takes place [67].

The other transport protein defective in some patients with cystinuria coded for by SLCA9 brings rBAT to the plasma membrane [68]. Mutations have been found in families with cystinuria other than type I. In a population of Libyan Jews homozygous for cystinuria Type III whose haplotype analysis was useful in the discovery of this gene a G693A substitution changed a valine to methionine (V17OM). The most common mutation was G105R [68].

An animal model in naturally cystinuric Newfoundland dogs has a stop codon in exon 2 or the canine gene for rBAT [69]. These dogs excrete over 57 mmol of cystine per mole creatinine (normal 6).

TREATMENT

The objective of treatment in cystinuria is the prevention of urinary lithiasis. Crystallization of cystine in urine and the formation of calculi can be minimized by dilution in larger urine volumes [70,71] or by doing something to alter the concentration of cystine, such as converting it to a more soluble compound. In order to obtain effective dilution very large amounts of oral fluid are required. It is particularly important for the patient to get up at night to urinate and drink more. In a patient excreting a gram of cystine, a urine volume of four liters is necessary to achieve a concentration of 250 mg/L. In practice, few adults and almost no children comply with an effective regimen. Alkalization of the urine is of no value; promotion of the solubility of cystine requires a urinary pH of 7.6, which is impossible to achieve physiologically.

For these reasons, penicillamine therapy [72,73] brought about a significant advance in management. Penicillamine ($\beta\beta$-dimethylcystine) forms a mixed disulfide with cysteine (Figure 70.7), which is considerably more soluble than cystine. Its oral administration to patients with cystinuria can reduce cystine concentrations in the urine to levels at which stones will not form (Figure 70.8). Doses of 1–2 g a day may be required to keep the excretion of cystine below 200 mg/g creatinine, at which level the formation of calculi should be prevented. Therapy in addition dissolves stones [74,75].

Penicillamine therapy is demanding because there are many side effects [76–84]. Reactions that have been thought

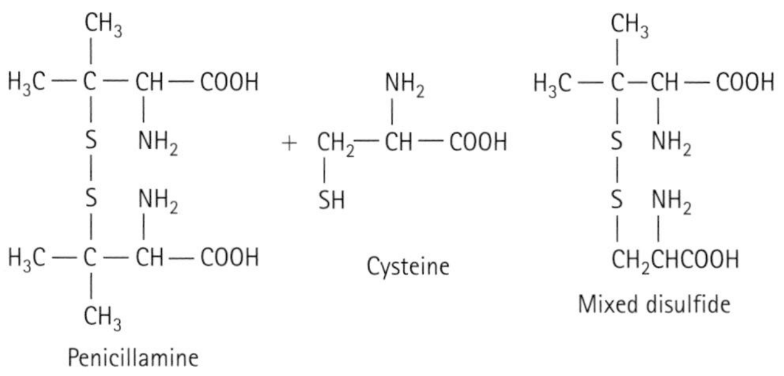

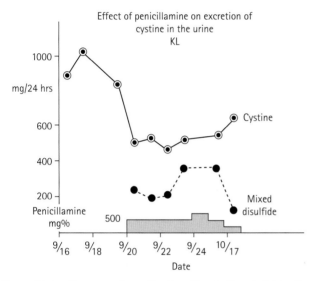

Figure 70.7 *Penicillamine and the formation of the cysteine-penicillamine disulfide.*

Figure 70.8 *Response of a cystinuric patient to the administration of penicillamine.*

Captopril is a sulfhydryl compound and it has been observed to lower urinary cystine, but to variable degree [89,90].

A variety of interventions may be necessary in patients who develop calculi. Infections should be treated with appropriate antibiotics. Lithotripsy is not as successful in cystinuria as in some other stone-forming diseases. Percutaneous lithotripsy may be effective, or may, by forming smaller units, make surgical lithotomy less formidable. Renal failure may lead to dialysis or renal transplantation [91].

to be allergic occur in as many as half the patients. They are manifested in skin eruptions and fever and some patients develop arthralgias [76]. These reactions are unlike conventional drug allergy in that with continued administration, often after reduced dosage, the reaction will subside, and treatment may then be maintained for many years [78]. More serious side effects such as nephrosis [77] or pancytopenia require the withdrawal of the drug. Thrombocytosis has also been observed [79]. A fatal Goodpasture syndrome has been reported in a patient with Wilson disease treated with penicillamine [80]. The compound has effects on collagen and some interesting dermatologic complications have been reported, including epidermolysis [81], pseudoxanthoma elasticum [82] and elastosis perforans serpiginosa [83]. Loss of taste sensation reflects the chelation of copper and is reversed by the administration of copper [84].

N-Acetylpenicillamine is also effective in the formation of mixed disulfides with cystine and appears to cause fewer side-effects [85,86]. Mercaptopropionylglycine [87,88] is effective, but it has some of the same side effects as penicillamine. It may be useful in a patient who can no longer tolerate penicillamine.

References

1 Wollaston WH. On cystic oxide: a new species of urinary calculus. *Trans R Soc London* 1810;**100**:223.
2 Berzelius JJ. Calculus urinaries.*Trait Chem* 1833;**7**:424.
3 Friedman E. Der Kreislauf des Schwefels in der Organischen Natur. *Ergebn Physiol* 1902;**1**:15.
4 Garrod AE. Inborn errors of metabolism. *Lancet* 1908;**2**: (Lecture I p 2; Lecture II p 73; Lecture III p 142; Lecture IV p 214).
5 Yeh HL, Frankl W, Dunn MS, *et al.* The urinary excretion of amino acids by a cystinuric subject. *Am J Med Sci* 1947;**214**:507.
6 Stein WH. Excretion of amino acids in cystinuria. *Proc Soc Exp Biol Med* 1951;**78**:705.
7 Dent CE, Senior B, Walshe JM. The pathogenesis of cystinuria II: Polarographic studies of the metabolism of sulphur-containing amino acids. *J Clin Invest* 1954;**33**:1216.
8 Arrow VK, Westall RG. Amino acid clearances in cystinuria. *J Physiol* 1958;**142**:141.
9 Foreman JW, Hwang SM, Segal S. Transport interactions of cystine and dibasic amino acids in isolated rat renal tubules. *Metabolism* 1980;**29**:53.
10 Segal S, McNamara PD, Pepe LM. Transport interaction of cystine and dibasic amino acids in renal brush border vesicles. *Science* 1977;**197**:169.
11 Dent CE, Rose GA. Amino acid metabolism in cystinuria. *Q J Med* 1951;**20**:205.
12 Kelly S. Cystinuria genotypes predicted from excretion patterns. *Am J Med Genet* 1978;**2**:175.
13 Pras E, Arber N, Aksentijevich I, *et al.* Localization of a gene causing cystinuria to chromosome 2p. *Nat Genet* 1994;**6**:415.
14 Calonge MJ, Gasparini P, Chillaron J, *et al.* Cystinuria caused by mutations in rBAT a gene involved in the transport of cystine. *Nat Genet* 1994;**6**:420.
15 Wright EM. Cystinuria defect expresses itself. *Nat Genet* 1994;**6**:328.
16 Bertran J, Werner A, Moore ML, *et al.* Expression cloning of a cDNA from rabbit kidney cortex that induces a single transport system for cystine and dibasic and neutral amino acid. *Proc Natl Acad Sci USA* 1992;**89**:5601.
17 Bisceglia L, Calonge MJ, Totaro A, *et al.* Localization by linkage analysis of the cystinuria type III gene to chromosome 19q131. *Am J Hum Genet* 1997;**60**:611.
18 Wartenfeld R, Golomb E, Katz G, *et al.* Exclusion of the SLC3A1 gene and mapping of a new locus on 19q. *Am J Hum Genet* 1997;**60**:617.
19 Fawcet NP, Nyhan WL. Cystinuria and dermatomyositis. *Clin Pediatr* 1970;**9**:727.
20 Renander A. The roentgen density of the cystine calculus. *Acta Radiol Suppl* 1941;**41**:35.
21 Hambraeus L, Lagergren C. Cystinuria in Sweden. VI Biophysical and roentgenological studies of urinary calculi from cystinurics. *J Urol* 1962;**88**:826.
22 Stephens AD. Cystinuria and its treatment: 25 years experience at St Bartholomew's Hospital. *J Inherit Metab Dis* 1989;**12**:197.
23 Millner DS. Cystinuria. *Endocr Metab Clin N Am* 1990;**19**:889.

24 Singer A. Cystinuria: A review of the pathophysiology and management. *J Urol* 1989;**142**:669.

25 Woolf LI. Large-scale screening for metabolic disease in the newborn in Great Britain: in *Phenylketonuria and Allied Metabolic Disorders* (eds JA Anderson, KF Swaiman). US Dept of Health Education and Welfare Children's Bureau, Washington DC;1967:50.

26 Turner B, Brown DA. Amino acid excretion in infancy and early childhood: a survey of 200 000 infants. *Med J Aust* 1972;**1**:62.

27 Levy HL, Shih VE, Madigan PM. Massachusetts metabolic disorders screening program. I Technics and results of urine screening. *Pediatrics* 1971;**49**:825.

28 Levy HL. Genetic screening: in *Advances in Human Genetics* Vol 4 (eds H Harris, K Hirschhorn). Plenum Press, New York;1973:1.

29 Harris H, Mittwoch U, Robson EB, Warren FL. Phenotypes and genotypes in cystinuria. *Ann Hum Genet* 1955;**20**:57.

30 Rosenberg LE. Genetic heterogeneity in cystinuria: in *Amino Acid, Metabolism and Genetic Variation* (ed. WL Nyhan). McGraw-Hill, New York;1967:341.

31 Rosenberg LE, Durant JL, Albrecht I. Genetic heterogeneity in cystinuria: evidence for allelism. *Trans Assoc Am Phys* 1966;**79**:284.

32 Morin CL, Thompson MW, Jackson SH, Sass-Kortsak A. Biochemical and genetic studies in cystinuria: observations on double heterozygotes of genotype I/II. *J Clin Invest* 1971;**50**:1961.

33 Lesch M, Nyhan WL. A familial disorder of uric acid metabolism and central nervous system function. *Am J Med* 1964;**36**:561.

34 Brand E, Harris MM, Biloon S. Cystinuria: excretion of a cystine complex which decomposes in the urine with the liberation of free cystine. *J Biol Chem* 1930;**86**:315.

35 Crawhall JC, Purkiss P, Watts RWE, Young EP. The excretion of amino acids by cystinuric patients and their relatives. *Ann Hum Genet* 1969;**33**:149.

36 Crawhall JC. Cystinuria diagnosis and treatment: in *Heritable Disorders of Amino Acid Metabolism* (ed. WL Nyhan) Wiley, New York;1974:593.

37 Purkiss P, Chalmers RA, Borud O. Combined iminoglycinuria and cystine and dibasic aminoaciduria in patients with propionic acidaemia and 3-methylcrotonylglycinuria. *J Inherit Metab Dis* 1980;**3**:85.

38 Delvalle JA, Merinero B, Garcia MJ, *et al.* Biochemical findings in a patient with neonatal methylmalonic acidaemia. *J Inherit Metab Dis* 1982;**5**:53.

39 Frimpter GW, Horwith M, Furth E, *et al.* Inulin and endogenous amino acid renal clearances in cystinuria: evidence for tubular secretion. *J Clin Invest* 1962;**41**:281.

40 Crawhall JC, Scowen EF, Thompson CJ, Watts RWE. The renal clearance of amino acids in cystinuria. *J Clin Invest* 1967;**46**:1162.

41 Kato T. Renal handling of dibasic amino acids and cystine in cystinuria. *Clin Sci Mol Med* 1977;**53**:9.

42 Lester FT, Cusworth DC. Lysine infusion in cystinuria: theoretical renal thresholds for lysine. *Clin Sci* 1973;**44**:99.

43 Robson EB, Rose GA. The effect of intravenous lysine on the renal clearances of cystine arginine and ornithine in normal subjects in patients with cystinuria and Fanconi syndrome and their relatives. *Clin Sci* 1957;**16**:75.

44 Frimpter GW. Cystathioninuria in a patient with cystinuria. *Am J Med* 1969;**46**:832.

45 King JS Jr, Wainer A. Cystinuria with hyperuricemia and methioninuria: biochemical study of a case. *Am J Med* 1967;**43**:125.

46 Frimpter GW. The disulfide of l-cysteine and l-homocysteine in urine of patients with cystinuria. *J Biol Chem* 1961;**236**:651.

47 Cox BD, Cameron JC. Homoarginine in cystinuria. *Clin Sci Mol Med* 1974;**46**:173.

48 Milne MD, London DR, Asatoor AM. Citrullinuria in cases of cystinuria. *Lancet* 1962;**2**:49.

49 McNamara PD, Pepe LM, Segal S. Cystine uptake by renal brush border vesicles. *Biochem J* 1969;**194**:443.

50 Milne MD, Asatoor AM, Edwards KDG, Loughridge LW. The intestinal absorption defect in cystinuria. *Gut* 1961;**2**:323.

51 Asatoor AM, Lacey BW, London DR, Milne MD. Amino acid metabolism in cystinuria. *Clin Sci* 1962;**23**:285.

52 Rosenberg LE, Durant JL, Holland JM. Intestinal absorption and renal extraction of cystine and cysteine in cystinuria. *N Engl J Med* 1965;**273**:1239.

53 Brand E, Cahill GF. Further studies on metabolism of sulfur compounds in cystinuria. *Proc Soc Esp Biol Med* 1934;**31**:1247.

54 Silk DB, Perrett D, Stephens AD, *et al.* Intestinal absorption of cystine and cysteine in normal human subjects and patients with cystinuria. *Clin Sci Mol Med* 1974;**47**:393.

55 Thier S, Fox M, Segal S, Rosenberg LE. Cystinuria: *in vitro* demonstration of an intestinal transport defect. *Science* 1964;**143**:482.

56 McCarthy CF, Borland JL, Lynch HJ, *et al.* Defective uptake of basic amino acids and l-cystine by intestinal mucosa of patients with cystinuria. *J Clin Invest* 1964;**43**:1518.

57 Thier S, Segal S, Fox M, *et al.* Cystinuria: defective intestinal transport of dibasic amino acids and cystine. *J Clin Invest* 1965;**44**:442.

58 Coicadan L, Heyman M, Grasset E, Desjeux JF. Cystinuria: reduced lysine permeability at the brush border of intestinal membrane cells. *Pediatr Res* 1980;**14**:109.

59 Goodyer PR, Clow C, Reade T, Girardin C. Prospective analysis and classification of patients with cystinuria identified in a newborn screening program. *J Pediatr* 1993;**122**:568.

60 McNamara PD, Rea CT, Segal S. Expression of rat jejunal cystine carrier in Xenopus oocytes. *J Biol Chem* 1991;**266**:986.

61 Wells R, Hediger MA. Cloning of a rat kidney cDNA that stimulates dibasic and neutral amino acid transport and has sequence similarity to glucosidases. *Proc Natl Acad Sci USA* 1992;**89**:5596.

62 Lee WS, Wells RG, Sabbah RV, *et al.* Cloning and chromosomal localization of a human kidney cDNA involved in cystine dibasic and neutral amino acid transport. *J Clin Invest* 1993;**91**:1959.

63 Bertran J, Werner A, Chillaron J, *et al.* Expression cloning of a human renal cDNA that induces high affinity of l-cystine shared with dibasic amino acids in Xenopus oocytes. *Am J Biol Chem* 1993;**268**:1482.

64 Magagnin S, Bertran J, Werner A, *et al.* Poly (A) + RNA from rabbit intestinal mucosa induces b0+ and y+ amino acid transport activities in Xenopus laevis oocytes. *J Biol Chem* 1992; **267**:15384.

65 Saadi I, Chen XZ, Hediger M, *et al.* Molecular genetics of cystinuria: mutation analysis of SLC3A1 and evidence for another gene in the type I (silent) phenotype. *Kidney Int* 1998;**54**:48.

66 Pras E, Golomb E, Drake C, *et al.* A splicing mutation (891 + 4A → G) in SLC3A1 leads to exon 4 skipping and causes cystinuria in a Moslem Arab family. *Hum Mutat* 1998;**1**:(suppl) S28.

67 Chillarón J, Estévez R, Samarzija I, *et al.* An intracellular trafficking defect in type I cystinuria rBAT mutants M467T and M467K. *J Biol Chem* 1997;**272**:9543.

68 The International Consortium of Cystinuria (Felivbadato L, *et al*). Non-type I cystinuria caused by mutations in SCL7A9 coding for a subunit (bo+ AT) of rBAT. *Nat Genet* 1999;**23**:52.

69 Casal ML, Giger U, Bovee KC, Patterson DF. Inheritance of cystinuria and renal defect in Newfoundlands. *J Am Vet Med Assoc* 1995;**207**:1585.

70 Dent CE, Friedmann M, Green H, Watson LCA. Treatment of cystinuria. *Br Med J* 1965;**1**:403.

71 Dent CE, Senior B. Studies on the treatment of cystinuria. *Br J Urol* 1955;**27**:317.

72 Crawhall JC, Scowen EF, Watts RWE. Effect of penicillamine on cystinuria. *Br Med J* 1963;**1**:585.

73 Crawhall JC, Scowen EF, Watts RWE. Further observations on use of d-penicillamine in cystinuria. *Br Med J* 1964;**1**:1411.

74 McDonald JE, Henneman PH. Stone dissolution *in vivo* and control of cystinuria with d-penicillamine. *N Engl J Med* 1965;**273**:578.

75 Crawhall JC, Scowen EF, Thompson CJ, Watts RWE. Dissolution of cystine stones during d-penicillamine treatment of a pregnant patient with cystinuria. *Br Med J* 1967;**1**:216.

76 Bartter FC, Lotz M, Thier S, *et al.* Cystinuria: combined clinical staff conference at the National Institutes of Health. *Ann Intern Med* 1965;**62**:796.

77 Fellers FX, Shahidi NT. The nephrotic syndrome induced by penicillamine therapy. *Am J Dis Child* 1959;**98**:669.

78 Corcos JM, Soler-Bechera J, Mayer K, *et al.* Neutrophilic agranulocytosis during administration of penicillamine. *JAMA* 1964;**189**:2654.

79 Fawcett NP, Nyhan WL, Anderson WW. Thrombocytosis during treatment of cystinuria with penicillamine. *JAMA* 1968;**203**:381.

80 Sternlieb I, Bennett B, Scheinberg IH. D-penicillamine-induced Goodpasture's syndrome in Wilson's disease. *Ann Intern Med* 1975;**82**:673.

81 Beer WE, Cooke KB. Epidermolysis bullosa induced by penicillamine. *Br J Dermatol* 1967;**79**:123.

82 Bolognia JL, Braverman I. Pseudoxanthoma-elasticum-like skin changes induced by penicillamine. *Dermatology* 1992;**184**:12.

83 Sahn EE, Maize JC, Garen PD, *et al.* D-penicillamine-induced elastosis perforans serpiginosa in a child with juvenile rheumatoid arthritis. *J Am Acad Dermatol* 1969;**20**:979.

84 Henkin RI, Keiser HR, Jaffe IA, *et al.* Decreased taste sensitivity after d-penicillamine reversed by copper administration. *Lancet* 1967;**16**:1268.

85 Stokes GS, Potts JT, Lotz M, Bartter F. A new agent in the treatment of cystinuria: N-acetyl-d-penicillamine. *Br Med J* 1968;**1**:283.

86 Stephens AD, Watts RWE. The treatment of cystinuria with N-acetyl-penicillamine a comparison with the results of d-penicillamine treatment. *Q J Med* 1971;**40**:335.

87 King JS. Treatment of cystinuria with α-mercapto-propionylglycine: a preliminary report. *Proc Soc Exp Biol Med* 1968;**129**:927.

88 Kinoshita K, Yachiku S, Kotake T, *et al.* Treatment of cystinuria with α-mercaptopropionylglycine (MPG). *Jap J Clin Med* 1972;**30**:232.

89 Perezella MA, Bullen GK. Successful treatment of cystinuria with captopril. *Am J Kidney Dis* 1993;**21**:504.

90 Dahlberg PJ, Jones JD. Cystinuria: failure of captopril to reduce cystine excretion. *Arch Intern Med* 1989;**149**:713.

91 Kelly S, Nolan DP. Letter to the editor. *JAMA* 1980;**243**:1897.

Cystinosis

MAJOR PHENOTYPIC EXPRESSION

Nephropathy progressive to renal failure; a Fanconi syndrome of glycosuria, phosphaturia and generalized amino aciduria leading to acidosis and rickets; inhibition of growth; fair skin, hair and irides; cystine crystals in bone marrow and other tissues; increased cellular lysosomal cystine; and defective adenosine triphosphate (ATP)-dependent lysosomal carrier mediated efflux of cystine resulting from abnormalities in cystinosin, a transmembrane lysosomal transporter.

INTRODUCTION

Cystinosis was first described in 1903 by Abderhalden [1] in a report of a patient in whose tissue deposits were identified chemically as cystine. Cystine deposits were also documented in the report of Lignac [2] in 1924 of three infants with rickets, shortness of stature and renal disease. Fanconi [3] in 1931 reported a child with rickets, dwarfism and glycosuria, and this picture of renal tubular defect has come to be known as the Fanconi syndrome, or the renal Fanconi syndrome to distinguish it from the Fanconi anemia. A patient with renal dwarfism, vitamin D-resistant rickets, spontaneous fractures, hypophosphatemia, acidosis and glycosuria was reported by de Toni [4] in 1933, and a similar patient was reported by Debré and colleagues [5] in 1934. Fanconi in 1936 [6] proposed that all of these patients constituted a syndrome of dwarfism and renal defect with glycosuria and hypophosphatemic rickets. The syndrome has been referred to as that of Lignac, Fanconi, De Toni and Debré, in various orders. The amino aciduria was documented by Dent [7]. This renal tubular abnormality may be seen in other conditions besides cystinosis. Its clear association with cystinosis was made by Franconi and Bickel [8,9].

Schneider and his colleagues [10,11] first characterized patients with cystinosis as having increased quantities of cystine in leukocytes and cultured fibroblasts. This provided a highly specific method of diagnosis. The lysosomal localization of the stored cystine was reported on the basis of electron microscopy by Patrick and Lake [12] and by Harms and Schneider on the basis of chemical fractionation [13]. The abnormality in cystine transport was discovered independently in 1982 by Steinherz, Tietze, Gahl, and colleagues [14] and by Jonas, Green and Schneider [15]. Isolated lysosomes from leukocytes or cultured lymphoblasts or fibroblasts of patients were also shown by Gahl and colleagues [16] and by Jonas, Smith and Schneider [17] to have defective transport of cystine out of the organelle. The efflux which is defective in cystinosis is linked to ATP, in a process in which a specific ATPase acts as a proton pump (Figure 71.1). This has been the protoype for other lysosomal transporters that are involved in human disease, such as those for cobalamin (Chapter 4) and sialic acid.

The gene for cystinosin was mapped to chromosome 7p13 in 1995 [18]. A number of mutations have been identified [19–21].

CLINICAL ABNORMALITIES

In classic cystinosis the patient appears normal at birth. The usual presentation is at 6 to 10 months-of-age with symptoms generated by renal tubular dysfunction. These patients have a classic renal Fanconi syndrome (Table 71.1) in which there is renal tubular deficiency in the reabsorption of glucose,

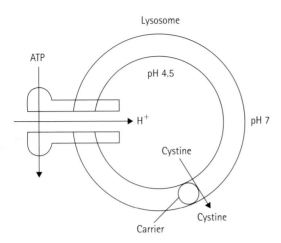

Figure 71.1 *Postulated lysosomal site of the defect in cystinosis in a cystine carrier (reprinted with permission from Nyhan WL: Abnormalities in Amino Acid Metabolism in Clinical Medicine, Appleton/Century/Crofts, Norwalk, Conn., 1984).*

Table 71.1 *Differential diagnosis of the renal Fanconi syndrome*

Cystinosis
Idiopathic
Hepatorenal tyrosinemia
Galactosemia
Wilson disease
Lowe syndrome
Glycogen storage disease (I, III)
Lysinuric protein intolerance

phosphate, amino acids and other organic acids, as well as of sodium, potassium, calcium, magnesium, bicarbonate and water [21–24]. The amino aciduria is a generalized amino-aciduria in which those amino acids usually found in the urine in moderate quantity, such as glycine, are excreted in very large amounts; those usually found in very small amounts, such as leucine, are excreted in moderate amounts; and the imino acids, such as proline, which are not normally found in urine are excreted in appreciable amounts.

Renal losses of phosphate lead to hypophosphatemia and rickets. Any of the clinical manifestations of rickets may develop, and roentgenograms reveal the typical cupped and frayed ends of the long bones. A thoracic rosary is characteristic. Alkaline phosphatase levels are increased. This is a form of vitamin D-resistant rickets in the sense that it develops in spite of the usual antirachitic doses of vitamin D, and does not respond to vitamin D in these amounts. Losses of sodium bicarbonate and potassium lead to chronic acidosis and hypokalemia. This is a proximal renal tubular acidosis. It is hyperchloremic, and a low serum bicarbonate is consistent with very great losses of bicarbonate. In normal individuals the sum of the urinary concentrations of sodium and potassium is lower than that of chloride (a negative urinary anion gap). In renal tubular acidosis their concentration is higher than that of chloride (positive urinary anion gap).

Growth retardation may be extreme. Patients may have tremendous polyuria and polydipsia. This makes these children highly vulnerable to dehydration, especially in the presence of otherwise minor infections, particularly gastrointestinal disease that interferes with fluid intake. In a patient in whom continued administration of large amounts of sodium bicarbonate is maintained, hypernatremic dehydration may occur. Symptomatic hypokalemia may present with recurrent episodes of weakness or prostration. Cardiovascular collapse and sudden death may occur. The patient with cystinosis may present initially with the picture of the Bartter syndrome [25–27]. There is proteinuria particularly of lower molecular height proteins (tubular proteinuria) [28], and protein excretion may reach 5 g a day. The renal tubular defect may lead to very great losses of free-carnitine [29], which is normally about 97 percent reabsorbed. Low levels of free-carnitine in the blood and muscle lead to deficient fatty acid oxidation, microvesicular fat in muscle and liver and clinical myopathy. Urinary tract calculi, of both urate and calcium oxalate, have been reported [30]. The increased excretion of calcium may lead to nephrocalcinosis [31,32].

Renal damage results from involvement of the glomeruli. Creatinine clearance decreases progressively. Uremia and renal failure are progressive, leading usually to death within the first 10 years of life. The mean age of renal death in 205 patients in Europe was 9.2 years [33].

Shortness of stature is typical in cystinosis. The process begins in the first year. By 8 years the height is at the 50th percentile for 4 years [34]. Bone age may be delayed [35]. Height and weight are similarly delayed; so the patient appears proportionate. Sparing of brain growth may give an appearance of relative macrocephaly.

Patients generally have a fair complexion and very fair hair (Figure 71.2). However, a dark skin color is not against the diagnosis. The disease has been seen in several non-Caucasian patients (Figure 71.3) including a black child [36]. Ability to sweat may be impaired [37] and this may lead to intolerance to heat. There may also be impaired production of tears and saliva.

A variety of ophthalmic abnormalities are seen in patients with cystinosis. Refractile crystalline bodies may be demonstrated by slit lamp examination of the cornea [38]. These birefringent refractile bodies are pathognomonic of cystinosis. The corneal deposits are not present at birth, but they may be found well before clinical nephropathy [39]. Ultimately, there may be a thickened cornea with a distinct haziness [40,41]. Corneal ulcers may occur [42]. Crystalline cystine has been identified in the conjunctiva by X-ray diffraction, as well as by biopsy [43]. Photophobia is a prominent and disturbing symptom. Patients with cystinosis also have a characteristic retinopathy [44]. The peripheral retina has a patchy pattern of hyperpigmentation and depigmentation, often in regular distribution, varying from about a tenth of a disc diameter to a fine, peppery size. Retinal changes, which are usually more marked temporally, may be the earliest clinical manifestation of the disease. The ability to keep patients alive longer with renal transplantation has permitted the development of much

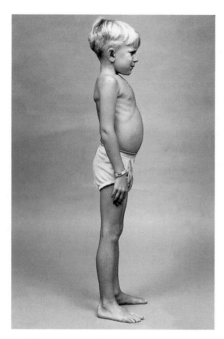

Figure 71.2   *W.B., a 7-year-old boy with advanced cystinosis had the characteristic very blond hair and pot belly. His height was 108 cm. (The illustration was kindly provided by Dr. Jerry Schneider of the University of California San Diego.)*

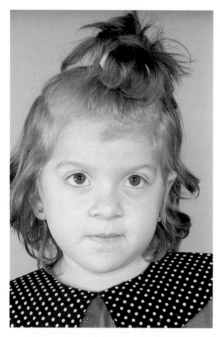

Figure 71.3   *R.D., a petite blond Arab girl with cystinosis. She was 4 years old and 83.6 cm tall (50th percentile for 21 months). Her weight was 12 kg. Cystine crystals were identified on skin biopsy and slit lamp examination of the cornea revealed refractile bodies characteristic of cystinosis.*

more marked ocular changes. Visual acuity is not usually impaired in children, but among those treated with renal transplantation and living into the third decade some can be legally blind.

Another late complication is hypothyroidism [45–47]. Atrophy of the gland results from cystine accumulation, and more than 70 percent of patients over 10 years of age need replacement therapy [48]. Thyroid stimulating hormone (TSH) may be elevated before the development of clinical hypothyroidism [49]. Some patients develop insulin-dependent diabetes mellitus [50]. Hypogonadism is common in adult males [51]. Puberty may be delayed in the female, but is ultimately normal, and one who had a renal transplantation had a normal pregnancy outcome [52]. Myopathy results from crystalline deposition in muscle, and this may be manifest in visible atrophy of muscles [53]. Symptoms may be aggravated by carnitine deficiency.

Impaired visual and spatial cognition has been recognized in cystinosis [54], but function is normal as is intelligence. There also may be late involvement of the central nervous system; [55,56], or cerebral atrophy visible on neuroimaging [57]. Some have had seizures, tremor, pyramidal signs or mental retardation [58,59]. Gait disturbance made one patient wheelchair bound, but neurological examination is usually normal [59].

Genetic heterogeneity has been defined clinically in cystinosis. A number of clinically variant phenotypes have been described. At the other extreme from classic nephropathic cystinosis is a benign or so-called adult variant in which patients develop neither nephropathy nor retinal symptomatology [60,61]. These patients have been identified by the presence of crystalline deposits in the cornea, bone marrow and leukocytes. Kidney biopsies, however, demonstrated no cystine crystals and the cystine content of the kidney was not elevated [61,62]. They may develop photophobia in middle age, but it is usually not severe. They do not have retinopathy.

Other patients have been described with phenotypes intermediate between the two [63–65]. These patients all have renal abnormalities, but they do not present until an older age. The Fanconi syndrome may be less than complete, and the glomerular disease may progress slowly. Among involved siblings in a family the phenotype tends to be quite similar. Overall, it is likely that there are a number of different variants. Photophobia and retinopathy are variable. Some patients have had some delay in growth, while others have grown normally.

Abnormal laboratory tests observed in patients with cystinosis include elevated sedimentation rates, platelet counts and cholesterol [35]. With the advent of uremia the patient may become anemic.

The pathology of the disease reflects the extensive deposition of cystine crystals throughout the tissues of the body. The disorder may be readily diagnosed by the examination of aspirated bone marrow for cystine crystals (Figure 71.4). Conjunctival biopsy has also been employed for this purpose. Crystals may also be demonstrated in the lymph nodes. Its deposition in the kidney leads to the nephropathy that characterizes the disease. This has the appearance of chronic interstitial nephritis, with glomerular endothelial proliferation, hyalinization and necrosis.

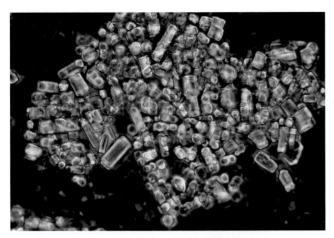

Figure 71.4 *Cystine crystals aspirated from the marrow of a patient with cystinosis. (The illustration was kindly provided by Dr. Jerry Schneider of the University of California San Diego.)*

GENETICS AND PATHOGENESIS

Cystinosis is transmitted by an autosomal recessive gene. Each of the forms of cystinosis follows this pattern of inheritance. Consanguinity has been observed. The incidence of the disease in North America is one per 100 000–200 000 births, but in France the incidence in Brittany is one in 26 000 [66].

The chemical hallmark of this disorder is the accumulation of large amounts of cystine in cells [10,11]. The measurement of cystine content in freshly isolated leukocytes or in cultured fibroblasts is diagnostic. The values in nephropathic cystinosis are 80–100 times the control value. In benign cystinosis, levels 30 times normal are found, and in the intermediate group the values tend to be intermediate, although there are exceptions [10,63,67]. Cystinotic fibroblasts in culture develop vacuoles when exposed to the mixed disulfide of penicillamine and cysteine, and this property may be useful in suggesting the diagnosis [68]. Within the cell the cystine is stored in the lysosomes [12,13].

Studies of cystine efflux from lysosomes have clarified the fundamental defect in cystinosis. When cultured cells are treated with cysteine-glutathione mixed disulfide or cystine dimethylester so that they accumulate large amounts of cystine, normal cells lose cystine progressively over 20 to 90 minutes, but cystinotic cells do not [14,15]. Lysosomes from freshly isolated normal leukocytes behaved *in vitro* like normal intact cells. They lose cystine progressively, while those isolated from cystinotic leukocytes do not [16]. There is a carrier-mediated lysosomal transport system for cystine, and it is defective in cystinosis. The process is energy related; the addition of 2,4-dinitrophenol to deplete normal cells of ATP inhibited the efflux of cystine. When ATP was added to lysosomes isolated from normal lysosomal fibroblasts, there was rapid, progressive efflux of cystine [17]. ATP had no effect on efflux from the lysosomes of cystinotic cells. Thus it is an ATP-linked efflux of cystine that is aberrant in cystinosis (Figure 71.1). In cystinosis

the ATPase was found to be normal as was lysosomal proton translocating activity [69], indicating that the defect was in the cystine carrier protein itself.

Heterozygotes may be detected by determining the cystine content of leukocytes or fibroblasts [10,11,67]. In nephropathic cystinosis the cells of heterozygotes display a mean cystine content 5 to 6 times the normal mean. Although these data have been obtained on both fibroblasts and leukocytes, the amount of variability encountered in fibroblasts is such that only the leukocyte assay is recommended. The clearance of cystine from leukocytes loaded with 35S-cystine dimethylester has been developed for the detection of heterozygosity [70]. Cystine efflux from isolated leukocyte lysosomes occurs at about half the normal maximal rate in heterozygotes [16].

Prenatal diagnosis on the basis of the content of cystine in cultured amniocytes or chorionic villus cells is a well established technique [71–73].

The gene for cystinosis, *CTNS*, codes for the transporter protein cystinosin [18–21]. It contains 12 exons over 23 kb of genomic DNA [19]. The protein contains 367 amino acids and has 7 transmembrane domains and 7 sites of potential glycosylation. It transports cystine and has appropriate kinetic properties [74].

More than 55 mutations have been identified [21]. The most common, found in 50 percent of nephropathic cystinosis patients from northern Europe, is a 57 kb deletion that removes the first 10 exons and is readily detectable by a multiplex polymerase chain reaction assay [19,20,75–77]. The mutation deletes expression of the protein, and displays a founder effect dating from 500 AD in Germany. The second most common nephropathic mutation, observed in 12 percent of American patients was a G753A, W138X stop mutation [19,21]. Mutations have been found in the promoter of the *CTNS* gene [78], including a $-295G \rightarrow C$ substitution in a patient with nephropathic cystinosis and two changes at -303, a T insertion and a $G \rightarrow T$ transition in two patients with ocular cystinosis. Some correlations of genotype and phenotype have been possible [78]. Mutational analysis may be used effectively in heterozygote detection and in prenatal diagnosis.

TREATMENT

Early diagnosis is a prerequisite for successful therapy. Glomerular damage, once caused, is not reversible.

Supportive therapy in nephropathic cystinosis is demanding. The renal tubular defect requires the provision of adequate amounts of water, sodium and potassium. Unrestricted access to salt and water is important. Polycitra, which contains 1 mEq of sodium and 1 mEq of potassium per milliliter, is convenient for electrolyte replacement [24]. In some patients whose potassium is normal, Bicitra (which contains only sodium citrate) or sodium bicarbonate may be used. The average dose is 45–60 mL/day. Rickets is treated with 10 000–15 000 units of vitamin D per day, or an equivalent amount of 1,25-dihydrocholecalciferol. Phosphate replacement permits

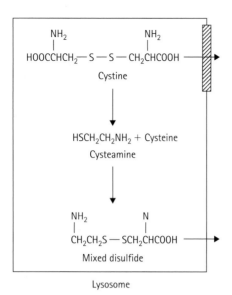

Figure 71.5 *The structure of cysteamine and its mechanism for depletion of stored cystine.*

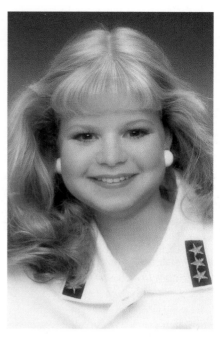

Figure 71.6 *W.G., an 18-year-old with cystinosis illustrating the efficiency of treatment with cysteamine since diagnosis of about one year-of-age. She has not had a renal transplantation and has continued to do well.*

reduction of the dose of vitamin D. In fact, healing of rickets may be obtained in this disorder using phosphate alone.

In the presence of intercurrent illness in which there is vomiting or diarrhea, a vigorous approach to parenteral fluid therapy is important. A patient with renal tubular acidosis receiving polycitra or sodium bicarbonate may present markedly dehydrated, but with a high concentration of sodium in the blood. It is important not to treat this volume-depleted patient as if nondehydrated sodium-intoxicated, gingerly using an administration of nonsodium-containing solutions calculated to lower the sodium gradually. Such an approach can readily lead to irreversible oligemic shock.

Treatment with carnitine rapidly reverses the low plasma levels of free-carnitine; however, muscle levels of carnitine may require years of treatment to reach the normal range [79,80]. Despite this, the muscle may still contain Oil Red-O staining lipid droplets. Doses employed have approximated 100 mg/kg per day.

Many patients with nephropathic cystinosis have been treated with renal transplantation [48,81]. Following transplantation growth does not usually improve, and visual disease and thyroid disease tend to progress. Nevertheless, it is clear that nephropathy does not develop in the transplanted kidney, and many patients have lived 10 years post-transplant. Hair color may darken following transplantation.

A variety of approaches have been undertaken to treat cystinosis using thiol compounds. Intracellular cystine can be lowered in cultured cells using a number of compounds. Most clinical experience is with cysteamine [82] (Figure 71.5). This compound with its neutral amino group readily enters the lysome, where it reacts with cysteine to form the mixed disulfide, whose structure is sufficiently like that of lysine to be transported out via the lysine transporter. Doses approximating 50–90 mg/kg per day have now been used for many years (Figure 71.6) with rewarding results [34,83]. Starting

dose is usually 10 mg/kg per day and increased by 10 per day until the target is reached. Depletion of stored cystine can be documented by analysis of leukocytes to be as much as 80 percent. Growth of treated children was 50–60 percent of the normal rate.

Renal tubular dysfunction, once established, does not improve, but it can be prevented. Glomerular function has been remarkably preserved [84]. With early treatment the prognosis for glomerular function is good. Tubular dysfunction still develops. Cysteamine will protect the thyroid obviating the need for thyroxine replacement therapy [85]. The taste and smell of cysteamine are quite disagreeable. Capsules of cysteamine bitartrate (Cystagon, Mylan) are preferred by those who can swallow capsules. Gastrointestinal symptoms are virtually the rule in patients treated with cysteamine; they are acid-related and improve with treatment with omeprazole (10–20 mg bid) [86]. A derivative, phosphocysteamine, is equally effective *in vitro* [87] and since it is odorless and tasteless it has advantages for human use. The two compounds can be used interchangeably. Neither is effective orally in managing the corneal disease, but cysteamine eye drops are remarkably effective if used 10–14 times a day [88].

References

1   Abderhalden E. Familiar Cystindiathese. *Z Physiol Chem* 1903;**38**:557.

2   Lignac GOE. Uber Storung des Cystinstoffwechsels bei Kindern. *Deutsch Arch Klin Med* 1924;**145**:139.

3   Fanconi G. Die nicht diabetischen Glykosurien und Hyperglykamien des altern Kindes. *Jahrb Kinderheilkd* 1931;**133**:257.

4 deToni G. Remarks on the relations between renal rickets (renal dwarfism) and renal diabetes. *Acta Paediatr* 1933;**16**:479.

5 Debré R, Marie J, Cletet F, Messimy R. Rachitisme tardif coexistent avec une nephrite chronique et une glycosurie. *Arch Med Enf* 1934;**37**:597.

6 Fanconi G. Der nephrotisch-glykosurische Zwergwuchs mit hypophosphatamischer Rachitis. *Dtsch Med Wochenschr* 1936;**62**:1169.

7 Dent CE. The amino-aciduria in Fanconi syndrome. A study making extensive use of techniques based on paper partition chromatography. *Biochem J* 1947;**41**:240.

8 Fanconi G, Bickel H. Die chronische aminoacidurie (aminosäurediabetes oder nephrotisch-glukosurischer zergwuchs) bei der glykogenose und der cystinkrankheit. *Helv Paediatr Acta* 1949;**4**:359.

9 Bickel H, Baar HS, Astley R. Cystine storage disease with aminoaciduria and dwarfism (Lignac-Fanconi Disease). *Acta Paed Uppsala* 1952;**42**:(suppl 90) 1.

10 Schneider JA, Bradley K, Seegmiller JE. Increased cystine in leukocytes from individuals homozygous and heterozygous for cystinosis. *Science* 1967;**157**:1321.

11 Schneider JA, Rosenbloom FM, Bradley KH, Seegmiller JE. Increased free-cystine content of fibroblasts cultured from patients with cystinosis. *Biochem Biophys Res Commun* 1967;**29**:527.

12 Patrick AD, Lake BD. Cystinosis: electron microscopic evidence of lysosomal storage of cystine in lymph node. *J Clin Pathol* 1968;**21**:571.

13 Harms E, Schneider JA. The lysosomal localization of free-cystine in normal cystinotic cells. *Clin Res* 1979;**27**:457A.

14 Steinherz R, Tietze F, Gahl WA, *et al.* Cystine accumulation and clearance by normal and cystinotic leukocytes exposed to cystine dimethyl ester. *Proc Natl Acad Sci USA* 1982;**79**:4446.

15 Jonas AJ, Greene AA, Smith ML, Schneider JA. Cystine accumulation and loss in normal heterozygous and cystinotic fibroblasts. *Proc Natl Acad Sci USA* 1982;**79**:4442.

16 Gahl WA, Bashan N, Tietze F, *et al.* Cystine transport is defective in isolated leukocyte lysosomes from patients with cystinosis. *Science* 1982;**217**:1263.

17 Jonas AJ, Smith ML, Schneider JA. ATP-dependent lysosomal cystine efflux is defective in cystinosis. *J Biol Chem* 1982;**257**:13185.

18 The Cystinosis Collaborative Research Group. Linkage of the gene for cystinosis to markers on the short arm of chromosome 17. *Nat Genet* 1995;**10**:246.

19 Town M, Jean G, Cherqui S, *et al.* A novel gene encoding an integral membrane protein is mutated in nephropathic cystinosis. *Nat Genet* 1998;**18**:319.

20 Forestier L, Jean G, Attard M, *et al.* Molecular characterization of CTNS deletions in nephropathic cystinosis: development of a PCR-based detection assay. *Am J Hum Genet* 1999;**65**:353.

21 Gahl WA, Thoene JG, Schneider JA. Cystinosis. *N Engl J Med* 2002;**347**:111.

22 Seegmiller JE, Friedmann T, Harrison HE, *et al.* Cystinosis, Combined Clinical Staff Conferences at the National Institutes of Health. *Ann Int Med* 1968;**68**:883.

23 Schulman JD. *Cystinosis*. DHEW Publication No (NIH) 72-249. US Government Printing Office, Washington DC;1973.

24 Gahl WA. Cystinosis coming of age. *Adv Pediatr* 1986;**33**:95.

25 Lebel M, Grose JH, Delage E, Crepin G. Syndrome de Bartter associéè une cystinose. Association des Médicin de la Langue Française du Canada Congrès annuel, October 1977.

26 Lemire J, Kaplan BS, Scriver CR. Presentation of cystinosis as Bartter's syndrome and conversion to Fanconi syndrome on indomethacin treatment. *Pediatr Res* 1978;**12**:544.

27 O'Regan S, Mongeau J-G, Robitaille P. A patient with cystinosis presenting with the features of Bartter syndrome. *Acta Pediatr Belg* 1980;**33**:51.

28 Waldmann TA, Mogielnicki RP, Strober W. The proteinuria of cystinosis: its pattern and pathogenesis: in *Cystinosis* (ed. JD Schulman). DHEW Publication, Washington DC;1972:55.

29 Bernardini I, Rizzo WB, Dalakas M, *et al.* Plasma and muscle free carnitine deficiency due to renal Fanconi syndrome. *J Clin Invest* 1985;**75**:1124.

30 Black J, Stapleton FB, Roy S, *et al.* Varied types of urinary calculi in a patient with cystinosis without renal tubular acidosis. *Pediatrics* 1986;**78**:295.

31 Saleem MA, Milford DV, Alton H, *et al.* Hypercalciuria and ultrasound abnormalities in children with cystinosis. *Pediatr Nephrol* 1995;**9**:45.

32 Theodoropoulous DS, Shawker TH, Heinrichs C, Gahl WA. Medullary nephrocalcinosis in nephropathic cystinosis. *Pediatr Nephrol* 1995;**9**:412.

33 Gretz N, Manz F, Augustin R, *et al.* Survival time in cystinosis. A collaborative study. *Proc Eur Dial Transplant Assoc* 1983;**19**:582.

34 Gahl WA, Reed GF, Thoene JG, *et al.* Cysteamine therapy for children with nephropathic cystinosis. *N Engl J Med* 1987;**316**:971.

35 Gahl WA, Kaiser-Kupfer MI. Complications of nephropathic cystinosis after renal failure. *Pediatr Nephrol* 1987;**1**:260.

36 Jonas AJ, Schneider JA. Cystinosis in a black child. *J Pediatr* 1982;**100**:934.

37 Gahl WA, Hubbard VS, Orloff J. Decreased sweat production in cystinosis. *J Pediatr* 1984;**104**:904.

38 Burki VE. Ueber die Cystinkrankheit im Kleinkindesalter unter besonderer Berucksichtigung des Augenbefundes. *Ophthalmologica* 1941;**101**:257.

39 Schneider JA, Wong V, Seegmiller JE. The early diagnosis of cystinosis. *J Pediatr* 1969;**74**:114.

40 Katz B, Melles RB, Schneider JA, Rao NA. Corneal thickness in nephropathic cystinosis. *Br J Ophthalmol* 1989;**73**:665.

41 Korn D. Demonstration of cystine crystals in peripheral white blood cells in a patient with cystinosis. *N Engl J Med* 1960;**262**:545.

42 Kaiser-Kupfer MI, Datiles MB, Gahl QA. Corneal transplant in a twelve-year-old boy with nephropathic cystinosis. *Lancet* 1987;**1**:331.

43 Frazier PD, Wong VG. Cystinosis: histologic and crystallographic examination of crystals in eye tissues. *Arch Ophthalmol* (Chicago) 1968;**80**:87.

44 Wong VG, Lietman PS, Seegmiller JE. Alterations of pigment epithelium in cystinosis. *Arch Ophthalmol* (Chicago) 1967;**77**:361.

45 Chan AM, Lynch MJG, Bailey JD, *et al.* Hypothyroidism in cystinosis. *Am J Med* 1970;**48**:678.

46 Burke JR, El-Bishti MM, Maisey MN, Chantler C. Hypothyroidism in children with cystinosis. *Arch Dis Child* 1978;**53**:947.

47 Czernichow P, Lenoir G, Roy M-P, *et al.* Atteintes thyroidiennes au cours de la cystinose. *Arch Fr Pediatr* 1978;**35**:930.

48 Gahl WA, Schneider JA, Thoene JG, Chesney R. Course of nephropathic cystinosis after age 10 years. *J Pediatr* 1986;**109**:605.

49 Lucky AW, Howley PM, Megyesi K, *et al.* Endocrine studies in cystinosis: compensated primary hypothyroidism. *J Pediatr* 1977;**91**:204.

50 Fivush B, Green OC, Porter CC, *et al.* Pancreatic endocrine insufficiency in posttransplant cystinosis. *Am J Dis Child* 1987;**141**:1087.

51 Chik CL, Friedman A, Merriam GR, Gahl WA. Pituitary-testicular function in nephropathic cystinosis. *Ann Intern Med* 1993;**119**:568.

52 Reiss RE, Kuwabara T, Smith ML, Gahl WA. Successful pregnancy despite placental cystine crystals in a woman with nephropathic cystinosis. *N Engl J Med* 1988;**319**:223.

53 Charnas LR, Luciano CA, Dalakas M, *et al.* Distal vacuolar myopathy in nephropathic cystinosis. *Ann Neurol* 1994;**35**:181.

54 Ballantyne AO, Trauner DA. Neurobehavioral consequences of a genetic metabolic disorder: visual processing deficits in infantile nephropathic cystinosis. *Neuropsychiatry Neuropsychol Behav Neurol* 2000;**13**:254.

55 Ehrich JHH, Stoeppler L, Offner G, Broedehl J. Evidence for cerebral involvement in nephropathic cystinosis. *Neuropadiatrie* 1979;**10**:128.

56 Ehrich JHH, Wolff G, Stoeppler L, *et al.* Psychosozial-intellektuelle entwicklung bei kindern mit infantiler zystinose und hirnatrophie. *Klin Padiatr* 1979;**191**:483.

57 Ehrich JHH, Stoeppler L, Offner G, Brodehl J. Evidence for cerebral involvement in nephropathic cystinosis. *J Neuropathol Exp Neurol* 1990;**49**:591.

58 Cochat P, Drachman R, Gagnadoux MF, *et al.* Cerebral atrophy and nephropathic cystinosis. *Arch Dis Child* 1986;**61**:401.

59 Fink JK, Brouwers P, Barton N, *et al.* Neurologic complications in long-standing nephropathic cystinosis. *Arch Neurol* 1989;**46**:543.

60 Lietman PS, Frazier PD, Wong VG, *et al.* Adult cystinosis – a benign disorder. *Am J Med* 1966;**40**:511.

61 Brubaker RF, Wong VG, Schulman JD, *et al.* Benign cystinosis: the clinical biochemical and morphologic findings in a family with two affected siblings. *Am J Med* 1970;**49**:546.

62 Dodd MG, Pusin SM, Green WR. Adult cystinosis: a case report. *Arch Ophthalmol* 1978;**96**:1054.

63 Goldman H, Scriver CR, Aaron K, *et al.* Adolescent cystinosis: comparisons with infantile and adult forms. *Pediatrics* 1971;**47**:979.

64 Aaron K, Goldman H, Scriver CR. Cystinosis: new observations: 1 Adolescent (type III) form 2 Correction of phenotypes *in vitro* with dithiothreitol: in *Inherited Disorders of Sulphur Metabolism* (eds NAJ Carson, DN Raine). Churchill Livingstone, Edinburgh;1971:150.

65 Spear GS, Slusser RJ, Schulman JD, Alexander F. Polykaryocytosis in the visceral glomerular epithelium in cystinosis with description of an unusual clinical variant. *Johns Hopkins Med J* 1971;**129**:83.

66 Bois E, Feingold J, Frenay P, Briard ML. Infantile cystinosis in France: genetics incidence geographic distribution. *J Med Genet* 1976;**13**:434.

67 Schneider JA, Wong V, Bradley KH, Seegmiller JE. Biochemical comparisons of the adult and childhood forms of cystinosis. *N Engl J Med* 1968;**279**:1253.

68 Schulman JE, Bradley KH. Cystinosis: selective induction of vacuolation in fibroblasts by L-cysteine-D-penicillamine disulfide. *Science* 1970;**169**:595.

69 Jonas AJ, Smith ML, Allison WS, *et al.* Proton translocating ATPase and lysosomal cystine transport. *J Biol Chem* 1983;**258**:11727.

70 Steinherz R, Tietze F, Triche T, *et al.* Heterozygote detection in cystinosis using leukocytes exposed to cystine dimenthyl ester. *N Engl J Med* 1982;**306**:1468.

71 Schneider JA, Bradley KH, Seegmiller JE. Transport and intracellular fate of cysteine-35S in leukocytes from normal subjects and patients with cystinosis. *Pediatr Res* 1968;**2**:441.

72 Schulman JD, Fujimoto WY, Bradley KH, Seegmiller JE. Identification of heterozygous genotype for cystinosis *in utero* by a new pulse-labeling technique: preliminary report. *J Pediatr* 1970;**77**:468.

73 Gahl WA, Dorfmann A, Evans MI, *et al.* Chorionic biopsy in the prenatal diagnosis of nephropathic cystinosis: in *First Trimester Fetal Diagnosis* (eds M Fraccaro, G Simmoni, B Brambti). Springer-Verlag;1985:260.

74 Kalatzis V, Cherqui S, Antignac C, Gasnier B. Cystinosin the protein defective in cystiniosis is a H^+-driven lysosomal cystine transporter. *EMBO J* 2001;**20**:5940.

75 Touchman JW, Anikster Y, Dietrich NL, *et al.* The genomic region encompassing the nephropathic cystinosis gene (CTNS): complete sequencing of a 200-kb segment and discovery of a novel gene within the common cystinosis-causing deletion. *Genome Res* 2000;**10**:165.

76 Anikster Y, Lucero C, Touchman JW, *et al.* Identification and detection of the common 65-kb deletion breakpoint in the nephropathic cystinosis gene (CTNS). *Mol Genet Metab* 1999;**66**:111.

77 Shotelersuk V, Larson D, Anikster Y, *et al.* CTNS mutations in an American-based population of cystinosis patients. *Am J Hum Genet* 1998;**63**:1352.

78 Phornphutkul C, Anikster Y, Huizing M, *et al.* The promoter of a lysosomal membrane transporter gene CTNS binds sp-1 shares sequences with the promoter of an adjacent gene CARKL and causes cystinosis if mutated in a critical region. *Am J Hum Genet* 2001;**69**:712.

79 Gahl WA, Bernardini I, Dalakas M, *et al.* Oral carnitine therapy in children with cystinosis and renal Fanconi syndrome. *J Clin Invest* 1988;**81**:549.

80 Gahl WA, Bernardini IM, Dalakas MC, *et al.* Muscle carnitine repletion by long-term carnitine supplementation in nephropathic cystinosis. *Pediatr Res* 1993;**34**:115.

81 Theodoropoulos DS, Krasnewich D, Kaiser-Kupfer MI, Gahl WA. Classic nephropathic cystinosis as an adult disease. *JAMA* 1993;**270**:2200.

82 Thoene JG, Oshima RG, Olson DL, Schneider JA. Cystinosis: intracellular cystine depletion by amino-thiols *in vitro* and *in vivo. J Clin Invest* 1976;**58**:180.

83 Reznik VM, Adamson M, Adelman RD, *et al.* Treatment of cystinosis with cysteamine from early infancy. *J Pediatr* 1991;**119**:491.

84 Kleta R, Bernardini I, Ueda M, *et al.* Long-term follow-up of well-treated nephropathic cystinosis patients. *J Pediatr* 2004;**145**:555.

85 Kimonis VE. Troendle J. Rose SR. *et al.* Effects of early cysteamine therapy on thyroid function and growth in nephropathic cystinosis. *J Clin Endocrinol Metab* 1995;**80**:3257.

86 Dohil R, Newbury RO, Sellers ZM, *et al.* The evaluation and treatment of gastrointestinal disease in children with cystinosis receiving cysteamine. *J Pediatr* 2003;**143**:224.

87 Thoene JG, Lemons R. Cystine depletion of cystinotic tissues by phosphocysteamine (WR638). *J Pediatr* 1980;**96**:1043.

88 Kaiser-Kupfer MI, Fujikawa L, Kuwabara T, *et al.* Removal of corneal crystals by topical cysteamine in nephropathic cystinosis. *N Engl J Med* 1987;**316**:775.

Hartnup disease

MAJOR PHENOTYPIC EXPRESSION

Cerebellar ataxia, pellagra-like photosensitive dermatosis, headaches, mental retardation, psychiatric abnormalities; a specific generalized amino aciduria in which small, neutral amino acids predominate but glycine is normal and amino acids are absent; and malabsorption of tryptophan which leads to indicanuria.

INTRODUCTION

Hartnup disease is a genetically determined disorder in which the renal tubular and intestinal transport of tryptophan and other ring-containing and neutral amino acids is impaired. It was named for the surname of the family in which the disorder was discovered [1,2].

Many patients with Hartnup disease are asymptomatic. The single constant phenotypic feature is the unusual aminoaciduria in which a large group of neutral α-amino acids are excreted in large quantities. The pattern was first recognized in paper partition chromatograms [1–3], but it is also clearly recognizable on electrophoresis (Figure 72.1) and on quantitative analysis of the amino acids of the urine in the amino acid analyzer (Figure 72.2). Deficient activity of a sodium-dependent transport system, which controls the absorption of these amino acids at the brush-border of the intestinal and renal epithelium, leads to the phenotype. The aminoaciduria is generalized, but it differs from the usual nonspecific generalized aminoaciduria in that glycine and the amino acids, proline and hydroxyproline, are not excreted in unusual quantity. The amino acids excreted in greatest quantity are those, excluding glycine, that are found in largest quantity in normal urine – alanine, glutamine, serine and histidine. Amino acids, many of them essential, which are excreted in very small quantities in normal urine but in prominent amounts in the urine of patients with Hartnup

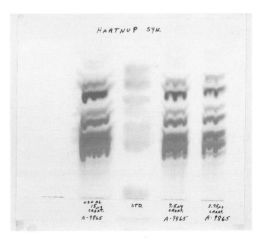

Figure 72.1 *High voltage electropherogram of the amino acids of the urine of a patient with Hartnup disease. The gross aminoaciduria is evident in the first column, in which the usual sample containing 15 μg creatinine was run. Column 2 were standards. The other two runs were with 7.5 and 3.75 μg of creatinine, respectively. The dark band at the top is histidine, the next glycine, followed by alanine, glutamine and serine.*

disease, include leucine, isoleucine, valine, threonine, phenylalanine, tyrosine and tryptophan. The tryptophanuria may be missed if the patient is studied only by column chromatography on the amino acid analyzer because tryptophan is destroyed by the conditions of analysis. Asparagine is also

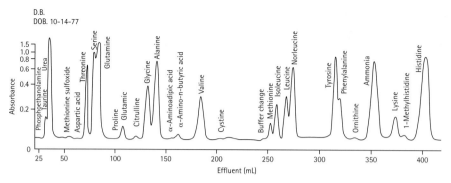

Figure 72.2 *Amino acid analyzer chromatogram of the urine of the same patient. The characteristic pattern is of the massive excretion of neutral monoaminomonocarboxylic acids including alanine, serine, threonine and histidine.*

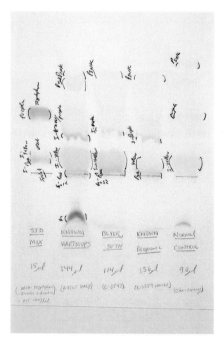

Figure 72.3 *High voltage electropherogram of indoles of the urine. Stained with Ehrlich reagent, the purple band among the standards on the left was tryptophan. The patient with Hartnup disease in lane 2 had a number of bands not observed in other patients.*

excreted in increased quantities, but this compound is not usually separated from glutamine by the amino acid analyzer. It is readily shown in paper chromatograms. The concentrations of these amino acids in the blood are normal or somewhat reduced [4].

A variety of indolyl derivatives of tryptophan is also found in the urine (Figure 72.3). The most prominent is indican. Patients have been reported to excrete as much as 400 mg of indoxylsulfate a day. They may also excrete increased amounts of indoxylglucuronide. Indolylacetic acid, indolylacetylglutamine and indolylacrogylycine are also excreted in abnormal amounts. The excretion of indoles in this disorder is a consequence of the failure of intestinal absorption of tryptophan, which is followed by bacterial metabolism in the intestine. The indolyluria can be suppressed by the oral administration of neomycin. Actually, all of the amino acids found in increased quantity in the urine are poorly absorbed in the intestine and are found in increased amounts in the feces [3]. Oral administration of each amino acid is followed by an abnormally low or delayed rise in its concentration in the plasma [5]. The defect in transport can also be demonstrated *in vitro* following intestinal biopsy [6]. In the presence of poor intestinal absorption of tryptophan, the excretions of nicotinic acid and its precursors in the kynurenin pathway are decreased.

CLINICAL ABNORMALITIES

The clinical manifestations of the disease appear to be the result of a deficiency of tryptophan that is a consequence of the defect in its absorption. Failure to thrive could be a reflection of failure to absorb other amino acids as well. A patient of ours failed to thrive despite what was described as a good appetite until the diagnosis was made and treatment initiated.

The most dramatic expression of the disease is with a red, scaly, pellagra-like dermatosis and cerebellar ataxia [1,2]. The rash has a predilection for exposed areas of the body and is clearly photosensitive. It can be extensive in patients with considerable exposure to ultraviolet light. Two patients [2] had hydroa vacciniforme, or vesiculobullous and erythematous photodermatosis with persistent scarring. The involved areas may remain depigmented. Some patients have had glossitis.

Ataxia may be seen in the absence of dermatosis and it may be episodic. During attacks the patient may be unsteady and walk with a wide-based gait. Our patient was developmentally slow, and his siblings were not; at 8 years he could readily be shown to be ataxic on finger to nose, heel to shin, or standing on one foot, and to have dysdiadochokinesia, despite good compliance with treatment. Intention tremor and nystagmus may be present. There may be diplopia. Some patients may have persistent headaches. The original patient was retarded in mental development, but this was not regularly seen in other involved members of the family. Nine of 39 reported patients [2] were mildly retarded. Others have been reported with retardation but no other symptoms [6].

In a recent study of 21 affected individuals identified through newborn screening, there were no differences in IQ or percentile levels of growth from those of 19 control siblings [7]. However, each of the two with poor academic performance scores encountered were in the Hartnup group, and two others in this group were considered to have learning difficulties. Two of these had clinical manifestations: in one it was described as a 'pellagrin' episode, in which an eczematoid eruption over the body and thighs associated with edema followed a prolonged episode of diarrhea; and in the other, there was somewhat impaired growth and intellectual development – his weight was in the third percentile and the IQ 97, but his two siblings scored 120. On the other hand, the disease does not seem to cause progressive mental defect, and some involved patients have been highly intelligent. The electroencephalogram may be abnormal.

Psychiatric symptoms may be dramatic, as in pellagra. The disorder may be discovered in patients with intermittent psychiatric abnormalities. Symptoms have ranged from mild emotional lability to severe delirium. Patients have been reported with delusions and with vivid hallucinations or depersonalization.

The disorder has been observed throughout the world, but until the advent of neonatal screening programs, such as the one in Massachusetts where the infant's urine is examined, it was rarely encountered in North America, where general levels of nutrition are high. This has led to the idea that marginal nutritional intake, especially of niacin or protein, may predispose an affected individual to the development of clinical manifestations. This issue and the greater requirements for growth could also explain the much more common occurrence of clinical manifestations in children than in adults. Certainly exposure to sunlight is important in the development of dermatological features of the phenotype. Sulfonamides have also been thought to be precipitating agents.

GENETICS AND PATHOGENESIS

The causative gene is rare and autosomal recessive. Consanguinity has been observed. The parents in the original family were first cousins [1]. Prevalence has been calculated from the Massachusetts-Quebec experience as 5.5 and 2.5 per 100 000 births [7]. One family of four siblings has been described in which the transport defect involved only the renal tubule, sparing the intestine [7]. A different phenotype was reported [8] in which a tissue-specific transport defect was confined to the intestine, but clearances of those amino acids excreted in excess are high, approaching the rate of glomerular filtration [9–11]. The occurrence of this pattern of abnormal transport indicated that these amino acids shared a common transporter. A sodium-dependent, neutral, amino acid transport system was characterized in mammalian cells by Christensen [12], who labelled it ASC. A cDNA has been identified and expressed which serves as a neutral amino acid transporter; the gene has been called ASCT1 [13]. It has been mapped to chromosome 19q13.3 [14]. It has not been studied in Hartnup disease.

TREATMENT

A plentiful intake of protein and supplemental nicotinic acid or nicotinamide appears to be prudent. We recommend a diet of 4 g protein/kg in childhood. Nicotinamide may be less likely than nicotinic acid to be accompanied by flushing. Doses of either compound are 40 to 300 mg q.d. Treatment has been observed to clear the skin and ameliorate ataxia or psychiatric symptoms. The aminoaciduria does not change. Experience has been reported with the use of oral tryptophan ethylester [15]. Lipid soluble esters of amino acids rapidly traverse intestinal membranes. Treatment with 20 mg/kg led to increased levels of tryptophan in blood and cerebrospinal fluid and improved weight gain.

References

1 Baron DN, Dent CE, Harris H, *et al.* Hereditary pellagra-like skin rash with temporary cerebellar ataxia constant renal amino aciduria and other bizarre features. *Lancet* 1956;**2**:421.

2 Jepson JB. Hartnup disease: in *The Metabolic Basis of Inherited Disease* (eds JN Stanbury, JB Wyngaarden, DS Fredrickson). McGraw-Hill, New York;1978:1563.

3 Scriver CR. Hartnup disease: a genetic modification of intestinal and renal transport of certain neutral alpha-amino acids. *N Engl J Med* 1965;**273**:530.

4 Cusworth DC, Dent CE. Renal clearances of amino acids in normal adults and in patients with aminoaciduria. *Biochem J* 1960;**74**:551.

5 Milne MD, Crawford MA, Girao CB, Loughridge LW. The metabolic disorder in Hartnup disease. *Q J Med* 1960;**29**:407.

6 Shih VE, Bixby EM, Alpers DH, *et al.* Studies of intestinal transport defect in Hartnup disease. *Gastroenterology* 1971;**61**:445.

7 Scriver CR, Mahon B, Levy HL, *et al.* The Hartnup phenotype: Mendelian transport disorder multifactorial disease. *Am J Hum Genet* 1987;**40**:401.

8 Hillman RE, Steward A, Miles JH. Amino acid transport defect in intestine not affecting kidney. *Pediatr Res* 1986;**20**:265A.

9 Jonxis JHP. Oligophrenia phenylpyruvica en de hartnupziekte. *Ned Tijdschr Geneeskd* 1957;**101**:569.

10 Tada K, Hirono H, Arakawa T. Endogenous renal clearance rates of free amino acids in prolinuric and Hartnup patients. *Tohoku J Exp Med* 1967;**93**:57.

11 Halvorsen S, Hygstedt O, Jagenburg R, Sjaastad O. Cellular transport of L-histidine in Hartnup disease. *J Clin Invest* 1969;**48**:552.

12 Christensen HN. Organic ion transport during seven decades. The amino acids. *Biochim Biophys Acta* 1984;**779**:255.

13 Arriza JL, Kavanaugh MP, Fairmon WA, *et al.* Cloning and expression of a human neutral amino acid transporter with structural similarity to the glutamate transporter gene family. *J Biol Chem* 1993;**268**:15329.

14 Kekuda R, Prasad PD, Fei Y-J, *et al.* Cloning of the sodium-dependent broad-scope neutral amino acid transporter B° from a human placental choriocarcinoma cell line. *J Biol Chem* 1996;**271**:18657.

15 Gleason WA, Butler JJ, Jonas AJ. Long term therapy of Hartnup disorder with tryptophan ethylester. *Pediatr Res* 1992;**31**:348A.

Histidinuria

MAJOR PHENOTYPIC EXPRESSION

Increased excretion of histidine in urine without histidinemia, and impaired intestinal absorption of histidine.

INTRODUCTION

Isolated histidinuria is a rare disorder of histidine transport. It has been reported in five individuals in four families [1–5]. There may be no other abnormalities, but four of the patients reported had some abnormality of the central nervous system.

CLINICAL ABNORMALITIES

Our patient [1] had a distinctive phenotype. He was moderately developmentally delayed and had bilateral neural hearing loss. He had a history of substantial neonatal hypoglycemia. In addition, he had a number of minor anomalies (Figures 73.1, 73.2). The shortness of the fifth fingers resulted from a short, rounded middle phalanx.

The other patients reported had a variety of abnormalities of the central nervous system. Two siblings had mild mental

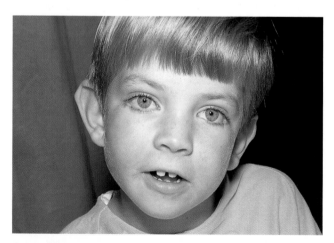

Figure 73.1 *D.B., an 8-year-old boy with histidinuria. External ears were large, protuberant and somewhat simple. The nasal bridge was broad and the philtrum long and smooth, and the upper lip was thin. He had bilateral nerve deafness. (This illustration and Figures 73.2 and 73.3 are reprinted with permission from the* American Journal of Human Genetics *[1].)*

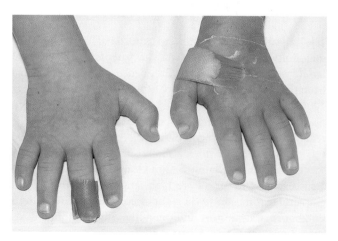

Figure 73.2 *The hands of D.B. illustrate the very small fifth fingers, which had only two horizontal creases, despite three phalanges on each hand. The first metacarpals were short.*

retardation [3]. Another was severely retarded and had microcephaly and spastic diplegia [4]. The fourth was intellectually normal, but he developed myoclonic seizures at the age of 13 years [2]. It appears unlikely that any of these abnormalities are consequences of abnormal transport of histidine; most probably they represent bias of ascertainment.

GENETICS AND PATHOGENESIS

Recessive inheritance seems likely, as the parents of all patients were normal, and there were siblings. The four patients were all male, and so X-linked inheritance is a possibility, but an autosomal gene is not ruled out. The consistent occurrence of abnormality of the central nervous system could represent the possibility of deletion of adjacent closely linked genes, or the pleiotropic effects of a single gene.

The hallmark of this disease is an elevated level of excretion of histidine in the urine. In our patient this was 276 mmol/mol creatinine. This was approximately twice the upper limit of normal for our laboratory. In another patient [4] the level was 1.5 times the upper limit of normal and 2.5 times the control mean. In the others, data were not reported in terms of creatinine excretion, but total 24-hour excretion was 2 to 3 times the control mean. In patients with histidinemia, urinary excretion was 7 times the control mean.

In contrast to patients with histidinemia, the patients tend to have low concentrations of histidine in plasma. In the patients reported [1–5] plasma concentrations ranged from 64 to 87 μmol/L. In our laboratory the normal range is 50–100 μmol/L, and the reported mean of 36 control subjects aged 3 to 10 years was 72 $\pm$ 19 [6]. Histidine concentration in the cerebrospinal fluid was normal in the patient in whom it was measured [4].

Intestinal absorption is, in our view, also low in these individuals. Figure 73.3 illustrates the response to oral loading in a patient. In these patients peak levels were not only lower; they were also achieved later than in controls.

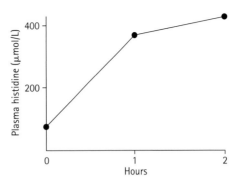

Figure 73.3   *Plasma concentrations of histidine in response to 100 mg/kg of oral histidine indicate impaired intestinal transport in the patient.*

TREATMENT

Treatment is not indicated for this abnormality in transport. Dietary sources of histidine are adequate to compensate and prevent symptoms of deficiency.

References

1   Nyhan WL, Hilton S. Histidinuria: defective transport of histidine. *Am J Med Genet* 1992;**44**:558.

2   Holmgren G, Hambraeus L, de Chateau P. Histidinemia and normo-histidinemic histinuria. *Acta Paediatr Scand* 1974;**63**:220.

3   Sabater J, Ferre C, Pulio M, Maya A. Histidinuria: a renal and intestinal histidine transport deficiency found in two mentally retarded children. *Clin Genet* 1976;**9**:117.

4   Kamoun PP, Parry P, Cathelineau L. Renal histidinuria. *J Inherit Metab Dis* 1981;**4**:217.

5   Scriver CR, Tenenhouse HS. Mendelian phenotypes as 'probes' of renal transport systems for amino acids and phosphate: in *Handbook of Physiology* Section 8: Renal Physiology (ed. E Windhager). Oxford University Press, New York;1992:1977.

6   Ghisolfi J, Augier D, Regnier C, Dalous A. Etude des variations physiologiques en fonction de l'age du taux des acides libres plasmatiques chez l'enfant normal. *Arch Franc Ped* 1973;**30**:951.

Menkes disease

MAJOR PHENOTYPIC EXPRESSION

Progressive early-onset cerebral degeneration; convulsions; depigmented, steel wool-like hair; bone lesions like those of scurvy; elongated, tortuous cerebral arteries; hypocupremia; diminished intestinal absorption of copper; increased concentrations of copper in intestinal mucosal cells and cultured fibroblasts; and defective activity of the copper-transporting adenosine triphosphatase (ATPase) (ATP7A).

INTRODUCTION

Menkes and colleagues [1] in 1962 described a disorder in five patients in which progressive cerebral deterioration was associated with characteristic abnormalities of the hair. The hair has been referred to as kinky [2], but it is anything but kinky. It is short and tends to stand on end, assuming a brush-like appearance (Figures 74.1, 74.2). It has been called steely hair by Danks [3]. It looks to us something like steel wool, but in Australia the wool of copper-deficient sheep has long been called steely. It was recognized in the initial report [1] that the disease was transmitted as an X-linked recessive trait. It was the recognition by Danks and colleagues [4,5] that the hair resembled the appearance of wool of copper-deficient sheep that led to their characterization of the disease as a disorder of copper transport. Copper deficiency in sheep leads to deficiency in the formation of cross-linking disulfide bonds in the keratin of the wool.

Abnormal transport of copper can be demonstrated in cultured fibroblasts which accumulate labeled copper, illustrating the failure of efflux also noted in intestinal cells [6,7]. The gene has been isolated from the Xq13 locus by three independent groups and shown to code for a copper-transporting P-type ATPase with six copper binding sites at the amino

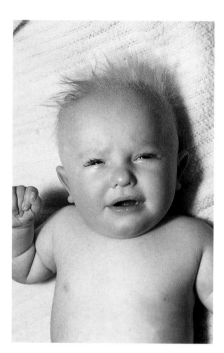

Figure 74.1 *J.E., an infant with Menkes disease. The hair was striking. (Illustrations of this patient were kindly provided by Dr. Marilyn Jones of UCSD and Children's Hospital and Health Center, San Diego.)*

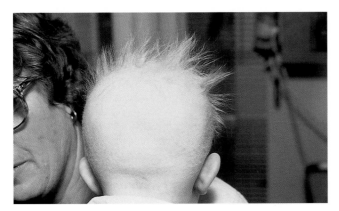

Figure 74.2 *J.E. In this view the unusual hair is seen even better.*

terminal end [8–10]. The ATPase, ATP7A is located on the trans-Golgi membrane of all human cells except hepatocyte. Thus in Menkes disease transport of copper from cytosol to Golgi is deficient, and enzymes that require copper and incorporate this copper in the Golgi are defective in activity because of the copper deficiency in the organelle [11–17]. Deletions in the gene were found early in patients with the disease [9], but a complete spectrum of mutation has been observed, most of them unique to an individual family [12–15].

CLINICAL ABNORMALITIES

The most important feature of the disease is its effect on the central nervous system. These patients usually appear normal at birth, although a number of them are born prematurely. There may be neonatal hypothermia and hyperbilirubinemia. The hair may be fine, but neonatal problems may resolve. The infants may grow and develop normally for 6–12 weeks, but vomiting, difficulty with feeding and poor weight gain are frequently encountered early. The onset of cerebral manifestations may be ushered in by seizures, or the patient may simply be noted to be apathetic, lethargic, or hypotonic and to display little interest in feedings. Rapid progressive neurologic deterioration ensues, with loss of milestones achieved. The ultimate state is flaccid hypotonia. There are few spontaneous movements and no contact with the environment. Seizures are generalized and frequent; and may be refractory to treatment. Myoclonic seizures may be seen as well as major motor seizures. Spastic quadriparesis may develop, and there may be opisthotonos and scissoring. Loss of visual ability and of hearing have been described.

The hair is a striking diagnostic feature (Figures 74.1–74.5) (Table 74.1). It tends to be short because hairs break off readily, especially at places of contact with the bed. It may be tangled and unkempt, looking stringy, or brush-like. It may be poorly pigmented, white or lackluster. Under the microscope the appearance may be that of pili torti (Figure 74.5) in which the hair shafts are twisted. They may also have the brush-like microscopic appearance of trichorrhexis nodosa or the segmental narrowing of monilethrix.

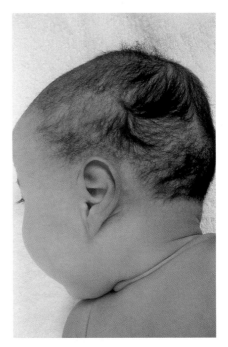

Figure 74.3 *N.S., an infant with Menkes disease. The hair had been cut; what was left was straight and wiry.*

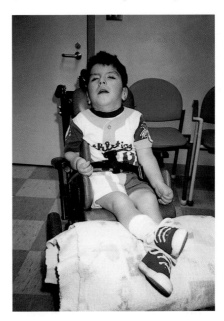

Figure 74.4 *R.E., a boy with Menkes disease. The hair was short and brittle and under the microscope displayed pili torti. He was globally delayed and spastic. The legs assumed a scissor position.*

The skin may appear pale or pasty, thick, or pudgy, especially in the cheeks. The jowels may sag, and there may be other signs of cutis laxa. The nasal bridge may be broad and there may be epicanthal folds. Hair of the eyebrows is also abnormal. Somatic growth is usually retarded.

The roentgenographic appearance of the bones is also characteristic. In addition to general osteoporosis in an irregular lucent trabecular pattern, there are spurs over flared

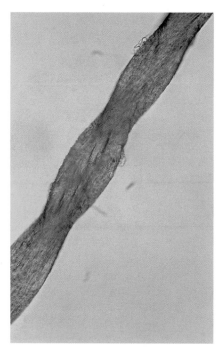

Figure 74.5 *Pili torti in the patient shown in Figure 74.3.*

Table 74.1 *Abnormalities of the hair*

Menkes disease, pili torti, trichorrhexis nodosa, monilethrix
Kinky hair, photosensitivity and mental retardation
Argininosuccinic aciduria
Pili torti – isolated, with deafness or with dental enamel hypoplasia, MIM 261900
Trichothiodystrophy – trichorrhexis nodosa, ichthyosis and neurologic abnormalities (Pollit syndrome) MIM 27550

Table 74.2 *Metabolic disease and stroke*

Stroke (conventional)	Metabolic stroke
Congenital disorders of glycosylation	Carbamyl phosphate synthase deficiency
Ethylmalonic aciduria	Glutaric acidemia type I
Fabry disease	Isovaleric acidemia
Homocystinuria	MELAS (Mitochondrial encephalomyopathy, lactic acidosis and stroke-like episodes)
Menkes disease	
α-Methylene tetrahydrofolate reductase deficiency	Methylcrotonyl CoA carboxylase deficiency
Purine nucleoside phosphorylase deficiency	Methylmalonic acidemia
	Ornithine transcarbamylase deficiency

metaphyseal areas that fracture and produce a scorbutic appearance [5,18]. Flaring of the ribs is like that seen in rickets and the ribs commonly fracture. Diaphyseal periosteal reaction along with fractures [19] may suggest a diagnosis of nonaccidental trauma [18]. This impression may be strengthened by finding subdural hematomas, which also occur in this disease [20]. Multiple wormian bones in the cranial sutures complete the characteristic roentgenographic picture [21].

Abnormalities of the electroencephalogram (EEG) are regularly seen. Multifocal spike patterns may eventually be replaced by a pattern of hypsarrhythmia. Visual and auditory evoked responses may disappear. Serial computed tomography (CT) scans in four patients [20] revealed a considerable variability in spite of similar general clinical courses. Early in the disease the scan may appear normal. Progressive abnormalities especially in the white matter have also been demonstrated by magnetic resonance imaging (MRI) [22]. Angiography reveals elongated and tortuous intracranial and visceral vessels. Multiple areas of localized narrowing are seen, and these abnormal changes in cerebral vessels may also be visualized by MRI. Diffuse cortical atrophy may be seen, or there may be multifocal areas of destruction of brain as a result of ischemic

infarction (Table 74.2). In some patients the rate of growth of the head falls off dramatically, resulting in microcephaly. Autopsy may reveal general cerebral and cerebellar atrophy, or loss of brain substance may be strikingly focal with evidence of infarction and later gliosis or cyst formation. These changes are consistent with the vascular abnormalities that characterize the disease [5,23,24]. The basic lesion appears to be a defect in the elastic fibers of the vessels; localized and similar changes are seen in the skin [23]. Much of the cerebral pathology may be secondary to the vascular abnormalities. Similar changes are seen in vessels in the viscera and extremities. Vessels may have localized areas of narrowing and dilatation. Vascular occlusion may occur anywhere. In one of our patients, thrombosis occluded both jugular veins in the neonatal period.

Connective tissue abnormality may also be evident in diverticulae of the bladder or ureters, and these may rupture or lead to urinary tract infections. Cystography may show a large, trabeculated bladder [25]. There may be umbilical hernia. Major gastrointestinal bleeding has been reported [26], arising from gastric polyps associated with underlying vascular ectasis and mucosal redundancy.

Most patients die between 3 and 12 months. Some survive until 3 years. A rare patient may survive as long as 12 years of age [25]. Two patients have been reported in whom there was a milder phenotype [17,27–29]. One presented at 2 years-of-age with ataxia and mild developmental delay [27]; changes in the bones were mild, but there was pili torti, and aortography indicated elongation and dilatation of the arteries. He was treated with parenteral copper, but it is not clear that it altered his disease [28]. By 14 years he was severely ataxic and had progressed slowly in school for his age. The other patient presented with recurrent urinary tract infection and diverticulae of the tract [29]. He had pili torti and mild ataxia; the facial appearance was that of Menkes disease, with loose skin and sagging jowels, and the joints were lax. Arteriography revealed only mild dilatation of vessels.

Another variant in which copper transport in fibroblasts is indistinguishable from Menkes disease is occipital horn disease

[30–38]. This disorder has been referred to as X-linked cutis laxa [30] and Ehlers-Danlos syndrome type IX [34]. It is characterized by cutis laxa, hernias and diverticulae of the bladder or ureters. Some patients have had chronic diarrhea [34]. Roentgenographic findings include the characteristic ossified occipital horns, which are palpable, hammer-like extensions pointing caudally on the sides of the foramen magnum. In addition, the lateral ends of the clavicles are broad and the cortices of long bones are wavy [34]. Intellect may be a little low.

The histopathology of Menkes disease is impressive for changes in the elastin lamina of the vessels, which are fragmented, disrupted or reduplicated [5]. The intima may be thickened. Electron microscopy suggests defective formation of elastin [39]. The cerebrum and cerebellum are notable for widespread neuronal loss and gliosis [1,39,40]. In muscle, iris and retina [41–43] there is mitochondrial disorganization, and ragged red fibers have been reported [42,43].

GENETICS AND PATHOGENESIS

Menkes disease and each of the variants are transmitted as X-linked recessive traits. Prevalence figures for Menkes disease have ranged from one in 35 000 in Melbourne [5] to one in 250 000 in Europe [16,43].

Mutant strains of mice have been studied that appear to be excellent models [44–49]. The brindled and blotchy mice (Mobr and Mobl) are determined by allelic mutations in genes on the X-chromosome. The genes in the mouse map close to the tabby locus and nearer to α-galactosidase and phosphoglycerate kinase [47,48]. Another (dappled) mutant is a pre-natal lethal (Modp). The macular mouse with the mutant mottled gene has been shown to have a C to T4223 change leading to serine 1382 proline in the transmembrane domain of the copper transporter [49]. Tissue distribution of expression was consistent with the pathology of Menkes disease.

The human gene is located at Xq13. It has been found to be large, spanning approximately 140 kb over 23 exons [8–10,51,52]. The coding sequence predicted a structure homologous with that of the P-type cation-transporting family of ATPase enzyme [50]. In addition to copper binding motifs it contains a dicysteine membrane spanning area. The mouse gene is expressed in most tissues. No mRNA was found in the Modp, a normal amount of normal message in Mobr and mottled, and structurally abnormal mRNA in Mobl. In patients with Menkes disease, greatly reduced or undetectable levels of mRNA have been frequently observed [8–10]. Deletions or rearrangements in the gene have been observed in almost half of these patients [9,13], and 1–2 percent have cytogenetically demonstrable abnormalities, such as translocations. Reduced levels of mRNA have also been observed in occipital horn syndrome [53], but Northern analysis of mRNA in most mild patients appeared normal [54]. Splicing mutations in milder patients suggest that some normal

protein is made. The gene codes for an 8 kb transcript that is expressed in all cells but those of the liver. The amino acid sequence of the Menkes protein is 55 percent identical to the Wilson protein and contains the same functional motifs. The synthesized polypeptide is N-glycosylated and localized to the trans-Golgi network.

The abnormal gene causes abnormal transport of copper. Altered handling of copper has been documented in cultured fibroblasts [6,7,55–60] in which copper content is abnormally high, accumulation of ^{64}Cu is elevated and efflux of ^{64}Cu to isotope-free medium is impaired.

Heterozygotes may be recognized by the abnormality in copper processing in cultured fibroblasts, but the result may be normal [6,55,57,61]. Cloning has revealed the presence of two cell populations [62]. Pili torti may also be recognized in some heterozygotes [63], and mosaic pigmentation of the skin has been observed in a black heterozygote [64].

The complete clinical expression of disease has been reported in a number of girls, in most of whom cytogenetic studies were normal [65–67]; one was the sister of an affected male [65]. In one the patient was a mosaic 45X/46XX [67]. Another girl had a balanced 2/X translocation in which the break point was at Xq13.2-13.3 and proximal to PGK-1 [68,69].

Prenatal monitoring has been carried out by the study of copper transport in cultured amniocytes or chorionic villus samples [6,70]. The method is tricky and very sensitive to conditions of culture and assay.

The immediate consequence of the basic defect is impaired absorption of copper because of failure of transfer into the secretory pathway causing accumulation of copper in cells of the intestine and of the blood–brain barrier and generalized deficiency of copper in the blood and central nervous system. Measured concentrations of copper in the blood are very low, and so are those of ceruloplasmin [4,5]. In normal individuals the serum contains over 12 μmol copper/L, while in most patients the levels were less than 6 μmol/L. Normal ceruloplasmin is over 20 mg/dL, while patients have less than 5 mg/dL. Over 80 percent of the copper in human plasma is in the form of ceruloplasmin. The copper contents of the liver and the brain are also low. Oral administration of copper indicates an absorptive abnormality in these patients. The content of copper in the intestinal mucosa is high [3,71], a clear index that the defect is in transport out of the intestinal cell. The generality of the transport defect is indicated not only by the abnormality in cultured fibroblasts, but also in the kidney, spleen, lung, muscle and pancreas [57]. In the case of an affected fetus, the placenta can also be shown to have a high content of copper, permitting confirmation of the prenatal diagnosis [72]. When the mutation is known, molecular analysis is the procedure of choice for prenatal diagnosis and heterozygote detection [73,74]. Red blood cell copper content is normal; there is no anemia or neutropenia, and the erythrocyte activity of superoxide dismutase is not reduced.

A shortage of copper in tissues leads to defective cross-linking of elastin and collagen, because lysyl oxidase is a copper-dependent enzyme, and lysyl oxidase activity is deficient in this syndrome [31,75–77]. The deficiency of this enzyme is consistent with the abnormalities in connective tissue in Menkes disease. It is because of the defect in lysyl oxidase that this disorder has been classified as Ehlers-Danlos syndrome type IX. Other copper-dependant enzymes are also deficient in activity. Deficiency of tyrosinase leads to the lack of pigmentation in these patients [77]. The abnormal hair results from defective bonding of disulfides in keratin [4,5]. Cytochrome oxidase deficiency has been demonstrated in mitochondria of patients with Menkes disease [78]. Elevated concentrations of lactic acid have been found in the cerebrospinal fluid. In a study of metabolites of collagen [19] urinary deoxypyridinoline was very low, and this has been proposed as a marker for the lysyloxidase deficiency in this disease.

TREATMENT

Treatment for this disease has been less than satisfactory. It is possible to administer sufficient copper intravenously or subcutaneously to bring concentrations of copper and ceruloplasmin in plasma and even liver to normal, and chronic therapy has been employed, but there has been no evident clinical influence on the course of the cerebral disease [79]. Concentrations of copper in the brain have not been brought to the normal range. Some success has been reported with copper-histidinate started soon after birth and continued for six and 15 years [80]; intellectual levels were at the lower end of the normal range, and there were abnormalities of hair and connective tissue. In a series of patients treated with subcutaneous copper histidinate, two patients treated from the first month for six and 16 years were judged to have done well neurologically [81]. Actually, the 16-year-old had an IQ of 87, but required a wheelchair because of extreme hypotonia and hyperextensibility of the joints. Five patients treated from the 2nd to 7th month did poorly. Histidine enhances the uptake of copper by cells from plasma. It is generally considered that the therapy should be offered to infants diagnosed early. Copper histidinate therapy has been initiated *in utero* [82]. It is clear that many effects of the disease begin *in utero*. Follow-up information is limited.

The mineral density of bone was reported to be improved in three patients treated with pamidronate intravenously for a year [83].

References

1   Menkes JH, Alter M, Steigleder GK, *et al.* A sex-linked recessive disorder with retardation of growth peculiar hair and focal cerebral and cerebellar degeneration. *Pediatrics* 1962;**29**:764.

2   French JH, Sherard EA. Studies of the biochemical basis of kinky hair disease. *Pediatr Res* 1967;**1**:206.

3   Danks DM, Cartwright E, Stevens BJ. Menkes' steely-hair (kinky-hair) disease. *Lancet* 1973;**1**:891.

4   Danks DM, Campbell PE, Walker-Smith J, *et al.* Menkes's kinky hair syndrome. *Lancet* 1972;**1**:1100.

5   Danks DM, Campbell PE, Mayne V, Cartwright E. Menkes's kinky hair syndrome. An inherited defect in copper absorption with widespread effects. *Pediatrics* 1972;**50**:188.

6   Horn N. Copper incorporation studies on cultured cells for prenatal diagnosis of Menkes' disease. *Lancet* 1976;**1**:1156.

7   Chan WY, Garnica AD, Rennert OM. Cell culture studies of Menkes kinky hair disease. *Clin Chim Acta* 1978;**88**:495.

8   Vulpe C, Levinson B, Whitney S, *et al.* Isolation of a candidate gene for Menkes disease and evidence that it encodes a copper-transporting ATPase. *Nat Genet* 1993;**3**:7.

9   Chelly J, Tumer Z, Tonnesen T, *et al.* Isolation of a candidate gene for Menkes disease that encodes a potential heavy metal binding protein. *Nat Genet* 1993;**3**:14.

10   Mercer JFB, Livingston J, Hall B, *et al.* Isolation of a partial candidate gene for Menkes disease by positional cloning. *Nat Genet* 1993;**3**:20.

11   Kodama H, Murata Y. Molecular genetics and pathophysiology of Menkes' disease. *Pediatr Int* 1999;**41**:430.

12   Zeynep T, Horn M. Menkes disease: recent advances and new aspects. *J Med Genet* 1997;**34**:265.

13   Das S, Levinson B, Whitney S, *et al.* Diverse mutations in patients with Menkes disease often lead to exon skipping. *Am J Hum Genet* 1994;**55**:883.

14   Tümer Z, Lund C, Tolshave J, *et al.* Identification of point mutations in 41 unrelated patients affected with Menkes disease. *Am J Hum Genet* 1997;**60**:63.

15   Gu YH, Kodama H, Murata Y, *et al.* ATP7A gene mutations in 16 patients with Menkes' disease and a patient with occipital horn syndrome. *Am J Med Genet* 2001;**99**:217.

16   Kaler SG. Menkes disease. *Adv Pediatr* 1994;**41**:263.

17   Kaler SG. Diagnosis and therapy of Menkes syndrome a genetic form of copper deficiency. *Am J Clin Nutr* 1998;**67**:(suppl)1029.

18   Adams PC, Strand RD, Bresnan MJ, Lucky AW. Kinky hair syndrome: serial study of radiological findings with emphasis on similarity to the battered child syndrome. *Radiology* 1974;**112**:401.

19   Kodama H, Sato E, Yanagawa Y, *et al.* Biochemical indicator for evaluation of connective tissue abnormalities in Menkes' disease. *J Pediatr* 2003;**142**:726.

20   Seay AR, Bray PF, Wing SD, *et al.* CT scans in Menkes disease. *Neurology* 1979;**29**:304.

21   Wesenberg RL, Gwinn JL, Barnes GR. Radiological findings in the kinky hair syndrome. *Radiology* 1969;**92**:500.

22   Blaser SI, Berns DH, Ross JS, *et al.* Serial MR studies in Menkes disease. *J Comput Assist Tomogr* 1989;**13**:113.

23   Oakes BW, Danks DM, Campbell PE. Human copper deficiency: ultrastructural studies of the aorta and skin in a child with Menke's syndrome. *Exp Mol Pathol* 1976;**25**:82.

24   Danks DM, Cartwright E, Campbell PE, Mayne V. Is Menkes' syndrome a heritable disorder of connective tissue? *Lancet* 1971;**2**:1089.

25   Gerdes AM, Tonnesen T, Pergament E, *et al.* Variability in clinical expression of Menkes syndrome. *Eur J Pediatr* 1988;**148**:132.

26   Kaler SG, Westman JA, Bernes SM, *et al.* Gastrointestinal hemorrhage associated with gastric polyps in Menkes disease. *J Pediatr* 1993;**122**:93.

27   Procopis P, Camakaris J, Danks DM. A mild form of Menkes' syndrome. *J Pediatr* 1981;**98**:97.

28   Danks DM. The mild form of Menkes disease: progress report on the original case. *Am J Med Genet* 1988;**30**:859.

29   Westman JA, Richardson DC, Rennert OM, Morrow G. Atypical Menkes steel hair disease. *Am J Med Genet* 1980;**30**:1280.

30   Byers PH, Siegel RC, Holbrook KA, *et al.* X-linked cutis laxa: Defective cross-link formation in collagen due to decreased lysyl oxidase activity. *N Engl J Med* 1980;**303**:61.

31 Peltonen L, Kuivanieni H, Palotie A, *et al.* Alterations of copper and collagen metabolism in the Menkes syndrome and a new subtype of Ehlers-Danlos syndrome. *Biochemistry* 1983;**22**:6156.

32 Kuivaniemi H, Peltonen L, Palotie A, *et al.* Abnormal copper metabolism and deficient lysyl oxidase activity in a heritable connective tissue disorder. *J Clin Invest* 1985;**69**:798.

33 Kuivaniemi H, Peltonen L, and Kivrikko KI. Type 1X Ehlers–Danlos syndrome and Menkes syndrome: the decrease in lysyl oxidase activity is associated with a corresponding deficiency in the enzyme protein. *Am J Hum Genet* 1985;**37**:798.

34 Sartoris DJ, Luzzatti L, Weaver DD, *et al.* Type 1X Ehlers–Danlos syndrome: a new variant with pathognomic radiographic features. *Radiology* 1984;**152**:665.

35 Proud VK, Mussell HG, Kaler SG, *et al.* Distinctive Menkes disease variant with occipital horns: delineation of natural history and clinical phenotype. *Am J Med Genet* 1996;**65**:44.

36 Willemse J, Van Den Hamer CJ, Prins HW, Jonker PL. Menkes' kinky hair disease. I Comparison of classical and unusual clinical and biochemical features in two patients. *Brain Dev* 1982;**4**:105.

37 Haas RH, Robinson A, Evans K, *et al.* An X-linked disease of the nervous system with disordered copper metabolism and features differing from Menkes' disease. *Neurology* 1982;**31**:852.

38 Mehes K, Petrovicz E. Familial benign copper deficiency. *Arch Dis Child* 1982;**57**:716.

39 Goto S, Hirano A, Rojas-Corona RR. A comparative immunocytochemical study of human cerebellar cortex in X-chromosome-linked copper malabsorption (Menkes' kinky hair disease) and granule cell type degeneration. *Neuropathol Appl Neurobiol* 1989;**15**:419.

40 Vuia O, Heye D. Neuropathologic aspects in Menkes' kinky hair disease (trichpoliodystrophy). *Neuropediatrics* 1974;**5**:329.

41 Seelenfreud MH, Gartner S, Vinger PF. The ocular pathology of Menkes' disease. *Arch Ophthalmol* 1968;**80**:718.

42 Morgello S, Peterson HD, Kahn LJ, Laufer H. Menkes kinky hair disease with 'ragged red' fibers. *Dev Med Child Neurol* 1988;**30**:812.

43 Tonnesen T, Kleijer WJ, Horn N. Incidence of Menkes disease. *Hum Genet* 1991;**86**:408.

44 Danks DM. Of mice and men, metals and mutations. *J Med Genet* 1986;**23**:99.

45 Danks DM. Copper transport and utilisation in Menkes' syndrome and in mottled mice. *Inorg Perspect Biol Med* 1977;**1**:73.

46 Hunt DM. Primary defect in copper transport underlines mottled mutants in the mouse. *Nature* 1974;**249**:852.

47 Phillips M, Camakaris J, Danks DM. A comparison of phenotype and copper distribution in blotchy and brindled mutant mice and in nutritionally copper-deficient controls. *Biol Trace Elem Res* 1991;**29**:11.

48 Brown RM, Camakaris J, Danks DM. Observation on the Menkes and brindled mouse phenotypes in cell hybrids. *Somat Cell Mol Genet* 1984;**10**:321.

49 Murata Y, Kodama H, Abe T, *et al.* Mutation analysis and expression of the mottled gene in the macular mouse model of Menkes disease. *Pediatr Res* 1997;**42**:436.

50 Silver S, Nucifora G, Chu L, Misra PK. Bacterial resistance ATPases: primary pumps for exporting toxic cations and anions. *Trends Biochem Sci* 1989;**14**:76.

51 Tümer Z, Vural B, Tønnesen T, *et al.* Characterization of the exon structure of the Menkes disease gene using vectorette PCR. *Genomics* 1995;**26**:437.

52 Dierick HA, Ambrosini L, Spencer J, *et al.* Molecular structure of the Menkes disease gene (ATP7A). *Genomics* 1995;**28**:462.

53 Levinson B, Gitschier J, Vulpe C, *et al.* Are X-linked cutis laxa and Menkes disease allelic? *Nat Genet* 1993;**3**:6.

54 Das S, Levinson B, Vulpe C, *et al.* Similar splicing mutations of the Menkes/Mottled copper-transporting ATPase gene in occipital horn syndrome and the blotchy mouse. *Am J Hum Genet* 1995;**56**:570.

55 Camakaris J, Danks DM, Ackland L, *et al.* Altered copper metabolism in cultured cells from human Menkes' syndrome and mottled mouse mutants. *Biochem Genet* 1980;**18**:117.

56 Beratis NG, Price P, LaBadie G, Hirschorn K. ^{64}Cu metabolism in Menkes' and normal cultured skin fibroblasts. *Pediatr Res* 1978;**12**:699.

57 Goka TJ, Stevenson RE, Hefferman PM, Howell RR. Menkes disease: a biochemical abnormality in cultured human fibroblasts. *Proc Natl Acad Sci USA* 1976;**73**:604.

58 Yamaguchi Y, Heiny ME, Suzuki M, Gitlin JD. Biochemical characterization and intracellular localization of the Menkes disease protein. *Proc Natl Acad Sci USA* 1996;**93**:14030.

59 Dierick HA, Adam AN, Escara-Wilke JF, Glover TW. Immunocytochemical localization of the Menkes copper transport protein (ATP7A) to the *trans* Golgi network. *Hum Mol Genet* 1997;**6**:409.

60 Petris MJ, Mercer JFB, Culvenor JG, *et al.* Ligand-regulated transport of the Menkes copper P-type ATPase efflux pump from the Golgi apparatus to the plasma membrane: A novel mechanism of regulated trafficking. *EMBO J* 1996;**15**:6084.

61 Horn N. Menkes' X-linked disease: heterozygous phenotypic uncloned fibroblast cultures. *J Med Genet* 1980;**17**:257.

62 Horn N, Mooy P, Berry C. Menkes X-linked disease. Two clonal cell populations in heterozygotes. *Clin Genet* 1986;**29**:258.

63 Moore CM, Howell RR. Ectodermal manifestations in Menkes disease. *Clin Genet* 1985;**28**:532.

64 Volpintesta EJ. Menkes' kinky hair syndrome in a black infant. *Am J Dis Child* 1974;**128**:244.

65 Iwakawa Y, Niwa T, Tomita J. Menkes' kinky hair syndrome; report on an autopsy case and his female sibling with similar clinical manifestations. *Brain Dev* 1979;**11**:260.

66 Barton NW, Dambrosia JM, Barranger JA. Menkes kinky-hair syndrome: report of a case in a female infant. *Neurology* 1983;**33**:154.

67 Gerdes AM, Tonnesen T, Horn N, *et al.* Clinical expression of Menkes syndrome in females. *Clin Genet* 1990;**38**:452.

68 Kapur S, Higgins JV, Delp K, Rogers B. Menkes syndrome in a girl with X-autosome translocation. *Am J Med Genet* 1987;**26**:503.

69 Verga V, Hall BK, Wang S, *et al.* Localization of the translocation breakpoint in a female with Menkes syndrome to Xq132-q133 proximal to PGK-1. *Am J Hum Genet* 1991;**48**:1133.

70 Tonnesen T, Horn N. Prenatal and postnatal diagnosis of Menkes disease an inherited disorder of copper metabolism. *J Inherit Metab Dis* 1989;**12**:207.

71 Danks DM, Cartwright E, Stevens BJ, Townley RRW. Menkes kinky hair disease: further definition of the defect in copper transport. *Science* 1973;**179**:1140.

72 Horn N. Menkes' X-linked disease: prenatal diagnosis of hemizygous males and heterozygous female. *Prenat Diagn* 1981;**1**:107.

73 Das S, Whitney S, Taylor J, *et al.* Prenatal diagnosis of Menkes disease by mutation analysis. *J Inherit Metab Dis* 1995;**18**:364.

74 Tümer Z, Tønnesen T, Böhamann J, *et al.* First trimester prenatal diagnosis of Menkes disease by DNA analysis. *J Med Genet* 1994;**31**:615.

75 Rowe DW, McGoodwin EB, Martin GR, Grahn D. Decreased lysyl oxidase activity in the aneurysm-prone mottled mouse. *J Biol Chem* 1977;**252**:939.

76 Royce PM, Camakaris J, Danks DM. Reduced lysyl oxidase activity in skin fibroblasts from patients with Menkes' syndrome. *Biochem J* 1980;**192**:579.

77 Holstein TJ, Fung RQ, Quevedo WC, Bienieki TC. Effect of altered copper metabolism induced by mottled alleles and diet on mouse tyrosinase. *Proc Soc Exp Biol Med* 1979;**162**:264.

78 Kodama H, Okabe I, Yanagisawa M, Kodama Y. Copper deficiency in the mitochondria of cultured skin fibroblasts from patients with Menkes syndrome. *J Inherit Metab Dis* 1989; **12**:386.

79 Williams DM, Atkin CL, Frens DB, Bray PF. Menkes' kinky hair syndrome: studies of copper metabolism and long-term copper therapy. *Pediatr Res* 1977;**11**:823.

80 Sherwood G, Sarkar B, Sass Kortsak A. Copper histidinate therapy in Menkes' disease: prevention of progressive neurodegeneration. *J Inherit Metab Dis* 1989;**12**:393.

81 Bidudhendra S, Lingertat-Walsh K, Clarke JTR. Copper-histidine therapy for Menkes disease. *J Pediatr* 1993;**123**:828.

82 Kaler SG, Miller RC, Wolf EJ, *et al. In utero* treatment of Menkes disease. *Pediatr Res* 1993;**33**:192A.

83 Kanumakala S, Boneh A, Zacharin M. Pamidronate treatment improves bone mineral density in children with Menkes disease. *J Inherit Metab Dis* 2002;**25**:391.

Wilson disease

MAJOR PHENOTYPIC EXPRESSION

Hepatocellular disease; neurologic degeneration; psychiatric disease; Kayser-Fleischer rings; renal tubular dysfunction with a distinctive aminoaciduria; reduced ceruloplasmin; increased copper in serum, urine and liver; reduced biliary excretion of copper and incorporation into ceruloplasmin; and an abnormal P-type adenosine triphosphate (ATP)ase transporter specific to liver (ATP7B).

INTRODUCTION

Wilson's definitive clinical and pathologic description of the disease was in 1912 [1]. The pathognomonic corneal ring was separately described by Kayser [2] and Fleischer [3] in 1902 and 1903, and it is likely that a number of earlier descriptions of progressive neurologic and hepatic disease represented the same syndrome; but Wilson's 211-page monograph was not only a landmark, it also predicted that the causative agent was a toxin. A year later the increased content of copper in the liver was reported by Rumpel [4]. This critical element was rediscovered between 1929 and 1945 [5–7] and led to an important series of observations and hypotheses that made this disease so amenable to precise early diagnosis and effective treatment today. Bennetts and Chapman [8] observed that deficiency of copper in lambs produced a fatal demyelinating disease. This led to the demonstration by Mandelbrotte and colleagues [9] that there was an increased urinary excretion of copper in Wilson disease. Cumings reported on the increased content of copper in brain, as well as liver [10], and proposed that 2,3-dimercaptopropanol (British Anti-Lewisite, BAL) might be therapeutic by chelation of accumulated copper. This was effective in removing copper, but not practical for the long-term therapy necessary. This problem was solved by the introduction of penicillamine therapy by Walshe in 1956 [11].

The rates of excretion of copper into the bile and its incorporation into ceruloplasmin were shown to be deficient in Wilson disease [12]. The gene has been mapped to chromosome 13q14.3 [13] and has been isolated [14–17]. It is smaller than the gene for Menkes disease, but the similarity of the two coding sequences indicates a P-type ATPase transporter with six copper-binding motifs. The function within the cell of the Wilson and Menkes ATPases is identical. The quite distinct phenotypes of the two diseases result from their very different tissue-specific expression. In Wilson disease the copper transporter functions only in hepatocytes to preserve copper homeostasis by regulating its excretion in the bile. When the function of the ATPase is impaired copper cannot be incorporated into ceruloplasmin, and it accumulates in liver, cornea, and brain, in each of which accumulated copper produces its characteristic toxic manifestations. Mutations in the gene have been delineated indicating considerable heterogeneity. The most common mutation, accounting for approximately 40 percent of Northern European alleles is H1069Q which changes as histidine residue conserved in all of the copper transporting p-type ATPases in a sequence SEHPL proximal to the ATP-binding domain [18,19].

CLINICAL ABNORMALITIES

The clinical manifestations of Wilson disease are highly variable. All patients go through an asymptomatic stage in which excessive amounts of copper are being deposited in the liver. The usual presentations are with hepatic disease or with neurologic disease, or both [20–24]. There are approximately equal numbers of each of these three groups. In some infants and children, presentation is with an acute hemolytic crisis [25,26]. In childhood the earliest manifestations of disease [27] are usually those of involvement of the liver [25,27–30]. Signs of hepatic dysfunction may present as early as 4 years-of-age [31], but seldom before. Most commonly the onset with hepatic symptoms occurs between 8 and 16 years [20,32–34]. This type of presentation is somewhat more common in the female. A neurologic picture is the more common presentation in the male [21]. Liver disease may manifest itself as asymptomatic hepatomegaly. This period may extend into adult life and during this time the patient may develop splenomegaly, or spider angiomata, especially on the dorsa of the hands. Serum transaminase levels are usually elevated. At the other extreme are children with a rapid fulminant course culminating in death from hepatic failure.

The diagnosis may not be suspected in patients dying of acute failure of the liver [35]. The initial episode may progress within weeks to hepatic insufficiency manifested by icterus, ascites, clotting abnormalities and disseminated intravascular coagulation [36–39]. This is followed by coma and renal failure. This outcome is more likely to occur in an adolescent or an adult. Such a patient may die acutely without a diagnosis of Wilson disease being made. It would be well to test such children for the diagnosis. Certainly, all children with chronic or recurrent liver disease should be investigated for Wilson disease. The true frequency of the disease is doubtless underestimated.

The initial clinical manifestation of hepatic disease may appear to be an acute hepatitis. Vomiting, anorexia, nausea and jaundice are common presenting complaints, and the episode may subside spontaneously. In the presence of splenomegaly, the diagnosis may appear to be infectious mononucleosis [40]. Alerting features are that in Wilson disease there is often an accompanying Coombs negative hemolytic anemia, which may be transient, and the serum concentration of uric acid is usually low.

Wilson disease can also present with a picture of chronic active hepatitis [41]. The patient may have malaise, fatigue or anorexia, along with hepatosplenomegaly. The serum concentration of albumin is low, and IgG and transaminase levels are high. The histologic picture on biopsy may be that of typical chronic active hepatitis. Any of these hepatic presentations may lead to cirrhosis, or the illness may be that of cirrhosis from the beginning [42]. The disease may be the cause in an adult with cirrhosis and no evidence of neurologic abnormality [43]. Weight loss, ascites or anasarca may be seen, as well as chronic jaundice, spider angiomata and epistaxis or other

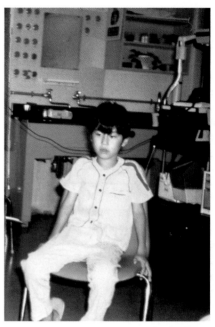

Figure 75.1   *A 9-year-old Japanese patient with Wilson disease. He presented with three episodes of acute hemolysis and was found to have a low level of ceruloplasmin. By 9 years-of-age he had a pronounced Kayser-Fleischer ring. (Illustration was kindly provided by Dr. M. Yoshino of Kurume University, Japan.)*

bleeding. Portal hypertension, hypersplenism or bleeding esophageal varices may occur. Patients may develop amenorrhea, delayed puberty or gynecomastia. Terminally there may be hepatic coma or a hepatorenal syndrome. Death may occur as early as 8 years-of-age [28] or in adulthood. It is easy to miss the underlying Wilson disease in any of these hepatic presentations. In order to make the correct diagnosis early it is important to have an index of suspicion [25,44,45]. Proper response to this suspicion is a readiness to assay for content of copper at the very first liver biopsy in a patient with liver disease [34].

Hemolytic anemia is a prominent feature of Wilson disease in childhood (Figure 75.1). Its presence along with hepatic disease may be useful in suggesting the diagnosis. However, some patients present with apparently isolated acute hemolytic anemia [25,26]. Of 18 patients younger than 21 years, two presented with acute hemolytic anemia, and nine were found to have hemolysis [25]. Of the seven asymptomatic patients, four were found to have hemolysis. The manifestations of hemolysis are reticulocytosis, depressed concentration of haptoglobin and high indirect bilirubin. Cholelithiasis may occur in children as well as adults [46] and may lead to abdominal pain.

The classic presentation of Wilson disease is with neurologic disease. The others of the classic triad are the corneal rings and hypoceruloplasminemia. Initial presentation with neurologic abnormality occurs in 40 percent of patients [28]. It was reported in 28 percent of children [25]. Neurologic disease may begin as early as 6 years-of-age and as late as 46 [28]. Manifestations are virtually all motor. Dysarthria, incoordination of voluntary movements and tremors at rest or on intention are the most common symptoms. Speech may be slurred, scanning, monotonous or indistinct. Involuntary movements may be choreiform or small twitches. Gait may be unsteady, lurching or staggering. Tone may increase, and rigidity about the mouth or legs may be a problem. Drooling may be embarrassing. Some patients have recurrent headaches; some have grand mal seizures.

The neurologic features of Wilson disease have been subclassified into two distinct but overlapping pictures.

- The dystonic form is characterized by rigidity and ultimately contractures and is seen in childhood, frequently associated with hepatic disease. A fixed, open-mouthed grin and a flapping tremor, and choreic or athetoid involuntary movements represent the classic lenticular degeneration [27].
- The other form, more commonly seen in adults, is called pseudosclerotic and is characterized largely by tremors. A tremulousness of action is characteristic [47].

Progression tends to be much slower in the pseudosclerotic form, while the dystonic form may progress to death within 4 years of onset. A pseudobulbar palsy may be the cause of death. Sensory abnormalities are lacking in Wilson disease.

Psychiatric presentations tend to be confusing, and they may occur even in children. Deterioration of intellectual function or abnormal behavior is unusual early, but usual later. Altered states of emotionality, deteriorating school performance, or even difficulty in swallowing, imperfect articulation, tremors and incoordination may lead to initial referral to a psychiatrist. Clumsiness and drooling may lead the patient to withdraw. Neurologic abnormalities developing later may be attributed to phenothiazine or other medication. Some type of organic dementia is ultimately an integral feature of untreated Wilson disease [28]. It may manifest itself as a learning disability or deterioration of performance in school, or at the other extreme the patient may be discovered among the inmates of a psychiatric institution with a diagnosis of schizophrenia [48]. The diagnosis should not be too difficult in the patient with full-blown dystonic neurologic manifestations, but in some patients neurologic features may be subtle or absent. Of course, in all of these patients there is the tell-tale corneal ring.

The Kayser-Fleischer ring (Figure 75.2) is a hallmark feature of the disease. It is always present, at least by slit lamp examination, in patients with neurologic or psychiatric manifestations of the disease [25], and can usually be seen with the naked eye. It is best to direct a light on the cornea from the side. The rings occur around the outer margin of the cornea as gray-green to red-gold pigmented rings. They represent the deposition of copper in the Descemet membrane; it is always advisable to confirm the localization by slit lamp, even in the presence of readily visualized rings. Rings do not always complete the circumferential circle, appearing sometimes as a crescent in the superior quadrant or at the upper and lower quadrants, sparing the side [49]. They are hardest

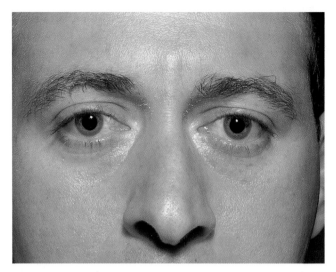

Figure 75.2   *The Kayser-Fleischer ring. The patient was an adult who had been admitted to an institution with a diagnosis of schizophrenia. The correct diagnosis was first suggested on the basis of the pattern of amino acids in the urine (Figure 75.3).*

to see in green-brown eyes. The rings are absent in more than 30 percent of children presenting with hepatic disease, and are usually absent in patients diagnosed while asymptomatic who are studied because they had affected siblings [49]. Rings may be absent in adults with isolated hepatic disease [40]. Some patients develop sunflower cataracts [49,50].

The bones may be affected in Wilson disease. Osteoporosis, osteomalacia or other abnormality occurs in over half of the patients [32,51,52]. There may be spontaneous fractures. Patients may have pain or stiffness in the joints, especially the knees; and early degenerative or osteoarthritis, with narrowing of the joint spaces and osteophyte formation, may be widespread. Brown pigmentation of the skin may develop, especially over the shins [53].

Renal stones are a relatively frequent complication of Wilson disease [54]. These may be the consequence of the renal tubular insufficiency that characterizes the disease and its inefficient acidification of the urine and hypercalciuria. There may be systemic acidosis and poor growth. Renal tubular disease is manifest at its most subtle by a generalized aminoaciduria, usually with special features that denote additional hepatic dysfunction (Figure 75.3). These include elevated levels of the sulfur-containing amino acids and tyrosine, but the cystine excretion appears to be more prominent than in the urine of patients with hepatic disease. In addition, there may be increased excretion of threonine and of citrulline [55]. Later, there is a full-blown Fanconi syndrome with glycosuria, phosphaturia, alkaline urine, renal tubular acidosis, hypercalciuria and osteomalacia or rickets. The excretion of large amounts of urate in the urine may lead to hypouricemia. Patients may develop diffuse nephrocalcinosis [28], and this may cause glomerular insufficiency and renal failure. Hypoparathyroidism has also been reported in Wilson disease [56] as has cardiac disease [57].

Laboratory evaluation of the patient with Wilson disease may reveal, in addition to the indices of renal dysfunction and the nonspecific abnormalities of hepatic disease or hemolytic anemia, a thrombocytopenia or neutropenia in a substantial number of patients [58]. Among specific diagnostic features of the disease a marked reduction in the level of ceruloplasmin is the most useful. This concentration is not always low, especially at times of active liver disease, because it is an acute phase reactant and rises with active hepatocellular disease [59]. A normal level of ceruloplasmin, especially in a young patient, does not rule out the disease. Diagnostic levels in patients range from 0 to 20 mg/dL. Normals are 20–40 mg/dL. In Wilson disease the serum concentration of nonceruloplasmin copper may be elevated. Its level in the urine is more greatly increased, and this may be very useful in diagnosis [9]. Urinary holoceruloplasmin has been suggested as a method for neonatal screening. Urine and blood should be collected in copper-free containers. The administration of penicillamine to increase the urinary excretion of copper may be useful diagnostically [28]. A dose of 10 mg/kg has been employed [60]. Normal adult individuals usually excrete a baseline level of less than 40 μg/24 h, and less than 600 μg/24 h with penicillamine, whereas patients may excrete 1000 μg/24 h untreated and 1500–3000 μg/24 h with penicillamine.

The most reliable test for the diagnosis of Wilson disease is the measurement of the level of copper in biopsied liver [35]. Errors can be avoided by the use of a disposable steel needle or a Menghini needle washed with ethylenediaminetetraacetic (EDTA) and rinsed with demineralized water, along with the use of five percent glucose in water, not saline, as propellant solution. Two cores of liver should be obtained as well as the tissue for histology in order to have 10–15 mg of liver for analysis. Patients with Wilson disease generally have over 250 μg of copper per gram of dry weight; normal individuals usually have less than 50 μg. In patients, levels are highest in young asymptomatic individuals with minimal histologic disease in whom the mean was over 1000 μg; levels decrease with age and the progression of cirrhosis, but even in older patients the mean approaches 500 μg/g. The biliary excretion of copper is abnormally low in Wilson disease. This is the normal route of excretion of dietary copper and its reduction is consistent with the accumulation of copper in the liver. Within the cell it is found in the lysosomes. In brain of Wilson patients dying of neurologic disease, concentrations of copper were significantly higher than in those of patients dying of hepatic involvement [61].

Differential diagnosis

It has been recognized for sometime that there were patients that had a phenotype quite different from Wilson disease who had very low levels of ceruloplasmin. It is now clear that these patients have aceruloplasminemia [62]. Patients have insulin-dependent diabetes, retinal degeneration and a neurodegenerative disease along with an absence or near absence of ceruloplasmin. Neurologic features include dysarthria, dystonia and dementia, and magnetic resonance imaging (MRI) reveals an accumulation of iron in the basal ganglia. There may be a microcytic anemia and elevated ferritin. Mutations in the ceruloplasmin gene have been identified.

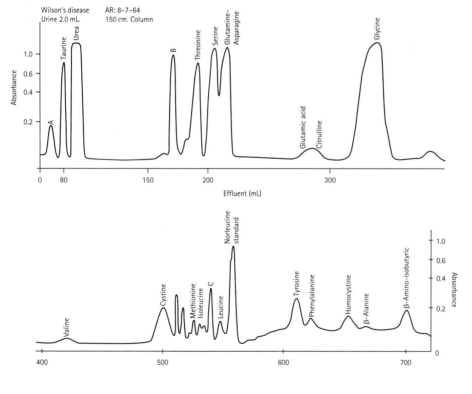

Figure 75.3 *Chromatographic pattern of the aminoaciduria of AR. In addition to the profile of a generalized renal aminoaciduria there were large amounts of cystine and methionine in the urine and the amount of tyrosine was considerably larger than that of phenalalanine.*

GENETICS AND PATHOGENESIS

Wilson disease is inherited in an autosomal recessive fashion [63]. The disorder has been observed frequently in siblings, and parental consanguinity has been observed. There are no clinical manifestations in heterozygotes, but some have low levels of ceruloplasmin [64]. The incidence of the disease has been estimated at one in 30 000 to 100 000 births, but a figure of one in 7000 has been estimated in Sardinia [24,65,66].

The fundamental defect in copper transport has been assessed by the intravenous injection of ^{64}Cu and measurement of the incorporation of copper into ceruloplasmin; this test reliably distinguishes patients with Wilson disease from normal individuals [28,67]. Normal individuals have a secondary rise in total serum radioactivity as ceruloplasmin is being synthesized, and this is absent in patients with Wilson disease, even when the concentration of ceruloplasmin is normal. The incorporation of ^{64}Cu into ceruloplasmin has been used to detect populations of heterozygotes [68], but it may not identify every individual heterozygote. The excretion of labeled copper after intravenous isotope has also been employed for this purpose [69].

In patients the biliary excretion of copper is markedly reduced [12]. Cultured fibroblasts from patients with Wilson disease have been reported [70] to have elevated intracellular concentrations of copper.

Following the mapping of the gene to q14.3 on chromosome 13, yeast artificial chromosomes (YACs) were prepared containing a 1–1.5 megabase region from this locus. Bull et al. [14] reasoned from the fact that the Menkes copper transporter gene was expressed in many tissues, but not the liver, consistent with the tissue distribution of copper in Menkes disease, but inconsistent with the fact that the liver is a major site of copper excretory transport, that there was a separate transporter for copper in the liver. Probes from the copper-binding domain of the Menkes gene were hybridized to the YACs, and a gene was isolated and designated Wcl with all the characteristics of a copper-transporting ATPase. The sequence of the gene has over 70 percent homology with the Menkes gene. These ATPases share a number of motifs, including MXCXXC, the copper-binding motif in the N terminus and a transmembrane CPC necessary for metal transfer across the membrane. The gene contains 21 exons over 60 kb.

In the study of patients with Wilson disease, two were found to be homozygous for a seven-base deletion (1950–1956) in the coding region [14]. The gene was cloned independently [15,16] and four mutations were identified: a C2142-to-A transversion which changed histidine 714 to glutamine, an A2744-to-G change converting asparagine 915 to serine, a C2237 deletion and a T2487 insertion, the latter two causing frameshifts. In at least 20 percent of alleles, a mutation could not be identified, suggesting upstream mutations regulating transcription [19]. A majority of patients are heterozygous for two mutations [71]. In addition to the common European mutation H1069Q, A778L has been shown to be common in

Asians [72,73]. In Sardinia, where the disease is common, 16 different mutations have been found, of which six are common, three deletions, an insertion and R778W and V1146M [66]. Expression studies have indicated that the H1069Q mutation causes defective folding of the protein, leading to mislocalization and degradation [74,75]. Knowledge of the mutation permits effective detection of heterozygotes and prenatal diagnosis.

TREATMENT

The availability of effective treatment for Wilson disease [11,76] has made even more important the early diagnosis of the disease. If the diagnosis is too long delayed, irreversible damage may occur. The best prognosis has been demonstrated by the treatment of asymptomatic patients [77].

D-Penicillamine (Figure 75.4), which chelates copper, is the treatment of choice [78]. It is usually given in adult doses of 1 g daily. Those under 10 years usually begin with 0.5 g daily. Children under 5 years may need less, but some have received up to 3 g daily. Treatment is initiated with a small test dose and then given by mouth four times a day, often in half the expected dose. The drug is given to the patient on an empty stomach, two or more hours before meals, to prevent chelation with food. Urinary copper is measured and dosage adjusted to obtain initial 24-hour rates of excretion over 2 mg per day.

Evidence of improvement may require weeks or more of therapy. Kayser-Fleischer rings regularly resolve. Even neurologic manifestations such as tremors, awkward gait, slurred speech and illegible writing may be expected to improve; but advanced dystonic rigidity or contractures are less likely to improve. Psychiatric symptomatology is likely to improve. Hepatic dysfunction is also likely to improve, generally dramatically. Of course, portal hypertension and advanced cirrhosis will not change, but even anasarca has been reversed. Fulminant hepatitis and hepatic failure have not been observed to develop in patients receiving maintenance treatment with penicillamine. However, both, and fatal outcomes, have been observed in patients in whom treatment was interrupted for nine months to three years [28]. Once improvement has been demonstrated, the dose is often reduced to one half.

Treatment with penicillamine is often not easy. Its administration is regularly complicated by skin rashes, fever and

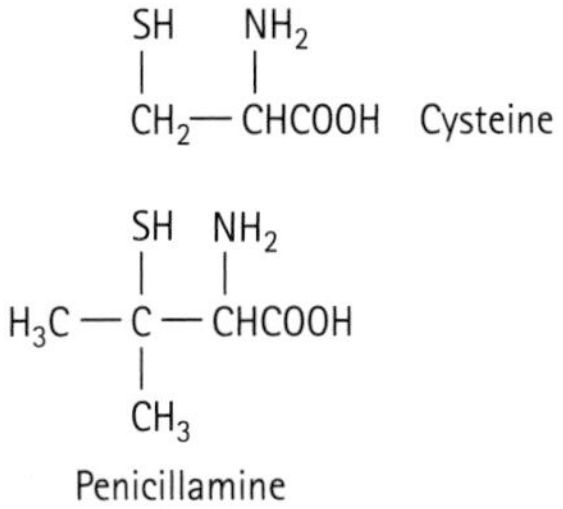

Figure 75.4 *Structure of penicillamine, illustrating its similarity to cysteine.*

thrombocytopenia or granulocytopenia. It is often possible to desensitize the patient by withdrawing the drug and reinstituting at 10–25 mg daily. Many patients require adjunctive prednisone, which can usually be withdrawn later without recrudescence of the reaction. Other more serious reactions requiring withdrawal of the drug are severe marrow depression, nephrotic syndrome and arthritis; so blood counts and urinalyses must be monitored regularly. A variety of skin lesions that have been reported include penicillamine dermatopathy, elastosis perforans serpiginnosa and pemphigoid lesions [76]. Many of the reactions can be handled by reduction of dosage, the addition of prednisone or both. Anaphylaxis requires its elimination. In patients who cannot be given penicillamine, triethylenetetramine hydrochloride (trientine) is an effective alternate chelator [79].

Zinc has also been employed in such patients, or as an adjunct to penicillamine. This is a different therapeutic mechanism. Zinc, given as acetate, decreases copper absorption by inducing metallothionine synthesis in mucosal cells [80,81].

Ammonium tetrathiomolybdate (TTM) is a copper chelator that was discovered as the cause of copper deficiency in sheep grazing on clover high in molybdenum. It is the most potent of the chelators used to treat Wilson disease [82,83]. It is particularly useful in those patients with very high copper burdens in whom neurologic deterioration occurs after the start of therapy with penicillamine. It is not recommended for children because it inhibits growth of bone.

The treatment of the desperately ill patient in an acute fulminant episode of hepatic disease is particularly demanding. The standard treatment has been peritoneal dialysis. In one patient penicillamine and albumin were added to the dialysate, which permitted the removal of large amounts of copper but did not prevent a fatal outcome [84]. Similar experience has been obtained with exchange transfusion, peritoneal dialysis or hemodialysis [28]. Plasmapheresis and hemofiltration may be more effective methods for removing copper [85]. Five patients survived severe hepatic decompensation following intensive medical therapy, including penicillamine, zinc, trientine and plasmapheresis [86]. TTM, because of its efficiency in removing large amounts of copper, may prove to be very useful in this acute situation.

Liver transplantation has been employed in a number of patients with Wilson disease, and it can be particularly effective in acute fulminant situations [65,87]. There have been some relatively long survivors in whom it is clear that the body burden of copper is decreased. The serum copper usually becomes normal within 6 months [88], and Kayser-Fleischer rings have progressively disappeared [89]. Liver transplantation was effective in the treatment of a 13-year-old girl with acute Wilson disease [90] whose hepatorenal failure was unresponsive to penicillamine, hemodialysis, plasmapheresis, cardiopulmonary support and total parenteral nutrition. For many patients, the variety of medical therapies available makes liver transplantation less desirable, but transplantation may be the only resource for patients with progressive hepatocellular disease that does not respond to medical therapy [65].

References

1   Wilson SAK. Progressive lenticular degeneration: a familial nervous disease associated with cirrhosis of the liver. *Brain* 1912;**34**:295.

2   Kayser B. Ueber einen Fall von angeborener grublicher Verfarbung der Kornea. *Klin Monatsbl Augenheilk* 1902;**40**:22.

3   Fleischer B. Zwei weitere Falle von grublicher Verfarbung der Kornea. *Klin Monatsbl Augenheilk* 1903;**41**:489.

4   Rumpel A. Uber Das Wesen und die Bedeutung der Leberveranderungen und der Pigmentierungen bei den damet verbundensen Fallen von Pseudosklerose zugleich ein Beitrag zur Lehre von der Pseudosklerose (Westphal-Strumpell). *Dtsch Z Nervenheilkd* 1913;**49**:54.

5   Vogt A. Kupfer und Silber aufgespeichert in Auge Leber Milz und Nieren als Symptom der Pseudosklerose. *Klin Monatsbl Augenheilk* 1929;**83**:417.

6   Haurowitz F. Ueber eine Anomalie des Kupferstoffwechsels Hoppe-Seylers. *Z Physiol Chemie* 1930;**190**:72.

7   Glaebrook AJ. Wilson's disease. *Edinb Med J* 1945;**52**:83.

8   Bennetts HW, Chapman FE. Copper deficiency in sheep in Western Australia: a preliminary account of the aetiology of enzootic ataxia of lambs and anaemia of ewes. *Aust Vet J* 1937;**13**:138.

9   Mandelbrotte BM, Stanier MW, Thompson RHS, Thruston MN. Studies on copper metabolism in demyelinating diseases of the central nervous system. *Brain* 1948;**71**:212.

10 Cumings JN. The copper and iron content of brain and liver in the normal and in hepato-lenticular degeneration. *Brain* 1948;**71**:410.

11 Walshe JM. Penicillamine. A new oral therapy for Wilson's disease. *Amer J Med* 1956;**21**:487.

12 Gibbs K, Walshe JM. Biliary excretion of copper in Wilson's disease. *Lancet* 1980;**2**:538.

13 Farrer LA, Bowcock AM, Hebert JM, *et al.* Predictive testing for Wilson disease using tightly linked and flanking DNA markers. *Neurology* 1991;**41**:992.

14 Bull P, Thomas GR, Rommens JM, *et al.* The Wilson disease gene is putative copper bind P-type ATPase similar to the Menkes gene. *Nat Genet* 1993;**5**:327.

15 Petrukhin K, Fischer SG, Pirastu M, *et al.* Mapping cloning and genetic characterization of the Wilson's disease region. *Nat Genet* 1993;**5**:338.

16 Tanzi RE, Putrukhin K, Chernov I, *et al.* Identification of the Wilson's disease gene; a copper transporting ATPase with homology to the Menkes disease gene. *Nat Genet* 1993;**5**:344.

17 Yamaguchi Y, Heiny ME, Gitlin JD. Isolation and characterization of a human liver cDNA as a candidate gene for Wilson disease. *Biochem Biophys Res Commun* 1993;**197**:271.

18 Petrukhin K, Lutsenko S, Chernov L, *et al.* Characterization of the Wilson disease gene encoding a P-type copper transporting ATPase: genomic organization alternative splicing and structure/function predicting. *Hum Mol Genet* 1994;**3**:1647.

19 Cox DW. Molecular advances in Wilson disease. *Prog Liver Dis* 1996;**14**:245.

20 Dobyns WB, Goldstein NP, Gordon H. Clinical spectrum of Wilson's disease (hepatolenticular degeneration). *Mayo Clin Proc* 1979;**54**:35.

21 Strickland GT, Leu M-L. Wilson's disease: clinical and laboratory manifestations in 40 patients. *Medicine* 1975;**54**:113.

22 Strickland GT, Frommer D, Leu M-L, *et al.* Wilson's disease in the United Kingdom and Taiwan. *Q J Med* 1973;**42**:619.

23 Arima M, Sano I. Genetic studies of Wilson's disease in Japan. *Birth Defects* 1968;**4**:54.

24 Giagheddu A, Demelia L, Puggioni G, *et al.* Epidemiologic study of hepatolenticular degeneration (Wilson's disease) in Sardinia (1902–1983). *Acta Neurol Scand* 1985;**72**:43.

25 Werlin SL, Grand RJ, Perman JA, Watkins JB. Diagnostic dilemmas of Wilson's disease: diagnosis and treatment. *Pediatrics* 1978;**62**:47.

26 Iser JH, Stevens BJ, Stening GF, *et al.* Hemolytic anemia of Wilson's disease. *Gastroenterology* 1974;**67**:290.

27 Denny-Brown D. Hepatolenticular degeneration (Wilson's disease): two different components. *N Engl J Med* 1964;**270**:1149.

28 Scheinberg IH, Sternlieb I. Wilson's Disease: Vol XXIII in the Series *Major Problems in Internal Medicine* (ed. H Lloyd, Jr Smith). WB Saunders Co, Philadelphia;1984.

29 Walshe JM, Cumings JN, (eds). *Wilson's Disease: Some Current Concepts.* Blackwell, Oxford;1961.

30 Owen CA Jr. *Wilson's Disease.* Noyes Publications, Park Ridge NJ;1981.

31 Arima M, Takeshita K, Yoshino K, *et al.* Prognosis of Wilson's disease in childhood. *Eur J Pediatr* 1977;**126**:147.

32 Sass-Kortsak A. Wilson's disease: a treatable cause of liver disease in children. *Pediatr Clin N Am* 1975;**22**:963.

33 Odievre M, Vedrenne J, Landriu P, Alagille D. Les formes hepatiques 'pures' de la maladie de Wilson chez l'enfant: A propos de dix observations. *Arch Franc Pediatr* 1974;**31**:215.

34 Danks DM, Stevens BJ. Diagnosis of Wilson's disease in children with liver disease: a report of two families. *Lancet* 1969;**1**:22.

35 Perman JA, Werlin SL, Grand RJ, Watkins JB. Laboratory measures of copper metabolism in the differentiation of chronic active hepatitis and Wilson's disease in children. *J Pediatr* 1979;**94**:564.

36 Roche-Sicot J, Benhamon J-P. Acute intravascular hemolysis and acute liver failure associated as a first manifestation of Wilson's disease. *Ann Intern Med* 1977;**86**:301.

37 Hamlyn AN, Gollan JL, Douglas AP, Sherlock S. Fulminant Wilson's disease with haemolysis and renal failure: copper studies and assessment of dialysis regimens. *Br Med J* 1977;**2**:660.

38 Adler R, Mahnovski V, Heuser ET, *et al.* Fulminant hepatitis: a presentation of Wilson's disease. *Am J Dis Child* 1977;**131**:870.

39 McCullough AJ, Fleming CR, Thistle JL, *et al.* Diagnosis of Wilson's disease presenting as fulminant hepatic failure. *Gastroenterology* 1983;**84**:161.

40 Silverberg M, Gellis SS. The liver in juvenile Wilson's disease. *Pediatrics* 1962;**30**:402.

41 Sternlieb I, Scheinberg IH. Chronic hepatitis as a first manifestation of Wilson's disease. *Ann Intern Med* 1972;**76**:59.

42 Lessner J, Bachmann H, Biesold D. Unteruchungen zur Wilsonhen Erkrankung in der DDR. *Z Ges Inn Med* 1980;**35**:136.

43 Danks DM, Metz G, Sewell R, Prewett IJ. Wilson's disease as a cause of cirrhosis in adults with no neurological abnormalities. *Br Med J* 1990;**301**:331.

44 Sternlieb I. Diagnosis of Wilson's disease. *Gastroenterology* 1978;**74**:787.

45 Cartwright GE. Diagnosis of treatable Wilson's disease. *N Engl J Med* 1978;**298**:1347.

46 Rosenfield N, Grand RJ, Watkins JB, *et al.* Cholelithiasis and Wilson's disease. *J Pediatr* 1978;**92**:210.

47 Boudin G, Pepin B. *Degenerescence Hepato-lenticulaire.* Masson, Paris;1959.

48 Beard AW. The association of hepatolenticular degeneration with schizophrenia. *Acta Psych Neurol Scand* 1959;**34**:411.

49 Wiebers DO, Hollenhorst RW, Goldstein NP. The ophthalmologic manifestation of Wilson's disease. *Mayo Clin Proc* 1977;**52**:409.

50 Cairns JE, Williams HP, Walshe JM. Sunflower cataract in Wilson's disease. *Br Med J* 1969;**3**:95.

51 Golding DN and Walshe JM. Arthropathy of Wilson's disease: study of clinical and radiological features in 32 cases. *Ann Rheumat Dis* 1977;**36**:99.

52 Canelas HM, Carvalho N, Scaff M, *et al.* Osteoarthropathy of hepatolenticular degeneration. *Acta Neurol Scand* 1978;**57**:481.

53 Leu ML, Strickland GT, Wang CC, Chen TSN. Skin pigmentation in Wilson's disease. *JAMA* 1970;**211**:1542.

54 Wiebers DO, Wilson DM, McLeod RA, Goldstain NP. Renal stones in Wilson's disease. *Am J Med* 1979;**67**:249.

55 Stein WH, Bearn AG, Furemoore S. The amino acid content of the blood and urine in Wilson's disease. *J Clin Invest* 1954;**33**:410.

56 Carpenter TO, Carnes DL Jr, Anast CS. Hypoparathyroidism in Wilson's disease. *N Engl J Med* 1983;**309**:873.

57 Hlubocka Z, Marecek Z, Linhart A, *et al.* Cardiac involvement in Wilson disease. *J Inherit Metab Dis* 2002;**25**:269.

58 Hoaglund HC, Goldstein NP. Hematologic (cytopenic) manifestations of Wilson's disease (hepatolenticular degeneration). *Mayo Clin Proc* 1978;**53**:498.

59 Walshe JM, Briggs J. Ceruloplasmin in liver disease: a diagnostic pitfall. *Lancet* 1962;**2**:263.

60 Frommer DH. Urinary copper excretion and hepatic copper concentration in liver disease. *Digestion* 1981;**21**:169.

61 Walshe JM, Gibbs KR. Brain copper in Wilson's disease. *Lancet* 1987;**2**:1030.

62 Harris ZL. Not all absent serum ceruloplasmin is Wilson disease: a review of aceruloplasminemia. *J Invest Med* 2002;**50**:236 (suppl).

63 Bearn AG. Genetic analysis of Wilson's disease. *Ann Hum Genet* 1960;**24**:33.

64 Gibbs K, Walshe JM. A study of the ceruloplasmin concentrations found in 75 patients with Wilson's disease their kinships and various control groups. *Q J Med* 1979;**48**:1.

65 Schilsky ML. Wilson disease: genetic basis of copper toxicity and natural history. *Semin Liver Dis* 1996;**16**:83.

66 Lovicu M, Dessi V, Zappu A, *et al.* Efficient strategy for molecular diagnosis of Wilson disease in the Sardinian population. *Clin Chem* 2003;**49**:496.

67 Sternlieb I, Schienberg IH. The role of radiocopper in the diagnosis of Wilson's disease. *Gastroenterology* 1979;**77**:138.

68 Sternlieb I, Morell AG, Bauer CD, *et al.* Detection of the heterozygous carrier of the Wilson's disease gene. *J Clin Invest* 1961;**40**:707.

69 Gibbs K, Hanka RA, Walshe JM. The urinary excretion of radiocopper in presymptomatic and symptomatic Wilson's disease heterozygotes and controls: its significance in diagnosis and management. *Q J Med* 1978;**47**:349.

70 Chan W-Y, Cushing W, Coffman MA, Rennert OM. Genetic expression of Wilson's disease in cell culture: a diagnostic marker. *Science* 1980;**208**:299.

71 Thomas GR, Forbes JR, Roberts EA, *et al.* The Wilson disease gene: spectrum of mutations and their consequences. *Nat Genet* 1995;**9**:210.

72 Kim EK, Yoo OJ, Song KY, *et al.* Identification of three novel mutations and a high frequency of the Arg778Leu mutation in Korean patients with Wilson disease. *Hum Mutat* 1998;**11**:275.

73 Chuang L-M, Wu H-P, Jang M-H, *et al.* High frequency of two mutations in codon 778 in exon 8 of the ATP7B gene in Taiwanese families with Wilson disease. *J Med Genet* 1996;**33**:521.

74 Payne AS, Kelly EJ, Gitlin JD. Functional expression of the Wilson disease protein reveals mislocalization and impaired copper-dependent trafficking of the common H1069Q mutation. *Proc Natl Acad Sci USA* 1998;**95**:10854.

75 La Fontaine SL, Firth SD, Camakaris J, *et al.* Correction of the copper transport defect of Menkes patient fibroblasts by expression of the Menkes and Wilson ATPases. *J Biol Chem* 1998;**273**:31375.

76 Scheinberg IH, Sternlieb I. The long term management of hepatolenticular degeneration (Wilson's disease). *Am J Med* 1960;**29**:316.

77 Sternlieb I, Scheinberg IH. Prevention of Wilson's disease in asymptomatic patients. *N Engl J Med* 1968;**278**:352.

78 Sternlieb I, Bennett B, Scheinberg IH. D-penicillamine-induced Goodpasture's syndrome in Wilson's disease. *Ann Intern Med* 1975;**82**:673.

79 Walshe JM. Copper chelation in patients with Wilson's disease. *Q J Med* 1973;**42**:441.

80 Lee D-Y, Brewer GJ, Wang Y. Treatment of Wilson's disease with zinc VII. Protection of the liver from copper toxicity by zinc-induced metallothionine in a rat model. *J Lab Clin Med* 1989;**114**:639.

81 Brewer GJ, Gretchen MH, Prasad AS, *et al.* Oral zinc therapy for Wilson's disease. *Ann Intern Med* 1983;**99**:3.

82 Gonneratne SR, Howell JMcC, Gawthorne JM. Intravenous administration of thiomolybdate for the prevention and treatment of chronic copper poisoning in sheep. *Br J Nutr* 1981;**46**:457.

83 Walshe JM. Tetrathiomolybdate (MoS4) as an anti-copper agent in man: in *Orphan Diseases and Orphan Drugs* (eds IH Scheinberg, JM Walshe). Manchester University Press, Manchester;1986:76.

84 De Bont B, Moulin D, Stein F, *et al.* Peritoneal dialysis with D-penicillamine in Wilson disease. *J Pediatr* 1985;**107**:545.

85 Danks DM. Penicillamine in Wilson's disease. *Lancet* 1982;**2**:435.

86 Silva Santos EE, Sarles J, Buts JP, Sokal EM. Successful medical treatment of severely decompensated Wilson disease. *J Pediatr* 1996;**128**:258.

87 Nazer H, Ede RJ, Mowat AP, Williams R. Wilson's disease: clinical presentation and use of prognostic index. *Gut* 1986;**27**:1377.

88 DiDonato M, Sarkar B. Copper transport and its alterations in Menkes and Wilson diseases. *Biochim Biophys Acta* 1997;**1360**:3.

89 Schoenberger M, Ellis PP. Disappearance of Kayser-Fleischer rings after liver transplantation. *Arch Ophthalmol* 1979;**97**:1914.

90 Sokol RJ, Francis PD, Gold SH, *et al.* Orthotopic liver transplantation for acute fulminant Wilson disease. *J Pediatr* 1985;**107**:549.

Mucopolysaccharidoses

76

Introduction to mucopolysaccharidoses

The mucopolysaccharidoses are genetically determined disorders in which acid mucopolysaccharides, known chemically as glycosaminoglycans, are stored in the tissues [1,2] and excreted in large quantities in the urine [3]. Storage in tissues leads to effects on a wide variety of systems and to remarkable changes in morphogenesis. Among these striking effects are the alterations in the appearance of the patient that are classically represented in the Hurler syndrome (Chapter 77). The elucidation of these disorders has provided clear evidence that even bizarre dysmorphic changes can be caused by single gene defects that interfere with body chemistry. They provide important models of the interaction of structure and function in humans. Mental retardation and early demise, prior to 10 years-of-age in the Hurler syndrome, are the most devastating consequences of mucopolysaccharide accumulation in the central nervous and cardiovascular systems. However, there is considerable variety of expression among patients with various individual mucopolysaccharidoses. Patients with some syndromes are intellectually normal, and some survive well into adult life. Research in this field has proceeded rapidly, so that it is now possible to delineate the molecular defect in each of the mucopolysaccharidoses.

Advances in the understanding of the mucopolysaccharidoses followed the growth of fibroblasts from these patients in cell culture and the recognition that there was phenotypic expression of the disease in the fibroblast. The elucidation of the molecular nature of the mucopolysaccharidoses represents a fascinating chapter in cell biology. Characterization of the mucopolysaccharidoses as disorders in the degradation of intracellular acid mucopolysaccharide began with the studies of Fratantoni, Hall and Neufeld [4] using ^{35}S-labeled sulfate. $^{35}SO_4$ is taken up by the cells of patients, just as it is by normal cells. However, in patients as opposed to controls, there is no turnover; these cells simply accumulate the label and keep it.

In what is now a landmark series of experiments, Fratantoni, Hall and Neufeld [5] mixed normal fibroblasts in culture with those of patients with Hurler or Hunter syndrome and found that the kinetics of $^{35}SO_4$ incorporation became normal. Furthermore, it was possible to restore normal kinetics in Hurler cells by mixing them with Hunter cells and vice versa. It was also found that the medium in which normal cells or Hunter cells had grown could correct the defect in Hurler cells. Corrective factors were soon identified for other mucopolysaccharidoses [6]. In fact, demonstration of two different corrective factors first permitted the distinction of Sanfilippo types A and B. On the other hand, fibroblasts from patients with Scheie syndrome could not be corrected by the factor from Hurler cells [7], indicating that the genes for these two conditions were allelic and represented different defects in the same enzyme protein. These studies in cell biology led directly to the identification of the enzymatic defects [8,9] (Table 76.1). They also laid the groundwork for current enzyme replacement therapy.

Hurler disease was originally classified by McKusick as mucopolysaccharidosis type I [1]. With the recognition of the enzyme defect in α-L-iduronidase and the fact that defective activity of the same enzyme was also the cause of the Scheie syndrome [8], the subclassifications IH for Hurler and IS for Scheie were employed. The classification of the mucopolysaccharidoses and a summary of their clinical biochemical characteristics are shown in Table 76.1. The seven types of mucopolysaccharidosis represent the deficiencies of ten specific enzymes. Prenatal diagnosis was initially carried out in Hurler and Hunter diseases by measuring labeled sulphate incorporation in cultured amniocytes [10].

The defect in the Hurler cell is in Aα-L-iduronidase [8,9,11] (see Figure 77.1, p. 504), and Hurler corrective factor has been shown to have iduronidase activity [8]. The Hurler corrective factor is a form of iduronidase that can be taken up by fibroblasts [12] because it contains the mannose-6-phosphate recognition marker, whereas the lower molecular weight enzyme purified from human kidney cannot. The gene for the enzymes defective in the mucopolysaccharidoses with the exception of the MPS IIIC enzyme have been mapped to their respective chromosomes [13] and cloned [14], and a number of mutations have been identified.

A suspected diagnosis of mucopolysaccharidoses is often pursued chemically by the documentation of increased amounts of mucopolysaccharide in the urine. However spot tests for mucopolysaccharide are unreliable and give false positive and negative results [15]. Semiqualitative and quantitative procedures may also be misleading [16]. If a diagnosis of a mucopolysaccharidoses is suspected, assay of the lysosomal enzymes should be performed. This is readily carried out in freshly isolated leukocytes. It can also be done on cultured fibroblasts.

Table 76.1 *Clinical and laboratory characteristics of the mucopolysaccharidoses*

Syndrome	MPS delegation	Inheritance	Mental retardation	Corneal clouding	Hepatosplenomegaly	Skeletal defect	Other clinical manifestations	Compound stored excreted	Defective enzyme
Hurler	I$_S$	Autosomal recessive	+	+	+	+	Coarse facial features, cardiac disease, motor weakness, hernia	Dermatan sulfate, heparan sulfate	α-L-iduronidase
Scheie *	I$_S$	Autosomal recessive	−	+	−	+	Coarse features, stiff joints	Dermatan sulfate, heparan sulfate	α-L-iduronidase
Hurler/Scheie	I$_{HS}$	Autosomal recessive	±	+	+	+	Phenotype intermediate	Dermatan sulfate, heparan sulfate	α-L-iduronidase
Hunter	II	X-linked recessive	+	−	+	+	Coarse features, weakness, aggressive behavior	Dermatan sulfate, heparan sulfate	Iduronate sulfatase
Sanfilippo Type A	III$_A$	Autosomal recessive	+	−	±	+	Mild somatic features, contrast with severity of cerebral disease	Heparan sulfate	Heparan N-sulfatase (sulfamidase)
Sanfilippo Type B	III$_B$	Autosomal recessive	+	−	±	+	Mild somatic features, contrast with severity of cerebral disease	Heparan sulfate	α-N-Acetylglucos-aminidase
Sanfilippo Type C	III$_C$	Autosomal recessive	+	−	±	+	Mild somatic features, contrast with severity of cerebral disease	Heparan sulfate	AcetylCoA:α-D-glucosaminide-N-acetyl transferase
Sanfilippo Type D	III$_D$	Autosomal recessive	+	−	±	+	Mild somatic features, contrast with severity of cerebral disease	Heparan sulfate	N-Acetyl-α-D-glucosaminide-6-sulfatase
Morquio A	IV$_A$	Autosomal recessive	±	+	−	+	Distinctive bone deformities, hypoplastic odontoid, thin enamel	Keratan sulfate	Galactose-6-sulfatase
Morquio B	IV$_B$	Autosomal recessive	±	+	+	+	Mild bone changes, hypoplastic odontoid	Keratan sulfate	β-Galactosidase
Maroteaux-Lamy	VI	Autosomal recessive	−	+	+	+	Severe bony deformities, valvular cardiac disease	Dermatan sulfate	N-Acetylgalactosamine-4-sulfatase (arylsulfatase B)
Sly	VII	Autosomal recessive	+	+	+	+	Coarse features	Dermatan sulfate, heparan sulfate, chondroitin-4-6-sulfates	β-Glucuronidase
IX	IX	Autosomal recessive	+	−	−	+	Periarticular soft tissue masses; short stature	Hyaluronan	Hyaluronidase

* The Scheie syndrome was initially designated mucopolysaccharidosis V. When it became evident that it was an allelic variant of MPS I, it was designated MPS I$_S$; MPS V has been left unused.

A common feature among the mucopolysaccharidoses is the roentgenographic appearance [17,18] known as dysostosis multiplex. This picture is best exemplified in Hurler disease. This is such a constant feature of the disease that roentgenographic search for the presence of dysostosis multiplex is an effective way to screen for the mucopolysaccharidoses. It is reliable in all but the Sanfilippo patients, and it is most dramatic in the Hurler patients. This picture is also seen in generalized GM_1 gangliosidosis (Chapter 90) and in the mucolipidoses (Chapters 84, 85). It is described in detail in Chapter 77, pp. 506–8.

References

1 McKusick VA. *Heritable Disorders of Connective Tissue* (4th edn). CV Mosby Co, St Louis;1972:521.

2 Brante G. Gargoylism. A mucopolysaccharidosis. *Scand J Clin Lab Invest* 1952;**4**:43.

3 Dorfman A, Lorincz AE. Occurrence of urinary mucopolysaccharides in the Hurler syndrome. *Proc Natl Acad Sci USA* 1957;**43**:443.

4 Fratantoni JC, Hall CW, Neufeld EF. The defect in Hurler's and Hunter's syndromes: faulty degradation of mucopolysaccharides. *Proc Natl Acad Sci USA* 1968;**60**:699.

5 Fratantoni JC, Hall CW, Neufeld EF. Hurler and Hunter syndromes. Mutual correction of the defect in cultured fibroblasts. *Science* 1968;**162**:570.

6 Neufeld EF, Cantz MJ. Corrective factors for inborn errors of mucopolysaccharide metabolism. *Ann NY Acad Sci* 1971;**179**:580.

7 Wiesmann U, Neufeld EF. Scheie and Hurler syndromes. Apparent identity of the biochemical defect. *Science* 1970;**169**:72.

8 Bach G, Friedman R, Weismann B, Neufeld EF. The defect in the Hurler and Scheie syndromes: deficiency of α-L-iduronidase. *Proc Natl Acad Sci USA* 1972;**69**:2048.

9 Matalon R, Cifonelli JA, Dorfman A. L-iduronidase in cultured human fibroblasts and liver. *Biochem Biophys Res Commun* 1971;**42**:340.

10 Fratantoni JC, Neufeld EF, Uhlendorf BW, Jacobson CB. Intrauterine diagnosis of the Hurler and Hunter syndrome. *N Engl J Med* 1969;**280**:686.

11 Matalon R, Dorfman A. Hurler's syndrome, an α-L-iduronidase deficiency. *Biochem Biophys Res Commun* 1972;**47**:959.

12 Shapiro LJ, Hall CE, Leder IG, Neufeld EF. The relationship of α-L-iduronidase and Hurler corrective factor. *Arch Biochem Biophys* 1976;**172**:156.

13 Scott HS, Ashton LJ, Eyre HJ, *et al.* Chromosomal localization of the human α-L iduronidase gene (IDUA) to 4 p 163. *Am J Hum Genet* 1990;**47**:802.

14 Scott HS, Guo X-H, Hopwood JJ, Morris CP. Structure and sequence of the human α-L-iduronidase gene. *Genomics* 1992;**13**:1811.

15 De Jong JGN, Hasselman JJF, van Landeghem AAJ, *et al.* The spot test is not a reliable screening procedure for mucopolysaccharidoses. *Clin Chem* 1991;**37**:572.

16 Thuy LP, Nyhan WL. A new quantitative assay for glycosaminoglycans. *Clin Chim Acta* 1992;**212**:17.

17 Caffey J. Gargoylism (Hunter-Hurler disease, dysostosis multiplex, lipochondrodystrophy). *Am J Roentgenol Radium Ther Nucl Med* 1952;**67**:715.

18 Grossman H, Dorst JP. The mucopolysaccharidoses and mucolipidoses: in *Progress in Pediatric Radiology* (ed. HJ Kauffman). Charger, Basel;1973:495.

77

Hurler disease/mucopolysaccharidosis type IH (MPSIH)/α-L-iduronidase deficiency

MAJOR PHENOTYPIC EXPRESSION

Coarse features, mental retardation, corneal clouding, hepatosplenomegaly, short stature, dysostosis multiplex and cardiac complications; widespread lysosomal storage of mucopolysaccharide, and excretion of dermatan sulfate and heparan sulfate; and deficiency of α-L-iduronidase.

INTRODUCTION

The Hurler syndrome is the classic or prototypic mucopolysaccharidosis (MPS). Hurler's original description was published in 1919 [1]. McKusick classified it as mucopolysaccharidosis I [2], and more recently as IH to distinguish it from the Scheie phenotype IS, or the intermediate Hurler-Scheie (IHS) picture. Modern molecular biology makes these distinctions less relevant, but we have continued to separate mucopolysaccharidosis I into two chapters because of the importance of these phenotypes and because these distinctions may have relevance to therapy.

The defect in the Hurler cell is in α-L-iduronidase [3–5] (Figure 77.1). The gene for α-L-iduronidase has been mapped to chromosome 4p16.3 [6] and has been cloned and sequenced [7]. A number of mutations has been identified, including at least two common alleles W402X and Q70X, accounting for over half the alleles in European patients [8–10]. Heterogeneity is also evident in different mutations in other ethnic groups [11,12].

CLINICAL ABNORMALITIES

Patients with Hurler syndrome appear normal at birth. They develop normally for some months, after which they begin to develop progressive disease. Patients may present first for repair of inguinal hernias or for chronic rhinitis [13]. The diagnosis is seldom suspected at that time. However, as the first year of life proceeds, the characteristic appearance develops. Nasal discharge tends to be persistent, as are recurrent respiratory infections and otitis. Breathing is noisy, as is snoring.

In the established syndrome the facial features are coarse (Figures 77.2–77.6). The head is large, bulging and scaphocephalic, and there may be hyperostosis of the sagittal sutures. Frontal bossing, prominent brow, wide-set prominent eyes with

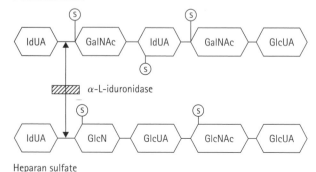

Dermatan sulfate

Heparan sulfate

Figure 77.1   *α-L-iduronidase, the site of the defect in Hurler and Scheie diseases. Dermatan sulfate and heparan sulfate accumulate when α-L-iduronidase activity is defective.*

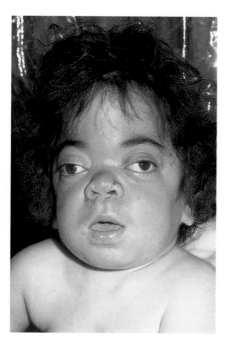

Figure 77.2   *D.D., a 6-year-old girl with Hurler disease. She was short (90 cm) at the age of 7 and had a relatively large head (55 cm). The facial features were coarse, the eyes were prominent and the nasal bridge depressed. There was frontal bossing. The abdomen was protuberant because of hepatosplenomegaly, and there was an umbilical hernia.*

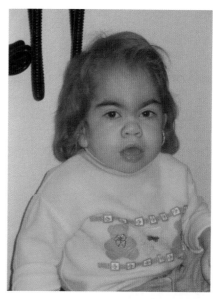

Figure 77.4   *S.C. This 2 yr and 10 month old with α-iduronidase deficiency had clearcut dysostosis multiplex, and her hand was the typical claw hand, but her facial features were subtle. The alae nasi and septum had begun to widen, and she was quite hirsute; corneas had begun to cloud.*

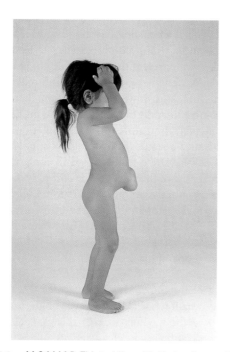

Figure 77.3   *M.O.M.M.R. This toddler with Hurler disease illustrates the evolution of the disease. The abdomen was protuberant and facial features coarse, but much less than in Figure 77.2.*

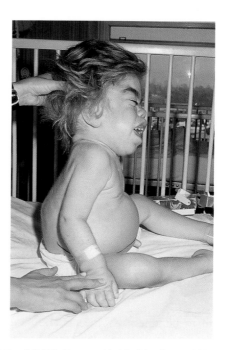

Figure 77.5   *B.R. This 5-year-old girl with advanced Hurler disease had massive hepatosplenomegaly and a gibbus.*

puffy-appearing lids and a depressed nasal bridge are characteristic. The face is flat, and the nose and nostrils wide and anteverted (Figures 77.2, 77.5, 77.6). The lips are large and thickened; the tongue is large and often protrudes through the open mouth (Figure 78.11). There is hypertrophy of the gums and the bony alveolar ridges; the teeth are small and widely spaced. Patients are generally hirsute. The hair is thick and coarse, the eyebrows bushy and the hairline low, and there is a large amount of forehead hair. Lanugo hair is plentiful. The skin is thick.

Clouding of the cornea is a hallmark of the syndrome (Figure 77.7). The cloudy cornea has a ground-glass appearance.

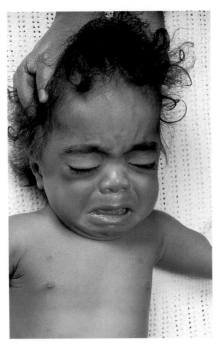

Figure 77.6 *G.A.N., an infant with pronounced stigmata of Hurler disease. The facial features were quite coarse as early as 5 months. Activity of α-L-iduronidase was undetectable.*

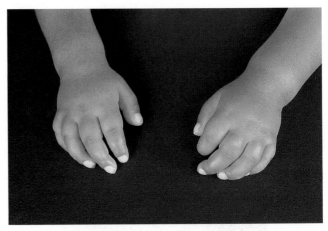

Figure 77.8 *The typical claw hands of a patient with Hurler disease. Limitation of motion is evident in the position of the digits.*

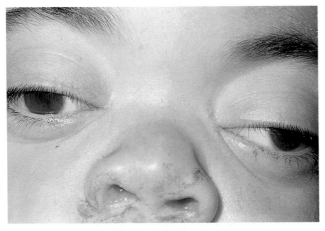

Figure 77.7 *D.D. The corneas were steamy.*

It may lead to blindness. Nystagmus and strabismus are occasionally seen. Some patients develop glaucoma [14]. Sensorineural or mixed conductive and neural deafness develops regularly.

Developmental delay may be evident within the first 12 months, but intellectual deterioration is progressive to a level of severe impairment. The peak of intellectual function may be about 2 to 4 years-of-age or earlier, after which there is a steady regression. Behavior is usually quite pleasant, and these are often lovable children despite their unusual appearance.

Shortness of stature is characteristic. Linear growth appears to stop at 2 to 3 years-of-age. Maximum height in one large series was 97 cm [13]; few exceed 100 cm. The neck is short,

and the large head appears to rest directly on the thorax. The lower rib cage flares. The back is kyphotic, and there is a gibbus in the lower thoracic or upper lumbar area (Figure 77.5). The joints become stiff, and mobility may be severely limited, especially at the elbows. The hands become broad, and the fingers stubby. This, and the limitation of extension and the position in flexion, produces the characteristic claw hand (Figure 77.8). The abdomen is protuberant. The liver and spleen become very large and very hard. Umbilical hernias are the rule, and inguinal hernias and hydroceles are common. Recurrence of a hernia is frequent following surgical repair.

Cardiac complications are prominent late features of the disease and often represent the cause of death. Some patients have been reported in whom acute cardiomyopathy and endocardial fibroelastosis were evident in the first year of life [15,16]. These are infantile cardiac manifestations. Later cardiac disease is valvular; murmurs, aortic regurgitation and mitral or tricuspid atresia result from storage of mucopolysaccharide in the valves. These features lead to congestive cardiac failure. Thickening of the valves of the coronary arteries leads to angina pectoris and myocardial infarction. Coronary angiography may underestimate the degree of involvement [17]. Patients may also die of pneumonia. They tolerate anesthesia very poorly [13].

The roentgenographic appearance of dysostosis multiplex in these patients is classic [18,19] (Figures 77.9–77.14). The shafts of all of the bones widen. The cortical walls become thickened externally during the first year of life, but later they become thin as the medullary cavity dilates. Lack of normal modeling and tubulation characterizes all of the bones (Figures 77.9, 77.10). Epiphyseal centers are poorly developed. The bones of the upper extremities become short and stubby (Figure 77.10) and taper toward the ends, often with enlargement of the mid-portions. The ends of the radius and ulna angulate toward each other (Figure 77.10). The roentgenographic appearance of the claw hand (Figure 77.9) of the patient with Hurler syndrome is pathognomonic of dysostosis multiplex. The metacarpals are broad at their distal ends

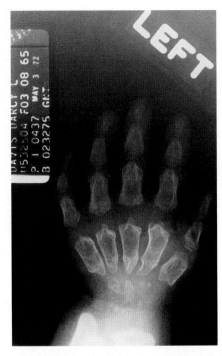

Figure 77.9 *D.D. Dysostosis multiplex is seen classically in the bones of the hand. The radial and ulnar articular surfaces are angulated toward each other. Marked irregularity and retarded ossification of the carpal bones are seen as well as coarsening of the trabeculae of the phalanges and metacarpals. The metacarpals are broadened at their distal ends and tapered at the proximal ends with a hook-like deformity. The phalanges, especially the distal ones, are short and the proximal and middle phalanges are characteristically thick and bullet-shaped.*

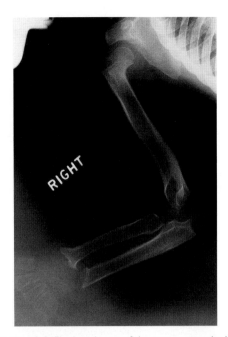

Figure 77.10 *D.D. The long bones of the upper extremity illustrate the lack of normal modeling and tubulation of the diaphyses, making these bones short and stubby. There was a varus deformity of the humerus. The ulnar semilunar notch was shallow and the radioulnar inclination abnormal.*

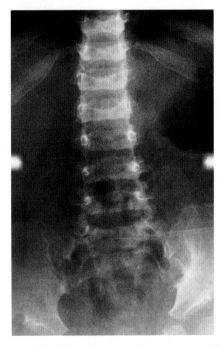

Figure 77.11 *D.D. The roentgenographic appearance of the ribs was classic. The spatulate shape is caused by a generalized widening of the ribs, which spares the relatively narrow proximal portions.*

and taper at their proximal ends. The phalanges are thickened and bullet-shaped. The lower extremities show moderate enlargement of the shaft. There may be coxa valga, small femoral heads and a poorly developed pelvis. The lower ribs are broad and spatulate (Figure 77.11). The clavicle is absolutely characteristic, while the lateral portion may be hypoplastic or even absent. The vertebrae are hypoplastic, scalloped posteriorly and beaked anteriorly, especially at the thoracolumbar junction (Figure 77.12). In this area there is anterior vertebral wedging, and this leads to the thoracolumbar gibbus, with typically a hooked-shaped vertebra at the gibbus. Hypoplasia of the odontoid may be present, and this can lead to atlantoaxial subluxation, as in Morquio disease (Chapter 81). The skull is large, the orbits shallow and the sella turcica shoe-shaped or J-shaped (Figures 77.13, 77.14).

Complications include cord compression, hydrocephalus and pigmentary degeneration of the retina. Death usually occurs by 10 years of age. At autopsy, the weight of the brain is increased, indicating that the increase in head size is a consequence of the storage of material. Thickening of the meninges is also seen. It is for this reason that some patients develop hydrocephalus. Pachymeningitis in the cervical area may also lead to myelitis or spinal nerve root compression.

Electron-microscopic examination of the brain reveals the presence of zebra bodies resembling those of Tay-Sachs disease (Chapter 91). These findings have been interpreted as indicating the accumulation of ganglioside in brain [20], and

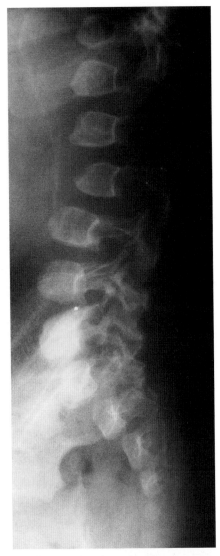

Figure 77.12 *Roentgenographic appearance of the spine of D.D. The antero-posterior distance was diminished in the vertebral bodies, and there was marked posterior scalloping. The pedicles of the lumbar spine were elongated. There was a marked thoracolumbar gibbus and inferior beaking of T12, L1 and L2.*

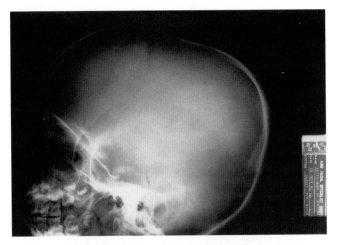

Figure 77.13 *S.M.Q. Roentgenogram of the skull illustrates the early appearance of the J-shaped sella turcica.*

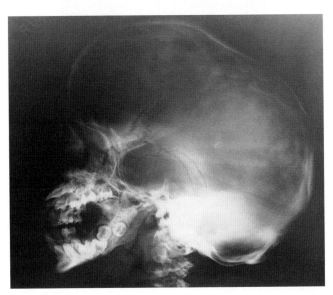

Figure 77.14 *Roentgenographic appearance of the skull of D.D. The very large cranium of both occipital and frontal areas was prominent. There was calcification of the choroid plexus of the left lateral ventricle. There was enormous enlargement of the sella and erosion of the clinoid processes. The mandibular rami were short, and there was increased angulation at the junction of the body and the varus, as well as flattening of the condyles.*

this has been documented chemically [21]. Large vacuolated cells are found in many tissues.

Characteristic granules (Reilly bodies) are found in the polymorphonuclear and other leukocytes (Figure 77.15). The mucopolysaccharide found in tissues such as the liver and spleen is dermatan sulfate [21,22]. Large quantities of dermatan sulfate and heparan sulfate are excreted in the urine. In Hurler syndrome these two compounds are excreted in an approximate ratio of 2:1. Mucopolysaccharide also accumulates in the brain. Metachromasia may be demonstrated in cultured fibroblasts by a pink stain with toluidine blue [23]. Quantitative analyses have revealed increased amounts of dermatan sulfate in fibroblasts of patients with Hurler syndrome [24,25].

GENETICS AND PATHOGENESIS

The Hurler syndrome is determined by an autosomal recessive gene. Parental consanguinity has commonly been reported. The incidence of the disease in a British Columbia survey was estimated at one in 144 000 births [26].

The molecular defect in Hurler disease is in the activity of α-L-iduronidase (Figure 77.1) [3,4,5]. This enzyme catalyzes the hydrolysis terminal iduronic acid residues of dermatan sulfate and heparan sulfate. The enzyme has been purified from human liver, kidney, and lung [27–29]. The cDNA

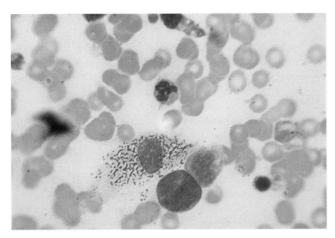

Figure 77.15   *Bone marrow illustrating the Reilly bodies of Hurler syndrome. The histiocytes in the center of the field were full of these inclusions. (This illustration was kindly provided by Dr. Faith Kung of the University of California San Diego.)*

codes a protein of 653 amino acids [30]. The protein exists as a monomer of 70 kDa minus the signal sequence [31]. There are six potential sites for N-glycosylation. It acquires mannose-6-phosphate, which permits targeting to lysosomes [31]. The deficient activity of enzyme is readily demonstrated in cultured fibroblasts and in leukocytes [32–35]. Residual activity of the enzyme has not been useful in distinguishing variants with phenotypes of greater or lesser severity, including the Scheie syndrome. Immunochemical studies have also not been helpful with these distinctions.

Carrier detection can be performed by assay of the enzyme in cultured fibroblasts or in freshly isolated leukocytes, in either of which activity of iduronidase is about half that of normal cells [36,37]. However, the ranges of activity in both normal and carrier populations are so great that it may be difficult to ascertain for certain that any individual is a non-carrier [38]. A positive identification of a carrier should be reliable. If the mutation in the proband is known, analysis of the DNA for heterozygosity in relatives is precise.

Prenatal diagnosis may be carried out [39] by assay of ^{35}S-mucopolysaccharide accumulation or the activity of iduronidase. In the ^{35}S assay, normal amniocytes behave just like fibroblasts, but iduronidase activity is much lower in amniocytes than in fibroblasts, and this could cause difficulties in distinguishing a heterozygote from an affected fetus. Prenatal diagnosis has also been accomplished by assay of iduronidase in chorionic villi [40], but activity is normally so very low in this material that great care is required.

The gene for iduronidase consists of 14 exons and approximately 19 kb. A large 13 kb intron separates the second and third exons [7]. There is a canine model of MPS I, and the canine gene for iduronidase has the same structure as the human gene [41]. The mutation in the model is a G to A transition in the donor splice site of intron 1, which leads to retention of this large intron in the RNA and premature termination of the intron-exon junction. A locus D4S111 linked to

Huntington disease on chromosome 4 has turned out to be the iduronidase gene [42].

The mutations that account for more than 50 percent of the alleles in populations of European origin change a tryptophan at position 402 and a glutamine at 70 to stop-codons; both yield no detectable functional protein [8,9,10]. Premature termination is also present at a deletion/insertion in exon 6 for which a Libyan Jewish patient with Hurler disease was homozygous [11]. Stop-codons resulting from changes of tyrosine 64 and glutamine 310 were found in Arab patients [12], as well as a threonine-to-proline change at 366 and a glycine-to-arginine change at 409. Among Japanese there are two common mutations, a 5 bp insertion between nts704 and 705, and R89Q which is seen in Caucasians, but uncommonly [43]. Homozygotes for all of these mutations except the Japanese missense mutation and compounds of any two of the others have a severe Hurler phenotype. Homozygosity for the first of these Japanese mutations conveyed a severe phenotype. Splice site mutations and deletions have also been observed [44]. In addition to the considerable mutational heterogeneity among MPSI patients, there are many polymorphic alleles consistent with common haplotype structure [45]. In homozygous setting null mutations and coding disruptions lead to the severe Hurler phenotype [45]; missense mutations are found that are individually characteristic of the H, HS or S phenotypes.

TREATMENT

The discovery of the MPS correcting factor capable of correcting the defective glycosaminoglycan catabolism in cultured cells raised the hope that these diseases might be treatable by transplantation or enzyme replacement therapy. The availability of animal models and recombinant enzyme with the mannose-6-phosphate recognition signal [46] as well as successes in the clinical management of Gaucher disease provided hope for successful enzyme replacement therapy. Recombinant iduronidase prepared in hamster cells administered to homozygous animals led to major improvement in storage in liver, spleen and kidney, but no improvement in brain, heart valves or cornea [46].

Enzyme replacement with human recombinant α-L-iduronidase has been reported [47,48] in 45 patients with MPSI. Patients were selected with Hurler-Scheie or Scheie phenotypes and given enzyme intravenously weekly for as long as 62 weeks. Hepatosplenomegaly decreased significantly in all patients. Liver size was normal in eight patients by 26 weeks. Growth in height and weight increased in prepubertal patients. Improvements were also notable in respiratory function and joint mobility as well as in the urinary excretion of glycosaminoglycans. The enzyme has now been approved by the FDA and is marketed as Aldurazyme (BioMarin/Genzyme). Corneal clouding did not change, and cardiac valvular disease did not appear altered. There is little likelihood that this approach would affect the brain.

Bone marrow transplantation [49] was followed by arrest or reversal of many of the peripheral features of the disease. It did not seem likely that this would appreciably affect the central nervous system, but longer-term follow-up of the results of bone marrow transplantation in Hurler disease [50] have documented resolution of hydrocephalus and, in four patients with normal IQs before the procedure, maintenance of intelligence for two to seven years post-transplantation. It appears clear that if performed early enough bone marrow transplantation will preserve cerebral function.

Magnetic resonance spectroscopy indicated high ratios of presumptive MPS to creatinine that did not fall after bone marrow transplantation [51]. Bone marrow transplantation appears not to improve the skeletal or ocular manifestations of the disease. In patients without a compatible donor, unrelated umbilical cord blood transplantation may be an option. It is possible that transplantation and enzyme replacement therapy may be complementary.

Supportive management includes shunting for hydrocephalus, surgical decompression for carpal tunnel syndrome, tonsillectomy and adenoidectomy for airway obstruction, and otitis media, hearing aids and visual aids. Inguinal hernias should be repaired. Cardiac valvular surgery may be indicated.

References

1 Hurler G. Ueber einen Typ multiplier Abartungen Vorwiegend am Skelettsystem. *Z Kinderheilk* 1919;**24**:220.
2 McKusick VA. *Heritable Disorders of Connective Tissue* (4th edn). CV Mosby Co, St Louis;1972:521.
3 Bach G, Friedman R, Weismann B, Neufeld EF. The defect in the Hurler and Scheie syndromes: deficiency of α-L-iduronidase. *Proc Natl Acad Sci USA* 1972;**69**:2048.
4 Matalon R, Cifonelli JA, Dorfman A. L-Iduronidase in cultured human fibroblasts and liver. *Biochem Biophys Res Commun* 1971;**42**:340.
5 Matalon R, Dorfman A. Hurler's syndrome, an α-L-iduronidase deficiency. *Biochem Biophys Res Commun* 1972;**47**:959.
6 Scott HS, Ashton LJ, Eyre HJ, et al. Chromosomal localization of the human α-L-iduronidase gene (IDUA) to 4 p 163. *Am J Hum Genet* 1990;**47**:802.
7 Scott HS, Guo X-H, Hopwood JJ, Morris CP. Structure and sequence of the human α-L-iduronidase gene. *Genomics* 1992;**13**:1811.
8 Bunge S, Kleijer WJ, Steglich C, et al. Mucopolysaccharidosis type I: identification of 8 novel mutations and determination of the frequency of the two common alpha-L-iduronidase mutations (W402X and Q70X) among European patients. *Hum Mol Genet* 1994;**3**:861.
9 Scott HS, Liyjens T, Hopwood JJ, Morris CP. A common mutation for mucopolysaccharidosis Type 1 associated with a severe Hurler phenotype. *Hum Mut* 1992;**1**:103.
10 Scott HS, Litjens T, Nelson PV, et al. α-L-Iduronidase mutations (Q70X and P533X) associated with severe Hurler phenotype. *Hum Mut* 1992;**1**:333.
11 Moskowitz SM, Tieu PT, Neufeld EF. A deletion/insertion mutation in the IDUA gene in a Libyan Jewish patient with Hurler syndrome (Mucopolysaccharidosis I). *Hum Mut* 1993;**2**:71.
12 Bach G, Moskowitz SM, Tieu PT, Neufeld EF. Molecular analysis of Hurler syndrome in Druze and Muslim Arab patients in Israel: multiple allelic mutations of the IDUA gene in a small geographic area. *Am J Hum Genet* 1993;**53**:330.
13 Leroy JG, Crocker C. Clinical definition of the Hurler–Hunter phenotypes. A review of 50 patients. *Am J Dis Child* 1966;**112**:518.
14 Nowaczyk MJ, Clarke JT, Morin JD. Glaucoma as an early complication of Hurler's disease. *Arch Dis Child* 1988;**63**:1091.
15 Donaldson MDC, Pennock CA, Berry PJ, et al. Hurler syndrome with cardiomyopathy in infancy. *J Pediatr* 1989;**114**:430.
16 Stephan MJ, Stevens EL Jr, Wenstrup RJ, et al. Mucopolysaccharidosis. I presenting with endocardial fibroelastosis of infancy. *Am J Dis Child* 1989;**143**:782.
17 Braunlin EA, Hunter DQ, Krivit W, et al. Evaluation of coronary artery disease in the Hurler syndrome by angiography. *Am J Cardiol* 1992;**69**:1487.
18 Caffey J. Gargoylism (Hunter–Hurler disease dysostosis multiplex lipochondrodystrophy). *Am J Roentgenol Radium Ther Nucl Med* 1952;**67**:715.
19 Grossman H, Dorst JP. The mucopolysaccharidoses and mucolipidoses: in *Progress in Pediatric Radiology* (ed. HJ Kauffman). Charger, Basel;1973:495.
20 McKusick VA. The nosology of the mucopolysaccharidoses. *Am J Med* 1969;**47**:730.
21 Dorfman A, Matalon R. The Hurler and Hunter syndromes. *Am J Med* 1969;**47**:691.
22 Muir H. The structure and metabolism of mucopolysaccharides. *Am J Med* 1969;**47**:673.
23 Danes BS, Bearn AG. Hurler's syndrome: demonstration of an inherited disorder of connective tissue in cell culture. *Science* 1965;**149**:989.
24 Matalon R, Dorfman A. Acid mucopolysaccharides in cultured human fibroblasts. *Lancet* 1969;**2**:838.
25 Matalon R, Dorfman A. Hurler's syndrome: biosynthesis of acid mucopolysaccharides in tissue culture. *Proc Natl Acad Sci USA* 1966;**56**:1310.
26 Lowry RB, Renwick DHG. Relative frequency of the Hurler and Hunter syndromes. *N Engl J Med* 1971;**284**:221.
27 Rome LH, Garvin AJ, Neufeld EF. Human kidney α-L-iduronidase: purification and characterization. *Arch Biochem Biophys* 1978;**189**:344.
28 Clemens PR, Brooks DA, Saccone GPT, Hopwood JJ. Human α-L-iduronidase. 1 Purification monoclonal antibody production and subunit molecular mass. *Eur J Biochem* 1985;**152**:21.
29 Schuchman EH, Guzman NA, Desnick RJ. Human α-L-iduronidase. 1 Purification and properties of the high uptake (higher molecular weight) and low uptake (processed) forms. *J Biol Chem* 1984;**259**:3132.
30 Scott HS, Anson DS, Orsborn AM, et al. Human α-L-iduronidase: cDNA isolation and expression. *Proc Natl Acad Sci USA* 1991;**88**:9695.
31 Myerowitz R, Neufeld EF. Maturation of α-L-iduronidase in cultured human fibroblasts. *J Biol Chem* 1981;**256**:3044.
32 Hall CW, Liebaers I, Di Natale P, Neufeld EF. Enzymic diagnosis of the genetic mucopolysaccharide storage disorders. *Methods Enzymol* 1978;**50**:439.
33 Kresse H, von Figura K, Klein U, et al. Enzymic diagnosis of the genetic mucopolysaccharide storage disorders. *Methods Enzymol* 1982;**83**:559.
34 Hopwood JJ, Muller V, Smithson A, and Baggett N. A fluorometric assay using 4-methylumbelliferyl a-L-iduronide for the estimation of α-L-iduronidase activity and the detection of Hurler and Scheie syndromes. *Clin Chim Acta* 1979;**92**:257.
35 Weissmann B. Synthetic substrates for α-L-iduronidase. *Methods Enzymol* 1978;**50**:141.
36 Hall CW, Neufeld EF. α-L-Iduronidase activity in cultured skin fibroblasts and amniotic fluid cells. *Arch Biochem Biophys* 1973;**158**:817.
37 Kelly TE, Taylor HA Jr. Leukocyte values of α-L-iduronidase in mucopolysaccharidosis I. *J Med Genet* 1976;**13**:149.

38 Shapiro LJ. Current status and future direction for carrier detection in lysosomal storage diseases: in *Lysosomes and Lysosomal Storage Diseases* (eds Callahan JW, Lowden JA). Raven Press, New York;1981:343.

39 Fratantoni JC, Neufeld EF, Uhlendorf BW, Jacobson CB. Intrauterine diagnosis of the Hurler and Hunter syndrome. *N Engl J Med* 1969;**280**:686.

40 Young EP. Prenatal diagnosis of Hurler disease by analysis of α-L-iduronidase in chorionic villi. *J Inherit Metab Dis* 1992;**15**:224.

41 Menon KP, Tieu PT, Neufeld EF. Architecture of the canine IDUA gene and mutation underlying canine mucopolysaccharidosis. *Genomics* 1992;**14**:763.

42 MacDonald ME, Scott HS, Whaley WL, *et al.* Huntington disease-linked locus D4S111 exposed as the α-L-iduronidase gene. *Somat Cell Mol Genet* 1991;**17**:421.

43 Yamagishi A, Tomatsu S, Fukuda S, *et al.* Mucopolysaccharidosis type I: identification of common mutations that cause Hurler and Scheie syndromes in Japanese populations. *Hum Mutat* 1996;**7**:23.

44 Scott HS, Bunge S, Gal A, *et al.* Molecular genetics of mucopolysaccharidosis type I: diagnostic clinical and biological implications. *Hum Mutat* 1995;**6**:288.

45 Li P, Wood T, Thompson JN. Diversity of mutations and distribution of single nucleotide polymorphic alleles in the human α-L-iduronidase (IDUA) gene. *Genet Med* 2002;**4**:420.

46 Shull RM, Kakkis ED, McEntee MF, *et al.* Enzyme replacement in a canine model of Hurler syndrome. *Proc Nat Acad Sci USA* 1994;**91**:12937.

47 Kakkis ED, Muenzer J, Tiller GE, *et al.* Enzyme-replacement therapy in mucopolysaccharidsosis I. *N Engl J Med* 2001;**344**:182.

48 Muenzer J, Clark LA, Kolodny EH, *et al.* Enzyme replacement therapy for MPS I: 36-week interim results of the phase 3 open-label extension study. Proc Annual Clin Genetic Meeting (ACMG). *Genet Med* 2003;34.

49 Krivit W, Peters C, Shapiro EG. Bone marrow transplantation as effective treatment of central nervous system disease in globoid cell leukodystrophy, metachromatic leukodystrophy, adrenoleukodystrophy, mannosidosis, fucosidosis, aspartylglucosaminuria, Hurler, Marteaux-Lamy and Sly syndromes, and Gaucher disease type III. *Curr Opin Neurol* 1999;**12**:167.

50 Whitley CB, Belani KG, Chang PN, *et al.* Long term outcome of Hurler syndrome following bone marrow transplantation. *Am J Hum Genet* 1993;**46**:209.

51 Takahashi Y, Sukegawa K, Aoki M, *et al.* Evaluation of accumulated mucopolysaccharides in the brain of patients with mucopolysaccharidoses by H-magnetic resonance spectroscopy before and after bone marrow transplantation. *Pediatr Res* 2001;**49**:349.

78

Scheie and Hurler–Scheie diseases/mucopolysaccharidosis IS and IHS/α-iduronidase deficiency

MAJOR PHENOTYPIC EXPRESSION

Scheie: stiffness of joints, corneal clouding, disease of the aortic valve, dystosis multiplex, normal intelligence. Hurler–Scheie: intermediate between Hurler and Scheie.

INTRODUCTION

Scheie, Hamprick and Barness [1], in 1962, described the phenotype as a 'forme fruste of Hurler's disease'. This was prescient, as it turned out that the phenotypes are allelic, both resulting from deficiency of the enzyme α-iduronidase (see Figure 77.1). It was the delineation of corrective factors by Fratantoni, Hall and Neufeld [2] that led to the clear recognition that the Hurler and Scheie genes were allelic, because sulfate accumulation in Hurler fibroblasts was not cross-corrected by Scheie cells, and vice versa [3], and Hurler–Scheie corrective factor was identified as α-l-iduronidase [4]. Both Hurler and Scheie fibroblasts contained no demonstrable α-iduronidase activity against substrate phenyl α-l-iduronide [5,6].

The intermediate Hurler–Scheie phenotype was first named on clinical grounds by McKusick [7], who postulated that Hurler IH and Scheie IH phenotypes represented homozygosity for one or the other allele and predicted that there would be compounds which expressed an intermediate phenotype that he called IH-S [7]. Actually it turns out that some of the intermediate phenotypes represent homozygosity for some specific mutations [8]. The cloning of the iduronidase gene on chromosome 4 [9] made it clear that there are many mutations and more to be discovered. Compounds are found even within each of the phenotypes, as are homozygotes. Among the latter with the H-S phenotype are P533R, which is the most common, and particularly common in Morocco [10] where it is the only mucopolysaccharidosis I (MPSI) mutation found to date, and A327P found in Italy and Brazil [11,12]. The Scheie phenotype was found in Brazil [11] and commonly in Japan [13] with homozygosity for R89Q.

CLINICAL ABNORMALITIES

Scheie disease

The Scheie phenotype has been of particular interest to ophthalmologists, because patients live long enough for the severe corneal clouding to affect vision. It is most dense on the periphery. The patient may first be aware early in the second decade, but it is diagnosable by slit lamp very early. There may also be pigmentary degeneration of the retina. Some patients develop glaucoma. Visual impairment may progress to blindness.

Abnormalities of the joints maybe evident early in childhood (Figure 78.1), at least by the age of 5 years. Joints are

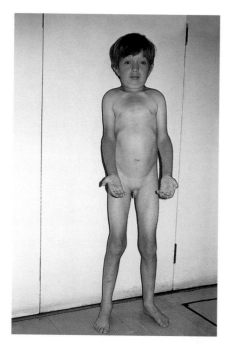

Figure 78.1   *A 7-year-old boy with Scheie disease illustrates the early claw hand deformities and gene valgum. (Illustration was kindly provided by Dr. Philip Benson.)*

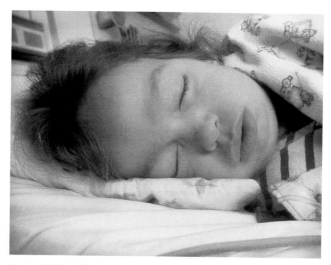

Figure 78.2   *C.L., a 13-year-old girl with Hurler–Scheie disease. Her face in repose showed clear evidence of mucopolysaccharide storage especially about the lips and nose. Corneas were slightly cloudy.*

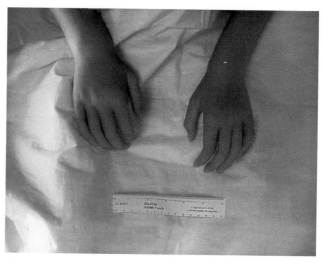

Figure 78.3   *C.L. She had the claw hand with considerable limitation of motion. There were also contractures at the shoulders and elbows, and she could not raise her hands above her head.*

stiff and angulated [14]. The claw hand may be identical to that of Hurler disease. Genu valgum is present early. There may be pes cavus and a stiff painful foot. Carpal tunnel syndrome is a common complication due to entrapment of the median nerve [15]. Distal interphalangeal acute angulation gives a trigger-finger appearance [15]. Degenerative arthritis of the hip has been reported [16] along with large femoral cysts and pathologic fracture, but this appears to be rare. Stature is normal.

Facial features may be somewhat coarse, but are often not recognizable as those of a mucopolysaccharidosis. Hypertrichosis is common, and so are inguinal hernias. Some patients develop deafness, and it can be progressive.

Life expectancy may be normal except in those that develop cardiac disease [17]. Aortic stenosis or regurgitation may be evident even early, but, as deposits of mucopolysaccharide increase on the valves and chordae tendinae, disability may develop [18–21]. Sleep apnea was reported in two brothers, 18 and 35 years-of-age, which was relieved by tracheostomy [22].

Neurologic manifestations are uncommon, but myelopathy has been reported as a consequence of cervical cord compression from thickened dura, the so-called pachymeningitis cervicalis [23,24]. This problem is more common in the H-S variants.

Hurler–Scheie disease

The clinical features of these patients are intermediate between those of the Hurler and Scheie phenotypes (Figures 78.2–78.11). Features may be coarse (Figure 78.2) or not, especially with time (Figure 78.11); an adult patient may have really grotesque features, having lived so much longer than a Hurler patient, and consequently had time to accumulate large amounts of mucopolysaccharide. Some patients have micrognathism, and this may contribute to a distinctive facial appearance [25]. Intellectual functions may be normal; some are mentally retarded. Survival to adulthood is common. Pregnancy has been reported [26]. Stature is short.

Clouding of the cornea is a regular feature of this disorder. In fact, only one patient has been reported with iduronidase deficiency in whom the corneas remained clear (to 14 years at the time of report) [27].

Hernias, stiffness of the joints and the classic claw hand (Figure 78.8) are seen uniformly; so is hepatosplenomegaly

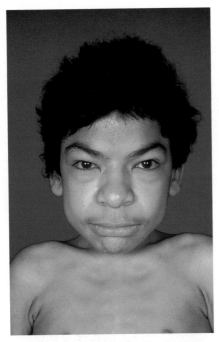

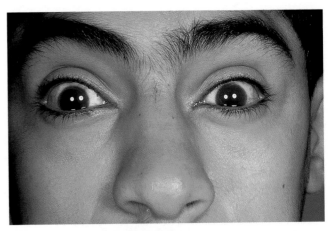

Figure 78.6   *H.Y. There was bilateral clouding of the cornea that ultimately led to corneal transplantation.*

Figure 78.4   *H.Y., a 16-year-old Saudi boy with α-iduronidase deficiency and the clinical phenotype of the Hurler–Scheie syndrome. Formal psychometric testing revealed the intelligence to be normal. He was short; height was 129 cm, and he had coarse facial features, including a large nose and thick lips and hirsutism.*

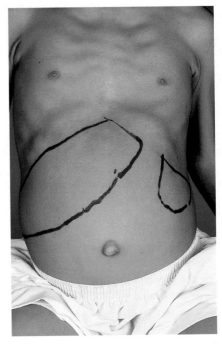

Figure 78.7   *H.Y. Liver and spleen were enlarged as outlined.*

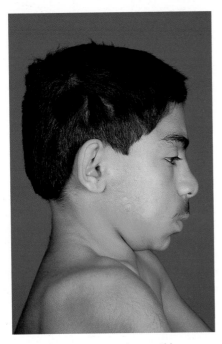

Figure 78.5   *H.Y. There was some micrognathism.*

(Figure 78.7). Lesions of the cardiac valves may cause cardiac failure and death. Myelopathy from cord compression is a frequent complication in this condition, as is hydrocephalus resulting from mucopolysaccharide deposition in the meninges

[28]. Increased intracranial pressure led to muscle weakness and spasticity attributed to obstruction of the basilar cisterns [28]. This patient presented first at 25 years-of-age with paranoia. Psychosis has also been observed in the Scheie syndrome. Another patient had marked destruction of the sella and the cribriform plate and spinal fluid rhinorrhea, as well as blindness from pressure on the optic nerves.

The pathologic appearance of the Hurler-Scheie and of the Scheie disease is that of widespread deposition of mucopolysaccharide [25,28]. The thickened dura may contain foamy macrophages and increased quantities of collagen. In MPS IS, cortical neurons have been reported as normal, while somatic cells are no different than those in MPS IH. In MPS IHS, changes in cortical neurons are less frequent than

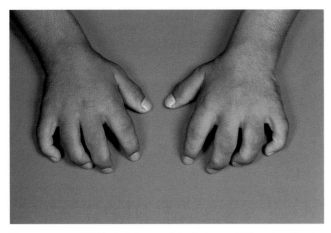

Figure 78.8 *H.Y. The hands were broad, short and flexed, and had a Hurler appearance. There was limitation of joint motion, which was progressive, and he had chronic joint pains.*

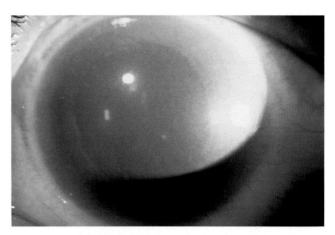

Figure 78.10 *A.M.A. The cornea was quite cloudy, and he had glaucoma. Two sisters had Hurler-Scheie disease and all had deficient activity of α-iduronidase. Parents were consanguineous.*

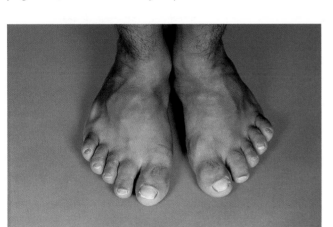

Figure 78.9 *H.Y. The feet were also short and broad.*

those seen in the anterior horn cells of the cord, in which there are typical concentric lamellar inclusions.

GENETICS AND PATHOGENESIS

The Scheie and Hurler-Scheie phenotypes are inherited in autosomal recessive fashion. The fundamental defect is in the α-L-iduronidase [5]. In general, it has not been possible to distinguish the Scheie from more severely affected individuals on the basis of residual enzyme in the usual assays with artificial substrates [29,30]. Some residual activity has been reported in a radioactive disaccharide assay [31], and others have found some activity in fibroblasts of Scheie patients when desulfated heparan was the substrate [32]. The Scheie disease has been estimated to occur at a frequency of one to 500 000 births in British Columbia [33].

It became clear that patients with the Hurler–Scheie phenotype have resulted from consanguineous matings [34,35], indicating that the phenotype may result from homozygosity for single mutant alleles rather than compounds of Hurler

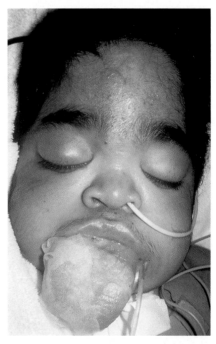

Figure 78.11 *A 22-year-old with Hurler–Scheie syndrome. Facial features were classic. The enormous tongue had led to respiratory obstruction and tracheotomy. The patient was in intensive care. Liver and spleen were greatly enlarged and he had typical trident hand.*

and Scheie alleles. Cell hybridization studies of all three phenotypes have led to failure of complementation [36]. These issues have been clarified by the definition of mutations. One patient with the Scheie phenotype has been found to have an allele with a G-to-A transition in intron 5 which creates a new acceptor splice site without losing the original site; thus some normal enzyme is produced [37,38], as demonstrated by enzyme assay of fibroblasts of the patient [39]. Compound heterozygosity for R89Q, which causes a mild phenotype when homozygous, and 704ins5, which causes a severe phenotype, produced an intermediate pattern of disease in Japanese patients.

TREATMENT

The supportive management and enzyme replacement set out in Chapter 77 is particularly appropriate for Scheie and Hurler–Scheie patients. Corneal transplantation has been successful [40,41]. Aggressive surgical treatment of glaucoma and carpal tunnel syndrome is also indicated. Cardiac valve replacement has also been successful in both IS and IH/IS patients [18,19]. Hydrocephalus requires shunting, and cervical cord decompression may be required.

References

1 Scheie HG, Hamprick GM Jr, Barness LH. A newly recognized form fruste of Hurler's disease (gargoylism). *Am J Ophthalmol* 1962;**53**:753.

2 Fratantoni JC, Hall CW, Neufeld EF. The defect in Hurler's and Hunter's syndromes: faulty degradation of mucopolysaccharides. *Proc Natl Acad Sci USA* 1988;**60**:699.

3 Weismann U, Neufeld EF. Scheie and Hurler syndromes: apparent identity of the biochemical defect. *Science* 1970;**169**:72.

4 Neufeld EF, Cantz MJ. Corrective factors for inborn errors of mucopolysaccharide metabolism. *Ann NY Acad Sci* 1971;**179**:580.

5 Bach G, Friedman R, Weismann B, Neufeld EF. The defect in the Hurler and Scheie syndromes: deficiency of α-L-iduronidase. *Proc Natl Acad Sci USA* 1972;**69**:2048.

6 Matalon R, Dorfman A. Hurler's syndrome and α-L-iduronidase deficiency. *Biochem Biophys Res Commun* 1972;**47**:959.

7 McKusick VA, Howell RR, Hussels IE, *et al*. Allelism nonallelism and genetic compounds among the mucopolysaccharidoses. *Lancet* 1972;**1**:993.

8 Li P, Wood T, Thompson JN. Diversity of mutations and distribution of single nucleotide polymorphic alleles in the human α-L-iduronidase (IDUA) gene. *Genet Med* 2002;**4**:420.

9 Schuchman EH, Astrin KH, Aula P, Desnick RJ. Regional assignment of the structural gene for α-L-iduronidase. *Proc Natl Acad Sci USA* 1984;**81**:1169.

10 Alif N, Hess K, Straczek J, *et al*. Mucopolysaccharidosis type I: characterization of a common mutation that causes Hurler syndrome in Moroccan subjects. *Ann Hum Genet* 1999;**63**:9.

11 Gatti R, DiNatale P, Villani GR, *et al*. Mutations among Italian mucopolysaccharidosis type I patients. *J Inherit Metab Dis* 1997;**20**:803.

12 Matte U, Leistner S, Lima L, *et al*. Unique frequency of known mutations in Brazilian MPS I patients. *Am J Med Genet* 2000;**90**:108.

13 Yamagishi A, Tomatsu S, Fukuda S, *et al*. Mucopolysaccharidosis type I: identification of common mutations that cause Hurler and Scheie syndrome in Japanese populations. *Hum Mutat* 1996;**7**:23.

14 Hamilton E, Pitt P. Articular manifestations of Scheie's syndrome. *Ann Rheum Dis* 1992;**51**:542.

15 MacDougal B, Weeks PM, Wray RC. Median nerve compression and trigger finger in the mucopolysaccharidoses and related diseases. *Plast Reconstr Surg* 1977;**59**:260.

16 Lamon JM, Trojak JE, Abbott MH. Bone cysts in mucopolysaccharidosis I S (Scheie syndrome). *Johns Hopkins Med J* 1980;**146**:73.

17 Dekaban AS, Constantopoulos G, Herman MM, Steusing JK. Mucopolysaccharidosis type V (Scheie syndrome). A postmortem study by multidisciplinary techniques with emphasis on the brain. *Arch Pathol Lab Med* 1976;**100**:237.

18 Pyeritz RE. Cardiovascular manifestations of heritable disorders of connective tissue: in *Progress in Medical Genetics* (eds Steinberg AG, Bearn AG, Motulsky AG, Childs B). Saunders, Philadelphia; 1983:191.

19 Butman SM, Karl L, Copelands JG. Combined aortic and mitral valve replacement in an adult with Scheie's disease. *Chest* 1989;**96**:209.

20 Horton WA, Schimke RN. A new mucopolysaccharidosis. *J Pediatr* 1970;**77**:252.

21 Emerit I, Maroteaux P, Vernant P. Deux observations de mucopolysaccharidose avec atteinte cardio-vasculare. *Arch Franc Pediatr* 1966;**23**:1075.

22 Perks WH, Cooper RA, Bradbury S, *et al*. Sleep apnoea in Scheie's syndrome. *Thorax* 1980;**35**:85.

23 Kennedy P, Swash M, Dean MD. Cervical cord compression in mucopolysaccharidosis. *Dev Med Child Neurol* 1973;**15**:194.

24 Paulson GW, Meagler JN, Burkhart J. Spinal pachymeningitis secondary to mucopolysaccharidosis: case report. *J Neurosurg* 1974;**41**:618.

25 Kajii T, Matsuda I, Oshaw AT, *et al*. Hurler-Scheie genetic compound (mucopolysaccharidosis IH-IS) in Japanese brothers. *Clin Genet* 1974;**6**:394.

26 Thompson JN, Finley SC, Lorincz AE, Finley WH. Absence of α-L-iduronidase activity in various tissues from two sibs affected with presumably the Hurler–Scheie syndrome: in *Disorders of Connective Tissue* (ed. D Bergsma). National Foundation-March of Dimes, New York;1975: Vol XI, 341.

27 Gardner RJM, Hay HR. Hurler's syndrome with clear corneas. *Lancet* 1974;**2**:845.

28 Winters PR, Harrod MJ, Molenich-Heetred SA, *et al*. α-L-iduronidase deficiency and possible Hurler–Scheie genetic compound: clinical pathologic and biochemical findings. *Neurology* 1976;**26**:1003.

29 Hall CW, Liebaers I, DiNatale P, Neufeld EF. Enzymic diagnosis of the genetic mucopolysaccharide storage disorders. *Meth Enzymol* 1978;**50**:539.

30 Dinatale P, Leder JG, Neufeld EF. A radio-active substrate and assay for α-L-iduronidase. *Clin Chim Acta* 1977;**77**:211.

31 Hopwood JJ, Muller V. Biochemical discrimination of Hurler and Scheie syndromes. *Clin Sci* 1979;**57**:265.

32 Matalon R, Deanching M. The enzymic basis for the phenotypic variation of Hurler and Scheie syndromes. *Pediatr Res* 1977;**11**:519.

33 Lowry RB, Renwick DHG. The relative frequency of the Hurler and Hunter syndromes. *N Engl J Med* 1971;**284**:221 (letter).

34 Jensen OA, Pedersen C, Schwartz M, *et al*. Hurler-Scheie phenotype: report of an inbred sibship with tapeto-retinal degeneration and electron-microscopic examination of the conjunctiva. *Ophthalmologica* 1978;**176**:194.

35 Kaibara H, Eguchi M, Shibata K, Takagishi K. Hurler–Scheie phenotype: a report of two pairs of inbred sibs. *Hum Genet* 1979;**53**:37.

36 Bach G, Moskowitz SM, Tieu PT, Neufeld EM. Molecular analysis of Hurler in Druze and Muslim Arab patients in Israel: multiple allelic mutations of the IDUA gene in a small geographic area. *Am J Hum Genet* 1993;**53**:330.

37 Scott HS, Litjens T, Nelson PV, *et al*. Identification of mutations in the α-L-iduronidase gene (IDUA) that cause Hurler and Scheie syndromes. *Am J Hum Genet* 1993;**53**:973.

38 Moskowitz SM, Tieu PT, Neufeld EF. Mutation in Scheie syndrome (MPS IS): a GtoA transition creates a new splice site in intron 5 of one IDUA allele. *Hum Mut* 1993;**2**:41.

39 Fortuin JJH, Kleijer WJ. Hybridization studies of fibroblasts from Hurler, Scheie and Hurler-Scheie compound patients: support for the hypothesis of allelic mutants. *Hum Genet* 1980;**53**:155.

40 Wraith JE, Alani SM. Carpal tunnel syndrome in the mucopolysaccharidoses and related disorders. *Arch Dis Child* 1990;**65**:962.

41 Pronicka E, Tylki-Szymanska A, Kwast O, *et al*. Carpal tunnel syndrome in children with mucopolysaccharidoses: needs for surgical tendons and median nerve release. *J Ment Defic Res* 1988;**32**:79.

79

Hunter disease/mucopolysaccharidosis type II (MPS II)/iduronate sulfatase deficiency

MAJOR PHENOTYPIC EXPRESSION

Coarse features, stiff joints, short stature, mental retardation, hepatosplenomegaly, cardiomegaly, nodular or thickened skin lesions especially over the scapular area, dysostosis multiplex, accumulation of dermatan sulfate and heparan sulfate, and defective activity of iduronate sulfatase.

INTRODUCTION

Hunter [1], in 1917, described two brothers with what is now known as mucopolysaccharidosis type II. Patients with the Hunter disease have clinical features similar to those of Hurler disease, although usually they are less severely affected. Patients have been classified clinically into mild and severe forms, although the two cannot be distinguished on the basis of enzyme activity. The advent of molecular analysis and extensive heterogeneity may make this classification obsolete. Patients with this disease were found, by Dorfman and Matalon [2] and by Muir [3], to excrete dermatan sulfate and heparan sulfate just like those with Hurler disease. It was in studies of Hunter and Hurler cells that Fratantoni, Hall and Neufeld [4] first found the correction factors from each that corrected the defective excess accumulation of sulfate in the other; thus Hurler cells could correct Hunter cells and vice versa, and the Hunter corrective factor would correct Hurler and other MPS cells, but not Hunter cells [5]. The Hunter factor was identified as iduronate sulfatase [6] (Figure 79.1), the enzyme that catalyzes the release of sulfate from the iduronate sulfate moieties of dermatan and heparan sulfates. This is the site of the molecular defect in Hunter disease. Thus the defect in MPS II is

in the first step in the enzymatic breakdown of these mucopolysaccharides.

The gene for iduronate sulfatase has been identified [7] and mapped to the X chromosome at position q28 [8–10]. A number of gross alterations in the gene have been found [7,11], as well as point mutations, especially at CpG dinucleotides [12,13].

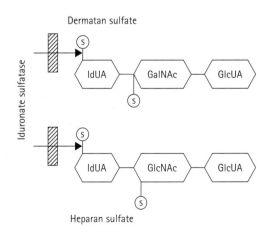

Figure 79.1 *Iduronate sulfatase, the site of the enzyme defect in Hunter disease. Both dermatan sulfate and heparan sulfate accumulate when activity is defective.*

CLINICAL ABNORMALITIES

Patients with Hunter disease present a broad spectrum of clinical activity; all of them have quite similar reduction in enzyme activity. Nevertheless, the disease has generally been subdivided into two groups, of severe and mild phenotypes, respectively [14–16].

Patients with the severe form may appear identical to those with Hurler disease (Figures 79.2, 79.3) except for the absence of cloudy corneas, but behavior is usually quite different.

Progression may be slower than in Hurler disease and the apparent onset may be later, often about 2 to 4 years-of-age. In the mild form (Figure 79.4) mental development may be normal, and lifespan may be long as in Scheie disease.

Hunter disease is distinguished from all other mucopolysaccharidoses by the presence of nodular or pebbly skin lesions (Figure 79.5), most characteristically over the scapular area, the upper arms or the lateral aspects of the thighs. The skin lesions are sometimes ivory in color. These lesions are not seen in any mucopolysaccharidosis except Hunter disease [17].

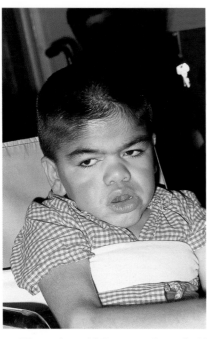

Figure 79.2 *C.T., a patient with Hunter syndrome. In this most severe form of the disease the features are quite coarse, the lips very thick, hirsutism prominent and the hands clawlike, as in Hurler disease. The corneas were clear.*

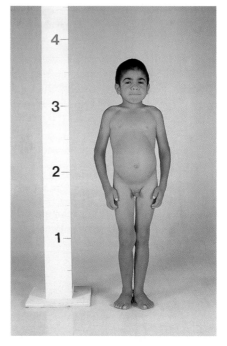

Figure 79.4 *A.M.A.Q., a 6-year-old boy with a milder expression form of Hunter disease. The hairline was low and the eyebrows bushy. The increased subcutaneous tissue was clearly evident in the anteverted nose, but features were less coarse than the patient in Figure 79.2. Limitation of joint motion was visible in the flexed elbows.*

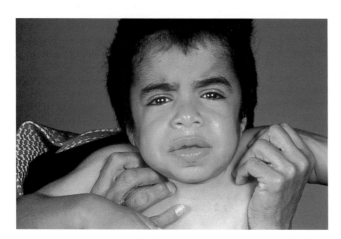

Figure 79.3 *A.D.F.S., an 8-year-old boy with Hunter disease. The facial features were quite coarse, the hairline low and the eyebrows abundant, and the lips were very full. Iduronate sulfatase activity was absent.*

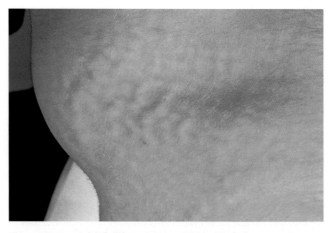

Figure 79.5 *A.D.F.S. The nodular or pebbly skin lesions constitute a cutaneous marker for the Hurler disease.*

As in other forms of mucopolysaccharidosis, chronic respiratory symptoms, rhinorrhea or stertorous breathing, or frequent upper respiratory infections and otitis media may be the earliest manifestations of disease. Presentation for hernia repair may be even earlier. Both inguinal and umbilical hernias are common. Mental development usually continues until at least 2 years-of-age.

Patients with the severe form of Hunter disease have the characteristic coarse features of mucopolysaccharidosis [18] (Figures 79.2, 79.3, 79.6, 79.7) The nose is flat, the nasal bridge depressed. The lips are thickened, the gums hypertrophic, and the tongue is large. Patients are generally hirsute and have low hairlines (Figures 79.2, 79.3). The superciliary ridges become very prominent. The head may appear disproportionately large. Stature is short, but this may not be as pronounced as in Hurler disease. Joints are stiff and mobility may become limited, or there may be contractures. Hearing loss is common; it may not be severe [19], but it tends to be progressive. The hands are broad and the fingers stubby. The clawhand appearance (Figures 79.6, 79.7) may be indistinguishable

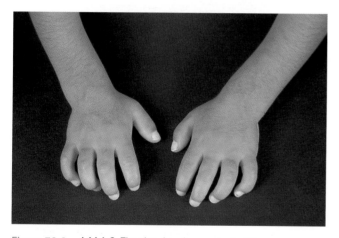

Figure 79.6   *A.M.A.Q. The claw hands were typical for mucopolysaccharidosis.*

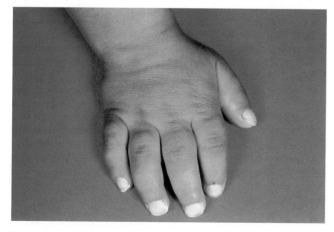

Figure 79.7   *The hand of A.D.F.S. was also typical.*

from that of Hurler patients. Patients tend to develop high coloration. The liver and spleen are large and hard.

Two important negative findings in the Hunter syndrome – the absence of a cloudy cornea and a gibbus [20] – distinguish it from Hurler syndrome. However, these patients may develop a rounded kyphosis and occasionally there is a severe kyphosis [21]. Corneal clouding may even be detected very late in the most severe forms of Hunter syndrome, but usually only with a slit lamp [22].

The voice is hoarse. Diarrhea may be a chronic problem; it may result from infiltration of the autonomic innervation of the intestine [23]. Retinitis pigmentosa may occur in this condition and retinal degeneration may cause blindness. Glaucoma may be a problem. Papilledema may be seen [24]; this is probably a consequence of pachymeningeal thickening, which may also lead to neurologic defects including quadriplegia from pressure on the cord [25]. It may also result in hydrocephalus [26]. Cerebral atrophy, which may also lead to ventricular enlargement, is seen regularly on computed tomography (CT) or magnetic resonance imaging (MRI) scan in severe Hunter disease [27–29], and there may be defective reabsorption of cerebrospinal fluid. Intracranial pressure may be increased.

Mental deterioration is progressive, but usually occurs at a slower rate than in Hurler disease. Rarely mental deterioration may be profound early in life.

The behavior of a patient with severe Hunter disease is often characteristic [19] and contrasts sharply with the sweet disposition of the Hurler patient. From 2–6 years-of-age the Hunter patient may develop primitive, uncontrolled activity in which he throws toys and seems to enjoy self-created noise. He is hyperkinetic. Rough, aggressive play may be dangerous to pets or younger siblings. These patients often are stubborn, fearless and unresponsive to discipline. Eating habits may be unusual, and pica is common. One patient developed lead poisoning. The management of such a child is difficult and admission to an institution is common.

Obstructive airway disease may result from infiltration of the vocal cords or trachea, or a large tongue. Tracheostomy may be necessary. Cardiac complications, such as congestive failure, result from valvular or myocardial infiltration. Coronary insufficiency may result from infiltration in the vessels. Thickened valves may be demonstrated by echocardiography. Some have pulmonary hypertension.

Most patients deteriorate progressively after 5 or 6 years-of-age. Physical activity decreases; gait may become unsteady; and speech deteriorates and ultimately is lost. Difficulty in ingesting solid food is progressive, and there is loss of weight. Respiratory infections become more frequent and more severe and may be the cause of death. Generalized seizures may occur in the final months of life. Death usually occurs by 15 years-of-age from respiratory or cardiac disease.

Patients with the milder forms of the disease may survive well into their sixties or beyond [30–33]. Intelligence may be preserved. Features may appear normal in childhood, or may be mildly coarse (Figure 79.4), but with time the appearance

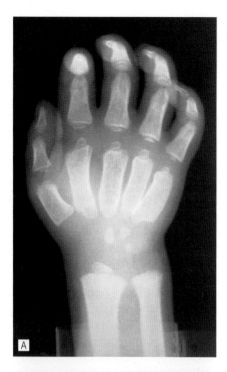

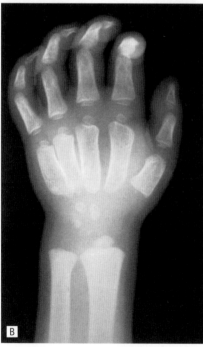

Figure 79.8   *A.M.A.Q. Roentgenograms of the hands illustrate the broadened phalanges and metacarpals as well as the fixed flexion deformities. The proximal ends of the metacarpals are tapered.*

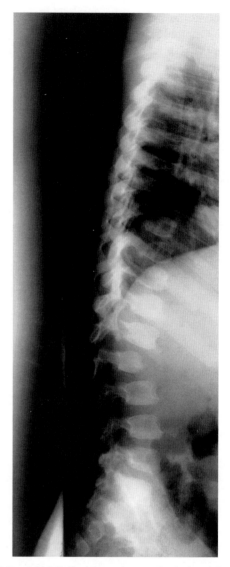

Figure 79.9   *A.M.A.Q. The L2 vertebra was beaked and displaced posteriorly.*

becomes increasingly recognizable. Joint stiffness may be an increasing problem, and patients may develop osteoarthritis. Carpal tunnel syndrome is common.

Hearing loss is regularly observed. Retinal dysfunction may be documented by electroretinography [34]. Chronic papilledema has been reported in the absence of increased intracranial pressure [35,36]. Hydrocephalus appears to be rare in the mild forms of Hunter disease [28]. Arachnoid cysts have been observed [37]. Spinal stenosis, especially cervical may cause cord compression [38].

Survival as long as 87 years has been observed [31], but death may occur in the second decade, even in the mild phenotypes. The cause may be cardiac disease, pulmonary infection, or airway obstruction.

The roentgenographic picture of all forms of the disease is that of dysostosis multiplex. The features may be quite similar to those of the Hurler disease, but they tend to be less dramatic (Figures 79.8–79.10). External thickening of the cortices of the bones may be seen early. With increasing age the cortical walls become thinner as the marrow cavities expand [39]. The skull is large and the sella shoe-shaped. The lower ribs are broad and spatulate. There is hypoplasia of the vertebrae and beaking of L2 (Figure 79.9). Large radiolucent areas

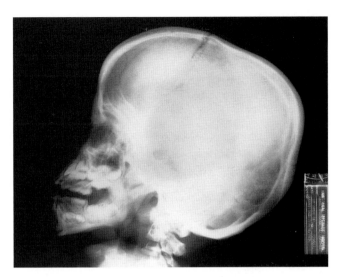

Figure 79.10 *The skull of A.M.A.Q. illustrates the thickened cranial vault.*

surrounding the unerupted teeth represent dentigenous cysts, not accumulation of mucopolysaccharide [40]. Smaller lucent lesions may be collections of collagen.

Fundamental to the clinical phenotype is the excessive intracellular accumulation of acid mucopolysaccharides. Large vacuolated cells containing metachromatic cytoplasmic material are present on histologic examination of many tissues. In the scapular nodules there is extracellular accumulation of metachromatic material [41]. Dermatan sulfate and heparan sulfate [2,14] are excreted in the urine in large and approximately equal amounts. Cultured fibroblasts show metachromatic staining and contain large amounts of mucopolysaccharide [2]. Hunter cells accumulate labeled sulfate in a typical mucopolysaccharidosis pattern.

GENETICS AND PATHOGENESIS

The Hunter disease is inherited as an X-linked recessive trait. Patients with specific mild or severe phenotypes closely resemble other affected members of an individual family. The incidence of the disease has approximated one in 100 000 male births in Great Britain and British Columbia [42–44], and one in 36 000 in Israel [45,46]. The disease has been recognized in a small number of female individuals. One had an X:5 autosome translocation in which the break point at the gene locus caused the disease, because the normal X was inactivated [47,48]. Others represented nonrandom inactivation of a normal X chromosome, including one of a pair of nonidentical twins [49–51].

The molecular defect is in the enzyme iduronate sulfatase [6,52,53] (Figure 79.1). The enzyme has been purified from human liver [54], placenta [55] and plasma [56]. The human cDNA codes for a polypeptide of 550 amino acids [10]. The enzyme [57], which removes the sulphate from the 2-position

of iduronic acid, is essential for the sequential degradation of heparan sulfate, which contains many sulfated iduronic acid residues, and dermatan sulfate, which contains a smaller number of such residues. The failure to degrade even a single sulfated uronic acid leads to the accumulation of the glycosaminoglycan. Enzymatic analysis for the activity of iduronate sulfatase fails to distinguish among the mild and severe clinical phenotypes; in all of them there is virtually complete absence of enzyme activity.

β-Galactosidase activity is diminished in the skin and other tissues of patients with the disease [58]. This abnormality, which also occurs in Hurler disease, is secondary to the primary defect, but it could relate to the accumulation of ganglioside and other lipids found in the brain of patients.

The diagnosis, once suspected clinically, has been confirmed by the quantitative assay of the excretion of total glycosaminoglycans in the urine, but the specific diagnosis depends on the assay for iduronate sulfatase, which can be carried out on serum, cells or tissues [59]. None of the screening tests for mucopolysaccharide in the urine is completely reliable.

Heterozygous female carriers of the Hunter gene have been recognized by cloning of fibroblasts followed by assessment of the accumulation of ^{35}S-mucopolysaccharide [60] or assay of iduronate sulfatase in individual hair roots [61,62]. Two clonal populations, one normal and the other abnormal, have been demonstrated using both of these techniques, as specified by the Lyon hypothesis. Demonstration of a major deletion in the gene provides a highly accurate and less demanding approach to carrier detection.

Prenatal diagnosis was initially carried out successfully by using sulfate incorporation in cultured amniocytes [63]. It is now done by assay of the enzyme in amniocytes or in amniotic fluid. It is recommended that the early information obtained from the fluid always be confirmed by assay of the cultured cells. Prenatal diagnosis has also been accomplished by assay of the enzyme in chorionic villus homogenates [64]. In the case of female fetuses, very low levels of enzyme may be found in either amniocytes or chorionic villus cells; therefore, it is important that karyotyping be carried out in all instances. In families in which the mutation is known, molecular methods are of choice for prenatal diagnosis and heterozygote detection.

The gene for iduronate sulfatase is very large. It contains nine exons over 24 kb [65,66]. Complete or partial deletions of the gene were identified in patients with the severe phenotype [57,67]. Among this population of patients with severe disease, deletions or rearrangements visible in Southern blots occur in about 20 percent [7,11,68–70]. It appears that this area is structurally susceptible to major alterations, because identical changes have been found in unrelated patients [66]. In addition, a number of missense and nonsense mutations have been identified [11–13,67,71–75]. Approximately half of the single base substitutions have occurred at CpG dinucleotides, suggesting independent origin in different families [76]. Codon R468 when changed to W led to mild disease in a patient in the US [13] and severe disease in a Japanese [70], typifying the problem of genotype phenotype correlation; it was also changed to Q, L and G in severely affected patients [13,77,78]. New mutation has been found to occur more frequently in the genesis of the heterozygous carrier than of the affected male [70,76].

TREATMENT

Specific treatment for this disease continues to be explored. Enzyme replacement therapy has not been effective to date. Bone marrow transplantation has been performed in this disease, but most experience is with MPS I (Chapters 77 and 78) [79]. It is not currently recommended in Hunter disease.

A variety of supportive measures are useful, especially in the milder forms of the disease, in which longer survival is associated with some painful complications. Shunting is important in the management of hydrocephalus. Hearing aids may aid in deafness. Physiotherapy is useful for the joint stiffness and the avoidance of contractures. Surgical decompression is carried out for carpal tunnel syndrome. Cardiac valvular status should be monitored by echocardiography. Tracheostomy or nasal continuous positive airway pressure may alleviate obstructive airway disease.

References

1   Hunter C. A rare disease in two brothers. *Proc R Soc Med* 1917;**10**:104.
2   Dorfman A, Matalon R. The Hurler and Hunter syndromes. *Am J Med* 1969;**47**:691.
3   Muir H. The structure and metabolism of mucopolysaccharidoses. *Am J Med* 1969;**47**:673.
4   Fratantoni JC, Hall CW, Neufeld EF. Hurler and Hunter syndromes I Mutual correction of the defect in cultured fibroblasts. *Science* 1968;**162**:570.
5   Cantz M, Chrambach A, Bach G, Neufeld EF. The Hunter corrective factor. *J Biol Chem* 1972;**247**:5456.
6   Bach G, Eisenberg F, Cantz M, Neufeld EF. The defect in the Hunter syndrome: deficiency of sulfoiduronate sulfatase. *Proc Natl Acad Sci USA* 1973;**70**:2134.
7   Palmieri G, Capra V, Romano G, *et al.* The iduronate sulfatase gene: isolation of a 12Mb YAC contig spanning the entire gene and identification of heterogeneous deletions in patients with Hunter syndrome. *Genomics* 1992;**12**:52.
8   Upadhyaya M, Sarfarazi M, Bamforth JS, *et al.* Localization of the gene for Hunter syndrome on the long arm of X-chromosome. *Hum Genet* 1986;**74**:39.
9   Le Guern E, Couillin P, Oberle I, *et al.* More precise localization of the gene for Hunter syndrome. *Genomics* 1990;**7**:358.
10 Wilson PJ, Morris CP, Anson DS, *et al.* Hunter syndrome: isolation of an iduronate-2-sulfatase cDNA clone and analysis of patient DNA. *Proc Natl Acad Sci USA* 1990;**87**:8531.
11 Wraith JE, Cooper A, Thornley M, *et al.* The clinical phenotype of two patients with a complete deletion of the iduronate-2-sulfatase gene (mucopolysaccharidosis type II Hunter syndrome). *Hum Genet* 1991;**87**:205.
12 Sukegawa K, Tomatsu S, Katsuyuki T, *et al.* Intermediate form of mucopolysaccharidosis type II (Hunter disease): a C1327 to T substitution in the iduronate sulfatase gene. *Biochem Biophys Res Commun* 1992;**183**:809.
13 Crotty PL, Braun SE, Anderson RA, Whitley CB. Mutation R468W of the iduronate-2-sulfatase gene in mild Hunter syndrome (mucopolysaccharidosis type II) confirmed by *in vitro* mutagenesis and expression. *Hum Mol Genet* 1992;**1**:755.
14 Spranger J. The systemic mucopolysaccharidoses. *Ergeb Inn Med Kinderheilkd* 1972;**32**:165.
15 Young ID, Harper PS, Archer IM, Newcombe RG. A clinical and genetic study of Hunter's syndrome. 1 Heterogeneity. *J Med Genet* 1982;**19**:401.
16 Young ID, Harper PS, Newcombe RG, Archer IM. A clinical and genetic study of Hunter's syndrome. 2 Differences between the mild and severe forms. *J Med Genet* 1982;**19**:408.
17 Prystowsky SD, Maumenee IH, Freeman RG, *et al.* A cutaneous marker in the Hunter syndrome: a report of four cases. *Arch Dermatol* 1977;**113**:602.
18 Young ID, Harper PS. The natural history of the severe form of Hunter's syndrome: a study based on 52 cases. *Dev Med Child Neurol* 1983;**25**:481.
19 Leroy JG, Crocker AC. Clinical definition of the Hurler–Hunter phenotypes. *Am J Dis Child* 1966;**112**:518.
20 McKusick VA. *Heritable Disorders of Connective Tissue.* 4th edn. CV Mosby Co, St Louis;1972:5556.
21 Benson PF, Button LR, Fensom AH, Dean MF. Lumbar kyphosis in Hunter's disease (MPSII). *Clin Genet* 1979;**16**:317.
22 Spranger J, Cantz M, Gehler J, *et al.* Mucopolysaccharidosis II (Hunter disease) with corneal opacities: report of two patients at the extremes of a wide clinical spectrum. *Eur J Pediatr* 1978;**129**:11.
23 Elsner B. Ultrastructure of the rectal wall in Hunter's syndrome. *Gastroenterology* 1970;**58**:856.
24 Young ID, Harper PS. Long-term complications in Hunter's syndrome. *Clin Genet* 1978;**16**:125.
25 Ballenger CE, Swift TR, Leshner RT, *et al.* Myelopathy in mucopolysaccharidosis type II (Hunter syndrome). *Ann Neurol* 1980;**7**:382.
26 Yatziv S, Epstein CJ. Hunter syndrome presenting as macrocephaly and hydrocephalus. *J Med Genet* 1997;**14**:445.
27 Gibbs DA. Computed tomography studies on patients with mucopolysaccharidoses. *Neuroradiology* 1981;**21**:9.
28 Van Aerde J, Plets C, van der Hauwaert L. Hydrocephalus in Hunter syndrome. *Acta Paediatr Belg* 1981;**34**:93.
29 Timms KM, Bondeson ML, Ansari-Lari MA, *et al.* Molecular and phenotypic variation in patients with severe Hunter syndrome. *Hum Mol Genet* 1997;**6**:479.
30 Young ID, Harper PS. Mild form of Hunter's syndrome: clinical delineation based on 31 cases. *Arch Dis Child* 1982;**57**:828.
31 Hobolth N, Pedersen C. Six cases of mild form of the Hunter syndrome in five generations. Three affected males with progeny *Clin Genet* 1978;**13**:121.
32 Differante NM, Nichols BL Jr. A case of the Hunter syndrome with progeny. *Johns Hopkins Med J* 1978;**130**:121.
33 Karpati G, Carpenter S, Eisan AA, *et al.* Multiple peripheral nerve entrapments: an unusual phenotypic variant of the Hunter syndrome (mucopolysaccharidosis II) in a family. *Arch Neurol* 1974;**31**:418.
34 Caruso RC, Kaiser-Kupfer MI, Muenzer J, *et al.* Electroretinographic findings in the mucopolysaccharidoses. *Ophthalmology* 1986;**93**:1612.
35 Beck M, Cole G. Disc oedema in association with Hunter's syndrome: ocular histopathological findings. *Br J Ophthalmol* 1984;**68**:590.
36 Beck M. Papilloedemas in association with Hunter syndrome. *Br J Ophthalmol* 1983;**67**:174.
37 Neuhauser EBD, Griscom NT, Gilles FH, Crocker AC. Arachnoid cysts in the Hurler–Hunter syndrome. *Ann Radiol* 1968;**11**:453.

38 Vinchon M, Cotten A, Clarisse J, et al. Cervical myelopathy secondary to Hunter syndrome in an adult. Am J Neuroradiol 1995;**16**:1402.

39 Caffey J. Gargoylism (Hunter-Hurler disease dysostosis multiplex lipochondrodystrophy). Am J Roentgenol Radium Ther Nucl Med 1952;**67**:715.

40 Lustmann J, Bimstein E, Yatziv S. Dentigerous cysts and radiolucent lesions of the jaw association with Hunter's syndrome. J Oral Surg 1975;**33**:679.

41 Freeman RG. A pathological basis for the cutaneous papules of mucopolysaccharidosis II (the Hunter syndrome). J Cutan Pathol 1977;**4**:673.

42 Young ID, Harper PS. Incidence of Hunter's syndrome. Hum Genet 1982;**60**:391.

43 Lowry RB, Renwick DHG. Relative frequency of the Hurler and Hunter syndromes. N Engl J Med 1971;**284**:221.

44 Lowry RB, Applegarth DA, Toone JR, et al. An update on the frequency of mucopolysaccharide syndromes in British Columbia. Hum Genet 1990; **85**:389.

45 Zlotogora J, Schaap T, Zeigler M, Bach G. Hunter syndrome in Jews in Israel: further evidence for prenatal selection favoring the Hunter allele. Hum Genet 1991;**86**:531.

46 Chakravarti A, Bale SJ. Differences in the frequency of X-linked deleterious genes in human populations. Am J Hum Genet 1983;**35**:1252.

47 Mossman J, Blunt S, Stephens R, et al. Hunter's disease in a girl: association with X:5 chromosomal translocation disrupting the Hunter gene. Arch Dis Child 1983;**58**:911.

48 Roberts SH, Upadhyaya M, Sarfarazi M, Harper PS. Further evidence localizing the gene for Hunter's syndrome to the distal region of the X-chromosome long arm. J Med Genet 1989;**26**:309.

49 Clarke JTR, Greer WL, Strasberg PM, et al. Hunter disease (mucopolysaccharidosis type II) associated with unbalanced inactivation of the X chromosome in a karyotypically normal girl. Am J Hum Genet 1991;**4**:289.

50 Clarke JTR, Wilson PJ, Morris CP, et al. Characterization of a deletion at Xq27-28 associated with unbalanced inactivation of the nonmutant X-chromosome. Am J Hum Genet 1992;**51**:316.

51 Winchester B, Young E, Geddes S, et al. Female twin with Hunter disease due to nonrandom inactivation of the X-chromosome: a consequence of twinning. Am J Med Genet 1992;**44**:834.

52 Sjoberg I, Fransson LA, Matalon R, Dorfman A. Hunter's syndrome: a deficiency of l-idurono-sulfate sulfatase. Biochem Biophys Res Commun 1973;**54**:1125.

53 Liebaers I, Neufeld EF. Iduronate sulfatase activity in serum lymphocytes and fibroblasts – simplified diagnosis of the Hunter syndrome. Pediatr Res 1976;**10**:733.

54 Bielicki J, Freeman C, Clements PR, Hopwood JJ. Human liver iduronate-2-sulphatase: purification characterization and catalytic properties. Biochem J 1990;**271**:75.

55 DiNatale P, Daniele A. Iduronate sulfatase from human placenta. Biochem Biophys Acta 1985;**839**:258.

56 Wasteson A, Neufeld EF. Iduronate sulfatase from human plasma. Methods Enzymol 1982;**83**:573.

57 Bielicki J, Freeman C, Clements PR, Hopwood JJ. Human liver iduronate-2-sulphatase. Purification, characterization and catalytic properties. Biochem J 1990;**271**:75.

58 Gerich JE. Hunter's syndrome Beta-galactosidase deficiency in skin. N Engl J Med 1969;**280**:799.

59 Yatziv S, Erickson RP, Epstein CJ. Mild and severe Hunter syndrome (MPSII) within the sibships. Clin Genet 1977;**11**:319.

60 Migeon BR, Sprenkle JA, Liebaers I, et al. X-linked Hunter syndrome: the heterozygous phenotype in cell culture. Am J Hum Genet 1977;**29**:448.

61 Yutaka T, Fluharty AL, Stevens RL, Kihara H. Iduronate sulfatase analysis of hair roots for identification of Hunter syndrome heterozygotes. Am J Hum Genet 1978;**30**:575.

62 Nwokoro N, Neufeld EF. Detection of Hunter heterozygotes by enzymatic analysis of hair roots. Am J Hum Genet 1979;**31**:42.

63 Fratantoni JC, Neufeld EF, Uhlendorf W, Jacobson CB. Intrauterine diagnosis of the Hurler and Hunter syndromes. N Engl J Med 1969;**280**:686.

64 Kleijer WJ, Van Diggelen OP, Janse HC, et al. First trimester diagnosis of Hunter syndrome on chorionic villi. Lancet 1984;**2**:472.

65 Flomen RH, Green EP, Bentley DR, Giannelli F. Determination of the organisation of coding sequences within the iduronate sulphate sulphatase (IDS) gene. Hum Mol Genet 1993;**2**:5.

66 Wilson PJ, Meaney CA, Hopwood JJ, Morris CP. Sequence of the human iduronate 2-sulfatase (IDS) gene. Genomics 1993;**17**:773.

67 Wilson PJ, Suthers GK, Callen DF. Frequent deletions at Xq28 indicate genetic heterogeneity in Hunter syndrome. Hum Genet 1991;**86**:505.

68 Steen-Bondeson ML, Dahl N, Tonnesen T, et al. Molecular analysis of patients with Hunter syndrome: implication of a region prone to structural alterations within the EDS gene. Hum Mol Genet 1992;**1**:195.

69 Bunge S, Steglich C, Beck M, et al. Mutation analysis of the iduronate 2-sulfatase gene in patients with mucopolysaccharidosis type II (Hunter syndrome). Hum Mol Genet 1992;**1**:335.

70 Beck M, Steglich C, Zabel B, et al. Deletion of the Hunter gene and both DXS466 and DXS304 in a patient with mucopolysaccharidosis type II. Am J Med Genet 1992;**44**:100.

71 Bunge S, Steglich C, Beck M, et al. Mutation spectrum of the iduronate-2-sulfatase gene in patients with Hunter syndrome. Am J Hum Genet 1992; **51**:A166.

72 Hopwood JJ, Bunge S, Morris CP, et al. Molecular basis of mucopolysaccharidosis type II: mutations in the iduronate 2-sulphatase gene. Hum Mutat 1993;**2**:435.

73 Muenzer J, Tutera M. Molecular analysis of iduronate sulfatase mutations in mucopolysaccharidosis II (Hunter syndrome). Am J Hum Genet 1992; **51**:A174.

74 Flomen RH, Green PM, Bentley DR, et al. Detection of point mutations and a gross deletion in six Hunter syndrome patients. Genomics 1992;**13**:543.

75 Froissant R, Maire I, Millat G, et al. Identification of idurontate sulfatase gene alterations in 70 unrelated Hunter patients. Clin Genet 1998; **53**:362.

76 Rathmann M, Bunge S, Beck M, et al. Mucopolysaccharidosis type II (Hunter syndrome): Mutation 'hot spots' in the iduronate-2-sulfatase gene. Am J Hum Genet 1996;**59**:1202.

77 Isogai K, Sukegawa K, Tomatsu S, et al. Mutation analysis in the iduronate-2-sulphatase gene in 43 Japanese patients with mucopolysaccharidosis type II (Hunter disease). J Inherit Metab Dis 1998;**21**:60.

78 Whitley CB, Anderson RA, Aronovich EL, et al. Caveat to genotype-phenotype correlation in mucopolysaccharidosis type II: discordant clinical severity of R468W and R468Q mutations of the iduronate-2-sulfatase gene. Hum Mutat 1993;**2**:235.

79 Krivit W, Shapiro E, Hoogerbrugge PM, Moser HW. State of the art review. Bone marrow transplantation treatment for storage diseases. Bone Marrow Transplant 1992;**10**:87.

80

Sanfilippo disease/mucopolysaccharidosis type III (MPS III)

MAJOR PHENOTYPIC EXPRESSION

Severe mental deterioration, mild skeletal dysostosis multiplex and urinary excretion of heparan sulfate. The Sanfilippo disease type A is due to a deficiency of heparan-N-sulfatase, type B to a deficiency of α-N-acetylglucosaminidase, type C to acetylCoA:α-glucosaminide acetyl transferase, and type D to N-acetylglucosamine-6-sulfatase.

INTRODUCTION

This disorder was first described by Harris [1] in 1961 with the report of a mildly retarded 6-year-old girl who had hepatosplenomegaly and a normal skeletal survey and excreted large amounts of heparan sulfate in the urine. Sanfilippo and colleagues [2,3] in 1962 and 1963 described eight children with a wide range in degree of mental retardation, all of whom had heparan sulfate mucopolysacchariduria. Some of these patients had similarities, in appearance and in roentgenographic findings, to patients with the Hurler and Hunter syndromes. The syndrome is characterized chemically by the exclusive excretion of heparan sulfate in the urine, which distinguishes it from all of the other mucopolysaccharidoses. It is also clinically unique in the disparity between the generally severe cerebral degeneration and the relatively mild effects on the skeleton, viscera and facial features [4].

Fibroblasts derived from patients with the Sanfilippo disease accumulate $^{35}SO_4$. The existence of more than one type of disease was first recognized through cross-correction studies [5]. Patients initially studied fell into two groups, and those of each group could correct the other. The correction factors are the enzymes whose activity is lacking in each of the types. In type A Sanfilippo cells, Kresse and Neufeld [6] found that the defective enzyme is heparan-N-sulfatase (Figures 80.1, 80.2). In type B the defect was found by O'Brien [7] and by von Figura and Kresse [8] to be in α-N-acetylglucosaminidase

(Figure 80.1). The latter group defined the acetyltransferase defect in type C [9] and the N-acetylglucosamine-6-sulfatase abnormality in type D disease [10]. The cDNA for this III D disease gene has been cloned [11] and mapped to chromosome 12q14 [12]. The cDNA for the IIIA enzyme was cloned and mapped to chromosome 17q25 [13]. The gene for IIIB was cloned and mapped to chromosome 17q21 [14]. A relatively small number of mutations, predominantly missense and private to an individual family has been found in the IIIA and IIIB genes [15,16].

CLINICAL ABNORMALITIES

The clinical features of each of the four Sanfilippo disease types are indistinguishable (Figures 80.3–80.10). Patients are characteristically normal in appearance at birth and appear to develop normally during the first year. They usually are referred after one or two years-of-age because of slowness in development or after three or four years because of delayed speech. They may have had difficulty in feeding, especially with solids, as well as repeated respiratory infections from the beginning. Mental retardation becomes progressively more obvious with time. These patients do not have abnormalities in linear growth, and muscle strength is good. Progressive degeneration occurs to a severe degree of mental incapacitation, although there is variability among patients. Skills learned during the

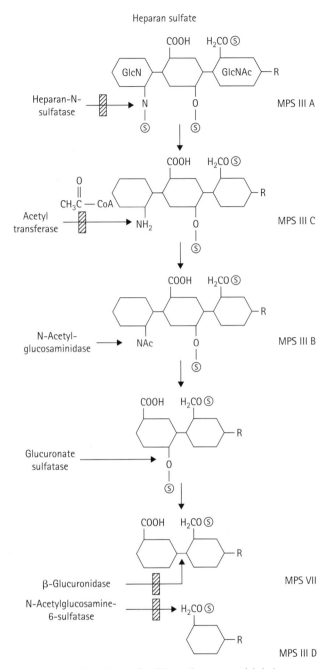

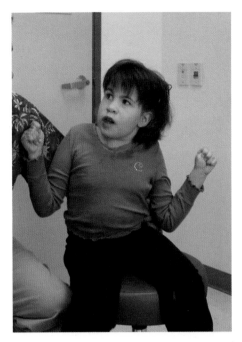

Figure 80.3   *C.F., an 11-year-old girl with Sanfilippo A disease. The thick alae nasi were clear evidence of mucopolysaccharide storage, but features were otherwise not coarse. She was quite hirsute and very hypertonic, as indicated by her hands. Liver was palpable at 4 cm.*

Figure 80.1   *The defect in Sanfilippo disease type A is in heparan-N-sulfatase, while in type B it is α-N-acetylglucosaminidase. In type C it is an acetyl transferase, and in type D it is N-acetylglucosamine-6-sulfatase. The phenotypes of the various types are indistinguishable.*

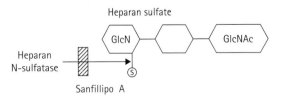

Figure 80.2   *Heparan sulfate accumulates in Sanfilippo disease.*

first years are lost, including speech and toilet training. Others never learn to speak, while speech in some is lost well after the first decade; some patients develop some impairment of hearing. Neurologic problems are progressive. The gait becomes clumsy and coordination poor. Deep tendon reflexes are accentuated. Purposeless athetoid-like movements may develop. The patient may drool constantly. There may be seizures, but anticonvulsant control is not difficult. Finally, the patient becomes bedridden and gastrostomy or nasogastric feeding is required. Death usually supervenes before the 20th birthday or even before the 10th [4], but survival into the third or fourth decade is possible [17].

Management of behavior may be a problem and may even be the presenting complaint. Behavior tends to become worse as, with age, patients become increasingly stubborn and withdrawn; many are hyperactive. Disorders of sleep and insomnia are common and some are up all night, at least on occasion. Chewing the bedclothes and sudden crying out are common. Inappropriate laughing or singing is less common. Patients may be aggressive, and temper tantrums occur. Patients may have pica and eat unusual objects. Interaction with other children may be difficult. They can be destructive and dangerous to siblings. The combination of aggressive behavior, profound dementia and normal physical strength is a daunting one. They often are so difficult to handle that admission to an institution is common [18]. Some patients have come to attention as adults with psychiatric disease, even of a type requiring admission to a closed ward [19]. Drug treatment of the behavior is seldom effective [20].

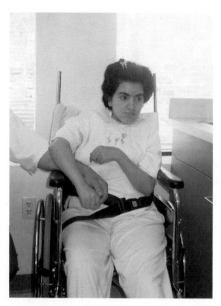

Figure 80.4 *C.L., a 21-year-old female with Sanfilippo A disease. She was thin, dystonic and wheelchair-bound.*

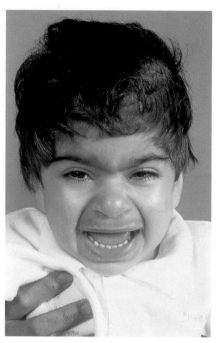

Figure 80.5 *R.G.Q., a 21-month-old girl with Sanfilippo disease type A. She was quite hirsute, and the facial features were somewhat coarse. The liver was palpable at 8 cm. Growth was normal, but she was developmentally delayed.*

There may be differences in the severity of disease in the different types. Adult onset of dementia and minimal somatic disease have been reported in type B [21]; while dementia is commonly observed by 6 years-of-age in type A [18]. In addition, early-onset progression tends to be more rapid in type A than in types B and C. However, there is considerable heterogeneity. A particularly severe type A disease has been reported [22] from the Cayman Islands. In both types A and B, severe and mild forms of the disease have been reported in the same sibship [23,24]. Type C severity may be intermediate between that of types A and B or may present in infancy [25]. Type D is rare, but also heterogenous [26–28].

The features of the patient with Sanfilippo disease usually become somewhat coarse (Figures 80.4–80.7), but often the patient is not recognizable as having a mucopolysacharidosis. In some the features are not recognizably coarse (Figures 80.9, 80.10). In our experience programs of screening of the urine for metabolic disease of unselected patients in institutions for the retarded are more likely to bring to light previously undiagnosed patients with this disorder than any other disease of metabolism.

The bridge of the nose may be slightly flattened and the lips somewhat thick. Many of the patients are hirsute; the eyebrows may be bushy and the hairline low. Some have had macrocephaly. The dull, rigid facies is a consequence of cerebral deterioration, as contrasted with the local tissue changes of Hurler disease. Some patients may have a mild limitation of joint mobility. Hepatosplenomegaly may be mild, especially in childhood; it is more often undetectable in adulthood. There is no gibbus, and the corneas are clear. Cardiac abnormalities have not usually been observed in these patients [17]; however, a patient has been reported [29] in whom there was severe incapacitating involvement of the mitral valve. Hernias may be a problem and may recur after correction. Hearing loss may

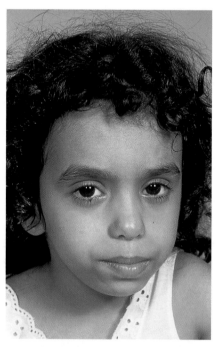

Figure 80.6 *G.G.Q., a 9-year-old girl with Sanfilippo disease, the sister of the patient in Figure 80.2. The history was of loss of developmental milestones, such as walking. She was very hirsute. There was no organomegaly. The calvaria was thickened, but she did not have dystosis multiplex. On follow-up by 16 years, she was profoundly retarded and spastic, had contractures and was unresponsive to social stimuli.*

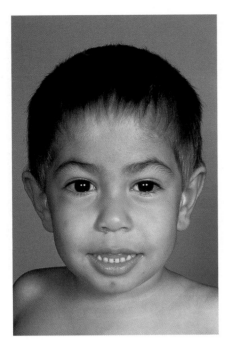

Figure 80.7   *H.M.Z., a 2½-year-old boy with Sanfilippo disease type B. The diagnosis was made because of a positive family history. Features were not coarse, but he was more hirsute than the unaffected members of the family. Development was slow; he had only a few words, but he had walked at 18 months.*

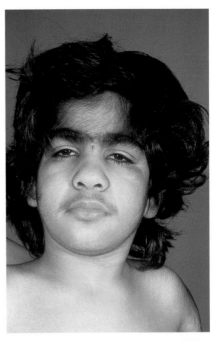

Figure 80.9   *H.R.I.H., a 12-year-old boy with Sanfilippo disease type B. He was hirsute and his facial features were coarse, especially about the nose and lips; mental deficiency was severe.*

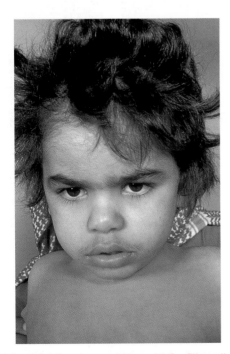

Figure 80.8   *A.R.A.Z., a 4-year-old boy with Sanfilippo disease type B. Mental deficiency increased progressively after 2 years-of-age, and facial features coarsened. Hirsutism was prominent. By 5 years, his cognitive mental age on the Bayley scale was 9 months, but motor performance was spared.*

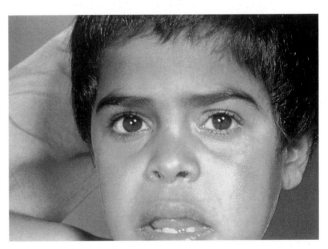

Figure 80.10   *A.S., a 6-year-old girl with Sanfilippo disease type D. She had progressive intellectual deterioration. She had no speech and autistic behavior, but facial features were unremarkable. Activity of N-acetylglucosamine-6-sulfatase was five percent of control.*

be progressive and severe. Watery diarrhea may be a recurrent problem in childhood. An early onset of puberty may be observed [30].

Roentgenographic findings are those of a mild dystosis multiplex [17] (Figures 80.11–80.13). Most patients with this syndrome have a thickening and increased density of the cranial vault in the posterior parietal and occipital areas [31] (Figure 80.12). The mastoids may be sclerotic. The sella turcica appears normal. There may be a biconvex appearance or an ovoid dysplasia of the thoracolumbar vertebrae, as well as platyspondyly (Figure 80.11). Among patients with dysostosis

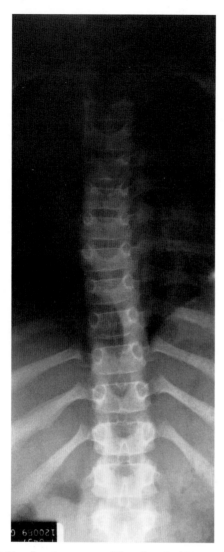

Figure 80.11 *Roentgenogram of the spine of a 16-year-old boy with Sanfilippo disease. There was mild platyspondyly, and the ribs were spatulate with posterior narrowing. This is consistent with dysostosis multiplex, but appreciably milder than those of other forms of mucopolysaccharidosis. Roentogenograms of his extremities were normal.*

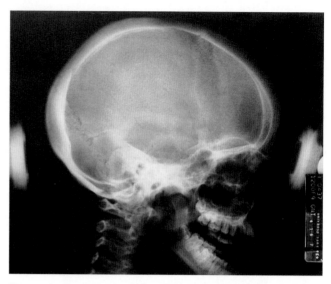

Figure 80.12 *Roentgenogram of the skull of the 16-year-old shows increase in thickness of the diploid space, especially posteriorly. This is characteristic of this disease. The sella turcica is normal.*

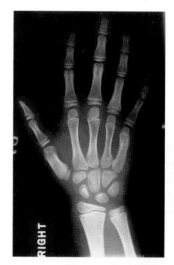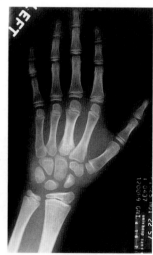

Figure 80.13 *Roentgenogram of the hands of the same 16-year-old looks normal. This highlights the difference in the bones of this disease, from those of disorders with more severe dysostosis multiplex.*

multiplex, those with this syndrome have the mildest bony changes. Those with I cell disease, or mucolipidosis II and Gm1 gangliosidosis, and Hurler disease have the most prominent bony changes. Computed tomography (CT) or magnetic resonance imaging (MRI) scans may reveal mild atrophy early, but this is progressive with the neurodegeneration.

Blood smears may reveal the presence of metachromatic inclusion bodies in the lymphocytes. They are characteristically coarser and sparser than those seen in Hurler disease. Inclusions may also be seen in cells of the bone marrow. Chondrocytes in cartilage biopsied from the iliac crest and the ribs have been reported to be vacuolated [32]. The diagnosis of a mucopolysaccharidosis is first made by the findings of increased quantities of mucopolysaccharide in the urine. In this disorder, it is heparan sulfate that is excreted in excess [33].

Patients with this disorder accumulate gangliosides in the brain [34,35] including Gm2 and Gm3 [34] or there may increased amounts of Gm1 [35]. The electron microscopic appearance of the neurons may be like those of Tay–Sachs disease [34] (Chapter 91). There may also be zebra bodies, and mucopolysaccharide may accumulate in the brain, as well as in the peripheral tissues.

GENETICS AND PATHOGENESIS

All four types of Sanfilippo syndrome are transmitted in an autosomal recessive fashion. Multiple affected siblings have been observed in several families, and consanguinity has been documented [18]. The frequency of the disease has been estimated at one in 24 000 in the Netherlands [18,36]. In this population and in Great Britain [37] the most frequent type was A. In the Cayman Islands there is a very high prevalence of Sanfilippo A disease [22]: the carrier frequency is 0.1. In Greece 10 of 11 patients reported were of type B [38].

The heparan sulfate molecule (Figure 80.1, p. 525) consists of a series of glucuronic acid and iduronic acid molecules alternating with glucosamine residues [39]. The amino nitrogen of the glucosamine moiety may be either sulfated or acetylated, and the 6-hydroxyl may be sulfated. The stepwise degradation of heparan sulfate provides the sites for the defects in the various forms of Sanfilippo disease. Heparan-N-sulfatase, the site of the defect in Sanfilippo disease type A [6,40,41], catalyzes the breakdown of the molecule by splitting off the sulfate groups linked to the amino group of glucosamine. The enzyme has been isolated and purified [42] and is formally a sulfamate sulfohydrolase. α-N-acetylglucosaminidase, the defective enzyme in type B, catalyzes heparan sulfate breakdown at the glucosamine to hexuronic acid linkage removing the N-acetylglucosamine generated by acetyl transfer in the IIIC reaction. This enzyme has been purified from human liver and urine, and the biosynthesis of the mature lysosomal enzyme has been elucidated [43–45]. In the sequential catabolism of heparan sulfate, removal of the sulfate in the reaction catalyzed by heparan-N-sulfatase exposes a terminal glucosamine moiety. This cannot be cleaved until it is acetylated, after which the reaction deficient in type B Sanfilippo disease comes into play. The acetylation is catalzyed by a specific N-acetyltransferase, and it is this reaction that is defective in type C Sanfilippo disease [9,46,47]. This is a two-step reaction in which the enzyme is first acetylated on the cytoplasmic side of the membrane and then transfers this acetyl group now inside the lysosome to a glucosamine. AcetylCoA does not cross the lysosomal membrane. Some patients with type C disease are defective in the second step and others in both steps [48–50].

The defective enzyme in type D Sanfilippo disease is in α-N-acetylglucosamine-6-sulfatase [50,51]. Glucosamine residues in heparan sulfate can be either N-sulfated or O-sulfated, and there are specific sulfatases for each residue. Defective activity of either leads to accumulation and to the Sanfilippo syndrome. The glucosamine-6-sulfatase has been purified [52] and its cDNA has been cloned [11]. Its structure is homologous to other sulfatases. Immunoprecipitation studies have demonstrated cross-reactive material in the Sanfilippo B-syndrome [53]. The enzyme is also involved in the degradation of keratan sulfate, but patients do not excrete keratan sulfate, because this block may be obviated by other enzymes. Patients excrete N-acetylglucosamine sulfate as well as heparan sulfate [54].

Within each of the forms there is not only interfamilial variability, but also intrafamilial variability [55,56]. Patients with all of the forms excrete heparan sulfate and no other glucosaminoglycan.

Detection of heterozygotes has been accomplished through enzyme assay [57] and by ^{35}S accumulation, which may be more reliable in distinguishing heterozygotes. Positive identification by enzyme assay is accurate, but there may be overlap, making identification of the normal noncarrier individual unreliable. When the mutation is known, molecular methods may be used for the detection of carriers.

Intrauterine diagnosis of the affected fetus has been accomplished in types A and B disease through assay of the relevant enzyme in amniotic cells in culture [58]. It may be useful to confirm the assay by assessment of ^{35}S accumulation, because some heterozygotes have very low levels of enzyme in the usual assays. Chorionic villus material has abundant enzyme activity and is available for the prenatal diagnosis of each of the forms of Sanfilippo disease [58–61].

The gene that encodes the heparan-N-sulfatase, defective in MPSIIIA, has 8 exons over 11 kb [13,62]. Among the early mutations identified was an 11bp deletion [13]. Some other deletions have been reported, but most mutations have been missense [15,16,63–66]. Among Australian, Dutch and German patients the most common mutations was R245H [64]. Among Polish patients it was R74C [65], S66W in Sardinians [65] and 1091delC in Spaniards [66].

The gene for the acetylglucosaminidase defective in MPSIIIB contains 6 exons over 8.5 kb [14]. A number of mutations have been identified [14,16,67,68]. A number of replacements of arginine by histidine or stop codon were found at CPG hotspots [14].

TREATMENT

There is no effective treatment for Sanfilippo patients. Enzyme replacement therapy has been attempted using partially purified enzyme, leukocytes and cultured fibroblasts [69], after which there may have been some changes in urinary mucopolysaccharides, but clinical benefit has not been evident. Bone marrow transplantation has been explored in Sanfilippo disease, as well as in other mucopolysaccharidoses, but results have not been impressive [70] in the Sanfilippo group, and the procedure is not recommended. The overwhelming experience with MPSIII is that transplantation of marrow or stem cells does not reverse the inexorable neurodegeneration of this disease. Loperamide hydrochloride may be useful in the management of diarrhea. The dose is 1–2 mg up to four times a day.

Behavioral modification may be useful in the management of problems of behavior. Otherwise, therapy is supportive.

References

1   Harris RC. Mucopolysaccharide disorder: a possible new genotype of Hurler's syndrome. *Am J Dis Child* 1961;**102**:741 (abstr).
2   Sanfilippo SJ, Good RA. Urinary acid mucopolysaccharides in the Hurler syndrome and Morquio's disease. *J Pediatr* 1962;**61**:296.

3   Sanfilippo SJ, Podosin R, Langer L, Good RA. Mental retardation associated with acid mucopolysacchariduria (heparitin sulfate type). *J Pediatr* 1963;**63**:837 (abstr).

4   Leroy JG, Crocker AC. Clinical definition of the Hurler-Hunter phenotypes. A review of 50 patients. *Am J Dis Child* 1966;**112**:518.

5   Kresse H, Wiesmann U, Gantz M, *et al*. Biochemical heterogeneity of the Sanfilippo syndrome: preliminary characterization of two deficient factors. *Biochem Biophys Res Commun* 1971;**42**:892.

6   Kresse H, Neufeld EF. The Sanfilippo A corrective factors. *J Biol Chem* 1972;**247**:2164.

7   O'Brien JS. Sanfilippo syndrome: profound deficiency of alpha-acetylglucosaminidase activity in organs and skin fibroblasts from type B patients. *Proc Natl Acad Sci USA* 1972;**69**:1720.

8   Von Figura K, Kresse H. The Sanfilippo B corrective factor: a N-acetyl-α-d-glucosaminidase. *Biochem Biophys Res Commun* 1972;**48**:262.

9   Klein U, Kresse H, von Figura K. Sanfilippo syndrome type C: deficiency of acetyl-CoA: α-glucosaminide N-acetyl-transferase in skin fibroblasts. *Proc Natl Acad Sci USA* 1978;**75**:5185.

10 Kresse H, Paschke E, von Figura K, *et al*. Sanfilippo disease type D: deficiency of N-acetylglucosamine 6-sulfate sulfatase required for heparan sulfate degradation. *Proc Natl Acad Sci USA* 1980;**77**:6822.

11 Robertson DA, Freeman C, Nelson PV, *et al*. Human glucosamine-6-sulfatase cDNA reveals homology with steroid sulfatase. *Biochem Biophys Res Commun* 1988;**157**:218.

12 Robertson DA, Callen DF, Baker EG, *et al*. Chromosomal localization of the gene for human glucosamine 6-sulphatase to 12q14. *Hum Genet* 1988;**79**:175.

13 Scott HS, Blanch L, Guo X-H, *et al*. Cloning of the sulphamidase gene and identification of mutations in Sanfilippo A syndrome. *Nat Genet* 1995;**11**:465.

14 Zhao HG, Li HH, Bach G, *et al*. The molecular basis of Sanfilippo syndrome type B. *Proc Nat Acad Sci USA* 1996;**93**:6101.

15 Blanch L, Weber B, Guo XH, *et al*. Molecular defects in Sanfilippo syndrome type A. *Hum Mol Genet* 1997;**6**:787.

16 Schmidtchen A, Greenberg D, Zhao HG, *et al*. NAGLU mutations underlying Sanfilippo syndrome type B. *Am J Hum Genet* 1998;**62**:64.

17 McKusick VA. *Heritable Disorders of Connective Tissue*. 4th edn. CV Mosby Co, St Louis;1972:521.

18 Van de Kamp JJP, Niermeijer MF, von Figura K, Giesberts MAH. Genetic heterogeneity and clinical variability in the Sanfilippo syndrome (types A, B and C). *Clin Genet* 1981;**20**:152.

19 Lindor NM, Hoffman A, O'Brien JF, *et al*. Sanfilippo syndrome type A in two adult sibs. *Am J Med Genet* 1994;**53**:241.

20 Nidiffer FD, Kelly TE. Developmental and degenerative patterns associated with cognitive behavioral and motor difficulties in the Sanfilippo syndrome: an epidemiological study. *J Ment Defic Res* 1987;**27**:185.

21 Van Schrojenstein-DeValk HMJ, van de Kamp HP. Follow-up on seven adult patients with mild Sanfilippo B disease. *Am J Med Genet* 1987;**28**:125.

22 Matalon R, Deanching M, ,Nakamura F, Bloom A. A recessively inherited lethal disease in a Caribbean isolate – a sulfamidase deficiency. *Pediatr Res* 1980;**14**:524.

23 McDowell GA, Cowan TM, Blitzer MG, Greene CL. Intrafamilial variability in Hurler syndrome and Sanfilippo syndrome type A: implications for evaluation of new therapies. *Am J Med Genet* 1965;**47**:1092.

24 Di Natale P. Sanfilippo B disease: a re-examination of a particular sibship after 12 years. *J Inherit Metab Dis* 1991;**14**:23.

25 Sewell AC, Pontz BF, Benischek G. Mucopolysaccharidosis type IIIC (Sanfilippo): early clinical presentation in a large Turkish pedigree. *Clin Genet* 1988;**34**:116.

26 Coppa GV, Giorgi PL, Felici L, *et al*. Clinical heterogeneity in Sanfilippo disease (mucopolysaccharidosis III) type D: presentation of two new cases. *Eur J Pediatr* 1983;**140**:130.

27 Kaplan P, Wolfe LS. Sanfilippo syndrome type D. *J Pediatr* 1987;**110**:267.

28 Siciliano L, Fiumara A, Pavone L, *et al*. Sanfilippo syndrome type D in two adolescent sisters. *J Med Genet* 1991;**28**:402.

29 Herd JK, Subramanian S, Robinson H. Type III mucopolysaccharidosis: report of a case with severe mitral valve involvement. *J Pediatr* 1973;**82**:1011.

30 Tylki-Szymanska A, Metera M. Precocious puberty in three boys with Sanfilippo A (mucopolysaccharidosis III A). *J Pediatr Endocrinol Metab* 1995;**8**:291.

31 Spranger J, Teller W, Kosenow W, *et al*. Die HS-mucopolysaccharidose von Sanfilippo (Polydystrophe oligophrenie). Bericht Uber 10 Patienten. *Z Kinderheilk* 1967;**101**:71.

32 Silberberg R, Rimoin DL, Rosenthal RE, Hasler MB. Ultrastructure of cartilage in the Hurler and Sanfilippo syndromes. *Arch Pathol* 1972;**94**:500.

33 Gordon BA, Haust MD. The mucopolysaccharidoses types I II and III: urinary findings in 23 cases. *Clin Biochem* 1970;**3**:302.

34 Wallace BJ, Kaplan D, Adachi M, *et al*. Mucopolysaccharidosis type III. Morphologic and biochemical studies of two siblings with Sanfilippo syndrome. *Arch Pathol* 1966;**82**:462.

35 Dekaban AS, Patton VM. Hurler's and Sanfilippo's variants of mucopolysaccharidosis. *Arch Pathol* 1971;**91**:434.

36 Van de Kamp JJP. The Sanfilippo syndrome: a clinical and genetical study of 75 patients in the Netherlands (doctoral thesis). S-Gravenhage, Rasmans JH,1979.

37 Whiteman P, Young E. The laboratory diagnosis of Sanfilippo disease. *Clin Chim Acta* 1970;**76**:139.

38 Beratis NG, Sklower SL, Wilbur L, Matalon R. Sanfilippo disease in Greece. *Clin Genet* 1986;**29**:129.

39 Roden L. Structure and metabolism of connective tissue proteoglycans: in *The Biochemistry of Glycoproteins and Proteoglycans* (ed. WJ Lennarz) Plenum Press, New York;1980:267.

40 Kresse H. Mucopolysacharidosis III A (Sanfilippo A disease): deficiency of heparin sulfamidase in skin fibroblasts and leucocytes. *Biochem Biophys Res Commun* 1973;**54**:1111.

41 Matalon R, Dorfman A. Sanfilippo A syndrome: sulfamidase deficiency in cultured skin fibroblasts and liver. *J Clin Invest* 1974;**54**:907.

42 Freeman C, Hopwood JJ. Human liver sulphamate sulphohydrolase. *Biochem J* 1986;**234**:83.

43 Von Figura K. Human a-N-acetylglucosaminidase. I Purification and properties. *Eur J Biochem* 1977;**80**:525.

44 Sasaki T, Sukegawa K, Masue M, *et al*. Purification and partial characterization of a-N-acetylglucosaminidase from human liver. *J Biochem* 1991;**110**:842.

45 Von Figura K, Hasilik A, Steckel F, van de Kamp J. Biosynthesis and maturation of a-N-acetylglucosaminidase in normal and Sanfilippo B fibroblasts. *Am J Hum Genet* 1984;**36**:93.

46 Bartsocas C, Grobe H, Vande Kamp JJP, *et al*. Sanfilippo type C disease clinical findings in four patients with a new variant of mucopolysaccharidosis III. *Eur J Pediatr* 1979;**130**:251.

47 Kresse H, von Figura K, Klein U. New biochemical subtype of the Sanfilippo syndrome: characterization of the storage material in cultured fibroblasts of Sanfilippo C patients. *Eur J Biochem* 1978;**92**:333.

48 Bame KJ, Rome LH. AcetylCoA: α-glucosaminide N-acetyl transferase from rat liver. *Methods Enzymol* 1987;**138**:607.

49 Bame KJ, Rome LH. Genetic evidence for transmembrane acetylation by lysosomes. *Science* 1986;**233**:1087.

50 Kresse H, Paschke E, von Figura K, *et al.* Sanfilippo disease type D; deficiency of N-acetylglucosamine-6-sulfatase required for heparan sulfate degradation. *Proc Natl Acad Sci USA* 1980;**77**:6622.

51 Freeman C, Hoopwood JJ. Human glucosamine-6-sulphatase deficiency. Diagnostic enzymology towards heparin-derived trisaccharide substrates. *Biochem J* 1992;**282**(pt2):605.

52 Freeman C, Clements PR, Hopwood JJ. Human liver N-acetylglucosamine-6-sulphate sulphatase. Purification and characterization. *Biochem J* 1987;**246**:347.

53 Von Figura K, Kresse H. Sanfilippo disease type B: presence of material cross reacting with antibodies against a-N-acetyl-glucosaminidase. *Eur J Biochem* 1976;**61**:581.

54 Fuchs W, Beck M, Kresse H. Intralysosomal formation and metabolic fate of N-acetylglucosamine 6-sulfate from keratan sulfate. *Eur J Biochem* 1985;**151**:551.

55 Andria G, Di Natale P, Del Giudice E, *et al.* Sanfilippo B syndrome (MPS III): mild and severe forms within the same sibship. *Clin Genet* 1979;**15**:500.

56 Van de Kamp JJP, van Pelt JF, Liem KO, *et al.* Clinical variability in Sanfilippo B disease: a report of six patients in two related sibships. *Clin Genet* 1976;**10**:279.

57 Toone JR, Applegarth DA. Carrier detection in Sanfilippo A syndrome. *Clin Genet* 1988;**33**:401.

58 Kleijer WJ, Janse HC, Vosters RPL, *et al.* First trimester diagnosis of mucopolysaccharidosis IIIA (Sanfilippo A disease). *N Engl J Med* 1986;**314**:185.

59 Di Natale P, Pannone N, D'Argenio G, *et al.* First trimester prenatal diagnosis of Sanfilippo C disease. *Prenat Diagn* 1987;**7**:603.

60 Poenaru L. First trimester prenatal diagnosis of metabolic diseases: a survey of countries from the European Community. *Prenat Diagn* 1987;**7**:333.

61 Nowakowski RW, Thompson JN, Taylor KB. Sanfilippo syndrome type D: a spectrophotometric assay with prenatal diagnostic potential. *Pediatr Res* 1989;**26**:462.

62 Karageorgos LE, Guo X-H, Blanch L, *et al.* Structure and sequence of the human sulphamidase gene. *DNA Res* 1996;**3**:269.

63 Weber B, Guo XH, Wraith JE, *et al.* Novel mutations in Sanfilippo A syndrome: implications for enzyme function. *Hum Mol Genet* 1997;**6**:1573.

64 Bunge S, Ince H, Steglich C, *et al.* Identification of 16 sulfamidase gene mutations including the common R74C in patients with mucopoly-saccharidosis type IIIA (Sanfilippo A). *Hum Mutat* 1997;**10**:479.

65 Di Natale P, Balzano N, Esposito S, Villani GR. Identification of molecular defects in Italian Sanfilippo A patients including 13 novel mutations. *Hum Mutat* 1998;**11**:313.

66 Montfort M, Vilageliu L, Garcia-Giralt N, *et al.* Mutation 1091delC is highly prevalent in Spanish Sanfilippo syndrome type A patients. *Hum Mutat* 1998;**12**:274.

67 Zhao HG, Aronovich EL, Whitley CB. Genotype-phenotype correspondence in Sanfilippo syndrome type B. *Am J Hum Genet* 1998;**62**:53.

68 Coll MJ, Antón C, Chabás A. Allelic heterogeneity in Spanish patients with Sanfilippo disease type B. Identification of eight new mutations. *J Inherit Metab Dis* 2001;**24**:83.

69 Munnich A, Saudubray JM, Hors-Cayla MC, *et al.* Letter to the Editor: Enzyme replacement therapy by transplantation of HLA-compatible fibroblasts in Sanfilippo syndrome: another trial. *Pediatr Res* 1982;**16**:259.

70 Shapiro EG, Lockman LA, Balthazor M, Krivit WJ. Neuropsychological outcomes of several storage diseases with and without bone marrow transplantation. *J Inherit Metab Dis* 1995;**18**:413.

81

Morquio syndrome/mucopolysaccharidosis type IV (MPS IV)/keratan sulfaturia

MAJOR PHENOTYPIC EXPRESSION

Shortness of stature, pectus carinatum, dorsolumbar kyphosis, odontoid hypoplasia, genu valgum, corneal clouding, dental anomalies, aortic valve disease and keratan sulfaturia. Activity of galactosamine-6-sulfate sulfatase is deficient in type A Morquio syndrome; lysosomal β-galactosidase is defective in type IV B.

INTRODUCTION

The syndrome was described by Morquio in 1929 [1] in four affected siblings in Uruguay who were the products of a marriage of first cousins of Swedish origin. In the same year Brailsford [2] described a similar patient in England. The excretion of keratan sulfate in the urine is the defining biochemical feature of patients with this disease and keratan sulfate has been documented to accumulate in tissues [3–5]. Defective degradation of keratan sulfate leads to its accumulation in those tissues in which it is normally abundant: cartilage, nucleus pulposus and cornea – tissues that are prominent in the clinical manifestation of the disease. Keratin sulphate consists of alternating galactose and N-acetylglucosamine residues; each may be sulphated. The molecular defect in type A or classic Morquio syndrome is in N-acetylgalactosamine-6-sulfatase. It is also a galactose-6-sulfatase responsible for the cleavage of the galactose-6-sulfate moieties of keratan sulfate [6–8] (Figure 81.1). This enzyme also catalyzes the removal of sulphate moieties from N-acetylgalatosamine-6-sulfate residues that are present in chondroitin-6-sulfate, and this leads to excretion in excess of chondroitin sulfate in Morquio syndrome.

In the sequential degradation of keratan sulfate, once the first sulfate has been cleaved, the terminal galactose is cleaved

in a reaction catalyzed by β-galactosidase. This is the enzyme that is defective in type B Morquio syndrome [9–12].

The gene for the galactose-6-sulfatase deficient in type A Morquio disease has been cloned [13] and mapped to

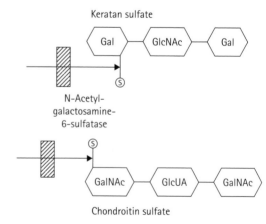

Figure 81.1 *N-Acetylgalactosamine-6-sulfatase and the degradation of keratan sulfate. This is the site of the defect in type A Morquio syndrome. The enzyme also hydrolyzes the sulfate from the N-acetylgalactosamine-6-sulfate moieties that occur in chondroitin-6-sulfate.*

chromosome 16q24.3 [14,15]. A number of mutations has been described [16–19]. The gene for the β-galactosidase defective in type B has been localized to chromosome 3p21-cen [20].

CLINICAL ABNORMALITIES

The clinical pictures in type A and type B are indistinguishable. In both there is considerable heterogeneity ranging from mild to severe including even hydrops fetalis phenotypes. The most characteristic features of this syndrome are skeletal deformities and shortness of stature, which is particularly short-trunked, though the long bones are also involved. The neck is short and the head appears to sit directly on the barrel chest,

which classically has a very pronounced pectus carinatum (Figures 81.2–81.6). The upper part of the sternum may be almost horizontal. There is also a pronounced genu valgum, and patients often have a semi-crouching stance. The joints are enlarged and prominent (Figures 81.7–81.12). On the other hand, as a result of ligamentous laxity there is usually extreme hypermobility and hyperextension of the joints, particularly at the wrists, where there may be marked ulnar deviation (Figure 81.9). Joints may become stiff with age. Pes planus is also seen.

These skeletal changes are not obvious during the first year of life because intrauterine growth and early extrauterine

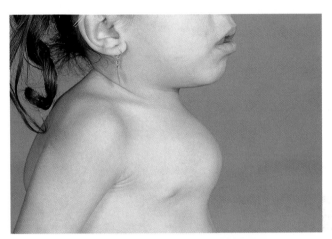

Figure 81.4   *M.K.M.T., a 4-year-old with Morquio type II disease. The prominent pectus is shown.*

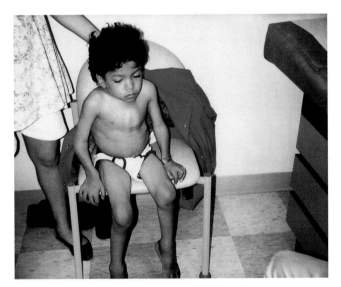

Figure 81.2   *F.D., a 10-year-old Honduran boy with Marquio syndrome. He was short and had a prominent pectus carnatum. The neck appeared very short.*

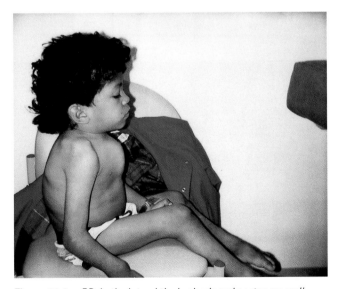

Figure 81.3   *F.D. In the lateral the kyphosis and pectus are well seen. There was irregular flaring at the rib cage.*

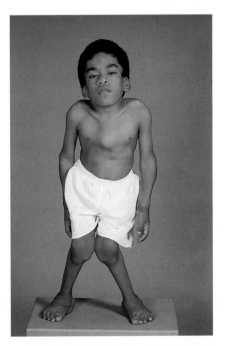

Figure 81.5   *A.B.V., a 12-year-old boy with Morquio disease. He had kyphosis, as well as a prominent manubrium and a small thoracic cage. He had marked genu valgum and flexion deformities of the hip. Activity of 2-N-acetylgalactosamine-6-sulfatase in fibroblasts was undetectable.*

development are normal. Prominence of the lower ribs may first bring the patient in for medical consultation at 12 to 18 months-of-age. Others first come to attention because of prominence of the sternum. Flat feet may be an early sign. In the second or third year, patients develop awkward gaits and retarded growth as skeletal deformities begin to be evident. The deformities are progressive and become exaggerated with age [21]. Patients with milder disease have presented in early adolescence with bilateral Legg-Perthes disease [22]. In similar fashion a 30-year-old was reported with severe hip disease [23]. Growth is markedly slowed after about 5 years-of-age. Maximal height of 85–100 cm is usually reached by 7 to 8 years-of-age. Diagnostic delay is the rule and the diagnosis may not be made until as late as 15 years [24,25].

These patients have fine corneal opacities, which usually are visible only on slit lamp examination, but may cause a hazy cloudiness of the cornea [3,26]. Glaucoma was observed in siblings in their thirties [27]. Progressive sensorineural or mixed deafness usually begins in the second decade and is present uniformly after 20 years [28].

The mouth tends to be broad, and there may be spacing between the teeth which may be small and flared [29,30]. The enamel is hypoplastic both in deciduous and in permanent teeth. The teeth develop a gray or yellowish color, and the enamel becomes flaky or fractured. Molars are tapered and often have sharp cusps. The teeth easily develop caries. In one series [31] dental changes were observed only in type A, not in type B.

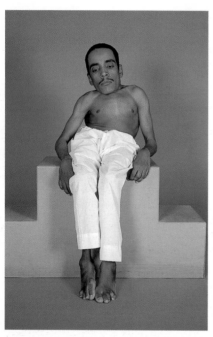

Figure 81.6   F.R.A.M., a 26-year-old with Morquio disease and a spastic tetraplegia, a consequence of cord compression at C1 and C2 and odontoid hypoplasia.

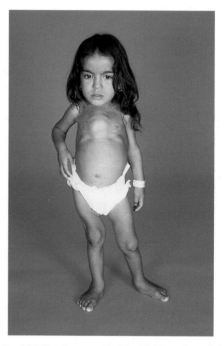

Figure 81.8   M.A.Z., a 3-year-old girl with Morquio and the typical pectus deformity, short neck and flat facies, as well as valgus deformities at the knees and ankles.

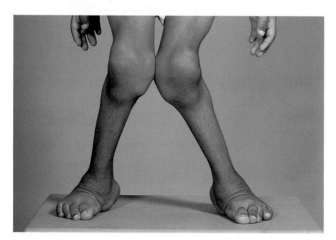

Figure 81.7   A.B.U. The genu valgum. The ankles and feet were quite broad.

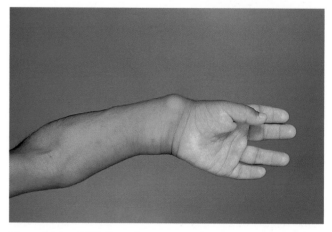

Figure 81.9   A.B.U. The wrists were very floppy, and he had poor grip strength.

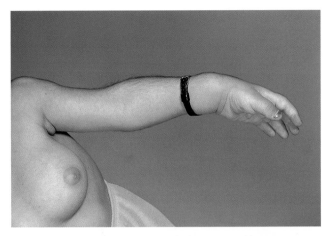

Figure 81.10   *A.B.A.O. The wrists of this 14-year-old were very floppy, and ulnar deviation was the result of the very short ulna.*

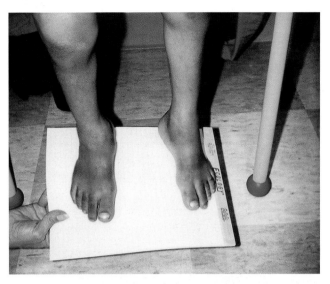

Figure 81.12   *F.D. The ankles and feet were also broadened.*

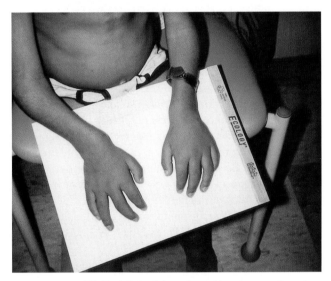

Figure 81.11   *F.D. The joints of the wrist and hand were enlarged.*

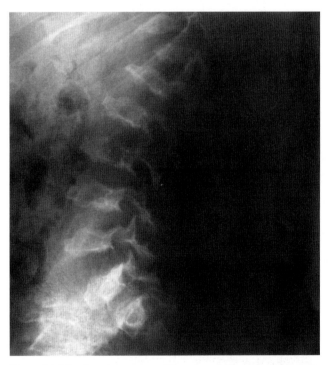

Figure 81.13   *Roentgenogram of the spine of a 5-year-old boy with Morquio syndrome. The vertebral bodies were very flat and beaked anteriorly. The second vertebra from the top was hypoplastic and displaced posteriorly. This is the genesis of the gibbus in this syndrome. (Illustration was kindly provided by Dr. David Rimoin, University of California, Los Angeles and Cedars of Lebanon Hospital, Los Angeles, California.)*

A regular later manifestation of the disease is aortic regurgitation [32]. Severe scoliosis may lead to cardiorespiratory complications. Three of Morquio's original patients died of pulmonary complications. Inguinal hernia is probably more common than in normal individuals.

The brain is normal and patients usually have normal intelligence. Ian Smith, a 3-feet-tall, 14-year-old with Morquio syndrome played the title role in the Disney film Simon Birch and speaks publicly in support of rare diseases. Facial features may be somewhat coarse, the chin prominent and the mouth wide. The neck is short (Figure 81.2).

Roentgenographic findings [33] in Morquio disease vary with the age of the patient. This is the only mucopolysaccharidosis in which there are no changes of dysostosis multiplex. The most characteristic and consistent finding is the universal platyspondyly or vertebra plana, which produces the short spine (Figure 81.13). The vertebral bodies are usually oval-shaped in the younger affected child, becoming flatter and more rectangular in later childhood and flat in the adult. The cervical spine is striking in that the odontoid process of C2 is either absent or hypoplastic [34]. The remainder of the cervical vertebrae are flat. The thoracic and lumbar vertebrae show flattening and anterior beaking or tonguing. L1 is often short, anteriorly wedged and displaced posteriorly, accounting for

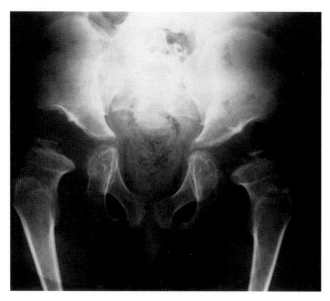

Figure 81.14   *Roentgenogram of the pelvis of the same patient. The capital femoral epiphyses were flattened and irregular. There was coxa valga. The lateral margins of the acetabula were hypoplastic, creating, in essence, large acetabula extending to the anterior superior iliac spine. (Illustration was kindly provided by Dr. David Rimoin.)*

the gibbus. Patients with this syndrome always have a marked coxa valga deformity (Figure 81.14). The pelvis is narrow. With age, the anterior portions of the ribs become wide and spatula-shaped. The sternum protrudes. The femoral head becomes progressively flattened and fragmented; it may be completely resorbed. The femoral neck initially loses its angle and later becomes thickened. The distal femur is wide, as is the proximal tibia. These changes contribute to the production of the genu valgum that is characteristic of this disease. The distal end of the humerus is wide and irregular, as are the proximal ulna and radius – changes similar to the corresponding bones of the lower extremities. The growth plates of the distal ulnae and radii are slanted toward each other, the ulna usually being somewhat shorter than the radius. The ossified carpal bones are small and may be reduced in number. The metacarpals are short, and their distal metaphyses are widened. Osteoporosis is common in the adult patient.

A very dangerous complication of the bony deformity in this syndrome is that the spinal cord may be compressed following atlantoaxial subluxation or dislocation [12,35–37]. This is a major cause of death. Manipulation of the head for intubation may be particularly risky in these patients for this reason and anesthesia should be planned with this problem in the forefront, but subluxation may occur even during sleep and lead to death. This propensity for subluxation is attributed to the hypoplasia of the odontoid process and to the general laxity of the ligaments. These features are present in all patients with the disease, who therefore sooner or later may all expect to experience a complication of compression of the spinal cord. Neurologic manifestations may include weakness and difficulty in walking, uselessness of the legs on awakening, or spastic

paraplegia. Loss of vibratory sensation in the lower extremities may be an early sign, and many patients have hyperactive deep tendon reflexes. Spinal cord compression may also occur at the level of the thoracolumbar gibbus. Subluxation of vertebra C2 to C3, as well as C1 to C2, has been observed [9] in type B patients. Conjunctival biopsy may show intracytoplasmic vacuoles indicating lysosomal storage [38]. Metachromatic granules may be seen in the polymorphonuclear leukocytes or cultured fibroblasts [39]. Storage vacuoles have been demonstrated in the skin and in chondrocytes [40]. There is minimal evidence of storage in the brain.

GENETICS AND PATHOGENESIS

Morquio syndrome is transmitted by autosomal recessive genes. It has been reported on several occasions that normal couples have produced multiple involved siblings. Parental consanguinity has been documented [21]. Prenatal diagnosis may be performed by the assay of either enzyme in cultured amniocytes or chorionic villus tissue [41].

Patients with Morquio disease characteristically have increased concentrations of keratan sulfate in the urine [42]. Levels of this acid mucopolysaccharide, which does not contain uronic acid, are often two to three times the normal amount. With age, the concentrations of this compound in urine decrease. A new developed immunoassay for keratan sulfate is capable of diagnostic assay of either blood or urine in any age group and permits distinction of mild and severe phenotypes [43]. Absence of keratansulfaturia has been documented in enzyme-proven type B [11] and type A [22,23,31,44,45] Morquio disease.

In Morquio type A the defective enzyme catalyzes the removal of 6-sulfate moieties from galactose, and from the N-acetylgalactosamine residues of chondroitin sulphate. This latter property gave the enzyme its name. N-acetylgalactosamine-6-sulfatase has been purified from human placenta [46] and the defective enzyme has been demonstrated in cultured fibroblasts and in brain [3,5,8]. Deficiency of the type A enzyme has been demonstrated in patients not excreting keratansulfate [47]. In five patients studied immunochemically, no cross-reacting material was demonstrated [48], but cross-reactive material has been demonstrated immunochemically in both Morquio type B and type A [49]. The full length of cDNA has been cloned and sequenced for human N-acetylgalactosamine-6-sulfatase [13], and transfection into deficient fibroblasts led to activity. The type A gene has 14 exons, and the sequence of 522 amino acids of the enzyme has considerable homology with other sulfatases, such as iduronate-2-sulfatase.

A considerable number and variety of mutations have been found in the Morquio type A gene, as well as some polymorphisms [50]. Most were missense point mutations, but there were a few nonsense and splice site mutations and small deletions. Insertions and large rearrangements were rare. Severe disease was present in patients with a T to C change at nucleotide 468 resulting in V138A and a C to T transition at 386 substituting a cysteine for arginine 386 [18]. A 2 base deletion 1342delCA was also associated with severe disease [51]. I113F was found to be a common missense mutation in Caucasian, particularly Irish patients [16,50]; so was T312S.

Some mutations in the β-galactosidase gene have been identified in genetic compounds [52,53]. Dependent on the mutation the phenotype can vary from that of severe GM_1 gangliosidosis (Chapter 93) to Morquio type B [54].

The diagnosis is best made by assay of cultured fibroblasts or leukocytes using a substrate derived from chondroitin-6-sulfate for the sulfatase [55,56] and using p-nitrophenyl or 4-methylumbelliferyl-β-galactoside for the β-galactosidase.

In addition to types A and B, there are other clinical examples of Morquio syndrome, usually mild, in which defects in neither of these enzymes can be detected. These are nonkeratansulfate-excreting patients [57]. The skeletal deformities and other symptoms in these patients are similar to those seen in Morquio syndrome, but less severe. There is platyspondyly, genu valgum, flat feet, pectus carinatum and flat, fragmented femoral heads.

TREATMENT

Surgical fusion of the cervical spine may be life-saving in the prevention of spinal cord compression [58]. Surgical decompression may be required for cord compression. There is a tendency for the prognosis to be better in females. Osteotomies may be useful in correction of the genu valgum [57,59]. Any surgery should be undertaken with caution because of the risk of atlantoaxial instability and because of the deformity of the chest and its effect on cardiopulmonary function [60]. Hearing aids may be useful [28]. The instability of the wrists, which makes working with the hands very difficult, may be improved by the use of wrist splints. Enzyme replacement therapy is under exploration in knockout mouse models.

References

1 Morquio L. Sur une form de dystrophie osseuse familiale. *Arch Med Enfants* 1929;**32**:129.

2 Brailsford JF. Chondro-osteo-dystrophy: roentgenographic and clinical features of a child with dislocation of vertebrae. *Am J Surg* 1929;**7**:404.

3 Maroteaux P, Lamy M. Opacities cornéennes et trouble métabolique dans la maladie de Morquio. *Rev Fr Etud Clin Biol* 1961;**6**:48.

4 Minami R, Katsuyuki A, Kudoh T, *et al.* Identification of keratan sulfate in liver affected by Morquio syndrome. *Clin Chim Acta* 1979;**93**:207.

5 Gadbois P, Moreau J, Laberge C. La maladie de Morquio dans la province de Quebec. *Union Med Can* 1973;**102**:602.

6 Matalon R, Arbogast B, Justice P, *et al.* Morquio's syndrome: deficiency of a chondroitin sulfate N-acetylhexosamine sulfate sulfatase. *Biochem Biophys Res Commun* 1974;**61**:759.

7 Singh J, Differrante NM, Nieves P, Tavella D. N-Acetylgalactosamine-6-sulfate sulfatase in man: absence of the enzyme in Morquio disease. *Clin Invest* 1976;**57**:1036.

8 Horwitz AL, Dorfman A. The enzymatic defect in Morquio's disease: the specificity of N-acetylhexosamine sulfatases. *Biochem Biophys Res Commun* 1978;**80**:819.

9 Tojak JE, Ho CH, Roesel RA, *et al.* Morquio-like syndrome (MPS IV B) associated with deficiency of β-galactosidase. *Johns Hopkins Med J* 1980;**146**:75.

10 Arbisser AI, Donnelly KA, Scott CI Jr, *et al.* Morquio-like syndrome with beta-galactosidase deficiency and abnormal hexosamine sulfatase activity: mucopolysaccharidosis IV B. *Am J Med Genet* 1977;**1**:195.

11 O'Brien JS, Gugler E, Giedion A, *et al.* Spondyloepiphyseal dysplasia corneal clouding normal intelligence and acid β-galactosidase deficiency. *Clin Genet* 1976;**9**:495.

12 Groebe H, Krins M, Schmidberger H, *et al.* Morquio syndrome (mucopolysaccharidosis IV B) associated with β-galactosidase deficiency: a report of two cases. *Am J Hum Genet* 1980;**32**:258.

13 Tomatsu S, Fukuda S, Masue M, *et al.* Morquio disease: isolation characterization and expression of full length DNA for human N-acetylgalactosamine-6-sulfatase. *Biochem Biophys Res Commun* 1991;**181**:677.

14 Masuno M, Tomatsu S, Nakashima Y, *et al.* Mucopolysaccharidosis IV A: assignment of the human N-acetylgalactosamine-6-sulfate sulfatase (GALNS) gene to chromosome 16q24. *Genomics* 1993;**16**:777.

15 Baker E, Guo X-H, Orsborn A, *et al.* The Morquio A syndrome (mucopolysaccharidosis IVA) gene maps to 16q243. *Am J Hum Genet* 1993;**52**:96.

16 Tomatsu S, Fukuda S, Cooper A, *et al.* Mucopolysaccharidosis IVA: identification of a common missense mutation I113F in the N-acetylgalactosamine-6-sulfate sulfatase gene. *Am J Hum Genet* 1995;**57**:556.

17 Hori T, Tomatsu S, Nakashima Y, *et al.* Mucopolysaccharidosis type IVA: common double deletion in the N-acetylgalactosamine-6-sulfatase gene (GALNS). *Genomics* 1995;**26**:535.

18 Tomatsu S, Fukuda S, Yamagishi A, *et al.* Mucopolysaccharidosis IVA: four new exonic mutations in patients with N-acetylgalactosamine-6-sulfate sulfatase deficiency. *Am J Hum Genet* 1996;**58**:950.

19 Tomatsu S, Fukuda S, Cooper A, *et al.* Two new mutations Q473X and N487S in a Caucasian patient with mucopolysaccharidosis IVA (Morquio disease). *Hum Mutat* 1995;**6**:195.

20 Shows TB, Scrafford-Wolff LR, Brown JA, Meisler M. Assignment of a β-galactosidase level (β-Gal-a) to chromosome 3 in man. *Cytogen Cell Genet* 1978;**22**:219.

21 McKusick VA. The mucopolysaccharidoses: in *Heritable Disorders of Connective Tissue* (4th edn) (VA McKusick). CV Mosby Co, St Louis;1972:583.

22 Hecht JT, Scott CI Jr, Smith TK, Williams JC. Mild manifestations of the Morquio syndrome (Letter). *Am J Med Genet* 1984;**18**:369.

23 Beck M, Glossl J, Grubisic A, Spranger J. Heterogeneity of Morquio disease. *Clin Genet* 1986;**29**:325.

24 Maroteaux P, Stanescu V, Stanescu R, *et al.* Heterogeneite des formes frustes de la maladie de Morquio. *Arch Franc Pediatr* 1982;**39**:761.

25 Holzgreve W, Grobe H, von Figura K, *et al.* Morquio syndrome: clinical findings in 11 patients with MPS IVA and 2 patients with MPS IVB. *Hum Genet* 1981;**57**:360.

26 Van Noorden GK, Zellweger H, Ponseti IV. Ocular findings in Morquio – Ullrich's disease. *Arch Ophthalmol* 1960;**64**:585.

27 Cahane M, Treister G, Abraham FA, Melamed S. Glaucoma in siblings with Morquio syndrome. *Br J Ophthalmol* 1990;**74**:382.

28 Reidner ED, Levin LS. Hearing patterns in Morquio's syndrome (mucopolysaccharidosis IV). *Arch Otolaryngol* 1977;**103**:518.

29 Northover H, Cowie RA, Wraith JE. Mucopolysaccharidosis type IVA (Morquio syndrome): A clinical review. *J Inherit Metab Dis* 1996;**19**:357.

30   Levin LS, Jorgenson RJ, Salinas CF. Oral findings in the Morquio syndrome (mucopolysaccharidosis IV). *Oral Surg Oral Med Oral Path* 1975;**39**:390.

31   Nelson J, Kinirons M. Clinical findings in 12 patients with MPS IV A (Morquio's disease): further evidence for heterogeneity Part II: dental findings. *Clin Genet* 1988;**33**:121.

32   John RM, Hunter D, Swanton RH. Echocardiographic abnormalities in type IV mucopolysaccharidosis. *Arch Dis Child* 1990;**65**:746.

33   Langer LO Jr, Carey LS. The roentgenographic features of the KS mucopolysaccharidosis of Morquio (Morquio-Brailsford's disease). *Am J Roentgenol Radium Ther Nucl Med* 1966;**97**:1.

34   Lipson SJ. Dysplasia of the odontoid process in Morquio's syndrome causing quadriparesis. *J Bone Joint Surg* 1977;**59**:340.

35   Blaw ME, Langer LO. Spinal cord compression in Morquio-Brailsford disease. *J Pediatr* 1969;**74**:593.

36   Hughes DG, Chadderton RD, Cowie RA, *et al.* MRI of the brain and craniocervical junction in Morquio's disease. *Neuroradiology* 1997;**39**:381.

37   Greenberg AD. Atlantoaxial dislocations. *Brain* 1968;**91**:655.

38   Scheie HG, Hambrick GW, Jr, Barnes LA. A newly recognized *forme fruste* of Hurler's disease (gargoylism). *Am J Ophthal* 1962;**53**:753.

39   Danes VS, Grossman H. Bone dysplasias including Morquio's syndrome studied in skin and fibroblast cultures. *Am J Med* 1969;**47**:708.

40   Koto A, Horwitz AL, Suzuki K, *et al.* The Morquio syndrome: neuropathology and biochemistry. *Ann Neurol* 1978;**4**:26.

41   Applegarth DA, Toone JR, Wilson RD, *et al.* Morquio disease presenting as hydrops fetalis and enzyme analysis of chorionic villus tissue in a subsequent pregnancy. *Pediatr Pathol* 1987;**7**:593.

42   Humbel R, Marchal C, Fall M. Diagnosis of Morquio's disease: a simple chromatographic method for the identification of keratosulfate in urine. *J Pediatr* 1972;**81**:107.

43   Tomatsu S, Okamura K, Taketani T, *et al.* Development and testing of new screening method for keratan sulfate in Mucopolysaccharidosis IVA. *Pediatr Res* 2004; **55**:592.

44   Nelson J, Thomas PS. Clinical findings in 12 patients with MPS IV A (Morquio's disease). Further evidence for heterogeneity Part III: odontoid dysplasia. *Clin Genet* 1988;**33**:126.

45   Nelson J, Broadhead D, Mossman J. Clinical findings in 12 patients with MPS IV A (Morquio's disease). Further evidence for heterogeneity Part I: Clinical and biochemical findings. *Clin Genet* 1988;**33**:111.

46   Glossl J, Truppe W, Kresse H. Purification and properties of N-acetyl-galactosamine-6-sulfate sulfatase from human placenta. *Biochem J* 1979;**181**:37.

47   Fujimoto A, Horwitz AL. Biochemical defect of non-keratan-sulfate-excreting Morquio syndrome. *Am J Med Genet* 1983;**15**:265.

48   Glossl J, Lembeck K, Gamse G, Kresse H. Morquio's disease type A: absence of material cross-reacting with antibodies against N-acetylgalactosamine-6-sulfate sulfatase. *Hum Genet* 1980;**54**:87.

49   van der Horst GTJ, Kleijer WJ, Hoogeveen AT, *et al.* Morquio B syndrome: a primary defect in beta-galactosidase. *Am J Med Genet* 1983;**16**:261.

50   Montano AM, Orii KO, Grubb JH, *et al.* Spectrums of mutations in mucopolysaccharidosis IVA (Morquio disease) gene. *Proc Jpn Soc Inherit Metab Dis* 1991;**44**:172.

51   Fukuda S, Tomatsu S, Masue M, *et al.* Mucopolysaccharidosis type IVA: N-acetylgalactosamine-6-sulfate sulfatase exonic point mutations in classical Morquio and mild cases. *J Clin Invest* 1992;**90**:1049.

52   Oshima A, Yoshida K, Shimmoto M, *et al.* Human beta-galactosidase gene mutations in Morquio B disease. *Am J Hum Genet* 1991;**49**:1091.

53   Ishii N, Oohira T, Oshima A, *et al.* Clinical and molecular analysis of a Japanese boy with Morquio B disease. *Clin Genet* 1995;**48**:103.

54   Suzuki Y, Oshima A. A beta-galactosidase gene mutation identified in both Morquio B disease and infantile G(M1) gangliosidosis (Letter). *Hum Genet* 1993;**91**:407.

55   Kresse H, von Figura K, Kelin U, *et al.* Enzymatic diagnosis of the genetic mucopolysaccharide storage disorders – an extension. *Meth Enzymol* 1982;**83**:(pt D) 559.

56   Glossl J, Kresse H. A sensitive procedure for the diagnosis of N-acetyl-galactosamine-6-sulfate sulfatase deficiency in classical Morquio's disease. *Clin Chem Acta* 1978;**88**:111.

57   Norum RA. Nonkeratosulfate-excreting Morquio's syndrome in four members of an inbred group: in *Skeletal Dysplasias, Clinical Delineation of Birth Defects.* Part IV, The National Foundation – March of Dimes, New York;1979:334.

58   Kopits SE, Perovic MN, McKusick VA, *et al.* Congenital atlantoaxial dislocations in various forms of dwarfism. *J Bone Joint Surg* 1972;**54A**:1349.

59   Kopits SE. Orthopedic complications of dwarfism. *Clin Orthop* 1976;**114**:153.

60   Jones AEP, Croley TF. Morquio syndrome and anesthesia. *Anesthesiology* 1979;**51**:261.

82

Maroteaux-Lamy disease/mucopolysaccharidosis VI (MPS VI)/N-acetylgalactosamine-4-sulfatase deficiency

---

MAJOR PHENOTYPIC EXPRESSION

Shortness of stature, limitation of joint motion and contractures, corneal clouding, hepatosplenomegaly, dysostosis multiplex, excretion of dermatan sulfate, and deficiency of N-acetylgalactosamine-4-sulfatase (arylsulfatase B).

INTRODUCTION

A distinct mucopolysaccharidosis was first recognized by Maroteaux, Lamy and colleagues [1] in 1963 as a syndrome in which patients displayed some of the features of the Hurler syndrome, but had normal intelligence [1,2]. Furthermore, the mucopolysaccharide found in the urine was predominantly dermatan sulfate. A number of variants have now been described in which the range of severity is quite broad.

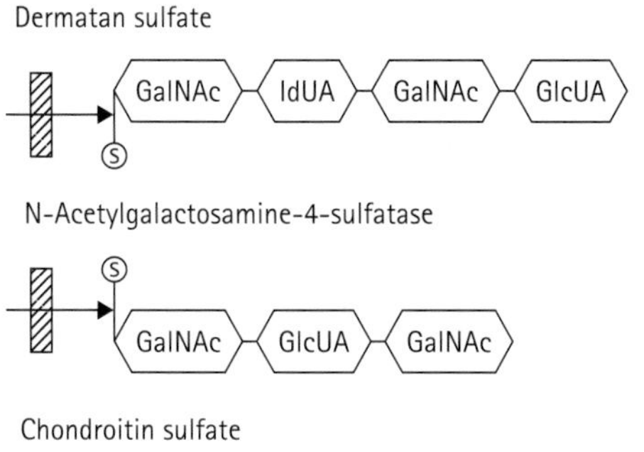

Dermatan sulfate

N-Acetylgalactosamine-4-sulfatase

Chondroitin sulfate

Figure 82.1 *Degradation of dermatan sulfate and chondroitin sulfate. N-acetylgalactosamine-4-sulfatase, the site of the defect of Maroteaux-Lamy syndrome, is active in the degradation of both glucosaminoglycans.*

The molecular defect (Figure 82.1) is in the enzyme N-acetylgalactosamine-4-sulfatase [3,4]. It catalyzes the removal of sulfate moieties from both dermatan sulfate and chondrioitin-4-sulfate. This protein is the Maroteaux-Lamy corrective factor [5]. The human cDNA has been cloned [6] and the gene has been mapped to chromosome 5q13-14 [7]. A variety of mutations have been identified [8,9].

CLINICAL ABNORMALITIES

The classic patient with the Maroteaux-Lamy syndrome develops impressively short stature [10,11]. The patient is often first brought to the physician at 2 to 3 years-of-age because of retarded growth. The problem involves both the trunk and the extremities. By this time the patient may be found to have the deformities and facial characteristics of a mucopolysaccharidosis (Figures 82.2–82.11). The facial features are recognizably coarse (Figures 82.2, 82.3, 82.6), but they are considerably more subtle than those of the patient with the Hurler syndrome. The breathing may be noisy from early infancy. A large head or prominent chest may be present at birth. There may be umbilical or inguinal hernias, and surgical repair may be required in the first years of life [10].

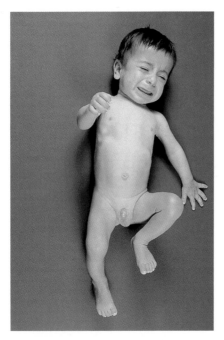

Figure 82.2   *T.S.M.G., a one-year-old Saudi Arabian boy with the Maroteaux-Lamy syndrome. He was very short. The facial features were coarse, but much less so than in Hurler syndrome or in most patients with Hunter syndrome.*

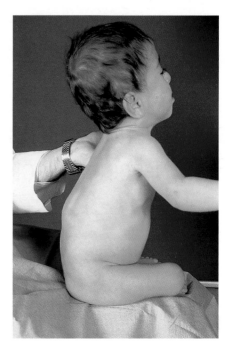

Figure 82.4   *T.S.M.G. In the lateral view, the gibbus is characteristic.*

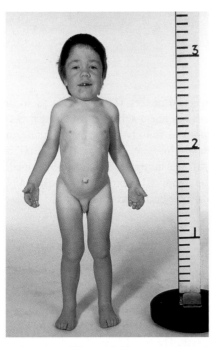

Figure 82.3   *A 7-year-old boy with Maroteaux-Lamy disease. Illustrated are the shortness of stature, somewhat coarse facies and genu valgum. He also had cloudy corneas. (Illustration was kindly provided by Dr. Philip Benson.)*

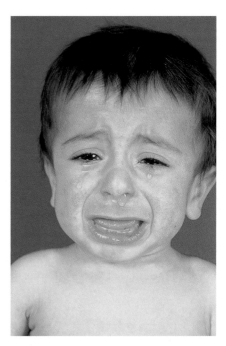

Figure 82.5   *Close-up of the face reveals coarse features, a flattened nasal bridge, and a large tongue.*

Ultimate height of 107–138 cm may be reached by 6 to 8 years, the age at which growth usually stops. The head appears larger than the body. The skin may appear tight. Hirsutism is common. There may be macroglossia and protrusion of the tongue. The typical appearance of the child with this disorder is of a short trunk, protuberant abdomen and lumbar lordosis.

Changes of the joints are progressive, and motion becomes increasingly limited. Genu valgum and a position of semiflexion of the knees are characteristic, giving the child a crouched stance. A claw-hand deformity develops that is typical of mucopolysaccharidosis (Figure 82.9). There may be flexion contractures of the fingers, as well as the knees and elbows.

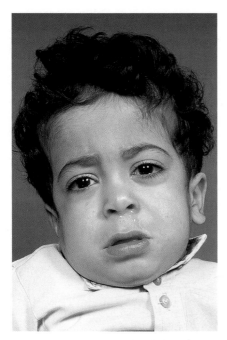

Figure 82.6   *T.S.M.G. at 18 months. The features were increasingly coarse.*

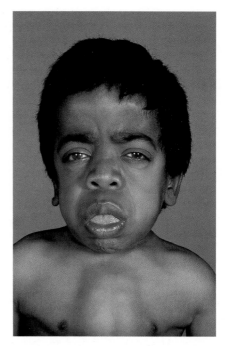

Figure 82.8   *H.A.H. Close-up of the face illustrates the low hair line, flat, coarse facies and macroglossia. He had bilateral corneal clouding.*

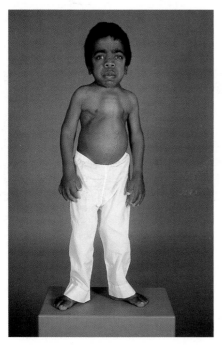

Figure 82.7   *H.A.H., a 9-year-old Saudi boy with Maroteaux-Lamy disease. Facial features were coarse. He was very short. The activity of arylsulfatase B in fibroblasts was four percent of control.*

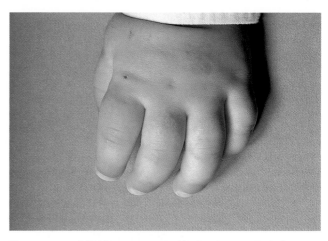

Figure 82.9   *T.S.M.G. at 18 months. The hand was typical of a mucopolysaccharidosis with broadening of the digits and claw-shaped contractures.*

The differential diagnosis may suggest mucolipidosis III (Chapter 85). A carpal tunnel syndrome may contribute to the limitation of hand motion. The subcutaneous tissues of the volar surfaces of the second to fourth fingers may be thickened, as in Dupuytren contractures [10]. Lumbar kyphosis and anterior protrusion of the sternum are also progressive.

Hepatomegaly is regularly observed in patients over 6 years-of-age, and splenomegaly is found in about half of the patients. Some patients have had frequent episodes of diarrhea.

Cardiac abnormality is an important component of this syndrome [12]. Murmurs heard indicate valvular involvement. The mitral and aortic valves become thickened, calcified and stenotic [13,14]. A murmur of aortic stenosis is frequently present [15–17], and mitral or aortic regurgitation may also be present. There may be right as well as left ventricular failure. An unusual presentation is with acute infantile cardiomyopathy [18,19]. Cardiac failure may be the cause of death, which usually occurs before 30 years-of-age in the classic form of

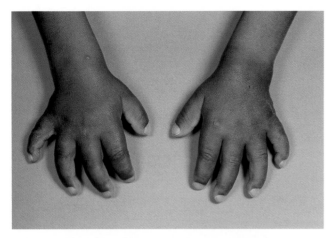

Figure 82.10   *H.A.H. at 9 years; the claw hand deformity was very prominent.*

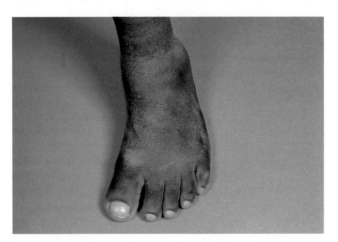

Figure 82.11   *H.A.H. The foot was also broad and the toes particularly wide.*

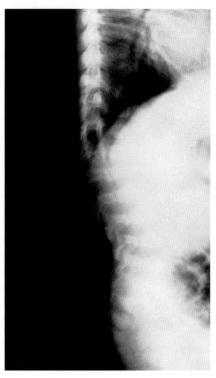

Figure 82.12   *T.S.M.G. Lateral roentgenogram of the spine. The vertebral body of L1 was hypoplastic and prominent anteriorly. The gibbus deformity was in this area.*

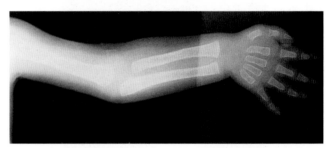

Figure 82.13   *T.S.M.G. Roentgenogram of the arm. The bones are all thickened and poorly modeled.*

the disease. Some have died of pulmonary infection. Another pulmonary complication is obstructive sleep apnea.

The corneas develop opacities at an early stage that are detectable by slit lamp examination and progressively become clinically cloudy. This is especially dense at the periphery and it may lead to visual impairment. Glaucoma was reported in four adult women [20]. Deafness is a regular feature, related at least in part to recurrent otitis media.

In contrast to most of the mucopolysaccharidoses, the Maroteaux-Lamy disease is characterized by normal intelligence. Two families have been reported in which there was mental retardation, but this may have had some other etiology [21,22].

On the other hand, neurologic complications occur frequently [23–26]. Hydrocephalus may result from pachymeningeal thickening. Ventricular shunting may be required. Myelopathy may result from cord compression following atlantoaxial subluxation. The dura may also be thickened in the cervical region, leading to insidious compression of the cord. The end result is spastic paraplegia [27]. Myelopathy due to compression may also result from developmental

abnormalities of the vertebral bodies and kyphoscoliosis [28]. Papilledema and progressive loss of vision may be a consequence of increased intracranial pressure [11]. Neurologic deterioration has been observed during pregnancy [24]. A complete lack of development of secondary sexual characteristics, as well as an unusual degree of dwarfism in a patient, suggested that the anterior pituitary was also affected.

Patients with milder variants may present with hip dysplasia resembling Legg-Perthes disease. Some present first as adults with disease of the hips [29].

Roentgenograms demonstrate the typical findings of dysostosis multiplex (Figures 82.12–82.14) [11]. Roentgenograms of the hand may in classic examples be indistinguishable from that of Hurler disease (Chapter 77). In some patients diaphyseal constriction may suggest Morquio disease (Chapter 81). The epiphyses are abnormal. Femoral heads may be

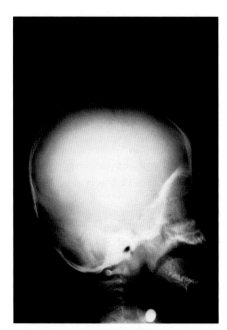

Figure 82.14   *T.S.M.G. Roentgenogram of the skull. The cranial vault was high and the sella J-shaped. Adenoid tissue was prominent.*

particularly dysplastic, and coxa valga is a regular occurrence. The iliac bodies tend to be small and constricted, and the wings flare. The acetabula are small and hypoplastic and the acetabular roofs are oblique. Ossification of the femoral head may be irregular, and this is the reason patients have been thought to have Legg-Perthes disease. The femoral necks may turn outward. Widening of the epiphyseal plates may resemble metaphyseal chondrodysplasia.

The long bones are short and thickened or distended (Figures 82.13) and the radius and ulna may be bowed. In addition, there may be a localized metaphyseal constriction. This may be particularly striking in the surgical neck of the femur. The ribs may be abnormally broad and short, but narrowed at the vertebral ends so that they resemble canoe paddles [11]. There may be oval radiolucencies in the tibial and distal femoral metaphyses, representing residual islands of cartilage. The first lumbar vertebra may be cuneiform. Beaking or anterior hypoplasia occurs typically in this vertebra and in T12; their posterior displacement causes a gibbus deformity. The odontoid may be quite hypoplastic. Along with macrocephaly, the large sella turcica may be omega or J-shaped (Figure 82.14). The calvaria may have a ground-glass appearance, and the mastoids may be sclerotic. Eruption of the teeth may be retarded [30,31]. The height of the mandible may be reduced, and teeth may be displaced so far toward its inferior border that the cortex of the mandible is nearly penetrated by the roots of the teeth.

Cytoplasmic inclusions are more prominent in the Maroteaux-Lamy syndrome than in any of the other mucopolysaccharidoses. They can be seen in 90–100 percent of granulocytes (Alder granules) [32] and as many as 50 percent of lymphocytes [10]. The inclusions are metachromatic.

Lysosomal inclusions are also seen in Kupffer cells and in hepatocytes [33], as well as in platelets [34], and in cells of the conjunctiva, cornea and skin [35]. Fibroblasts may contain large, clear, juxtanuclear inclusions. Large quantities of dermatan sulfate are excreted in the urine, but the total mucopolysaccharide in the urine may be normal [30]; so screening tests for urinary mucopolysaccharidosis may be misleading.

GENETICS AND PATHOGENESIS

The inheritance of this disorder is autosomal recessive. Multiple affected siblings and normal parents have been observed in a number of families, and consanguinity has been documented [10,36]. The site of the defect is in the activity of N-acetyl-galactosamine-4-sulfatase (Figure 82.1, p. 539), which is coded for by a gene on chromosome 5 at position q13-14 [6].

N-acetyl-galactosamine-4-sulfatase catalyzes the hydrolysis of the sulfate from moieties of N-acetylgalactosamine-4-sulfate which occur in dermatan sulfate. The moieties are also found in chondroitin-4-sulfate. Defective activity in this hydrolysis may account for some of the abnormalities in the joints, but chondroitin sulfate is not found in the urine because it can be degraded by hyaluronidase. The enzyme is also known as arylsulfatase B. The human enzyme has been purified [37,38]. Its biosynthesis and processing involve the phosphorylation of mannose moieties and proteolysis in the classic lysosomal enzyme pattern [39,40].

It was initially demonstrated, using artificial substrate, that this enzyme was deficient in Maroteaux-Lamy disease [6,41–44]. The enzyme also has uridine diphospho-N-acetyl-galactosamine-4-sulfate sulfohydrolase activity [44].

cDNAs for the human [4,5] and feline [45] enzymes have been cloned. The human monomeric protein contains 533 amino acids, including a 46 amino acid signal peptide. There is considerable homology with other sulfatases.

Correlation of clinical severity with the amount of residual enzyme activity has not been possible, but over 20 percent of normal activity is consistent with a normal phenotype [46]. The disorder has been diagnosed prenatally by enzyme assay [47]. Heterozygosity may also be demonstrated by assay of arylsulfatase B activity [48].

Analysis of the nature of mutation promises to permit better correlation of genotype with phenotype. Southern blot analysis of genomic DNA of 17 patients revealed no deletions or rearrangements [49]. A majority of patients were compound heterozygotes for two mutations. Homozygous deletion of a base, DG238, was found in a patient with a severe disease [9]. Severe disease was also present in a patient with different deletions on the 2 alleles [50]. A similar degree of severity was found in a patient with a missense conversion of cystine 117 to arginine [8], while the more conservative conversion of glycine 137 to valine was found in a patient with an intermediate phenotype [51]. Two different frameshift mutations led to stop codons in a child with severe disease [50].

Mild disease was found in a patient with two mutant alleles, one a leucine 266 to proline change, and the other a cysteine 405 to tyrosine [7].

TREATMENT

Surgical corrective procedures may be useful in the management of carpal tunnel syndrome, the hips or the cornea. Laminectomy and removal of the thickened dura has led to improvement in myelopathy [27]. Replacement of aortic and mitral valves has been successful [14].

Bone marrow transplantation was carried out in a 13-year-old girl with normal intelligence who had advanced cardiac failure and obstructive apnea, requiring oxygen during sleep and a tracheotomy [52]. Following successful engraftment, urinary excretion of mucopolysaccharide decreased, as did hepatosplenomegaly. Cardiopulmonary function became normal. Visual acuity improved, though the cloudy appearance of the cornea was unchanged. There was no obvious change in the dysostosis multiplex. Bone marrow transplantation has also been carried out in a feline model of the syndrome in which arylsulfatase B activity was deficient [53–55]. Corneal clouding of these animals disappeared. A model in rats has also been established [56] which should facilitate experimental therapy. Needle biopsy of the liver in human transplanted patients has revealed clearing of Kupffer cells and hepatocytes of stored glycosaminoglycan [57].

References

1 Maroteaux P, Leveque B, Maruie J, Lamy M. Une nouvelle dysostose avec élimination urinaire de chondroitine sulfate B. *Presse Med* 1963;**71**:1849.

2 Maroteaux P, Lamy M. Hurler's disease Morquio's disease and related mucopolysaccharidoses. *J Pediatr* 1965;**67**:312.

3 Matalon R, Arbogast B, Dorfman A. Deficiency of chondroitin sulphate N-acetylgalactosamine 4-sulfate sulfatase in Maroteaux–Lamy syndrome. *Biochem Biophys Res Commun* 1974;**61**:1450.

4 O'Brien JS, Cantz M, Spranger J. Maroteaux–Lamy disease (mucopolysaccharidosis VI) subtype A: deficiency of N-acetylgalactosamine-4-sulfatase. *Biochem Biophys Res Commun* 1974;**60**:1170.

5 Barton RW, Neufeld EF. A distinct biochemical deficit in the Maroteaux–Lamy syndrome (mucopolysaccharidosis VI). *J Pediatr* 1972;**80**:114.

6 Schuchman EH, Jackson CE, Desnick RJ. Human arylsulfatase B: MOPAC cloning nucleotide sequence of a full-length cDNA and regions of amino acid identity with arylsulfatases A and C. *Genomics* 1990;**6**:149.

7 Litjens T, Baker EG, Beckmann KR, *et al.* Chromosomal localization of ARSB the gene for human N-acetylgalactosamine-4-sulphatase. *Hum Genet* 1989;**82**:67.

8 Jin WD, Jackson CE, Desnick RJ, Schuchman EH. Mucopolysaccharidosis type VI: identification of three mutations in the arylsulfatase B gene of patients with the severe and mild phenotypes provides molecular evidence for genetic heterogeneity. *Am J Hum Genet* 1992;**50**:795.

9 Litjens T, Morris CP, Robertson EF, *et al.* An N-acetylgalactosamine-4-sulfatase mutation (DG238) results in a severe Maroteaux–Lamy phenotype. *Hum Mut* 1992;**1**:397.

10 Spranger JW, Koch F, McKusick VA, *et al.* Mucopolysaccharidosis VI (Maroteaux–Lamy's disease). *Helv Paediatr Acta* 1970;**25**:337.

11 McKusick VA. *Heritable Disorders of Connective Tissue.* CV Mosby, St Louis;1972:611.

12 Krovetz LJ, Schiebler GL. Cardiovascular manifestations of the genetic mucopolysaccharidoses: in *Clinical Delineation of Birth Defects.* XIII Cardiovascular System (ed. D Bergsma). Williams and Wilkins Co, Baltimore;1972.

13 Tan CT, Schaff HV, Miller FA Jr, *et al.* Valvular heart disease in four patients with Maroteaux–Lamy syndrome. *Circulation* 1992;**85**:188.

14 Marwick TH, Bastian B, Hughes CF, Bailey BP. Mitral stenosis in the Maroteaux–Lamy syndrome: a treatable cause of dyspnea. *Postgrad Med J* 1992;**68**:287.

15 Di Ferrante N, Hyman BH, Klish W, *et al.* Mucopolysaccharidosis VI (Maroteaux–Lamy disease): clinical and biochemical study of a mild variant case. *Johns Hopkins Med J* 1974;**135**:42.

16 Glober GA, Tanaka KR, Turner JA, Liu CK. Mucopolysaccharidosis an unusual case of cardiac valvular disease. *Am J Cardiol* 1968;**22**:133.

17 Wilson CS, Mankin HT, Pluth JR. Aortic stenosis and mucopolysaccharidosis. *Ann Intern Med* 1980;**92**:496.

18 Miller G, Partridge A. Mucopolysaccharidosis Type VI presenting in infancy with endocardial fibroelastosis and heart failure. *Pediatr Cardiol* 1983;**4**:61.

19 Hayflick S, Rowe S, Kavanaugh-McHugh A, *et al.* Acute infantile cardiomyopathy as a presenting feature of mucopolysaccharidosis VI. *J Pediatr* 1992;**120**:269.

20 Cantor LB, Disseler JA, Wilson FM II. Glaucoma in the Maroteaux–Lamy syndrome. *Am J Ophthalmol* 1989;**108**:426.

21 Taylor HR, Hollows FC, Hopwood JJ, Robertson EF. Report of mucopolysaccharidosis occurring in Australian aborigines. *J Med Genet* 1978;**15**:455.

22 Vestermark S, Tonnesen T, Andersen MS, Guttler F. Mental retardation in a patient with Maroteaux–Lamy. *Clin Genet* 1987;**31**:114.

23 Goldberg MF, Scott CI, McKuscik VA. Hydrocephalus and papilledema in the Maroteaux–Lamy syndrome (mucopolysaccharidosis type VI). *Am J Ophthalmol* 1970;**69**:969.

24 Sostrin RD, Hasso AN, Peterson DI, Thompson JR. Myelographic features of mucopolysaccharidosis: a new sign. *Radiology* 1977;**125**:421.

25 Peterson DI, Bucchus A, Seaich L, Kelly TE. Myelopathy associated with Maroteaux–Lamy syndrome. *Arch Neurol* 1975;**32**:127.

26 Upton ARM, McComas AJ. The double crush in nerve-entrapment syndromes. *Lancet* 1973;**2**:359.

27 Young R, Kleinman G, Ojemann RG, *et al.* Compressive myelopathy in Maroteaux–Lamy syndrome: clinical and pathological findings. *Ann Neurol* 1980;**8**:336.

28 Wald SL, Schmidek HH. Compressive myelopathy associated with type VI mucopolysaccharidosis (Maroteaux–Lamy syndrome). *Neurosurgery* 1984;**14**:83.

29 Tonnesen T, Gregersen HN, Guttler F. Normal MPS excretion but dermatan sulphaturia combined with a mild Maroteaux–Lamy phenotype. *J Med Genet* 1991;**28**:499.

30 Grossman H, Dorst JP. The mucopolysaccharidoses: in *Progress in Pediatric Radiology* (ed. H Kaufman). Vol IV. Year Book Medical Publishers, Chicago;1972:495.

31 Worth HM. The Hurler's syndrome; a study of radiologic appearances in the jaws. *Oral Surg* 1966;**22**:21.

32 Alder A. Ueber konstitutionell bedingte Granulationsveraenderungen der Leukocyten. *Dtsch Arch Klin Med* 1939;**183**:372.

33 Tondeur M, Neufeld EF. The mucopolysaccharidoses: biochemistry and ultrastructure: in *Molecular Pathology* (eds RA Good, SB Day, JJ Yunis). Charles C Thomas, Springfield;1975:600.

34   Levy LA, Lewis JC, Sumner TE. Ultrastructures of Reilly bodies (metachromatic granules) in Maroteaux-Lamy syndrome (mucopolysaccharidosis VI): a histochemical study. *Am J Clin Pathol* 1980;**73**:416.

35   Quigley HA, Kenyon KR. Ultrastructural and histochemical studies of a newly recognized form of systemic mucopolysaccharidosis (Maroteaux-Lamy syndrome mild phenotype). *Am J Ophthalmol* 1974;**77**:809.

36   Slot G, Burgess GL. Gargoylism. *Proc R Soc Med* 1937;**31**:1113.

37   McGovern MM, Vine DT, Haskins ME, Desnick RJ. Purification and properties of feline and human arylsulfatase B isozymes: evidence for feline homodimeric and human monomeric structures. *J Biol Chem* 1982;**257**:12605.

38   Gibson GJ, Saccone GTP, Brooks DA, *et al.* Human N-acetylgalactosamine-4-sulphate sulphatase: purification monoclonal antibody production and native and subunit M values. *Biochem J* 1987;**248**:755.

39   Steckel F, Hasilik A, von Figura K. Biosynthesis and maturation of arylsulfatase B in normal and mutant cultured human fibroblasts. *J Biol Chem* 1983;**258**:14322.

40   Taylor JA, Gibson GJ, Brooks DA, Hopwood JJ. Human N-acetylgalactosamine-4-sulphatase biosynthesis and maturation in normal Maroteaux-Lamy and multiple-sulphatase-deficiency fibroblasts. *Biochem J* 1990;**268**:379.

41   Fluharty AL, Stevens RL, Sander DL, Kihara H. Arylsulfatase B deficiency in Maroteaux-Lamy syndrome cultured fibroblasts. *Biochem Biophys Res Commun* 1974;**59**:455.

42   Shapira E, De Gregorio RP, Matalon R, Nadler HL. Reduced arylsulfatase B activity of the mutant enzyme protein in Maroteaux-Lamy syndrome. *Biochem Biophys Res Commun* 1975;**62**:448.

43   Stumpf DA, Austin JH, Crocker AC, Lafrance M. Mucopolysaccharidosis Type VI (Maroteaux-Lamy syndrome): arylsulfatase B deficiency in tissues. *Am J Dis Child* 1973;**126**:747.

44   Fluharty AL, Stevens RL, Fung D, *et al.* Uridine diphospho-N-acetylgalactosamine-4-sulfate sulfohydrolase activity of human arylsulfatase B and its deficiency in the Maroteaux-Lamy syndrome. *Biochem Biophys Res Commun* 1975;**64**:955.

45   Jackson CE, Yuhki N, Desnick RJ, *et al.* Feline arylsulfatase B (ARSB): isolation and expression of the full length cDNA sequence comparison with human ARSB and gene localization to feline chromosome A1. *Genomics* 1992;**14**:403.

46   Brooks DA, McCourt PAG, Gibson GJ, *et al.* Analysis of N-acetylgalactosamine-4-sulfatase protein and kinetics in mucopolysaccharidosis type VI patients. *Am J Hum Genet* 1991;**48**:710.

47   Van Dyke DL, Fluharty AL, Schafer IA, *et al.* Prenatal diagnosis of Maroteaux-Lamy syndrome. *Am J Med Genet* 1981;**8**:235.

48   Beratis NG, Turner BM, Weiss R, Hirschhorn K. Arylsulfatase B deficiency in Maroteaux-Lamy syndrome: cellular studies and carrier identification. *Pediatr Res* 1975;**9**:475.

49   Litjens T, Brooks DA, Peters C, *et al.* Identification expression and biochemical characterization of N-acetylgalactosamine-4-sulfatase mutations and relationship with clinical phenotype in MPS-VI patients. *Am J Hum Genet* 1996;**58**:1127.

50   Isbrandt D, Hopwood JJ, von Figura K, Peters C. Two novel frameshift mutations causing premature stop codons in a patient with the severe form of Maroteaux-Lamy syndrome. *Hum Mutat* 1996;**7**:361.

51   Wicker G, Prill V, Brooks D, *et al.* Mucopolysaccharidosis VI (Maroteaux-Lamy syndrome). An intermediate clinical phenotype caused by substitution of valine for glycine at position 137 of arylsulfatase. B *J Biol Chem* 1991;**266**:27386.

52   Krivit W, Pierpont ME, Ayaz K, *et al.* Bone-marrow transplantation in the Maroteaux-Lamy syndrome (muco-polysaccharidosis type V1). Biochemical and clinical status 24 months after transplantation. *N Engl J Med* 1984;**311**:1606.

53   Wenger D, Casper PW, Thrall MA, *et al.* Bone marrow transplantation in the feline model of arylsulfatase B deficiency: in *Bone Marrow Transplantation for Lysosomal Storage Diseases* (eds W Krivit, NW Paul). March of Dimes Birth Defects Foundation, New York;1986: Original Article Series, Vol 22, 1, p 177.

54   Jezyk PF, Haskins ME, Patterson DF, *et al.* Mucopolysaccharidosis in a cat with arylsulfatase B deficiency: a model of Maroteaux-Lamy syndrome. *Science* 1977;**198**:834.

55   Haskins ME, Jezyk PF, Patterson DF. Mucopolysaccharide storage disease in three families of cats with arylsulfatase B deficiency: leukocyte studies and carrier identification. *Pediatr Res* 1979;**13**:1203.

56   Yoshida M, Noguchi J, Ikada H, *et al.* Arylsulfatase B-deficient mucopolysaccharidosis in rats. *J Clin Invest* 1993;**91**:1099.

57   Resnick JM, Krivit W, Snover DC, *et al.* Pathology of the liver in mucopolysaccharidosis: light and electron microscopic assessment before and after bone marrow transplantation. *Bone Marrow Transplant* 1992;**10**:273.

83

Sly disease/β-glucuronidase deficiency/ mucopolysaccharidosis VII (MPS VII)

MAJOR PHENOTYPIC EXPRESSION

Short stature, coarse facies; hepatosplenomegaly; kyphoscoliosis and vertebral anomalies, including odontoid hypoplasia; mental retardation; dystosis multiplex; increased excretion of glycosaminoglycans; and deficiency of β-glucuronidase.

INTRODUCTION

Sly and colleagues [1] reported, in 1973, a patient with what they recognized as a distinct mucopolysaccharidosis in whom the activity of lysosomal β-glucoronidase was deficient. Complementation studies by Quinton and colleagues [2] on fibroblasts derived from the patient had revealed this disease to be different from any previously encountered mucopolysaccharidosis. Subsequently, a small number of patients has been described. A considerable variation in clinical expression has been observed [3]. The classic infantile form is similar to Hurler disease, but much milder presentations occur. At the extreme end of the spectrum is the acute fetal or neonatal form characterized by hydrops fetalis [4].

Mucopolysacchariduria in this condition may be mild. The defective enzyme (Figure 83.1), β-glucuronidase [1], catalyzes the removal of glucuronic acid residues that occur in dermatan sulfate and heparan sulfate; it is also active against chondroitin 4- or 6-sulfates, but these compounds are not stored or excreted in the urine, because of the activity of hyaluronidase [5].

β-Glucuronidase was a key enzyme in the development of current understandings of lysosomal enzyme processing. It was in studies of this enzyme that the mannose-6-phosphate recognition marker was first identified [6]. Full-length

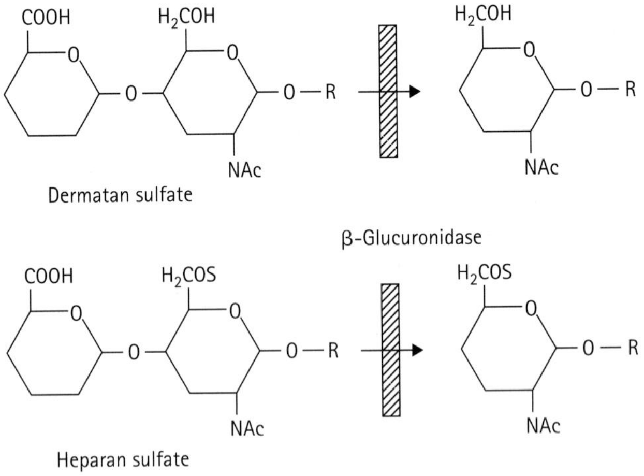

Figure 83.1 *The β-glucuronidase reaction. In addition to the removal of glucuronic acid residues from dermatan sulfate and heparan sulfate, the enzyme catalyzes this reaction with the chondroitin sulfates.*

cDNAs from the human and rodent genes have been cloned, sequenced and expressed; they encode polypeptides of 651 and 648 amino acids, respectively [7,8]. The gene is 21kb in length and contains 12 exons [9]. It is located at chromosome 7q21-22 [10]. The mutation has been defined in the initial patient [11] and a small number of others [11–13].

CLINICAL ABNORMALITIES

The original patient [1] was characterized by shortness of stature, relatively severe skeletal abnormalities as compared with other mucopolysaccharidoses and relatively mild impairment of cognitive function. He was first seen at 7 weeks for metatarsus adductus and recognized as having unusual facial features. The nasal bridge was depressed, the nostrils were anteverted, the maxillae prominent, and the eyes were wide and had epicanthal folds. The abdomen was protuberant and the liver palpable 4 cm below the costal margin. The spleen was at 3 cm. There was a long diastasis recti and an umbilical hernia. There was puffy skin over the dorsa of the hands and feet. A thoracolumbar gibbus had already developed. Short stature had been evident at 18 months, and the head circumference reached the 98th percentile by 5 months. The gibbus increased, and he developed a pigeon breast with a sharp angle between the body of the sternum pointing forward and the xyphoid pointing backward. He developed bilateral inguinal hernias. Hepatomegaly increased.

Developmental milestones and neurologic examination were normal for 2 years. By 3 years, retardation, especially in speech, was evident, but it appeared to be nonprogressive. Orthopedic problems progressed and walking became painful. He died suddenly at 20 years of age, but autopsy did not reveal the cause – a relatively common occurrence in patients with odontoid hypoplasia and other problems about the neck.

This classic presentation [1,14–19] of a moderately severe Hurler-like mucopolysaccharidosis with modest mental retardation (Figures 83.2, 83.3) represents a relatively uncommon intermediate presentation of MPS VII. There are appreciably milder forms, and the most severe prenatal or neonatal forms appear to be the most common. Clouding of the cornea became evident in the index patient by 8 years-of-age, but in others it has been evident earlier. It can usually be readily demonstrated by slit lamp examination.

Most patients have had frequent upper respiratory infections, and pneumonia has occurred in some. Hernias, shortness of stature [1], relative macrocephaly and coarse features are regularly observed. Most have had gingival hyperplasia. Gibbus deformity has regularly been reported.

Joint contractures have been observed and also hydrocephalus [16], concomitants of a classic mucopolysaccharidosis. Some have had dislocated hips [18]. Camptodactyly has been noted at birth along with absence of distal phalangeal creases, indicating prenatal onset. All have had hepatosplenomegaly. Developmental delay has been mild to moderate.

A severe example of this phenotype [3] died at 2½ years after a course characterized by marked inhibition of growth, hepatosplenomegaly of neonatal onset, corneal clouding, by 7 months, and gingival hypertrophy. Icterus, recurrent diarrhea and hypoalbuminemia may have been unrelated consequences of giant cell hepatitis and carbohydrate intolerance.

The most severe phenotype, a neonatal or fetal form [4,20–27] is typified by nonimmune hydrops fetalis

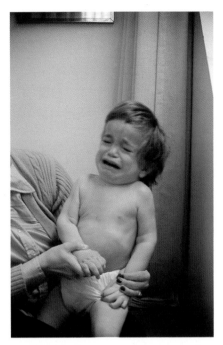

Figure 83.2   *T.M., a boy with mucopolysaccharidosis VII had the classic phenotype. Facial features were coarse. He had hepatosplenomegaly, a gibbus and bilateral inguinal hernia, and developed hydrocephalus [16]. (This illustration and Figure 83.3 were kindly provided by Dr. Kenneth Lyons Jones of UCSD.)*

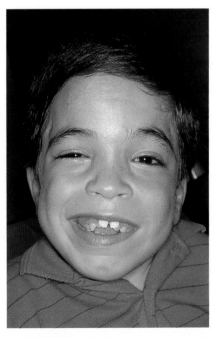

Figure 83.3   *T.M. With time the features were coarser. There was marked gingival hyperplasia. He died at 15 years-of-age.*

(Figure 83.4) The metabolic differential diagnosis of hydrops fetus is shown in the Appendix (p. 759). Three reports were of fetal death, and family histories of hydropic or neonatal patients indicate an increase in spontaneous abortions [26].

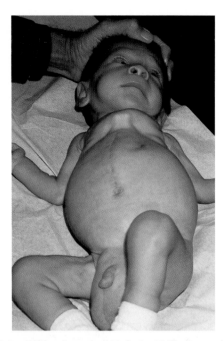

Figure 83.4   *W.M., a 6-week-old infant with Sly disease. He had fetal and neonatal ascites evident at birth and macrocephaly. There was prominent subcutaneous tissue visible in the nares. Liver and spleen were enlarged, and he had bilateral inguinal hernias. He had a gibbus and a prominent manubrium.*

This is a distinct presentation for a mucopolysaccharidosis recognizable *in utero* or at least at birth. Dystosis multiplex is present at birth in these patients. The facies is coarse. There is pitting neonatal edema, ascites and hepatosplenomegaly. Talipes equinovarus has been reported and congenital dislocation of the hip [4]. Cardiomyopathy may be progressive [4]. Death may occur in the first six months.

A number of patients have also been reported with milder manifestations with onset after 4 years-of-age or much later and with skeletal manifestations predominating [5,17,26,28–30]. One was 14-years-old at the time of report [3] and was well except for hypertension and fibromuscular dysplasia causing narrowing of the aorta and femoral arteries. Height was normal, and dysostosis multiplex of ribs and spine was very mild. Speech therapy was required at 3 years. Another patient [28] appeared normal at 11 years except for bilateral club feet, which had been surgically corrected, and frequent upper respiratory infections in childhood. Intelligence was tested as normal. A 13-year-old girl [29] had normal height, moderate mental retardation, a short neck and protruding sternum, corneal clouding, dysplastic hips and vertebral abnormalities. There was no hepatosplenomegaly. Another variant was described [30] as an oligosymptomatic 20-year-old male despite severe skeletal dysplasia. It is clear from these observations that there is a very wide spectrum of clinical phenotypes.

Dysostosis multiplex (Chapter 77) has been present in roentgenograms of patients with β-glucuronidase deficiency, especially those with the classic and neonatal forms. The skull is large and the sella J-shaped. The ribs are spatulate [1,3,16].

Vertebrae are shortened and anteriorly beaked, and there may be odontoid hypoplasia [1,3,16]. Dysplasia of the hips is associated with hypoplastic ilia [1,3,16,18]. Proximal metacarpals are pointed [1,16].

Coarse lamellar Alder-Reilly inclusions are seen in peripheral granulocytes [1,30,31] and also in the bone marrow. Pathological examination has revealed vacuolated hepatocytes; electron microscopy has shown cytoplasmic membrane-bound vesicles [18]. The stored material stains with alcian blue, and this staining may be seen in cultured fibroblasts, which also display metachromasia.

Glycosaminoglycan excretion is usually moderately increased in this condition [1,3,18] but screening tests for mucopolysaccharide excretion may be normal [16], and some adult patients have not had increased glycosaminoglycan excretion. The material has been shown to consist of dermatan sulfate and heparan sulfate [3,18].

GENETICS AND PATHOGENESIS

The disorder is transmitted in an autosomal recessive fashion via mutant genes on chromosome 7 [10]. Its incidence has been estimated at in 300 000 live births in British Columbia [32]. The molecular defect is in the enzyme β-glucuronidase. (EC 3.2.1.31) [1,33]. Cultured fibroblasts from patients accumulate sulfated mucopolysaccharide when incubated with $^{35}SO_4$, and this abnormality is corrected by the addition of bovine liver β-glucuronidase to the medium [33]. Identity of the corrective factor and the glucuronidase was demonstrated by coelectrophoresis in polyacrylamide gel. Virtually complete deficiency has been demonstrated with a variety of synthetic substrates in leukocytes and in fibroblasts [33]. It has also been detected in serum [18]. The enzyme is a tetramer of 75 kDa subunits [34]. It is synthesized as a precursor protein and processed at the carboxyl end by the loss of the signal peptide [33]. Immunochemical studies have indicated the presence of cross-reacting material (CRM) in patients with the disease [35]. The measurement of enzyme activity has not correlated well with the degree of severity of phenotype.

Reduced levels of enzyme were found in the leukocytes of parents [1]. Prenatal diagnosis is available by the assay of cultured amniocytes or chorionic villus material. In families in which the mutation is known, this is the method of choice for prenatal diagnosis and for carrier detection.

The human and murine gene have considerable homology in the coding region for the mature protein. Alternate splicing of the human gene leads to 2 types of cDNA [9], the shorter one containing a large deletion in exon 6. A pseudodeficiency allele was defined in the study of a pseudodeficient mother of a child who carried a mutation, L176F [36]. The mother had greatly reduced levels of β-glucuronidase without evident clinical effect and a substitution of asparagine for aspartic acid, D152N. The existence of pseudodeficiency greatly complicates prenatal diagnosis by enzyme assay, and also heterozygote detection [37].

In the index patient, there was a compound of two alleles, a missense tryptophan 627 to cysteine and a nonsense arginine 256 to stop [11]. In two Japanese patients mutations at two CpG sites have been identified: alanine 619 to valine [12] and arginine 382 to cysteine [13]. Four more mutations described in two Caucasian patients [38] were a 38 bp deletion at positions 1642–1679 in exon 10 caused by a single base change that generated a new splice site; and three point mutations – proline 148 to serine, tyrosine to cysteine, and tryptophan 507 to a stop-codon. A prenatally diagnosed patient with hydrops fetalis [39] was found [13] to have a C to T transition that led to a substitution of cysteine for arginine 382. In studies of 21 patients with hydrops fetalis or early severe disease [40] 19 different mutations were reported.

TREATMENT

Specific treatment such as bone marrow transplantation (BMT) has not been reported in humans, but success has been obtained in neonatal mice, as contrasted with adult mice with β-glucuronidase deficiency [41]. Enzyme replacement initiated at birth followed by BMT at 5 weeks was highly successful in this model [42]. This deficiency has also been found in a dog model [42], which has been reported to more closely mimic the human clinical disease and enzyme deficiency than the mouse, in which activity is 20 percent of control. The availability of animals should be useful for the development of gene transfer. Among approaches to gene therapy affected murine fibroblasts were transfected with a retroviral vector containing human β-glucuronidase cDNA and implanted into mice; there was expression of enzyme *in vivo* and disappearance of lysosomal storage in the liver and spleen [43].

Supportive treatment should include attention to potential cervical instability – for example, during anesthesia. Corneal transplantation may be useful in older patients in whom vision is impaired. Physiotherapy is useful for joint stiffness and the preservation of function.

References

1 Sly WS, Quinton BA, McAlister WH, Rimoin DL. β-glucuronidase deficiency: report of clinical radiologic and biochemical features of a new mucopolysaccharidosis. *J Pediatr* 1973;**82**:249.

2 Quinton BA, Sly WS, McAlister WH, *et al*. β-glucuronidase deficiency: a new mucopolysaccharide storage disease: in *Society for Pediatric Research*. Atlantic City NJ;1971:198 (abstr).

3 Beaudet AL, DiFerrante NM, Ferry GD, *et al*. Variation in the pheno-typic expression of β-glucuronidase deficiency. *J Pediatr* 1975;**86**:388.

4 Nelson A, Peterson L, Frampton B, Sly WS. Mucopolysaccharidosis VII β-glucuronidase deficiency presenting as nonimmune hydrops fetalis. *J Pediatr* 1982;**101**:574.

5 Lee JES, Falk RE, Ng WG, Donnel GN. β-Glucuronidase deficiency: a heterogeneous mucopolysaccharidosis. *Am J Dis Child* 1985;**139**:57.

6 Kaplan A, Achord DT, Sly WS. Phosphohexosyl components of a lysosomal enzyme are recognized by pinocytosis receptors on human fibroblasts. *Proc Natl Acad Sci USA* 1977;**74**:2026.

7 Oshima A, Kyle JW, Miller RD, *et al*. Cloning sequencing and expression of cDNA for human glucuronidase. *Proc Natl Acad Sci USA* 1987;**84**:685.

8 Nishimura Y, Rosenfeld MG, Kreibich G, *et al*. Nucleotide sequence of rat preputial β-glucuronidase cDNA and *in vivo* insertion of its encoded polypeptide in microsomal membranes. *Proc Natl Acad Sci USA* 1986;**83**:7292.

9 Miller RD, Hoffmann JW, Powell PP, *et al*. Cloning and characterization of the human β-glucuronidase gene. *Genomics* 1990;**7**:280.

10 Speleman F, Vervoort R, Van Roy N, *et al*. Localization by fluorescence *in situ* hybridization of the human functional beta-glucuronidase gene (GUSB) to 7q1121-q1122 and two pseudogenes to 5p13 and 5q13. *Cytogenet Cell Genet* 1996;**72**:53.

11 Shipley JM, Klinkenberg M, Wu BM I. Mutational analysis of a patient with mucopolysaccharidosis type VII and identification of pseudogenes. *Am J Hum Genet* 1993;**52**:517.

12 Tomatsu S, Sukegawa K, Ikedo Y, *et al*. Molecular basis of mucopolysaccharidosis type VII: replacement of Ala619 in β-glucuronidase with Val. *Gene* 1990;**89**:283.

13 Tomatsu S, Fukuda S, Sukegawa K, *et al*. Mucopolysaccharidosis type VII: characterization of mutations and molecular heterogeneity. *Am J Hum Genet* 1991;**48**:89.

14 Sly WS. The mucopolysaccharidoses: in *Metabolic Control and Disease* (eds Bondy PK, Rosenberg LE). WB Saunders Co, Philadelphia;1980:545.

15 Guibaud P, Maire I, Goddon R, *et al*. Mucopolysaccharidose Type VII par deficit en β-glucuronidase. Etude d'une famille. *J Genet Hum* 1979;**27**:29.

16 Hoyme HE, Jones KL, Higginbottom MC, O'Brien JS. Presentation of mucopolysaccharidosis VII (beta-glucuronidase deficiency) in infancy. *J Med Genet* 1981;**18**:237.

17 Sewell AC, Gehler J, Mittermaier G, Meyer E. Mucopolysaccharidosis type VII (β-glucuronidase deficiency): a report of a new case and a survey of those in the literature. *Clin Genet* 1982;**21**:366.

18 Gehler J, Cantz M, Tolksdorf M, *et al*. Mucopolysaccharidosis VII: β-glucuronidase deficiency. *Humangenetik* 1974;**23**:149.

19 Beighton P, McKusick VA. *Heritable Disorders of Connective Tissue*. 5th ed. CV Mosby, St Louis;1993.

20 Wilson D, Melnik E, Sly W, Makesbery WR. Neonatal β-glucuronidase deficiency mucopolysaccharidosis (MPS VII): autopsy findings. *J Neuropathol Exp Neurol* 1982;**41**:344.

21 Irani D, Kim HS, El-Hibri H, *et al*. Postmortem observations on beta-glucuronidase deficiency presenting as hydrops fetalis. *Ann Neurol* 1983;**14**:486.

22 Kagie MJ, Kleijer WJ, Huijmans JGM, *et al*. Beta-glucuronidase deficiency as a cause of fetal hydrops. *Am J Med Genet* 1992;**42**:693.

23 Stangenberg M, Lingman G, Roberts G, Ozand P. Mucopolysaccharidosis VII as a cause of fetal hydrops in early pregnancy. *Am J Med Genet* 1992;**15**:142.

24 Machin GA. Hydrops revisited: literature review of 1414 cases published in 1980s. *Am J Med Genet* 1989;**34**:366.

25 Molyneux AJ, Blair E, Coleman N, Daish P. Mucopolysaccharidosis type VII associated with hydrops fetalis: histopathological and ultrastructural features with genetic implications. *J Clin Pathol* 1997;**50**:252.

26 Vervoort R, Islam MR, Sly WS, *et al*. Molecular analysis of patients with beta-glucuronidase deficiency presenting as hydrops fetalis or as early mucopolysaccharidosis VII. *Am J Hum Genet* 1996;**58**:457.

27 Nelson J, Kenny B, O'Hara D, *et al*. Foamy changes of placental cells in probable beta glucuronidase deficiency associated with hydrops fetalis. *J Clin Pathol* 1993;**46**:370.

28 Danes BS, Degnan M. Different clinical and biochemical phenotypes associated with β-glucuronidase deficiency: in *Skeletal Dysplasias* (ed. D Bergsma). Birth Defects, Ser X, No 12, National Foundation – March of Dimes, New York;1974:251.

29 Pfeiffer RA, Kresse H, Baumer N, Sattinger E. Beta-glucuronidase deficiency in a girl with unusual clinical features. *Eur J Pediatr* 1977;**126**:155.

30 de Kremer RD, Givogri I, Argarana CE, *et al.* Mucopolysaccharidosis type VII (beta-glucuronidase deficiency): a chronic variant with an oligosymptomatic severe skeletal dysplasia. *Am J Med Genet* 1992;**44**:145.

31 Gitzelmann R, Wiesmann UN, Spycher MA, *et al.* Unusually mild course of beta-glucuronidase deficiency in two brothers (mucopolysaccharidosis VII). *Helv Paediatr Acta* 1978;**33**:413.

32 Lowry RB, Renwick DH. Relative frequency of the Hurler and Hunter syndromes. *N Engl J Med* 1971;**284**:221.

33 Hall CW, Cantz M, Neufeld EF. A β-glucuronidase deficiency mucopolysaccharidosis: studies in cultured fibroblasts. *Arch Biochem Biophys* 1973;**155**:32.

34 Erickson AH, Blobel G. Carboxyl-terminal proteolytic processing during biosynthesis of the lysosomal enzymes β-glucuronidase and cathepsin D. *Biochemistry* 1983;**22**:5201.

35 Bell CE Jr, Sly WS, Brot FE. Human β-glucuronidase deficiency mucopolysaccharidosis; identification of cross-reactive antigen in cultured fibroblasts of deficient patients by enzyme immunoassay. *J Clin Invest* 1977;**59**:97.

36 Vervoort R, Islam MR, Sly W, *et al.* A pseudodeficiency allele (D152N) of the human beta-glucuronidase gene. *Am J Hum Genet* 1995;**57**:798.

37 Vervoort R, Gitzelmann R, Bosshard N, *et al.* Low beta-glucuronidase enzyme activity and mutations in the human beta-glucuronidase gene in mild mucopolysaccharidosis type VII pseudodeficiency and a heterozygote. *Hum Genet* 1998;**102**:69.

38 Yamada S, Tomatsu S, Sly WS, *et al.* Four novel mutations in muco-polysaccharidosis type VII including a unique base substitution in exon 10 of the beta-glucuronidase gene that creates a novel 5'-splice site. *Hum Mol Genet* 1995;**4**:651.

39 Lissens W, Dedobbeleer G, Foulon W, *et al.* Beta-glucuronidase deficiency as a cause of prenatally diagnosed non-immune hydrops fetalis. *Prenatal Diag* 1991;**11**:405.

40 Vervoort R, Buist NRM, Kleijer WJ, *et al.* Molecular analysis of the beta-glucuronidase gene: novel mutations in mucopolysaccharidosis type VII and heterogeneity of the polyadenylation region. *Hum Genet* 1997; **99**:462.

41 Sands MS, Barker JE, Vogler C, *et al.* Treatment of mucopolysaccharidosis type VII by syngeneic bone marrow transplantation in neonates. *Lab Invest* 1993;**68**:676.

42 Haskins ME, Desnick RJ, Di Ferrante N, *et al.* β-Glucuronidase deficiency in a dog: a model of human mucopolysaccharidosis VII. *Pediatr Res* 1984;**18**:980.

43 Moullier P, Bohl D, Heard JM, Danos O. Correction of lysosomal storage in the liver and spleen of MPS VII mice by implantation of genetically modified skin fibroblasts. *Nature Genet* 1993;**4**:154.

PART 1

Mucolipidoses

I-cell disease/mucolipidosis II

MAJOR PHENOTYPIC EXPRESSION

Coarse features, shortness of stature, progressive developmental retardation, limitation of joint motion, dysostosis multiplex, cytoplasmic inclusions in fibroblasts, deficient intracellular activity of many hydrolases, and elevated activity of these enzymes in serum because of defective post-translational modification of acid hydrolases, a consequence of the fundamental defect in N-acetylglucosaminyl-(GlcNAc) 1-phosphotransferase.

INTRODUCTION

I-cell disease was first described by Leroy and Demars in 1967 [1]. Cultured fibroblasts derived from the skin of their two patients contained striking cytoplasmic inclusions visible by phase contrast microscopy (Figure 84.1). The patients resembled those with Hurler syndrome, but they presented earlier, did not usually have cloudy corneas, and they did not have increased urinary excretion of mucopolysaccharides. Leroy and colleagues [2] named the disorder I-cell disease, the 'I' indicating inclusions. It has since been designated a mucolipidosis [3], because of the coexistence of abnormalities typical of both mucopolysaccharidoses and sphingolidoses. Leroy [4] has proposed the designation of these disorders as oligosaccharidoses, since large quantities of oligosaccharides are excreted in the urine [5]. The molecular defect has now been defined in N-acetylglucosaminyl-1-phosphotransferase [6] (Figure 84.2) (GlcNAc phosphotransferase). The same enzyme is defective in mucolipidosis III (Chapter 85). These two disorders represent a unique mechanism of disease in which the basic defect is in the processing of lysosomal enzymes to permit their recognition and uptake into cells [7].

GlcNAc phosphotransferase has a 3 subunit structure – $\alpha_2\beta_2\gamma_2$ – that is coded for by 2 genes, one for the α and β subunits and another for the γ [8]. The $\alpha/\beta B$ gene is located on chromosome 12p [9]. The γ gene is on 16p [10]. Patients with mucolipidosis II have been found to have no α/β mRNA,

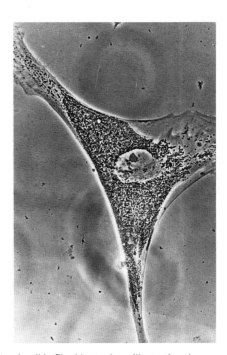

Figure 84.1 *I-cell in fibroblast culture illustrating the characteristic cytoplasmic inclusions. (Courtesy of Dr. Jules Leroy, The State University of Antwerp, Belgium.)*

while reduced amounts were found in patients with mucolipidosis III [9], although the 22 exons of the gene could be amplified. In other families with mucolipidosis III a mutation

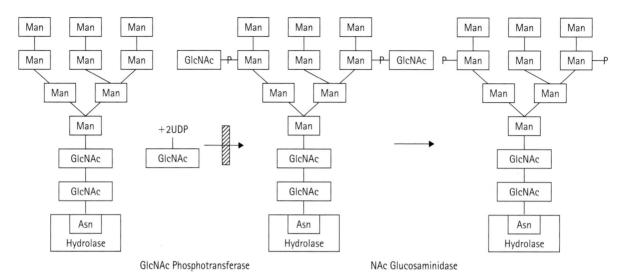

Figure 84.2 *N-acetylglucosamine (GlcNAc) phosphotransferase, the site of the defect in I-cell disease and in mucolipidoses III. The pathway for phosphorylating the acid hydrolase enzymes is shown as a two-step reaction, which ultimately forms the mannose-6-phosphate recognition site that targets the enzyme for cellular uptake. Abbreviations employed in addition to GlNAc:UDP-GlcNAc for uridine diphosphate-GlcNAc; Man, mannose; and Asn to indicate the linkage of the oligosaccharide to an asparagine residue of the enzyme protein.*

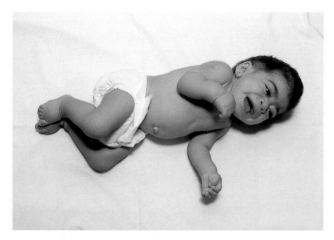

Figure 84.3 *F.S.Y. A 19-month-old female infant with I-cell disease. She was small and developmentally delayed. She had an umbilical hernia. An inguinal hernia was repaired at 4 months. The liver was palpable 2 cm below the costal margin. Her sister had the disease.*

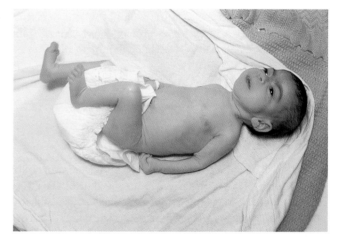

Figure 84.4 *F.S.Y. The features were coarse. The nasal bridge was depressed. She was hirsute and the hairline was low. The head was small.*

was found in the γ gene, a cytosine insertion at codon 167, which causes a frameshift and a premature termination [10].

CLINICAL ABNORMALITIES

The typical phenotype of the patient with I-cell disease is that of an earlier-onset Hurler syndrome [2,11–13] (Figures 84.3–84.11). Findings present at birth include dislocation of the hips, hernias and talipes equinovarus, as well as coarse features [14]. Neonatal cholestatic jaundice has also been reported in an infant with I-cell disease [15].

Retardation of psychomotor development is profound and progressive. Patients do not learn to sit, walk, roll over or speak.

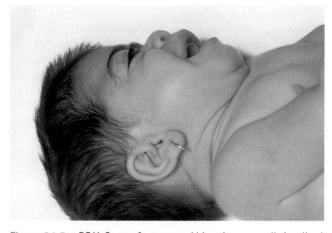

Figure 84.5 *F.S.Y. Coarse features and hirsutism are well visualized in profile.*

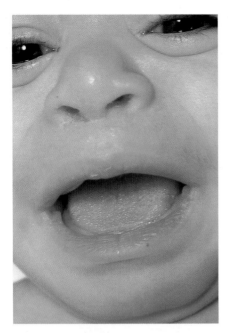

Figure 84.6   *F.S.Y. She had gingival hypertrophy. Corneas were not cloudy. The tongue appeared large.*

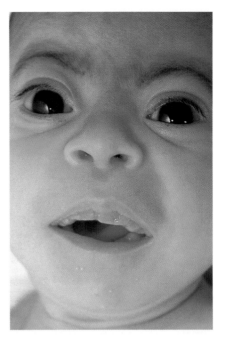

Figure 84.8   *A.S.Y. She already had coarse features and gingival hypertrophy. The corneas were clear.*

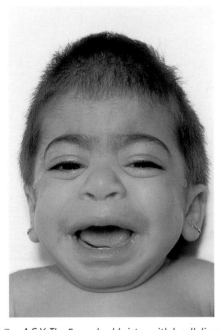

Figure 84.7   *A.S.Y. The 5-week-old sister with I-cell disease. In addition, she had congenital heart disease. She had delayed linear growth and the head was small.*

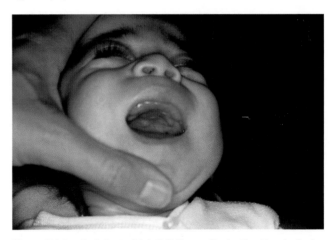

Figure 84.9   *An infant with I-Cell disease illustrating the gingival hyperplasia. (Illustration was kindly provided by Dr. Philip Benson.)*

The IQ is very low. Retardation of linear growth is impressive: most patients reach a maximal height of 0.74–0.76 m by 2 years-of-age. In contrast in Hurler disease, the final height is 1.0–1.1 m. Coarse features are evident very early, and features are progressively coarser as additional mucopolysaccharide is deposited in bones and soft tissues. The ears are thick and firm. The skin is thick, smooth and firm; it may be so tight that it cannot be pinched. The forehead is high and narrow with a prominent metopic ridge (Figures 84.10). There are epicanthal folds and puffy eyelids. The bridge of the nose is flat, the tip of the nose wide and the nostrils are anteverted. The filtrum is long. The corneas are characteristically clear, but slit lamp examination may reveal a fine granularity [16], and there may be corneal opacity [17]. There is very prominent gingival hypertrophy [18] (Figure 84.9) – this is a difference from Hurler disease. The voice is hoarse.

Limitation of joint motion is characteristic and contractures may develop at the hips, knees, shoulders, elbows and fingers. The claw-hand deformity may be identical to that of the Hurler patient. The hands tend to deviate in an ulnar direction. There is a dorso-lumbar kyphosis and a lumbar gibbus. The abdomen is protuberant and may contain a pronounced diastasis recti and an umbilical hernia. Inguinal hernias are common in males. Hepatomegaly is minimal, and splenomegaly is slight or absent.

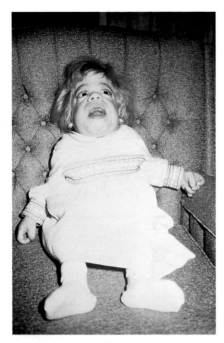

Figure 84.10   *A 7-year-old girl with I-cell disease. This was the original patient studied by Dr. Jules Leroy [1]. By this age, she had flexion contractures of the fingers, hips and knees. Her height of 30 inches was equivalent to that of a 1-year-old. Facial features were quite like those of a patient with the Hurler disease, but the corneas were clear. (Illustration provided by Dr. Leroy of Antwerp, Belgium.)*

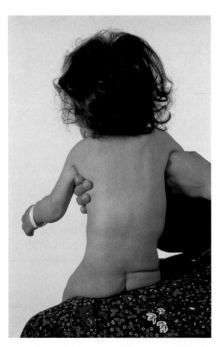

Figure 84.11   *Infant with kyphosis, a manifestation of I-cell disease. (Illustration was kindly provided by Dr. Philip Benson.)*

A nasal discharge is usually present. Respiratory infections and otitis media are common. Cardiomegaly may be present early in life [19]. Most patients die between 2 and 8 years-of-age, usually of pneumonia or congestive cardiac failure

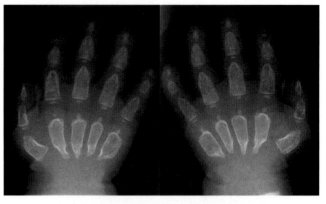

Figure 84.12   *Roentgenogram of the hand of a 1-month-old patient with I-cell disease illustrates the typical appearance of dysostosis multiplex. The phalanges were short and thick. The metacarpals were broad distally, and tapered proximally. The bones had a coarse trabecular pattern.*

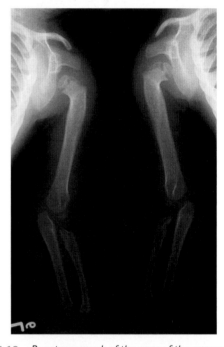

Figure 84.13   *Roentgenograph of the arms of the same patient illustrate the thick bone with poor modeling. The radius and ulna were angulated toward each other.*

[20,21]. Longer survivors may turn out to be examples of mucolipidosis III.

Roentgenographic features are those of dysostosis multiplex (Figures 84.12–84.14). They appear at an early age and are similar to those of GM_1 gangliosidosis (Chapter 90) or Hurler disease (Chapter 77). Skeletal changes are present at birth and may be extreme in infancy. Extensive periosteal new bone function produces cloaking and loss of tubulation of the long bones [11]. Premature synostosis of the cranial sutures may be observed as early as 1 month-of-age [22]. Changes in the bones are progressive. The long bones are short, wide and thick. The distal radius and ulna tilt toward

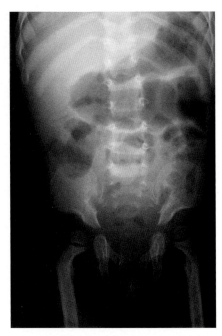

Figure 84.14   *Roentgenograph of the same patient illustrates the broadened spatulate ribs.*

each other. Bullet-shaped proximal phalanges are associated with proximal pointing of metacarpals and widening of their distal ends. The ribs are broad and spatulate. The vertebral bodies are short and rounded, and there is anterior inferior breaking at L1 and D12. The proximal tibia and fibula may be deeply notched [16].

At necropsy there may be thickening of the endocardium and myocardium and of the coronary arteries and aorta. The cytoplasmic inclusions in skin fibroblasts (Figure 84.1, p. 553) are large, dark granules which fill the cytoplasm [1,17,23,24]. Vacuolated lymphocytes may be seen in the blood or bone marrow [25] and vacuolated hepatocytes or hepatic mesenchymal cells are found [24], as well as storage in renal glomerular and tubular epithelium. Typical histologic changes have been seen in a 15-week-old fetus [26] and a placenta at 14 weeks [27]. The inclusions are sudanophilic and positive for acid phosphatase. The nervous system may appear normal, but lamellar bodies have been observed in spinal ganglia nerves [28] and anterior horn cells [29]. Cardiac muscle is histologically normal: the valves are thickened, and contain vacuolated fibroblasts [29,30].

GENETICS AND PATHOGENESIS

Cells of patients with I-cell disease are characterized by deficient activity of a large number of lysosomal enzymes [12,31–33]. These include β-glucuronidase, β-galactosidase, α-mannosidase, α-fucosidase, N-acetyl-β-d-galactosiaminidase and arylsulfatase-A. Wiesmann and colleagues [31] found that the activities of the same lysosomal enzymes were high in the medium surrounding cultured I-cell fibroblasts. High

levels of activity of lysosomal enzymes are also found in the serum of patients with I-cell disease [34]. These include hexosaminidase A and B and α-galactosidase. These patients do not have excessive excretion of urinary mucopolysaccharides.

The key to these unusual findings was provided by the observation of Hickman and Neufeld [35] that in I-cell disease there is a defect in the uptake and intracellular location of lysosomal enzymes. I-cells absorb purified normal lysosomal enzyme perfectly well, but lysosomal enzymes derived from I-cell patients are not effectively taken up by normal cells [35]. Lysosomal enzymes such as hexosaminidase A are taken up into cells by absorptive pinocytosis. The uptake of these enzymes by cells is a function of the carbohydrate moieties of the enzyme proteins, because oxidation by sodium metaperiodate interferes with uptake without affecting catalytic activity. These enzymes are normally secreted from cells, after which they must be specifically recognized and taken up. The I-cell mutation interferes with formation of the carbohydrate recognition site on the hydrolases. The recognition marker on lysosomal acid hydrolase enzymes is mannose-6-phosphate [36]. Normal cells incorporate ^{32}P into newly synthesized lysosomal enzymes; fibroblasts from patients with I-cell disease do not [37,38]. This led to the hypothesis that the defect in I-cell disease was in the biosynthesis of the phosphomannosyl signal that binds to receptors responsible for targeted uptake of the enzymes. The phosphorylation of the enzymes takes place in a two-step process in which N-acetylglucosaminylphosphate is added to mannose residues of the exposed oligosaccharide of the glycoprotein enzyme [7,39–41] (Figure 84.2).

The enzyme which catalyzes the first reaction is UDP-N-acetylglucosamine:lysosomal enzyme-N-acetylglucosamine-1-phosphotransferase, or N-acetylglucosaminyl phosphotransferase (GlcNAc phosphotransferase) [6,42–47]. Fibroblasts from patients with I-cell disease are almost completely deficient in the activity of this enzyme [6,45]. The other enzyme required for the biosynthesis of the mannose-6-phosphate recognition site is a glucosaminidase that catalyzes the removal of the N-acetylglucosamine residue, exposing the mannose-6-phosphate groups [48]. It is formally called N-acetyl-glucosamine-1-phosphodiester-α-N-acetyl-glucosaminidas. Its activity is normal or elevated in fibroblasts of patients with I-cell disease. The biosynthesis of lysosomal enzymes takes place in the endoplasmic reticulum, and the enzyme is transported through the Golgi complex, where the transfer of the N-acetylglucosaminylphosphate to the mannose site occurs prior to transport to the lysosome [49]. As a result of the primary defect in GlcNAc phosphotransferase in I-cell disease this process breaks down, and a number of secondary effects occur, such as the deficiency of a number of lysosomal hydrolases. This leads to the storage of a variety of material such as complex lipids and mucopolysaccharides. I-cell lysosomes also accumulate cystine, much like those of patients with cystinosis [50,51]. In addition, these cells accumulate sialic acid [52]. Patients with mucolipidosis III, or pseudo-Hurler polydystrophy, have defective activity of the GlcNAc phosphotransferase enzyme (Chapter 85).

Diagnosis is generally made by assay of lysosomal enzymes in cultured fibroblasts, where there is a distinct deficiency [30,53] or in the plasma or serum where there is as much as a 10- to 20-fold increase in enzyme activity [31]. Assay of fibroblasts or plasma for glycosylasparaginase has been reported [54] as useful for the diagnosis of I-cell disease. The diagnosis can also be made by assay of the GlcNAc phosphotransferase in leukocytes or cultured fibroblasts [55,56]. Substrates are commercially available.

Heterogeneity in the mucolipidoses was documented first in studies of complementation. Instances were reported of complementation between ML II and ML III fibroblasts which is consistent with the enzyme subunit structure and the fact that there are two genes [57]. The α/β gene contains 20 exons and 80kb [9]. The precursor molecule that is its product undergoes post translational cleavage to yield the 928 amino acid α unit and the 328 amino acid β unit. The γ gene codes for a protein of 281 amino acids [10]. There are 23 asparagine-linked glycosylation sites among the subunits. Among patients with mucolipidosis II mutations studied appear to have been small deletions or point mutations because amplification of the individual α/β exons revealed them to be present, although there was no mRNA [9]. The γ gene was transcribed normally.

I-cell disease is transmitted as an autosomal recessive. Multiple siblings, both male and female, have been reported from families with normal parents. Consanguinity has been documented [3,16]. Abnormal inclusions have been found in the fibroblasts of some phenotypically normal parents [2]. Obligate heterozygotes have been found to have intermediate levels of the GlcNAc phosphotransferase enzyme in leukocytes and cultured fibroblasts [55,56]. Prenatal diagnosis of I-cell disease has been carried out by the demonstration of high levels of multiple acid hydrolases in amniotic fluid or their deficiency in cultured amniocytes, as well as by demonstrating accumulation of ^{35}S mucopolysaccharide [26,58–60]. One affected fetus has been diagnosed on the basis of hexosaminidase assay of maternal serum [61]. A boy has been described [61] with an atypical form of I-cell disease: he was found to be a mosaic in whom two populations of fibroblasts were demonstrated, one with the characteristic morphology and enzyme defect of I-cell disease, and the other normal.

TREATMENT

Symptomatic treatment (for example, of respiratory infection) is helpful. The natural history is of uniform fatality. Two patients have been treated with bone marrow transplantation [62,63] with limited improvement.

References

1   Leroy JG, Demars RI. Mutant enzymatic and cytological phenotype in cultured human fibroblasts. *Science* 1967;**157**:804.

2   Leroy JG, Demars RI, Opitz JM. I-cell disease: in *Proc First Conference on Clinical Delineation of Birth Defects.* Original Article Series Vol V, No 4. The National Foundation, New York;1969:174.

3   Spranger JW, Wiedemann HR. The genetic mucolipidoses. *Humangenetik.* 1970;**9**:113.

4   Leroy JG. The oligosaccharidoses: proposal of a new name and a new classification for the mucolipidoses: in *Dysmorpholgy* (eds Nyhan WL, Jones KL). Birth Defects Original Article Series, Vol 18, No 3B. The National Foundation, New York;1982:3.

5   Strecker G, Peers MC, Michalski JC, *et al.* Structure of nine sialyloligosaccharides accumulated in urine of eleven patients with three different types of sialidosis. *Eur J Biochem* 1977;**75**:391.

6   Reitman ML. Varki AM. Kornfeld S. Fibroblasts from patients with I-cell disease and pseudo-Hurler polydystrophy are deficient in uridine 5' diphosphate-N-acetylglucosamine:glycoprotein N-acetylglucosaminyl-phosphotransferase activity. *J Clin Invest* 1981;**67**:1574.

7   Creek KE, Sly WS. The role of the phosphomannosyl receptor in the transport of acid hydrolases to lysosomes: in *Lysosomes in Biology and Pathology* (eds Dingle JR, Dean RT, Sly W). Elsevier/North Holland, New York;1984:63.

8   Bao M, Booth JL, Elmendorf BJ, Canfield WM. Bovine UDP-N-acetylglucosamine: Lysosmal-enzyme N-acetylglucosamine-1-phosphotransferase: I Purification and subunit structure. *J Biol Chem* 1996;**271**:31437.

9   Canfield W, Bao M, Pan J, *et al.* Mucolipidosis II and mucolipidosis IIIA are caused by mutations in the GlcNAc-phosphotransferace α/β gene on chromosome 12. *Am J Hum Genet* 1998;**63**:A15.

10 Raas-Rothschild A, Cormier-Daire V, Bao M, *et al.* Truncation of the UDP-N-acetylglucosamine: Lysosomal enzyme N-acetylglucosamine-1-phosphotransferase γ-subunit gene causes variant mucolipidosis III (pseudo-Hurler polydystrophy). *J Clin Invest* 2000;**105**:673.

11 Leroy JG, Spranger JW, Feingold M, *et al.* I-cell disease: a clinical picture. *J Pediatr* 1971;**79**:360.

12 Leroy JG, Spranger JW. I-cell disease. *N Eng J Med* 1970;**283**:598.

13 Luchsinger U, Buhler EM, Mehes K, Hirt HR. I-cell disease. *N Engl J Med* 1970;**282**:1374 (Letter).

14 Cipolloni C, Boldrini A, Dontiee E, *et al.* Neonatal mucolipidosis II (I-cell disease): clinical radiological and biochemical studies in a case. *Helv Paediatr Acta* 1980;**35**:85.

15 Hochman JA, Treem WR, Dougherty F, Bentley RC. Mucolipidosis II (I-cell disease) presenting as neonatal cholestasis. *J Inherit Metab Dis* 2001;**24**:603.

16 Blank E, Linder D. I-cell disease (mucolipidosis II): a lysosomopathy. *Pediatrics* 1974;**54**:797.

17 deMontis G, Garnier P, Thomassin N, *et al.* La mucolipidose Type II (maladie des cellules a inclusions). Etude d'un cas et revue de la literature. *Ann Pediatr* 1972;**19**:369.

18 Taylor NG, Shuff RY. I-cell disease: An unusual cause of gingival enlargement. *Br Dent J* 1994;**176**:106.

19 Spritz RA, Doughty RA, Spackman TJ, *et al.* Neonatal presentation of I-cell disease. *J Pediatr* 1978;**93**:954.

20 Okada S, Owada M, Sakiyama T, *et al.* I-cell disease: Clinical studies of 21 Japanese cases. *Clin Genet* 1985;**28**:207.

21 Satoh Y, Sakamoto K, Fujibayashi Y, *et al.* Cardiac involvement in mucolipidosis: importance of non-invasive studies for detection of cardiac abnormalities. *Jpn Heart J* 1983;**24**:149.

22 Patriquin HB, Kaplan P, Kind HP, Giedion A. Neonatal mucolipidosis I (I-cell disease) clinical and radiologic features in three cases. *Am J Roentgenol* 1977;**129**:37.

23 Hanai J, Leroy JG, O'Brien JS. Ultrastructure of cultured fibroblasts in I-cell disease. *Am J Dis Child* 1971;**122**:34.

24 Kenyon KR, Sensebrenner JA, Wylie RG. Hepatic ultrastructure and histochemistry in mucolipidosis II (I-cell disease). *Pediatr Res* 1973;**7**:560.

25 Rapola J, Autio S, Aula P, Nanto V. Lymphocytic inclusions in I-cell disease. *J Pediatr* 1974;**85**:88.

26 Aula P, Rapola J, Autio S, *et al.* Prenatal diagnosis and fetal pathology of I-cell disease (mucolipidosis type II). *J Pediatr* 1975;**87**:221.

27 Rapola J, Aula P. Morphology of the placenta in fetal I-cell disease. *Clin Genet* 1977;**11**:107.

28 Nagashima K, Sakakibara K, Endo H, *et al.* I-cell disease (mucolipidosis II): pathological and biochemical studies of an autopsy case. *Acta Pathol Jpn* 1977;**27**:251.

29 Martin JJ, Leroy JG, Van Eygen M, Ceuterick C. I-cell disease: a further report on its pathology. *Acta Neuropathol (Berl)* 1984;**64**:234.

30 Martin JJ, Leroy JG, Farriaux JP, *et al.* I-cell disease (mucolipidosis II). *Acta Neuropathol (Berl)* 1975;**33**:285.

31 Wiesmann UN, Lightbody J, Vasella F, Herschkowitz NN. Multiple lysosomal enzyme deficiency due to enzyme leakage? *N Engl J Med* 1971;**284**:109.

32 Wiesmann UN, Herschkowitz NN. Studies on the pathogenic mechanism of I-cell disease in cultured fibroblasts. *Pediatr Res* 1974;**8**:965.

33 Leroy JG, Ho MW, MacBrinn MC, *et al.* I-cell disease; biochemical studies. *Pediatr Res* 1972;**6**:752.

34 Wiesmann UN, Vasella F, Hershkowitz NN. I cell disease. Leakage of lysosomal enzymes into extracellular fluids. *N Engl J Med* 1971;**28**:1090.

35 Hickman S, Neufeld EF. A hypothesis for I-cell disease: defective hydrolases that do not enter lysosomes. *Biochem Biophys Res Commun* 1972;**49**:992.

36 Natowicz MR, Chi MY-Y, Lowry OH, Sly WS. Enzymatic identification of mannose 6-phosphate on the recognition marker for receptor-mediated pinocytosis of β-glucuronidase by human fibroblasts. *Proc Natl Acad Sci USA* 1979;**76**:4322.

37 Hasilik A, Heufeld EF. Biosynthesis of lysosomal enzymes in fibroblasts; phosphorylation of mannose residues. *J Biol Chem* 1980;**255**:4946.

38 Bach G, Barga R, Cantz M. I-cell disease: deficiency of extracellular hydrolase phosphorylation. *Biochem Biophys Res Commun* 1979;**91**:476.

39 Tabas I, Kornfeld S. Biosynthetic intermediates of β-glucuronidase contain high mannose oligosaccharides with blocked phosphate residues. *J Biol Chem* 1980;**255**:6633.

40 Varki A, Kornfeld S. Structural studies of phosphorylated high mannose-type oligosaccharides. *J Biol Chem* 1980;**255**:10847.

41 Hasilik A, Klein U, Waheed A, *et al.* Phosphorylated oligosaccharides in lysosomal enzymes: identification of a-N-acetylglucosamine (1) phospho (6)mannose diester groups. *Proc Natl Acad Sci USA* 1980;**77**:7074.

42 Reitman ML, Kornfeld S. Lysosomal enzyme targeting: N-acetylglucosaminylphosphotransferase selectively phosphorylates native lysosomal enzymes. *J Biol Chem* 1981;**256**:11977.

43 Waheed A, Hasilik A, Von Figura K. UDP-N-acetylglucosamine:lysosomal enzyme precursor N-acetylglucosamine-1-phosphotransferase: partial purification and characterization of the rat liver Golgi enzyme. *J Biol Chem* 1982;**257**:12322.

44 Lang L, Reitmen M, Tang J, *et al.* Lysosomal enzyme phosphorylation: recognition of a protein-dependent determinant allows specific phosphorylation of oligosaccharides present on lysosomal enzymes. *J Biol Chem* 1984;**259**:14663.

45 Hasilik A, Waheed A, Von Figura K. Enzymatic phosphorylation of lysosomal enzymes in the presence of UDP-N-acetylglucosamine. Absence of the activity in I-cell fibroblasts. *Biochem Biophys Res Commun* 1981;**98**:761.

46 Waheed A, Pohlmann R, Hasilik A, Von Figura K. Subcellular location of two enzymes involved in the synthesis of phosphorylated recognition markers in lysosomal enzymes. *J Biol Chem* 1981;**256**:4150.

47 Reitman ML, Kornfeld S. UDP-N-acetylglucosamine:glycoprotein N-acetyl-glucossamine-1-phosphotransferase. Proposed enzyme for the phosphorylation of the high mannose oligosaccharide units of lysosomal enzymes. *J Biol Chem* 1981;**256**:4275.

48 Varki A, Sherman N, Kornfeld S. Demonstrations of the enzymatic mechanisms of a-N-acetyl-d-glucosamine-1-phosphodiester N-acetylglucosaminidase (formerly called a-N-acetyl-glucosaminyl-phosphodiesterase) and lysosomal-N-acetylglucosaminidase. *Arch Biochem Biophys* 1983;**222**:145.

49 Fischer HD, Gonzalez-Noriega A, Sly WS, Morre DJ. Phosphomannosyl-enzyme receptors in rat liver. Subcellular distribution and role in intracellular transport of lysosomal enzymes. *J Biol Chem* 1980;**255**:9608.

50 Greene AA, Jonas AJ, Harms E, *et al.* Lysosomal cystine storage in cystinosis and mucolipidosis type II. *Pediatr Res* 1985;**19**:1170.

51 Tietze F, Rome LH, Butler JD. Impaired clearance of free cystine from lysosome-enriched granular fractions of I-cell disease fibroblasts. *Biochem J* 1986;**237**:9.

52 Vladutiu GD, Fike RM, Amigone VT. Influence of sialic acid on cell surface properties in I-cell disease fibroblasts. *In Vitro* 1981;**17**:588.

53 Hall CW, Liebaers I, DiNatale P, Neufeld EF. Enzymatic diagnosis of the genetic mucopolysaccharide storage disorders. *Methods Enzymol* 1978;**50**:439.

54 Ylikangas PK, Mononen IT. Glycosylasparaginase as a marker enzyme in the detection of I-cell disease. *Clin Chem* 1988;**44**:2543.

55 Varki A, Reitman ML, Vannirt S, *et al.* Demonstration of the heterozygous state for I-cell disease and psuedo-Hurler polydystrophy by assay of N-acetyl-glucosaminylphosphotransferase in white blood cells and fibroblasts. *Am J Hum Genet* 1982;**34**:717.

56 Mueller OT, Little LE, Miller AL, *et al.* I-cell disease and pseudo-Hurler polydystrophy: heterozygote detection and characteristics of the altered N-acetylglucosaminephosphotransferase in genetic variants. *Clin Chim Acta* 1985;**150**:175.

57 Mueller OT, Honey NK, Little LE, *et al.* Mucolipidosis II and III: the genetic relationship between two disorders of lysosomal enzyme biosynthesis. *J Clin Invest* 1983;**72**:1016.

58 Hujing F, Warren RJ, McLeod AGW. Elevated activity of lysosomal enzymes in amniotic fluid of a fetus with mucolipidosis II (I-cell disease). *Clin Chim Acta* 1973;**44**:453.

59 Matsuda I, Arashum S, Mitsuyama T, *et al.* Prenatal diagnosis of I-cell disease. *Hum Genet* 1975;**30**:69.

60 Gehler J, Cantz M, Stoeckenius M, Spranger J. Prenatal diagnosis of mucolipidosis II (I-cell disease). *Eur J Pediatr* 1976;**122**:201.

61 Hug G, Bove KE, Soukup S, *et al.* Increase serum hexosaminidase in a woman pregnant with a fetus affected by mucolipidosis II (I-cell disease). *N Engl J Med* 1984;**311**:988.

62 Kurobane I, Inoue S, Gotoh YH, *et al.* Biochemical improvement after treatment by bone marrow transplantation in I-cell disease. *Tohoku J Exp Med* 1986;**150**:63.

63 Imaizumi M, Gushi K, Kurobane I, *et al.* Long-term effects of bone marrow transplantation for inborn errors of metabolism: a study of four patients with lysosomal storage diseases. *Acta Paediatr Jpn* 1994;**36**:30.

Mucolipidosis III/psuedo-Hurler polydystrophy/ N-acetyl-glucosaminyl-I-phosphotransferase deficiency

MAJOR PHENOTYPIC EXPRESSION

Joint pain, stiffness, contractures; shortness of stature; malocclusion, gingival hypertrophy; aortic diastolic murmur; dysostosis multiplex, and deficiency of GLcNAc phosphotransferase.

INTRODUCTION

Mucolipidosis II and III reflect multiple deficiencies of many lysosomal hydrolases that require post-translational processing to form the recognition site that permits their cellular uptake. The fundamental defect is in N-acetylglucosaminyl-l-phosphotransferase (GlcNAc phosphotransferase) [1] (Figure 84.2, p. 554). The lysosomal enzyme substrates for this enzyme are glycoproteins containing reactive mannose molecules and in the reaction a GlcNAc phosphate is linked to the mannose; a subsequent phosphodiesterase reaction cleaves off the GlcNAc, leaving the mannose phosphate recognition site. Patients with I-cell disease, or mucolipidosis II, have complete deficiency of this enzyme, while patients with mucolipidosis III have varying amounts of residual activity of the enzyme. Variable patterns of clinical phenotype in mucolipidosis III reflect the considerable variation in enzyme activity as well as its effect on so very many lysosomal enzymes. The extent of the phenotypic variability has doubtless not yet been defined.

It is now clear that there is genetic heterogeneity in mucolipidosis III. Two genes code for the three subunits of GlcNAc phosphotransferase, α/β and γ [2,3]. Abnormalities in both genes have been found in different patients with mucolipidosis III.

CLINICAL ABNORMALITIES

Mucolipidosis III shares many of the clinical manifestations of the classic mucopolysaccharidoses. In fact the roentgenographic characteristics are those of a florid dysostosis multiplex.

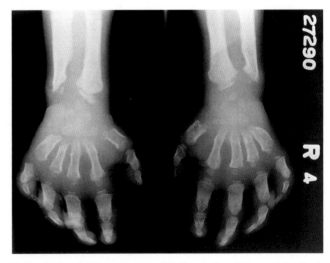

Figure 85.1 *Roentgenogram of the hand of an 11-year-old patient with mucolipidosis Type III. The picture was that of an extreme degree of dysostosis multiplex.*

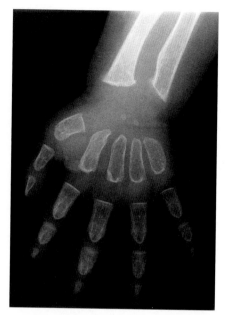

Figure 85.2   *Roentgenogram of hand of a 10-month-old infant with mucolipidosis III. There was extreme osteopenia with a fine inner reticular pattern. The phalanges were bullet-shaped. The metacarpals were broad at their distal ends and tapered proximally. The radius and ulna were angulated toward each other.*

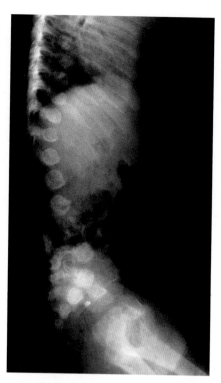

Figure 85.4   *Roentgenographic appearance of the broad spatulate ribs and spine of a patient with mucolipidosis III.*

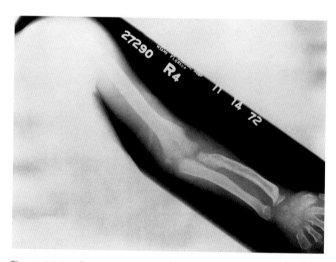

Figure 85.3   *Roentgenogram of the radius and ulna of a patient with mucolipidosis III.*

(Figures 85.1–85.5). The films of one of our patients [4] were kept in the teaching file of a medical school department of radiology as exemplifying Hurler disease. The disease was originally described [5] as pseudo-Hurler polydystrophy. There is however no mucopolysacchariduria. The long bones are short and thick. The distal radius and ulna tilt toward each other. The proximal phalanges are bullet-shaped and the metacarpals are broad distally and pointed proximally. The ribs are broad and spatulate. Vertebral bodies are short and Ll and T12 may be anteriorly beaked (Figures 85.4, 85.5). There may be early craniosynostosis (Figure 85.6). In other patients the skull may be normal. There may be hypoplasia of the

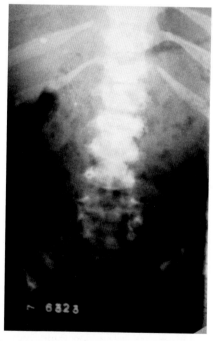

Figure 85.5   *Roentgenographic appearance of the broad spatulate ribs and spine of another patient with mucolipidosis III.*

odontoid. Degenerative changes of the joints, especially the proximal femoral areas, may be characteristic.

Patients usually present between 2 and 4 years-of-age with symptoms referable to the joints [4]. Pain is severe enough to awaken them from sleep. Tenderness and early progressive

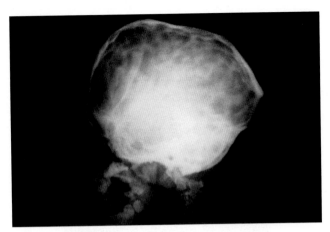

Figure 85.6 *Roentgenogram of the skull of same patient illustrates the shape and beaten silver appearance of premature craniosynostosis.*

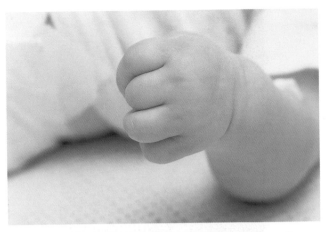

Figure 85.8 *The hand of the infant shows periarticular swelling and limitation of joint motion.*

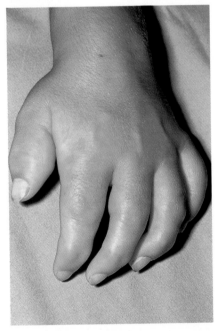

Figure 85.7 *The claw hand deformity may be identical to that of Hurler syndrome.*

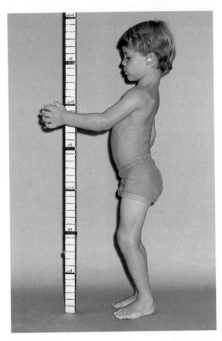

Figure 85.9 *An 11-year-old boy with mucolipidosis III. Contractures of the knees and hips and exaggerated lordosis give a bent position.*

stiffness and limitation of motion may lead to a presumptive diagnosis of juvenile rheumatoid arthritis, but the sedimentation rate remains normal [6]. All of the joints may be involved, and most patients develop some contractures. The claw hand that results by 6 years-of-age may be indistinguishable from that of the patient with Hurler disease (Figures 85.7, 85.8). A carpal tunnel syndrome may develop. Contractures of the knees, hips and elbows are in flexion, leading to a jockey-like appearance (Figure 85.9). These changes lead regularly to shortness of stature (Figure 85.10), but this may be variable. Females may be taller and less severely affected than males [7,8]. Progressive destructive changes in the hip may

lead to a waddling gait and compromised mobility. Rarely, isolated involvement of the hip and spine may be the only clinical manifestations [9]. Late effects are destruction of the femoral heads and of vertebral bodies.

The facial features may also be sufficiently coarse to suggest a diagnosis of mucopolysaccharidosis (Figures 85.10–85.13), but in some patients the face may appear normal (Figure 85.9). Hirsutism may be prominent and there may be synophris. The appearance of the mouth may be characteristic, with gingival hypertrophy and crowding of teeth with malocclusion (Figures 85.14–85.15). Gingival hypertrophy is always seen in I-cell disease (mucolipidosis II). The skin may become

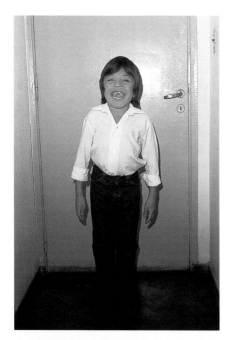

Figure 85.10   *A 10-year-old boy with mucolipidosis was short and had limitation of motion at the elbows, knees and hands.*

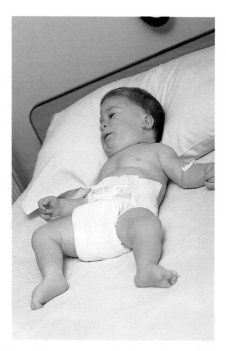

Figure 85.12   *R.V., a 1-month-old infant with mucolipidosis III. She was developmentally delayed and had coarse features. The position of the legs was in treatment of bilateral dislocations of the hips.*

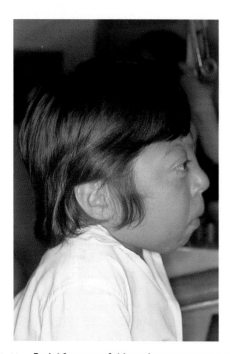

Figure 85.11   *Facial features of this patient were coarse and the eyes prominent.*

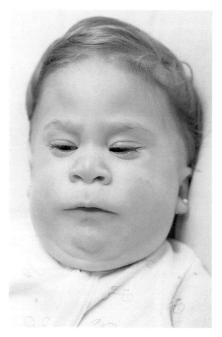

Figure 85.13   *Close-up of the face illustrates the coarse features indicative of storage of mucopolysaccharide within the skin, illustrated for example in the nose.*

thickened. The corneas may appear normal, but steaminess of the cornea may require a slit lamp for visualization, or it may be evident to the naked eye, as in Hurler or Maroteaux-Lamy syndromes. In some, slit lamp examination may be normal. Hyperopic astigmatism and mild retinopathy have also been described [10]. Intelligence may be normal [4], but most patients with mucolipidosis III have some limitation in

cognitive function. IQ levels of 70 to 90 are commonly encountered. In contrast, patients with I-cell disease have degrees of retardation incompatible with walking or talking. Infiltration of the endocardium may lead to aortic regurgitation and its characteristic diastolic murmur by the end of the first decade,

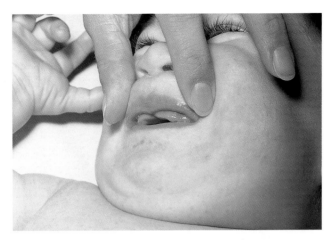

Figure 85.14 *The hyperplasia of the gums was well delineated by 10 months; it had been noted by the parents at birth. The gingiva was also cleft.*

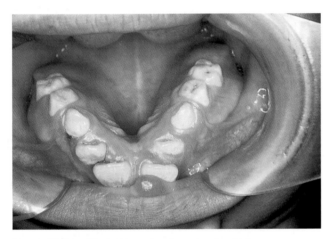

Figure 85.15 *Gingival hypertrophy and malocclusion were prominent features in this patient.*

but symptoms of cardiac insufficiency are rare. The liver is only moderately enlarged [11]. Some patients have inguinal hernias. Intelligence is usually to some extent compromised, but not severely [4,8]. Life expectancy is appreciably better than in mucolipidosis II, and survival to adulthood is not uncommon [8,12].

The histologic characteristic of these mucolipidoses is the appearance of cytoplasmic inclusion bodies [8]. These dense bodies, seen in cultured fibroblasts on phase microscopy (Chapter 84, p. 553), are the inclusions that gave I-cell disease its first name. Inclusions or vacuolation may be seen in other cells, such as biopsied cornea, bone marrow cells or lymphocytes [13,14].

GENETICS AND PATHOGENESIS

Specific biochemical diagnosis is often first suggested when fibroblasts or lymphocytes are assayed for the activity of lysosomal hydrolase enzymes. Defective activity is demonstrable

for a number of different enzymes, such as hexosaminidase, glucuronidase and arylsulfatase A [8]. Activities of the same enzymes are high in the media in which the cells are grown [15], which suggested at first that the cells were leaky. These same enzymes may be found in high levels of activity in the serum of patients. Activities may be 100-fold the normal level for some enzymes. The reason for this is not leaky cells but abnormal lysosomal enzymes, which are normally secreted and then avidly taken up. Mucolipidosis III enzymes cannot be taken up by normal cells while enzymes from normal cells are taken up normally by mucolipidosis cells [16]. This is because normal enzymes have the mannose-6-phosphate recognition marker that is essential for normal transport of the enzyme, and those of mucolipidosis patients are deficient in this phosphomannosyl signal (see Figure 84.2, p. 554). Activities of β-glucosidase in fibroblasts of patients are normal, because this enzyme is targeted to lysosomes by a phosphorylation-independent mechanism [17].

The enzyme that catalyzes the initial phosphorylation of mannose residues in the glycoprotein enzymes is formally UDP-N-acetylglucosamine:lysosomal enzyme-N-acetylglucosamine-l-phosphtransferase; because its other substrate is UDP-N-acetylglucosamine, we have shortened this to GlcNAc phosphotransferase. Somatic cell hybridization studies have revealed distinct complementation groups [18,19], which are now referred to as groups A, B and C. Group A is the most common; many I-cell patients also fit into this group [20]. Group C is uncommon and group B is rare. In the phosphotransferase assay, which utilizes a-methylmannoside as acceptor, patients with mucolipidosis III in the complementation group C have normal activity [21,22]. Those of groups A and B display defective activity against all substrates. The enzyme normally has two distinct functions: recognition of and affinity for the lysosomal enzyme protein, and catalytic phosphorylation of mannose residues. In parallel, studies with lysosomal enzymes as substrates and methylmannoside substrate have elucidated the existence of two distinct groups of patients: one in which activity against both is deficient, and the other in which activity against α-methylmannoside is normal but phosphorylation of lysosomal enzymes is impaired. This would be consistent with specific interference with recognition versus defect in catalytic function [23].

The α/β gene has been mapped to chromosome 12p [2]. The γ gene has been mapped to 16p [3]. Some patients with mucolipidosis III have been found to have abnormalities in the α/β gene, because there is reduced transcription to mRNA [2]. In other families with mucolipidosis III a mutation was found in the γ gene [3]. This insertion of a cytosine at codon 167 leads to a frame shift and a premature termination 107 bp downstream [3].

Genetic transmission is autosomal recessive, as it is in I-cell disease. Consanguinity has been observed [7]. Heterozygotes have been reported to have intermediate levels of GlcNAc phosphotransferase in leukocytes and cultured fibroblasts [21]. Prenatal diagnosis should be possible by assay of the enzyme in cultured amniocytes or chorionic villus cells.

TREATMENT

Supportive orthopedic management and physiotherapy may be useful, especially for abnormalities in the hips. It is recommended that hip surgery is delayed until after puberty. Surgical correction of carpal tunnel syndrome is useful. Intravenous pamidronate has been reported [24] to reduce bone pain and improve mobility, but biochemical, histological and roentgenographic evidence of bone resorption did not improve.

References

1 Reitman ML, Varki A, Kornfeld S. Fibroblasts from patients with I-cell disease and pseudo-Hurler polydystrophy are deficient in uridine 5'-diphosphate-N-acetylglucosamine: glycoprotein acetylglucosaminylphosphotransferase activity. *J Clin Invest* 1981;**67**:1574.

2 Canfield W, Bao M, Pan J, *et al*. Mucolipidosis II and mucolipidosis IIIA are caused by mutations in the GlcNAc-phosphotransferase α/β gene on chromosome **12**. *Am J Hum Genet* 1998;63:A15.

3 Raas-Rothschild A, Cormier-Daire V, Bao M, *et al*. Truncation of the UDP-N-acetylglucosamine: Lysosomal enzyme N-acetylglucosamine-1-phosphotransferase y-subunit gene causes variant mucolipidosis III (pseudo-Hurler polydystrophy). *J Clin Invest* 2000;**105**:673.

4 O'Brien JS, Nyhan WL, Shear C, *et al*. Clinical and biochemical expression of a unique mucopolysaccharidosis. *Clin Genet* 1976;**9**:399.

5 Maroteaux P, Lamy M. Les dysplasies spondylo-epiphysaires genotypiques. *Semin Hop Paris* 1958;**34**:1685.

6 Brik R, Mandel H, Aiziil A, *et al*. Mucolipidosis III presenting as a rheumatological disorder. *J Rheumatol* 1993;20:133.

7 Ward C, Singh R, Slade C, *et al*. A mild form of mucolipidosis type III in four Baluch siblings. *Clin Genet* 1993;**44**:313.

8 Kelly TE, Thomas GH, Taylor HA Jr, *et al*. Mucolipidosis III (pseudo-Hurler polydystrophy): clinical and laboratory studies in a series of 12 patients. *Johns Hopkins Med J* 1975;**137**:156.

9 Freisinger P, Padovani JC, Maroteaux P. An atypical form of mucolipidosis III. *J Med Genet* 1992;**29**:834.

10 Traboulsi M, Maumenee IH. Ophthalmologic findings in mucolipidosis III (pseudo-Hurler polydystrophy). *Am J Ophthalmol* 1986;**102**:592.

11 McKusick VA. Mucolipidosis III (the mucopolysaccharidoses): in *Heritable Disorders of Connective Tissue*. 4th edn. C V Mosby, St Louis;1972:652.

12 Umehara F, Matsumoto W, Kuriyama M, *et al*. Mucolipdosis III (pseudo-Hurler polydystroophy): Clinical studies in aged patients in one family. *J Neurol Sci* 1997;**146**:167.

13 Taylor HA, Thomas GH, Miller CS, *et al*. Mucolipidosis III (pseudo-Hurler polydystrophy): Cytological and ultrastructural observations of cultured fibroblast cells. *Clin Genet* 1973;**4**:388.

14 Stein H, Berman ER, Lioni N, *et al*. Pseudo-Hurler polydystrophy (mucolipidosis III): A clinical biochemical and ultrastructural study. *Isr J Med Sci* 1974;**10**:463.

15 Wiesemann UN, Lightbody J, Vassella F, Hersch-Kowitz NN. Multiple lysosomal enzyme deficiency due to enzyme leakage? *N Engl J Med* 1971;**284**:109.

16 Hickman S, Neufeld EF. A hypothesis for I-cell disease: Defective hydrolases that do not enter lysosomes. *Biochem Biophys Res Commun* 1972;**49**:992.

17 Aerts JMFG, Schram AW, Strijland A, *et al*. Glucocerebrosidase, a lysosomal enzyme that does not undergo oligosaccharide phosphorylation. *Biochem Biophys Acta* 1988;**964**:303.

18 Honey NK, Mueller OT, Little LB, *et al*. Mucolipidosis III is genetically heterogeneous. *Proc NatlAcad Sci USA* 1982;**79**:7420.

19 Gravel RA, Gravel YA, Miller AL, Lowden JA. Genetic complementation analysis of I-cell disease and pseudo-Hurler polydystrophy. in *Lysosomes and Lysosomal Storage Diseases* (eds JW Callahan, JA Lowden). Raven Press, New York;1981:289.

20 Mueller OT, Honey NK, Little LB, *et al*. Mucolipidosis II and III. The genetic relationships between two disorders of lysosomal enzyme biosynthesis. *J Clin Invest* 1983;**72**:1016.

21 Varki A, Reitman ML, Vannirt S, *et al*. Demonstration of the heterozygous state for I-cell disease and pseudo-Hurler polydystrophy by assay of N-acetyl-glucosaminylphosphotransferase in white blood cells and fibroblasts. *Am J Hum Genet* 1982;**34**:717.

22 Mueller OT, Little LB, Miller AL, *et al*. I-cell disease and pseudo-Hurler polydystrophy: Heterozygote detection and characteristics of the altered N-acetyl-glucosamine-phosphotransferase in genetic variants. *Clin Chim Acta* 1985;**150**:176.

23 Varki AP, Reitman ML, Kornfeld S. Identification of a variant of mucolipidosis III (pseudo-Hurler polydystrophy): A catalytically active N-acetyl-glucosaminylphosphotransferase that fails to phosphorylate lysosomal enzymes. *Proc Natl Acad Sci USA* 1981;**78**:7773.

24 Robinson C, Baker N, Noble J, *et al*. The osteodystrophy of mucolipidosis type III and the effects of intravenous pamidronate treatment. *J Inherit Metab Dis* 2002;**25**:681.

PART 12

Disorders of cholesterol and
neutral lipid metabolism

Familial hypercholesterolemia

MAJOR PHENOTYPIC EXPRESSION

Xanthomas, coronary artery disease, hypercholesterolemia, elevated concentration of low density lipoprotein (LDL) cholesterol in plasma, and defective LDL receptor activity.

INTRODUCTION

Familial hypercholesterolemia is an important model disease. The fundamental defect is an abnormality in a receptor molecule [1]. The study of this disease, especially in the homozygous form, has provided insights into the regulation of the metabolism of cholesterol. This has led to practical approaches to the management of the more common heterozygous disease and other forms of hypercholesterolemia. Familial hypercholesterolemia makes for compelling evidence of the causal relationship between elevated levels of cholesterol in the blood and coronary atherosclerosis.

The disease is dominantly expressed in heterozygotes, who develop coronary artery disease after the age of 30 years. In homozygotes the concentrations of cholesterol in the blood are enormous; coronary artery disease develops in childhood. The genetics were worked out by Khachadurian [2] in Lebanon, where an unusual number of homozygotes and a very high incidence of consanguinity have been observed. Variation at a single gene locus leads to three distinct phenotypes: homozygous affected, heterozygous, and homozygous normal.

The relationship between familial hypercholesterolemia and LDL was established by the studies of Gofman [3] and of Frederickson [4] and their colleagues. The nature of the fundamental defect in the receptor, its variety and the nature of mutation have been laid out in the elegant work of Brown and Goldstein [1,5,6] (Figure 86.1). LDL cholesterol is taken up by cells after binding of the LDL to its receptor in coated pits on the cell surface, which then undergo endocytic internalization. When receptor is defective, LDL cholesterol cannot be removed from the plasma, levels are very high and the clinical consequences ensue.

Five types of defects have been established.

- In the most common, class 1, no immunoprecipitable (CRM) receptor protein is found.
- In class 2, the protein cannot be transported to the endoplasmic reticulum and the Golgi complex.
- In class 3, the receptor does not properly bind LDL.
- In class 4, the receptor does not cluster in the coated pits and bound LDL is not internalized.
- In class 5 the receptors bind and internalize in coated pits but are unable to release the LDL in the endosome and recycle it.

The disease is caused by mutations in the *LDLR* gene. The gene has been mapped to the short arm of chromosome 19, at p13.1-13.3. A very large number of mutations have been defined and there are now two websites (http://www.ucl.ac.uk/fh/ and http://www.umd.necker.fr) [7–10]. The most common, Class 1 mutations (Table 86.1) are null alleles in the sense that there is no immunoprecipitable receptor protein [11]. Mutations have been defined in each of the four classes. Homozygous individuals may have two identical mutant alleles, or they may be compound heterozygotes, who inherited a different allele from each parent.

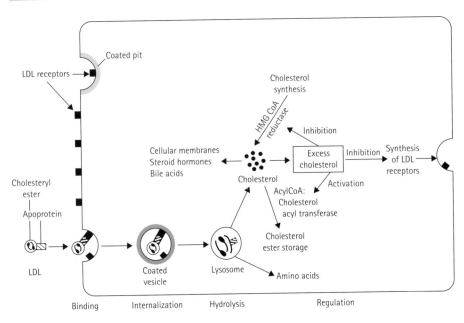

Figure 86.1 *The LDL receptor and its role in the regulation of the metabolism of cholesterol.*

Table 86.1 *Classes of mutation of the LDL receptor*

Class	Defect	Binding of LDL	Internalization
1	Synthesis	Absent	—
2	Transport to Golgi	Absent or reduced	—
			Normal
3	Binding of LDL	Reduced or absent	Normal
			—
4	Clustering in coated pits	Normal	Defective
5	Discharge in endosome (recycling)	Normal	Normal

CLINICAL ABNORMALITIES

Homozygous familial hypercholesterolemia

Hypercholesterolemia is present from birth in heterozygotes as well as homozygotes, but homozygotes have severe hypercholesterolemic disease [12]. Their cholesterol concentrations range from 600 to 1200 mg/dL (15–30 mmol/L) [13–15]. The first clinical manifestation is usually the appearance of xanthomas (Figures 86.2–86.7). Xanthomas may be flat (planar), tuberous or tendinous. Xanthomatous deposits are particularly common over the Achilles tendon and the extensor tendons of the hands. Tuberous xanthomas are seen over the elbows, knees and elsewhere. Subperiosteal xanthomas may be seen below the knee at the tibial tuberosity and at the elbow. Trauma appears to influence the local occurrence of these lesions. Cutaneous xanthomas may be bright orange or yellow and they are prominent over the buttocks and the hands. The interdigital web between the first and second fingers is a favorite site. Xanthomas sometimes occur on the tongue or the buccal mucosa. An arcus about the cornea is regularly seen in homozygotes prior to the age of 10 years (Figure 86.8).

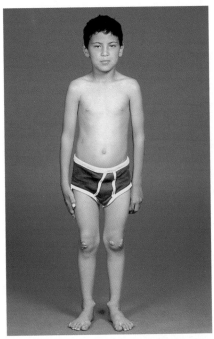

Figure 86.2 *M.A.S., a 12-year-old Egyptian boy with homozygous familial hypercholesterolemia. In addition to multiple xanthomas, he had severe aortic stenosis and died in an attempt at surgical correction. He had a 9-year-old affected brother, and the parents were first cousins.*

The most significant clinical consequence of familial hypercholesterolemia is the occurrence of severe atherosclerosis in the aorta and coronary arteries because LDL-derived cholesterol is deposited also in arterial atheromatous plaques [16]. Peripheral and cerebral vessels are also involved. Plaques contain abundant deposits of lipid in the extracellular space and in large foamy cells. Disease of the heart tends to be rapidly progressive. Patients may have clinical angina as early as 5 years-of-age. Myocardial infarctions have been recorded as

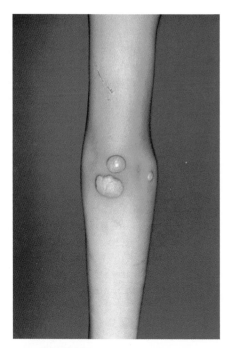

Figure 86.3   *M.A.S. Xanthomas over the elbow.*

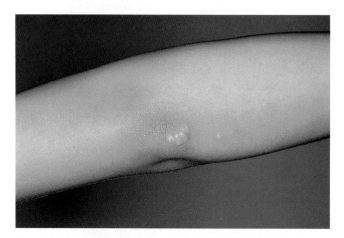

Figure 86.4   *M.A.S. Cutaneous xanthomas over the knee.*

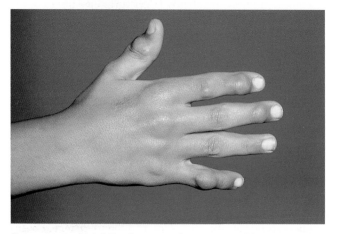

Figure 86.5   *M.A.S. Tendinous xanthomas were evident over each metacarpophalangeal joint, the distal interphalangeal joints of the first, second and third fingers, and the proximal interphalangeal joints of the second and fifth fingers.*

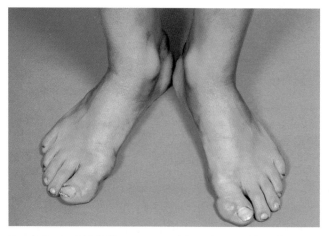

Figure 86.6   *M.A.S. There were medial xanthomas of both feet.*

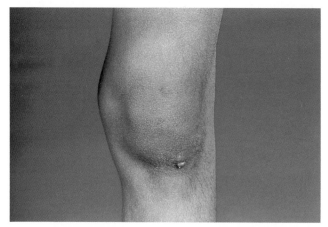

Figure 86.7   *B.A.S.J., a 7-year-old with homozygous familial hypercholesterolemia. There were xanthomas over the Achilles tendon and the elbows, as well as the knees, from the age of 3 years.*

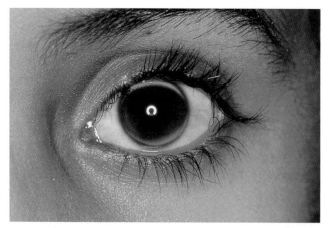

Figure 86.8   *B.A.S.J. At 7 years the arcus senilis was well developed.*

early as 18 months and 3 years-of-age. Most patients have died of this disease by 30 years-of-age [15,17].

There is evidence of genetically determined phenotypic variation in that homozygotes who have no LDL receptor function tend to have more relentless disease (with a mean age at death of 11 years) than those with defective receptors with some function (only one of 26 patients had died by the time of the report [18] and he was 23 years old). There is also evidence that other genes or factors modify the expression of the disease. In one family of two sibs with the identical mutation in the LDL receptor gene, one died at 3 years but the other was asymptomatic until 14 years [19]. In an effort to enhance the assessment of risk of vascular disease, a cholesterol-year score has been developed at the National Institutes of Health, similar to the pack-years score for cigarette smokers. By multiplying the number of years a patient has had a certain level of cholesterol (mg/dL), a score is achieved which in a series of 11 consecutive homozygous patients correlated very well with the development of angina [20].

Xanthomatous deposits are also found on the endocardium and on the mitral and aortic valves, leading to regurgitation and stenosis [21,22]. The aortic valve hemodynamics may be indistinguishable from rheumatic or calcific aortic stenosis [2,23,24]. A diagnosis of acute rheumatic fever may also be suspected, on the basis of migratory painful joints and an elevated sedimentation rate, which patients may also have [25,26]. Recurrent attacks of arthritis or tenosynovitis occur in the ankles, wrists and proximal interphalangeal joints [22,26,27]. These symptoms tend to last for 3 to 12 days and subside spontaneously. The elevated sedimentation rate may be present in the absence of arthritis, or absent when joint symptoms are present [26]. There may also be a two-fold elevation of the plasma concentration of fibrinogen.

Heterozygous familial hypercholesterolemia

In heterozygotes, concentrations of cholesterol in the blood range from 270 to 550 mg/dL (7 to 14 mmol/L [28]; mean levels approximate 350 mg/dL (9 mmol/L) [13,14,29,30]. Levels of triglycerides are usually normal [29]. Phospholipids are slightly elevated: they are more consistently elevated in homozygotes [31]. The increased cholesterol content of the plasma is entirely in the LDL fraction [3,4,32]. The normal concentration of LDL cholesterol is 110 ± 25 mg/dL. In heterozygotes the mean levels reported [13] were 241 ± 60, whereas in homozygotes the mean was 625 ± 160 mg/dL. Levels of high density lipoprotein (HDL) cholesterol tend to be a bit lower in both heterozygotes and homozygotes than in normals. In the absence of hypertriglyceridemia, an elevated level of cholesterol in the blood indicates that LDL cholesterol level is elevated.

Heterozygotes usually develop xanthomas by the time of death [29]. They occur typically over tendons such as the Achilles. Heterozygotes regularly develop xanthelasma, the palpebral xanthoma that is rarely seen in homozygotes. People with normal concentrations of cholesterol may also develop xanthelasma [3]. The corneal arcus is also seen in people with normal lipid metabolism. In heterozygotes, it is found in 10 percent by 30 years-of-age and in 50 percent of those over 30 [32].

Clinical manifestations of coronary artery disease appear in heterozygotes as early as the fourth decade [33]. Its pattern is much more variable than in homozygotes. Mean age at death in males was 55 and in females 64 years [34]. The probability of a coronary event was 16 percent by the age of 40 and 52 percent by the age of 60 in males [35]. In females the probability was 33 percent by the age of 60.

GENETICS AND PATHOGENESIS

The fundamental defect in familial hypercholesterolemia is in the LDL receptor [36–38] (Figure 86.1). There are a number of allelic gene mutations in a locus on the short arm of chromosome 19, which is placed at p13.1 to 13.3 [39]. Heterozygotes are found in a frequency of one in 500 [40]. This appears to be the most common single gene disease in humans and it is seen throughout the world. It is expressed as dominant in heterozygotes. Homozygotes have two abnormal copies of the gene.

Cultured cells require cholesterol for survival: it is a necessary component of the plasma membrane of the cells. Amounts in excess of what is required are stored as cholesterol ester. Mammalian cells grown in serum utilize its LDL rather than synthesizing the compound [41]. The critical component in the uptake of cholesterol from LDL is the highly specific receptor that binds the apoprotein B-100 of the LDL [42,43].

LDL is a large, spherical particle with an oily core made up of many cholesterol molecules in ester linkage to fatty acids. There is a hydrophilic phospholipid coat in which one large protein (apoprotein B-100) is embedded. This apoprotein is recognized and bound by the receptor, which is an acidic glycoprotein. The receptor has been solubilized and purified to homogeneity. Its apparent molecular weight is 160 kDa [44–46]. It is synthesized as a precursor with an apparent molecular weight of 120 kDa and 30 minutes after synthesis it is converted to the apparently larger form and inserted into the plasma membrane.

LDL is taken up or internalized by a process termed receptor-mediated endocytosis [47–49]. The receptors are found in coated pits of the plasma membrane, where the surface is indented (Figure 86.1). Pits, containing bound LDL, invaginate and pinch off to form coated vesicles, which migrate to lysosomes and fuse with them. There, hydrolysis takes place to yield free cholesterol.

Intracellular cholesterol regulates its own intracellular concentration by means of an elegant system of feedback controls [50]. Some is required in the synthesis of cell surface membranes and in specialized cells such as the adrenal and liver, and some is converted to steroid hormones and bile acids. Excess may be stored as cholesterol ester, and the enzyme catalyzing this, acylCoA:cholesterol acyltransferase (ACAT), is activated by cholesterol [51]. The rate-limiting step in intracellular cholesterol synthesis is catalyzed by

3-hydroxy-3-methylglutaryl-CoA (HMG CoA) reductase. Regulation occurs at this level in that cholesterol suppresses the synthesis of this enzyme, thus turning off cholesterol biosynthesis [52]. The third regulatory process is a turning off by cholesterol of the synthesis of LDL receptors [53]. This prevents entry of additional LDL and the overloading of cells with cholesterol.

These considerations have relevance to the pathogenesis of atherosclerosis and coronary artery disease in normal individuals who do not have a defect in the LDL receptor. The consumption of a diet rich in dairy products, eggs and animal meats provides enough cholesterol to overload the system and turn off the synthesis of LDL receptors. This protects the cell against too much cholesterol, but then excessive amounts of LDL accumulate in the blood and cholesterol is laid down in atherosclerotic plaques.

The LDL receptor is a cell-surface glycoprotein containing both N-linked and O-linked oligosaccharide chains [54]. The protein is synthesized in the endoplasmic reticulum and then migrates to the Golgi complex; in the process the mannose-rich portion of the precursor protein is reduced and O-linked sugars, including sialic acid, are added to the core N-acetyl-galactosamine [54]. Next the receptor moves to the cell surface to cluster in the coated pits, which are lined by a surface protein, clathrin [55]. The coated pits invaginate to form endocytic vesicles, which fuse to form endosomes. The pH in the endosome falls, and LDL dissociates from the receptor which then returns to the surface ready to initiate another cycle of LDL binding and transport.

The gene contains 18 exons spanning 45 kb. The mRNA is 5.3 kb; it codes for a protein of 860 amino acids [56]. The very large number of mutations so far identified have fallen into 5 classes representing the 5 phenotypic groups [11,54,57–66]. Class 1 mutations are null alleles which produce no immuno-precipitable protein. At least one Class 1 allele was found in over half of 128 fibroblast lines studied. Among 32 of these alleles studied, 12 had large deletions [11] recognizable on Southern blots. Four French-Canadian homozygotes were found to have a deletion over 10 kb involving the promoter and exon 1 [58]. A different 5 kb deletion of exons 13–15 leads to a truncated mRNA but no protein [59]. In patients with two null alleles there is no immunoprecipitable protein and receptors cannot be seen electron microscopically [11,47].

In Class 2 mutations the proteins synthesized fail to be transported to the Golgi and the receptors accumulate intra-cellularly. These, too, are relatively common. Two of them were small deletions in exon 4. Deletion in exon 4 is the mutation for the Watanabe rabbit (WHHL), an animal model for familial hypercholesterolemia [60,61]. These rabbits have less than five percent of the normal number of LDL receptors, and high circulating levels of LDL and cholesterol, and they develop atherosclerosis and infarctions by 2 years-of-age. A nonsense mutation in which a single nucleotide substitution produces a stop codon that leads to a truncated protein has been called the Lebanese allele and has been found in several

unrelated Arab patients [62]. A majority of class 2 mutants are leaky in the sense some transport remains.

In Class 3 mutations the proteins are synthesized and they are transported normally, but their structure is altered so that they fail to bind the LDL properly. Levels of binding activity range from two to 30 percent of normal. Three mutations documented included two deletions and a duplication; the former do not bind LDL, indicating deletion in the ligand binding domain, while the product of the duplication binds reduced quantities of LDL [54]. Differential effects on binding are illustrated by FH Paris-1 in which deletion of exon 5 leads to binding of VLDL, but not LDL [58], while FH French Canadian 3 binds neither [67].

Class 4 mutations are altered in their ability to cluster in the coated pits, and consequently they fail to internalize bound LDL. These defects are rare, but interesting. Among mutations identified early there were two deletions, an insertion, a non-sense mutation, and a missense mutation [63]. The stop codon in the nonsense mutation leaves only two of the normal 50 amino acids in the cytoplasmic domain. The insertion adds eight amino acids in this domain and the missense mutation changes a tyrosine to a cysteine at the 80th amino acid of this domain [64]. These observations suggested that this area is critical for binding to a protein as a requirement for movement into the clathrin-coated pits. This was the first evidence that clustering in the pits was required for transport into cells. The two deletions appear to constitute a different subclass of defects in which the membrane spacing domain is altered and the truncated receptors are largely secreted into the medium of cultured cells [63].

Class 5 mutations code for receptors that cannot discharge the ligand in the endosome and thus cannot recycle to the cell surface. The receptor is then degraded. Deletion of exons 7–14 in FH Osaka-2 leads to this phenotype [68]. A small number of mutations have been found in the promotor [69–71].

Prenatal diagnosis of homozygous familial hypercholesterolemia has been made [72] by assay of LDL receptor activity in cultured amniocytes. In a series of pregnancies at risk, one was homozygous affected, two were heterozygotes, and one was normal. Prenatal diagnosis of an affected fetus has also been made by fetal blood sampling and analysis of cholesterol [73]. If the mutation is known, it is likely that molecular diagnosis would be the procedure of choice. Heterozygosity for the Lebanese mutation has been documented in chorionic villus material [74].

Heterozygosity has been diagnosed in cord blood [12] as well as prenatally, but the assay of cord blood is not a reliable method of screening the general public. Even at a year of age, when the methodology is more accurate, family study would be required to determine that an elevated level of LDL cholesterol is caused by familial hypercholesterolemia. Defective LDL receptor function can be documented in cultured fibroblasts or lymphocytes [73]. DNA based diagnosis is feasible in populations in which a particular mutation is common.

TREATMENT

Homozygotes

Transplantation of the liver has been performed in a 6-year-old child [75] with homozygous disease. The LDL receptors of the transplanted liver removed cholesterol from the plasma at a near normal rate and effectively reversed the abnormal concentrations. In another patient successfully transplanted, lesions in the coronary arteries regressed, as did xanthomas [20]. Experience with a small number of other patients confirmed dramatic fall in plasma LDL [76–78].

Homozygotes are generally resistant to the drugs and diet that are effective in heterozygotes, but those with some functional receptor activity may respond. The most practical and effective approach to the treatment of most homozygotes has been the removal of LDL by plasmapheresis or LDL apheresis [20,79]. These procedures lower blood concentrations of cholesterol appreciably, and xanthomas have been observed to regress, as have lesions in the coronary arteries, which were limiting flow. Currently this appears to be the treatment of choice [80,81]. Lowering of cholesterol levels has also been reported following portacaval anastomosis [82].

Gene therapy has been undertaken in homozygous familial hypercholesterolemia [83]. In this *ex vivo* technique, hepatocytes are isolated from the patient and grown in culture, transfected with the normal gene and reinjected into the portal circulation. The procedure is effective in lowering cholesterol in the WHHL rabbit, and a human protocol has been approved. Results to date have been disappointing.

Heterozygotes

Two major approaches have been developed for the treatment of heterozygotes. These patients have one normal LDL receptor gene that is known to be under feedback control. The first group of drugs to be employed is anion-binding resins such as cholestyramine and colestipol [84]. They prevent the recycling of bile acids and thus stimulate the synthesis of LDL receptors and lower LDL cholesterol concentrations by 15 to 20 percent. This was enough to reduce the incidence of myocardial infarctions by 20 percent in a 10-year prospective study [36]. This approach is limited by the fact that the cell also responds to cholesterol deprivation by induction of HMG CoA reductase synthesis and by increasing *de novo* synthesis of cholesterol, which inhibits the synthesis of new LDL receptors.

The development of drugs that inhibit cholesterol biosynthesis by inhibiting HMG CoA reductase has provided a systematic approach to treatment by combination with bile acid sequestration. The first of these drugs was mevastatin (Compactin), a compound isolated from Penicillium [85] that has a side chain resembling mevalonic acid. A more potent inhibitor isolated from Aspergillus differs in structure only in the substitution of a methyl for hydrogen group and

is called mevinolin or lovastatin [86]. Both compounds lower blood levels of LDL and cholesterol and significantly increase LDL receptors. Combined therapy with cholestyramine and mevinolin lowers LDL cholesterol levels by 50 to 60 percent [87]. Currently lovastatin and chemically modified natural statins (pravastatin and simvastatin) or synthetic statins (fluvastatin, cerivastatin, and atorvastatin) are in use in human therapy, not only for FH heterozygotes but for many others with hypercholesterolemia [88]. These drugs lower LDL cholesterol. They are not without side-effects, including hepatic toxicity and myopathy, which may manifest as rhabdomyolysis. The addition of nicotinic acid to the regimen may further improve the effect on levels of cholesterol [87]. A prudent diet for these patients is one low in cholesterol and saturated fat.

References

1 Brown MS, Goldstein JL. Familial hypercholesterolemia: model for genetic receptor disease. *Harvey Lect Ser* 1979;**73**:163.

2 Khachadurian AK. The inheritance of essential familial hypercholesterolemia. *Am J Med* 1964;**37**:402.

3 Gofman JW, Rubin L, McGinley JP, Jones HB. Hyperlipoproteinemia. *Am J Med* 1954;**17**:514.

4 Frederickson DS, Levy RI, Lees RS. Fat transport in lipoproteins: an integrated approach to mechanisms and disorders. *N Engl J Med* 1967;**276**: 34, 94, 148, 215, 273.

5 Goldstein JL, Brown MS. Binding and degradation of low density lipoprotein by cultured human fibroblasts: comparison of cells from a normal subject and from a patient with homozygous familial hypercholesterolemia. *J Biol Chem* 1974;**249**:5153.

6 Rader DJ, Cohen J, Hobbs HH. Monogenic hypercholesterolemia: new insights in pathogenesis and treatment. *J Clin Invest* 2003;**111**:1795.

7 Day INM, Whittall RA, O'Dell SD, *et al*. Spectrum of LDL receptor gene mutations in heterozygous familial hypercholesterolemia. *Hum Mutat* 1997;**10**:116.

8 Wilson DJ, Gahan M, Haddad L, *et al*. A World Wide Web site for low-density lipoprotein receptor gene mutations in familial hypercholesterolemia: Sequence-based tabular and direct submission data handling. *Am J Cardiol* 1998;**81**:1509.

9 Varret M, Rabes J-P, Collod-Beroud G, *et al*. Software and database for the analysis of mutations in the human LDL receptor gene. *Nucleic Acids Res* 1997;**25**:172.

10 Varret M, Rabes J-P, Thiart R, *et al*. LDLR database (second edition): New additions to the database and the software and results of the first molecular analysis. *Nucleic Acids Res* 1998;**26**:248.

11 Hobbs HH, Lettersdorf E, Goldstein JL, *et al*. Multiple crm-mutations in familial hypercholesterolemia: evidence for 13 alleles including four deletions. *J Clin Invest* 1988;**81**:909.

12 Kwiterovich PO Jr, Levy RI, Frederickson DS. Neonatal diagnosis of familial type II hyperlipoproteinaemia. *Lancet* 1973;**1**:118.

13 Kwiterovich PO Jr, Frederickson DS, Levy RI. Familial hypercholesterolemia (one form of familial type II hyperlipoproteinemia). A study of its biochemical genetic and clinical presentation in childhood. *J Clin Invest* 1974;**53**:1237.

14 Khachadurian AK. A general view of clinical and laboratory features of familial hypercholesterolemia (type II hyperbetalipoproteinemia). *Protides Biological Fluids* 1971;**19**:315.

15 Khachadurian AK, Uthman SM. Experiences with the homozygous cases of familial hypercholesterolemia. A report of 52 patients. *Nutr Metab* 1973;**15**:132.

16   Buja LM, Kovanen PT, Bilheimer DW. Cellular pathology of homozygous familial hypercholesterolemia. *Am J Pathol* 1979;**97**:327.

17   Stefel HC, Baker SG, Sandler MP, *et al.* A host of hypercholesterolaemic homozygotes in South Africa. *Br Med J* 1980;**281**:633.

18   Goldstein JL, Brown MS. The LDL receptor defect in familial hypercholesterolemia: implications for pathogenesis and therapy. *Med Clin North Am* 1982;**66**:335.

19   Hobbs HH, Brown MS, Russell DW, *et al.* Deletion in LDL receptor gene occurs in majority of French Canadians with familial hypercholesterolemia. *N Engl J Med* 1987;**317**:734.

20   Hoeg JM. Familial hypercholesterolemia. What the zebra can teach us about the horse. *JAMA* 1994;**271**:543.

21   Maher JA, Epstein FH, Hand EA. Xantho-matosis and coronary heart disease: necropsy study of two affected siblings. *Arch Intern Med* 1958;**102**:137.

22   Schettler FC. Essential familial hypercholesterolemia: in *Atherosclerosis* (eds Schettler FG, Boyd GS). Elsevier, Amsterdam;1969:543.

23   Haitas B, Baker SG, Meyer TE, *et al.* Natural history and cardiac manifestations of homozygous familial hypercholesterolaemia. *Q J Med* 1990;**76**:731.

24   Beppu S, Minura Y, Sakakibara H, *et al.* Supravalvular aortic stenosis and coronary ostial stenosis in familial hypercholesterolemia: Two-dimensional echocardiographic assessment. *Circulation* 1983;**67**:878.

25   Khachadurian AK. Migratory polyarthritis in familial hypercholesterolemia (type II hyperlipoproteinemia). *Arthritis Rheum* 1968;**11**:385.

26   Khachadurian AK. Persistent elevation of the erythrocyte sedimentation rate (ESR) in familial hypercholesterolemia. *J Med Liban* 1967;**20**:31.

27   Rooney PJ, Third J, Madkour MM, *et al.* Transient polyarthritis associated with familial hyperbetalipoproteinemia. *Q J Med* (New Series) 1978;**47**:249.

28   Brown MS, Goldstein JL. Familial hypercholesterolemia: genetic biochemical and pathophysiologic considerations. *Adv Intern Med* 1975;**20**:273.

29   Schrott HG, Goldstein JL, Hazzard WR, *et al.* Familial hypercholesterolemia in a large kindred. Evidence for a monogenic mechanism. *Ann Intern Med* 1972;**76**:711.

30   Nevin NC, Slack H. Hyperlipidaemic xanthomatosis. II Mode of inheritance in 55 families with essential hyperlipidaemia and xanthomatosis. *J Med Genet* 1968;**5**:9.

31   Slack J, Mills GL. Anomalous low density lipoproteins in familial hyperbetalipoproteinaemia. *Clin Chim Acta* 1970;**29**:15.

32   Frederickson DS, Levy RI. Familial hyperlipoproteinemia: in *The Metabolic Basis of Inherited Disease,* 3rd ed (eds JB Stanbury, JB Wyngaarden, DS Frederickson) McGraw-Hill, New York;1972:545.

33   Slack J. Risks of ischaemic heart-disease in familial hyperlipoproteinaemic states. *Lancet* 1969;**2**:1380.

34   Heiberg A. The risk of atherosclerotic vascular disease in subjects with xanthomatosis. *Acta Med Scand* 1975;**198**:249.

35   Stone NJ, Levy RI, Frederickson DS, Veter J. Coronary artery disease in 116 kindred with familial type II hyperlipoproteinemia. *Circulation* 1974;**49**:476.

36   Brown MS, Goldstein JL. How LDL receptors influence cholesterol and atherosclerosis. *Sci Am* 1984;**251**:58.

37   Brown MS, Goldstein JL. Receptor-mediated endocytosis: insights from the lipoprotein receptor system. *Proc Natl Acad Sci USA* 1979;**76**:3330.

38   Brown MS, Goldstein JL. Receptor-mediated control of cholesterol metabolism. *Science* 1976;**181**:150.

39   Lindgren V, Luskey KL, Russell DW, Francke U. Human genes involved in cholesterol metabolism: chromosomal mapping of the loci for the low density lipoprotein receptor and 3-hydroxy-3-methylglutaryl-coenzyme A reductase with cDNA probes. *Proc Natl Acad Sci USA* 1985;**82**:8567.

40   Slack J. Inheritance of familial hypercholesterolemia. *Atherosclerosis Rev* 1979;**5**:35.

41   Goldstein JL, Brown MS. The LDL pathway in human fibroblasts: a receptor-mediated mechanism for the regulation of cholesterol metabolism. *Curr Top Cell Regul* 1976;**11**:147.

42   Brown MS, Goldstein JL. Familial hypercholesterolemia: defective binding of lipoproteins to cultured fibroblasts associated with impaired regulation of 3-hydroxy-3-methylglutaryl coenzyme A reductase activity. *Proc Natl Acad Sci USA* 1974;**71**:788.

43   Mahley RW, Innerarity TL, Pitas RE, *et al.* Inhibition of lipoprotein binding to cell surface receptors of fibroblasts following selective modification of arginyl residues in arginine-rich and B-apoproteins. *J Biol Chem* 1977;**252**:7279.

44   Schneider WJ, Basu SK, McPhaul MJ, *et al.* Solubilization of the low density lipoprotein receptor. *Proc Natl Acad Sci USA* 1979;**76**:5577.

45   Schneider WJ, Goldstein JL, Brown MS. Partial purification and characterization of the low density lipoprotein receptor from bovine adrenal cortex. *J Biol Chem* 1980;**255**:11442.

46   Schneider WJ, Beisiegel U, Goldstein JL, Brown MS. Purification of the low density lipoprotein receptor an acidic glycoprotein of 164 000 molecular weight. *J Biol Chem* 1982;**257**:2664.

47   Anderson RGW, Goldstein JL, Brown MS. Localization of low density lipoprotein receptors on plasma membrane of normal human fibroblasts and their absence in cells from a familial hypercholesterolemia homozygote. *Proc Natl Acad Sci USA* 1976;**73**:2434.

48   Anderson RGW, Brown MS, Goldstein JL. Role of the coated endocytic vesicle in the uptake of receptor-bound low density lipoprotein in human fibroblasts. *Cell* 1977;**10**:351.

49   Orci L, Carpenter J-L, Perrelet A, *et al.* Occurrence of low density lipoprotein receptors within large pits on the surface of human fibroblasts as demonstrated by freeze-etching. *Exp Cell Res* 1978;**113**:1.

50   Brown MS, Goldstein JL. A general scheme for the regulation of cholesterol metabolism in mammalian cells: in *Disturbances in Lipid and Lipoprotein Metabolism* (eds JM Dietschy, AM Gotto, J Ontko). American Physiological Society, Bethesda MD;1978:173.

51   Goldstein JL, Dana SE, Brown MS. Esterification of low density lipoprotein in human fibroblasts and its absence in homozygous familial hyper-cholesterolemia. *Proc Natl Acad Sci USA* 1974;**71**:4288.

52   Brown MS, Dana SE, Goldstein JL. Regulation of 3-hydroxy-3-methylglutaryl coenzyme A reductase activity in cultured human fibroblasts: comparison of cells from a normal subject and from a patient with homozygous familial hypercholesterolemia. *J Biol Chem* 1974;**24**:789.

53   Brown MS, Goldstein JL. Regulation of the activity of the low density lipoprotein receptor in human fibroblasts. *Cell* 1975;**6**:307.

54   Tolleshaug H, Goldstein JL, Schneider WJ, *et al.* Post-translational processing of the LDL receptor and its genetic disruption in familial hypercholesterolemia. *Cell* 1982;**30**:715.

55   Brown MS, Goldstein JL. A receptor-mediated pathway for cholesterol homeostasis. *Science* 1986;**232**:34.

56   Yamamoto T, Davis CG, Brown MS, *et al.* The human LDL receptor: A cysteine-rich protein with multiple Alu sequences in its Mrna. *Cell* 1984;**39**:27.

57   Hobbs H, Brown MS, Goldstein JL. Molecular genetics of the LDL receptor gene in familial hypercholesterolemia. *Hum Mut* 1992;**1**:445.

58   Hobbs HH, Brown MS, Goldstein JL, Russell DW. Deletion of exon encoding cysteine-rich repeat of LDL receptor alters its binding specificity in a subject with familial hypercholesterolemia. *J Biol Chem* 1986;**261**:13114.

59   Lehrman MA, Russell DW, Goldstein JL, Brown MS. Exon-Alu recombination deletes 5 kilobases from low density lipoprotein receptor gene producing null phenotype in familial hypercholesterolemia. *Proc Natl Acad Sci USA* 1986;**83**:3679.

60 Watanabe Y. Serial inbreeding of rabbits with hereditary hyperlipidemia (WHHL-Rabbit). Incidence and development of atherosclerosis and xanthoma. *Atherosclerosis* 1980;36:261.

61 Yamamoto T, Bishop RW, Brown MS, *et al*. Deletion in cysteine-rich region of LDL receptor impedes transport to cell surface in WHHL rabbit. *Science* 1986;**232**:1230.

62 Lehrman MA, Schneider WJ, Brown MS, *et al*. The Lebanese allele at the LDL receptor locus: nonsense mutation produces truncated receptor that is retained in endoplasmic reticulum. *J Biol Chem* 1987;**262**:401.

63 Lehrman MA, Russell DW, Goldstein JL, Brown MS. Alu-Alu recombination deletes splice acceptor sites and produces secreted LDL receptor in a subject with familial hypercholesterolemia. *J Biol Chem* 1987;**262**:3345.

64 Davis CG, Lehrman MA, Russell DW, *et al*. The JD mutation in familial hypercholesterolemia: substitution of cysteine for tyrosine in cytoplasmic domain impedes internalization of LDL receptors. *Cell* 1986;**45**:15.

65 Kajinami K, Mabuchi H, Inazu A, *et al*. Novel gene mutations at the low density lipoprotein receptor locus: FH-Kanazawa and FH-Okayama. *J Intern Med* 1990;**227**:247.

66 Day INM, Whittall RA, O'Dell SD, *et al*. Spectrum of LDL receptor gene mutations in heterozygous familial hypercholesterolemia. *Hum Mutat* 1997;**10**:116.

67 Leitersdorf E, Tobin EJ, Davignon J, Hobbs HH. Common low-density lipoprotein receptor mutations in the French Canadian population. *J Clin Invest* 1990;**85**:1014.

68 Miyake Y, Tajima S, Funahashi T, Yamamoto A. Analysis of a recycling-impaired mutant of low density lipoprotein receptor in familial hypercholesterolemia. *J Biol Chem* 1989;**264**:16584.

69 Jensen LG, Jensen HK, Nissen H, *et al*. An LDL receptor promoter mutation in a heterozygous FH patient with dramatically skewed ratio between the two allelic mRNA variants. *Hum Mutat* 1996;**7**:82.

70 Koivisto U-M, Palvimo JJ, Janne OA, Kontula K. A single-base substitution in the proximal Sp1 site of the human low density lipoprotein receptor promoter as a cause of heterozygous familial hypercholesterolemia. *Proc Natl Acad Sci USA* 1994;**91**:10526.

71 Sun X-M, Neuwirth C, Wade DP, *et al*. A mutation (T-45C) in the promoter region of the low-density-lipoprotein (LDL)-receptor gene is associated with a mild clinical phenotype in a patient with heterozygous familial hypercholesterolaemia (FH). *Hum Mol Genet* 1995;**4**:2125.

72 Brown MS, Kovanen PT, Goldstein JL, *et al*. Prenatal diagnosis of homozygous familial hypercholesterolaemia: expression of a genetic receptor disease *in utero*. *Lancet* 1978;**1**:526.

73 De Gennes JL, Daffos F, Dairou F, *et al*. Direct fetal blood examination for prenatal diagnosis of homozygous familial hypercholesterolemia. *Arteriosclerosis* 1985;**5**:440.

74 Reshef A, Meiner V, Dann EJ, *et al*. Prenatal diagnosis of familial hypercholesterolemia caused by the 'Lebanese' mutation at the low density lipoprotein receptor locus. *Hum Genet* 1992;**89**:237.

75 Bilheimer DW, Goldstein JL, Grundy SM, *et al*. Liver transplantation to provide low-density-lipoprotein receptors and lower plasma cholesterol in a child with homozygous familial hypercholesterolemia. *N Engl J Med* 1984;**311**:1658.

76 Valdivielso P, Escolar JL, Cuervas-Mons V, *et al*. Lipids and lipoprotein changes after heart and liver transplantation in a patient with homozygous familial hypercholesterolemia. *Ann Intern Med* 1988;**108**:204.

77 Barbir M, Khaghani A, Kehely A, *et al*. Normalisation of lipoproteins including Lp(a) after liver-heart transplantation in homozygous familial hypercholesterolaemia. *Q J Med* 1992;**85**:807.

78 Téllez de Peralta G, Burgos Lázaro R. Transplantes multiorgánicos. *Rev Esp Cardiol* 1995;**48**:46.

79 Thompson GR, Lowenthal R, Myant NB. Plasma exchange in the management of homozygous familial hypercholesterolaemia. *Lancet* 1975;**1**:1208.

80 Gordon BR, Kelsey SF, Dau PC, *et al*. Long-term effects of low-density lipoprotein apheresis using an automated dextran sulfate cellulose adsorption system. *Am J Cardiol* 1998;**81**:407.

81 Tatami R, Inoue N, Itoh H, *et al*. Regression of coronary atherosclerosis by combined LDL-apheresis and lipid-lowering drug therapy in patients with familial hypercholesterolemia: a multicenter study. *Atherosclerosis* 1992;**95**:1.

82 Bilheimer DW, Stone NJ, Grundy SM. Metabolic studies in familial hypercholesterolaemia: evidence for a gene-dosage effect *in vivo*. *J Clin Invest* 1975;**64**:1420.

83 Wilson JM, Chowdury JR. Prospects for gene therapy of familial hypercholesterolemia. *Mol Biol Med* 1990;**7**:223.

84 Grundy SM. Treatment of hypercholesterolemia by interference with bile acid metabolism. *Arch Intern Med* 1972;**130**:638.

85 Endo A, Kuroda M, Tanzawa K. Competitive inhibition of 3-hydroxy-3-methylglutaryl coenzyme A reductase by ML-236A and ML-236B fungal metabolites, having hypocholesterolemic activity. *FEBS Lett* 1976;**72**:323.

86 Alberts AW, MacDonald JS, Till AE, Tobert JA. Lovastatin. *Cardiovasc Drug Rev* 1989;**7**:89.

87 Hoeg JM, Maher MB, Zech LA, *et al*. Effectiveness of mevinolin on plasma lipoprotein concentrations type II hyperlipoproteinemia. *Am J Cardiol* 1986;**57**:933.

88 Malloy MJ, Kane JP, Kunitake ST, Tun P. Complementarity of colestipol, niacin and lovastatin in treatment of severe familial hypercholesterolemia. *Ann Intern Med* 1987;**107**:616.

Mevalonic aciduria

MAJOR PHENOTYPIC EXPRESSION

Failure to thrive; diarrhea and malabsorption; psychomotor retardation; cataracts; retinal dystrophy; hypotonia; hepatosplenomegaly and lymphadenopathy; ataxia; recurrent crises of fever, arthralgia and skin eruption; hyperimmunoglobulin D (IgD); mevalonic aciduria; and defective activity of mevalonic acid kinase.

INTRODUCTION

Mevalonic aciduria was discovered in 1986, the first inborn error in the biosynthesis of cholesterol and nonsterol isoprenoid compounds [1]. It results from a deficiency of the activity of mevalonate kinase (Figures 87.1, 87.2). The disorder is recognized by organic acid analysis of the urine via gas chromatography/mass spectrometry (GCMS). This compound can easily be missed [2].

Mevalonic acid (Figure 87.3) is 3-hydroxy-3-methyl-5-hydroxypentanoic acid. The compound spontaneously cyclizes to form the lactone under the acidic conditions usually employed in liquid partition chromatography, extraction and other forms of preparation for organic acid analysis. The lactone does not open up under conditions of formation of trimethylsilyl (TMS) derivatives. The mono-TMS derivative of the lactone is formed under acid conditions and the tri-TMS derivative of mevalonic acid is formed after treatment

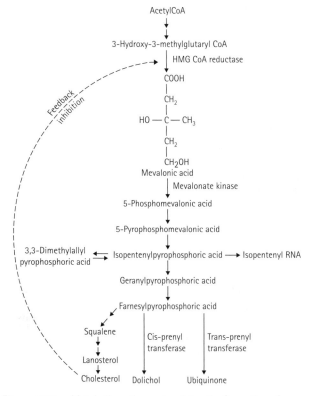

Figure 87.2 *Metabolic pathways involving the formation of mevalonic acid and its role in the synthesis of cholesterol, dolichol and ubiquinone.*

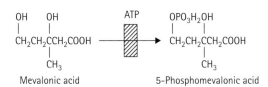

Figure 87.1 *Mevalonate kinase, the site of the defect in mevalonic aciduria.*

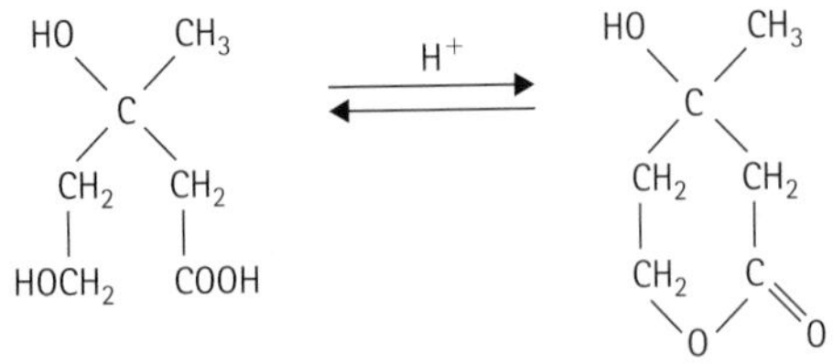

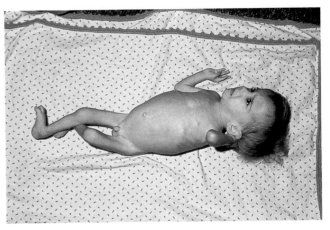

Figure 87.3 *Structure of mevalonic acid and its lactone.*

with alkali. Methylation of the acid followed by formation of the TMS derivative provides the best approach to identification. The development of a stable isotope dilution GCMS assay for mevalonic acid has facilitated quantification of the compound in body fluids [2].

In the mevalonate kinase reaction (Figures 87.1, 87.2) the 5-hydroxy group of 3-R-mevalonic acid is phosphorylated to yield mevalonic-5-phosphate. The cDNA for the human enzyme has been cloned and localized to chromosome 12q24 [3]. A small number of mutations have been defined [3–5].

CLINICAL ABNORMALITIES

Less than 20 patients have been reported [6,7], but varying degrees of clinical severity have been observed, and the spectrum of phenotypes has been enlarged [8–11]. The most severely affected have died in infancy [1,8] or childhood [9]. Less severely impaired patients have had developmental delay, ataxia and hypotonia. Most have had recurrent crises of fever, tender lymphadenopathy, increase in liver and spleen size, arthralgia and a morbilliform eruption. Acute phase reactants, the erythrocyte sedmentation rate, C-reactive protein and leukocytosis, as well as creatine kinase (CK) and transaminases, are elevated. It has recently been recognized that patients with the hyperimmunoglobulin D and periodic fever syndrome (HIDS) have mevalonic aciduria [12,13]. Mutations in the mevalonate kinase gene have been found in patients with HIDS indicating that HIDS is a milder, allelic form of mevalonic aciduria [14,15]. An even milder presentation was observed in a 5-year-old with cerebellar ataxia and retinal dystrophy and no febrile crises or hyperimmunoglobulin D elevation [7].

Our first patient [1] presented with severe failure to thrive, diarrhea and hepatosplenomegaly, a picture that led to referral to gastroenterologists. At 19 months his weight, height and head circumference were 4 to 8 SD below the mean for age. He had little or no subcutaneous fat (Figures 87.4, 87.5). He died at 21 months [6]. Failure to thrive was present in nearly all of the early reported patients: it was described as severe in two [1,16], moderate in five and mild in two [6]. The two most severely affected had gastrointestinal symptoms suggesting intolerance to cows' milk. Hepatosplenomegaly was notable in five patients.

Psychomotor retardation has been characteristic of each of the patients described. It was of such severity in the most

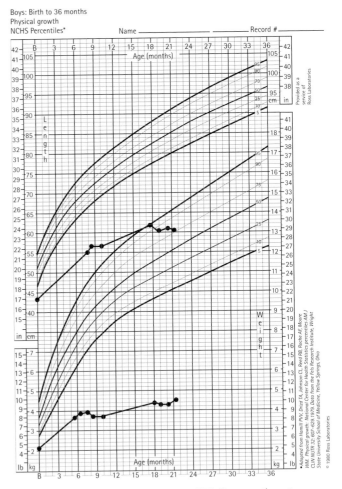

Figure 87.4 *Z.W., a 22-month-old with mevalonic aciduria. He was tiny and had virtually no subcutaneous fat. The penis was very small.*

Figure 87.5 *Anthropometric data on Z.W. illustrate the extreme failure to thrive.*

severely affected patients that no social interaction was possible [1,6,8,9]. Two siblings [16] had IQs of 60 and 65; in two others [6] IQs were 77 and 82, and in the least severe patient [17,18] the IQ was 85. Intellectual impairment has appeared to be nonprogressive. In contrast, ataxia and dysarthria

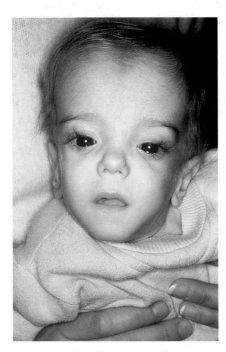

Figure 87.6   *Close-up of the face revealed the prominent forehead and the low-set ears, as well as the long philtrum and thin lips.*

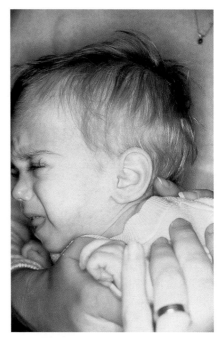

Figure 87.7   *Profile illustrates the dolichocephaly and mild hypognathia. This ear was larger than the other.*

developed after the second year of life in a majority of the patients surviving that long and became progressively more prominent. Imaging of the central nervous system revealed progressive cerebellar atrophy [7]. Deep tendon reflexes may be accentuated, and a crossed response may be elicited. There may be cortical thumbs and incomplete extension at the elbows and knees.

Hypotonia is observed regularly, and some patients have appeared to have myopathy. In one of the least severely affected patients [17] the complete picture was of static myopathy, borderline mental retardation and severe ataxia in a 12-year-old. Myopathy became more severe during febrile crises. One patient developed cardiomyopathy and heart block and required artificial ventilation for two weeks. Two patients had febrile convulsions at 1 and 2 years of age.

Cataracts were observed in a number of patients [11,16]. Two others [6] developed uveitis and retinitis pigmentosa, which became worse with crises. Retinal dystrophy may take the form of bone-spicule retinitis pigmentosa or may be more subtle, thinned vessels and uneven retinal surface and abnormal electroretinogram, and there may be optic atrophy [7].

Dysmorphic features were described in all but a few patients [7,17], but were described as subtle in four [6]. The characteristic picture (Figures 87.6, 87.7) is of dolichocephaly with frontal bossing, posteriorly rotated low-set ears, antimongoloid slanting of the eyes, a small mouth and jaw and thin lips. One patient [1] had a small penis and a congenital hydrocele. In this boy closure of fontanelles and sutures was delayed; by 19 months they were all widely patent. A third fontanelle may be present.

Malabsorption was documented by an increase in quantified stool fat in two patients studied [6]. Biopsies of the duodenum revealed no abnormalities. Bile acids were found to be in normal concentration in serum, urine and feces [6] and studies of the pool size, fractional turnover rates and rates of synthesis of bile acids appeared to be normal [19].

Electroencephalograms were done in eight patients, five of which were normal and three showed generalized slowing. Neuroimaging was most striking for the presence of cerebellar atrophy [6,7]. In one patient, a normal magnetic resonance image (MRI) at 1½ years when he was presymptomatic was followed over the next three years by the parallel development of severe ataxia and cerebellar atrophy. In some patients there was also some cortical atrophy. Neuropathologic examination in one patient confirmed loss of cerebellar mass, including the entire vermis. Histology of the muscle was consistent with atrophy. Myopathy or hypotonia may lead to kyphoscoliosis.

The recurrent crises of fever have been associated with vomiting and diarrhea. Careful search has failed to reveal infectious agents. They occurred up to 25 times per year and averaged four to five days in duration. Four patients died during crises. Some have had arthralgia, subcutaneous edema and a cutaneous eruption during the crisis.

Most patients with HIDS exhibit only the recurrent febrile crises and do not have neurologic abnormalities or dysmorphic features [20]. On the other hand elevated levels of IgD have been found in 100 percent of patients with the classic mevalonic aciduria phenotype [7], and they rise during acute febrile crises [13]; so do the acute phase reactants.

Anemia may be sufficiently severe that a number of blood transfusions are required [8]. Some degree of anemia was present in five of the nine patients on whom this information was available. The serum cholesterol concentration may be normal or slightly reduced. Abnormal levels were reported in four patients, but two of these also had normal levels on occasion [6]. The creatinine kinase levels in plasma were markedly elevated in a majority of patients. Values as high as 3000 and 7520 IU/L have been recorded. The highest levels were in the course of acute crises, but the peak elevation followed the peak of symptoms by 2–4 days. The level of CK was positively correlated with the urinary excretion of mevalonic acid. Transaminases (AST and ALT) were also elevated in a majority of patients. Metabolic acidosis is not a feature of this disease.

GENETICS AND PATHOGENESIS

The disorder is autosomal recessive in nature. Two affected offspring were observed in four families, and the sex distribution has been equal [6]. Furthermore, activity of mevalonate kinase intermediate between patient and control was found in lymphocytes freshly isolated from both the father and mother of patients [1,2]. Prenatal diagnosis of an affected fetus was carried out in a subsequent pregnancy of the index patient by analyzing the amniotic fluid for mevalonic acid. The pregnancy was terminated and the diagnosis confirmed by assay of the enzyme in fetal tissues.

The molecular defect in mevalonic aciduria is in the enzyme mevalonate kinase (Figure 87.1, p. 577). In the usual assay, ^{14}C-labeled mevalonic acid and adenosine triphosphate (ATP) are converted to labeled mevalonate phosphate and pyrophosphate [1,2,21,22]. Control fibroblast lysates displayed a mean activity of 1380 pmol/min/mg protein. Lysates of fibroblasts derived from the patient had activities of 0–4 percent of the control mean. In lymphoblasts, activity in the patients was 1–2 percent of the control mean. The enzyme is also active in freshly isolated lymphocytes and defective activity has been documented in lymphocytes of patients [1]. The level of residual activity has correlated poorly with clinical phenotype; the mildest phenotype reported had 0.4 percent of control activity in fibroblasts [7]. In nine heterozygotes mean activity in lymphoblasts was 47 percent and in seven, activity in fibroblasts was 67 percent of the control mean.

The localization of the gene was more finely defined to 12q24 and narrowed to a 9 cm region [15]. A missense mutation has been identified in the index patient with mevalonic aciduria [3], an A to C change at nucleotide 902 causing a change of asparagine 301 to threonine (N301T). He was a compound of this mutation and another considered to have been inherited from his mother. Two patients in another family with a relatively mild phenotype were homozygous for a G to A change at 1000 yielding a change from alanine 334 to threonine [4,7]. Another patient was homozygous for I268T [5]. The patient with the mildest phenotype [7] was a compound of A334T and 72insT [7]. In patients with HIDS, 4 missense mutations and a 92bp deletion were identified [14,15]. One mutation (V337I) was found in nearly all of the patients studied, usually compound. Enzyme activity was

reduced in all, but not completely deficient. Four novel mutations were found [23] in a cluster: L243I, L264F, L265P and L268T, the last found in a Mennonite family. Bacterial expression assay confirmed the enzyme-deficient nature of these mutations.

In the presence of the metabolic block, mevalonic acid accumulates in body fluids. Quantitative analysis of the urine of 10 patients revealed a massive excretion ranging from 900 to 56 000 mmol/mol creatinine, while normal subjects excrete a mean of 0.16 mmol/mol creatinine. Excretions of 900–1700 mmol/mol creatinine were found in patients with milder disease. Plasma concentrations in patients have ranged from 30 to 540 μmol/L; the control mean was 0.026 μmol/L. Mevalonic acid clearance by the kidney is very efficient and it appears to involve active renal tubular secretion. A patient with a low level of mevalonic aciduria (51–69 mmol/mol creatinine) was found to have a relatively large amount of residual activity of the enzyme [21].

The pathogenesis of the clinical manifestations of mevalonic aciduria is not clear. Mevalonic acid occupies a unique place in intermediary metabolism. It is an important precursor in the biosynthesis of cholesterol and other sterols, dolichol, and ubiquinone, as well as nonsterol isoprenes involved in the formation of membranes, the glycosylation of proteins, the respiratory chain and the replication of DNA [24,25] (Figure 87.2, p. 577). The enzyme is present in peroxisomes as well as the cytosol.

The pathway is regulated via feedback inhibition by cholesterol of the synthesis of mevalonic acid at the 3-hydroxy-3-methylglutaryl-CoA (HMG CoA) reductase step. When cholesterol, which is ingested or derived from plasma low density lipoproteins (LDL), down-regulates HMG CoA reductase, nonsterol isoprenoid synthesis is preserved by inhibition of squalene synthetase and more distal enzymes, further limiting the incorporation of farnesylpyrophosphate into cholesterol. The initial enzymes in the nonsterol branches of the pathway have a very high affinity for farnesylpyrophosphate [24,26].

Provision of exogenous cholesterol was without evident effect on patients, indicating (along with their relatively normal levels of cholesterol) that the clinical disease is not a consequence of a shortage of cholesterol. On the other hand, a direct test of the hypothesis that mevalonic acid itself was toxic, by inhibition of HMG CoA reductase with lovastatin, resulted in a severe clinical crisis with rhabdomyolysis [6]. These observations have focused on the possibility of diminished synthesis of a nonsterol isoprenoid product of the pathway.

Ubiquinone concentrations in plasma were found to be reduced in four of six patients studied. Levels were consistently below the control range, though not very far below. Ubiquinone is important for cardiac and muscular function. Concentrations of leukotirene E4 in the urine of patients were found to be highly elevated [6,27]. Furthermore, in the two patients given lovastatin there was a further 20 percent reduction in ubiquinone.

The recognition that this defect causes HIDS could provide clues as to the pathogenesis of these diseases. Studies of

$2^{14}C$-mevalonate in rats indicated a difference in metabolism in brain and skin where there was formation of labeled fatty acids palmitate and stearate, through a postulated shunt mechanism, from liver where there was no labeling of fatty acids [28]. It has become clear that the elevated levels of leukotrienes and IgD are secondary [7]. In addition the febrile crises appear to diminish with increasing age.

TREATMENT

Effective treatment has not as yet been devised. Trials of supplemental cholesterol, bile acids and inhibitors of HMG CoA reductase have not been therapeutic. Corticosteroid therapy appears to ameliorate acute crises [6] and a trial of long-term intermittent steroid treatment is in progress. Supplementation with ubiquinone may be of interest.

References

1 Hoffmann G, Gibson KM, Brandt IK, et al. Mevalonic aciduria. An inborn error of cholesterol and non-sterol isoprene biosynthesis. N Engl J Med 1986;**314**:1610.

2 Hoffmann GF, Sweetman L, Bremer HJ, et al. Facts and artefacts in mevalonic aciduria: development of a stable isotope dilution GCMS assay for mevalonic acid and its application to physiologic fluids, tissue samples, prenatal diagnosis and carrier detection. Clin Chim Acta 1991;**198**:209.

3 Schafer BL, Bishop RW, Kratunis VJ, et al. Molecular cloning of human mevalonic kinase and identification of a missense mutation in the genetic disease mevalonic aciduria. J Biol Chem 1992;**267**:13229.

4 Hinson DD, Chambliss KL, Hoffmann GF, et al. Identification of an active site alanine in mevalonate kinase through characterization of a novel mutation in mevalonate kinase deficiency. J Biol Chem 1997;**272**:26756.

5 Houten SM, Wanders RJ, Waterham HR. Biochemical and genetic aspects of mevalonate kinase and its deficiency. Biochim Biophys Acta 2000;**1529**:19.

6 Hoffmann GF, Charpentier C, Mayatepek E, et al. Clinical and biochemical phenotype in 11 patients with mevalonic aciduria. Pediatrics 1993;**91**:915.

7 Prietsch V, Mayatepek E, Krastel H, et al. Mevalonate kinase deficiency: Enlarging the clinical and biochemical spectrum. Pediatrics 2003;**111**:258.

8 de Klerk JBC, Duran M, Dorland L, et al. A patient with mevalonic aciduria presenting with hepatosplenomegaly congenital anaemia thrombocytopenia and leukocytosis. J Inherit Metab Dis 1988;**2**:233.

9 Kozich V, Gibson KM, Zeman J, et al. Mevalonic aciduria. J Inherit Metab Dis 1991;**14**:265.

10 Mancini J, Philip N, Chabrol B, et al. Mevalonic aciduria in 3 siblings: A new recognizable metabolic encephalopathy. Pediatr Neurol 1993;**9**:243.

11 Cenedella RJ, Sexton PS. Probing cataractogenesis associated with mevalonic aciduria. Curr Eye Res 1998;**17**:153.

12 Di Rocco M, Caruso U, Waterham HR, et al. Mevalonate kinase deficiency in a child with periodic fever and without hyperimmunoglobinaemia D. J Inherit Metab Dis 2001;**24**:411.

13 Tsimaratos M, Kone-Paut I, Divry P, et al. Mevalonic aciduria and hyper-IgD syndrome: two sides of the same coin? J Inherit Metab Dis 2001;**24**:413.

14 Houten SM, Kuis W, Duran M, et al. Mutations in MVK encoding mevalonate kinase cause hyperimmunoglobulinaemia D and periodic fever syndrome. Nat Genet 1999;**22**:175.

15 Drenth JP, Cuisset L, Grateau G, et al. Mutations in the gene encoding mevalonate kinase cause hyper-IgD and periodic fever syndrome. International Hyper-IgD Study Group. Nat Genet 1999;**22**:178.

16 Divry P, Rolland MO, Zabot MT, et al. Mevalonic kinase deficiency in 2 siblings. Society for the Study of Inborn Errors of Metabolism. Proceedings of the 29th Annual Symposium, London, Sept 1991:146 (abstr).

17 Berger R, Smit GPA, Schierbeek H, et al. Mevalonic aciduria: an inborn error of cholesterol biosynthesis? Clin Chim Acta 1985;**152**:219.

18 Gibson KM, Hoffmann G, Nyhan W, et al. Mevalonate kinase deficiency in a child with cerebellar ataxia, hypotonia and mevalonic aciduria. Eur J Pediatr 1988;**148**:250.

19 Gibson KM, Stellaard F, Hoffmann GF, et al. Bile acid metabolism in three patients with mevalonic aciduria due to mevalonate kinase deficiency. Clin Chim Acta 1993;**217**:217.

20 Drenth JP, Haagsma CJ, van der Meer JW. Hyperimmunoglobulinemia D and periodic fever syndrome. The clinical spectrum in a series of 50 patients. International Hyper-IgD Study Group. Medicine (Baltimore) 1994;**73**:133.

21 Gibson KM, Hoffmann GF, Sweetman L, Buckingham B. Mevalonate kinase deficiency in dizygotic twin with mild mevalonic aciduria. J Inherit Metab Dis 1997;**20**:391.

22 Hoffmann GF, Brendel SU, Scharfschwerdt SR, et al. Mevalonate kinase assay using DEAE-cellulose column chromatography for first-trimester prenatal diagnosis and complementation analysis in mevalonic aciduria. J Inherit Metab Dis 1992;**15**:738.

23 Hinson DD, Ross RM, Krisans S, et al. Identification of a mutation cluster in mevalonate kinase deficiency including a new mutation in a patient of Mennonite ancestry. Am J Hum Genet 1999;**65**:327.

24 Brown MS, Goldstein JL. Multivalent feedback regulation of HMG CoA reductase, a control mechanism coordinating isoprenoid synthesis and cell growth. J Lipid Res 1980;**21**:505.

25 Surani MA, Kimber SJ, Osborn JC. Mevalonate reverses the developmental arrest of preimplantation mouse embryos by Compactin, an inhibitor of HMB CoA reductase. J Embryol Exp Morph 1983;**75**:205.

26 Faust JR, Goldstein JL, Brown MS. Synthesis of ubiquinone and cholesterol in human fibroblasts: regulation of a branched pathway. Arch Biochem Biophys 1979;**192**:86.

27 Frenkel J, Willemsen MA, Weemaes CM, et al. Increased urinary leukotriene E(4) during febrile attacks in the hyperimmunoglobulinaemia D and periodic fever syndrome. Arch Dis Child 2001;**85**:158.

28 Edmond J, Popják G. Transfer of carbon atoms from mevalonate to n-fatty acids. J Biol Chem 1974;**249**:66.

88

Lipoprotein lipase deficiency/type I hyperlipoproteinemia

MAJOR PHENOTYPIC EXPRESSION

Creamy appearance of fasting plasma, episodic abdominal pain, pancreatitis, eruptive xanthomas, lipemia retinalis, hepatosplenomegaly, increased concentration of triglycerides in plasma, hyperchylomicronemia, type I hyperlipoproteinemia and deficient activity of lipoprotein lipase.

INTRODUCTION

Some of the clinical characteristics of familial hyperchylomicronemia were recognized as early as 1932 in the report by Burger and Grutz [1] of an 11-year-old boy, the product of a first-cousin mating, in whom cutaneous xanthomas and hepatosplenomegaly were associated with creamy fasting plasma. Holt and colleagues [2] in 1939 reported two siblings with gross hyperlipemia. The proband had severe attacks of abdominal pain. The defect in lipoprotein lipase in postheparin plasma was defined by Havel and Gordon [3] in 1960 in a study of three siblings with fasting hyperchylomicronemia. The initial patient of Holt *et al.* [2] was followed by Knittle and Ahrens [4] and shown by Frederickson and colleagues [5] to have defective activity of postheparin lipoprotein lipase (EC 3.1.1.3) activity. The enzyme requires a cofactor, apolipoprotein CII, and catalyzes the hydrolysis of the triglycerides of chylomicrons. Deficiency of the apoenzyme or the cofactor can cause clinical lipoprotein lipase deficiency. The gene for lipoprotein in lipase has been mapped to chromosome 8p22 [6], and it contains 10 exons over 30 kb [7]. A number of mutations have been identified.

CLINICAL ABNORMALITIES

The earliest recognition of this disorder is often fortuitous. The lactescence of blood, plasma or serum (Figure 88.1) is observed in a routine sample drawn for some other purpose. In fact, the obtaining of blood samples is so common in developed countries that it is surprising most patients are not recognized in this way. The disorder may be evident as early as 2 days (Figures 88.2–88.5), 8 days [8] and 1 month [9].

At the other extreme, asymptomatic patients have been discovered in the course of screening family members. The blood looks like cream of tomato soup. The characteristic appearance of an excess of chylomicrons in the blood is demonstrated by permitting the plasma to stand 18–24 hours at 4°C (Table 88.1). The chylomicrons appear as a creamy layer on top and the infranatant layer is clear. In types III, IV and V hyperlipoproteinemia both layers are turbid, while in type II the plasma is clear throughout. A supernatant creamy layer is also seen in type V. The convention for these observations and for quantitative studies of lipid concentrations is that blood samples are obtained after a 12–14-hour fast. In addition, the individual should not have gained or lost weight unusually for two weeks previously, received an unusual diet,

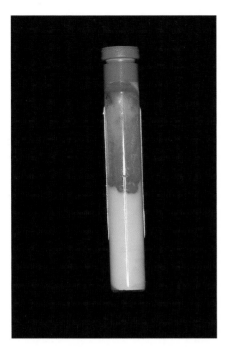

Figure 88.1   *Whole blood of an untreated patient with lipoprotein lipase deficiency. The sample appeared virtually uniformly creamy. With standing for 18 hours or more at 4°C, plasma of these patients displays a layer of cream above and a clear layer below.*

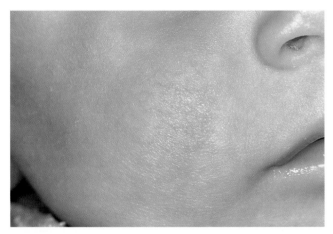

Figure 88.2   *J.L., a 2½-month-old infant with Type I hyperlipoproteinemia. The face at the time of admission revealed a roughened patch on the cheek containing tiny, pearly xanthomata. These disappeared promptly after dietary lowering of triglyceride concentrations. The patient was admitted because of abdomen distension and found to have a hepatic mass, which was removed and was a benign hemangio-endothelioma.*

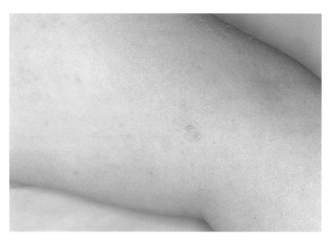

Figure 88.3   *J.L. Two xanthomata that appeared on the leg after poor compliance with diet.*

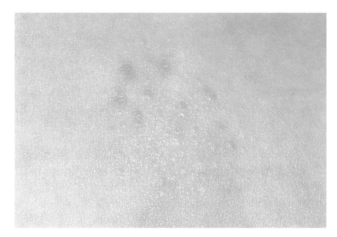

Figure 88.4   *A group of xanthomata on the skin of the same patient.*

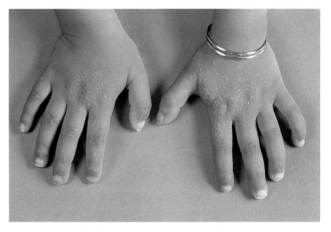

Figure 88.5   *Small but plentiful xanthomata characterize lipoprotein lipase deficiency in this 4-year-old patient with advanced cutaneous disease. Triglycerides ranged from 2000 to 4000 mg/dL.*

or taken any drugs known to affect lipid concentrations. The period of fasting is usually modified in young infants, although our infant withstood a 24-hour fast without hypoglycemia or other complication.

The most common clinical presentation is with acute, recurrent episodes of abdominal pain [10–12]. The age at which this symptomatology begins is quite variable, but it ultimately occurs in virtually all individuals with this disorder. It may occur first in infancy, somewhat later in mid-childhood [11], or not until 20 [9] or 25 years-of-age. Pains may vary from mild apparently infantile colic to severe peritonitis. They may be quite disabling. They are often generalized or mid-epigastric,

Table 88.1 *Lipoprotein patterns characteristic of inherited hyperlipidemias*

Type current designation	Lipoprotein patterns				Appearance of plasma[a]	Lipid concentration		
	Chylomicrons	VLDL	LDL	HDL		Cholesterol	Triglycerides	Chol/Tri ratio
I Hyperchylomicronemia	Increased	N or Sl. ↑	N or ↓	N or ↓	Creamy on top	N or Sl. ↑	↑	<0.2
II Familial hypercholesterolemia	Absent	N (IIa) ↑(IIb)	↑	N	Clear, or slightly turbid	↑	N	>1.5
III 'Broad' or 'floating beta' disease	Absent	B-VLDL[b]	Abn.[b]	N	Turbid, or faint layer of cream	↑	↑	Variable; May = 1
IV Familial hyper-pre-β-lipoproteinemia	Absent	↑	N	N	Turbid, no layer of cream	↑ or N		Variable
V Familial hyper-pre-β-lipoproteinemia and hyperchylomicronemia	Increased	↑	N	N	Creamy on top, turbid below	↑		0.15–0.6

a. After standing for 18–24 hours at 4°C.
b. LDL of abnormal lipid composition.
Abbreviations include: HDL, high density lipoprotein; LDL, low density lipoprotein; VLDL, very low density lipoprotein, Abn, abnormal; N, normal; Sl, slightly.

but may be localized, especially to the right or left upper quadrant. Narcotic dependence has been observed. Pain may be associated with spasm, rigidity or rebound tenderness. There may also be fever and leukocytosis, and this presentation has led to surgical intervention. Usually a milky exudate in the peritoneal cavity is the only finding. The viscera may appear pale or fatty. Pains may be accompanied by anorexia and abdominal distension, or by vomiting, or diarrhea [13].

Acute attacks are always associated with hyperlipemia. In a patient being successfully managed they may follow dietary indiscretion or noncompliance. They are especially likely to follow the resumption of a normal diet in an individual who had reduced triglyceride levels by dietary restriction. They may also follow intercurrent infection, and attacks have been related to alcohol. Pregnancy may severely exacerbate symptoms [9] and so may oral contraceptive agents. Many patients learn to regulate their dietary intake of fat in a manner sufficient to eliminate the occurrence of abdominal pains [11].

Acute pancreatitis is a well recognized complication of hyperchylomicronemia [9,14,15]. This may cause severe abdominal pain radiating to the back or shoulders and prostration, hypotension, sweating and shock. It may lead to complete pancreatic necrosis, but does not lead to calcification. Pancreatitis may be fatal [9]. Necrotizing pancreatitis may be recognized at surgery [14], and pancreatic pseudocysts may be found [9], as well as extensive mesenteric fat necrosis and multiple adhesions. The serum amylase level may be very high. On the other hand, the diagnosis of pancreatitis in these patients may be complicated by the fact that the turbid plasma of the patient with hyperchylomicronemia may interfere with the determination of amylase activity in the serum [16,17]. Normal amylase values have been observed in patients documented at laparotomy to have pancreatitis [18].

These problems may be overcome by serial dilution of the serum if the lactescence is recognized and a true elevation demonstrated [16], or probably better by examination of amylase in the urine, especially the amylase/creatinine clearance

ratio [17]. Pancreatitis has been clearly related to the presence of hyperlipemia [2,14], and dietary reduction of serum triglyceride levels is successful in preventing further attacks. In fact, attacks of pancreatitis appear to occur only when serum concentrations of triglycerides exceed 1000 mg/dL [15], and morbidity and mortality are rare when levels are under 2000 mg/dL [18]. The association between hyperchylomicronemia and pancreatitis is so close that patients with diagnosed pancreatitis or recurrent abdominal pain should be screened for hyperlipemia. In 45 patients with acute pancreatitis examined prospectively, 10 were found to have hyperlipoproteinemia [15]. Certainly, infants and children with pancreatitis and patients with familial pancreatitis should be examined for hyperchylomicronemia.

Hepatosplenomegaly is the rule in type I hyperlipoproteinemia [19]. It may be particularly prominent in infants and children. It is clearly related to fat intake, and the size of these organs can decrease within 24 to 48 hours of the initiation of the fat-free diet. Generally, some enlargement remains even with long-term dietary management. Occasionally, pains have been related to the spleen, and the spleen may be quite hard. It also recedes in size with reduction in the intake of fat. Fat embolism may occur in hyperlipemic individuals, and a variety of complications such as seizures, transient paralysis or gastrointestinal hemorrhage have been attributed to such aggregations of chylomicrons. In one patient what appeared to be splenic infarcts were seen on angiography, but at surgery the patient had pancreatitis and the removed spleen contained foam cells, but no infarcts [20]. Foam cells have been observed on needle biopsy of the liver [14] representing storage of lipid in macrophages and Kupffer cells.

Among early manifestations in 14 infants with the onset of symptoms prior to 1 year-of-age were irritability in seven, lower intestinal bleeding in two, splenomegaly in one, pallor or anemia in four [21]. In this series one additional patient came to light because of a positive family history, and another was discovered fortuitously. The intestinal bleeding stopped

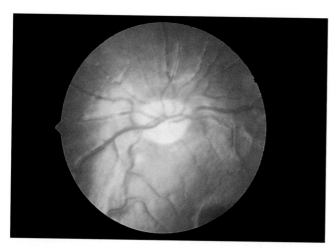

Figure 88.6   *Lipemia retinalis in a patient with lipoprotein lipase deficiency.*

with institution of a low fat diet. Each patient had lactescent plasma at presentation.

Cutaneous eruptive xanthomas (Figures 88.3–88.5) have been observed in about 50 percent of patients with type I hyperlipoproteinemia [19]. They cluster preferentially over the buttocks, proximal portions of the extremities and extensor surfaces, but they may occur anywhere, including the skin of the face. Lesions have been seen on the mucous membranes, including the hard palate and tonsils or fauces. They appear as nodules 1–5 mm in diameter. They may be yellow or have a yellow center, but they may not. They may be erythematous; they tend to be flat. They may coalesce to form larger plaques. However, patients with this disease do not develop tendinous, tuberous or planar xanthomas, or xanthelasma. The lesions are usually neither painful nor pruritic. They may occur within days of the elevation of plasma triglyceride levels over 2000 mg/dL and have been described as early as the first weeks of life [12]. They may fade rapidly on dietary reduction of these levels, but complete disappearance may take as long as three weeks. Histologically, these are chylomicrons filling macrophages [22].

Lipemia retinalis (Figure 88.6) is seen occasionally, but is characteristic of long-standing hyperlipemia. The entire fundus may have a pale or salmon cast, and there may be an increased light reflex over the vessels. The arteries and veins may appear milky-white. There may rarely be white deposits of lipid in the retina; and disturbances of circulation such as microaneurysms and hemorrhages have been reported [23,24].

It is of interest that patients with type I hyperlipoproteinemia do not appear to be at risk for premature atherosclerotic disease. The numbers of autopsied patients have been small, but none have had appreciable atherosclerotic change at ages ranging from 24 to 42 years-of-age [9]. Certainly, there has been no clinical evidence of coronary artery disease or cerebral vascular disease.

Some patients have been anemic [21], and one patient has been reported with persistent thrombocytopenia, leukopenia

and occasional anemia [25]. Bruising has been reported in another [26]. One patient [2] had chronic leg ulcers. A group of five patients has been reported with an unusual problem of intermittent swelling of the scrotum, and swelling, along with blueness or mottling, of the legs [11]. Surgical exploration of the scrotum revealed a milky effusion in the tunica vaginalis.

These patients, unlike those with many forms of hypertriglyceridemia, do not have abnormal glucose tolerance curves, and they do not have hyperuricemia. Secondary diabetes or pancreatic exocrine insufficiency may develop after many attacks of pancreatitis.

The very high plasma lipid may produce artefactual lowering of the values of many plasma solutes, determined in the routine clinical chemistry laboratory. The degree of error is approximately one percent for each 0.9 g triglyceride/dL [27]. Thus, in a patient with triglyceride of 10 000 mg/dL, an 11 percent reduction would yield a sodium concentration value of 129 mEq/L for a true sodium concentration of 145 mEq/L in fat-free plasma water. The importance of recognizing this issue is that such patients should not be treated for hyponatremia. On the other hand lipemia may spuriously elevate levels of hemoglobin and bilirubin [28].

GENETICS AND PATHOGENESIS

Lipoprotein lipase deficiency is autosomal recessive in inheritance. Occurrence in a number of siblings has been reported [2], as has consanguinity [8]. Lipoprotein lipase activity of about 50 percent of normal has been reported in adipose tissue of parents of patients with deficiency [29]. Low levels of a lipolytic activity have also been observed in postheparin plasma of relatives [30], but heterozygosity cannot always be demonstrated by assay of the plasma [12]. Heterozygotes may have hypertriglyceridemia [29], but fasting levels of triglycerides are usually normal [29,31]. In fact, it has been demonstrated by careful study of an extended pedigree [12] that hypertriglyceridemia of many genetic and other causes is so common in adults that the finding of an elevated concentration of triglycerides in a parent or relative cannot be equated with heterozygosity for lipoprotein lipase deficiency.

Analysis of the lipids of the plasma in patients reveals markedly elevated concentrations of triglycerides. In the untreated patient, levels usually range from 1000 to 4000 mg/dL but may be as high as 15 000 mg/dL [27]. Triglycerides constitute 80–95 percent of chylomicrons. Concentrations of cholesterol are normal or moderately elevated. It is only when the triglycerides are very high that the cholesterol rises; the ratio of the cholesterol to triglyceride is always less than 0.2 in type I hyperlipoproteinemia, and often less than 0.1.

Lipoprotein electrophoresis yields a characteristic chylomicron band at the origin. The type I pattern can be demonstrated by electrophoresis or ultracentrifugation as consisting exclusively, or nearly so, of chylomicrons (Table 88.1). The very low density lipoproteins (VLDL) are normal or slightly increased and the LDL and HDL are usually depressed. Treatment with a low fat, high carbohydrate diet usually leads, as chylomicrons fall, to an increase toward normal of LDL and increased levels of VLDL, but those of HDL remain low. The diagnosis of type I hyperlipoproteinemia is often confirmed by the elimination of fat from the diet, after which the chylomicrons disappear from the blood within a few days and triglyceride concentrations fall to 200–400 mg/dL. Most pediatric patients with hyperchylomicronemia have type I hyperlipoproteinemia. Most patients with type V are adults. However, childhood type V hyperlipoproteinemia has been reported [32], and patients with classic lipoprotein lipase deficiency sometimes have a type V pattern with time. Incubation of plasma in three percent polyvinylpyrrolidone will separate chylomicrons from other lipoproteins and is thus useful for the diagnosis of hyperchylomicronemia.

The definitive diagnosis of the classic type I disease requires demonstration of the molecular defect in the activity of the enzyme lipoprotein lipase [33–35]. This enzyme catalyzes the hydrolysis of glycerolester bonds in circulating triglycerides at the vascular endothelial surface in tissues, especially adipose. The enzyme is released by the intravenous administration of 60–100 units/kg heparin and is assayed in plasma obtained 10–15 minutes later. The enzyme requires the specific plasma cofactor, apoprotein C-II. It is inhibited by protamine. Concentrations of enzyme in patients are usually less than 10 percent of control levels and may approximate zero. Heparin was originally observed [36,37] to clear postprandial lipemia in dogs. *In vitro* addition to plasma does not reproduce this effect; injection *in vivo* releases the lipase.

Defective activity of the enzyme may be documented in postheparin plasma or in adipose tissue. Heparin also releases hepatic lipase into plasma. This enzyme has little activity against chylomicrons, and so it created no problem in the original assay of Havel and Gordon [3], but most modern assays are done with artificial emulsions of triglycerides. Selective assay requires inhibition of the lipoprotein lipase with protamine or concentrated saline and calculating the difference from total lipolytic activity [38], inhibition of the hepatic lipase by specific antiserum [31], or chromatographic separation of two enzymes [39]. In classic lipoprotein lipase deficiency, patients have marked triglyceridemia and virtually always have clinical symptoms before puberty, and they have defective enzyme activity in every tissue studied [40]. The enzyme may be measured in adipose tissue obtained by needle aspiration, which is of advantage because it does not contain hepatic lipase, but the assay must be done immediately thereafter. In patients with classic deficiency the activity in adipose tissue is defective whether the patient is in the fed or fasted state [41].

Some individuals have been observed in whom there was a partial deficiency of the enzyme [40]. A form of familial dominantly inherited hyperchylomicronemia has been reported in which there was a circulating inhibitor of lipoprotein lipase activity [42]. Another patient has been described [43] in whom a transient deficiency of lipoprotein lipase led to an attack of acute pancreatitis.

The enzyme is a homodimeric glycoprotein with identical 60 kDa subunits [44]. In many patients with deficient enzyme activity an immunochemically detectable protein is present, but a few patients have had no lipase protein [45]. The first of these was in a patient with no enzyme activity or cross-reactive material who had a 6 kb deletion involving exons 3 to 5 on one allele and a 2 kb deletion in exon 6 on the other [46,47]. No mRNA could be found in adipose tissue.

The cDNA for the human enzyme codes for a mature protein of 448 amino acids. There is alternate splicing in adipose tissue, which produces two mRNAs [48,49]. The mRNA is found in muscle, kidney, adrenal, intestine and neonatal liver, as well as adipose tissues, but it is not found in adult liver.

Since the patient with the 6 kb deletion a number of mutations have been identified, a majority of them missense [50–52], but coding for very reduced or absent enzyme activity. A point mutation in exon 5 was found to account for the majority of alleles in the French-Canadian population, where prevalence is the highest in the world [53,54]. A C-to-T transition at nucleotide 875 led to a change from proline 207 to leucine. Dot blot analysis is available. Missense mutations have been found in 28 instances. Stop-codons have been produced by five single-base changes. A 3 kb deletion in exon 9 has been reported [55] and two splice site defects have occurred in intron 2 [56,57]. The majority of missense mutations have been in exon 5, and in exons 4 and 6, areas of considerable homology among lipases. Some mutations have converted hydrophobic residues to less hydrophobic amino acids.

Phenotypic expression in heterozygotes was reported [58] in a pedigree of a proband homozygous for a mutation, G to A at position 818 leading to a glycine 188 to glutamic acid substitution which resulted in an immunoreactive but nonfunctional enzyme. Heterozygotes had increased plasma triglyceride, VLDL cholesterol and apolipoprotein B and decreased LDL and HDL cholesterol, clearly distinguished from noncarriers only after 40 years-of-age.

Differential diagnosis – apolipoprotein

C-II DEFICIENCY

A distinct molecular abnormality in the lipoprotein lipase enzyme complex has been defined as a deficiency in the apolipoprotein C-II activator of the complex [59–65]. These patients tend to present clinically later than those with classic lipoprotein lipase deficiency, in post-adolescence or adult life. The nature of the defect was suggested in the first patient who had displayed hyperlipemia and no activity of lipoprotein lipase, when the concentration of triglycerides fell sharply following a transfusion of blood for anemia. It was demonstrated that his plasma completely lacked apo C-II.

Patients with this disorder have had abdominal pains and pancreatitis. None have been described with xanthomas or hepatomegaly [62]. A few have had splenomegaly, and about half have had anemia. The pattern of hyperchylomicronemia is the same as in classic lipoprotein lipase deficiency [61]. The deficiency has most often been documented by the assay of lipoprotein lipase in the presence and absence of apo C-II or normal plasma. It can be assayed directly by electrophoresis of the tetramethylurea-soluble apoproteins on polyacrylamide gel.

The two molecularly defined genetic disorders, apo C-II deficiency and lipoprotein lipase deficiency, are rare. The most common causes of milky plasma are acquired and they are secondary to such disorders as diabetes, nephrosis or alcoholism. Some have been associated with systemic lupus erythematosus, malignant histiocytosis or lymphoma. In addition, there are clearly familial examples of hypertriglyceridemia and patients with typical symptomatic type I hyperlipoproteinemia [13] in whom no molecular defect can be defined. Of 123 patients studied for hypertriglyceridemia, 110 were acquired, and eight fell into this latter category [33]. Only five had an abnormality in lipoprotein lipase, and these studies were done in the laboratory most of us rely on for assays for lipoprotein lipase.

In apo C-II deficiency, biochemical data are consistent with pedigree information and an autosomal recessive mode of transmission [63]. The gene for apo C-II has been mapped to chromosome 19 [64] and contains four exons spanning 3.3 kb [66]. Patients to date have been homozygous for a single mutation and are often products of a consanguinous mating. The nature of mutation has been defined in many of the small number of kindreds so far described [51]. In four, single-base change has led to a stop-codon [66–71], and in one there was a single-base substitution in the methionine initiation codon [71]. A donor splice mutation intron 2 [72] rounds out this group, none of whom had demonstrable apo C-II protein on immunoassay. Four frame shift mutations would be expected to lead to truncated proteins; two of them had no detectable protein [73–78].

TREATMENT

The dietary restriction of the intake of fat has a dramatic effect in clearing hyperchylomicronemia and the avoidance of all of the manifestations of the disease. The argument for treatment is the substantial morbidity and mortality from pancreatitis. This should be eliminated along with the abdominal pains if concentrations of triglycerides are kept below 2000 mg/dL [79]. Most recommendations [27] are to keep levels below 1000 or even 750 mg/dL. It is generally agreed that symptoms will not occur at these levels. Both saturated and unsaturated fats must be restricted. Overall restriction should be to less than 15 percent of the calories from fats. In adults, diets containing less than 50 g of fat a day are usually sufficient. A value of 0.5 g/kg is useful in initiating therapy in children. An exception to restriction of fats is medium-chain triglycerides, which do not contribute to chylomicrons [80]. Diets extremely low in fat are well tolerated and consistent with normal growth and development (Figure 88.7).

Triglyceride levels should be studied throughout the day, not simply after an overnight fast. The regimen should ensure

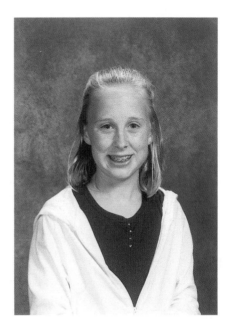

Figure 88.7 *L.S., a 12-year-old girl with lipoprotein lipase deficiency. She had had episodes of pancreatitis, but she was well despite a lifelong severe restriction of the intake of fat.*

compliance around the clock. No single meal should contain more than 20 g of fat. At the same time, deficiency of essential fatty acids must be avoided. The management of an infant or child with type I hyperlipoproteinemia can be very difficult. Triglyceride levels may rise suddenly from a few hundred to several thousand mg/dL following a single fat-filled meal [3]. Agents known to increase concentrations of triglycerides, include alcohol, estrogens, diuretics, isotretinoin, Zoloft and β-adrenergic blockers. Extreme dietary fat restriction during pregnancy has resulted in normal offspring.

Management of the acute abdominal pain requires vigilance about the diagnosis of pancreatitis and recognition that amylase values may be normal. The treatment of pancreatitis should follow the usual conservative regimen, with the additional precept that fat should be eliminated. In a neonate with chylomicronemia and congestive cardiac failure, triglyceride levels of 38 000 mg/dL were reduced to normal by plasmapheresis, and cardiac function became normal [81]. The treatment of apo C-II deficiency should generally be the same as that of lipoprotein lipase deficiency. An episode of pancreatitis may be successfully treated in apo C-II deficiency by the infusion of normal human plasma.

References

1 Burger M, Grutz O. Uber Hepatosplenomegale Lipoidose mit Xanthomatosen Veranderungen in Haut und Schleimhaut. *Arch Dermatol Syph* 1932;**166**:542.

2 Holt LE Jr, Aylward FX, Timbres HG. Idiopathic familial lipemia. *Bull Johns Hopkins Hosp* 1939;**64**:279.

3 Havel RJ, Gordon RS Jr. Idiopathic hyperlipemia: metabolic studies in an affected family. *J Clin Invest* 1960;**39**:1777.

4   Knittle JL, Ahrens EH Jr. Carbohydrate metabolism in two forms of hyperglyceridemia. *J Clin Invest* 1964;**43**:485.

5   Fredrickson DS, Ono K, David LL. Lipolytic activity of postheparin plasma in hyperglyceridemia. *J Lipid Res* 1963;**4**:24.

6   Sparks RS, Zollner S, Klisak I, *et al.* Human genes involved in lipolysis of plasma lipoproteins: mapping of loci for lipoprotein lipase to 8p22 and hepatic lipase to 15q21. *Genomics* 1987;**1**:138.

7   Deeb SS, Peng R. Structure of the human lipoprotein lipase gene. *Biochemistry* 1989;**28**:4131.

8   Sadan N, Drucker MM, Arger I, *et al.* Type I hyperlipoproteinemia in an 8-day-old infant. *J Pediatr* 1977;**90**:775.

9   De Gennes JL, Menage JJ, Truffert MJ. Hyperglyceridemie exogene (hyperchylomicronemie) essentielle de type I: etude clinique et évolutive de cinq observations. *Nour Presse Med* 1972;**1**:1835.

10 Bloomfield AL, Shenson B. The syndrome of idiopathic hyperlipemia with crises of violent abdominal pain. *Stanford Med Bull* 1947;**5**:185.

11 Deckelbaum RJ, Dupont C, LeTarte J, Pencharz P. Primary hypertriglyceridemia in childhood. *Am J Dis Child* 1983;**137**:396.

12 Wilson DA, Edwards CO, Chan IF. Phenotypic heterogeneity in the extended pedigree of a proband with lipoprotein lipase deficiency. *Metabolism* 1983;**32**:1107.

13 Burton BK, Nadler HL. Primary type I hyperlipoproteinemia with normal lipoprotein lipase activity. *J Pediatr* 1977;**90**:777.

14 Klatskin G, Gordon M. Relationship between relapsing pancreatitis and essential hyperlipemia. *Am J Med* 1952;**12**:3.

15 Farmer RG, Winkelman EI, Brown HB, Lewis LA. Hyperlipoproteinemia and pancreatitis. *Am J Med* 1973;**54**:161.

16 Fallat RW, Vester JW, Glueck CJ. Suppression of amylase activity by hypertriglyceridemia. *JAMA* 1973;**224**:1331.

17 Lesser PB, Warshaw AL. Diagnosis of pancreatitis masked by hyperlipemia. *Ann Intern Med* 1975;**82**:795.

18 Brunzell JD, Schrott HG. The interaction of familial and secondary causes of hypertriglyceridemia: role in pancreatitis. *Trans Assoc Am Physicians* 1973;**86**:245.

19 Lees RS, Wilson DE, Schonfeld G, Fleet S. The familial dyslipoproteinemias: in *Progress in Medical Genetics.* Vol 9. (eds AG Steinberg, AG Bearn) Grune and Stratton, New York;1973:237.

20 Ferrans VJ, Roberts WC, Levy RI, Fredrickson DS. Chylomicrons and the formation of foam cells in type I hyperlipoproteinemia. A morphologic study. *Am J Pathol* 1973;**70**:253.

21 Feoli-Fonseca JC, Levy E, Godard M, Lambert M. Familial lipoprotein lipase deficiency in infancy: clinical biochemical and molecular study. *J Pediatr* 1998;**133**:417.

22 Parker F, Bagdade JD, Odland GF, Bierman EL. Evidence for the chylomicron origin of lipids accumulating in diabetic eruptive xanthomas: a correlative lipid biochemical histochemical and electron microscopic study. *J Clin Invest* 1970;**49**:2172.

23 Moreau PG, Pichon P, Rifle G. Manifestations chorioretiniennes des hyperlipidemies. La retinopathie hyperlipidemique a propos de 44 observations. *Sem Hop* 1970;**46**:3467.

24 Henkens HE, Houtsmuller AJ, Bos PJM, Crone RA. Fundus changes in primary hyperlipaemia. *Ophthalmologica* 1976;**173**:190.

25 Romics L. Hypertriglyceridemia associated with thrombocytopenia and lipoprotein lipase deficiency. *Ann Intern Med* 1981;**95**:660.

26 Potter JM, MacDonald WB. Primary type I hyperlipoproteinaemia – a metabolic and family study. *Aust NZ J Med* 1979;**9**:688.

27 Brown WV, Baginsky ML, Ehnholm C. Primary type I and type V hyperlipoproteinaemia: in *Hyperlipidemia: Diagnosis and Therapy* (eds BM Rifkind, RI Levy). Grune and Stratton, New York;1977:93.

28 Shah PC, Patel AR, Rao KR. Hyperlipemia and spuriously elevated hemoglobin levels. *Ann Intern Med* 1975;**82**:382.

29 Harlan WR Jr, Winesett PS, Wasserman AJ. Tissue lipoprotein lipase in normal individuals and in individuals with exogenous hypertriglyceridemia and the relationship of this enzyme to assimilation of fat. *J Clin Invest* 1967;**46**:239.

30 Tohshin G, Ohkubo H, Mochizuki Y, *et al.* Primary type I hyperlipoproteinemia: significance of lipoprotein lipase and hepatic triglyceride lipase activity in heterozygotes of patients with familial lipoprotein lipase deficiency. *J Pediatr* 1983;**102**:405.

31 Huttunen JK, Ehnholm C, Kinnunen PKJ, Nikkila EA. An immunochemical method for selective measurement of two triglyceride lipases in human postheparin plasma. *Clin Chim Acta* 1975;**63**:335.

32 Kwiterovich PO, Farah JR, Brown WV, *et al.* The clinical biochemical and familial presentation of type V hyperlipoproteinemia in childhood. *Pediatrics* 1977;**59**:513.

33 Brunzel JD, Bierman EL. Chylomicronemia syndrome. Interaction of genetic and acquired hypertriglyceridemia. *Med Clin N Am* 1982;**66**:455.

34 Nilsson-Ehle P. Measurements of lipoprotein lipase activity: in *Lipoprotein Lipase* (ed. Borensztajn J). Evener Publishers, Chicago;1987:59.

35 Iverius P-H, Ostlund-Lindqvist A-M. Preparation characterization and measurement of lipoprotein lipase. *Methods Enzymol* 1986;**129**:691.

36 Hahn PF. Abolishment of alimentary lipemia following injection of heparin. *Science* 1943;**98**:19.

37 Eckel RH. Lipoprotein lipase: A multifunctional enzyme relevant to common metabolic diseases. *N Engl J Med* 1989;**320**:1060. Erratum: *N Engl J Med* 1990;**322**:477.

38 Ehnholm C, Shaw W, Greten H, Brown WV. Purification from human plasma of a heparin-released lipase with activity against triglyceride and phospholipids. *J Biol Chem* 1975;**250**:6756.

39 Boberg J, Augustin J, Baginsky ML, *et al.* Quantitative determination of hepatic and lipoprotein lipase activities from human postheparin plasma. *J Lipid Res* 1977;**18**:544.

40 Brunzell JD, Chait A, Nikkila EA, *et al.* Heterogeneity of primary lipoprotein lipase deficiency. *Metabolism* 1980;**29**:624.

41 Goldberg AP, Chait A, Brunzell JD. Postprandial adipose tissue lipoprotein lipase activity in primary hypertriglyceridemia. *Metabolism* 1980;**29**:223.

42 Brunzell JD, Miller NE, Alaupovic P, *et al.* Familial chylomicronemia due to a circulating inhibitor of lipoprotein lipase activity. *J Lipid Res* 1983;**24**:12.

43 Goldberg IJ, Paterniti JR Jr, Franklin BH, *et al.* Transient lipoprotein lipase deficiency with hyperchylomicronemia. *Am J Med Sci* 1983;**286**:28.

44 Olivecrona T, Bengtsson G, Osborne JC Jr. Molecular properties of lipoprotein lipase: effects of limited trypsin digestion on molecular weight and secondary structure. *Eur J Biochem* 1982;**124**:629.

45 Brunzell JD, Iverius P-H, Scheibel MS, *et al.* Primary lipoprotein lipase deficiency: in *Lipoprotein Deficiency Syndromes* (eds A Angel, J Frohlich). Plenum Press, New York;1986:227.

46 Langlois S, Deeb S, Brunzell JD, *et al.* A major insertion accounts for a significant proportion of mutations underlying human lipoprotein lipase deficiency. *Proc Natl Acad Sci USA* 1989;**86**:948.

47 Devlin RH, Deeb SS, Brunzell JD, Hayden MR. Partial gene duplication involving exon-Alu interchange results in lipoprotein lipase deficiency. *Am J Hum Genet* 1990;**46**:112.

48 Enerback S, Bjursell G. Genomic organization of the region encoding guinea pig lipoprotein lipase; evidence for exon fusion and unconventional splicing. *Gene* 1989;**84**:391.

49 Kirchgessner TG, Chaut JC, Heinzman C, *et al.* Organization of the human lipoprotein gene and evolution of the lipase family. *Proc Natl Acad Sci USA* 1989;**86**:9647.

50 Stenson PD, Ball EV, Mort M, *et al.* Human Gene Mutation Database (HGMD). *Hum Mutat* 2003;**21**:577. Web site: http://archive.uwcm.ac.uk/ uwcm/mg/ hgmd0.html (accessed December 2004)

51 Santamarina-Fojo S. Genetic dyslipoproteinemias: Role of lipoprotein lipase and apolipoprotein C-II. *Curr Opin Lipido* 1992;**3**:186.

52 Henderson H, Ma Y, Kastelein J, *et al*. Identification of the molecular defects underlying chylomicronemia in the majority of 75 separate probands with LPL deficiency. *Clin Res* 1991;**39**:336A (abstr).

53 Bernstein R, Bocian M, Bengtsson U, Wasmuth J. Clinical application of fluorescent *in situ* hybridization techniques. *Clin Res* 1991;**39**:96A.

54 Ma Y, Henderson HE, Ven Murthy MR, *et al*. A mutation in the human lipoprotein lipase gene as the most common cause of familial chylomicronemia in French Canadians. *N Engl J Med* 1991;**324**:1761.

55 Benlian P, Loux N, De Gennes JL, *et al*. A homozygous deletion of exon 9 in the lipoprotein lipase gene causes type I hyperlipoproteinemia. *Arteriosclerosis* 1991;**11**:1465.

56 Gotoda T, Yamada N, Murase T, *et al*. Occurrence of multiple aberrantly spliced mRNAs upon a donor splice site mutation that causes familial lipoprotein lipase deficiency. *J Biol Chem* 1991;**266**:24757.

57 Hata A, Emi M, Luc G, *et al*. Compound heterozygote for lipoprotein lipase deficiency: Ser®Thr244 and transition in 3 splice site of intron 2(AG®AA) in the lipoprotein lipase gene. *Am J Hum Genet* 1990;**47**:721.

58 Wilson DE, Emi M, Iverius P-H, *et al*. Phenotypic expression of heterozygous lipoprotein lipase deficiency in the extended pedigree of a proband homozygous for a missense mutation. *J Clin Invest* 1990;**86**:735.

59 Breckenridge WC, Little JA, Steiner G, *et al*. Hypertriglyceridemia associated with deficiency of apolipo-protein C-II. *N Engl J Med* 1978;**298**:1265.

60 Stalenhoef AFH, Casparie AF, Demacker PNM, *et al*. Combined deficiency of apolipoprotein C-II and lipoprotein lipase in familial hyperchylomicronemia. *Metabolism* 1981;**30**:919.

61 Fellin R, Baggion G, Poli A, *et al*. Familial lipoprotein lipase and apolipoprotein C-II deficiency. Lipoprotein and apoprotein analysis, adipose tissue and hepatic lipoprotein lipase levels in seven patients and their first degree relatives. *Atherosclerosis* 1983;**49**:55.

62 Little JA, Cox D, Breckenridge WC, McGuire VM. Introduction to deficiencies of apolipoproteins CII and EIII with some associated clinical findings: in *Atherosclerosis V* (eds AM Gotto Jr, LC Smith, B Allen). Springer-Verlag, New York;1980: 671.

63 Miller NE, Rao SN, Alaupovic P, *et al*. Familial apolipoprotein C II deficiency: plasma lipoproteins and apolipoproteins in heterozygous and homozygous subjects and the effects of plasma infusion. *Eur J Clin Invest* 1981;**11**:69.

64 Humphries SE, Berg K, Gill L, *et al*. The gene for apolipoprotein C-II is closely linked to the gene for apolipoprotein E on chromosome 19. *Clin Genet* 1984;**26**:389.

65 Fellin R, Baggio G, Poli A, *et al*. Familial lipoprotein lipase and apolipoprotein C-II deficiency: lipoprotein and apoprotein analysis, adipose tissue and hepatic lipoprotein lipase levels in seven patients and their first degree relatives. *Atherosclerosis* 1983;**49**:55.

66 Wei C-F, Tsao Y-K, Robberson DL, *et al*. The structure of the human apolipoprotein C-II gene: electron microscopic analysis of RNA:DNA hybrids complete nucleotide sequence and identification of 5′ homologous sequences among lipoprotein genes. *J Biol Chem* 1985;**260**:15211.

67 Baggio G, Manzato E, Gabelli C, *et al*. Apolipoprotein C-II deficiency syndrome: clinical features lipoprotein characterization lipase activity and correction of hypertriglyceridemia after apo lipoprotein C-II administration in two affected patients. *J Clin Invest* 1986;**77**:520.

68 Crepaldi G, Fellin R, Baggio G, *et al*. Lipoprotein and apoprotein adipose tissue and hepatic lipoprotein lipase levels in patients with familial chylomicronemia, and their immediate family members: in *Atherosclerosis V* (eds AM Gotto Jr, LC Smith, B Allen). Springer-Verlag, New York;1980:250.

69 Crepaldi G, Fellin R, Baggio G, *et al*. Lipoprotein and apoprotein adipose tissue and hepatic lipoprotein lipase levels in patients with familial chylomicronemia, and their immediate family members: in *Atherosclerosis V* (eds AM Gotto Jr, LC Smith, B Allen). Springer-Verlag, New York;1980:250.

70 Fojo SS, De Gennes JL, Chapman J, *et al*. A nonsense mutation in the apolipoprotein C-II$_{Padova}$ gene in a patient with apolipoprotein C-II deficiency. *J Clin Invest* 1989;**84**:1215.

71 Fojo SS, De Gennes JL, Chapman J, *et al*. An initiation codon mutation in the apo C-II gene (apo C-II$_{Paris}$) of a patient with a deficiency of apolipoprotein C-II. *J Biol Chem* 1989;**264**:20839.

72 Fojo SS, Beisiegel U, Beil U, *et al*. Donor splice site mutation in the apolipoprotein (apo) C-II gene (apo C-II$_{Hamburg}$) of a patient with apo C-II deficiency. *J Clin Invest* 1988;**82**:1489.

73 Fojo SS, Stalenhoef AF, Marr K, *et al*. A deletion mutation of the apo C-II gene (apo C-II$_{Nijmegen}$) of a patient with a deficiency of apolipoprotein C-II. *J Biol Chem* 1988;**263**:17913.

74 Yamamura T, Sudo H, Ishikawa K, Yamaoto A. Familial type I hyperlipoproteinemia caused by apolipoprotein C-II deficiency. *Atherosclerosis* 1979;**34**:53.

75 Matsuoka N, Shirai K, Johnson JD, *et al*. Effects of apolipoprotein C-II (apo C-II) on the lipolysis of very low density lipoproteins from apo C-II deficient patients. *Metabolism* 1981;**30**:818.

76 Connelly PW, Maguire GF, Hofmann T, Little JA. Structure of apolipoprotein C-II Toronto, a nonfunctional human apolipoprotein. *Proc Natl Acad Sci USA* 1987;**84**:270.

77 Connelly PW, Maguire CF, Little JA. Apolipoprotein CII$_{St Michael}$ familial apolipoprotein CII deficiency associated with premature vascular disease. *J Clin Invest* 1987;**80**:1597.

78 Xiong WJ, Li W-H, Posner I, *et al*. No severe bottleneck during human evolution: evidence from two apolipoprotein C-II deficiency alleles. *Am J Hum Genet* 1991;**48**:383.

79 Brunzell JD, Schrott HG. The interaction of familial and secondary causes of hypertriglyceridemia: Role in pancreatitis. *Trans Assoc Am Physicians* 1973;**86**:245.

80 Furman RH, Howard RP, Brusco OJ, Alaupovic P. Effects of medium chain length triglyceride (MCT) on serum lipids and lipoproteins in familial hyperchylomicronemia (dietary fat induced lipemia) and dietary carbohydrate-accentuated lipemia. *J Lab Clin Med* 1965;**66**:912.

81 Bartuli A, Landolfo A, Pirozzi N, *et al*. Severe chylomicronemia syndrome (CHS) with neonatal onset successful treatment of cardiac failure with plasmapharesis. *J Inherit Metab Dis* 2002;**25**:161 (suppl 1).

Lipid storage disorders

89

Fabry disease

MAJOR PHENOTYPIC EXPRESSION

Angiokeratomas of the skin, episodic pain in the extremities, hypohidrosis, corneal and lenticular opacities, postprandial pain and diarrhea, neuropathy, renal disease, coronary and cerebral vascular disease, accumulation of glycosphingolipids with a terminal galactose, and deficiency of ceramide trihexosidase (α-galactosidase A).

INTRODUCTION

Fabry disease was first described in 1898 independently by Anderson [1] in England and Fabry [2] in Germany. The latter name has become its designation [3], possibly because Fabry continued to publish information about his patient over a 32-year period [4]. Anderson and Fabry each recognized the systemic nature of the disease but, as dermatologists, their focus was on the cutaneous angiokeratomas by which the patient is so readily recognized. The disease is also known as angiokeratoma corporis diffusum universale [5–7]. It was first noted to be X-linked by Opitz and colleagues in 1965 [7]. The disorder was appropriately classified as a glycosphingolipidosis following the isolation and characterization by Sweeley and Klionsky [8] of the Fabry lipid as galactosylgalactosylglucosylceramide (Figure 89.1). The molecular defect was demonstrated by Brady and colleagues [9] as an inability to cleave the terminal galactose from this ceramide trihexoside; thus the defective activity is ceramide trihexosidase (Figure 89.1). The defective enzyme was shown by Kint [10] by means of an artificial substrate to be an α-galactosidase. It is referred to as α-galactosidase A to distinguish it from the α-N-acetyl-galactosaminidase which is deficient in Schindler disease and is also an α-galactosidase (B). The gene is on the X chromosome at Xq22.1 [11]; the gene has been cloned and its sequence determined [12–14]. A large number and variety of mutations have been defined.

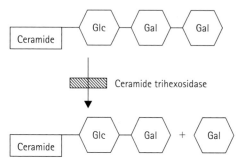

Figure 89.1 *The enzyme ceramide trihexosidase is the site of the defect in Fabry disease. The reaction which cleaves a terminal galactose is an Q-galactosidase.*

CLINICAL ABNORMALITIES

The initial symptom is usually pain occurring often within the first 10 years of life (Table 89.1). It may be excruciating, has a burning quality and tends to occur intermittently [15]. Pain is most often noted in the fingers and toes, or the hands and feet. There may be associated tingling acroparasthesias [16,17]. An attack may be brief or may last for weeks. It may be induced by exposure to extreme heat or cold, fatigue or emotional stress. It may be associated with elevated body temperature and an elevated erythrocyte sedimentation rate, and patients have been diagnosed as having rheumatoid arthritis

Table 89.1 *Clinical signs and symptoms of Fabry disease at different ages*

Age	Signs
Childhood	Pain in extremities, fever, Fabry crisis
Adolescence	Angiokeratomas
Adulthood	Central nervous system symptoms
	Myocardial and pulmonary disease
Middle age	Renal failure, lymphedema

Figure 89.3 *Angiokeratomas of the skin.*

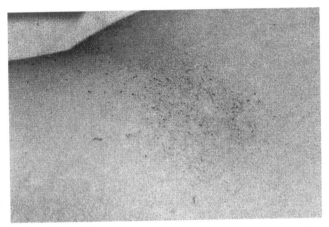

Figure 89.2 *Angiokeratomas of the skin. These red-purple macules or maculopapules may feel hyperkeratotic. They are prominent on the hips, buttocks and scrotum.*

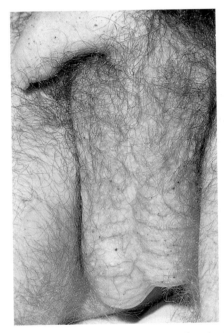

Figure 89.4 *Angiokeratomas of the scrotum and penis of a 31-year-old man.*

or rheumatic fever [18,19]. Degeneration of the interphalangeal joints may lead to deformities. Abdominal or back pain may suggest appendicitis or renal colic [20]. Narcotics may not provide relief. Crises of pain are self-limited, disappearing spontaneously, only to return later. Pains may decrease in frequency and severity with age, and some older patients have no history of pain. Patients may also have recurrent episodes of fever.

It is the appearance of the skin lesions in adolescence or later that usually permits the diagnosis [5,21]. These lesions are dark red punctate macules that do not blanch with pressure (Figures 89.2–89.4). They occur in clusters and may be mistaken for petechiae. With time some become papular and may feel rough to touch. There is some tendency for bilaterally symmetric distribution. The areas of most common involvement are the scrotum and buttocks, but they are also seen on the hips, back and thighs in a bathing-trunks distribution. The oral mucosa may also be involved. Microscopically the skin lesions are angiectatic lesions in the dermis with keratotic build-up superficially. These angiokeratomas are not usually symptomatic, but occasionally large lesions on the scrotum may bleed. The hands or feet or just the tips of the toes or fingers may be bright red, and sensitive to touch. Lymphedema may also be seen in the legs. Hypohidrosis or even absence of sweating is another dermatologic manifestation of the disease. Sweat pores may appear reduced. Patients are intolerant of heat and flush with exercise. One of our

patients responded to hot weather by filling rubber boots with water and sloshing around in them, as well as soaking his head in cold water.

Ocular lesions [22,23] regularly include dilated tortuous venules of the conjunctivae (Figure 89.5). Similar dilatation may be seen in the vessel of the retina. Corneal opacities develop in males and in some heterozygous females. The diagnosis can be made by slit lamp examination, in which the typical cream-colored interior, whorl-like opacities are visualized. Corneal opacities have been seen as early as 6 months-of-age [24]. Cataracts of the posterior capsule of the lens are pathognomonic [22]. The ocular lesions result from the deposition of glycosphingolipid and do not usually impair vision. As the disease progresses, the retinal changes of uremia may be found. Visual loss has been observed following central retinal artery occlusion [25]. Some patients display edema of the

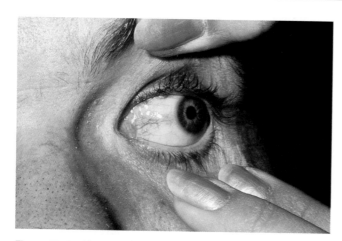

Figure 89.5 *Tortuous, dilated, telangiectatic vessels of the conjunctiva. This man also had fine telangiectases of the facial skin.*

eyelids, in the absence of renal disease [22,24]. Neurosensory hearing loss may develop [18].

Gastrointestinal manifestations may be prominent [26]. In some patients they may be the only complaints for years. There may be postprandial pain or diarrhea. Infiltration of autonomic nerve cells and mucosal cells with lipid may interfere with peristalsis. Diverticula may develop, and rupture of a diverticulum is a surgical emergency.

The long-term complications of Fabry disease are consequences of the accumulation of glycosylsphingolipid in endothelial cells. The most regular concomitant of vascular dysfunction is chronic renal disease. The earliest manifestation is proteinuria, which usually occurs in the fourth decade. Hypertension is common. Examination of the urine may reveal red cells, casts and birefringent lipid globules forming maltese crosses within and outside cells, best seen under polarizing microscopy. Renal function gradually deteriorates, leading to renal failure. This usually occurs by the fifth decade, but may occur as early as 21. The concentration of creatinine in the blood increases linearly with time [18,27]. Polyuria is a manifestation of defective concentrating ability [28]. Prior to the development of programs of hemodialysis, many hemizygotes died before 40 years-of-age [29].

Cardiac manifestations of vascular disease include myocardial ischemia or infarction. Cardiac symptoms include shortness of breath, angina or syncope resulting from arteriovenous (AV) block or ventricular outflow obstruction. Coronary occlusion or cerebral vascular disease often occurs before the age of 25 years [28,30,31]. Cardiac enlargement and myocardial failure may result from infiltration of the myocardium or the valves with lipid [30,31]. Arrhythmias are also common. The PR interval is shortened [32]. Echocardiography may show increased thickness of the interventricular septum and the posterior wall of the left ventricle [33].

Cerebrovascular manifestations may be transient ischemic attacks, strokes, seizures, hemiplegia, or aphasia. They result from infiltration and obstruction of cerebral vessels [34]. Magnetic resonance imaging (MRI) or proton magnetic

resonance spectroscopy (MRS) imaging may reveal cerebrovascular disease [34,35]. Some patients have had psychotic manifestations [36]. Abnormal cutaneous thermal sensation is common [34]. Elevated threshold for the detection of cold precedes that of warmth. Auditory and vestibular dysfunction increase with time [34].

Dyspnea on exertion is common, and airway obstruction may result from infiltration of bronchial epithelial cells [37]. Pulmonary function tests may show impairment. Other manifestations include lymphedema of the legs [38], priapism [39] and anemia [16]. Death usually results from uremia or from vascular disease of the heart or brain.

Heterozygous females have clinical manifestations with such frequency that the disease may be considered an X-linked dominant [40]. In a series of 20 heterozygotes none were asymptomatic [40,41]. All but two had pain or burning either chronically or in Fabry crises. Ten had lymphedema and 11 angiokeratomata. Typical corneal lesions were seen in 14. MRI revealed multifocal infarcts or white matter disease. In a series of 60 obligate carriers, studied largely by questionnaire, serious or debilitating consequences were found in 30 percent and hypohidrosis in 33 percent, while pains occurred in 70 percent [41]. Cardiac involvement, especially left ventricular hypertrophy and valvular abnormalities were found to be common in a series of 35 female patients, and they progressed with age [42].

The pathology of Fabry disease consists of the widespread deposition of glycosphingolipid. Vacuoles are seen in a wide variety of cells, especially the endothelium of the blood vessels [43,44]. Electronmicroscopy reveals a concentric or lamellar structure of the lysosomal inclusions.

GENETICS AND PATHOGENESIS

Fabry disease is an inborn error of glycosphingolipid metabolism transmitted in an X-linked character [7] which is far from fully recessive; the level of expression in the heterozygote ranges from asymptomatic to severity equal to that of the hemizygote.

The defective activity of α-galactosidase leads to the accumulation of glycosphingolipids that have a terminal α-galactosyl moiety [8,45]. The most prominent is ceramide trihexoside (Figure 89.1), which is also known as globotriasylceramide [Gal(α1→4)Gal(β1→4)Glc(β1-1′)ceramide]. Galabiosylceramide, a compound in which ceramide is linked to two galactose moieties, is also found in large quantities in tissues such as kidney [23,46]. The blood group B antigenic glycosphingolipid also contains a terminal galactose and, hence, it accumulates in Fabry patients with B or AB blood types [47].

The basic defect in Fabry disease is an inability to degrade these glycosphingolipids because of defective activity of the enzyme that catalyzes the hydrolysis of the terminal galactose moieties [9]. The activity of α-galatosidase in most hemizygous males is less than three percent of normal, but as much

Fabry's disease
W. Kindred-La Jolla, 1970

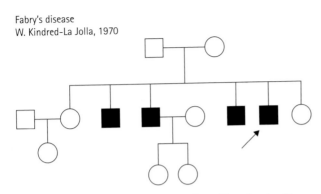

Figure 89.6   *Pedigree of a family with four affected males. The pattern is of X-linked recessive inheritance.*

as 20 percent of normal activity has been observed [48]. Studies with antibody against the enzyme have usually shown no cross-reactive material [49,50]. α-Galactosidase is synthesized as a 50 kDa precursor protein, transported to the lysosome in a mannosphosphate receptor-dependent processing and cleaved to a mature 46 kDa enzyme [51]. Study of this sequence in cells of classic Fabry patients has indicated considerable variation: no enzyme precursor synthesized; precursor, but no mature proteins as a consequence of protein instability; and normal-appearing mature protein with no catalytic activity [51].

The gene for α-galactosidase has been localized to Xq22.1 [11]. X-linked inheritance was first established by pedigree analysis (Figure 89.6). Two populations of cells – one with normal galactosidase activity and the other defective – were shown by cloning of cultured fibroblasts [52]. The cDNA for the gene for α-galactosidase has been cloned and sequenced [12,53], and this has permitted delineation of the nature of a number of mutations. The gene has seven exons. Major gene rearrangement detected by Southern hybridization included five deletions and a duplication [54,55]. A number of smaller deletions and insertions have been identified, many of which led to frameshifts and premature termination. Most mutations in Fabry hemizygotes are not detected in this way. Mutations altering the processing of the mRNA transcript have been observed. Single nucleotide missense mutations have been identified in a majority of families [55–57], and most have been found only in a single family. However a high frequency of mutation was observed at 14 CpG dinucleotides in the coding sequence. More than 300 mutations have been found in patients with Fabry disease [58]. Among them two novel mutations, 1277delAA(del2) and 1284delACTT(del4) in the 3' terminus, obliterated the termination codon and generated multiple transcripts, most of them inactive [58].

Fabry disease is the most common lysosomal storage disease after Gaucher disease. The prevalence of heterozygous carriers in the United Kingdom was estimated at 1 in 339 000 females [41]. Heterozygote detection has been carried out by enzyme assay of cultured fibroblasts after cloning [52] and cell sorting, but these methods are not practical for clinical use. The assay of the enzyme in individual hair roots [59] is more convenient but still labor intensive. In a family in which the mutation has been identified, this can be employed for precise identification of heterozygosity.

Prenatal diagnosis has been accomplished by the demonstration of deficient α-galactosidase activity in cultured amniotic fluid cells [60]. A microtechnique for α-galactosidase has been developed for prenatal diagnosis which requires small numbers of cultured amniocytes [61]. Diagnosis has also been made prenatally by chorionic villus sampling [62]. The identification of the molecular nature of mutation in a family permits this molecular technique to be used for prenatal diagnosis.

TREATMENT

Prevention and amelioration of the painful crises of the disease have been difficult, but diphenylhydantoin has been shown to be helpful; chronic low dosage has been employed (200–300 mg qd) [17]. Carbamazepine may also be helpful, and the combination of the two drugs may be particularly useful [63]. Gabapentin (Neurontin) has been recommended for this purpose [64]. Doses employed in adults have ranged from 100 mg bid to 300 mg bid, or 15–60 mg/kg in children. Neurotropin, an extract of inflamed skin of vaccinia inoculated rabbits was reported to be as effective as carbamazepine in the usual leg pains; neither were effective in episodic colicky pain, but treatment with both eliminated it [65].

Chronic hemodialysis has been the mainstay of management of renal failure. Many patients have received kidney transplants following renal failure [65–68]. This solves the problem of renal failure, but does not alter the accumulation of lipid in other tissues. Some transplanted patients have survived long enough to die of cardiac disease. Enzyme replacement therapy with purified α-galactosidase [69] has been extended to trials with recombinant human enzyme, which have demonstrated safety and efficacy [70–72]. It is clear that treatment reverses the storage in lysosomes, which causes the disease. The product has been approved by the USFDA and the European Agency for the Evaluation of Medicinal Products. It is marketed in the US as Fabrazyme. Optimal dosage has yet to be determined. Doses employed have been 0.2 [71]–1.0 [72] mg/kg [intravenously every 2 weeks for 20 to 22 weeks]. Two products have been approved in Europe. They should have equal efficacy as neither mRNA is edited [73].

Activation of mutant enzymes by compounds such as 1-deoxygalactonojirimycin are being explored in novel approaches to the treatment of glycosphingolipidoses [74,75]. This compound is an inhibitor of lysosomal α-galactosidase, but in low doses it serves as an activator increasing activity in mutant enzymes up to 14 times. These compounds have been referred to as chemical chaparones, because they accelerate transport and maturation of the enzyme molecule.

Another approach is substrate deprivation. Compounds such as D-*erythro*-1-ethylenedeoxyphenyl-2-palmitylamino-3-pyrrolidino-propanol (d-t-EtDO-P4) reduce accumulation of globotriosylceramide in tissues of murine Fabry models [76] by inhibiting the sphingolipid glucosyltransferase involved in their synthesis.

References

1 Anderson W. A case of angiokeratoma. *Brit J Dermatol* 1898;**10**:113.

2 Fabry J. Ein Beitrag zur Kenntnis der Purpura haemorrhagica nodularis (Purpura papulosa hemorrhagica Hebrae). *Arch Dermatol Syph* 1898;**43**:187.

3 Aerts JMFG, Beck M, Cox TM. Fabry disease, new insights and future perspectives. *J Inherit Metab Dis* 2001;**24**:1 (suppl 2).

4 Fabry J. Weiterer Beitrag zur Klinik des Angiokeratoma naeviforme (Naevus angiokeratosus). *Dermatol Schnschr* 1930;**90**:339.

5 Johnston AW, Weller SDV, Warland BJ. Angiokeratoma corporis diffusum. *Arch Dis Child* 1968;**43**:73.

6 Wallace RD, Cooper WJ. Angiokeratoma corporis diffusim universale (Fabry). *Am J Med* 1965;**39**:656.

7 Opitz JM, Stiles FCD, von Gemmingen G, *et al.* The genetics of angiokeratoma corporis diffusum (Fabry's disease) and its linkage with Xg(a) locus. *Am J Hum Genet* 1965;**17**:325.

8 Sweeley CC, Klionsky B. Fabry's disease: classification as a sphingolipidosis and partial characterization of a novel glycolipid. *J Biol Chem* 1963;**238**:3148.

9 Brady RO, Gal AE, Bradley RM, *et al.* Enzymatic defect in Fabry's disease – ceramidetrihexosidase deficiency. *N Engl J Med* 1967;**276**:1163.

10 Kint JA. Fabry's disease α-galactosidase deficiency. *Science* 1970;**167**:1268.

11 Shows TB, Brown JA, Haley LL, *et al.* Assignment of alpha-galactosidase (alpha-GAL) gene to the q22-qter region of the X chromosome in man. *Cytogenet Cell Genet* 1978;**22**:541.

12 Bishop DF, Calhoun DH, Bernstein HS, *et al.* Human α-galactosidase A: Nucleotide sequence of a cDNA clone encoding the mature enzyme. *Proc Natl Acad Sci USA* 1986;**83**:4859.

13 Bishop DF, Kornreich R, Desnick RJ. Structural organization of the human alpha-galactosidase A gene: Further evidence for the absence of a 3′ untranslated region. *Proc Natl Acad Sci USA* 1988;**85**:3903.

14 Kornreich R, Desnick RJ, Bishop DF. Nucleotide sequence of the human α-galactosidase A gene. *Nucleic Acids Res* 1989;**17**:3301.

15 Wise D, Wallace HJ, Jellinek EH. Angiokeratoma corporis diffusum: a clinical study of eight affected families. *Q J Med* 1962;**31**:177.

16 Bagdale JD, Parker F, Ways PO, *et al.* Fabry's disease: a correlative clinical morphologic and biochemical study. *Lab Invest* 1968;**18**:681.

17 Lockman LA, Hunnighake DB, Krivit W, Desnick RJ. Relief of pain of Fabry's disease by diphenyl-hydantoin. *Neurology* 1971;**23**:871.

18 Pyeritz RE, Bender WL, Lipford ED III. Anderson-Fabry disease. *Johns Hopkins Med J* 1982;**150**:181.

19 Sheth KJ, Bernhard GC. The arthropathy of Fabry disease. *Arth Rheum* 1979;**22**:781.

20 Rahman AN, Simcone FA, Hackel DB, *et al.* Angiokeratoma corporis diffusum universale (hereditary dystopic lipidosis). *Trans Assoc Am Physicians* 1961;**74**:366.

21 Frost P, Spaeth GL, Tanaka Y. Fabry's disease – glycolipid lipidosis. Skin manifestations. *Arch Intern Med* 1966;**117**:440.

22 Sher NA, Letson RD, Desnick RJ. The ocular manifestations in Fabry's disease. *Arch Ophthalmol* 1979;**97**:671.

23 Brady RO. Ophthalmologic aspects of lipid storage diseases. *Ophthalmology* 1978;**85**:1007.

24 Spaeth GL, Frost P. Fabry's disease: its ocular manifestations. *Arch Ophthalmol* 1965;**74**:760.

25 Sher NA, Reiff W, Letson RD, Desnick RJ. Central retinal artery occlusion complicating Fabry's disease. *Arch Opthalmol* 1978;**96**:315.

26 Rowe JW, Gilliam JI, Warthin TA. Intestinal manifestations of Fabry's disease. *Ann Intern Med* 1974;**81**:628.

27 Mitch WE, Walser M, Buffington GA, Lemann JR. A simple method of estimating progression of chronic renal failure. *Lancet* 1976;**2**:1326.

28 Parkinson JE, Sunshine A. Angiokeratoma corporis diffusum universale (Fabry) presenting as suspected myocardial infarction and pulmonary infarcts. *Am J Med* 1961;**31**:951.

29 Colombi A, Kostyal A, Bracher R, *et al.* Angiokeratoma corporis diffusum-Fabry's disease. *Helv Med Acta* 1967;**34**:67.

30 Becker AR, Schoorl R, Balk AG, van der Heider RM. Cardiac manifestations of Fabry's disease. *Am J Cardiol* 1975;**36**:829.

31 Desnick RJ, Blieden L, C Sharp HL, *et al.* Cardiac valvular anomalies in Fabry disease. *Circulation* 1976;**54**:818.

32 Mehta J. Electrocardiographic and vectorcardiographic abnormalities in Fabry's disease. *Am Heart J* 1977;**93**:699.

33 Bass JL, Shrivastava S, Grabowski GA, *et al.* The M-mode echocardiogram in Fabry's disease. *Am Heart J* 1980;**100**:807.

34 Morgan SH, Rudge P, Smith SJ, *et al.* The neurological complications of Anderson-Fabry disease (alpha-galactosidase A deficiency) – Investigation of symptomatic and presymptomatic patients. *Q J Med* 1990;**75**:491.

35 Moumdjian R, Tampieri D, Melanson D, Ethier R. Anderson-Fabry disease: a case report with MR, CT and cerebral angiography. *Am J Neuroradiol* 1989;**10**:S69.

36 Liston EH, Levine MD, Philippart M. Psychosis in Fabry disease and treatment with phenoxybenzamine. *Arch Gen Psychiatry* 1973;**29**:402.

37 Rosenberg DM, Ferrans VJ, Fulmer JD, *et al.* Chronic airflow obstruction in Fabry's disease. *Am J Med* 1980;**68**:898.

38 Gemignani F, Pietrini Y, Tagliavini F, *et al.* Fabry's disease with familial lymphedema of the lower limbs. *Eur Neurol* 1979;**18**:84.

39 Funderburk SJ, Philippart M, Dale G, *et al.* Priapism after phenoxybenzamine in a patient with Fabry's disease. *N Engl J Med* 1974;**290**:630.

40 Whybra C, Kampmann CO, Willers I, *et al.* Anderson-Fabry disease: clinical manifestations of disease in female heterozygotes. *J Inherit Metab Dis* 2001;**24**:715.

41 MacDermot KD, Homes A, Miners AH. Anderson-Fabry disease: clinical manifestations and impact of disease in a cohort of 60 obligate carrier females. *J Med Genet* 2001;**38**:769.

42 Kampmann C, Baehner F, Whybra C, *et al.* Cardiac manifestations of Anderson-Fabry disease in heterozygous females. *J Am Coll Cardiol* 2002;**40**:1668.

43 Pompen AWM, Ruiter M, Wyers JJG. Angiokeratoma corporis diffusum (universale) Fabry, as a sign of an unknown internal disease: two autopsy reports. *Acta Med Scand* 1947;**128**:234.

44 Scriba K. Zur Pathogenese des Angiokeratoma corporis diffusum Fabry mit cardiovasorenalem Symptomenkomplex. *Verh Deutsch Ges Pathol* 1950;**34**:221.

45 Schibanoff JM, Kamoshita S, O'Brien JS. Tissue distribution of glycosphingolipids in a case of Fabry's disease. *J Lipid Res* 1969;**10**:515.

46 Christenson-Lou HO. A biochemical investigation of angiokeratoma corporis diffusum. *Acta Pathol Microbiol Scand* 1966;**68**:332.

47 Wherret JR, Hakimori S. Characterization of a blood group B glycolipid accumulating in the pancreas of a patient with Fabry's disease. *J Biol Chem* 1973;**218**:3046.

48 Romeo G, Urso M, Pisacane A, *et al.* Residual activity of α-galactosidase A in Fabry's disease. *Biochem Genet* 1975;**13**:615.

49 Beutler E, Kuhl W. Purification and properties of human alpha-galatosidases. *J Biol Chem* 1972;**247**:7195.

50   Beutler E, Kuhl W. Absence of cross-reactive antigen in Fabry disease. *N Engl J Med* 1973;**289**:694.

51   Lemansky P, Bishop DF, Desnick RJ, *et al*. Synthesis and processing of α-galactosidease A in human fibroblasts. Evidence for different mutations in Fabry disease. *J Biol Chem* 1987;**262**:2062.

52   Romeo G, Migeon BR. Genetic inactivation of the alpha-galactosidase locus in carriers of Fabry's disease. *Science* 1970;**170**:180.

53   Calhoun DH, Bishop DF, Bernstein HS, *et al*. Fabry disease: isolation of a cDNA clone encoding human a-galactosidase A. *Proc Natl Acad Sci USA* 1985;**82**:7364.

54   Bernstein HS, Bishop DF, Astrin KH, *et al*. Fabry disease: gene rearrangements and a coding region point mutation in the a-galactosidase A gene. *J Clin Invest* 1989;**83**:1390.

55   Eng CM, Resnick-Silverman LA, Niehaus DJ, *et al*. Nature and frequency of mutations in the a-galactosidase A gene causing Fabry disease. *Am J Hum Genet* 1993;**53**:1186.

56   Eng CM, Desnick RJ. Molecular basis of Fabry disease: mutations and polymorphisms in the human α-galactosidase A gene. *Hum Mutat* 1994;**3**:103.

57   Eng CM, Ashley GA, Burgert TS, *et al*. Fabry disease: Thirty-five mutations in the α-galactosidase A gene in patients with classic and variant phenotypes. *Mol Med* 1997;**3**:174.

58   Yasuda M, Shabbeer J, Osawa M, Desnick RJ. Fabry disease: Novel α-galactosidase A 3'-terminal mutations result in multiple transcripts due to aberrant 3'-end formation. *Am J Hum Genet* 2003;**73**:162.

59   Beaudet A, Caskey CT. Detection of Fabry's disease heterozygotes by hair root analysis. *Clin Genet* 1978;**13**:251.

60   Brady RO, Uhlendorf BW, Jacobson CB. Fabry's disease: antenatal diagnosis. *Science* 1971;**172**:174.

61   Galjaard H, Niermeijer MF, Hahnemann N, *et al*. An example of rapid prenatal diagnosis of Fabry's disease using microtechniques. *Clin Genet* 1974;**5**:368.

62   Kleijer WJ, Hussaarts-Odijk LM, Sacks ES, *et al*. Prenatal diagnosis of Fabry's disease by direct analysis of chorionic villi. *Prenat Diagn* 1987;**7**:283.

63   Lenoir G, Rivron M, Gubler MC, *et al*. La maladie de Fabry. Traitement du syndrome acrodyniforme par la carbamazepine. *Arch Fr Pediatr* 1977;**34**:704.

64   Germain DP. Fabry's disease (alpha-galactosidase-A deficiency): recent therapeutic innovations. *J Soc Biol* 2002;**196**:183.

65   Inagaki M, Ohno K, Ohta S, *et al*. Relief of chronic burning pain in Fabry disease with neurotropin. *Pediatr Neurol* 1990;**6**:211.

66   Clarke JTR, Guttmann RD, Wolfe LS, *et al*. Enzyme replacement therapy for renal allotransplantation in Fabry's disease. *N Engl J Med* 1972;**287**:1215.

67   Schweitzer EJ, Drachenberg CB, Bartlett ST. Living kidney donor and recipient evaluation in Fabry's disease. *Transplantation* 1992;**54**:924.

68   Desnick RJ, Dean KJ, Grabowski GA, *et al*. Enzyme therapy XII: enzyme therapy in Fabry's disease – differential enzyme and substrate clearance kinetics of plasma and splenic a-galactosidase isozymes. *Proc Natl Acad Sci USA* 1979;**76**:5326.

69   Friedlaender MM, Kopolovic J, Rubinger D, *et al*. Renal biopsy in Fabry's disease eight years after successful renal transplantation. *Clin Nephrol* 1987;**27**:206.

70   Desnick RJ, Brady R, Barranger J, *et al*. Fabry disease an under-recognized multisystemic disorder: expert recommendations for diagnosis management and enzyme replacement therapy. *Ann Int Med* 2003;**138**:338.

71   Schiffmann R, Kopp JB, Austin HA III, *et al*. Enzyme replacement therapy in Fabry disease. *JAMA* 2001;**27**:43.

72   Wilcox WR, Banikazemi M, Guffon N, *et al*. Long-term safety and efficacy of replacement therapy for Fabry disease. *Am J Hum Genet* 2004;**75**:65.

73   Blom D, Speijer D, Linthorst GE, *et al*. Recombinant enzyme therapy for Fabry disease: absence of editing of human α-galactosidase A mRNA. *Am J Hum Genet* 2003;**72**:23.

74   Ogawa Y, Nanba E, Ohno K, *et al*. A new therapeutic approach to β-galactosidosis: galactose analog compounds of low molecular weight restore mutant human β-galactosidases expressed in enzyme-deficient knockout mouse fibroblasts. *Proc Jpn Soc Inherit Metabol Dis* 2001;**44**:238.

75   Asano N, Ishii S, Kizu H, *et al*. *In vitro* inhibition and intracellular enhancement of lysosomal α-galactosidase A activity in Fabry lymphoblasts by 1-deoxygalactonojirimycin and its derivatives. *Eur J Biochem* 2000;**267**:4179.

76   Abe A, Gregory S, Lee L, *et al*. Reduction of globotriaosylceramide in Fabry disease mice by substrate deprivation. *J Clin Invest* 2000;**105**:1563.

90

GM₁ gangliosidosis/β-galactosidase deficiency

MAJOR PHENOTYPIC EXPRESSION

Cerebral degenerative disease of infantile onset combining features of a mucopolysaccaridosis including dysostosis multiplex and hepatosplenomegaly with those of a neurolipidosis, including cherry red macular spots; accumulation of the ganglioside GM₁ in the brain and viscera and of mucopolysaccharides in viscera; and deficiency of acid β-galactosidase.

Variants with late infantile, juvenile or adult forms have progressive neurologic degeneration. Defects in same enzyme cause Morquio B disease, in which there is a mild Morquio phenotype.

INTRODUCTION

Infantile GM₁ or generalized gangliosidosis is a lysosomal storage disease in which GM₁ ganglioside (Figure 91.1, p. 610) accumulates in the brain and viscera [1–5]. The resultant cerebral degenerative disease is a devastating one, and affected patients usually die before 2 years-of-age. This was the first of the GM₁ gangliosidoses to be described [5], and it is the most common. It has also been referred to as type 1, but as increasing genetically determined variation becomes evident, it is less appropriate to number these disorders. A spectrum of considerable differences in phenotype appears to reflect different degrees of residual enzyme activity resulting from different mutations. It has been practical clinically to consider the GM₁ gangliosidosis broadly as infantile, juvenile, or adult.

Defective activity of β-galactosidase (EC 3.2.1.23) (Figure 90.1) was first discovered by Okada and O'Brien [6]. Recognition of the enzyme abnormality led to the elucidation of later onset forms of GM₁ gangliosidosis [7–9]. Spondyloepiphyseal dysplasia and normal intelligence in a Morquio-like syndrome were also found in patients with deficiency of the same β-galactosidase enzyme [10–12].

The gene for β-galactosidase has been assigned to chromosome 3p21.33[13]. The human placental cDNA was cloned by Oshima *et al.* [14], and found to have a coding sequence of 2031 nucleotides encoding a protein of 677 amino acids. A number of mutations has been found in GM₁ gangliosidosis [15,16], and in Morquio B disease [17,18], and these very different phenotypes are allelic.

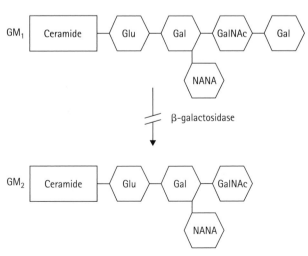

Figure 90.1 *Lysosomal acid β-galactosidase. The site of the defect in GM₁ gangliosidosis.*

CLINICAL ABNORMALITIES

Infantile GM₁ gangliosidosis

Classic GM₁ gangliosidosis differs from most of the other storage diseases in that abnormalities are present from birth. The first symptoms are facial edema, pitting edema of the extremities or ascites, and motor retardation, evident in poor sucking and appetite and failure to thrive. Some infants present with hydrops fetalis [19,20]. In a patient with transient fetal ascites examination of the macroscopically normal placenta revealed vacuolated cells, and enzyme analysis confirmed the diagnosis of GM₁ gangliosidosis. The infant is hypotonic and hypoactive. The facial features may be coarse, even very early, and the expression is dull. There is frontal bossing, downy hirsutism over the forehead, a depressed nasal bridge, large, low-set ears, and an increased distance between the nose and the upper lip (Figures 90.2–90.4). Patients have hypertrophy of the gums and a large tongue [3–5]. A cherry red macular spot (Figure 90.5) is visible bilaterally in about half the patients [21]. Nystagmus may be present. The cornea may show mild or absent clouding, but a true cloudy cornea has been reported in one patient [22]. Hepatomegaly is prominent, and the spleen may be palpable.

By 8 months-of-age the infant may be able to hold up his head, but he cannot sit or crawl. He may follow objects with his eyes and even reach for them, but his grasp is poor. Movements are uncoordinated. The infant rarely smiles and appears uninterested in his environment. His cry is weak. Parents may say he is a good baby, meaning that he sleeps a lot and is immobile much of the day. Hepatomegaly is uniformly found after 6 months, and splenomegaly is seen in 80 percent of patients. Coarse features are accentuated. Macrocephaly may develop,

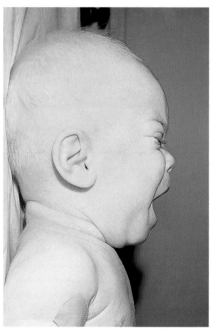

Figure 90.3 *C.D. Lateral view of the face illustrates the coarse features. The ear is low-set and the nasal bridge depressed. The prominent maxillary area is characteristic. (Courtesy of Dr. John S. O'Brien, University of California San Diego.)*

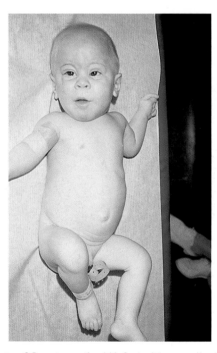

Figure 90.2 *C.D., a 4-month-old infant with generalized GM₁ gangliosidosis. Features were coarse. Frontal bossing, a depressed nasal bridge, and low-set ears can be seen. (Courtesy of Dr. John S. O'Brien, University of California San Diego.)*

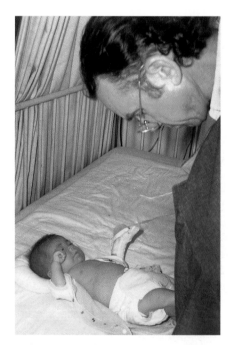

Figure 90.4 *A 4-month-old Japanese baby with GM₁ gangliosidosis. Features were a little coarse. There was frontal bossing and a depressed nasal bridge.*

but it is less frequent and less prominent than in Tay-Sachs disease. Deep tendon reflexes become hyperactive, and hyperacusis may develop [3,23,24]. Muscle weakness progresses, and there may be a head lag on elevating the shoulders. Early hypotonia is replaced by spasticity. Deep tendon reflexes are exaggerated, and pyramidal tract signs are evident. After the first year, deterioration is rapid. Convulsions are frequent, and swallowing is so poor that tube feeding is required. Recurrent pneumonias complicate the course. By 16 months the patient is blind and deaf and has decerebrate rigidity. Optic atrophy is seen and the retina may be edematous [25]. Flexion contractures develop, and there is no response to stimuli. Death usually follows pneumonia by 2 years-of-age. Angiokeratomas have been described in this disease as early as 10 months [26]. We have seen a patient with a single lesion on a leg. They may be widely scattered, but do not cluster as in Fabry disease, and they have not been observed on the penis or scrotum.

An unusual presentation has been observed in infants with GM$_1$ gangliosidosis [27–29], suggesting that this disorder should be included in the differential diagnosis of cardiomyopathy. Each developed congestive cardiac failure. Awareness that this disorder may present in this fashion should facilitate early diagnosis in such patients.

The skeletal manifestations of the disease are also progressive. The fingers are short and stubby. The joints are stiff and limited in motion. There are flexion contractures of the fingers, especially the fifth. The wrists and ankles become enlarged. Flexion contractures also occur at the elbows and knees. The dorsolumbar kyphosis may be a prominent gibbus. The characteristic picture is that of a mucopolysaccharidosis, but in some patients these features may be subtle, and patients with severe neurodegeneration may not have recognizable dysmorphic features [30].

Roentgenographic findings are usually those of an early and very severe dysostosis multiplex. These changes are similar to those of I-cell disease (Chapter 84), and they are usually earlier in onset and more severe than those of Hurler syndrome (Chapter 77) [3,31,32]. The long tubular bones are shortened and widened in midshaft, tapering distally and proximally (Figure 90.6). Subperiosteal new bone formation is characteristic. The consequent cloaking of the already widened bones is particularly evident in the humerus, and the pinching-off of the end of the bones is striking. The distal ends of the radius and ulna tilt obliquely toward each other. Middle and proximal phalanges are widened. The metacarpals are short and broad and taper proximally. The carpal centers are hypoplastic. The lumbar vertebrae are hypoplastic and beaked anteriorly at the site of the kyphosis (Figure 90.7). The ribs are thickened and spatula-like. The ilia are flared. The sella turcica is shallow and elongated, giving it a shoe-shaped appearance. Bone age is retarded [33].

Neuroimaging may show white matter changes followed by loss of white matter and atrophy [34]. Increased signal has been seen in the basal ganglia [35], and basal ganglia calcification has been reported [8]. The electroencephalogram (EEG) may be normal early on [33], but later there is evidence of dysthymia [36,37]. Visual evoked potentials are abnormal [36].

Neuronal lipidosis is prominent on histologic examination of the brain. The ballooned neurons look exactly like those of Tay-Sachs disease [38,39]. Indeed, electron microscopy shows identical lamellar cytoplasmic inclusion bodies in the neurons. These membranous cytoplasmic bodies also may be seen in retinal ganglion cells [21]. In viscera such as the liver there is histiocytosis, and vacuoles may be present in both hepatocytes and histiocytes that stain with periodic acid-Schiff. A characteristic lesion is the cytoplasmic vacuolation and ballooning of the renal glomerular epithelial cells [4], seen only in this disorder and in Fabry disease (Chapter 89). Lysosomal inclusions in the epithelial cells of the skin may aid in the diagnosis [40]. There are vacuolated lymphocytes

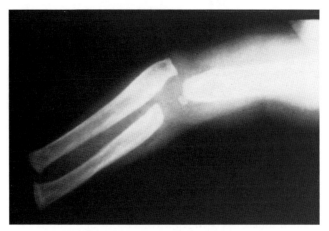

Figure 90.6   *C.D. Roentgenograms of the arm at 7 months. The picture was that of advanced dysostosis multiplex. The bones were short and had prominent midshaft thickening. The distal ends of the radius and ulna had begun to point toward each other. The distal end of the humerus showed the characteristic pinched-off appearance. The changes in the bones in this syndrome are just like those of Hurler syndrome, but in this disease they are prominent much earlier in life. (Courtesy of Dr. John S. O'Brien, University of California San Diego.)*

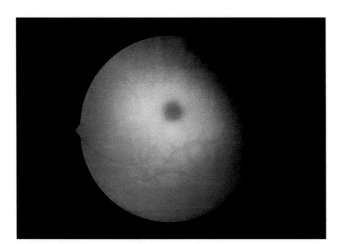

Figure 90.5   *Cherry red macular spot in an infant with GM$_1$ gangliosidosis.*

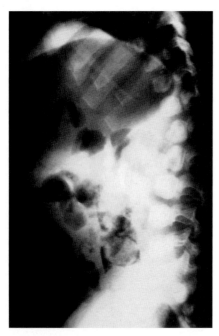

Figure 90.7   *C.D. Roentgenogram of the spine at 7 months. The vertebral bodies were hypoplastic. There was anterior breaking of L1 and L2. (Courtesy of Dr. John S. O'Brien, University of California San Diego.)*

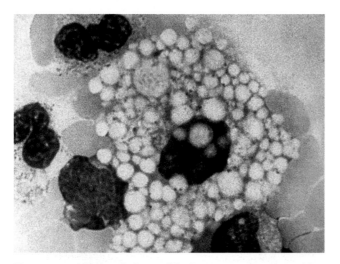

Figure 90.8   *Histiocytic foam cell in the marrow of a patient with GM₁ gangliosidosis.*

in the peripheral blood and foamy histiocytes in the bone marrow (Figure 90.8).

Mucopolysacchariduria usually has not been detected, but keratan sulfate has been reported in excess in the urine [39]. The ganglioside that accumulates in the brain and in the viscera in generalized gangliosidosis is the GM₁ ganglioside [3,5,41]. It is the major monosialoganglioside of normal brain. Its structure is galactosyl(1→3)-N-acetylgalactosaminyl-(1→4)-[(2→3)-N-acetylneuraminyl]-galactosyl-(1→4)-glycosyl-(1→1)-[2-N-acyl]-sphingosine. Thus, it is a trihexoside with an N-acetylneuraminic acid side chain. It differs from the Tay-Sachs, or GM₂, ganglioside in the presence of the terminal

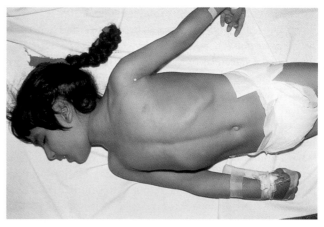

Figure 90.9   *M.S., a 9-year-old Saudi girl with juvenile GM₁ gangliosidosis. She is shown in an essentially decerebrate posture. Early development was normal, and she walked at less than 1 year, but shortly thereafter began to lose milestones. Seizures began at 4 years. There were no coarse or dysmorphic features in contrast to classic GM₁ gangliosidosis. There was no dysostosis multiplex. β-Galactosidase activity in fibroblasts was 1.7 percent of control.*

galactose on GM₁. This ganglioside is present in 10 times normal amounts in the cerebral gray matter of patients with GM₁ gangliosidosis. Mucopolysaccharides also are stored in peripheral tissues [41]. The magnitude of the storage is similar to that in Hurler disease, but the mucopolysaccharides stored differ, in that they more closely resemble keratan sulfate. It appears reasonable that the abnormalities of bone are caused by the mucopolysaccharide storage and that cerebral degeneration is a consequence of the storage of ganglioside in the brain.

Other genetic variants

LATE INFANTILE/JUVENILE GM₁ GANGLIOSIDOSIS

GM₁ ganglioside also accumulates in the brain in patients with onset in late infancy or childhood [38,42–45]. In chronic adult GM₁ gangliosidosis it is found only in the caudate and the putamen [46].

Patients with the late infantile/juvenile disease have progressive cerebral deterioration, but it begins later than in the classic form, often at about 1 year-of age [47]. Onset may be with ataxia. There may be incoordination or frequent falling and generalized muscular weakness. Speech, if present, is lost. Thereafter mental and motor deterioration may progress rapidly. Patients develop spasticity and rigidity, and they have seizures, which may be a major problem in management. They exhibit myoclonus, sound-induced myoclonus and myoclonic seizures [45]. They usually die between 3 and 7 years-of-age in a state of decerebrate rigidity.

Phenotypic expression may be quite variable in these patients. The facial appearance may be coarse in late infantile patients. It may be quite normal in juvenile patients (Figures 90.9–90.14). Similarly, hepatosplenomegaly may be present

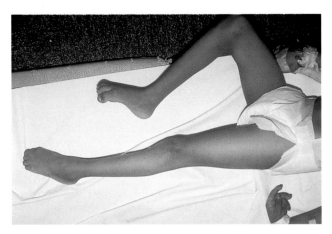

Figure 90.10   *M.S. The legs were in a tonic neck response. They were very spastic and deep tendon reflexes were exaggerated. Plantar reflexes were down. There were vacuolated histiocytes in the marrow.*

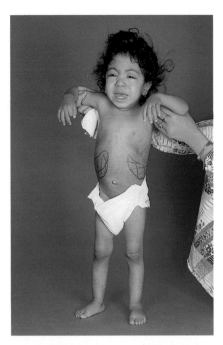

Figure 90.12   *A.M.A.Q. Hepatosplenomegaly. The pigmentation was also present over the abdomen.*

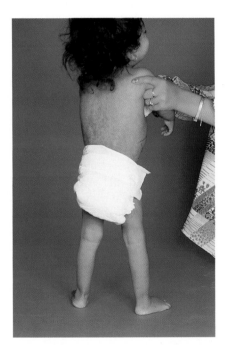

Figure 90.11   *A.M.A.Q. The hyperpigmented areas appeared to be diffuse Mongolian spots.*

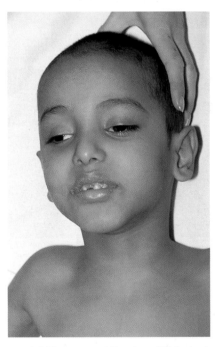

Figure 90.13   *A.S. The 7-year-old brother of M.S. also had juvenile GM₁ gangliosidosis. He lay in bed in decerebrate posture with rigid arms and legs. He showed no interest in his surroundings, but was conscious. There was no coarsening of the features.*

(Figure 90.12), but is usually absent[46]. There may be internal strabismus or nystagmus. There are usually no cherry red spots or other fundoscopic findings, although blindness may occur later; and atypical cherry red spots were reported in one patient [48]. Many widely disseminated Mongolian spots were seen in one patient (Figures 90.11, 90.12). Extensive Mongolian spots have also been reported in some infantile patients [49–51].

EEG may be abnormally slow or show spike discharges. Neuroimaging reveals cerebral atrophy [45]. Patients have vacuolated cells in the bone marrow. Sea blue histiocytes have been reported [45]. Membranous cytoplasmic bodies are found in the neuronal cytoplasm, and large amounts of GM_1

ganglioside accumulate in the brain [42]. Keratosulfaturia has been described [42].

CHRONIC/ADULT GM1 GANGLIOSIDOSIS

The adult form of GM_1 gangliosidosis storage disease presents with progressive cerebellar dysarthria, progressive ataxia,

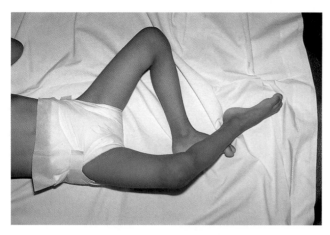

Figure 90.14 *A.S. The legs were spastic in flexion and extension and deep tendon reflexes were accentuated.*

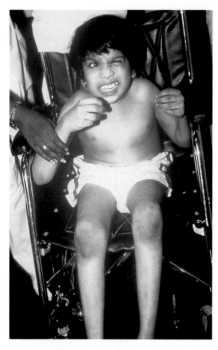

Figure 90.15 *J.A.H., an 11-year-old boy with Morquio Type B disease. He and his affected brother were severely retarded. Facial features were coarse. (This illustration was kindly provided by Dr. Philip Benson.)*

myoclonus and spasticity [9,52,53]. Dystonia is a major manifestation in many patients [54–56]. Intellectual impairment may be mild, but there is usually loss of function over time. There may be abnormalities of gait or speech. These patients do not have cherry red spots. Rare patients have cherry red spots and progressive disease [57]. They do not have dysmorphic features, suggesting storage of mucopolysaccharide. In one patient onset was at 2 to 3 years-of-age with unsteadiness of gait, and at 5 he was thought to have cerebral palsy. Dystonia began at 6 years and was extreme by 15. He died at 27 years-of-age. Pathologic changes were largely confined to the basal ganglia, where there was intraneuronal storage and

accumulation of GM₁ ganglioside [56]. Seizures are uncommon, and vision is preserved. Kyphosis and moderate flattening of vertebral bodies has been reported [53] as well as flattening of the femoral heads.

MORQUIO B DISEASE

A very different clinical phenotype has been described in which there is severe skeletal dysplasia without neurologic involvement [11,58,59](Figure 90.15). This condition is also referred to as mucopolysaccharidosis IV B, as well as Morquio syndrome type B [11,60]. One patient presented at 20 years-of-age with pain in the hip and was found to have progressive dysplasia of the pelvis and the femoral heads [58]. She had vertebral platyspondyly and modeling abnormalities of the vertebral bodies like those seen in hereditary spondyloepiphyseal dysplasia. A different variant was reported [60] in which a brother and sister had typical clinical and roentgenographic features of Morquio disease, but had atypical mental regression. In these patients a severe deficiency has been found in the activity of β-galactosidase in cultured fibroblasts and in leukocytes.

GENETICS AND PATHOGENESIS

GM₁ gangliosidosis and all of the β-galactosidase variants are transmitted in an autosomal recessive fashion. In any family in which multiple patients are seen, each one virtually always has the same phenotype. However, phenotypic variation within a family has been reported [61]. A risk of recurrence of 25 percent in siblings is consistent with observed data [2,3]. The rate of consanguinity in reported families has been high. There is no ethnic predominance for the common classic infantile forms, or most of the other variants, but the adult form has been reported predominantly from Japan.

Detection of the heterozygous carrier has been accomplished by the assay of the enzyme in leukocytes [62], and heterozygotes as a group can be distinguished from normals by enzyme assay in a statistically significant fashion; however, overlap with normals makes detection potentially unreliable in any individual in which a normal value is obtained. When the mutation is known, carrier detection is highly reliable [54]. In adult type Japanese families the I51T mutation has been useful for this purpose [54].

Intrauterine diagnosis by assay of β-galactosidase in cultured amniocytes or chorionic villus cells is an established procedure [63–65]. Rapid prenatal diagnosis has been accomplished by the direct analysis of galactosyloligosaccharides in amniotic fluid using high performance liquid chromatography [66]. Rapid enzymatic diagnosis is also available by microchemical assay [67].

The mutations causing each type of GM₁ gangliosidosis are allelic. Somatic cell hybridization has failed to reveal evidence of complementation [68,69]. The fundamental defect in all of the GM₁ gangliosidoses is the nearly complete activity of the lysosomal acid β-galactosidase [6]. The enzyme is synthesized

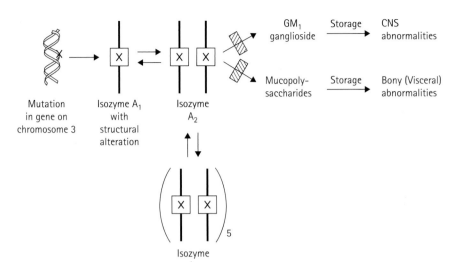

Figure 90.16 *Model of the pathogenesis of the phenotypes of GM₁ gangliosidosis. The phenotypic effect of a single gene mutation results from the effects of a single enzyme on multiple substrates.*

as an 8 kD protein which is processed to a 64 kD monomeric protein which contains 7.5 percent carbohydrate [70,71].

The precursor protein is coded for by a gene on chromosome 3 (3p21.33) [13,72,73]. The 64 kD monomer aggregates to a homopolymer of about 700 kDa, a process that is promoted by association with a 32 kDa protein coded for by a gene originally mapped to chromosome 22 [74] which increases stability in the presence of proteases. It is this 32 kD protein that is the defect in galactosialidosis, protective protein/cathepsin A (PPCA), and it is actually located on chromosome 22q13.1 [75] (Chapter 101). Different forms of β-galactosidase have been separated electrophoretically or isolated, representing monomer, dimer and multimer. The enzyme hydrolyzes the terminal galactose of GM₁ (Figure 90.1, p. 599). It also cleaves a terminal galactose from asialoGM₁, lactosylceramide, keratan sulfate, lactose and a variety of oligosaccharides. It does not cleave galactocerebroside, which is cleaved by galactocerebroside β-galactosidase (EC 3.2.1.46), the enzyme that is deficient in Krabbe disease (Chapter 97).

In GM₁ gangliosidosis the deficiency of the enzyme may be demonstrated using artificial substrate such as *p*-nitrophenylgalactoside and 4-methylumbelliferylgalactoside. It also may be done using isolated GM₁ ganglioside. The activity of this enzyme is markedly deficiency when GM₁ ganglioside or galactose-containing glycoprotein is used as substrate [75,76]. The enzyme is markedly deficient in liver and brain [68] and virtually inactive in leukocytes [77] or cultured fibroblasts [78]. GM₁ ganglioside β-galactosidase activities have been reported as less than 0.1 percent of normal [67]. Normal amounts of immuno-cross-reactive material have been found [75]. The activity of residual enzyme is not different in infantile and juvenile forms of GM₁ gangliosidosis [42]. Patients with juvenile GM₁ gangliosidosis have considerably more activity when tested against GM₁ ganglioside [6] than patients with the infantile disease. Higher levels, 5 to 10 percent of control activity have been reported in adult GM₁ gangliosidosis [16,54].

Impaired degradation of keratan sulfate from shark cartilage was shown to be deficient in fibroblasts of patients with GM₁ gangliosidosis [79]. In patients with Morquio B disease activities of 5–10 percent [58] and less than five percent [80] have been reported with actually varying activity against varying substrates. Activity against keratan sulfate was undetectable in these patients [12]. Qualitative differences in pH optima and in thermolability have been observed among variants [81].

β-Galactosidase splits the terminal galactose from GM₁ converting it to GM₂. It also cleaves galactose [76] from the mucopolysaccharides that accumulate in the viscera of patients. Thus, the storage of both ganglioside and mucopolysaccharide may be seen as direct consequences of the deficiency of the galactosidase.

The pleiotropic effect of the single mutation that gives rise to the GM₁ gangliosidosis phenotype conforms to a one gene one polypeptide enzyme multiple substrates model (Figure 90.16). The A₁ enzyme is a monomer that spontaneously dimerizes to form A₂, which can reversibly be formed from the A₃ [69,70,75]. The A₁ isozyme is heterocatalytic, cleaving galactose from many galactoconjugates, among which the GM₁ ganglioside and mucopolysaccharide are two. Different phenotypes in which bone or cerebral manifestations predominate could result from different mutations that selectively affect the catalytic activity for one or another set of substrates. Patients have been described [58] in whom there is relatively normal activity against the peripheral galactose-containing glycoconjugates and little or none against GM₁, and the phenotype is of rapid neurologic degeneration without bony abnormalities. Similarly, patients with the Morquio type B phenotype have severe skeletal dysplasia without neurologic abnormalities [11,58,59].

The direct consequences of the defective enzymatic activity against the various subtrates are the accumulation of ganglioside in brain and keratan sulfate in bone and tissues. In addition, galactose-containing oligosaccharides accumulate

Table 90.1 *Mutations in the gene for β-galactosidase*

Exon	Amino acid	DNA
2	Arg49 → Cys	CGC → TGC
3	Gly123 → Arg	GGG → AGG
3	Duplication-stop codon	288–310
6	Arg201 → Cys	CGG → TGC
	Arg208 → Cys	CGG → TGC
9	Tyr316 → Cys	TAT → TGT
11–12	Duplication	1103–1267
14	Arg457 → Ter	CGA → TGA
	Arg482 → His	CGE → CAC
15	Gly494 → Cys	GGT → TGT
15	Lys577 → Arg	AAG–AGG

Late infantile/juvenile GM₁ gangliosidosis		
6	Arg201 → Cys	GCG → TGC
16	Glu632 → Gly	GAA → GGA

Chronic adult GM₁ gangliosidosis		
2	Ile51 → Thr	ATC → ACC
2–3	Thr82 → Met	ACG → ATG
14	Arg457 → Gln	CGA → CAA

Morquio B disease		
8	Trp273 → Leu	TGG → CTG
14	Arg482 → Cys	CGC → CGT
15	Trp509 → Cys	TGG → TGT

in the viscera and are excreted in the urine, which can be very useful in diagnosis [14–17,21,32,42,70,82–87]. The variety of oligosaccharides excreted is great. The most abundant are similar to partially degraded erythrocyte glycoprotein [70]. They are all galacto-oligosaccharides that contain a terminal galactose in β-1-4 linkage to N-acetylglucosamine [83,87]. This is in contrast to GM₁ ganglioside, in which the linkage of the terminal galactose is 1→3 to N-acetylgalactosamine. In the most sensitive method [86], which employs the high performance liquid chromatography of oligosaccharides made radioactive by reaction with tritium-labeled sodium borohydride, the infantile phenotype could be distinguished from the juvenile by an increase of 3- to 10-fold higher levels of oligosaccharides and especially higher concentrations in the higher molecular weight compounds. Patients with adult onset disease had levels 130- to 180-fold lower than those with infantile onset disease and no high molecular weight oligosaccharides. Three fractions were present in the infantile but not in the juvenile patients, suggesting an ability of the juvenile patients to cleave compounds not cleavable in the infantile form [85].

The cloning of the human gene for β-galactosidase [14] has permitted elucidation of the molecular biology of the β-galactosidase deficiencies. The gene contains 16 exons. Mutations have been found in examples of each of the clinical phenotypes. Most have been missense mutations, and the majority of patients studied have been Japanese [14–17,54]

(Table 90.1). In general, mRNA is normal in size and quantity in late infantile, adult and Morquio B phenotypes, and reduced or absent in infantile patients. In an infantile patient with reduced but detectable mRNA a point mutation led to a change from arginine 49 to cysteine (R49C) [15]. In another infantile patient arginine 457 was changed to a stop codon [15]. Among these patients, two duplications were found [16,17,88]; that in exon 3 led to a premature termination. The other led to an abnormally large mRNA. R208C has been found relatively commonly in American infantile patients [89], and R482H in Italian patients with this phenotype [90]. In four juvenile Japanese patients, all were found to have a mutation of arginine 201 to cystine [15], while six adult patients all had the isoleucine 51 to threonine mutation (I51T). This mutation [15] creates a Bsu36I restriction site in exon 2 that is useful for diagnosis and genetic analysis [54]. Some compounds of two mutant genes have been observed. In Morquio B disease 3 missense mutations have been identified; all three individuals in two families were genetic compounds [17]. W273L has been relatively common in Caucasian patients with the Morquio B phenotype [17]. In general among compounds, the allele with the higher residual activity determines the clinical phenotype [89].

TREATMENT

Effective treatment has not yet been developed. The availability of animal models, in both cats [91] and dogs [92], as well as sheep and cattle provides subjects for the exploration of experimental approaches to therapy. Allogenic bone marrow transplantation in an affected Portuguese water dog was without effect on clinical course or enzyme activity despite engraftment. Amniocyte transplantation was without effect in a patient with Morquio B disease. Trihexyphenidyl appeared to modulate dystonia in a patient with the adult phenotype [93]. Gene transfer is under study in experimental animals.

Among promising approaches to therapy, substrate reduction with the iminosugar N-butyldeoxygalactonojirimycin (Zavesca®) has been shown [94] to reduce significantly cerebral storage of GM₁ ganglioside in β-galactosidase-deficient knockout mice. Another approach is chaperone therapy: N-octyl-4-epi-β-valienamine (NOEV) is an inhibitor of lysosomal β-galactosidase, but in low concentration it restored enzyme activity in cultured human fibroblasts expressing the mutations R201C and R201H [95]. In addition, oral administration for a week enhanced enzyme activity in the brain of a mouse model of juvenile GM₁ gangliosidosis expressing the R201C mutant protein and reduced histochemically detected GM₁ in brain. It is thought that the effects of NOEV represent chaperone function which would be expected to function in the case of milder variables whose enzyme is synthesized with normal or near normal enzyme activity, but fails in normal transport to the lysosome.

References

1. O'Brien JS. Gangliosode storage diseases. An updated review. *J Neurol Sci* 1981;**3**:219.

2. Sandhoff K, Christomanou H. Biochemistry and genetics of gangliosidoses. *Hum Genet* 1979;**50**:107.

3. O'Brien J. Generalized gangliosidosis. *J Pediatr* 1969;**75**:167.

4. Landing BH, Silverman FN, Craig JM, et al. Familial neurovisceral lipidosis. *Am J Dis Child* 1964;**108**:503.

5. O'Brien JS, Stern MB, Landing BH, et al. Generalized gangliosidosis. *Am J Dis Child* 1965;**109**:338.

6. Okada S, O'Brien JS. Generalized gangliosidosos: beta-galactosidase deficiency. *Science* 1968;**160**:1002.

7. O'Brien JS, Ho MW, Veath ML, et al. Juvenile GM$_1$-gangliosidosis: clinical, pathological, chemical and enzymatic studies. *Clin Genet* 1972;**3**:411.

8. Lowden JA, Callahan JW, Norman MG. Juvenile GM$_1$-gangliosidosis. Occurrence with absence of two β-galactosidase components. *Arch Neurol* 1974;**31**:200.

9. Suzuki Y, Nakamura N, Fukuoka K, et al. β-Galactosidase deficiency in juvenile and adult patients. Report of six Japanese cases and review of literature. *Hum Genet* 1977;**36**:219.

10. O'Brien JS, Gugler E, Giedion A, et al. Spondyloepiphyseal dysplasia, corneal clouding, normal intelligence and acid β-galactosidase deficiency. *Clin Genet* 1976;**9**:495.

11. Arbisser AI, Donnelly KA, Scott CI, et al. Morquio-like syndrome with β-galactosidase deficiency and normal hexosamine sulfatase activity: mucopolysaccharidosis IVB. *Am J Med Genet* 1977;**1**:195.

12. van der Horst GTJ, Kleijer WJ, Hoofgeveen AT, et al. Morquio B syndrome: a primary defect in β-galactosidase. *Am J Med Genet* 1983;**16**:261.

13. Shows TB, Scrafford-Wolff L, Brown JA, and Meisler M. Assignment of a beta-galactosidase gene (beta-GAL-alpha) to chromosome 3 in man. *Cytogenet Cell Genet* 1978;**22**:219.

14. Oshima A, Tsuji A, Nagao Y, et al. Cloning, sequencing, and expression of cDNA for human beta-galactosidase. *Biochem Biophys Res Commun* 1988;**157**:238.

15. Nishimoto J, Nanba E, Inui K, et al. GM$_1$-gangliosidosis (genetic beta-galactosidase deficiency): identification of four mutations in different clinical phenotypes among Japanese patients. *Am J Hum Genet* 1991;**49**:566.

16. Yoshida K, Oshima A, Shimmoto M, et al. Human beta-galactosidase gene mutations in G(M$_1$)-gangliosidosis: a common mutation among Japanese adult/chronic cases. *Am J Hum Genet* 1991;**49**:435.

17. Oshima A, Yoshida K, Shimmoto M, et al. Human beta-galactosidase gene mutations in Morquio B disease. *Am J Hum Genet* 1991;**49**:1091.

18. Suzuki Y, Oshima A. A β-galactosidase gene mutation identified in both Morquio B disease and infantile GM$_1$-gangliosidosis. *Hum Genet* 1993;**91**:407.

19. Stone DL, Sidransky E. Hydrops fetalis: lysosomal storage disorders in extremis. *Adv Pediatr* 1999;**46**:409.

20. Tasso MJ, Martinez-Gutierrez A, Carrascosa C, et al. GM$_1$-gangliosidosis presenting as nonimmune hydrops fetalis: a case report. *J Perinat Med* 1996;**24**:445.

21. Emery JM, Green WR, Wyllie RG, Howell RR. GM$_1$ gangliosidosis. *Arch Ophthalmol* 1971;**85**:177.

22. Barbarik A, Benson PF, Fenson AH, Barrie H. Corneal clouding in GM$_1$ generalized gangliosidosis. *Br J Ophthalmol* 1976;**60**:565.

23. Hooft C, Senesael L, Delbeke MJ, et al. The GM$_1$-gangliosidosis (Landing disease). *Eur Neurol* 1969;**2**:225.

24. Feldges A, Muller HJ, Buhler E, Stalder G. GM$_1$-gangliosidosis. I. Clinical aspects and biochemistry. *Helv Paediatr Acta* 1973;**28**:511.

25. Hubain P, Adam E, Dewelle A, et al. Etude d'une observation de gangliosidose à GM$_1$. *Helv Paediatr Acta* 1969;**24**:337.

26. Beratis NG, Varvarigou-Frimas A, Beratis S, Sklower SL. Angiokeratoma corporis diffusum in GM$_1$ gangliosidosis, type 1. *Clin Genet* 1989;**36**:59.

27. Rosenberg H, Frewen TC, Li MD, et al. Cardiac involvement in diseases characterized by β-galactosidase deficiency. *J Pediatr* 1985;**106**:78.

28. Kohlschutter A, Sieg K, Schuylte FJ, et al. Infantile cardiomyopathy and neuromyopathy with beta-galactosidase deficiency. *Europ J Pediat* 1982;**139**:75.

29. Benson PF, Babarik A, Brown SP, Mann TP. GM1-generalized gangliosidosis variant with cardiomegaly. *Postgrad Med J* 1976;**52**:159.

30. Fricker H, O'Brien JS, Vassella F, et al. Generalized gangliosidosis: acid β-gangliosidase deficiency with early onset, rapid mental deterioration and minimal bone dysplasia. *J Neurol* 1976;**12**:329.

31. Caffey J. Gargoylism (Hunter-Hurler disease, dysostosis multiplex, lipochondrodystrophy): prenatal and neonatal bone lesions and their early postnatal evolution. *Bull Hosp Joint Dis* 1951;**12**:38.

32. Spranger JW, Langer LEO, Wiedemann HR. GM$_1$ gangliosidosis: in *Bone Dysplasias: An Atlas of Constitutional Disorders of Skeletal Development.* (JW Spranger, LEO Langer, HR Wiedemann) W.B. Saunders Co, Philadelphia;1974:171.

33. Suzuki K, Suzuki K, Chen GC. Morphological, histochemical and biochemical studies on a case of systemic late infantile lipidosis (generalized gangliosidosis). *J Neuropathol Exp Neurol* 1968;**27**:15.

34. Curless RG. Computed tomography of GM$_1$ gangliosidosis. *J Pediatr* 1984;**105**:964.

35. Kobayashi O, Takashima S. Thalamic hyperdensity on CT in infantile GM$_1$-gangliosidosis. *Brain Dev* 1994;**16**:472.

36. Harden A, Martinovic Z, Pampiglione G. Neurophysiological studies in GM$_1$-gangliosidosis. *Ital J Neurol Sci* 1982;**3**:201.

37. Pampiglione G, Harden A. Neurophysiological investigations in GM$_1$ and GM$_2$-gangliosidosis. *Neuropediatrics* 1984;**15**(suppl):74.

38. Gonatas NK, Gonatas J. Ultrastructural and biochemical observations on a case of systemic late infantile lipidosis and its relationship to Tay-Sachs disease and gargoylism. *J Neuropathol Exp Neurol* 1965;**24**:318.

39. Severi F, Magrini U, Tettamanti G, et al. Infantile GM$_1$ gangliosidosis. Histochemical, ultrastructural and biochemical studies. *Helv Paediatr Acta* 1971;**26**:192.

40. O'Brien JS, Bernett J, Veath ML, Paa D. Lysosomal storage disorders: diagnosis by ultrastructural examination of skin biopsies. *Arch Neurol* 1975;**32**:592.

41. Suzuki K. Cerebral GM$_1$ gangliosidosis: Chemical pathology of visceral organs. *Science* 1968;**159**:1471.

42. Wolfe LS, Calahan J, Fawcett JS, et al. GM$_1$ gangliosidosis without chondrodystrophy or visceromegaly. *Neurology* 1970;**20**:23.

43. Singer HS, Schafer IA. Clinical and enzymatic variations in GM$_1$ generalized gangliosidosis. *Am J Hum Genet* 1972;**24**:454.

44. Patton VM, Dekaban AS. GM$_1$ gangliosidosis and juvenile cerebral lipidosis. *Arch Neurol* 1971;**24**:529.

45. Generoso G, Gascon MD, Ozand PT, Erwin RE. GM$_1$ gangliosidosis type 2 in two siblings. *J Child Neurol* 1992;**7**:41.

46. Owman T, Sjöblad S, Gohlin J. Radiographic skeletal changes in juvenile GM$_1$ gangliosidosis. *Fortschr Röntgenstr* 1980;**132**:692.

47. Derry DM, Fawcett JS, Andermann F, Wolfe LS. Late infantile systemic lipidosis. Major monosialogangliosidosis. Delineation of two types. *Neurology* 1968;**18**:340.

48. Takamoto K, Beppu H, Hirose K, Uono M. Juvenile β-galactosidase deficiency – a case with mental deterioration, dystonic movement, pyramidal symptoms, dysostosis and cherry red spot. *Clin Neurol* (Tokyo) 1980;**20**:339.

49. Weissbluth M, Esterly NB, Caro WA. Report of an infant with GM$_1$ type I and extensive and unusual mongolian spots. *Br J Dermatol* 1981;**104**:195.

50. Selsor LC, Lesher JLJ. Hyperpigmented macules and patches in a patient with GM$_1$ type 1 gangliosidosos. *J Am Acad Dermatol* 1990;**20**:878.

51 Esterly NB, Weissbluth M, Caro WA. Mongolian spots and GM₁ type 1 gangliosidosis. *J Am Acad Dermatol* 1990;**22**:320.

52 Stevenson RE, Taylor HA and Parks S. β-Galactosidase deficiency: prolonged survival in three patients following early central nervous deterioration. *Clin Genet* 1978;**13**:305.

53 Wenger DA, Sattler M, Mueller OT, *et al.* Adult GM₁ gangliosidosis: clinical and biochemical studies on two patients and comparison to other patients called variant or adult GM₁ gangliosidosis. *Clin Genet* 1980;**17**:323.

54 Yoshida K, Oshima A, Sakuraba H, *et al.* GM₁-gangliosidosis in adults: clinical and molecular analysis of 16 Japanese patients. *Ann Neurol* 1992;**31**:328.

55 Goldman JE, Katz D, Rapin I, *et al.* Chronic GM₁ gangliosidosis in presenting as dystonia: I. Clinical and pathological features. *Ann Neurol* 1981;**9**:465.

56 Kobayashi T, Suzuki K. Chronic GM₁ gangliosidosis in presenting as dystonia; II. Biochemical studies. *Ann Neurol* 1981;**9**:476.

57 Yamamoto A, Adachi S, Kawamura S, *et al.* Localised β-galactosidase deficiency. Occurrence in cerebellar ataxia with myoclonus epilepsy and macular cherry-red spot – a new variant of GM₁-gangliosidosis? *Arch Intern Med* 1974;**134**:627.

58 Groebe H, Krins M, Schmidberger H, *et al.* Morquio syndrome (mucopolysaccharidoses IV B) associated with β-galactosidase deficiency. Report of two cases. *Am J Hum Genet* 1980;**32**:258.

59 van Gemund JJ, Giesberts MA, Eerdmans RF *et al.* Morquio-B disease, spondyloepiphyseal dysplasis associated with acid β-galactosidase deficiency. Report of three cases in one family. *Hum Genet* 1983;**64**:50.

60 Giugliani R, Jackson M, Skinner SJ, *et al.* Progressive mental regression in siblings with Morquio disease Type B (mucopolysaccharidosis IV B). *Clin Genet* 1987;**32**:313.

61 Farrell DF, Ochs U. GM₁: Phenotypic variation in a single family. *Ann Neurol* 1981;**9**:225.

62 Singer HS, Schafer IA. White cell β-galactosidase activity. *N Engl J Med* 1970;**282**:571.

63 Lowden JA, Cutz E, Conen PE, *et al.* Prenatal diagnosis of GM₁ gangliosidosis. *N Engl J Med.* 1973;**288**:255.

64 Kaback MM, Sloan HR, Sonneborn M, *et al.* GM₁ gangliosidosis type I in utero: detection and fetal manifestations. *J Pediatr* 1973;**82**:1037.

65 Booth CW, Gerbie AB, Nadler HL, Intrauterine diagnosis of GM₁ gangliosidosis, type 2. *Pediatrics* 1973;**52**:521.

66 Warner TG, Robertson AD, Mock AK, *et al.* Prenatal diagnosis of GM₁ gangliosidosis by detection of galactosyl-oligosaccharides in amniotic fluid with high performance liquid chromatography. *Am J Hum Genet* 1983;**35**:1034.

67 Kleijer WJ, Van der Veer E, Niermeijer MF. Rapid prenatal diagnosis of GM₁-gangliosidosis using microchemical methods. *Hum Genet* 1976;**33**:299.

68 Norden AGW, O'Brien JS. Ganglioside GM₁ β-galactosidase: studies in human liver and brain. *Arch Biochem Biophys* 1973;**159**:383.

69 Norden AGW, Tennant LL, O'Brien JS. GM₁ ganglioside A; purification and studies of the enzyme from human liver. *J Biol Chem* 1974;**249**:7969.

70 Frost RG, Holmes EW, Norden AGW, O'Brien JS. Characterization of purified human liver acid β-galactosidases A₂ and A₃. *Biochem J* 1978;**175**:181.

71 D'Azzo A, Hoogeveen A, Reuser ADJ, *et al.* Molecular defect in combined β-galactosidase and neuroaminidase deficiency. *Proc Natl Acad Sci USA* 1982;**79**:4535.

72 Shows T, Scrafford-Wolff LR, Brown JA, Meisler MH. GM₁ gangliosidosis: chromosome 3 assignment of the β-galactosidase gene. *Somatic Cell Genet* 1979;**5**:147.

73 Takano T, Yamanouchi Y. Assignment of human β-galactosidase-A gene to 3p21.33 by fluorescence *in situ* hybridization. *Hum Genet* 1993;**92**:403.

74 Hoogeveen AT, Verheijen FW, Galjaard H. The relationship between human lysosomal β-galactosidase and its protective protein. *J Biol Chem* 1983;**258**:12143.

75 O'Brien JS. Molecular genetics of GM₁ β-gangliosidosis: *Clin Genet* 1975;**8**:303.

76 Macbrinn MC, Okada S, Ho MW, *et al.* Generalized gangliosidosis: impaired cleavage of galactose from a mucopolysaccharide and a glycoprotein. *Science* 1969;**163**:946.

77 Singer HS, Nankervis GA, Schafer IA. Leukocyte beta-galactosidase activity in the diagnosis of generalized GM₁ gangliosidosis. *Pediatrics* 1972;**49**:352.

78 Sloan HR, Uhlendorf W, Jacobson CB, Frederickson DS. β-Galactosidase in tissue culture derived from human skin and bone marrow: enzyme defect in GM₁ gangliosidosis. *Pediatr Res* 1969;**3**:532.

79 Yutaka T, Okada S, Kato T, Yabuuchi H. Impaired degradation of keratan sulfate in GM₁-gangliosidosis. *Clin Chim Acta* 1982;**125**:233.

80 Beck M, Petersen EM, Spranger J, Beighton P. Morquio's disease type B (β-galactosidase deficiency) in three siblings. *S Afr Med J* 1987;**72**:704.

81 Pinsky L, Powell E, Callahan J. GM₁-gangliosidosis types 1 and 2: enzymatic differences in cultured fibroblasts. *Nature* 1970;**228**:1093.

82 Wolfe LS, Senior RG, Ng Y, Kin NMK. The structures of oligosaccharides accumulating in the liver of GM₁ gangliosidosis, type 1. *J Biol Chem* 1974;**249**:1828

83 Strecker G, Montreuil JG. Glycoproteins et glycoproteinoses. *Biochemie* 1979;**61**:1199.

84 Yamashito K, Ohkura T, Okada S, *et al.* Urinary oligosaccharides of GM₁ gangliosidosis. Different excretion patterns in the urine of type 1 and type 2 subgroups. *J Biol Chem* 1981;**256**:45789.

85 Ohkura T, Yamashito K, Kobata Q. Urinary oligosaccharides of GM₁-gangliosidosis. Structure of oligosaccharides excreted in the urine of type 1 but not in the urine of type 2 patients. *J Biol Chem* 1981;**256**:8485.

86 Warner TG, Robertson AD, O'Brien JS. Diagnosis of GM₁ gangliosidosis based on defect in the urinary oligosaccharides with high performance liquid chromatography. *Clin Chim Acta* 1983;**127**:313.

87 Holmes Z, O'Brien JS. Separation of glycoprotein derived oligosaccharides by thin-layer chromatography. *Anal Biochem* 1979;**93**:167.

88 Oshima A, Yoshida K, Ishizaki A, *et al.* GM₁-gangliosidosis: tandem duplication within exon 3 of β-galactosidase gene in an infantile patient. *Clin Genet* 1992;**41**:235.

89 Boustany R-M, Qian W-H, Suzuki K. Mutations in acid β-galactosidase cause GM₁-gangliosidosis in American patients. *Am J Hum Genet* 1993;**53**:881.

90 Mosna G, Fattore S, Tubiello G, *et al.* A homozygous missense arginine to histidine substation at position 482 of the β-galactosidase in an Italian infantile GM₁-gangliosidosis patient. *Hum Genet* 1992;**90**:247.

91 Baker HJ, Lindsay JR. Feline GM₁-gangliosidosis. *Am J Pathol* 1974;**74**:649.

92 Read DH, Harrington DD, Kenan TW, Hinsman EJ. Neuronal visceral GM₁ gangliosidosis in a dog with β-gangliosidase deficiency. *Science* 1976;**194**:442.

93 Ushiyama M, Hanyu N, Ikeda S, Yanagisawa N. A case of type III (adult) GM₁-gangliosidosis that improved markedly with trihexyphenidyl. *Clin Neurol (Tokyo)* 1986;**26**:221.

94 Kasperzyk JL, El-Abbadi MM, Hauser EC, *et al.* N-butyldeoxygalactonojirimycin reduces neonatal brain ganglioside content in a mouse model of GM₁ gangliosidosis. *J Neurochem* 2004;**89**:645.

95 Matsudo J, Suzuki O, Oshima A, *et al.* Chemical chaperone therapy for brain pathology in GM₁-gangliosidosis. *Proc Nat Acad Sci USA* 2003;**100**:15912.

Tay-Sachs disease/hexosaminidase A deficiency

MAJOR PHENOTYPIC EXPRESSION

Infantile cerebral and retinal degeneration with cherry red macular spots, hyperacusis, macrocephaly, storage of GM_2 ganglioside in the brain, and deficiency of hexosaminidase A.

INTRODUCTION

Tay-Sachs disease has been described as the prototype of the lysosomal storage disorders [1]. It represents a paradigm for the success of research in biochemical genetics not only in providing precise molecular understanding of the nature of disease but also in the practical community-based control of a genetic disease.

The disease was first described by Tay [2] in 1881 in an infant in whom a cherry macular spot was associated with delayed development. Sachs [3] defined the clinical entity, which he called a familial amaurotic idiocy [4]. The enzymatic defect was discovered in 1969 by Okada and O'Brien [5]. The deficiency in hexosaminidase A results in a failure to cleave the terminal N-acetylgalactosamine (GalNAc) from the GM_2 ganglioside (Figure 91.1). The development of methodology for the rapid, relatively easy quantification of the A isozyme has permitted accurate identification of heterozygous carriers of the gene and prenatal diagnosis, permitting a public health approach to human genetics and the virtual prevention of the birth of affected children in the population at highest risk [6,7].

The various disorders of ganglioside GM_2 storage are summarized in Table 91.1. All are progressive cerebral degenerative diseases. The cherry red macular spot is a prominent feature in all of the early infantile presentations, all of which are fatal in infancy. All of these diseases are autosomal recessive. Neuronal lipidosis is a common histologic feature and results from the storage of ganglioside. Deficiency of lysosomal hydrolase activity provides in each a molecular explanation for the disease in which storage of GM_2 ganglioside results from failure to cleave its terminal GalNAc. There are three types of GM_2 gangliosidosis. Sandhoff disease (Chapter 92) has been referred to as the O variant to indicate that neither hexosaminidase A nor hexosaminidase B is active. In this classification Tay-Sachs disease was termed the B variant, since only the B isozyme is active; in what was called the AB variant both enzymes are active and the defect is in the GM_2 activator (Chapter 93).

Hexosaminidase A is a heterodimer containing the α and β subunits. Hexosaminidase B is composed of two β subunits. Cultured cells of patients with Tay-Sachs disease lack the α chain. The genes for the α and β chains have been cloned and the locus for the α chain and for Tay-Sachs disease is on chromosome 15q23 [8]. The gene is common in Ashkenazi Jews. A considerable number and variety of mutations have been described, most in patients with the classic infantile phenotype [9,10]. The most frequent mutation in the Ashkenazi Jewish population is a four-nucleotide insertion in exon 11, which introduces a frame shift and a downstream premature termination signal that results in a deficiency of mRNA.

CLINICAL ABNORMALITIES

Patients with Tay-Sachs disease appear normal at birth, although storage of GM_2 ganglioside has been demonstrated

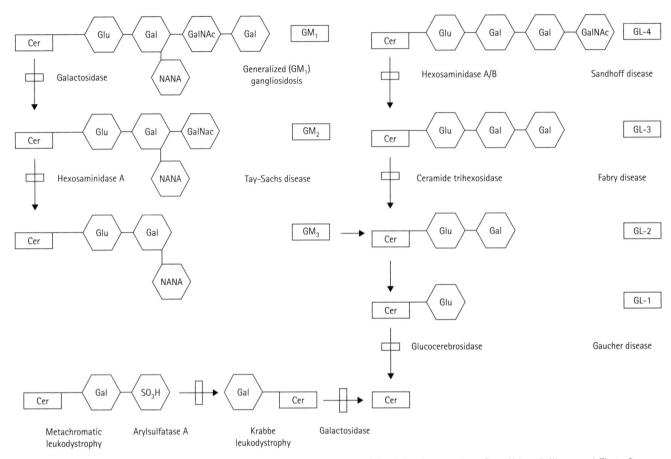

Figure 91.1 *Metabolic pathways of glycosphingolipid metabolism. The site of the defect in a number of conditions is illustrated. That of Tay-Sachs disease is in hexosaminidase A, which catalyzes the removal of N-acetyl-galactosamine from the GM$_2$ lipid to produce GM$_3$. Abbreviations used are* Cer, ceramide; Glu, glucose; Gal, galactose; NANA, N-acetyl-neuraminic acid; and GalNac, N-acetylgalactosamine.

Table 91.1 *GM$_2$ ganglioside storage diseases*

Disorder	Age at onset	Age at death (y)	Enzyme defect	Carrier detection	Prenatal diagnosis
Tay-Sachs disease	3–6 months	2–4	Hexosaminidase A	+	Established
Sandhoff disease	3–6 months	2–4	Hexosaminidase A and B	+	Established
AB variant	3–6 months		Activator	+	Possible
Juvenile GM$_2$ gangliosidosis	2–6 years	5–15	Hexosaminidase A	+	Possible
Adult GM$_2$ gangliosidosis	2 years–adulthood	Variable	Hexosaminidase A	+	Possible

even in the fetus [11]. Infants continue to appear alert and healthy until about 6 months-of-age. The onset of clinical disease may be between birth and 10 months-of-age [12]. The earliest clinical manifestation may be an exaggerated startle response to sound, in which the arms and legs extend. This usually is present by 1 month-of-age, but it may not be appreciated early, since it can be seen in some normal babies, usually disappearing in about 4 months. In contrast, in the baby with Tay-Sachs disease this hyperacusis becomes more prominent. It is brought on even by very gentle sound stimuli. It may be accompanied by clonus.

Parents may notice motor weakness as the first clinical sign. By 8 months-of-age the baby may look sleepy or less alert. The infant may begin to sit less well or to begin to lose head control.

Physical examination at this stage reveals hypotonia. This is progressive. By 1 year-of-age few of these patients can sit without support. The usual developmental milestones are lost or never attained. There may be nystagmus and a fixed, staring or roving gaze. Examination of the fundus reveals the typical cherry red spot in the macula (Figure 91.2). This is usually present as early as 2 months-of-age and has been demonstrated by retinal photography as early as the first days of life. In looking for this it is important to remember that the white degeneration of the macula is larger and more impressive than the red foveal spot in the middle. Together they look very much like a fried egg. Lipid storage in the ganglion cells obscures the choroidal vessels behind. In the fovea, where ganglion cells are few in number, vascularity of the choroid is seen as the red spot. With

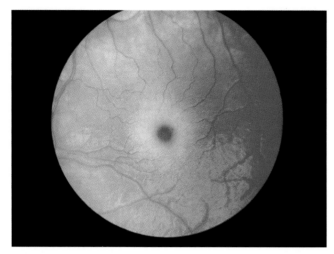

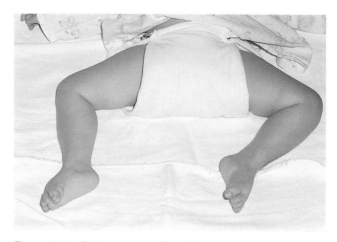

Figure 91.2 *The cherry red spot. Photograph of the fundus of an infant with Tay-Sachs disease.*

Figure 91.4 *The lower extremities of the same patient were flaccid.*

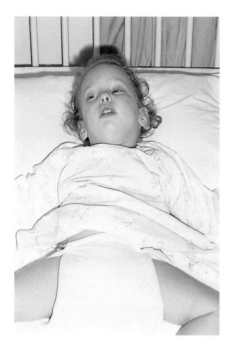

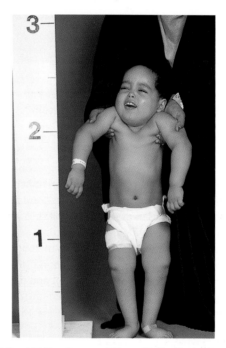

Figure 91.3 *A.S., a 2-year-old patient with Tay-Sachs disease. He was blind and decerebrate at this time. Hexosaminidase A activity was absent.*

Figure 91.5 *M.A.S., a 2-year-old boy with Tay-Sachs disease. He was hypotonic but had increased deep tendon reflexes and positive Babinski responses. He had hyperacusis and was blind.*

time the spot may become darker or brownish in color. Opaque white streaks may develop along the vessels.

Cerebral and macular degeneration is rapidly progressive. The infant becomes blind, rigid and decerebrate by 12 to 18 months (Figure 91.3), and usually must be fed by tube because swallowing is ineffective. The extremities may be flaccid (Figure 91.4), but muscle tone is usually increased, and there is hyperreflexia (Figures 91.5, 91.6) and opisthotonos. Convulsions and myoclonic jerks are common. Seizures almost invariably occur after 1 year-of-age but they are not difficult to control with anticonvulsant medication. Electroencephalograph (EEG) abnormalities are relatively mild but become progressive after

the first year [13]. The electroretinogram is normal but visual evoked potentials disappear.

Patients often have a doll-like facial appearance (Figure 91.3) with clear, translucent skin, long eyelashes, fine hair and delicate pink coloring. After about 15 months the head size usually enlarges. By this time there is decerebrate posturing, difficulty with swallowing and secretions, and vegetative unresponsiveness. The brain weight at the time of death may be 50 percent heavier than normal. This is a consequence of glial proliferation and of lipid storage. There is no hepatosplenomegaly or other peripheral evidence of storage disease.

Death usually results from aspiration and pneumonia; usually by 2 to 4 years-of-age. Pathologic changes are restricted to

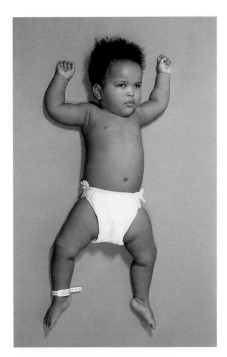

Figure 91.6 *F.H.S., a 16-month-old girl with Tay-Sachs disease. She was hypotonic but hyper-reflexic and had bilateral ankle clonus and positive Babinski responses. Pupils reacted poorly to light, and she had bilateral cherry red spots.*

the nervous system, where the neurons are swollen, or 'ballooned', displacing the nucleus toward the periphery [14]. This picture may be seen in neurons of the autonomic system and rectal mucosa as well as in the cerebral cortex. 'Meganeurites' have been described among cortical neurons [15]. Electron microscopy of the neuron reveals lamellar membranous cytoplasmic bodies [16]. These inclusions are round concentric layers of accumulated ganglioside cholesterol and phospholipid in lysosomes. Pathologic changes can be demonstrated by electron microscopic study of biopsied skin [17,18]. As axonal degeneration proceeds in the brain there is secondary demyelination and cortical gliosis. Membranous cytoplasmic bodies have been found in fetal brain as early as 12 weeks [19].

A certain amount of genetic heterogeneity has been established among GM_2 gangliosidoses [20–22]. The first to be appreciated was Sandhoff disease (Chapter 92), in which there is deficiency of both hexosaminidases A and B and a phenotype indistinguishable from that of Tay-Sachs disease. This is also true of GM_2 activator deficiency (Chapter 93).

A more indolent phenotype referred to as juvenile GM_2 gangliosidosis has an onset at about 2 years-of-age with ataxia and incoordination. Speech is lost and deterioration is progressive to spasticity and decerebrate rigidity. Activity of hexosaminidase A is deficient but not to the degree seen in Tay-Sachs disease [20,23]. A less severe form of GM_2 gangliosidosis has been referred to as adult or chronic GM_2 gangliosidosis [24]. This and the juvenile phenotype represent parts of a spectrum of genetically determined variants, ranging from the classic infantile Tay-Sachs phenotype to adult disease that

progresses so slowly intellect is hardly affected. The advent of molecular biology and the very extensive documentation of mutation make most of these clinical classifications obsolete.

Prominent features in variant patients are distal or proximal muscle atrophy, pes cavus or foot drop, as well as spasticity, dystonic movements, dysarthria, and ataxia. The overall picture may be reminiscent of spinocerebellar degeneration [24,25]. Some patients [26] have been clinically normal when first diagnosed on the basis of low enzyme activity, but later have developed difficulties of speech and gait. Others have been studied [27,28] in whom clinical manifestations have not been observed. Psychotic disease has been common in adult onset GM_2 gangliosidosis [29,30]. Response to antipsychotic medication has been poor. Some patients have been observed with problems of supranuclear gaze [31], raising the differential diagnosis of Niemann-Pick type C disease (Chapter 96).

An assay has been developed [23] in which fibroblasts of the various phenotypes have had activities of hexosaminidase A that correlated well with the clinical picture. In this assay patients with Tay-Sachs disease displayed 0.1 percent of control activity, the late-infantile or so-called juvenile 0.5 percent, and the adult GM_2 gangliosidosis 2–4 percent. The clinically asymptomatic individuals with low hexosaminidase activity had 11–20 percent of control activity.

GENETICS AND PATHOGENESIS

Tay-Sachs disease is transmitted as an autosomal recessive disease. The gene frequency in Ashkenazi Jews has been calculated to be approximately one in 30 [6]. This would predict an annual incidence of one in 4000 births with Tay-Sachs disease among parents from this population. These frequencies were so high that it became practical to undertake programs of prevention through heterozygote detection. Gene frequency in non-Jews has been calculated to be one in 300 [6,32]. The disease is also common in some isolates in Switzerland [33] and in French descendants in Eastern Quebec and Southern Louisiana [34].

The GM_2 ganglioside stored in Tay-Sachs disease is an acidic glycosphingolipid with a terminal hexosamine, GalNAc [35–38] (Figure 91.1). The ganglioside, which is normally present in very small amounts, is increased 100 to 1000 times in Tay-Sachs disease. The sphingolipids all contain the long-chain base sphingosine, which has the following structure:

$$CH_3(CH_2)_{12}CH = CH - \underset{\underset{OH}{|}}{CH} - \underset{\underset{OH}{\|}}{CH} - \underset{\underset{NH2}{\|}}{CH} - CH_2OH$$

This compound is acylated with long-chain fatty acids on the amino group on carbon 2 to form ceramide, which makes up the base unit of all of the sphingolipids. In the gangliosides, as well as in the cerebrosides and glycolipids, a sugar is linked glucosidically to carbon 1. In the parent ganglioside, GM_1, the glycolipid that accumulates in generalized gangliosidosis, ceramide is linked successively to glucose; to galactose, to which N-acetylneuraminic acid is attached; to N-acetylgalactosamine; and to galactose. This terminal galactose is cleaved by a β-galactosidase, which is defective in generalized GM$_1$ gangliosidosis, to yield the Tay-Sachs lipid, GM$_2$ [36]. This is normally converted to GM$_3$ by cleavage of the terminal GalNAc. The amounts of GM$_2$ storage in the brain in variant patients tend to be less than in Tay-Sachs disease [39,40].

The defect in hexosaminidase A represents a failure to hydrolyze this terminal aminosugar from the GM$_2$ ganglioside. It was first demonstrated by Okada and O'Brien [5] by starch gel electrophoresis which separated hexosaminidase activity into two components, designated A and B, the former (A) of which was absent in patients with Tay-Sachs disease. The A enzyme is more heat-labile and negatively charged than the B isozyme [38]. The diagnosis is made by measuring total and heat-stable hexosaminidase activity in serum, using artificial methylumbelliferyl N-acetylgalactosamine or N-acetylglucosamine substrate whose product of cleavage is the fluorigenic 4-methylumbelliferone [41]. The heat-labile enzyme is hexosaminidase A, and its activity is represented by the difference in activity before and after denaturation. The enzyme can also be measured in freshly isolated leukocytes, tears and cultured fibroblasts or amniotic fluid cells [42]. In Tay-Sachs disease the activity of hexosaminidase A is virtually zero [5,21,43]. Assays have also employed [20,21] the natural substrate ganglioside GM$_2$.

Cross-reacting material (CRM) was demonstrated using antibodies prepared against human placental hexosaminidase A and the α-subunit of kidney and liver extracts of some patients with Tay-Sachs disease [44], but most are CRM-negative. The gene for the α subunit of hexosaminidase A contains 14 exons over 35 kb and 5′ regulatory elements (TATA) and 3′ untranslated areas [45]. Very many mutations have been documented [6,10,46–50] spanning all 14 exons. Twenty-one of these occur at CpG dinucleotide sites, which are known to be mutagenic hot spots and which account for more than one-third of human polymorphisms and disease mutations [47,48]. Even within the classic Tay-Sachs infantile phenotype almost 100 different mutations have been reported [6,9,10]. Deletions in sections, frameshifts and stop codons are found in this phenotype.

Two mutations account for 93 percent of the mutant alleles in the Ashkenazi Jewish population of North America [9,46] (Table 91.2). In addition to the 4 bp insertion, 1278ins4, the other common deletion in this population is a splice site inversion in intron 12. A G-to-C change in the first nucleotide of the intron leads to several abnormally spliced mRNAs. The other common mutation is the French Canadian mutation, a 7.6 kb deletion in exon 1 and flanking sequences in a population in which the frequency of the disease has been similar to that of the Ashkenazi Jewish population [51].

All of the other mutations are rare and have been found generally in compounds except in consanguineous families. The Δ Phe 304 or 305 represents deletion of one of two adjacent

Table 91.2 *Mutations in the hexosaminidase A gene in Tay-Sachs disease*

Mutation	Population	Frequency
+TATC 1278ius4	Ashkenazi Jewish	80%
+IVS 12 (G →C)	Ashkenazi Jewish	15%
G269S	Ashkenazi Jewish	Most late onset
910 del TTC	Moroccan Jewish	Most of that population
−IVS 5-1G →T	Japanese	Most of that population
+IVS 7 (G →A)	French Canadian	Rare
+IVS 9+1(G →A)	Celtic, French, Pennsylvania Dutch	Rare
ΔPhe304 or 305	Moroccan, Jewish, Irish, French	Rare
−IVS4 (G →T)	Armenian, Black	Rare
C deletion 1510	Italian	Rare
A →G, exon 1	American Black	Rare
G436 deletion (exon 4)	American Black	Rare
C →T 409 (exon 3)	American non-Jewish, Caucasian	Rare

Assembled from data reported by Kaback *et al.* [6].

phenylalanine moieties [48]. The mutation found in two unrelated black American families [49] was an interesting one in which a G-to-T transversion in the invariant AG of the acceptor splice site of intron 4 interfered with splicing. An A-to-G transition in exon 1 found in a black American family changed the initiating methionine to a valine. Of the last two mutations in Table 91.2, C to T409 creates a termination codon, and deletion of G436 frameshift leads to a termination codon. Some interesting mutations interfere with the assembly or processing of a synthesized α subunit. R504C and R504H are secreted, and not retained in early compartments but fail to associate with β subunits to form the enzyme [48,52].

The mutations associated with the later-onset phenotypes of GM$_2$ gangliosidosis have generally been single-base substitutions, leading to a single amino acid change [6]. Many have been found in compounds. In one [53] a mutation, G570A led to alternate splicing in which a certain amount of normal mRNA was made, while in most of the mRNA exon 5 was missing. The adult-onset phenotype in Jewish populations results in a glycine 269 to serine change [54].

Heterozygous carriers of the gene have intermediate activities of hexosaminidase A in their serum or plasma [41]. These values average 65 percent of those of normal. Screening for heterozygosity should be done prior to the development of pregnancy, since this may cause a false positive result in the serum assay. The issue can be resolved by assay of leukocytes.

The heat denaturation assay has been automated and employed in mass screening for heterozygotes throughout the world [55–57]. Such programs have shown that the disease can be virtually eliminated in those at highest risk [6]. Between 1971 and 1992 almost a million people were screened for heterozygosity in 17 countries (Table 91.3). Of these over 36 000 carriers were detected and 1000 couples at risk were identified because both were carriers. Considering couples identified by

Table 91.3 *Prevention of Tay-Sachs disease (1971–1992, showing >90% reduction in the disease in Jewish population (1970–1993)*

Group	Number	
Total screened	9.53×10^6 (seven countries)	
Carriers identified	36 418	
Couples at risk	1056	
Pregnancies monitored	2415*	
Affected fetuses	469	
Aborted	451	
Normal offspring born	1881	
Births per year with Tay-Sachs:		
Prior to 1969	100 (US and Canada)	(80% Jewish)
1980	13	(80% non-Jewish)
1985–1992	3–10	(85% non-Jewish)

* Prior offspring as well as heterozygote screening (1969–1992).

screening and also those identified because of prior offspring, 2416 pregnancies were monitored and 469 affected fetuses were found, of which all but 18 were aborted. More important than the prevention of all these patients with Tay-Sachs disease, almost 2000 normal offspring were born to these couples at risk. When this program began, 50 to 100 infants with Tay-Sachs disease were born annually in the United States and Canada, 80 percent of whom were Jewish. In the past 20 years the incidence has varied between three and 10 annually, of whom 85 percent were non-Jewish. This represents a 90 percent reduction in the incidence of Tay-Sachs disease in the Jewish population of the two countries.

Tay-Sachs disease can be detected prenatally [11]. The enzyme is reliably assayed in cultured amniotic fluid cells or chorionic villus material [6,58]. Tay-Sachs is the metabolic disease most frequently diagnosed prenatally [6]. Early pitfalls or misdiagnoses have been eliminated by regular use of cultured amniotic fluid cells for assay, prior establishment that both parents are heterozygotes [59] and the use of ultrasonography to rule out the presence of twinning. Even so, there have been a few misdiagnoses, all attributable to such laboratory errors as mix-ups of samples.

Testing of potential heterozygotes by enzyme assay with synthetic substrates has uncovered the existence of pseudodeficiency genes that can result in a healthy person who has no hexosaminidase A activity in this assay. Approximately 35 percent of non-Jewish persons identified as heterozygotes by enzyme assay are pseudodeficiency carriers [60]. Many of the individuals have been identified to have a mutation substituting tryptophan 247 for arginine [61]. The existence of the pseudodeficiency allele makes it essential to do mutational analysis in couples at risk because both have been identified as carriers by enzyme analysis. There is no risk if one or both carry the pseudodeficiency allele. In families in which mutation has been identified, analysis for mutation can be employed for heterozygote detection and prenatal diagnosis [62].

TREATMENT

Specific treatment has not been developed. Skilled supportive care should be provided for the family and the patient should be made as comfortable as possible.

References

1   Kaback MM, O'Brien JS. Tay-Sachs: prototype for prevention of genetic disease. *Hosp Pract* 1973;**8**:107.

2   Tay W. Symmetrical changes in the region of the yellow spot in each eye of an infant. *Trans Ophthalmol Soc UK* 1881;**1**:1155.

3   Sachs B. On arrested cerebral development with special reference to its pathology. *J Nerv Ment Dis* 1887;**14**:541.

4   Sachs B. A family form of idiocy generally fatal associated with early blindness. *J Nerv Ment Dis* 1896;**21**:475.

5   Okada S, O'Brien JS. Tay-Sachs disease: generalized absence of a b-d-N-acetylhexosaminidase component. *Science* 1969;**165**:698.

6   Kaback M, Lim-Steele J, Dabholkar D, *et al.* Tay-Sachs disease-carrier screening, prenatal diagnosis and the molecular era. An international perspective 1970 to 1993. *JAMA* 1993;**270**:2307.

7   Kaplan F. Tay-Sachs disease carrier screening: a model for prevention of genetic disease. *Genet Test* 1998;**2**:271.

8   Gilbert F, Kucherlapati R, Creagan RP, *et al.* Tay-Sachs and Sandhoff's diseases: the assignment of genes for hexosaminidases A and B to individual human chromosomes. *Proc Natl Acad Sci USA* 1975;**72**:263.

9   Paw BH, Tieu PT, Kaback MM, *et al.* Frequency of three Hex A mutant alleles among Jewish and non-Jewish carriers identified in a Tay-Sachs screening program. *Am J Hum Genet* 1990;**47**:698.

10 Triggs-Raine BL, Feigenbaum ASJ, Natowicz M, *et al.* Screening for carriers of Tay-Sachs disease among Ashkenazi Jews: a comparison of DNA-based and enzyme-based tests. *N Engl J Med* 1990;**323**:6.

11 O'Brien JS, Okada S, Fillerup DL, *et al.* Tay-Sachs disease: prenatal diagnosis. *Science* 1971;**172**:61.

12 Volk BW (ed). *Tay-Sachs Disease.* Grune and Stratton, New York;1964.

13 Pampiglione G, Privett G, Harden A. Tay-Sachs disease: neurophysiological studies in 20 children. *Develop Med Child Neurol* 1974;**16**:201.

14 Volk BS, Schneck L, Adachi M. Clinic pathology and biochemistry of Tay-Sachs disease: in *Textbook of Neurology* (eds PJ Vinken, GW Bruyn) North-Holland, Amsterdam;1970;**10**:385.

15 Purpura DP, Suzuki K. Distortion of neuronal geometry and formation of aberrant synapses in neuronal storage disease. *Brain Res* 1976;**116**:1.

16 Terry RD, Weiss M. Studies in Tay-Sachs disease. II Ultrastructure of the cerebrum. *J Neuropathol Exp Neurol* (Berl) 1973;**24**:43.

17 Martin JJ, Jacobs K. Skin biopsy as a contribution to diagnosis in late infantile amaurotic idiocy with curvilinear bodies. *Eur Neurol* 1973; **10**:281.

18 O'Brien JS, Bernett J, Veath ML, Paa D. Lysosomal storage disorders: diagnosis by ultrastructural examination of skin biopsy specimens. *Arch Neurol* 1975;**32**:592.

19 Myrianthopoulos N, Aronson S. Reproductive fitness and selection: in *Tay-Sachs Disease and Inborn Errors of Sphingolipid Metabolism* (eds S Aronson, B Volk). Pergamon Press, New York;1967.

20 O'Brien JS, Norden AGW, Miller AL, *et al.* Ganglioside GM₂ N-acetyl-b-d-galactosaminidase and asialo GM₂ (GA2) N-acetyl-b-d-galactosaminidase: studies in human skin fibroblasts. *Clin Genet* 1977;**11**:171.

21 O'Brien JS, Tennant LL, Veath ML, *et al.* Characterization of unusual hexosaminidase A-deficient human mutants. *Am J Hum Genet* 1978;**30**:602.

22 Sandhoff K, Christomanou H. Biochemistry and genetics of gangliosidoses. *Hum Genet* 1979;**50**:107.

23 Conzelmann E, Kytzia H-J, Navon R, Sandhoff K. Ganglioside GM_2 N-acetyl-b-d-galactosaminidase activity in cultured fibroblasts of late-infantile and adult GM_2 gangliosidosis patients and of healthy probands with low hexosaminidase level. *Am J Hum Genet* 1983;**35**:900.

24 Rapin I, Suzuki K, Suzuki K, Valsamis M. Adult (chronic) GM_2 gangliosidosis. Atypical spinocerebellar degeneration in a Jewish sibship. *Arch Neurol* 1976;**33**:120.

25 Kaback M, Miles J, Yaffe M, *et al*. Hexosaminidase A (Hex-A) deficiency in early adulthood: a new type of GM_2 gangliosidosis. *Am J Hum Genet* 1978;**30**:31A.

26 Navon R, Argov Z, Brandt N, Sandbank U. Adult GM_2 gangliosidosis in association with Tay-Sachs disease: a new phenotype. *Neurology* 1981;**31**:1397.

27 Dreyfus JC, Poenaru L, Svennerholm L. Absence of hexosaminidase A and B in a normal adult. *N Engl J Med* 1975;**292**:61

28 Dreyfus JC, Poenaru L, Vilbert M, *et al*. Characterization of a variant of b-hexosaminidase: 'Hexosaminidase Paris'. *Am J Hum Genet* 1977;**29**:287.

29 Navon R, Argov Z, Frisch A. Hexosaminidase A deficiency in adults. *Am J Med Genet* 1986;**24**:179.

30 Argov Z, Navon R. Clinical and genetic variations in the syndrome of adult GM_2 gangliosidosis resulting from hexosaminidase. A deficiency. *Ann Neurol* 1984;**16**:14.

31 Renshaw PF, Stern TA, Welch C, *et al*. Electroconvulsive therapy treatment of depression in a patient with adult GM_2-gangliosidosis. *Ann Neurol* 1992;**31**:342.

32 Petersen GM, Rotter JI, Cantor RM, *et al*. The Tay-Sachs disease gene in North American Jewish populations: geographic variations and origin. *Am J Hum Genet* 1983;**35**:1258.

33 Hanhart E. Uber 27 Sippen mit infantiler amaurotischer Idiotie (Tay-Sachs). *Acta Genet Med Gemellol* 1954;**3**:331.

34 Brzustowicz LM, Lehner T, Castilla LH, *et al*. Genetic mapping of chronic childhood-onset spinal muscular atrophy to chromosome 5q112-133. *Nature* 1990;**344**:540.

35 Klenk E. Uber die ganglioside eine neue Gruppe von zuckerhaltigen Gehirnlipoiden. *Z Physiol Chem* 1942;**273**:76.

36 Svennerholm L. Chemical structure of normal human brain and Tay-Sachs gangliosidoses. *Biochem Biophys Res Commun* 1962;**9**:436.

37 Svennerholm L. Ganglioside metabolism: in *Comprehensive Biochemistry* (eds Florkin M, Stotz EH). American Elsevier Publishing Co Inc, Amsterdam;1970;**18**:201.

38 Robinson D, Stirling JL. N-Acetyl-b-glucosaminidases in human spleen. *Biochem J* 1968;**107**:301.

39 Suzuki K, Rapin I, Suzuki Y, Ishii N. Juvenile GM_2-gangliosidosis: clinical variant of Tay-Sachs disease or a new disease. *Neurology* 1970;**20**:190.

40 Jatzkewitz H, Pilz H, Sandhoff K. The quantitative determination of gangliosides and their derivatives in different forms of amaurotic idiocy. *J Neurochem* 1965;**12**:135.

41 O'Brien JS, Okada S, Chen A, Fillerup DL. Tay-Sachs disease: detection of heterozygotes and homozygotes by serum hexosaminidase assay. *N Engl J Med* 1970;**283**:15.

42 Srivastava SK. Tay-Sachs and Sandhoff disease: in *Practical Enzymology of the Sphingolipidoses* (eds RH Glew, SP Peters). Alan R Liss, New York;1977:217.

43 Okada S, Veath ML, Leroy J, O'Brien JS. Ganglioside GM_2 storage diseases: hexosaminidase deficiencies in cultured fibroblasts. *Am J Hum Genet* 1971;**23**:55.

44 Srivastava SK, Ansari NH, Hawkins LA, Wiktorowicz JE. Demonstration of cross-reacting material in Tay-Sachs disease. *Biochem J* 1979;**179**:657.

45 Proia RL, Saravia E. Organization of the gene encoding the human beta-hexosaminidase alpha-chain. *J Biol Chem* 1987;**262**:5677.

46 Akli S, Boue J, Sandhoff K, *et al*. Collaborative study of molecular epidemiology of Tay-Sachs disease in Europe. *Eur J Hum Genet* 1993;**1**:229.

47 Barker D, Schafer M, White R. Restriction sites containing CpG show a higher frequency of polymorphism in human DNA. *Cell* 1984;**36**:131.

48 Paw BH, Wood LC, Neufeld EF. A third mutation at the CpG dinucleotide of codon 504 and a silent mutation at codon 506 of the HEX A gene. *Am J Hum Genet* 1991;**48**:1139.

49 Mules EH, Dowling CE, Petersen MB, *et al*. A novel mutation in the invariant AG of the acceptor splice site of intron 4 of the b-hexosaminidase a-subunit gene in two unrelated American Black GM_2-gangliosidosis (Tay-Sachs disease) patients. *Am J Hum Genet* 1991;**48**:1181.

50 Mules EH, Hayflick S, Miller CS, *et al*. Six novel deleterious and three neutral mutations in the gene encoding the a-subunit of hexosaminidase A in non-Jewish individuals. *Am J Hum Genet* 1992;**50**:834.

51 Myerowitz R, Hogikyan ND. Different mutations in Ashkenazi Jewish and non-Jewish French Canadians with Tay-Sachs disease. *Science* 1986;**232**:1646.

52 Paw BH, Moskowitz SM, Uhrhammer N, *et al*. Juvenile GM_2 gangliosidosis caused by substitution of histidine for arginine at position 499 or 504 of the alpha-subunit of beta-hexosaminidase. *J Biol Chem* 1990;**265**:9452.

53 Akli S, Chelly J, Mezard C, *et al*. A 'G' to 'A' mutation at position-1 of a 5' splice site in a late infantile form of Tay-Sachs disease. *J Biol Chem* 1990;**265**:7324.

54 Paw BH, Kaback MM, Neufeld EF. Molecular basis of adult-onset and chronic GM_2 gangliosidoses in patients of Ashkenazi Jewish origin: substitution of serine for glycine at position 269 of the alpha-subunit of beta-hexosaminidase. *Proc Natl Acad Sci USA* 1989;**86**:2413.

55 Kaback MM, Zeiger RS. Heterozygote detection in Tay-Sachs disease: a prototype community screening program for the prevention of genetic disorders: in *Sphingolipidoses and Allied Disorders* (eds BW Volk, SM Aronson). Plenum Press, New York;1972:613.

56 Kaback MM. Thermal fractionation of serum hexosaminidase: approaches to heterozygote detection and diagnosis of Tay-Sachs disease: in *Methods in Enzymology* (ed. V Ginsberg). Academic Press, New York;1972:862.

57 Lowden JA, Skomorowski MA, Henderson F, Kaback MM. Automated assays of hexosaminidases in serum. *Clin Chem* 1973;**19**:1345.

58 Grebner EE, Wapner RJ, Barr MA, Jackson LG. Prenatal Tay-Sachs diagnosis by chorionic villi sampling. *Lancet* 1983;**2**:286.

59 O'Brien JS. Pitfalls in the prenatal diagnosis of Tay-Sachs disease: in *Tay-Sachs Disease: Screening and Prevention* (eds M Kaback, D Rimoin, JS O'Brien). Alan R Liss, New York;1977:283.

60 Cantor RM, Lim JS, Roy C, Kaback MM. Sandhoff disease heterozygote detection: a component of population screening for Tay-Sachs disease carriers. I Statistical methods. *Am J Hum Genet* 1985;**37**:912.

61 Triggs-Raine BL, Mules EH, Kaback MM, *et al*. A pseudodeficiency allele common in non-Jewish Tay-Sachs carriers: implications for carrier screening. *Am J Hum Genet* 1992;**51**:793.

62 Triggs Raine BL, Archibald A, Gravel RA, Clarke JT. Prenatal exclusion of Tay-Sachs disease by DNA analysis. *Lancet* 1990;**335**:1164.

Sandhoff disease/GM$_2$ gangliosidosis/deficiency of hexosaminidase A and B/hex-B subunit deficiency

MAJOR PHENOTYPIC EXPRESSION

Progressive cerebral degeneration starting at 6 months-of-age, blindness, cherry red macular spots, hyperacusis, accumulation of GM$_2$ ganglioside, and deficiency of hexosaminidase A and B (Hex-A and Hex-B), resulting from mutation in the gene for Hex-B.

INTRODUCTION

The clinical phenotype of Sandhoff disease may be indistinguishable from that of Tay-Sachs disease (Chapter 91), but there may be hepatosplenomegaly in Sandhoff disease. The distinction between the two conditions was delineated by Sandhoff *et al.* [1] in 1968 in a patient who was unusual in that he stored ganglioside not only in the brain but also in other viscera. In contrast to patients with Tay-Sachs disease, the activity of total hexosaminidase was found to be deficient [1]. Hexosaminidase B is a glycoprotein homopolymer with four identical subunits; its structure is designated $\beta_2\beta_2$ [2,3]. Hexosaminidase A is a heteropolymer of α and β subunits. Activity of the Hex-A and Hex-B isozymes are defective because of a defective β subunit. The disease has also been referred to as GM$_2$ gangliosidosis (variant O). The Hex-B gene is located on chromosome 5q13 [4]. Heterogeneity has been observed in the mutations in the gene for Hex-B [5]. Most mutations lead to the most severe infantile onset phenotype. The causative mutations in these patients tend to be deletions, nonsense mutations, or splice site mutations. The most common is a 16 kb deletion that includes the promoter, exons 1 to 5 and part of the intron [6].

CLINICAL ABNORMALITIES

It has often not been possible to distinguish Sandhoff disease from Tay-Sachs disease clinically [2,3,7–9]. The disorder tends to be suspected in non-Jewish patients with the Tay-Sachs phenotype. Individual patients appear normal at birth and appear to develop normally (Figures 92.1–92.9) until 4–9 months-of-age, when signs of motor weakness and hypotonia begin to become evident. Abilities that have been learned are progressively lost. These might include the ability to grasp objects or to sit, crawl or hold up the head. Patients never learn to walk. Many of these infants have doll-like faces with long eyelashes and fine hair, pale translucent skin and pink coloring. Cherry red macular spots (Figures 92.10, 92.11) are seen bilaterally. Blindness is progressive and optic atrophy develops. Patients develop hyperacusis, or an exaggerated startle response to noise, which may be seen even quite early. The size of the head increases abnormally. Seizures are common; they develop some months after the onset of clear neurologic abnormality. They may be generalized or myoclonic. The electroencephalogram (EEG) also becomes progressively more abnormal. Visual loss is progressive and visual evoked potentials abnormal. Spasticity develops, and mental deterioration continues until the patient

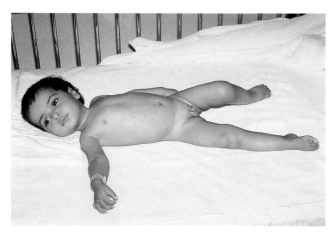

Figure 92.1   *S.O., a 13-month-old with Sandhoff disease in the tonic neck reflex position. He was spastic and hyper-reflexic. Babinski's were positive bilaterally, and he had ankle clonus. The neck was hypotonic.*

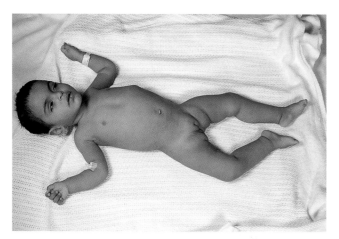

Figure 92.2   *T.O. There was no evidence of coarse features. Activities of hexosaminidase A and B were virtually completely deficient.*

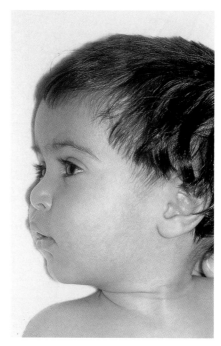

Figure 92.3   *T.O. at 18 months. Regression had begun after 6 months and all milestones were lost. She had an exaggerated startle to noise.*

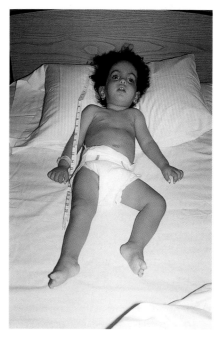

Figure 92.4   *M.O. A 17-month-old with Sandhoff disease. She was flaccid and apathetic. Head circumference was increased and she had acoustic myoclonus to slight sound, as well as myoclonic and tonic seizures. Leukocyte hexosaminidase activity was zero.*

is rigid, decerebrate and completely blind. Computed tomography (CT) scan may reveal the Turkish moustache sign (Figure 92.12). Alimentation requires tube feeding. Death usually occurs between the ages of 1 and 4 years, most often from bronchopneumonia or aspiration.

At autopsy the visceral organs may be somewhat heavier than those of patients with Tay-Sachs disease [7]. Visceral storage may be evident in lipid-laden histiocytes [2]. Some patients may have clinical hepatosplenomegaly, but most do not. Renal tubular cells show lipid deposits. Foamy histiocytes may be seen in bone marrow aspirates. In the brain there is a typical neuronal lipidosis. Membranous cytoplasmic bodies seen by electronmicroscopy are identical to those characteristic of Tay-Sachs disease. Vacuolated cells and lamellar inclusions are demonstrable by conjunctival biopsy.

A small number of variant later onset forms of Sandhoff disease have been observed. They have variously been referred to as juvenile, subacute or adult – chronic, but now that there

are molecular distinctions it is likely that there will be a spectrum of phenotype. The majority of these variants present between 2 and 10 years-of-age, most often with ataxia or incoordination [10–15]. There may be choreoathetosis or dystonia.

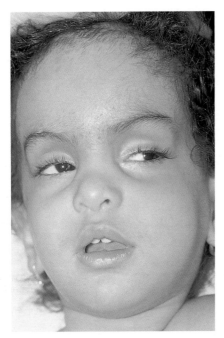

Figure 92.5   *M.O. The vacant facial expression. She had bilateral cherry red spots.*

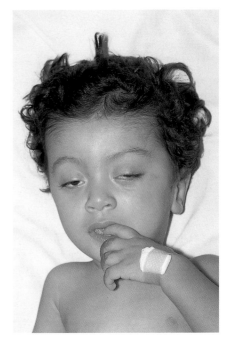

Figure 92.7   *A.M.H. This 14-month-old boy with Sandhoff disease had a similar facial appearance, cherry red macular spots, acoustic myoclonus and no detectable leukocyte hexosaminidase activity.*

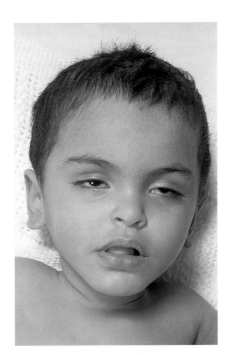

Figure 92.6   *T.O., indicating the similar facial expression.*

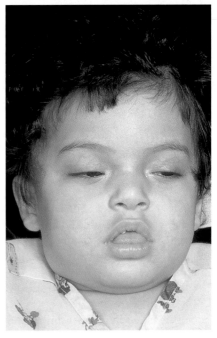

Figure 92.8   *M.S.O., an 11-month-old with Sandhoff disease had a similar facial appearance and cherry red spots.*

Neurodegeneration is progressive, and seizures and spasticity develop. There may be cherry red spots, or more commonly retinitis pigmentosa and optic atrophy. By 10–15 years the patient is blind and decerebrate, as in the infantile patient, and death shortly ensues. One patient referred to as having a juvenile form of Sandhoff disease [11] developed slurred speech, ataxia and some mental deterioration at 5 years-of-age. By 10 he had spasticity, but the optic fundi were normal.

Adult onset patients may have psychiatric symptoms. Ataxia and an apparent spinocerebellar picture may be evident [10–15]. Dysarthria may be severe. The disorder may be very slowly progressive. In late onset patients typical membranous cytoplasmic bodies have been reported in the myenteric plexus [16].

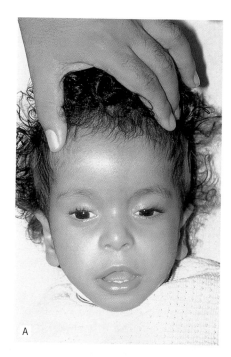

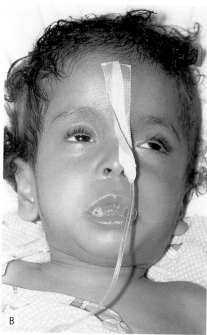

Figure 92.9 A and B   *A boy with Sandhoff disease at 18 and 19 months indicating the change in expression with progressive degeneration. He was blind and had cherry red spots at the time of the first photograph.*

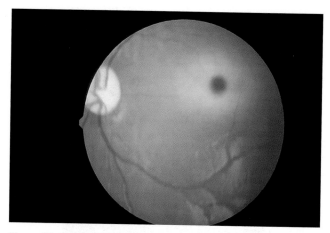

Figure 92.10   *S.O. The cherry red spot.*

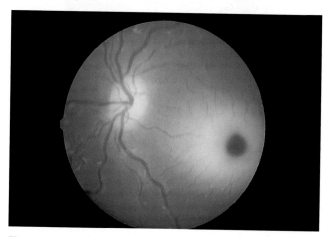

Figure 92.11   *T.O. The cherry red spot of an 18-month-old with Sandhoff disease. A cousin died at 17 months with a similar picture. Two brothers married two sisters. Hexosaminidase activity of both parents was in the heterozygote range.*

patients also accumulate globoside, the common neutral glycolipid of erythrocyte and renal membranes, which has the same amino terminal sugar as GM_2 ganglioside, N-acetyl galactosamine, in extraneural tissues, especially the liver, kidney and spleen [17–20]. In the brain there is storage of GM_2; in addition the asialo derivative of GM_2 (GA_2) accumulates, and this too is a difference from Tay-Sachs disease. Globoside may be demonstrated in urinary sediments and plasma [18]. The stored compounds are all structurally related. The asialo derivative differs from GM_2 in the absence of the N-acetylneuraminic side chain, whereas globoside contains an extra galactose moiety. GA_2 is found in the brain in Sandhoff disease in amounts 100 times normal [17]. Oligosaccharides and glycopeptides, which have a glycosidically-bound N-acetylhexosamine, accumulate in various tissues, and they are excreted in the urine [21,22], providing a readily accessible approach to diagnosis.

The Sandhoff disease is characterized by the lack not only of hexosaminidase A, but also of hexosaminidase B [7,20–24]. The enzyme defect has been demonstrated with natural substrates, including GM_2, GA_2 and globoside, as well as with the

GENETICS AND PATHOGENESIS

Patients with Sandhoff disease accumulate GM_2 ganglioside in the brain [1]. The amounts found are 100–300 times the normal concentrations and quite similar to those of Tay-Sachs disease. In contrast to patients with Tay-Sachs disease, these

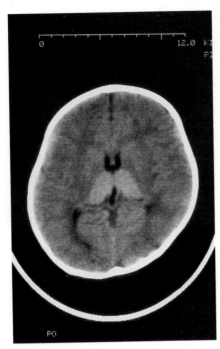

Figure 92.12 *CT scan of the brain of a patient with Sandhoff disease indicating the Turkish moustache sign.*

artificial substrates nitrophenylacetylglucosaminide and 4-methylumbelliferyl-N-acetylglucosamine [1,7]. The deficiency is present in all tissues of the body. It is readily assessed in serum, leukocytes and cultured fibroblasts [17]. In the classic infantile patients the activity of each enzyme is about 1–3 percent of normal [17]. Distinctions among the variant GM$_2$ gangliosidoses cannot be done well using the usual assays with artificial substrate, because there is a poor correlation between severity of clinical phenotype and degree of enzyme residual activity [25].

Each of the Hex-A and Hex-B enzymes has a molecular weight of about 100 000. The subunits are about 25 000 daltons. Both hexosaminidases cleave the lipids globoside and GA$_2$, but only hexosaminidase A hydrolyzes GM$_2$. The β chain is coded for on chromosome 5, while the α chain is determined by a locus on chromosome 15. Cells from patients with Sandhoff disease lack the β chains [26]. In some examples of Sandhoff disease the residual hexosaminidase in liver has been shown to have an increased Km, and pH optimum, indicating that there is a structural gene alteration [23]. In somatic cell hybrids there was independent segregation of hexosaminidase A and B, consistent with their loci on two different chromosomes [27,28]. Hybridization of fibroblasts from a patient with Tay-Sachs disease with those of a patient with Sandhoff disease revealed complementation in which hexosaminidase activity appeared, although it was present in neither parental strain [29]. Correction of hexosaminidase A activity represented provision of the α subunit from the Sandhoff fibroblasts and the β unit from the Tay-Sachs cells to form a hybrid heteropolymer [29–31].

Sandhoff disease is transmitted as an autosomal recessive trait. The gene for the disease appears to be unusually prevalent

in Lebanon [32]. It is also high in an area north of Cordoba in Argentina [33]. In Saudi Arabia [34] it is one of four frequently encountered lysosomal storage diseases. Unlike the others, Sandhoff disease was tribal in the sense that half of the patients were of one large tribe. In California there is an increased frequency among Hispanic people of Mexican or Central American origin [35]. Most recent estimates [36] of carrier frequency have yielded a frequency of one in 278 for carriers of the Sandhoff gene in non-Jews and one in 500 in Jews. This would yield a frequency of infants born with the disease of one in 300 000 non-Jews and one in a million Jews.

The Hex-B gene contains 14 exons and spans approximately 45 Kb [37,38]. There is extensive homology with the Hex-A gene, as there is between the two α and β proteins. The mutations observed in Sandhoff disease have been heterogeneous [11,37–39]. Some yield subunits that are cross-reacting material (CRM) positive; others are CRM negative. In the classic infantile Sandhoff disease there have been a number of partial deletions; there may be normal or reduced amount of mRNA, but the activity of hexosaminidase A is always essentially undetectable [5]. In a patient with later onset at 5 years [11] whose variant was referred to as hexosaminidase Paris [40–42] hexosaminidase B activity was deficient, but there was preservation of some activity of hexosaminidase A. Another variant had considerable activity of both isozymes in serum but marked reduction in tissues [38]. In general among the so-called juvenile variants hexosaminidase A activity has been expressed at one to three percent of control [43].

Mutations identified in classic infantile patients have usually been major alterations [44]. In addition to the 16 kb deletion involving the promoter and exons 1 to 5 [6], a 50 kb deletion was found in a single family [45]. At least one splicing mutation led to almost complete absence of mRNA.

Among later onset patients, many were compound heterozygotes, such as I207V and Y456S [46]. In a family in which there was compound heterozygosity for P417L and the severe 16 kb deletion which, when homozygous, leads to the classic infantile disease, there was late onset presentation in the 51-year-old proband and four asymptomatic patients, 51 to 61 years-of-age [47]. In the hexosamidase Paris, the Hex-B minus, Hex-A plus phenotype, a duplication straddling intron 13 and exon 14 generated an alternative splice site and caused an in-frame insertion of 18 nucleotides for the mRNA. The second allele was not known. The 16 kb deletion has been observed in French and French Canadian patients. Among the Argentine patients, there were two null mutations, a G to A transition (IVS 2 + 1) and a four base deletion (784del4) [48].

Detection of heterozygous carriers is possible by enzyme assay, which reveals amounts of hexosaminidase A and B in leukocytes, skin, cultured fibroblasts and serum that are intermediate between normal and patient concentrations [49–53]. Heterozygotes have been reported [9] in whom the activity of the A isozyme was present, but the B isozyme was less than 20 percent of normal. In heterozygotes the B isozyme was more thermolabile than normal [53], indicating the presence of a heteropolymer containing mutant and normal β chains. Intrauterine diagnosis has been accomplished by assay of cultured amniocytes [54–56]. The detection of N-acetylgalactosaminyloligosaccharides in amniotic fluid has been used for prenatal diagnosis, as it has in the urine for postnatal diagnosis [57,58]. In a family in which the mutation is known, mutational analysis is the method of choice for prenatal diagnosis and for heterozygote detection.

TREATMENT

The treatment of Sandhoff disease is entirely supportive, but a variety of experimental approaches to therapy are being explored. An animal model for Sandhoff disease in cats and a knock out mouse permit rational studies of therapy [59,60,61]. These include enzyme replacement, bone marrow transplantation and gene therapy. In the mouse, bone marrow transplantation prolonged lifespan from 4–5 months to 8 months and appeared to slow neurologic degeneration, but there was no improvement in storage of glycolipid in brain or neuronal pathology [61]. Bone marrow transplantation in a patient with Sandhoff disease appeared to be without beneficial effect [62].

Substrate deprivation therapy in which an inhibitor lowers the synthesis of glycosphingolipid has been employed in the Sandhoff mouse, with N-butyldeoxynojirimycin (NB-DNJ), an inhibitor of glucosylceramide synthase [63]. Treatment prolonged lifespan and reduced storage of GM_2 and GA_2 in brain. It is expected that treatment would be of greater utility in later-onset phenotypes, rather than in the infantile form of the disease. Therapy should potentially be of use in all three forms of GM_2 gangliosidosis (Chapters 92 and 93), Gaucher disease (Chapter 94), GM_1 gangliosidosis (Chapter 90) and Fabry disease (Chapter 89).

References

1   Sandhoff K, Andreae U, Jatzkewitz H. Deficient hexosaminidase activity in an exceptional case of Tay-Sachs disease with additional storage of kidney globoside in visceral organs. *Life Sci* 1968;**7**:283.

2   Sandhoff K. Sphingolipidoses. *J Clin Path* 1974;**27**:(suppl 8) 94.

3   Sandhoff K, Christomanou H. Biochemistry and genetics of gangliosidoses. *Hum Genet* 1979;**50**:107.

4   Fox MF, DuToit DL, Warnich L, Retief AE. Regional localization of alpha-galactosidase (GLA) to Xpter q22 hexosaminidase B (HEXB) to 5q13 → qter and arylsulfatase B (ARSB) to 5pter → q13. *Cytogenet Cell Genet* 1984;**38**:45.

5   O'Dowd BF, Klavins MH, Willard HF, *et al.* Molecular heterogeneity in the infantile and juvenile forms of Sandhoff disease (O-variant GM_2 gangliosidosis). *J Biol Chem* 1986;**261**:12680.

6   Neote K, McInnes B, Mahuran DJ, Gravel RA. Structure and distribution of an Alu-type deletion mutation in Sandhoff disease. *J Clin Invest* 1990;**86**:1524.

7   Sandhoff K, Harzer K, Wassle W, Jatzkewitz H. Enzyme alterations and lipid storage in three variants of Tay-Sachs disease. *J Neurochem* 1971;**18**:2469.

8   Dolman CL, Chang E, Duke RJ. Pathologic findings in Sandhoff disease. *Arch Pathol* 1973;**96**:272.

9   Costa TR, Pampols T, Gonzalez-Sastre F, *et al.* Enfermedad de Sandhoff (Gangliosidosis GM_2 tipo II) Presentacion de un case con estudio clinico y bioquimico Investigacion de portadores. *Ann Exp Pediat* 1984;**20**:146.

10 Johnson WG. The clinical spectrum of hexosaminidase deficiency disease. *Neurology* 1981;**31**:1453.

11 MacLeod PM, Wood S, Jan JE, *et al.* Progressive cerebellar ataxia psychomotor retardation and hexosaminidase deficiency in a 20-year-old child: juvenile Sandhoff disease. *Neurology* 1977;**27**:571.

12 Brett EM, Ellis RB, Haas L, *et al.* Late onset GM_2 gangliosidosis: clinical pathological and biochemical studies in eight patients. *Arch Dis Child* 1973;**48**:775.

13 Wood S, MacDougall BG. Juvenile Sandhoff disease: some properties of the residual hexosaminidase in cultured fibroblasts. *Am J Hum Genet* 1976;**28** 489

14 Kolodny E, Raghavan S. Hexosaminidase mutations not of the Tay-Sachs type produce unusual clinical variants. *Trends Neurosci* 1983;**6**:16.

15 Navon R. Molecular and clinical heterogeneity of adult GM_2 gangliosidosis. *Dev Neurosci* 1991;**13**:295.

16 Rubin M, Karpati G, Wolfe LS, *et al.* Adult onset motor neuronopathy in the juvenile type of hexosaminidase A and B deficiency. *J Neurol Sci* 1988;**87**:103.

17 Okada S, McCrea M, O'Brien JS. Sandhoff's disease (GM_2 gangliosidosis type 2): clinical chemical and enzyme studies in five patients. *Pediatr Res* 1972;**6**:606.

18 Krivit W, Desnick RJ, Lee J, *et al.* Generalized accumulation of neutral glycosphingolipids with GM_2 ganglioside accumulation in the brain. *Am J Med* 1972;**52**:763.

19 Snyder PD, Krivit W, Sweeley CC. Generalized accumulation of neutral glycosphingolipids with GM_2 ganglioside accumulation in the brain. *J Lipid Res* 1972;**13**:128.

20 Sandhoff K, Harzer K. Total hexosaminidase deficiency in Tay-Sachs disease (variant O): in *Lysosomes and Storage Diseases* (eds HG Hers, F Van Hoof). Academic Press, New York;1973:345.

21 Cantz M, Kresse H. Sandhoff disease: defective glycosaminoglycan catabolism in cultured fibroblasts and its correction by β-N-acetylhexosaminidase. *Eur J Biochem* 1974;**47**:581.

22 Strecker G, Montreuil J. Glycoproteins et glycoproteinoses. *Biochemie* 1979;**61**:1199.

23 Tateson R, Bain AD. GM_2 gangliosidoses. Consideration of the genetic defects. *Lancet* 1971;**2**:612.

24 Suzuki Y, Jacob JC, Suzuki K, Kutty KM. GM_2 gangliosidosis with total hexosaminidase deficiency. *Neurology* 1971;**21**:313.

25 Geiger B, Arnon R. Chemical characterization and subunit structure of human N-acetylhexosaminidases A and B. *Biochemistry* 1976;**15**:3484.

26 Proia RL, Neufeld EF. Synthesis of β-hexosaminidase in cell-free translation and intact fibroblasts: an insoluble precursor a-chain in a rare form of Tay-Sachs disease. *Proc Natl Acad Sci USA* 1982;**79**:6360.

27 Gilbert F, Kucherlapati R, Creagan RP, *et al.* Tay-Sachs and Sandhoff's diseases: the assignment of genes for hexosaminidases A and B to individual human chromosomes. *Proc Natl Acad Sci USA* 1975;**72**:263.

28 Lalley PA, Rattazzi MC, Shows TB. Human β-d-N-acetyl-hexosaminidase A and B: expression and linkage relationships in somatic cell hybrids. *Proc Natl Acad Sci USA* 1974;**71**:1569.

29 Thomas GH, Taylor HA, Miller CS, *et al.* Genetic complementation after fusion of Tay-Sachs and Sandhoff cells. *Nature* 1974;**250**:580.

30 Galjaard H, Hoogeveen A, De Wit-Verbeak HA, *et al.* Tay-Sachs and Sandhoff's disease: intergenic complementation after somatic cell hybridization. *Exptl Cell Res* 1974;**87**:444.

31 Srivastava SK, Beutler E. Studies on human β-d-acetyl-hexosaminidase. III Biochemical genetics of Tay-Sachs and Sandhoff's disease. *J Biol Chem* 1974;**249**:2054.

32 Der Karloustian VM, Khoury MJ, Hallal R, *et al.* Sandhoff disease: a prevalent form of infantile GM$_2$ gangliosidosis in Lebanon. *Am J Hum Genet* 1981;**33**:85.

33 De Kremer RD, De Levstein IM. Enfermedad de Sandhoff O gangliosidosis GM$_2$, tipo 2. Alta frequencia del gen en una poblacion criolla. *Medicina* (Buenos Aires) 1980;**40**:55.

34 Ozand PT, Gascon G, Al Aqeel A, *et al.* Prevalence of different types of lysosomal storage diseases in Saudi Arabia. *J Inherit Metab Dis* 1990;**13**:849.

35 Cantor RM, Roy C, Lim JST, Kaback MM. Sandhoff disease heterozygote detection: a component of population screening for Tay-Sachs disease carriers. II Sandhoff disease gene frequencies in American jewish and non-Jewish populations. *Am J Hum Genet* 1987;**41**:16.

36 Kaback M. *Summary of Worldwide Tay-Sachs Disease Screening and Detection.* University of California, Los Angeles;1988.

37 Proia RL. Gene encoding the human beta-hexosaminidase beta chain: extensive homology of intron placement in the alpha- and beta-chain genes. *Proc Natl Acad Sci USA* 1988;**85**:1883.

38 Neote K, Bapat B, Dumbrille Ross A, *et al.* Characterization of the human HEXB gene encoding lysosomal beta-hexosaminidase. *Genomics* 1988;**3**:279.

39 Lane AB, Jenkins T. Two variant hexosaminidase β-chain alleles segregating in a South African family. *Clin Chim Acta* 1978;**87**:219.

40 Dreyfus JC, Peonaru L, Svennerholm L. Absence of hexosaminidase A and B in a normal adult. *N Engl J Med* 1975;**292**:61.

41 Dreyfus JC, Poenaru L, Vibert M, *et al.* Characterization of a variant of β-hexosaminidase: 'Hexosaminidase Paris'. *Am J Hum Genet* 1977;**29**;287.

42 Dlott B, D'Azzo A, Quon DVK, Neufeld EF. Two mutations produce intron insertion in mRNA and elongated beta-subunit of human beta hexosaminidase. *J Biol Chem* 1990;**265**:17921.

43 Conzelmann E, Kytzia H-J, Navon R, Sandhoff K. Ganglioside GM$_2$ N-acetyl-b-d-galactosaminidase activity in cultured fibroblasts of late-infantile and adult GM$_2$ gangliosidosis patients and of healthy probands with low hexosaminidase levels. *Am J Hum Genet* 1983;**35B**;900.

44 Neufeld EF. Natural history and inherited disorders of a lysosomal enzyme beta-hexosaminidase. *J Biol Chem* 1989;**264**:10927.

45 Zhang ZX, Wakamatus N, Akerman BR, *et al.* A second large deletion in the HEXB gene in a patient with infantile Sandhoff disease. *Hum Mol Genet* 1995;**4**:777.

46 Banerjee P, Siciliano L, Oliveri D, *et al.* Molecular basis of an adult form of beta-hexosaminidase B deficiency with motor neuron disease. *Biochem Biophys Res Commun* 1991;**181**:108.

47 McInnes B, Potier M, Wakamatsu N, *et al.* An unusual splicing mutation in the HEXB gene is associated with dramatically different phenotypes in patients from different racial backgrounds. *J Clin Invest* 1992;**90**:306.

48 Brown CA, McInnes B, De Kremmer RD, Mahuran DJ. Characterization of two HEXB gene mutations in Argentinean patients with Sandhoff disease. *Biochim Biophys Acta* 1992;**1180**:91.

49 Harzer K. Inheritance of the enzyme deficiency in three neuro lipidoses: variant O of Tay-Sachs disease (Sandhoff's disease), classic Tay-Sach's disease and metachromatic leukodystrophy. Identification of the heterozygous carriers. *Humangenetik* 1973;**20**:1.

50 Harzer K, Sandhoff K, Schall H, Kollman F. Enzymatische untersuchungen im blut von ubertragern einer variante der Tay-Sach'schen erkrankung (variante O). *Klin Wschr* 1971;**49**:1189.

51 Kolodny EH. Sandhoff's disease: studies on the enzyme defect in homozygotes and detection of heterozygotes: in *Sphingolipidoses and Allied Disorders* (eds BW Volk, SM Aronson). Plenum Press, New York;1972:321.

52 Lowden JA, Ives EJ, Keene DL, *et al.* Carrier detection in Sandhoff's disease. *Am J Hum Genet* 1978;**30**:38.

53 Lowden JA. Evidence for a hybrid hexosaminidase isoenzyme in heterozygotes for Sandhoff disease. *Am J Hum Genet* 1979;**31**:281.

54 Desnick RJ, Krivit W, Sharp HL. *In utero* diagnosis of Sandhoff's disease. *Biochem Biophys Res Commun* 1973;**51**:20.

55 Kaback MM, Howell RR. Heterozygote detection and prenatal diagnosis of lysosomal diseases: in *Lysosomes and Storage Diseases* (eds HG Hers, F Van Hoof). Academic Press, New York;1973:599.

56 Harzer K, Stengel-Rutkowski S, Gley EO, *et al.* Prenatale diagnose der GM$_2$ gangliosidose type 2 (Sandhoff–Jatzkowitz–Krankheit). *Dtsch Med Wschr* 1975;**100**:106.

57 Warner TG, De Kremer RD, Applegarth D, Mock AK. Diagnosis and characterization of GM$_2$ gangliosidosis type II (Sandhoff disease) by analysis of the accumulating N-acetyl-glucosaminyl oligosaccharides with high performance liquid chromatography. *Clin Chim Acta* 1986;**154**:151.

58 Warner TG, Turner MW, Toone JR, Applegarth D. Prenatal diagnosis of infantile GM$_2$ gangliosidosis type II (Sandhoff disease) by detection of N-acetylglucosaminyl-oligosaccharides in amniotic fluid with high-performance liquid chromatography. *Prenat Diagn* 1986;**6**:393.

59 Cork LC, Munnell JF, Lorenz MD, *et al.* GM$_2$ ganglioside storage disease in cats with b-hexosaminidase deficiency. *Science* 1977;**196**:1014.

60 Bikker H, Van Den Berg FM, Wolterman RA, *et al.* Demonstration of a Sandhoff disease-associated autosomal 50-kb deletion by filed inversion gel electrophoresis. *Hum Genet* 1989;**81**:287.

61 Norflus F, Tifft CJ, McDonald MP, *et al.* Bone marrow transplantation prolongs life span and ameliorates neurologic manifestations in Sandhoff disease mice. *J Clin Invest* 1998;**101**:1881.

62 Hoogerbrugge PM, Brouwer OF, Bordigoni P, *et al.* Allogeneic bone marrow transplantation for lysosomal storage disease. The European Group for Bone Marrow Transplantation. *Lancet* 1995;**345**:1398.

63 Jeyakumar M, Butters TD, Cortina-Borja M, *et al.* Delayed symptom onset and increased life expectancy in Sandhoff-disease mice treated with N-butyldeoxynojirimycin. *Proc Natl Acad Sci USA* 1999;**96**:6388.

93

GM$_2$ activator deficiency/GM$_2$ gangliosidosis – deficiency of the activator protein

MAJOR PHENOTYPIC EXPRESSION

Progressive cerebral degeneration indistinguishable clinically from Tay-Sachs disease, with blindness, cherry red macular spots, hyperacusis, accumulation of GM$_2$ ganglioside, and deficiency of the GM$_2$ activator.

INTRODUCTION

GM$_2$ activator deficiency was discovered in 1978 [1] by Conzelmann and Sandhoff in a patient who accumulated GM$_2$ ganglioside but was not deficient in hexosaminidase A activity. The disorder has been referred to as the AB variant of GM$_2$ gangliosidosis [2], with Tay-Sachs and Sandhoff diseases there are now three nonallelic variants that cause GM$_2$ gangliosidosis.

The GM$_2$ activator protein is one of a family of sphingolipid activator proteins (SAPs) which though nonenzymatic are required for sphingolipid degradation [3]. The GM$_2$ activator forms a 1:1 water-soluble complex with lipid substrates [4]; it also interacts specifically with the hexosaminidase A enzyme [5] and in these ways promotes the catalytic degradation of GM$_2$ ganglioside. The gene for the activator protein is located on chromosome number 5 [6] at q31 [6,7]. Each of the point mutations described to date leads to premature degradation of the activator protein and storage of GM$_2$ ganglioside [8–12].

CLINICAL ABNORMALITIES

The clinical phenotype of this disease is identical to that of Tay-Sachs disease [13–17]. In some patients onset and progress may be a little slower than in the classic Tay-Sachs patient. Patients appear normal at birth and develop normally for the first 6 months, then they begin to lose acquired milestones. Neurologic degeneration is rapidly progressive. Tendon reflexes are brisk and the Babinski response positive. Patients may become macrocephalic. By 1 year they are usually blind, rigid and decerebrate (Figures 93.1, 93.2). They

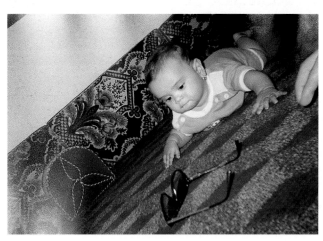

Figure 93.1 *Early photograph of the girl in Figure 93.2 documenting unremarkable early development, which appeared normal at both 6 and 10 months. The parents were first cousins.*

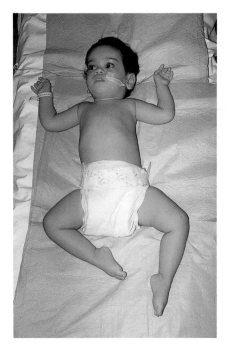

Figure 93.2   *A 2-year-old Saudi girl with GM$_2$ gangliosidosis on the basis of deficiency of the activator protein. Her appearance was reminiscent of a Dresden china doll. She had developed well for 8 months and then regressed. At 2, she was blind and lay in a frog-leg position. Tone was increased and reflexes brisk. Babinski responses were positive.*

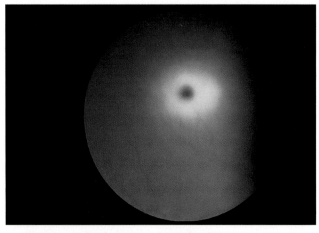

Figure 93.3   *The cherry red or reddish black spot of macular degeneration. The activator protein was studied by Dr. Sandhoff, who found no immunoprecipitable material and no utilization of the GM$_2$ ganglioside by cultured fibroblasts.*

have typical hyperactive startle responses to noise. Cherry red spots are readily visible in the ocular fundi (Figure 93.3). Seizures are common. One patient [12] had hepatomegaly, but no others had any suggestion of visceral storage. Death usually supervenes by 1 to 4 years-of-age.

Gross pathological examination of the brain has been described as normal [13–15,17]. Histologic examination reveals typical neuronal storage throughout the brain along with demyelination of the subcortical white matter. Golgi preparations reveal increased numbers and size of meganeurites and atrophy of the perisomatic dendritic system [18]. Electron microscopy reveals the typical lamellar membranous cytoplasmic bodies in neurons, as in Tay-Sachs disease. Some neurons have zebra bodies and other inclusions. Inclusions in glial cells provide a difference from Tay-Sachs disease [15].

GENETICS AND PATHOGENESIS

In contrast to Tay-Sachs disease, patients studied to date have all been non-Jewish. Inheritance appears to be autosomal recessive. Our patient was the product of a first-cousin mating. Spanish parents were also first cousins [12]. Knowledge of the mutation should permit prenatal diagnosis and heterozygote detection.

Mutation at the GM$_2$ activator locus has been observed to result in extreme reduction of the activator protein [19]. Amounts of cross-reacting material (CRM) have ranged from 0 to 5 percent of control. The protein found in one patient's fibroblasts was appreciably larger, at 26 kDa, than the normal activator protein. In this respect it resembled the precursor form of the protein [20], and it was secreted into the medium.

The disease has generally been suspected when assay of hexosaminidase A or A and B with the usual artificial substrates gives normal results in a patient with otherwise typical infantile GM$_2$ gangliosidosis [1,17,21]. Degradation of the natural GM$_2$ ganglioside requires the activator protein. The hexosaminidase isozymes A and B are present in normal or elevated amounts [22].

The GM$_2$ activator protein is a small, acidic, monomeric protein containing 162 amino acids [23–25]. It is synthesized as a larger precursor protein and cleaved to the mature form; it is a glycoprotein containing a carbohydrate chain linked to the N of asparagine 32 [20,24], and it is situated in the lysosomes [19]. The activator binds to substrate and hexosaminidase A, which then catalyzes the cleavage of the oligosaccharides of GM$_2$ and the glycolipid GA$_2$ [26].

The concentration of the activator, and the presence of a deficient content can be determined by an enzyme-linked immunoassay [25]. Detection of CRM positive mutant proteins must be detected by assay of the degradation of GM$_2$ by fibroblasts [27].

The cDNA for the activator protein has been isolated and sequenced [28,29]. It contains 4 exons over approximately 2.4 kb [30]. Among mutations identified, a T-to-C transition at nucleotide 412 resulted in substitution of an arginine for cysteine at position 107 [8,9]. Transfection of cells with the mutant cDNA yielded low levels of the activator protein, indicating that the mutation is responsible for the disease phenotype. A Saudi patient was homozygous for a 3 bp deletion, which deleted lysine 88 [12]. A Spanish patient was homozygous for a single base deletion which caused a frameshift [12]. Expression of the cDNA in *E. coli* yielded a carbohydrate-free fusion protein that was taken up by cells and restored the activity of mutant fibroblasts to degrade GM$_2$ ganglioside [30]. This should permit the isolation of quantities of protein that would permit X-ray crystallography. It raises the possibility of therapy.

TREATMENT

Only supportive treatment is available.

References

1   Conzelmann E, Sandhoff K. AB variant of infantile GM$_2$-gangliosidosis: Deficiency of a factor necessary for stimulation of hexosaminidase A-catalyzed degradation of ganglioside GM$_2$ and glycolipid GA2. *Proc Natl Acad Sci USA* 1978;**75**:3979.

2   Sandhoff K, Harzer K, Wassle W, Jatzkewitz H. Enzyme alterations and lipid storage in three variants of Tay-Sachs disease. *J Neurochem* 1971;**18**:2469.

3   Sonderfeld S, Conzelmann E, Schwarzmann G, *et al.* Incorporation and metabolism of ganglioside GM$_2$ in skin fibroblasts from normal and GM$_2$ gangliosidosis subjects. *Eur J Biochem* 1985;**149**:247.

4   Conzelmann E, Burg J, Stephan G, Sandhoff K. Complexing of glycolipids and their transfer between membranes by the activator protein for lysosomal ganglioside GM$_2$ degradation. *Eur J Biochem* 1982;**123**:455.

5   Kytzia H-J, Sandhoff K. Evidence for two different active sites on human hexosaminidase A: Interaction of GM2 activator protein with hexosaminidase A. *J Biol Chem* 1985;**260**:7568.

6   Burg J, Conzelmann E, Sandhoff K, *et al.* Mapping of the gene coding for the human GM$_2$ activator protein to chromosome 5. *Ann Hum Genet* 1985;**49**:41.

7   Heng HH, Xie B, Shi XM, *et al.* Refined mapping of the GM$_2$ activator protein (GM$_{2A}$) locus to 5q313-331 distal to the spinal muscular atrophy locus. *Genomics* 1993;**18**:429.

8   Schroder M, Schnabel D, Suzuki K, Sandhoff K. A mutation in the gene of a glycolipid-binding protein (GM$_2$ activator) that causes GM$_2$-gangliosidosis variant AB. *FEBS Lett* 1991;**290**:1.

9   Xie B, Wang W, Mahuran DJ. A Cys138-to-Arg substitution in the GM$_2$ activator protein is associated with the AB variant form of GM$_2$ gangliosidosis. *Am J Hum Genet* 1992;**50**:1046.

10 Xie B, Rigat B, Smijanic-Georgijev N, *et al.* Biochemical characterization of the Cys138Arg substitution associated with the AB variant form of GM$_2$ gangliosidosis: Evidence that Cys138 is required for the recognition of the GM$_2$ activator/GM$_2$ ganglioside complex by beta-hexosaminidase A. *Biochemistry* 1998;**37**:814.

11 Schroder M, Schnabel D, Hurwitz R, *et al.* Molecular genetics of GM$_2$-gangliosidosis AB variant: A novel mutation and expression in BHK cells. *Hum Genet* 1993;**92**:437.

12 Schepers U, Glombitza GJ, Lemm T, *et al.* Molecular analysis of a GM$_2$-activator deficiency in two patients with GM$_2$-gangliosidosis AB variant. *Am J Hum Genet* 1996;**59**:1048.

13 Goldman JE, Yamanaka T, Rapin I, *et al.* The AB-variant of GM$_2$ gangliosidosis. Clinical biochemical and pathological studies of two patients. *Acta Neuropathol (Berl)* 1980;**52**:189.

14 Kolodny EH, Pruszkow IW, Moser HW, *et al.* GM$_2$ gangliosidosis without deficiency in the artificial substrate cleaving activity of hexosaminidase A and B. *Neurology* 1973;**23**:427.

15 De Baeque CM, Suzuki K, Rapin I, *et al.* GM$_2$ gangliosidosis AB variant. Clinico-pathological study of a case. *Acta Neuropathol (Berl)* 1975;**33**:207.

16 Sakuraba H, Itoh K, Shimmoto M, *et al.* GM$_2$ gangliosidosis AB variant – Clinical and biochemical studies of a Japanese patient. *Neurology* 1999;**52**:372.

17 Hechtman P, Gordon BA, Ng Ying Kim NMK. Deficiency of the hexosaminidase A activator protein in a case of GM$_2$ gangliosidosis; variant AB. *Pediatr Res* 1982;**16**:217.

18 Purpura DP. Ectopic dendritic growth in mature pyramidal neurons in human ganglioside storage disease. *Nature* 1978;**276**:520.

19 Banerjee A, Burg J, Conzelmann E, *et al.* Enzyme-linked immunosorbent assay for the ganglioside GM$_2$-activator protein. Screening of normal human tissues and body fluids of tissues of GM$_2$ gangliosidosis, and for its subcellular localization. *Hoppe-Seyler's Z Physiol Chem* 1984;**365**:347.

20 Burg J, Banerjee A, Sandhoff K. Molecular forms of GM$_2$-activator protein. A study on its biosynthesis in human skin fibroblasts. *Biol Chem Hoppe-Seyler* 1985;**366**:887.

21 Hirabayashi Y, Li Y-T, Li S-C. The protein activator specific for the enzymic hydrolysis of GM$_2$ ganglioside in normal human brain and in brains of three types of GM$_2$ gangliosidosis. *J Neurochem* 1983;**40**:168.

22 Conzelmann E, Sandhoff K, Nehrkorn H, *et al.* Purification, biochemical and immunological characterization of hexosaminidase A from variant AB of infantile GM$_2$ gangliosidosis. *Eur J Biochem* 1978;**84**:27.

23 Conzelmann E, Sandhoff K. Purification and characterization of an activator protein for the degradation of glycolipids GM$_2$ and GA$_2$ by hexosaminidase A. *Hoppe-Seyler's Z Physiol Chem* 1979;**360**:1837.

24 Furst W, Schubert J, Machleidt W, *et al.* The complete amino-acid sequences of human ganglioside GM$_2$-activator protein and cerebroside sulfate activator protein. *Eur J Biochem* 1990;**19**:709.

25 Wu YY, Sonnino S, Li YT, Li SC. Characterization of an alternatively spliced GM$_2$ activator protein, GM$_2$A protein. An activator protein which stimulates the enzymatic hydrolysis of *N*-acetylneuraminic acid, but not *N*-acetylgalactosamine, from GM$_2$. *J Biol Chem* 1996;**271**:10611.

26 Meier EM, Schwarzmann G, Furst W, Sandhoff K. The human GM$_2$ activator protein. *J Biol Chem* 1991;**266**:1879.

27 Leinekugel P, Michel S, Conzelmann E, Sandhoff K. Quantitative correlation between the residual activity of β-hexosominidase A and arylsulfatase A and the severity of the resulting lysosomal storage disease. *Hum Genet* 1992;**88**:513.

28 Schroder M, Klima H, Nakano T, *et al.* Isolation of a cDNA encoding in the human GM$_2$ activator protein. *FEBS Lett* 1989;**251**:197.

29 Klima H, Tanaka A, Schnabel D, *et al.* Characterization of full-length cDNA and the gene coding for the human GM$_2$-activator protein. *FEBS Lett* 1991;**289**:260.

30 Klima H, Klein A, Van Echten G, *et al.* Over-expression of a functionally active human GM$_2$-activator protein in *Escherichia coli. Biochem J* 1993;**292**:571.

Gaucher disease

MAJOR PHENOTYPIC EXPRESSION

Type 1

Splenomegaly, pancytopenia, hepatomegaly, bony pain, fractures, avascular necrosis.

Type 2

Acute neuronopathic: Early infantile onset, hypertonicity, seizures, trismus, retroflexion of the head; splenomegaly; hepatomegaly; rapid neurologic deterioration and death between 1 and 24 months.

Type 3

Subacute neuronopathic: Splenomegaly, hepatomegaly; childhood onset of neurologic manifestations – ataxia, spastic paraparesis, seizures, ophthalmoplegia; death in childhood or adulthood if untreated.

All Types

Accumulation glucocerebroside (glycosylceramide) and defective activity of lysosomal acid β-glucosidase.

INTRODUCTION

Gaucher disease is the most common of the lysosomal storage diseases. It was first described in 1882 by Gaucher [1], then a French medical student. He identified the pathognomonic cells, which are now known as Gaucher cells, in a 32-year-old woman with massive enlargement of the spleen. The eponym Gaucher disease was first employed by Brill in 1905 [2]. This phenotype, now referred to as type 1, was recognized in the 1950s to be common in Ashkenazi Jews [3,4]. Two other types of disease are known (Table 94.1). The acute neuronopathic early infantile, type 2, disease was described in 1927 [5]. In 1959, a Type 3, subacute neuronopathic disease was described in an isolated population in Northern Sweden [6]; this slowly progressive neurologic disease is referred to as the Norrbottnian form, after the place of origin of the initial patients. Actually, each of the forms of the disease is panethnic.

Recognition of Gaucher disease as a reticuloendothelial storage disease was as early as 1907 [7], and in 1924 the stored material was identified as lipid and characterized as a cerebroside [8,9]. Identification of the sugar in this cerebroside as glucose was reported by Aghion in 1934 in his thesis for the doctorate of philosophy [10] (Figure 94.1). The molecular defect in glucocerebrosidase (Figure 94.2) was described in 1965, independently by Brady and colleagues [11], and by Patrick [12]. The defective enzyme is a lysosomal acid β-glucosidase, active in catalyzing the release of glucose from a number of substrates in addition to glucosylceramide. There is an activator of the enzyme, saposin C, which has a low molecular weight [13]. The gene for β-glucosidase is located

Table 94.1   *Clinical presentations of Gaucher disease*

	Type 1	Type 2	Type 3
Onset	Infants Child/Adulthood	3–6 months	Childhood
Neurodegeneration	Absent	++++	++→++++
Survival	6–80 + years	<2 Years	2nd to 4th decade
Splenomegaly	++++	++	++
Hepatomegaly	++	+	+
Fractures – bone crises	+	−	+
Ethnic predilection	Ashkenazi	Panethnic	Norrbottnian Swedish

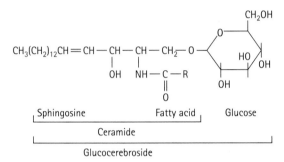

Figure 94.1   *Structure of glucocerebroside, the Gaucher lipid.*

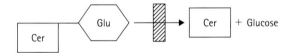

Figure 94.2   *β-Glucocerebrosidase, the site of the defect in Gaucher disease.*

on chromosome 1q21 [14]. The cDNA has been cloned and a number and variety of mutations have been identified [15–17]. The type 1 disease provides an interesting therapeutic model because enzyme replacement therapy has been quite successful [18]. Bone marrow transplantation may be curative.

CLINICAL ABNORMALITIES

Type 1

There is considerable heterogeneity of clinical expression. As many as 25 percent of affected individuals may be asymptomatic or have splenomegaly discovered incidental to an examination well into adult life, even into the eighth and ninth decades [19–22]. Severely affected individuals with Type 1 disease may die in the first or second decade. The spleen may be massively enlarged.

The initial clinical manifestation is usually painless splenomegaly [23,24]. The spleen may be massively enlarged (Figures 94.3, 94.4). It may be so large as to interfere with the

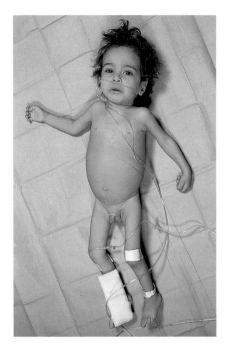

Figure 94.3   *F.T.H. A 2-year-old Saudi patient with Gaucher disease. Abdominal distention had been progressive and associated with weakness and failure to thrive. The liver was palpable 12 cm below the right costal margin. The spleen had been removed. β-Glucosidase activity of fibroblasts was 9 μmol/mg/hr or 5 percent of control.*

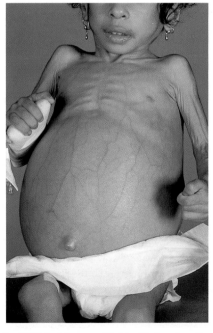

Figure 94.4   *Z.Y.A.A. A 3-year-old girl with Gaucher disease. The abdomen was enormous and the patient emaciated. The liver was palpated at 20 cm and the spleen at 17 cm below the costal margins. Hemoglobin was 6 g/dL and platelet count 45 × 10³ per mm³. β-Glucosidase activity was 1 μmol/hr/mg cells or 6 percent of control.*

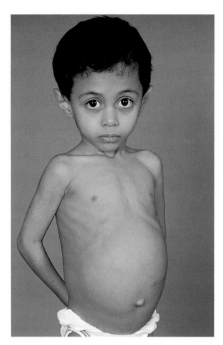

Figure 94.5   *H.F.B. A 4-year-old Saudi boy with Gaucher disease. The spleen had been removed, but the abdomen was distended by the enormous liver. In addition, he was thin, short and wasted. Enzyme activity was 12 percent of control.*

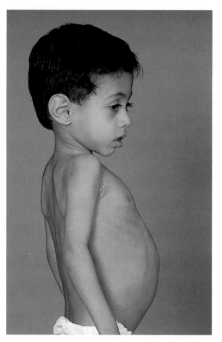

Figure 94.6   *H.F.B. Lateral view highlights the abdominal distention. Parents were first cousins. IQ was 93. Treatment was initiated with ceredase (glucocerebrosidase).*

intake of food into the stomach or to cause dispareunia. Splenic infarcts may occur. A large infarction may produce the picture of an acute abdomen, along with hyperuricemia. Radionuclide scans may be helpful in the diagnosis of the splenic infarcts.

The liver is also enlarged (Figures 94.4–94.7), usually less than the spleen, but it maybe as large or larger than the spleen (Figure 94.4) and it may be particularly prominent in splenectomized patients (Figure 94.5–94.7). The large liver is usually not associated with liver disease, but there may be elevated transaminases, cirrhosis, esophageal varices or hepatic failure [25–27]. Hepatic infarction may present as an acute abdominal catastrophe with a Budd-Chiari syndrome. One patient we saw was left with a large palpable notch in the center of the hepatic outline.

Thrombocytopenia is a common hematological manifestation of Gaucher disease [26]. It may be accompanied by leukopenia and anemia, the full picture of hypersplenism and resolves with splenectomy [28]. Late hematological dysfunction in splenectomized patients may result from replacement of normal marrow with Gaucher cells. There may be bleeding, petechiae and easy bruising.

Skeletal manifestations may be the chief or only complaint in some patients. Most patients have some bony abnormality. In many patients, they take the form of acute crises of pain, tenderness, redness and swelling, mimicking acute osteomyelitis or the thrombotic crises of sickle cell disease.

There may be fever, leukocytosis and elevation of the erythrocyte sedimentation rate. The diagnosis is best confirmed by technetium radionuclide scan [29]. Pyogenic osteomyelitis is rare in Gaucher disease and usually follows some invasive

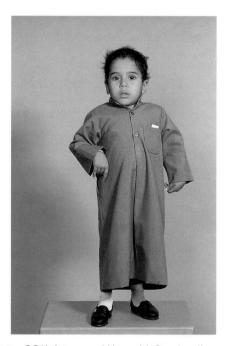

Figure 94.7   *S.S.H. A 3-year-old boy with Gaucher disease. The abdominal enlargement caused by the hepatomegaly is evident even with the patient fully clothed. β-Glucosidase activity was 5 percent of control. He had a splenectomy and had recently had successful bone marrow transplantation.*

procedure on bone; therefore surgical diagnostic procedures are not recommended for crises [30].

Areas of focal destruction of bone, osteonecrosis or avascular necrosis occur in the absence of acute crises, especially in the area of the femoral head [31]. A child with hip pain

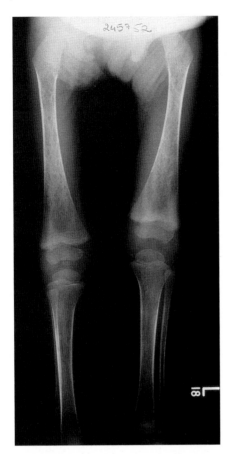

Figure 94.8   *Roentgenogram of the lower extremities of a patient with Gaucher disease illustrates the osteoporosis and enlargement of the width particularly of the femur leading to an Erlenmeyer flask appearance.*

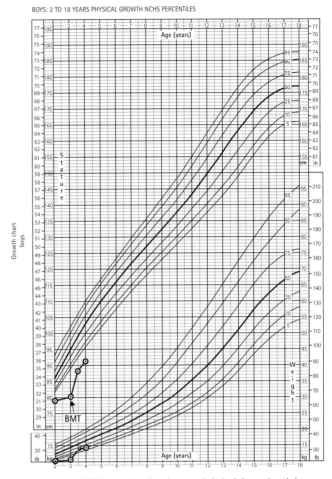

Figure 94.9   *S.S.H. Acceleration in growth in height and weight following bone marrow transplantation. Adapted from Hamill* et al. *Physical growth: National Center for Health Statistics percentiles.* Am J Clin Nutr *1979; 32: 607–29.*

maybe thought to have Legg-Calve-Perthes disease [32]. Pathologic fracture is common. Some degree of osteoporosis is the rule in this disease. Compression fracture of vertebral bodies is a common complication [31,33–35], and there may be radicular or spinal cord compression or kyphoscoliotic deformity. Roentgenograms reveal osteoporosis of the spine and compression fractures [36]. Magnetic resonance imaging (MRI) is more effective than conventional radiography or computed tomography (CT) scanning in evaluating the spine and effects on the cord and also in assessing areas of avascular necrosis [37]. The most common skeletal feature of Gaucher disease is the loss of modeling and increased width that leads to the Erlenmeyer flask appearance of the femur [38] (Figure 94.8). In addition, areas of severe loss of bone density may alternate with areas of osteosclerosis and focal infarctions.

Growth and development may be altered drastically in Gaucher disease (Figure 94.9). Pubertal development may also be delayed. In addition to the effects of anemia, splenic enlargement and chronic disease, resting energy expenditure is increased about 44 percent [39].

Pulmonary infiltration may also occur [40] (Figure 94.10) and may lead to pulmonary failure. There may also be right to left intrapulmonary shunting of blood. Fingers may be clubbed. The skin may show yellow or brown pigmentation and a propensity to tan [41]. Patients with Gaucher disease appear to be susceptible to cancer, especially lymphoproliferative diseases [42]. The nervous system is by definition spared in Type 1 disease, but a number of secondary complications do affect the nervous system in addition to the complications of vertebral disease. These include cerebral fat emboli secondary to skeletal disease, neuropathy and hematomyelia secondary to bleeding [42]; a case was reported with lumbosacral cauda equina syndrome secondary to an intrathecal sacral cyst, apparently the result of subdural hemorrhage [43].

A few patients with Type 1 Gaucher disease have been found to develop parkinsonian symptoms [44], with onset typically in the fourth decade and a limited responsiveness to therapy. There has not been any association with genotype, but in several cases there was a family history of parkinsonism [45]. In a study of tissue from patients with parkinsonism, alterations in glucocerebrosidase were found in 12 out of 57 individuals [46]. Overall, although the association between parkinsonism and Gaucher disease remains to be explained, it appears that

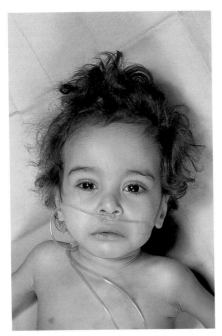

Figure 94.10   *F.T.H. Involvement of the lung was documented by biopsy. The patient was oxygen-dependent. Roentgenogram revealed virtually completely opaque lung fields with air bronchograms.*

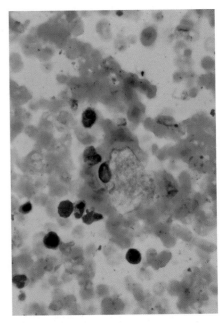

Figure 94.11   *Gaucher cells. In this power the size relative to leukocytes and erythrocytes is evident.*

deficiency of glucocerebrosidase confers predisposition to development of parkinsonism.

Type 2

Infants with acute neuronopathic Gaucher disease appear normal at birth, although splenomegaly maybe found in the first three months, and they usually develop some early milestones. Early evidence of neurologic disease may be unusual irritability, a lack of alertness, apparent weakness in holding up the head, oculomotor apraxia or a fixed strabismus [24,47]. Neurodegenerative disease appears in six months and proceeds rapidly to a classic picture of spasticity and opisthotonus, with trismus, strabismus and hyperextension of the neck [47]. There may be seizures, bulbar signs or involuntary choreoathetoid movements. Visual fixation may be absent as well as visual evoked response (VER). Atrophy may be evident on the MRI of the brain. Death usually results from apnea, aspiration pneumonia or respiratory failure at an average age of 18 months. Autopsy reveals neuronal degeneration and neuronophagia.

A subtype of infants with this type of Gaucher disease has a rapid fulminant neonatal onset course [47,48]. Death may occur as early as 2 months-of-age. This disorder is reminiscent of the disease in mice homozygous for a null glucocerebrosidase allele [49] who die within 24 hours. Infants with Gaucher disease may present with lamellar ichthyosis, which may take the form of the collodion baby [50–52]. Presentation of Gaucher disease with non-immune hydrops fetalis [53] may represent the same process. Perinatal-lethal Gaucher disease with hydrops, ichthyosis, and fetal akinesia sequence has been associated with particularly severe mutations [54].

Type 3

In the classic Norrbottnian form of disease [55,56], the patient's early manifestations may lead to a diagnosis of Type 1 Gaucher disease. The neurologic keynote finding is myoclonus of cerebral origin [57,58]. Multifocal jerky movements are widespread in the muscles and occur at rest or with movement. The electroencephalogram (EEG) may reveal spike discharges [59]. With time there are generalized grand mal seizures [60,61]. Careful examination of the eyes discloses deficits in saccadic velocities, progressive with time to paralysis of lateral gaze [62,63]. There may be slow upward looping of the eyes [64]. As the disease progresses ataxia and spasticity appear. There may be dementia.

A group of patients in whom paralysis of horizontal supranuclear gaze is the major neurologic sign have been considered as subgroup of type 3 [47,63]. They may have mild cognitive impairment [65]. These patients often have aggressive systemic manifestations. Some authors have subdivided Type 3 patients into groups, for example designating those with progressive myoclonic epilepsy and dementia, and a poorer prognosis, as type 3a [63], but there are clearly unidentified genetic modifiers which determine prognosis [66]. When untreated, death in Type 3 patients characteristically occurs in childhood or adolescence from pulmonary or hepatic disease, and in those with progressive myoclonic epilepsy, neurologic deterioration may cause death in adulthood despite treatment.

Diagnosis

The diagnosis is often first made clinically by the recognition of Gaucher cells (Figures 94.11, 94.12) in a bone marrow aspirate or biopsied tissue. These cells are large lipid-laden macrophages with foamy cytoplasm. The fibrillary pattern is quite different from that of Niemann-Pick cells. Electron microscopy reveals tubular structures. These cells are widely dispersed in tissues. The diagnosis may be suspected by the presence of elevated activity of acid phosphatase in plasma [67], a high level of ferritin [68], angiotensin-converting enzyme [69], and particularly chitotriosidase, which is induced in activated macrophages, and is very significantly elevated in most cases of Gaucher disease [69].

Definitive diagnosis requires the assay of acid β-glucosidase. This can be done in leukocytes or cultured fibroblasts [70–72]. Enzyme assay is not useful in distinguishing the various types of Gaucher disease.

GENETICS AND PATHOGENESIS

Gaucher disease is inherited in an autosomal recessive fashion. Most patients are of Type 1, and this is most common in Ashkenazi Jews, in whom the incidence has been estimated at between 1 in 640 [24] and 1 in 855 [73]. This is the most prevalent genetic disorder in that population.

The gene for acid β-glucosidase has been cloned and linked to chromosome 1q21 [14,17,74]. It contains 11 exons and is approximately 7 kb in length. The cDNA is about 2.5 kb [16,75]. More than 200 mutations have been defined in patients with Gaucher disease [76,77]. Four are common enough to account for over 96 percent of the Ashkenazi Jewish patients [78,79] (Table 94.2). The A to G transition at

position 1226 which causes an asparagine to serine substitution at amino acid 370 (N370S) [80] is the major cause of the disease in this population. The next most frequent is the frameshift mutation at 84GG [81], a mutation which leads to no enzyme protein. The point mutation which changes a leucine to proline at 444 (L444P) and the splice junction mutation at IVS2 + 1 account for most of the rest of mutations in this population [17,28].

Heterozygote detection is sometimes possible by enzyme analysis, but it is not reliable because of overlap with the normal population. In Jewish populations heterozygote detection may be carried out by genotyping. This is less useful in non-Jewish populations; about 25 percent of these patients carry the N370S mutation and 35 percent the L444P mutation, and the rest are unidentified or rare.

Some correlations of phenotype with genotype have emerged from increasing information on the nature of mutation in Gaucher disease. The N370S mutation appears relatively conservative and a majority of patients who carry this mutation have relatively mild disease. Homozygosity for this mutation excludes neuronopathic disease, but even a single 370 allele in a compound leads to an absence of neurologic disease [76]; compounds tend to have more severe somatic disease than 370 homozygotes. The Norrbottnian population of Gaucher patients in Northern Sweden are homozygous for the L444P mutation and have type 3 disease of variable severity [82]. The L444P mutation is also found in other populations, and though it is associated with severe somatic symptoms and generally with neurologic symptoms, in some patients neuronopathic symptoms may be absent [63]. The 84GG frameshift leads to severe disease and no enzyme activity, as does the IVS2 + 1 mutation in intron 2 [28,78,82].

An index of complexity, and the power of molecular techniques to unravel it, is a family [83] in which two children died of type 2 disease, and a son had relatively indolent type 1 disease. The mother and son had similarly low levels of β-glucosidase, while the father's level was consistent with heterozygosity. Molecular analysis revealed the mother, asymptomatic at 62 years, and the son to be S370N/L444P compounds. The father was heterozygous L444P/normal. It was assumed that the infants who died by 1 year-of-age had inherited two L444P alleles.

The consequence of defective activity of acid β-glucosidase is the accumulation of glycosylceramide (Figure 94.1, p. 668). In ceramide there is a long chain fatty acid amide linkage at the carbon 2 of sphingosine. Glycosphingolipids with longer oligosaccharide moieties are successively degraded

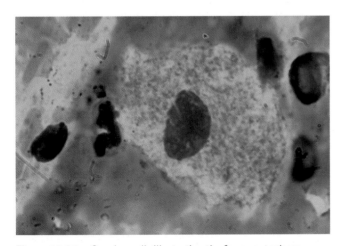

Figure 94.12 *Gaucher cells illustrating the foamy cytoplasm.*

Table 94.2 *Common mutations in Gaucher disease*

cDNA no.	Amino acid no.	Nucleotide substitution	Amino acid substitution	Type of mutation
1226	370	A → G	Asn Ser	Point mutation
84		G → GG		Frameshift insertion
1448	444	T → C	Leu Pro	Point mutation
IVS2 + 1		G → A		Splice junction mutation

(Chapter 91, p. 609) to glycosylceramide. The amounts of this compound stored in Gaucher disease are enormous. Deacylated glycosylsphingosine has also been found in tissues of patients [84]. It is thought that the accumulated compounds are toxic to certain tissues.

TREATMENT

Among the earliest approaches to provide a source of active enzyme in Gaucher disease was the use of bone marrow transplantation [85] (Figure 94.9). The procedure may be essentially curative in type 1 disease, but there is a considerable risk of mortality from the procedure. It certainly raises the possibility that gene therapy in which the normal gene is introduced into the patient's hematopoietic cells will one day be an option.

Meanwhile, enzyme replacement therapy has become a major advance in the management of this disease. Gaucher disease was the first lysosomal storage disease for which this approach became available. The major breakthrough in permitting successful therapy was the recognition that lipid-laden macrophages have a mannose-receptor [86]; modifying the glycoprotein glucocerebrosidase to expose a terminal mannose permits the enzyme to attach to and be incorporated into the macrophage [47,87]. A modified form of the enzyme purified from human placenta was approved for treatment in 1991 under the name Ceredase (algucerase), and then in 1994 a form of human glucocerebrosidase produced in cultured Chinese hamster ovary cells was approved in 1994 under the name Cerezyme (imiglucerase).

Clinical responses have been clearly evident in hematological (anemia and thrombocytopenia), visceral and even (with longer courses of treatment) bony disease. Decrease in organ size is evident within six months. Bone pains diminish or disappear and at least in children roentgenograms of the bones have improved after years of treatment. Growth and development regularly improve. The treatment is expensive. There is still some controversy as to dose. The dose generally employed is 60 U/kg every two weeks [47] but 30 U/kg every two weeks maybe just as effective [88]. Success has also been reported with 2.3 U/kg three times a week [89]. Practical considerations of intravenous access and demands on the patient's time have made the larger, less frequent dosing more popular. It is possible that maintenance requirements for enzyme will be lower after the initial removal of accumulated glycolipid. Another approach, called substrate reduction therapy, is possible with an inhibitor of ceramide glucosyltransferase, and the agent N-butyldeoxynojirimycin was approved in 2004 (miglustat) for adult patients with Gaucher disease for whom intravenous enzyme replacement is not practical [90,91].

It is generally agreed that enzyme replacement is not effective in Type 2 disease, while in the Type 3 disease systemic improvement is accompanied by no change in cerebral manifestations [92]. Piracetam may be helpful in the management of myoclonus [93].

A variety of supportive measures may be rendered unnecessary by the early use of enzyme replacement. There is in general no longer a place for splenectomy, but it might be considered in a patient with extensive thrombocytopenia or cardiopulmonary symptoms from a massive spleen. Hip replacement is the preferred modality for avascular necrosis. Replacement of other joints may be necessary. The avoidance of injury to bone especially in sports is prudent. The frequency and severity of crises of bone pain and fractures were reported to improve in patients treated with biphosphonates [94], which are analogues of pyrophosphate that bind to hydroxyapatite, inhibiting resorption. A placebo-controlled trial of alendronate showed significant benefit as an adjuvant to enzyme replacement, with improvement in bone density and bone mineral content within 18 months [95].

References

1   Gaucher PCE. De l'epithelioma primitif de la rate, hypertrophie idiopathique de la rate sans leucemie. Thesis. Paris, 1882.

2   Brill NE, Mandelbaum FS, Libman E. Primary splenomegaly-Gaucher type. Report on one of few cases occurring in a single generation of one family. *Am J Med Sci*;**129**:491.

3   Fried K. Gaucher's disease among the Jews of Israel. Proceedings of the Fourth Meeting of the Israel Genetics Circle. *Bull Res Counc Isr* 1958;**7B**:213.

4   Fried K. Population study of chronic Gaucher's disease. *Isr J Med Sci* 1973;**9**:1396.

5   Oberling C, Woringer P. La maladie de Gaucher chez la nourrison. *Rev Fr Pediatr* 1927;**3**:475.

6   Hillborg PO. Morbus Gaucher: Norbotten. *Nord Med* 1959;**61**:303.

7   Marchand F. Uber sogenannte idiopathische Splenomegalie (Typus Gaucher). *Munch Med Wochenschr* 1907;**54**:1102.

8   Epstein E. Beitrag zur Chemie der Gaucherschen Krankheit. *Hoppe-Seyler's Z Physiol Chem* 1924;**271**:211.

9   Lieb H. Der Zucker im Cerebrosid der Milz bei der Gaucher Krankheit. *Hoppe-Seyler's Z Physiol Chem* 1924;**271**:211.

10 Aghion A. La maladie de Gaucher dans l'enfance. Thesis. 1934.

11 Brady RO, Kanfer JN, Shapiro D. Metabolism of glucocerebrosides. II. Evidence of an enzymatic deficiency in Gaucher's disease. *Biochem Biophys Res Commun* 1965;**18**:22.

12 Patrick AD. A deficiency of glucocerebrosidase in Gaucher's disease. *Biochem J* 1965;**97**:17c.

13 Ho MW, O'Brien JS. Gaucher's disease: deficiency of 'acid'-glucosidase and reconstitution of enzyme activity *in vitro*. *Proc Natl Acad Sci USA* 1971;**68**:2810.

14 Barneveld RA, Keijzer W, Tegelaers FP, *et al.* Assignment of the gene coding for human beta-glucocerebrosidase to the region q21-q31 of chromosome 1 using monoclonal antibodies. *Hum Genet* 1983;**64**:227.

15 Ginns EI, Choudary PV, Martin BM, *et al.* Isolation of cDNA clones for human beta-glucocerebrosidase using the lambda gt11 expression system. *Biochem Biophys Res Commun* 1984;**123**:574.

16 Sorge J, West C, Westwood B, Beutler E. Molecular cloning and nucleotide sequence of human glucocerebrosidase cDNA. *Proc Natl Acad Sci USA* 1985;**82**:7289.

17 Tsuji S, Choudary PV, Martin BM, *et al.* A mutation in the human glucocerebrosidase gene in neuronopathic Gaucher's disease. *N Engl J Med* 1987;**316**:570.

18 Barton NW, Brady RO, Dambrosia JM, *et al*. Replacement therapy for inherited enzyme deficiency – macrophage-targeted glucocerebrosidase for Gaucher's disease. *N Engl J Med* 1991;**324**:1464.

19 Berrebi A, Wishnitzer R, der-Walde U. Gaucher's disease: unexpected diagnosis in three patients over seventy years old. *Nouv Rev Fr Hematol* 1984;**26**:201.

20 Brinn L, Glabman S. Gaucher's disease without splenomegaly. Oldest patient on record, with review. *NY State J Med* 1962;**62**:2346.

21 Chang-Lo M, Yam LT, Rubenstone AI. Gaucher's disease. Review of the literature and report of twelve new cases. *Am J Med Sci* 1967;**254**:303.

22 Beutler E. Gaucher's disease in an asymptomatic 72-year-old *JAMA* 1977;**237**:2529.

23 Matoth Y, Fried K. Chronic Gaucher's disease; clinical observations on 34 patients. *Isr J Med Sci* 1965;**1**:521.

24 Kolodny EH, Ullman MD, Mankin HJ, *et al*. Phenotypic manifestations of Gaucher disease: clinical features in 48 biochemically verified type 1 patients and comment on type 2 patients. *Prog Clin Biol Res*;**95**:33.

25 Morrison AN, Lane M. Gaucher's disease with ascites: a case report with autopsy findings. *Ann Intern Med* 1955;**42**:1321.

26 Javett SN, Kew MC, Liknaitsky D. Gaucher's disease with portal hypertension: case report. *J Pediatr* 1966;**68**:810.

27 James SP, Stromeyer, FW Stowens DW, Barranger JA. Gaucher disease: hepatic abnormalities in 25 patients. *Prog Clin Biol Res* 1982;**95**:131.

28 Beutler E, Gelbart T, Kuhl W, *et al*. Mutations in Jewish patients with Gaucher disease. *Blood* 1992;**79**:1662.

29 Katz K, Mechlis-Frish S, Cohen IJ, *et al*. Bone scans in the diagnosis of bone crisis in patients who have Gaucher disease. *J Bone Joint Surg Am* 1991;**73**:513.

30 Lachiewicz PF. Gaucher's disease. *Orthop Clin North Am* 1984;**15**:765.

31 Amstutz HC, Carey EJ. Skeletal manifestations and treatment of Gaucher's disease: review of twenty cases. *J Bone Joint Surg Am* 1966;**48**-A:670.

32 Kenet G, Hayek S, Mor M, *et al*. The 1226G (N370S) Gaucher mutation among patients with Legg-Calve-Perthes disease. *Blood Cells MolDis* 2003;**31**:72.

33 Goldblatt J, Sacks S, Beighton P. The orthopedic aspects of Gaucher disease *Clin Orthop* 1978;**137**:208.

34 Hermann G, Goldblatt J, Desnick RJ. Kummell disease: delayed collapse of the traumatised spine in a patient with Gaucher type 1 disease. *Br J Radiol* 1984;**57**:833.

35 Raynor RB. Spinal-cord compression secondary to Gaucher's disease. Case report. *J Neurosurg* 1962;**19**:902.

36 Katz K, Sabato S, Horev G, *et al*. Spinal involvement in children and adolescents with Gaucher disease. *Spine* 1993;**18**:332.

37 Rosenthal DI, Scott JA, Barranger J, *et al*. Evaluation of Gaucher disease using magnetic resonance imaging. *J Bone Joint Surg Am* 1986;**68**:802.

38 Mankin HJ, Doppelt SH, Rosenberg, AE Barranger JA. Metabolic bone disease in patients with Gaucher's disease: in: *Metabolic Bone Disease and Clinically Related Disorders*, (eds LV Aviali and SM Krane) 2nd Edn. Philadelphia: WB Saunders, 1990:730–752.

39 Barton DJ, Ludman MD, Benkov K, *et al*. Resting energy expenditure in Gaucher's disease type 1: effect of Gaucher's cell burden on energy requirements. *Metabolism* 1989;**38**:1238.

40 Schneider EL, Epstein CJ, Kaback MJ, Brandes D. Severe pulmonary involvement in adult Gaucher's disease. Report of three cases and review of the literature. *Am J Med* 1977;**63**:475.

41 Goldblatt J, Beighton P. Cutaneous manifestations of Gaucher disease. *Br J Dermatol* 1984;**111**:331.

42 Grewal RP, Doppelt SH, Thompson MA, *et al*. Neurologic complications of nonneuronopathic Gaucher's disease. *Arch Neurol* 1991;**48**:1271.

43 Hamlat A, Saikali S, Lakehal M, *et al*. Cauda equina syndrome due to an intra-dural sacral cyst in type-1 Gaucher disease. *Eur Spine J* 2004;**13**:249.

44 Neudorfer O, Giladi N, Elstein D, *et al*. Occurrence of Parkinson's syndrome in type I Gaucher disease. *Q J Med* 1996;**89**:691.

45 Tayebi N, Walker J, Stubblefield B, *et al*. Gaucher disease with parkinsonian manifestations: does glucocerebrosidase deficiency contribute to a vulnerability to parkinsonism? *Mol Genet Metab* 2003;**79**:104.

46 Lwin A, Orvisky E, Goker-Alpan O, *et al*. Glucocerebrosidase mutations in subjects with parkinsonism. *Mol Genet Metab* 2004;**81**:70.

47 Sidransky E, Ginns EI. Clinical heterogeneity among patients with Gaucher's disease. *JAMA* 1993;**269**:1154.

48 Martin BM, Sidransky E, Ginns EI. Gaucher's disease: advances and challenges. *Adv Pediatr* 1989;**36**:277.

49 Tybulewicz VL, Tremblay ML, LaMarca ME, *et al*. Animal model of Gaucher's disease from targeted disruption of the mouse glucocerebrosidase gene. *Nature* 1992;**357**:407.

50 Lui K, Commens C, Choong R, Jaworski R. Collodion babies with Gaucher's disease. *Arch Dis Child* 1988;**63**:854.

51 Lipson AH, Rogers M, Berry A. Collodion babies with Gaucher's disease – a further case. *Arch Dis Child* 1991;**66**:667.

52 Girgensohm H, Kellner H, Südhof H. Angeborener Morbus Gaucher bei Erythroblastose und Gefassverkalkung. *Klin Wochenschr* 1954;**32**:57.

53 Sun CC, Panny S, Combs J, Gutberlett R. Hydrops fetalis associated with Gaucher disease. *Pathol Res Pract* 1984;**179**:101.

54 Mignot C, Gelot A, Bessieres B, *et al*. Perinatal-lethal Gaucher disease. *Am J Med Genet* 2003;**120A**:338.

55 Erikson A. Gaucher disease – Norrbottnian type (III). Neuropaediatric and neurobiological aspects of clinical patterns and treatment. *Acta Paediatr Scand Suppl* 1986;**326**:1.

56 Dreborg S, Erikson A, Hagberg B. Gaucher disease – Norrbottnian type I. General clinical description. *Eur J Pediatr* 1980;**133**:107.

57 Miller JD, McCluer R, Kanfer JN. Gaucher's disease: neurologic disorder in adult siblings. *Ann Intern Med* 1973;**78**:883.

58 King JO. Progressive myoclonic epilepsy due to Gaucher's disease in an adult. *J Neurol Neurosurg Psychiatry* 1975;**38**:849.

59 Vinken PJ, Bruyn GW, Klawans HL (eds). *Handbook of Clinical Neurology*, vol 5: extrapyramidal disorders. Amsterdam: Elsevier, 1986.

60 Tripp JH, BD Lake, E Young, *et al*. Juvenile Gaucher's disease with horizontal gaze palsy in three siblings. *J Neurol Neurosurg Psychiatry* 1977;**40**:470.

61 Grover WD, Tucker SH, Wenger DA. Clinical variation in two related children with neuronopathic Gaucher disease. *Ann Neurol* 1978;**3**:281.

62 Sidransky E, Tsuji S, Stubblefield BK, *et al*. Gaucher patients with oculomotor abnormalities do not have a unique genotype. *Clin Genet* 1992;**41**:1.

63 Patterson MC, Horowitz, M Abel RB, *et al*. Isolated horizontal supranuclear gaze palsy as a marker of severe systemic involvement in Gaucher's disease. *Neurology* 1993;**43**:1993.

64 Cogan DG, Chu FC, Reingold D, Barranger J. Ocular motor signs in some metabolic diseases. *Arch Ophthalmol* 1981;**99**:1802.

65 Erikson A, Karlberg J, Skogman AL, Dreborg S. Gaucher disease (type III): intellectual profile. *Pediatr Neurol* 1987;**3**:87.

66 Park JK, Orvisky E, Tayebi N, *et al*. Myoclonic epilepsy in Gaucher disease: genotype-phenotype insights from a rare patient subgroup. *Pediatr Res* 2003;**53**:387.

67 Lam KW, Li CY, Yam LT, *et al*. Comparison of prostatic and nonprostatic acid phosphatase. *Ann NY Acad Sci* 1982;**390**:1.

68 Zimran A, Kay A, Gelbart T, *et al*. Gaucher disease. Clinical, laboratory, radiologic, and genetic features of 53 patients. *Medicine* (Baltimore) 1992;**71**:337.

69 Cabrera-Salazar MA, O'Rourke E, Henderson N, *et al*. Correlation of surrogate markers of Gaucher disease. Implications for long-term follow up of enzyme replacement therapy. *Clin Chim Acta* 2004;**344**:101.

70 Beutler E, Kuhl W. The diagnosis of the adult type of Gaucher's disease and its carrier state by demonstration of deficiency of beta-glucosidase activity in peripheral blood leukocytes. *J Lab Clin Med* 1970;**76**:747.

71 Beutler E, Kuhl W, Trinidad F, *et al.* Beta-glucosidase activity in fibroblasts from homozygotes and heterozygotes for Gaucher's disease. *Am J Hum Genet* 1971;**23**:62.

72 Ho MW, Seck J, Schmidt D, *et al.* Adult Gaucher's disease: kindred studies and demonstration of a deficiency of acid-glucosidase in cultured fibroblasts. *Am J Hum Genet* 1972;**24**:37.

73 Beutler E, Nguyen NJ, Henneberger MW, *et al.* Gaucher disease: gene frequencies in the Ashkenazi Jewish population. *Am J Hum Genet* 1993;**52**:85.

74 Shafit-Zagardo B, Devine EA, Smith M, *et al.* Assignment of the gene for acid beta-glucosidase to human chromosome 1. *Am J Hum Genet* 1981;**33**:564.

75 Tsuji S, Choudary PV, Martin BM, *et al.* Nucleotide sequence of cDNA containing the complete coding sequence for human lysosomal glucocerebrosidase. *J Biol Chem* 1986;**261**:50.

76 Brady RO, Barton NW, Grabowski GA. The role of neurogenetics in Gaucher disease. *Arch Neurol* 1993;**50**:1212.

77 Zhao H, Keddache M, Bailey L, *et al.* Gaucher's disease: identification of novel mutant alleles and genotype-phenotype relationships. *Clin Genet* 2003;**64**:57.

78 Beutler E. Gaucher disease: new molecular approaches to diagnosis and treatment. *Science* 1992;**256**:794.

79 Strom CM, Crossley B, Redman JB, *et al.* Molecular screening for diseases frequent in Ashkenazi Jews: lessons learned from more than 100 000 tests performed in a commercial laboratory. *Genet Med* 2004;**6**:145.

80 Tsuji S, Martin BM, Barranger JA, *et al.* Genetic heterogeneity in type 1 Gaucher disease: multiple genotypes in Ashkenazic and non-Ashkenazic individuals. *Proc Natl Acad Sci USA* 1988;**85**:2349.

81 Beutler E, Gelbart T, Kuhl W, *et al.* Identification of the second common Jewish Gaucher disease mutation makes possible population-based screening for the heterozygous state. *Proc Natl Acad Sci USA* 1991;**88**:10544.

82 Dahl N, Lagerstrom M, Erikson A, Pettersson U. Gaucher disease type III (Norrbottnian type) is caused by a single mutation in exon 10 of the glucocerebrosidase gene. *Am J Hum Genet* 1990;**47**:275.

83 Shahinfar M, Wenger DA. Adult and infantile Gaucher disease in one family: mutational studies and clinical update. *J Pediatr* 1994;**125**:919.

84 Nilsson O, Svennerholm L. Accumulation of glucosylceramide and glucosylsphingosine (psychosine) in cerebrum and cerebellum in infantile and juvenile Gaucher disease. *J Neurochem* 1982;**39**:709.

85 Hobbs JR. Experience with bone marrow transplantation for inborn errors of metabolism. *Enzyme* 1987;**38**:194.

86 Ashwell G, Morell AG. The role of surface carbohydrates in the hepatic recognition and transport of circulating glycoproteins. *Adv Enzymol Relat Areas Mol Biol* 1974;**41**:99.

87 Barton NW, Furbish FS, Murray GJ, *et al.* Therapeutic response to intravenous infusions of glucocerebrosidase in a patient with Gaucher disease. *Proc Natl Acad Sci USA* 1990;**87**:1913.

88 Pastores GM, Sibille AR, Grabowski GA. Enzyme therapy in Gaucher disease type 1: dosage efficacy and adverse effects in 33 patients treated for 6 to 24 months. *Blood* 1993;**82**:408.

89 Figueroa ML, Rosenbloom BE, Kay AC, *et al.* A less costly regimen of alglucerase to treat Gaucher's disease. *N Engl J Med* 1992;**327**:1632.

90 Cox TM, Aerts JM, Andria G, *et al.* The role of the iminosugar N-butyldeoxynojirimycin (miglustat) in the management of type I (non-neuronopathic) Gaucher disease: a position statement. *J Inherit Metab Dis* 2003;**26**:513.

91 Pastores GM, Barnett NL. Substrate reduction therapy: miglustat as a remedy for symptomatic patients with Gaucher disease type 1. *Expert Opin Investig Drugs* 2003;**12**:273.

92 Bembi B, Zanatta M, Carrozzi M, *et al.* Enzyme replacement treatment in type 1 and type 3 Gaucher's disease. *Lancet* 1994;**344**:1679.

93 Obeso JA, Artieda J, Rothwell JC, *et al.* The treatment of severe action myoclonus. *Brain* 1989;**112** (Pt 3):765.

94 Samuel R, Katz K, Papapoulos SE, *et al.* Aminohydroxy propylidene bisphosphonate (APD) treatment improves the clinical skeletal manifestations of Gaucher's disease. *Pediatrics* 1994;**94**:385.

95 Wenstrup RJ, Bailey L, Grabowski GA, Moskovitz J, *et al.* Gaucher disease: alendronate disodium improves bone mineral density in adults receiving enzyme therapy. *Blood* 2004;**104**:1253.

Niemann-Pick disease

MAJOR PHENOTYPIC EXPRESSION

Type A

Hepatosplenomegaly, neurologic degeneration, failure to thrive, cherry red macular spot, foam cells in bone marrow, storage of sphingomyelin and deficiency of lysosomal acid sphingomyelinase.

Type B

Hepatosplenomegaly, pulmonary infiltration, foam cells, storage of sphingomyelin and deficiency of sphingomyelinase.

INTRODUCTION

The disease was first described by Niemann in 1914 [1] in an infant with hepatosplenomegaly who died at 18 months after progressive neurologic deterioration and was found to have large foam cells in the liver and spleen. Pick's contribution [2,3] was to distinguish this disorder from Gaucher disease on the basis of the appearance of the foam cells. Phenotypic variation became apparent with additional reports [4,5], especially of adults with hepatosplenomegaly, but no neurologic abnormality in what has come to be called type B [6]. In 1934 the stored lipid was identified by Klenk [7] as sphingomyelin (Figure 95.1). Brady et al. in 1966 [8] identified the deficiency of sphingomyelinase (EC 3.1.4.12) (Figure 95.2) as the cause of Niemann-Pick disease. The deficiency was also readily documented in a type B patient [9].

The discovery of the enzyme permitted the categorization of other patients classified as Niemann-Pick disease who

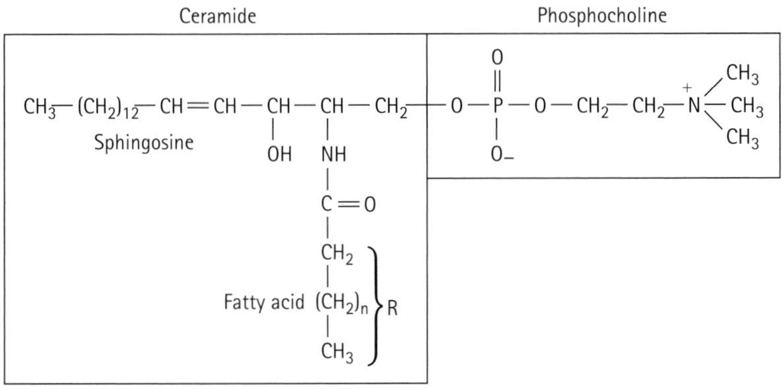

Figure 95.1   *The structure of sphingomyelin.*

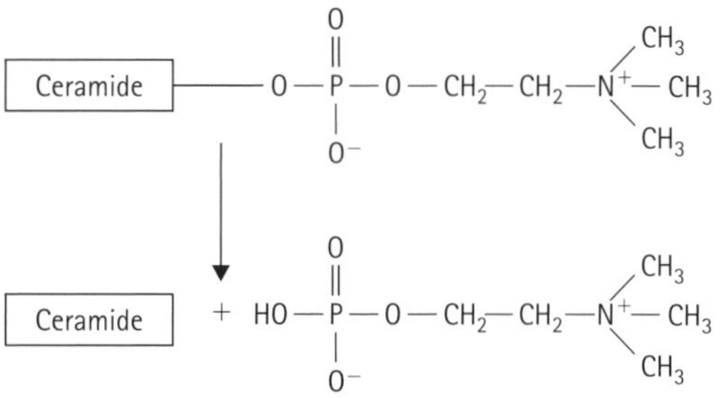

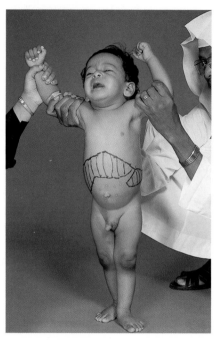

Figure 95.2 *The sphingomyelinase reaction, the site of defect in Niemann-Pick disease.*

clearly did not have sphingomyelinase deficiency as their molecular etiology, such as type C (Chapter 96). The separation of type C is an important distinction, but now that the nature of mutation has begun to be defined, separation into types A and B begins to appear artificial. There are certainly some very distinct phenotypes among the deficiencies of sphingomyelinase; soon the genotype for each will be known. It is already clear that there are quite distinct genotypes. Type A disease is relatively rare except in Ashkenazi Jews [5,10,36]; in whom type B is quite rare. Various phenotypes of type B are found commonly in Arabs, Turks and Portuguese [11]. Somatic cell hybridization indicated clearly that types A and B represented allelic variation in a single gene [12] and that type C was different. Molecular studies were confirmatory.

The cDNA for sphingomyelinase has been cloned and sequenced [13,14]. The gene has been mapped to chromosome 11 p15.1-p15.4 [15]. A number of mutations have been identified in both type A and type B patients [11,16,17]. Distinct mutations have been found in the ethnic groups in which Niemann-Pick disease is common.

CLINICAL ABNORMALITIES

Type A

The acute infantile form of Niemann-Pick disease usually presents first with massive enlargement of the liver and spleen [5,6,10,18–20] (Figures 95.3–95.5). Some patients have neonatal edema and hydrops fetalis may occur [21]. The liver and spleen may be enlarged at birth, and storage of lipid has been documented in liver, brain, kidney and placenta prior to birth [18,22,23]. Placental enlargement has been shown by ultrasound [24] and it is thought that storage in the placenta may lead to fetal loss [18]. The abdomen is protuberant. The liver seems always to be enlarged out of proportion to the spleen, in contrast to Gaucher disease (Chapter 94).

We have seen Niemann-Pick patients with hepatosplenomegaly whose history was that the spleen was not palpable early. Transaminases aspartate transaminase (AST) and alanine transaminase (ALT) are elevated, at least at times [25]. The

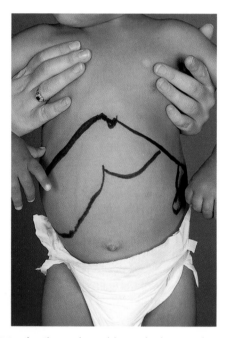

Figure 95.3 *A patient with infantile Niemann-Pick disease. The hepatosplenomegaly is outlined.*

Figure 95.4 *Another patient with massive hepatosplenomegaly due to Niemann-Pick disease.*

alkaline phosphatase is also usually elevated. The cholesterol may be elevated in addition. There may be prolonged neonatal jaundice, and episodes of unexplained jaundice later. We have seen patients who presented in early infancy with acute jaundice, abnormal liver function tests and hepatomegaly, suggesting a diagnosis of acute hepatocellular disease rather than a lipid storage disease. We have also seen a patient in whom two liver biopsies had been done in another institution and

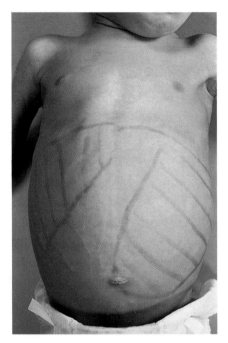

Figure 95.5 *Massive hepatosplenomegaly in an 11-month-old infant with Niemann-Pick disease. Abdominal distension was noted at birth. He had jaundice and acholic stools at 6 months, and repeated pulmonary infections.*

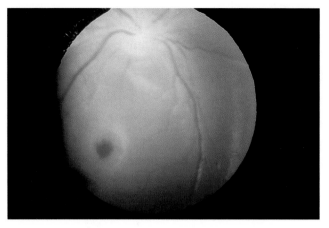

Figure 95.6 *The cherry red macular degeneration in a 10-month-old with Niemann-Pick disease.*

appearance, the macular halo syndrome, or melting snow appearance [31–34]. The electroretinogram is abnormal.

Brownish-yellow discoloration may develop in the skin [35]. Xanthomas have been described, particularly on the face and arms [5,10,36]. Most patients develop osteoporosis. A hypochromic, microcytic anemia may be followed with time by thrombocytopenia or granulocytopenia. The terminal episode may be with asphyxia or pneumonia.

Type B

Type B patients represent quite a varied spectrum, from those diagnosed in infancy because of hepatomegaly or hepatosplenomegaly to those first detected in adulthood, as expected for a variety of different mutations. Nevertheless, the type A phenotype is much more common and accounts for about three-fourths of all patients. We suspect that among the type B patients there are a number of distinct phenotypes that are beginning to correlate with genotype.

What we think of as the classic type B patient is an adult or older adolescent who comes to attention because of splenomegaly found incidentally on physical examination [37–39] (Figures 95.7, 95.8). Some of these patients have had sea-blue histiocytes in marrow [37] or tissues [39] and this type has been called the Lewis variant [37]. Such patients may have elevation of the serum level of acid phosphatase. The King Faisal series now includes 35 patients. Pancytopenia may result from hypersplenism, and splenectomy may be required. Splenic rupture has been described [37]. Patients have been described in whom there were no neurological abnormalities well into adult life [5,39–41]. This may be one phenotype.

Others with a relatively mild phenotype may have some neurologic features. Extrapyramidal signs were reported in one family [42]. Mental retardation was reported in unrelated patients at 9 and 18 years [43]. A number of patients have been reported with cerebellar ataxia [18,42,43]. Some of these may have been patients with Niemann-Pick type C disease. Patients have had cherry red spots or other grayish macular

interpreted as fatty metamorphosis. At least one patient with Niemann-Pick disease was thought on biopsy to have glycogenosis [26]. Jaundice is a common terminal finding and some patients have developed disseminated intravascular coagulopathy. There may be lymphadenopathy.

By 6 months episodes of respiratory distress occur, which may require oxygen. Some episodes are clear-cut infections, such as bronchiolitis or pneumonia, but in others infection is not obvious. Some patients have had noisy respirations and rhinorrhea from birth [27]. Chest film may reveal diffuse interstitial infiltrates in a reticular or finely nodular pattern [28]. Patients may also have unexplained fevers.

Failure to thrive is evident by 8 to 9 months of age. Weight gain stops, but increase in linear growth may not stop until 15 to 18 months of age, and so the patient looks increasingly cachectic. Anorexia may be complicated by vomiting, and there may be some diarrhea [29,30] or constipation.

Neurologic involvement may be first evidenced in a failure to achieve milestones, such as sitting, but some have developed normally for 6 months [27], or as long as a year [6]. Progression of disease occurs with loss of milestones achieved. Patients may appear weak or hypotonic. Deep tendon reflexes are exaggerated. Neurologic degeneration is progressive to a spastic, rigid state in which there appears to be no consciousness of the environment. Seizures are not common; the electroencephalograph (EEG) is usually normal. Cherry red or cherry black (dependent on the pigment of the patient) macular spots (Figure 95.6) are seen in about 50 percent of the patients. Sometimes there is a sprinkled salt appearance around the macula, a gray granular

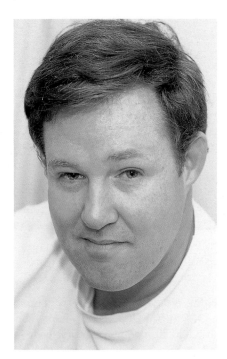

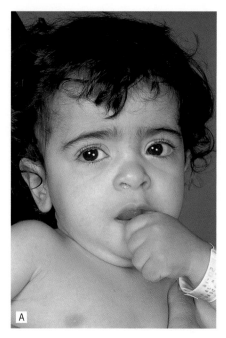

Figure 95.7 *A 39-year-old man with Lewis variant of Niemann-Pick disease. The spleen was palpable 6 cm below the costal margin. The liver was at 4 cm. Sphingomyelinase activity of fibroblasts was 18 percent of control.*

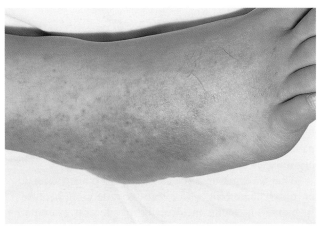

Figure 95.8 *Brownish pigment on the dorsal and lateral ankle correlated with a loss of vibratory sensation in the area.*

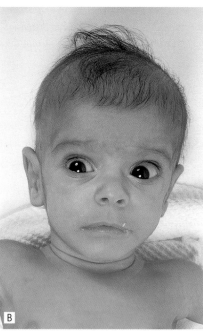

Figure 95.9 *Four Saudi infants (A–D) with Niemann-Pick disease illustrating some similarity of facial features. Patients tend to lose adipose tissue over the forehead and about the orbits; the nasal bridge is spared, giving the appearance of a crest of tissue.*

pigmentation about the macula, often with no other neurologic manifestation [31,32,39,44–47]. Evidence of abnormal neural storage has been observed despite absence of neurologic abnormalities [48]. Two sisters without mental retardation had inclusion bodies in exons and Schwann cells of rectal biopsies, and vacuolated macrophases in the cerebrospinal fluid (CSF) [48].

Some others that have been included in Type B have had quite severe, and early-onset disease. We think of this as the Saudi variant [49,50]. Early symptoms are failure to thrive and abdominal distension. On examination the spleen is huge (Figures 95.3–95.5). The liver may be just as huge or even more

so. They have been said not to have neurodegenerative disease, but they all have cherry red macular spots (Figure 95.6). Furthermore, two patients who survived infancy and bone marrow transplantation went on to develop white matter changes in the central nervous system (CNS) and neurological manifestations. The facial appearance may develop similarities (Figure 95.9).

Patients are hypotonic and developmentally delayed. One patient at 20 months could sit, but could not crawl or stand

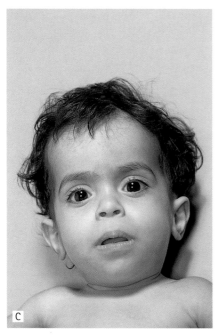

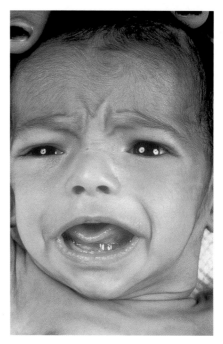

Figure 95.10   *Another Saudi infant with Niemann-Pick disease, illustrating a more advanced degree of emaciation of the face. The eyes appear sunken.*

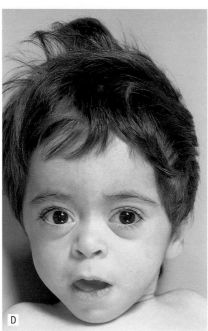

Figure 95.9   (*Continued*).

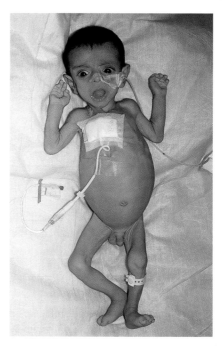

Figure 95.11   *This Saudi infant illustrates the extreme emaciation and the large abdomen resulting from organomegaly.*

[50]. She could speak two or three words. Cachexia is prominent early (Figures 95.10, 95.11). Most of these patients die by 3 years-of-age. Terminal events include bleeding, anemia and thrombocytopenia, often requiring daily transfusion of platelets, and hepatic failure. In a series of Saudi patients, some of whose pictures are shown in this chapter, five died between 18 and 36 months; one survivor to 4.5 years had had a bone marrow transplantation. Pulmonary infiltration is evident in roentgenograms as miliary nodular lesions [50]. Pulmonary function may be abnormal, and there may be complicating pneumonia. Liver function tests, alanine amino-transferase and aspartate amino transferase may be elevated, along with triglycerides. Abdominal ultrasound documents the hepatosplenomegaly.

Other patients may have hepatic or pulmonary disease. Liver disease, either biliary cirrhosis [51], or cirrhosis, may be life-threatening, and portal hypertension and ascites may develop

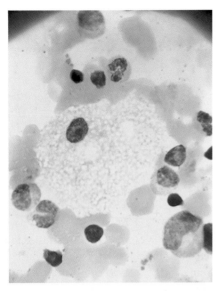

Figure 95.12   *The Niemann-Pick foam cells of the bone marrow.*

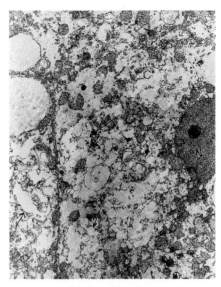

Figure 95.13   *Electron microscopy of biopsied liver of an infant with classic infantile Niemann-Pick disease and deficiency of sphingomyelinase. Hepatocytes were large and pale. Electron microscopy, with the nucleus on the right, illustrates many irregular rounded membrane-bound lucent areas. These are considered to have contained lipid, which was extracted ($\times$ 10 000).*

[52]. This latter picture was reported in an otherwise adult-type disease [52]. Pulmonary disease has also been reported in adult type disease [53]. In addition to the diffuse infiltration seen on roentgenograms, there may be exertional dyspnea and decreased pO_2 because of diminished diffusion. Bronchopneumonia may develop, and/or cor pulmonale [53].

In a series of Type B patients in the US, in whom sphingomyelinase deficiency and the mutation were documented, height and weight were usually low; 39 percent and 21 percent were below the fifth percentile for height and weight, and these correlated with large organ volumes [54]. Bone age was also behind 2.5 years.

Common pathological features

The pathognomonic feature of all patients with deficiency of sphingomyelinase is the foam cell (Figure 95.12). This large (20–90 μ) cell or macrophage is most commonly first detected in the bone marrow aspirate. As a reticuloendothelial cell it is found widely in these patients' spleen, liver, lymph nodes and lungs. In stained preparations the cells have a foamy appearance that results from the stored material, which stains positively with stains for lipids. The lipid droplets are uniform in size, and the appearance has been called honeycomb-like or mulberry-like. The cytoplasm of these cells stains blue with Wright stain, which gives rise to the sea-blue histiocyte designation [37]. It is clear now that sea-blue histiocytes, once thought to represent a distinct disease [55,56] are seen in sphingomyelinase deficiency [39]. On electron microscopy (Figures 95.13, 95.14), foam cells have small eccentric nuclei and membrane-bound lucent areas from which storage material has been dissolved. There may be granular material, whorls or lamellae. There may be infiltration in the gastrointestinal tract, which might account for intestinal symptoms and failure to thrive, and diagnosis has been made by rectal biopsy. Storage is seen in

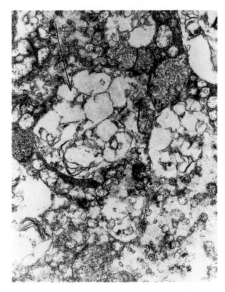

Figure 95.14   *In higher magnification ($\times$ 33,000) the lucent inclusions contained fragments of membranes and granular material.*

neuronal cells and axons, and cerebral atrophy and neuroaxonal dystrophy are characteristic of type A disease.

GENETICS AND PATHOGENESIS

Niemann-Pick disease is transmitted as an autosomal recessive disease. The disease has been seen widely throughout the population of the world. The frequency of type A is much higher in Ashkenazic Jewish populations in which type B disease is rare.

The molecular defect is in the enzyme sphingomyelinase (Figure 95.2, p. 636) [8,9]. The enzyme was first purified from rat liver [57]. It cleaves the phosphocholine moiety from sphingomyelin. It is a lysosomal enzyme with a pH optimum about 4.5 and a molecular weight of approximately 70 kDa [58,59]. The cDNA predicts a protein monomer of 64 kDa; if the 6 potential glycosylations were filled the molecular weight would be 72–74 kDa. There are a number of sphingomyelinase activator proteins (SAPs), but they do not appear to be required for enzymatic activity.

The defect has been demonstrated in tissues such as liver, kidney and brain [60,61], cultured fibroblasts [40,62,63] and leukocytes [64,65]. Patients with type A and type B are defective in the same enzyme. Clinical diagnosis is generally based on the assay of leukocytes or fibroblasts. In general, in type A patients there is less than five percent of control activity, and often activity is undetectable. In type B disease activity is variable and may be higher, up to 10 percent of control [40,59,61], but it may also be zero in type B. Residual activity is not a reliable index of clinical severity.

In order to approximate physiological conditions more closely, a number of investigators have explored intact cell assays in which ^{14}C-labeled or fluorescent natural substrate was taken up and transported to lysosomes and then hydrolyzed [40,63–65]. In these studies substantial hydrolysis of sphingomyelin was demonstrable in type B cells, while very little occurred in those of type A.

Heterozygotes for types A and B disease generally have enzyme activity that is intermediate between those of homozygotes and normal [12,66]. In fact some heterozygotes have had splenomegaly or foam cells in the marrow. On the other hand heterozygote detection may not be reliably excluded, because of overlap with the normal range.

Prenatal diagnosis has been undertaken by enzyme analysis in cultured amniocytes [40] and chorionic villus material [67], and a number of affected fetuses have been detected [68]. The intact cell assay with labeled sphingomyelin has also been effectively employed with cultured amniocytes [40].

The nature of the enzyme defect leads to the accumulation of sphingomyelin in tissues. This phospholipid is composed of the sphingosine C-18 base with a long-chain fatty acid in amide linkage, forming the ceramide moiety, linked to choline monophosphate (Figure 95.1, p. 635). Levels in affected patients are enormously increased, especially in tissues rich in reticuloendothelial cells [69,70]. Type A patients accumulate sphingomyelin in the brain [20,71], while type B patients generally do not [20]. There is also storage of cholesterol in the liver of patients [69], and this tends to be more in tissues of type A than of type B patients. The other compound that accumulates in the viscera is bis(monacylglycero)phosphate [72].

The molecular genetics of Niemann-Pick disease proceeded rapidly once the gene was sequenced and DNA probes became available. Three common mutations were found in Ashkenazic

type A patients [15,73,74] that account for 92 percent of the mutant alleles studied [16]. Two are point mutations in exons 6 and 2, R496L (an arginine to leucine change) and L302P (a leucine to proline). The third is a single-base deletion in exon 2 that creates a frameshift (fsP 330) that leads to a stop-codon. The R496L mutation occurred at a CpG dinucleotide, where mutation is common. The two point mutations have been found in patients homozygous for each and in compounds. The R496L mutation has been found in only one of 20 non-Jewish, type A patients; the other two mutations in none. Interestingly, each of the common type A mutations, R476L, L302P and FsP330 has been found along with a type B mutation in Ashkenazi patients with a type B phenotype [11,17], underscoring the artificiality of these old classifications. A small number of mutations have been identified in non-Jewish type A patients, each unique to the family in which it was found [75–78]. Four were single-base substitutions; one a nonsense mutation; one was a single-base deletion which caused a frameshift; and one was a splice site change. Two of the point mutations were in adjacent codons in exon 3.

Among type B patients a three-base deletion removing an arginine at 608 (ΔR608) [11,17] was found in about 12 percent of a large population of type B patients. In homozygous form, patients had mild disease. It also predicts mild disease in compounds with other genes, including the five Ashkenazic Jewish type B patients who carried type A genes in the other allele. This mutation was found in approximately 90 percent of North African Arabs with splenomegaly [79]. In the study of growth restriction in type B children [54] the children homozygous for ΔR608 were of normal height and weight. The S436R (a serine to arginine) also was associated with mild disease in a 19-year-old Japanese patient [76]. L137P, A196P and R474W were also associated with mild disease [11].

Expression studies [73,75] indicated that the ΔR608 and other mutations found in milder type B phenotype expressed considerable catalytic activity, while mutations that caused premature stop-codons expressed no catalytic activity in COS cells.

Among the Saudi Arabian patients some 85 percent of alleles carried the two mutations H421Y and K576N [11]; 11 patients were homozygous for the former and two for the latter. These mutations led to early onset and early demise. All had pulmonary disease.

Niemann-Pick type B is relatively common in Turkish patients, in whom 3 mutations L137P, FsP189 and L549P accounted for about 75 percent of the alleles [11]. L137P was consistent with quite mild disease in homozygotes and heterozygotes. The A196P mutation, found to be common in patients of Scottish heritage appeared to convey mild disease even when in compound with a null mutation.

The phenotype-genotype correlations are useful in counseling the parents of newly diagnosed patients, at least in the populations where mutations are common. They are also useful for prenatal diagnosis and carrier detection in any family in which the precise mutation is known, or in an ethnic group in which a small number of mutations is common.

TREATMENT

A variety of transplantations have been made, including liver and amniotic cells, without evident change. Bone marrow transplantation has been reported as being without effect on the neurologic picture of the type A disease [80]. However, it should be of considerable advantage in type B patients because in type B [81] and in type A patients it has been observed that liver and spleen size decreased following transplantation, and improvement in lung infiltration was documented roentgenographically. Both enzyme replacement and gene therapy are under active exploration, and animal models of sphingomyelinase deficiency are available.

References

1   Niemann A. Ein unbekanntes Krankheitsbild. *Jahrb Kinderheilkd* 1914;**79**:1.

2   Pick L. Uber die lipoidzellige Splenohepatomegalie typus Niemann-Pick als Stoffwecheslerkrankung. *Med Klin* 1927;**23**:1483.

3   Pick L. Il Niemann-Pick's disease and other forms of so-called xanthomatoses. *Am J Med Sci* 1933;**185**:601.

4   Pflander U. La maladie de Niemann-Pick dans le cadre des lipidoses. *Schweiz Med Wochenschr* 1946;**76**:1128.

5   Crocker AC, Farber S. Niemann-Pick disease: a review of eighteen patients. *Medicine (Baltimore)* 1958;**37**:1.

6   Crocker AC. The cerebral defect in Tay-Sachs disease and Niemann-Pick disease. *J Neurochem* 1961;**7**:69.

7   Klenk E. Uber die Natur der Phosphatide der Milz bei Niemann-Pickchen Krankheit. *Z Physiol Chem* 1934;**229**:151.

8   Brady RO, Kanfer JN, Mock MB, Frederickson DS. The metabolism of sphingomyelin. Il Evidence of an enzymatic deficiency in Niemann-Pick disease. *Proc Natl Acad Sci USA* 1966;**55**:366.

9   Schneider PB, Kennedy EP. Sphingomyelinase in normal human spleens and in spleens from subjects with Niemann-Pick disease. *J Lipid Res* 1967;**8**:202.

10 Schettler G, Kahlke W. *Niemann-Pick Disease*. Springer-Verlag, New York;1967.

11 Simonaro CM, Desnick RJ, McGovern MM, *et al.* The demographics and distribution of type B Niemann-Pick disease: novel mutations lead to new genotype/phenotype correlations. *Am J Hum Genet* 2002;**71**:1413.

12 Besley GTN, Hoogeboom AJM, Hoogeveen A, *et al.* Somatic cell hybridization studies showing different gene mutations in Niemann-Pick variants. *Hum Genet* 1980;**54**:409.

13 Quintern L, Schuchman EH, Levran O, *et al.* Isolation of cDNA clones encoding human acid sphingomyelinase. Occurrence of alternatively spliced transcripts. *EMBO J* 1989;**8**:2469.

14 Schuchmann EH, Levran O, Desnick RJ. Structural organization and complete nucleotide sequence of the gene encoding human acid sphingomyelinase. *Genomics* 1992;**12**:197.

15 Pereira L, Desnick RJ, Adler D, *et al.* Regional assessment of the human acid sphingomyelinase gene by PCR analysis of somatic cell hybrids and *in situ* hybridization to 11p151–p154. *Genomics* 1991;**9**:229.

16 Levran O, Desnick RJ, Schuchman EH. Niemann-Pick disease: a common mutation in Ashkenazi Jewish individuals results in the type A and B forms. *Proc Natl Acad Sci USA* 1991;**88**:3748.

17 Levran O, Desnick RJ, and Schuchman EH. Niemann-Pick type B disease: identification of a single codon deletion in the acid sphingomyelinase gene and genotype/phenotype correlations in Type A and B patients. *J Clin Invest* 1991;**88**:806.

18 Frederickson DS, Sloan HR. Sphingomyelin lipidoses: Niemann-Pick disease: in *The Metabolic Basis of Inherited Disease* (eds JB Stanbury, JB Wyngaarden, DS Frederickson). 3rd edn. McGraw Hill, New York;1972:783.

19 Elleder M, Jirasek A. International symposium on Niemann-Pick disease. *Eur J Pediatr* 1983;**140**:90.

20 Spence M, Callahan J. *Sphingomyelin-Cholesterol Lipidoses: The Niemann-Pick Group of Diseases,* Vol 2. 6th ed. McGraw-Hill, New York;1989.

21 Meizner I, Levy A, Carmi R, Robinson C. Niemann-Pick disease associated with nonimmune hydrops fetalis. *Am J Obstet Gynecol* 1990;**163**:128.

22 Schneider EL, Ellis WG, Brady RO, *et al.* Prenatal Niemann-Pick disease: biochemical and histologic examination of a 19-gestational-week fetus. *Pediatr Res* 1972;**6**:720.

23 Sarrut S, Belamich P. Etude du placenta dans trois observations de dyslipidosie a revelation neonatale *Arch Anat Cytol Pathol* 1983;**31**:187.

24 Schoenfeld A, Abramovici A, Klibanski C, Ovadia J. Placental ultrasonographic biochemical and histochemical studies in human fetuses affected with Niemann-Pick disease type A. *Placenta* 1985;**6**:33.

25 Tamaru J, Iwasaki I, Horie H, *et al.* Niemann-Pick disease associated with liver disorders. *Acta Pathol Jap* 1985;**35**:1267.

26 Smith WE, Kahler SG, Frush DP, *et al.* Hepatic storage of glycogen in Niemann-Pick disease type B. *J Pediatr* 2001;**138**:946.

27 Balint JH, Nyhan WL, Lietman P, Turner PH. Lipid patterns in Niemann-Pick disease. *J Lab Clin Med* 1961;**58**:548.

28 Grunebaum M. The roentgenographic findings in the acute neuronopathic form of Niemann-Pick disease. *Br J Radiol* 1976;**49**:1018.

29 Dinari G, Rosenbach Y, Grunebaum M, *et al.* Gastrointestinal manifestations of Niemann-Pick disease. *Enzyme* 1980;**25**:407.

30 Yamano T, Shimada M, Okada S, *et al.* Ultrastructural study of biopsy specimens of rectal mucosa: its use in neuronal storage diseases. *Arch Pathol Lab Med* 1982;**106**:673.

31 Cogan DG, Kuwabara T. The sphingolipidoses and the eye. *Arch Ophthalmol* 1968;**79**:437.

32 Cogan DG, Chu FC, Barranger JA, Gregg RE. Macular halo syndrome. Variant of Niemann-Pick disease. *Arch Opthalmol* 1983;**101**:1698.

33 Lipson MH, O'Donell J, Callahan JW, *et al.* Ocular involvement in Niemann-Pick disease Type B. *J Pediatr* 1986;**108**:582.

34 Matthews JD, Weiter JJ, Kolodney EH. Macular halos associated with Niemann-Pick type B disease. *Ophthalmology* 1986;**93**:933.

35 Markini MK, Gergen P, Akhtar M, Ghandour M. Niemann-Pick disease: report of a case with skin involvement. *Am J Dis Child* 1982;**136**:650.

36 Maurer LE. Niemann-Pick's disease a report of four cases. *Rocky Mtn Med J* 1941;**38**:460.

37 Blankenship RM, Greenburg BR, Lucas RN, *et al.* Familial sea-blue histiocytes with acid phosphatemia. A syndrome resembling Gaucher disease: the Lewis variant. *JAMA* 1973;**225**:54.

38 Chan WC, Lai KS, Todd D. Adult Niemann-Pick disease – a case report. *J Pathol* 1977;**121**:177.

39 Dawson PG, Dawson G. Adult Niemann-Pick disease with sea-blue histiocytes in the spleen. *Hum Pathol* 1982;**13**:1115.

40 Vanier MT, Rousson R, Garcia I, *et al.* Biochemical studies in Niemann-Pick disease. III *In vitro* and *in vivo* assays of sphingomyelin degradation in cultured skin fibroblasts and amniotic fluid cells for the diagnosis of the various forms of the disease. *Clin Genet* 1985;**27**:20.

41 Landas S, Foucar K, Sando GN, *et al.* Adult Niemann-Pick disease masquerading as sea-blue histiocyte syndrome: report of a case confirmed by lipid analysis and enzyme assays. *Am J Hematol* 1985;**20**:391.

42 Elleder M, Cihula J. Niemann-Pick disease (variation in sphingomyelinase deficient group): neurovisceral phenotype (A) with an abnormally protracted

clinical course and variable expression of neurological symptomatology in three siblings. *Eur J Pediatr* 1981;**140**:323.

43 Sogawa H, Horino K, Nakamura F, *et al*. Chronic Niemann-Pick disease with sphingomyelinase deficiency in two brothers with mental retardation. *Eur J Pediatr* 1978;**128**:235.

44 Hammersen G, Oppermann HC, Harms E, *et al*. Oculo-neural involvement in an enzymatically proven case of Niemann-Pick disease type B. *Eur J Pediatr* 1979;**137**:77.

45 Shah MD, Desai AP, Jain MK, *et al*. Niemann-Pick disease type B with oculoneural involvement. *Indian Pediatr* 1983;**20**:521.

46 Harzer K, Ruprecht KW, Seuffer-Schulze D, Jans U. Morbus Niemann-Pick type B: Enzymatisch Gesichert mit unerwarteter retinaler Beiteligung. *Albrecht Von Graefes Arch Klin Ophthalmol* 1978;**206**:79.

47 Lowe D, Martin F, Sarks J. Ocular manifestations of adult Niemann-Pick disease: a case report. *Aust NZ J Ophthalmol* 1986;**14**:41.

48 Takada G, Satoh W, Komatsu K, *et al*. Transitory type of sphingomyelinase deficient Niemann-Pick disease: clinical and morphological studies and follow-up of two sisters. *Tohoku J Exp Med* 1987;**153**:27.

49 Al-Essa MA, Ozand PT. Lysosomal storage disease. *Atlas of Common Lysosomal and Peroxisomal Disorders* (MA Alessa, PT Ozard). King Faisal Specialist Hospital and Research Centre, Riyadh;1999:1.

50 Roy D, Oqiel SA. What's your diagnosis? *Ann Saudi Med* 2001;**21**:127.

51 Conolly CE, Kennedy SM. Primary biliary atresia and Niemann-Pick disease. *Hum Pathol* 1984;**15**:97 (letter).

52 Tassoni JP, Fawaz KA, Johnson DE. Cirrhosis and portal hypertension in a patient with adult Niemann-Pick disease. *Gastroenterology* 1991;**100**:567.

53 Lever AML, Ryder JB. Cor pulmonale in adult secondary to Niemann-Pick disease. *Thorax* 1983;**38**:873.

54 Wasserstein MP, Larkin AE, Glass RB, *et al*. Growth restriction in children with type B Niemann-Pick disease. *J Pediatr* 2003;**142**:424.

55 Bloom W. Splenomegaly (type Gaucher) and lipoid-histiocytosis (type Niemann). *Am J Pathol* 1925;**1**:595.

56 Bloom W. The histogenesis of essential lipoid histiocytosis (Niemann-Pick disease). *Arch Pathol* 1928;**6**:827.

57 Kanfer JN, Young OM, Shapiro D, Brady RO. The metabolism of sphingomyelin. I Purification and properties of a sphingomyelin-cleaving enzyme from rat liver tissue. *J Biol Chem* 1966;**241**:1081.

58 Quintern LE, Weitz G, Nehrkorn H, *et al*. Acid sphingomyelinase from human urine. Purification and characterization. *Biochim Biophys Acta* 1987;**922**:323.

59 Quintern LE, Zenk TS, Sandhoff K. The urine from patients with peritonitis as a rich source for purifying human acid sphingomyelinase and other lysosomal enzymes. *Biochim Biophys Acta* 1989;**1003**:121.

60 Callahan JW, Khalil M. Sphingomyelinases in human tissues. III Expression of Niemann-Pick disease and other lysosomal storage diseases. *Biochim Biophys Acta* 1975;**754**:82.

61 Gatt S, Dinur T, Kopolvic J. Niemann-Pick disease: presence of the magnesium-dependent sphingomyelinase in brain of infantile form of the disease. *J Neurochem* 1978;**30**:917.

62 Brady RO. The abnormal biochemistry of inherited disorders of lipid metabolism. *Fed Proc* 1973;**32**:1660.

63 Kudoh T, Velkoff MA, Wenger DA. Uptake and metabolism of radioactively labeled sphingomyelin in cultured skin fibroblasts from controls and patients with Niemann-Pick disease and other lysosomal storage diseases. *Biochim Biophys Acta* 1983;**754**:82.

64 Kampine JP, Brady RO, Kanfer JN. Diagnosis of Gaucher's disease and Niemann-Pick disease with small samples of venous blood. *Science* 1967;**155**:86.

65 Zitman D, Chazan S, Klibansky C. Sphingomyelinase activity levels in human peripheral blood leukocytes using [3H] sphingomyelin as substrate: study of heterozygotes and homozygotes for Niemann-Pick disease variants. *Clin Chim Acta* 1978;**86**:37.

66 Gal AE, Brady RO, Hibbert SR, Pentchev PG. A practical chromogenic procedure for the detection of homozygotes and heterozygous carriers of Niemann-Pick disease. *N Engl J Med* 1975;**293**:632.

67 Vanier MT, Boue J, Dumaz Y. Niemann-Pick disease Type B: first-trimester prenatal diagnosis on chorionic villi and biochemical study of a foetus at 12 weeks of development. *Clin Genet* 1985;**28**:348.

68 Maziere JC, Maziere C, Hosli P. An ultramicrochemical assay for sphingomyelinase: rapid prenatal diagnosis of a fetus at risk for Niemann-Pick disease. *Monogr Hum Genet* 1978;**9**:198.

69 Vanier MT. Biochemical studies in Niemann-Pick disease. I Major sphingolipids in liver and spleen. *Biochim Biophys Acta* 1983;**750**:178.

70 Rao BG, Spence MW. Niemann-Pick disease: lipid analyses and studies on sphingomyelinases. *Ann Neurol* 1977;**1**:385.

71 Besley GTN, Elleder M. Enzyme activities and phospholipid storage patterns in brain and spleen samples from Niemann-Pick disease variants: a comparison of neuropathic and non-neuropathic forms. *J Inherit Metab Dis* 1986;**9**:59.

72 Rouser G, Kritchevsky G, Yamamoto A, *et al*. Accumulation of a glycerolphospholipid in classical Niemann-Pick disease. *Lipids* 1968;**3**:287.

73 Levran O, Desnick RJ, Schuchman EH. A common missense mutation (L302P) in Ashkenazi Jewish Type A Niemann-Pick disease patients. Transient expression studies demonstrate the causative nature of the two common Ashkenazi Jewish Niemann-Pick disease mutations. *Blood* 1992;**80**:2081.

74 Levran O, Desnick RJ, Schuchman EH. Type A Niemann-Pick disease: a frame-shift mutation in the acid sphingomyelinase gene (fsP330) occurs in about 8 percent of Ashkenazi Jewish alleles. *Hum Mut* 1993;**2**:213.

75 Takahashi T, Suchi M, Desnick RJ, *et al*. Identification and expression of five new mutations in the acid sphingomyelinase gene which cause types A and B Niemann-Pick disease. Molecular evidence for genetic heterogeneity in the neuronopathic and non-neuronopathic forms. *J Biol Chem* 1992;**267**:1255.

76 Takahashi T, Desnick RJ, Takada G, Schuchman EH. Identification of a missense mutation (S436R) in the acid sphingomyelinase gene from a Japanese patient with type B Niemann-Pick disease. *Hum Mut* 1992;**1**:70.

77 Ferlinz K, Hurwitz R, Sandhoff K. Molecular basis of acid sphingomyelinase deficiency in a patient with Niemann-Pick disease Type A. *Biochem Biophys Res Commun* 1991;**179**:1187.

78 Levran O, Desnick RJ, Schuchman EH. Identification of a 3′ acceptor splice site mutation (g2610c) in the acid sphingomyelinase gene of patients with types A and B Niemann-Pick disease. *Hum Mol Genet* 1993;**2**:205.

79 Vanier MT, Ferlinz K, Rousson R, *et al*. Deletion of arginine (608) in acid sphingomyelinase is the prevalent mutation among Niemann-Pick disease type B patients from North Africa. *Hum Genet* 1993;**92**:325.

80 Bayeuer E, August CS, Kaman N, *et al*. Bone marrow transplantation for Niemann-Pick disease (Type 1A). *Bone Marrow Transplant* 1992;**10**:83.

81 Vellodi A, Hobbs JR, O'Donnel NM, *et al*. Treatment of Niemann-Pick disease type B by allogenic bone marrow transplantation. *BMJ* 1987;**295**:1375.

96

Niemann-Pick type C disease/cholesterol-processing abnormality

MAJOR PHENOTYPIC EXPRESSION

Paralysis of vertical gaze, ataxia, dystonia, hypotonia, prolonged neonatal icterus, hepatosplenomegaly, dementia, foam cells, lysosomal storage of cholesterol in viscera, and impaired cellular esterification of cholesterol.

INTRODUCTION

Niemann-Pick type C was first described in the review by Crocker and Farber [1] of their 18 patients with Niemann-Pick disease; the classic features of paralysis of upward gaze, ataxia, dystonia, spasticity and seizures were clearly described in one of the patients, all of whom had the characteristic foam cells and storage of sphingomyelin. They classified Niemann-Pick into types A and B (Chapter 95), C and D, which is now known to be a variant of C, described in a French-Acadian isolate in Nova Scotia [2]. When the defect in sphingomyelinase was found in types A and B by Brady and his colleagues [3], it became evident that this enzyme was normal in type C [4]. Pentchev and colleagues [5,6] discovered defective esterification of exogenous cholesterol in the mutant BALB/c mouse. This group then showed that the same faulty regulation of cholesterol processing and storage was present in cultured fibroblasts from patients with Niemann-Pick type C disease [7]. The study of complementation in somatic cell hybrids indicated that type D was allelic with type C on one gene, and clearly separate from types A and B [8].

Complementation studies of type C indicated the presence of two complementation groups [9,10]. In 95 percent of a small number of patients studied the gene (NPC1) has been mapped to chromosome 18q11–12 [11,12]. The smaller group of patients considered to have a defective NPC2 gene [10] have been reported [13] to have abnormalities in the gene HE1 on chromosome 14q24.3, which codes for a lysosomal cholesterol-binding protein [14]. A number of mutations in the NPC1 gene have been found [12].

In Niemann-Pick type C disease the trafficking of lipid within the cell leads to accumulation of unesterified cholesterol in lysosomes and late endosomes. The NPC1 protein, which is defective in this disease, is a multifunctional protein, normally situated in a unique late endosomal compartment that becomes enriched with low density lipoprotein (LDL) cholesterol [15,16]. It is thought that this protein facilitates the transport of cholesterol from late endosomes to the Golgi, endoplasmic reticulum and plasma membrane [17–19]. Ultimately, one would hope that this disease would be known by a name that more closely reflects the fundamental defect.

CLINICAL ABNORMALITIES

The classic patient with this disease appears normal at birth, and while some patients may have neonatal manifestations of hepatosplenomegaly, jaundice or hepatic dysfunction, isolated splenomegaly may be the only manifestation for as long as seven years before neurologic signs become apparent [20]. The usual onset is with neurological manifestations between the ages of 3 and 13 years [21] (Figures 96.1–96.3).

There may be a tremor, clumsiness, or progressive ataxia. School performance may suffer, as ability to concentrate is lost. On examination, the key finding is vertical supranuclear ophthalmoplegia [22] (Figures 96.4–96.6). Impairment of upward gaze may be the first clinical finding. Downward gaze may also be impaired. Speech is dysarthric. Dystonia develops with posturing on movement and becomes progressively more pronounced and generalized [23]. Seizures may develop and may be difficult to control. Neurologic dysfunction is progressive. Opthalmoplegia may ultimately be complete. Hepatosplenomegaly may be detected in childhood (Figures 96.1–96.3), but with growth this organomegaly may recede. An unusual, not common feature, referred to as gelastic cataplexy may manifest in nods of the head or may be a complete collapse in response to a humerous stimulus [24,25]. The sudden loss of postural tone may lead to falls and injury. Abnormal behavior may progress to dementia or psychosis. The patient becomes wheelchair-bound, and then bedridden. Some have become blind. Early hypotonia may be displaced by spasticity or rigidity. Dysphagia develops, and drooling and aspiration pneumonia. Death may ensue for these reasons or inanition.

The disease is highly variable in presentation and accordingly difficult to recognize and often diagnosed late. Among the earliest onset, most severe disease, some patients have presented with progressive hepatic dysfunction leading to death well before the onset of neurologic disease [26–29]. Patients have also been reported with fetal ascites [30,31]; most died in infancy; this disease has been listed as the

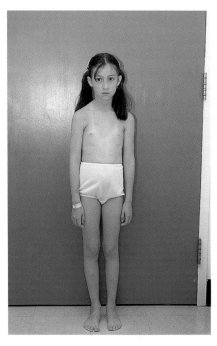

Figure 96.2   *G.C., a 9-year-old Costa Rican girl with Niemann-Pick disease type C. The first symptom was a tremor at 7 years. She then developed ataxia. She had paralysis of upward gaze and weakness of peripheral muscles. Liver and spleen were not enlarged.*

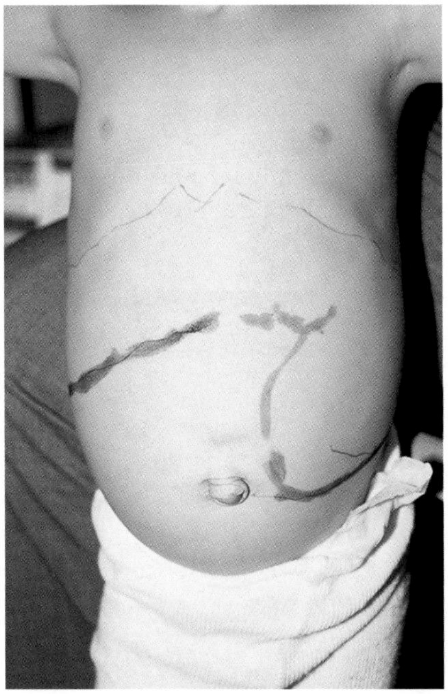

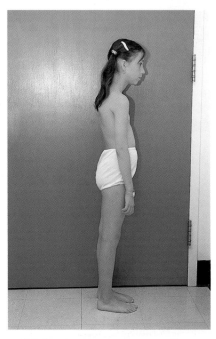

Figure 96.1   *A 3-year-old with Niemann-Pick disease Type C. Illustrated is the hepatomegaly and even more massive splenomegaly. Early development was slow, but she walked by 2 years; by 3 years she could no longer walk. She was hypertonic. She died at 5 years. (Illustration kindly provided by Dr. Philip Benson.)*

Figure 96.3   *G.C. Development was at 7 years. Storage material was evident in conjunctival cells, and typical Niemann-Pick cells were found in the marrow. Cultured fibroblasts were examined by Dr. Roscoe Brady who found defective transport of cholesterol out of the golgi and lysosomes.*

second most common cause of liver disease in the UK, after α-1-antitrypsin deficiency (Chapter 106) [32]. Of four patients, two died of hepatic failure and another from respiratory failure with foam cells in the interstitial tissue of the lungs [33]. One child presented at 4 months with respiratory manifestations [20].

Some patients have had delayed development from infancy [25,34–36], but neurodegeneration began at about 3 years. Others have had hypotonia.

A variety of hepatic presentations has been observed. The most common is neonatal cholestatic jaundice [21] and this usually disappears spontaneously early, but there may be prolonged, severe jaundice with elevated conjugated bilirubin [37]. Neonatal jaundice has been reported with early-onset rapidly progressive neurologic disease [38]. Others have developed hepatic failure in the absence of neurologic disease.

A number of late-onset or adult presentations have also been reported [22,39–45]. Some of the patients have had exclusively psychiatric symptoms, psychosis or progressive

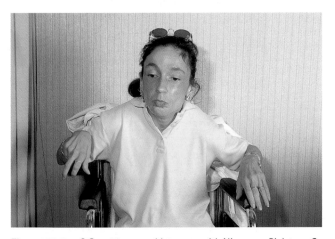

Figure 96.4 *G.S., a 29-year-old woman with Niemann-Pick type C disease. She was wheelchair-bound, athetoid, dystonic and dysphagic. She had expressive aphasia. A sibling had died at 32 years-of-age, and ballooned cells were found in the brain and other organs.*

cognitive loss and dementia. Most adults have developed paralysis of vertical gaze, but some have not, and some have complained that their eyes became stuck on looking up. Others have developed ataxia and pyramidal and extrapyramidal signs, and the neurologic picture of the classic disease [45]. One patient was described as mimicking multiple sclerosis [46]. Cerebral atrophy may be evident on neuroimaging. Some have had neonatal hepatitis and then seemed to be well until the development of psychotic symptoms in adolescence or adulthood [44]. A past history of splenomegaly may be another clue to the nature of the disease. Some adults have had a non-neuropathic presentation [44,45], including a man whose large spleen was ruptured in a traffic accident at 46 years and found to contain foam cells [45]; four years later he was asymptomatic and had a normal neurologic examination. In a search for criteria to aid early diagnosis neonatal head circumference was assessed in 21 patients [46]. The mean head circumference was statistically lower in patients than controls, but in only approximately half was head circumference at birth below the third percentile.

The phenotype of patients with NPC2 disease appears to be indistinguishable clinically or biochemically from the more common type 1 disease, but severe pulmonary involvement has been observed [46].

The diagnosis of a neurolipidosis is usually made on the basis of the characteristic foam cells. The usual source is a bone marrow aspirate [22,47,48]. Sea-blue histiocytes may be seen [47], as well as the foam cells (Fig. 95.10). The cells stain with periodic acid-Schiff stain, and strongly so with the Schultz stain for cholesterol and the acid phosphatase stain [48–53]. Foam cells may be found on conjunctival biopsy and skin biopsy [54]. In the electron microscope, there are numerous concentric electron-dense inclusions and electron-lucent vacuoles [39,49,50,55].

Pathologic examination indicates the presence of foamy storage cells, particularly in the liver, spleen, tonsils and lymph nodes [51,52]. Early infantile onset disease is associated with an appearance of giant cell hepatitis and cholestasis [26,29,38,39].

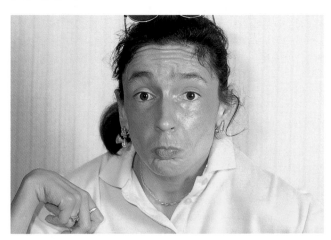

Figure 96.6 *G.S. Ophthalmoplegia also involved inability of downward gaze. The hand illustrates the athetoid movement induced by the effort. She could still move her gaze to each side.*

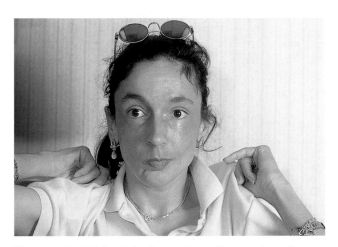

Figure 96.5 *G.S. Paralysis of upward gaze. She was attempting to look up at the examiner's fingers.*

Storage in neurons is seen widely in the cerebrum, the cerebellum and the retina [50,56–58], and the brain is atrophic. Lamellar inclusions may resemble the membranous cytoplasmic bodies of the gangliosidoses or zebra bodies. Crystalline structures were observed [59] in a 20-week-old fetus, suggesting crystalline cholesterol. Similar structures were found in a murine model of the disease [60].

GENETICS AND PATHOGENESIS

Niemann-Pick type C is an autosomal recessive lysosomal storage disease [61]. Despite considerable clinical variability, one complementation group represents a majority of the patients [9,10,61]. The gene was mapped to chromosome 18 (q11–12) [11]. In a study of 32 unrelated patients [10], 27 fell into this NPC1 group. Five patients fell into the second NPC2 group. Patients in the first group illustrated the entire spectrum of disease. In general, phenotypes within any family were quite similar, except that fatal neonatal disease was found in families in which others had classic neurologic disease [61].

The disease has been seen widely throughout the world [62]. A genetic isolate of French Acadians in Nova Scotia was originally called type D [2]. In their county the incidence was one percent and carrier frequency was 10–26 percent [63]. Another isolate was found in Hispanic-Americans in south Colorado [47]. In France and England the disease was found to be as frequent as Niemann-Pick types A and B combined [64].

The NPC1 gene contains 25 exons over 47 kb [65]. It predicts a protein of 1278 amino acids [12]. The protein appears to be a permease which acts as a transmembrane efflux pump [14]. It has extensive homology to other proteins, including the murine ortholog, and to patched, the defect in the basal cell nevus syndrome [66], which is also related to the sonic hedgehog signalling pathway; and to proteins involved in cholesterol homeostasis. Eight mutations were originally found in five patients, two deletions, one insertion and five missense mutations. In Japan mutations identified included two splicing abnormalities [67]. In the Nova Scotian French isolate the defect was a missense mutation [68]. A considerable number and variety of unique mutations have now been found [69]. The only common Caucasian mutation, I1061T, when homozygous leads to a juvenile neurological phenotype [70]. This mutation has been found in the Hispanic-American isolate in Colorado and New Mexico. In most populations compound heterozygosity is the rule rather than the exception [71].

Animal models of Niemann-Pick type C disease have been found: a feline and two murine models [5,6,72]. The mice are ataxic and have typical foam cells like those of human patients. There is marked cerebellar Purkinje cell loss.

The fundamental defect in the mice and in humans is in the transportation system for cholesterol in cells [5–7]. Cultured fibroblasts of patients and affected mice are deficient in their ability to make cholesteryl esters from endocytically taken-up exogenous LDL cholesterol [6]. This leads to lysosomal

accumulation of cholesterol [7,73–75]. The enzymes involved in cholesterol esterification, such as acyl-CoA:cholesterol acyl transferase (ACAT), are normal in these cells, and treatment of the cells with 25-hydroxycholesterol reverses the abnormality of cellular regulation of exogenous cholesterol [76].

The abnormality is conveniently demonstrated with filipin, a fluorescent probe that detects unesterified cholesterol [77]. Following LDL uptake by type C cells, the lysosomal vacuoles light up; this is the procedure that has facilitated complementation studies [10]. Endogenously synthesized cholesterol is processed normally because it does not end up in lysosomes [17]. These observations served to focus attention on systems for transport out of lysosomes.

The diagnosis of Niemann-Pick type C disease is currently made in cultured fibroblasts by demonstration of both impaired cholesterol esterification and the positive filipin test for accumulation of free-cholesterol [78–80]. A considerable amount of heterogeneity has been observed in these tests, ranging from mild to severe changes [81]. A majority of patients (86 percent) have cholesterol esterification rates less than 10 percent of normal [79]. Some are very mildly affected and some intermediate, but correlations of this biochemistry with phenotype have not been clear. Assay by filipin staining is more broadly effective, particularly in the diagnosis of variant patients [21,79]. It is also more specific, because abnormal esterification occurs in other disorders, such as I cell disease (Chapter 84), familial cholesterolemia (Chapter 86) and acid lipase deficiency (Chapter 98).

An aid to diagnosis may be obtained by assay of the activity of chitotriosidase [44]. This activity is significantly increased in Gaucher disease [82]. It may be moderately elevated in Niemann-Pick type C disease and some other lysosomal storage diseases, but it may be normal too [44].

Heterozygote detection is unreliable, although some have foamy cells in marrow or skin biopsies [83,84] and intermediate levels of cholesterol esterification are found in about half of obligate heterozygotes [21,79,80,85]. Prenatal diagnosis has been carried out by biochemical testing in cultured amniocytes and chorionic villus cells [86,87]. Thirteen affected fetuses were found in 37 pregnancies at risk [87]. Only the families with the most severe chemical expression appear to be reliable candidates for biochemical prenatal diagnosis. The extensive molecular heterogeneity makes mutational analysis formidable, except in population isolates or in families in which the mutation is known. In these instances this is the method of choice for heterozygote detection and prenatal diagnosis [69,71].

The adenosine triphosphatase (ATP)-binding cassette transporter A1 (ABACA1) is also up regulated in response to increase cellular cholesterol, leading to high density lipoprotein (HDL) particle formation. Mutations in this ABACA1 lead to increased intracellular cholesterol and very low levels of HDL in Tangier disease [88]. Mutations in NPC1 appear to impair also the regulation and activity of ABACA1 [89]. Fibroblasts from patients with NPC disease were shown to have decreased efflux of labeled LDL-cholesterol mediated by apolipoprotein

A-I. These fibroblasts also displayed diminished ABCA1 mRNA and protein in both basal and cholesterol stimulated states. Furthermore 17 of 21 patients studied had low levels of HDL-cholesterol. This observation can provide another diagnostic aid in evaluating children for NPC disease.

Despite the large and increasing body of knowledge about the metabolism and transport of cholesterol and other lipids, the pathogenesis of the neurologic features of Niemann-Pick type C disease remains obscure [90]. Experience with cholesterol-lowering drugs and bone marrow transplantation in man and even combined liver and bone marrow transplantation in the mouse model, none of which were effective in influencing the neurodegeneration [91,92], indicated clearly that the central nervous system is autonomous from the rest of the body. Liver transplantation in a 7-year-old cirrhotic girl restored hepatic function, but failed to reverse neurologic deterioration [93]. A variety of lipids in addition to cholesterol accumulate in the brains of patients with this disease. These include GM2 and GM3 gangliosides, glucosylceramide and lactosylceramide. There is neuronaxonal dystrophy and neurofibrillary tangles, like those of Alzheimer disease. In Niemann-Pick type C lipid rafts, which occur in the lipid bilayer of the plasma membranes of glia and neurons, accumulate because of defective egress. Approaches to reduce the accumulation of sphingolipid by inhibiting its synthesis have been underway in murine models, and human trials are planned. N-butyldeoxynojirimycin inhibits the synthesis of GM2 ganglioside [94] and has resulted in reduced ganglioside accumulation in brain, reduced Purkinje cell loss and modest delay in neurologic disease and death. Similarly breeding affected mice with mice carrying a mutation in the transferase gene that inhibits synthesis of GM2, GA1 and GA2 indicated that these lipids are not the cause of the neuropathology [95].

TREATMENT

Specific treatment is not available. The promise of gene therapy was raised by successful prevention of neurodegeneration and extension of life span in homozygous npc⁻ mice by overexpression of the NPC1 gene targeted to the CNS [96].

Seizures may be controlled with the usual anticonvulsant agents. Protryptilene and clomipramine are useful in cataplexy and sleep problems [97,98]. Dystonia and tremor may respond to anticholinergic drugs. Supportive care including physical and occupational therapy is important. Support groups are available in the US and in Europe.

References

1 Crocker AC, Farber S. Niemann-Pick disease: a review of eighteen patients. *Medicine (Baltimore)* 1958;**37**:1.

2 Crocker AC. The cerebral defect in Tay-Sachs disease and Niemann-Pick disease. *J Neurochem* 1961;**7**:69.

3 Brady RO, Kanfer HJN, Mock MB, Frederickson DS. The metabolism of sphingomyelin. II Evidence of an enzymatic deficiency in Niemann-Pick disease. *Proc Natl Acad Sci USA* 1966;**55**:366.

4 Schneider PB, Kennedy EP. Sphingomyelinase in normal human spleens and in spleens from subjects with Niemann-Pick disease. *J Lipid Res* 1967;**8**:202.

5 Pentchev PG, Gal AE, Boothe AD, et al. A lysosomal storage disorder in mice characterized by dual deficiency of sphingomyelinase and glucocerebroside. *Biochem Biophys Acta* 1980;**619**:669.

6 Pentchev PG, Comly ME, Kruth HS, et al. The cholesterol storage disorder of the mutant BALB/c mouse. A primary genetic lesion closely linked to defective esterification of exogenously derived cholesterol and its relationship to human type C Niemann-Pick disease. *J Biol Chem* 1986;**261**:2792.

7 Pentchev PG, Comly ME, Kruth HS, et al. Group C Niemann-Pick disease: faulty regulation of low-density lipoprotein uptake and cholesterol storage in cultured fibroblasts. *FASEB J* 1987;**1**:40.

8 Besley GT, Hoogeboom AJ, Hoogeveen A, et al. Somatic cell hybridisation studies showing different gene mutations in Niemann-Pick variants. *Hum Genet* 1980;**54**:409.

9 Steinberg SJ, Ward CP, Fensom AH. Complementation studies in Niemann-Pick disease type C indicate the existence of a second group. *J Med Genet* 1994;**31**:317.

10 Vanier MT, Duthel S, Rodriguez-Lafrasse C, et al. Genetic heterogeneity in Niemann-Pick C disease: a study using somatic cell hybridization and linkage analysis. *Am J Hum Genet* 1996;**58**:118.

11 Carstea ED, Polymeropoulos MH, Parker CC, et al. Linkage of Niemann-Pick disease type C to human chromosome 18. *Proc Natl Acad Sci USA* 1993;**90**:2002.

12 Carstea ED, Morris JA, Coleman KG, et al. Niemann-Pick C1 disease gene: homology to mediators of cholesterol homeostasis. *Science* 1997;**277**:228.

13 Naureckiene S, Sleat DE, Lackland H, et al. Identification of HE1 as the second gene of Niemann-Pick C disease. *Science* 2000;**209**:2298.

14 Davies JP, Chen FW, Ioannou YA. Transmembrane molecular pump activity of Niemann-Pick C1 protein. *Science* 2000;**290**:2295.

15 Neufeld EB, Wastney M, Patel S, et al. The Niemann-Pick C1 protein resides in a vesicular compartment linked to retrograde transport of multiple lysosomal cargo. *J Biol Chem* 1999;**274**:9627.

16 Garver WS, Heidenreich RA, Erickson RP, et al. Localization of the murine Niemann-Pick C1 protein to two distinct intracellular compartments. *J Lipid Res* 2000;**41**:673.

17 Liscum L, Ruggiero RM, Faust JR. The intracellular transport of low density lipoprotein-derived cholesterol is defective in Niemann-Pick type C fibroblasts. *J Cell Biol* 1989;**108**:1625.

18 Garver WS, Krishnan K, Gallagos JR, et al. Niemann-Pick C1 protein regulates cholesterol transport to the trans-Golgi network and plasma membrane caveolae. *J Lipid Res* 2002;**43**:579.

19 Wojtanik KM, Liscum L. The transport of low density lipoprotein-derived cholesterol to the plasma membrane is defective in NPC1 cells. *J Biol Chem* 2003;**278**:14850.

20 Imrie J, Wraith JE. Isolate splenomegaly as the presenting feature of Niemann-Pick disease type C. *Arch Dis Child* 2000;**84**:427.

21 Vanier MT, Wenger DA, Comley ME, et al. Niemann-Pick disease group C: clinical variability and diagnosis based on defective cholesterol esterification. A collaborative study on 70 patients. *Clin Genet* 1988;**33**:331.

22 Grover WD, Naiman JL. Progressive paresis of vertical gaze in lipid storage disease. *Neurology* 1982;**32**:1295.

23 Longstreth WT, Daven JR, Farrell DF, et al. Adult dystonic lipidosis: clinical histologic and biochemical findings of a neurovisceral storage disease. *Neurology* 1982;**32**:1295.

24 Denoix C, Rodriguez-Lafrasse C, Vanier MT, *et al*. Cataplexie révélatrice d'une forme atypique de la maladie de Niemann-Pick type C. *Arch Fr Pediatr* 1991;**48**:31.

25 Miyake S, Inoue H, Ohtahara S, *et al*. A case of Niemann-Pick disease type C with narcolepsy syndrome. *Rinsho Shinkeigaku* 1983;**23**:44.

26 Rutledge JC. Case 5 Progressive neonatal liver failure due to type C Niemann-Pick disease. *Pediatr Pathol* 1989;**9**:779.

27 Gonzalez de Dios J, Fernandez Tejada E, Diaz Fernandez MC, *et al*. Estada actual de la enfermedad de Niemann-Pick: valoracion de seis casos. *An Esp Pediatr* 1990;**32**:143.

28 Guibaud P, Vanier MT, Malpeuch G, *et al*. Forme infantile précoce cholestatique rapidement mortelle de la sphingomyelinase de type C. A propos de deux observations. *Pediatric* 1979;**43**:103.

29 Jaeken J, Proesmans W, Eggermont E, *et al*. Niemann-Pick type C disease and early cholestasis in three brothers. *Acta Paediatr Belg* 1980;**33**:43.

30 Maconochie JK, Chong S, Mieli-Vergani G, *et al*. Fetal ascites: an unusual presentation of Niemann-Pick disease type C. *Arch Dis Child* 1989;**64**:1391.

31 Manning DJ, Price WI, Pearse RG. Fetal ascites: an unusual presentation of Niemann-Pick disease type C. *Arch Dis Child* 1990;**65**:335.

32 Mieli-Vergani G, Howard ER, Mowat AP. Liver disease in infancy: A 20-year perspective. *Gut* 1991;**Suppl**:S123.

33 Pin I, Pradines S, Pincemaille O, *et al*. Forme réspiratoire mortelle de maladie de Niemann-Pick type C. *Arch Fr Pediatr* 1990;**47**:373.

34 Fensom AH, El Kalla S, Bizzari R, *et al*. Clinical presentation and diagnosis of Niemann-Pick disease type C. *Emirates Med J* 1990;**8**:215.

35 Wiedemann H-R, Debuch H, Lennert K, *et al*. Uber eine infantil-juvenile subchronisch verlaufende, den Sphingomyelinosen (Niemann-Pick) anzureihende Form der Lipidosen-ein neuer Typ? Klinische pathohistologische elektronmikroskopische und biochemische Untersuchengen. *Z Kinderheilkd* 1972;**112**:187.

36 Harzer K, Schlote W, Peiffer J, *et al*. Neurovisceral lipidosis compatible with Niemann-Pick disease type C: morphological and biochemical studies of a late infantile case and enzyme and lipid assays in a prenatal case of the same family. *Acta Neuropathol (Berl)* 1978;**43**:97.

37 Coleman RJ, Robb SA, Lake BD, *et al*. The diverse neurological features of Niemann-Pick disease Type C: a report of two cases. *Mov Disord* 1988;**3**:295.

38 Higgins JJ, Paterson MC, Dambrosia JM, *et al*. A clinical staging classification for type C Niemann-Pick disease. *Neurology* 1992;**42**:2286.

39 Ashkenazi A, Yarom G, Gutman A, *et al*. Niemann-Pick disease and giant cell transformation of the liver. *Acta Paediatr Scand* 1971;**60**:285.

40 Elleder M, Jirasek A, Vik J. Adult neurovisceral lipidosis compatible with Niemann-Pick disease type C. *Virchows Arch* 1983;**A401**:35.

41 Wherrett JR, Rewcastle NB. Adult neurovisceral lipidosis. *Clin Res* 1969;**17**:665.

42 Houroupian DS, Yang SS. Paired helical filaments in neurovisceral lipidosis (juvenile dystonic lipidosis). *Ann Neurol* 1978;**4**:404.

43 Hulette CM, Earl NL, Anthony DC, Crain BJ. Adult onset Niemann-Pick disease type C presenting with dementia and absent organomegaly. *Clin Neuropathol* 1990;**1**:293.

44 Imrie J, Vijayaraghaven S, Whitehouse C, *et al*. Niemann-Pick disease type C in adults. *J Inherit Metab Dis* 2002;**25**:491.

45 Fensom AH, Grant AR, Steinberg SJ. Case report: an adult with a non-neuronopathic form of Niemann-Pick C disease. *J Inherit Metab Dis* 1999;**22**:84.

46 Schofer O, Mischo B, Puschel W, *et al*. Early-lethal pulmonary form of Niemann-Pick type C disease belonging to a second rare genetic complementation group. *Eur J Pediatr* 1998;**157**:45.

47 Wenger DA, Barth G, Githens JH. Nine cases of sphingomyelin lipidosis a new variant in Spanish-American children. Juvenile variant of Niemann-Pick disease with foamy and sea blue histiocytes. *Am J Dis Child* 1977;**131**:955.

48 Neville BGR, Lake BD, Stephens R, Sanders MD. A neurovisceral storage disease with vertical supranuclear ophthalmoplegia and its relationship to Niemann-Pick disease. A report of nine patients. *Brain* 1973;**96**:97.

49 Martin JJ, Lowenthal A, Ceuterick C, Vanier MT. Juvenile dystonic lipidosis (variant of Niemann-Pick type C). *J Neurol Sci* 1984;**66**:33.

50 Gilbert EF, Callahan J, Viseskul C, Opitz JM. Niemann-Pick disease type C. Pathological, histochemical, ultrastructural and biochemical studies. *Eur J Pediatr* 1981;**136**:263.

51 Elleder M, Jirasek A, Smid F, *et al*. Niemann-Pick disease type C with enhanced glycolipid storage. Report on further case of so-called lactosylceramidosis. *Virchows Arch* 1984;**A402**:307.

52 Philipart M, Martin L, Martin JJ, Menkes JH. Niemann-Pick disease. Morphologic and biochemical studies in the visceral form with later central nervous system involvement (Crocker's type C). *Arch Neurol* 1969;**20**:227.

53 Elleder M, Jirasek A, Smid F. Niemann-Pick disease (Crocker's type C). *Acta Neuropathol (Berl)* 1975;**133**:191.

54 Arsenio-Nunes ML, Goutieres F. Morphological diagnosis of Niemann-Pick disease type C by skin and conjunctival biopsies. *Acta Neuropathol (Berl)* 1981;**7**:204.

55 Merin S, Livni N, Yatziv S. Conjunctival ultrastructure in Niemann-Pick disease type C. *Am J Ophthalmol* 1980;**90**:708.

56 Pellissier JF, Hassoun J, Gambarelli D, *et al*. Maladie de Niemann-Pick type 'C' de Crocker. Etude ultrastructural d'un cas. *Acta Neuropathol (Berl)* 1976;**34**:65.

57 Palmer M, Green WR, Maumenee IH, *et al*. Niemann-Pick disease – type C. Ocular histopathologic and electronmicroscopic studies. *Arch Ophthalmol* 1985;**103**:817.

58 Elleder M, Jirasek A, Smid F, *et al*. Niemann-Pick disease type C. Study on the nature of cerebral storage process. *Acta Neuropathol (Berl)* 1985;**66**:325.

59 Dumontel C, Girod C, Dijoud F, *et al*. Fetal Niemann-Pick disease type C: ultrastructural and lipid findings in liver and spleen. *Virchows Arch A Pathol Anat Histopathol* 1993;**422**:253.

60 Higashi Y, Pentchev PG, Murayama S, Suzuki K. Pathology of Niemann-Pick type C: Studies of murine mutants: in *Neuropathology in Brain Research* (ed. F Ikuta). Amsterdam: Elsevier Science;1991:85.

61 Vanier MT, Pentchev P, Rodriguez-Lafrasse C, Rousson R. Niemann-Pick disease type C: an update. *J Inherit Metab Dis* 1991;**14**:580.

62 Vanier MT, Wenger DA, Comly ME, Rousson R, Brady RO, Pentchev PG. Niemann-Pick disease group C: clinical variability and diagnosis based on defective cholesterol esterification: a collaborative study on 70 patients. *Clin Genet* 1988; **33**:331–348.

63 Winsor EJT, Welch JP. Genetic and demographic aspects of Nova Scotia Niemann-Pick disease (type D). *Am J Hum Genet* 1978;**30**:530.

64 Vanier MT, Rodriguez-Lafrasse C, Rousson R, *et al*. Type C Niemann-Pick disease: biochemical aspects and phenotypic heterogeneity. *Dev Neurosci* 1991;**13**:307.

65 Morris JA, Zhang D, Coleman KG, *et al*. The genomic organization and polymorphisms analysis of the human Niemann-Pick C1 gene. *Biochem Biophys Res Commun* 1999;**261**:493.

66 Johnson RL, Rothman AL, Xie J, *et al*. Human homolog of patched a candidate gene for the basal cell nevus syndrome. *Science* 1996;**272**:1668.

67 Yamamoto T, Nanba E, Ninomiya H, *et al*. NPC1 gene mutations in Japanese patients with Niemann-Pick disease type C. *Hum Genet* 1999;**105**:10.

68 Greer WL, Riddell DC, Gillan TL, *et al*. The Nova Scotia (type D) form of Niemann-Pick disease is caused by a G3097 → T transversion in NPC1. *Am J Hum Genet* 1998;**63**:52.

69 Patterson M. Niemann-Pick disease type C: in *GeneClinics: Clinical Genetic Information Resource* [database online]. University of Washington, Seattle. Available at *www.geneclinics.org* (accessed November 2004).

70   Millat G, Marcais C, Rafi MA, *et al*. Niemann-Pick C1 disease: the I1061T substitution is a frequent mutant allele in patients of Western European descent and correlates with a classic juvenile phenotype. *Am J Hum Genet* 1999;**65**:1321.

71   Kaminski WE, Klünemann HH, Ibach B, *et al*. Identification of novel mutations in the NPC1 gene in German patients with Niemann-Pick C disease. *J Inherit Metab Dis* 2002;**25**:385.

72   Morris MD, Bhuvaneswaran C, Shio H, Fowler S. Lysosome storage disorder in NCTR-BALB/c mice. I Description of the disease and genetics. *Am J Pathol* 1982;**108**:140.

73   Butler JD, Comly ME, Kruth HS. Niemann-Pick variant disorders: comparison of errors of cellular cholesterol homeostasis in group D and group C fibroblasts. *Proc Natl Acad Sci USA* 1987;**84**:556.

74   Sokol J, Blanchette-Mackie J, Kruth HS, *et al*. Type C Niemann-Pick disease. Lysosomal accumulation and defective intracellular mobilization of low density lipoprotein cholesterol. *J Biol Chem* 1988;**263**:3411.

75   Blanchette-Mackie EJ, Dwyer NK, Amende LM. Type-C Niemann-Pick disease: low density lipoprotein uptake is associated with premature cholesterol accumulation in the Golgi complex and excessive cholesterol storage in lysosomes. *Proc Natl Acad Sci USA* 1988;**85**:8022.

76   Liscum L, Faust JR. Low density lipoprotein (LDL)-mediated suppression of cholesterol synthesis and LDL uptake is defective in Niemann-Pick fibroblasts. *J Biol Chem* 1987;**262**:17002.

77   Severs NJ, Robeneck H. Detection of micro-domains in biomembranes. An appraisal of recent developments in freeze-fracture cytochemistry. *Biochem Biophys Acta* 1983;**737**:373.

78   Vanier MT, Suzuki K. Niemann-Pick diseases. In: *Neurodystrophies and Neurolipidoses* Moser HW, Vinken PJ, Bruyn GW (eds) Vol 66. Handbook of Clinical Neurology. Amsterdam: Elsevier Science, 1996:133.

79   Vanier MT, Rodriguez-Lafrasse C, Rousson R, *et al*. Type C Niemann-Pick disease: spectrum of phenotypic variation in disruption of intracellular LDL-derived cholesterol processing. *Biochim Biophys Acta* 1991;**1096**:328.

80   Roff CF, Goldin E, Comly ME, *et al*. Niemann-Pick type C disease: deficient intracellular transport of exogenously derived cholesterol. *Am J Hum Genet* 1992;**42**:593.

81   Argoff CE, Comly ME, Blanchette-Mackie J, *et al*. Type C Niemann Pick disease: cellular uncoupling of cholesterol homeostasis is linked to severity of disruption in the intracellular transport of exogenously derived cholesterol. *Biochem Biophys Acta* 1991;**1096**:319.

82   Guo Y, He W, Boer AM, *et al*. Elevated plasma chitotriosidase activity in various lysosomal storage disorders. *J Inherit Metab Dis* 1995;**18**:717.

83   Frank V, Lasson V. Ophthalmoplegic neuro-lipidosis storage cells in heterozygotes. *Neuropediatrics* 1985;**16**:3.

84   Ceuterick C, Martin JJ. Niemann-Pick disease type C. Skin biopsies in parents. *Neuropediatrics* 1986;**17**:111.

85   Kruth HS, Comly ME, Butler JD, *et al*. Type C Niemann-Pick disease. Abnormal metabolism of low density lipoprotein in homozygous and heterozygous fibroblasts. *J Biol Chem* 1986; **261**:16769.

86   Vanier MT, Rousson RM, Mandon G, *et al*. Diagnosis of Niemann-Pick disease type C on chorionic villus cells. *Lancet* 1989;**1**:104.

87   Vanier MT, Rodriguez-Lafrasse C, Rousson R, *et al*. Prenatal diagnosis of Niemann-Pick type C disease: current strategy from an experience of 37 pregnancies at risk. *Am J Hum Genet* 1992;**51**:111.

88   Bodzioch M, Orsó E, Klucken J, *et al*. The gene encoding ATP-binding cassette transporter 1 is mutated in Tangier disease. *Nat Genet* 1999;**22**:347.

89   Choi HY, Karten B, Chan T, *et al*. Impaired ABCA1-dependent lipid efflux and hypoalphalipoproteinemia in human Niemann-Pick type C disease. *J Biol Chem* 2003. In press (MS304553200).

90   Vincent I, Bu B, Erickson RP. Understanding Niemann-Pick type C disease: a fat problem. *Curr Opin Neurol* 2003;**16**:155.

91   Hsu YS, Hwu WL, Huang SF, *et al*. Niemann-Pick disease type C (a cellular cholesterol lipidosis) treated by bone marrow transplantation. *Bone Marrow Transplant* 1999;**24**:103.

92   Yasumizu R, Miyawaki S, Sugiura K, *et al*. Allogenic bone marrow-plus-liver transplantation in the C57BL/KsJ SPM/SPM mouse, an animal model of Niemann-Pick disease. *Transplantation* 1990;**49**:759.

93   Gartner JC, Bergman I, Malatack JJ, *et al*. Progression of neurovisceral storage disease and supra-nuclear ophthalmoplegia following orthotopic liver transplantation. *Pediatrics* 1986;**77**:104.

94   Zervas M, Somers KL, Thrall MA, *et al*. Critical role for glycosphingolipids in Niemann-Pick disease type C. *Curr Biol* 2001;**11**:1283.

95   Liu Y, Wu YP, Wada R, *et al*. Alleviation of neuronal ganglioside storage does not improve the clinical course of the Niemann-Pick C disease mouse. *Hum Mol Genet* 2000;**9**:1087.

96   Loftus SK, Erickson RP, Walkley SU, *et al*. Rescue of neurodegeneration in Niemann-Pick C mice by a prion-promoter-driven Npc1 cDNA transgene. *Hum Mol Genet* 2002;**11**:3107.

97   Kandt RS, Emerson RG, Singer HS, *et al*. Cataplexy in variant forms of Niemann-Pick disease. *Ann Neurol* 1982;**12**:284.

98   Philipart M, Engel J, Zimmerman EG. Gelastic cataplexy in Niemann-Pick disease group C and related variants without generalized sphingomyelinase deficiency. *Ann Neurol* 1983;**14**:492.

97

Krabbe disease/galactosylceramide lipidosis/ globoid cell leukodystrophy

MAJOR PHENOTYPIC EXPRESSION

Rapidly progressive central nervous system degenerative disease, characterized by spastic quadriplegia, blindness, deafness, peripheral neuropathy and pseudobulbar paralysis; diffuse demyelination; massive infiltration with multinucleated globoid cells; deficiency of galactosylceramide β-galactosidase.

INTRODUCTION

The syndrome was first described by Krabbe in 1916 [1]. He reported five patients, of whom four represented two sets of siblings. All were normal at birth, but had rapidly progressive neurologic deterioration from an early onset at 4–6 months until death by age of 1.5–2 years. In addition to a detailed description of clinical features of the disease, he clearly documented the pathognomonic neuropathologic features of the disorder, including the accumulation of large multinucleated globoid cells in the white matter. Chemical analysis documented the accumulation of cerebroside in these cells [2,3] and the induction of globoid cells uniquely by the intracerebral administration of galactocerebroside [4,5]. The enzymatic defect (Figure 97.1) was discovered in 1970 by Suzuki and colleagues [6,7], in galactosylceramidase (galactosylceramide-β-galactosidase) (EC 3.2.1.46). The cDNA has been cloned [8], and the gene was mapped to chromosome 24q24.3–32.1 [9,10]. A considerable number of mutations have been identified [11]. A single mutation, a 30 kb deletion (502Tdel) accounts for a large number of Northern European, US and Mexican patients [12,13].

CLINICAL ABNORMALITIES

Patients with this disease appear normal at birth, and they develop normally for the first few months. The first symptoms

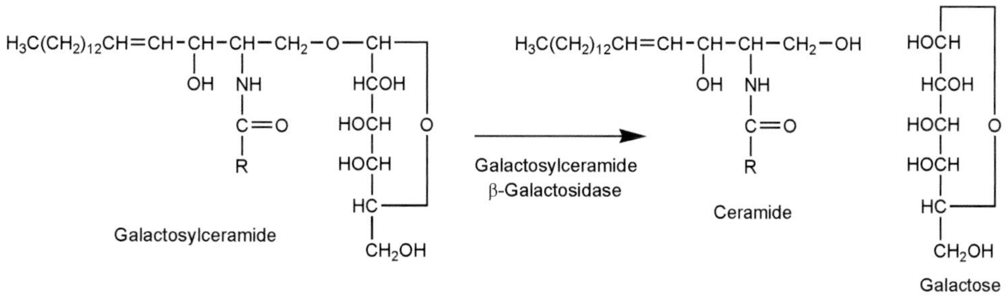

Figure 97.1 *The structure of the galactocerebroside, galactosylceramide and the reaction catalyzed by its β-galactosidase. This is the site of defect in the Krabbe disease.*

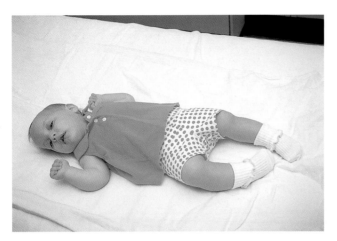

Figure 97.2   *S.A., a 10-month-old infant with Krabbe disease. This was a modified tonic neck reflex. She was very irritable and hypertonic. Deep tendon reflexes were exaggerated. She had begun to have trouble handling her secretions.*

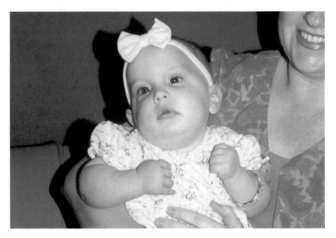

Figure 97.4   *S.A. at 9 months. The expression was blank and the fists clenched.*

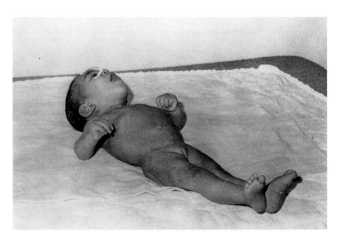

Figure 97.5   *M.C., a 9-month-old infant with far advanced manifestations of the Krabbe disease. The body was stiff throughout and the hands clenched.*

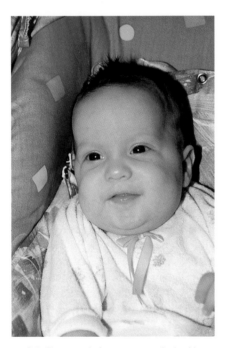

Figure 97.3   *S.A. The same infant at 5 months had begun to manifest developmental delay, but appeared alert and happy. Bifrontal diameter was narrow.*

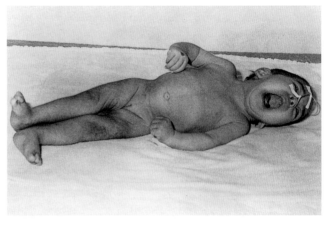

Figure 97.6   *This view at 9 months illustrated the spasticity, opisthotonus, and clenching of the hands.*

usually appear between 3 and 6 months-of-age [1,2]. The earliest manifestations are often irritability and bouts of crying or screaming without apparent cause. The neurodegeneration is then rapidly progressive (Figures 97.2–97.6). Universal rigidity of the muscles is the most typical appearance of the patients with this disease. Fists are clenched and the legs extended. An occasional patient is stiff from birth and there may be irritability and twitching [14,15]. Vomiting may be an early symptom [16].

Patients are hypersensitive to sound, light or touch, and these stimuli set off screaming and rigidity. There may be unexplained fever or convulsive seizures [1,17]. Some retardation or regression of psychomotor development may be evident early. The level of protein in cerebrospinal fluid is elevated at the time of first symptomatology [16], and electrophoresis indicates increase in albumin and decrease in β-globulins. In the second stage of progression [17] the patient is rigid, in opisthotonos, with the head bent well back. The upper extremities are flexed at the elbows, and the hands are clenched. The lower extremities are usually extended at the hips, knees and ankles, and they are adducted so much that they cross. This may ultimately become the patient's constant position. Deep tendon reflexes are diminished. Motor and mental deterioration are rapid. Mild pallor may be seen in the optic discs, and the pupillary response to light may be sluggish. Convulsive seizures may be tonic, clonic or myoclonic.

The third stage, by 9–12 months [17], is one of decerebrate blindness, deafness and flaccidity (Figures 97.5 and 97.6). These patients lose all contact with their surroundings and require tube feeding. Death occurs around 2 years-of-age, usually from aspiration pneumonia. Frequent vomiting may lead to malnutrition, as well as aspiration and pneumonia. One patient was admitted to hospital at 8 weeks with failure to thrive, feeding problems and weakness [15]; there were seizures, and deterioration was rapid to death at 15 weeks. Recurrent fever of unknown origin is common. The stiffness of the muscles is always greater in the lower extremities.

These patients often have microcephaly but macrocephaly has been observed [18–21], as has hydrocephalus [22]. They have no hepatosplenomegaly or bony abnormalities. One patient had ichthyosis [20].

Peripheral neuropathy may not be recognized clinically, but the knee jerks may be observed to disappear [1,18,23–25]. A segmental demyelination of the peripheral nerves is seen [26] and nerve conduction velocity is decreased [21,23]. In one patient, diagnosed prenatally, neurologic examination was normal in the neonatal period, but deep tendon reflexes were absent by 5 weeks [27]. By 7 weeks, peripheral nerve conduction velocity was abnormal. Psychomotor development was normal for 2 months; weakness of neck muscles was first found at 3 weeks. Elevation of the protein concentration of the cerebrospinal fluid (CSF) may be helpful in suggesting the diagnosis. The electrophoretic pattern of the CSF protein in which albumin and α-globulin are increased, while β- and γ-globulin are decreased, is also seen in metachromatic leukodystrophy.

Nonclassic or late-onset forms of Krabbe galactosylceramide lipidosis have been recognized increasingly since the advent of enzymologic diagnosis [28–33]. Heterogeneity of phenotype has been considerable. Most have presented by 10 years-of-age, but in others neurologic signs developed between 10 and 20 years [29,34,35]. In the late infantile group of patients in whom the onset was between 6 months and 3 years [36], the manifestations and progression were little different from the classic disease and death usually ensued within two years of onset. In a second group, in whom the onset was 3 to 8 years [36], the progression was slower and none had died in the period of follow-up, which was as long as seven years. Some were developmentally delayed before the onset of deterioration [31,32,37]; some had seizures [38–40]; two had hemiparesis, progressive in one to tetraplegia [41]. Onset with ataxia has been observed [31,32]. Adult patients have been described in

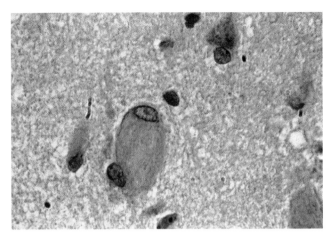

Figure 97.7 *The globoid cell that is the hallmark of the Krabbe disease. Section was taken from the brain of M.C.*

whom onset was between 10 and 35 years-of-age. The CSF protein is abnormal in the late infantile patients, but may be normal or only slightly elevated in juvenile or adult patients [34,35,42]. Adult onset patients are being increasingly reported [33,43] with progressive spastic paraparesis or peripheral neuropathy. Others have had dementia.

In classic Krabbe disease and its variants, neuroimaging usually indicates diffuse cerebral atrophy [44–46]. The scan may be normal early in the disease [47]. Diffuse hypodensity of the white matter has also been described [48]. Plaque-like high intensity T2 signal has been observed in periventricular and cerebellar white matter in three patients [49].

The electroencephalograph (EEG) is disorganized and slow [14,18,20], and there are paroxysmal discharges. There may be asymmetry [19]. The electromyogram (EMG) may be abnormal and there may be fibrillations [18,23,24]. Motor nerve conduction velocity is regularly decreased [18,23,25]. The patient may have hyperactive deep tendon reflexes, while electrophysiologic studies indicate a prominent peripheral neuropathy [24,50]. Among adult patients nerve conduction may be normal [34], or there may be EMG evidence of demyelinating neuropathy [35]. Visual or auditory evoked responses (VER, BAER) may be abnormal [35,51]. BAER responses are abnormal early while VER abnormalities occur later [52].

The neuroanatomic pathology of Krabbe disease is characterized by an extreme hardness or sclerosis of the white matter. Prior to the availability of enzymatic assay, the diagnosis was often established antemortem, by biopsy of brain, which revealed diffuse loss of myelin, astrocytic gliosis and the hallmark finding of a massive infiltration with the multinucleated globoid cells (Figure 97.7) in the white matter [1,19,53,54]. These large irregular cells range from 20 to 50 microns in diameter and contain as many as 20 nuclei. The ultrastructure of the globoid cells reveals abnormal tubular crystalloid inclusions [14,18,21,54]. The same inclusions are seen in globoid cells produced in rats, by intracerebral injection of galactocerebroside [55]. These observations suggested that the cells accumulate galactosylceramide, and this has been documented by chemical analysis [2]. Peripheral nerves appear grossly thick and chalk-white [18,26]. Histologically, there is endoneural fibrosis and complete loss or thinning of myelin sheaths [25].

GENETICS AND PATHOGENESIS

The disease is transmitted as an autosomal recessive trait [56]. Multiple sibs have been reported with normal parents. In Krabbe's original report there were two sets of siblings [1]. Parental consanguinity has also been observed. There is no ethnic preponderance and the disorder has been seen throughout the world. It appears to be common in Scandinavia, where the incidence in Sweden was calculated to be 1.9 per 100 000 births [56], and in Japan where the estimate was one in 100 000 to 200 000. The parents of patients have been found to have enzyme activity that is distinctly lower than normal and higher than in patients [57]. However, carrier detection is not always reliable, because values in some carriers may overlap the normal range. Prenatal diagnosis of an affected fetus was first reported in 1971 [58]. It is now possible by enzymatic assay of chorionic villus material, as well as amniocytes. It is recommended that enzyme assay be done on parents before prenatal diagnosis is undertaken to avoid a false positive in the case of a very low value in a heterozygote. Once the mutation is known molecular diagnosis may be done for heterozygosity and prenatal diagnosis.

The structure of galactosylceramide is shown in Figure 97.1, p. 651. Cerebrosides are monohexosyl ceramides in which the sugar is glycosidically linked to the C-1 of ceramide. Galactosylceramide is the characteristic cerebroside of myelin and of the central nervous system. The compound is normally degraded to ceramide and galactose by the lysosomal enzyme galactosylceramide β-galactosidase [6]. In patients, the level of activity has been documented to be 5–10 percent normal in brain, liver, spleen and kidney [6,7]. The assay is conveniently and reliably done on leukocytes or cultured fibroblasts [59]. Enzymatic diagnosis with the natural substrate is demanding and should be done in an experienced laboratory [57,60].

A mutant allele has been reported [61] in which the galactosidase activity overlaps that of patients with Krabbe disease. The proband of the first family was a healthy public health nurse who had volunteered as a control in a study of Krabbe disease. Her leukocyte enzyme activity was consistently lower than 10 percent of control. The presence of this new allelic gene could lead to a misdiagnosis of Krabbe disease, especially *in utero*. The situation could be like that of the Duarte variant for galactose-1-phosphate uridyltransferase, in which compound variants have been observed who were heterozygous for both the gene for galactosemia and that for the Duarte variant. These findings reinforce the recommendation to establish the enzymatic profile in parents before undertaking a prenatal diagnosis. Enzymatic assay does not distinguish infantile from late onset forms of the disease. Methodology has been developed for dried blood spots in which the product is assayed by tandem mass spectrometry, which permits newborn screening [62].

The twitcher mouse has an autosomally recessively determined deficiency of galactosylceramide β-galactosidase and is an interesting model for Krabbe disease [63]. Other models have been found in West Highland and Cairn terriers, sheep and monkeys. In the mouse the gene has been mapped to chromosome 12 [64].

The cDNA for the GALC gene contains 3795 base pairs and codes for 669 amino acids [8]. There are 5′ and 3′ untranslated regions. Expression has been documented by transfer to COS-1 cells.

A rapid test of genomic DNA for the common 502T/del mutation has been developed [13]. In Holland this accounts for 50 percent of mutant alleles [65]. Two other mutations, C1538T and A1652C, are relatively common in patients of European ancestry [11,65]. In Israel homozygosity for T1748G (I5835) is found in the Druze population, and C1582T (D528N) in Arab Muslim patients [11]. Among late onset patients G809A is relatively common. A polymorphism, T1637C, which reduces activity slightly, is found on one allele and a disease-causing mutation, such as 502T/del or G809A on the other in some late onset patients [66].

The pathogenesis of disease in galactosylceramide lipidosis is not clear. It is an unusual lipid storage disease, in that the stored substrate accumulates only in globoid cells. Storage cannot be demonstrated in lysosomes. The disease in the mouse differs in that inclusions are seen, and the cerebroside accumulates in both kidney and lymphocytes.

In both mouse and man, levels of psychosine increase in brain and peripheral nerves [67,68]. This compound, galactosylsphingosine, which differs from the cerebroside in the absence of the fatty acid, is not present in large amounts, but it is essentially absent from normal brain. The terminal galactose is cleaved from this compound, too, by the enzyme that is defective in Krabbe disease. Psychosine is a natural detergent and highly toxic [69]. Oligodendroglia appear to be selectively destroyed by psychosine formed within them.

TREATMENT

Effective specific treatment has not yet been devised. Bone marrow transplantation has been performed in a few late-onset patients without clear evidence of efficacy [29,70,71], although stabilization of some late-onset patients appears to have been accomplished by hematopoietic stem cell transplantation [72]. The cloning of the gene and the availability of animal models provide avenues for the study of gene therapy.

References

1   Krabbe K. A new familial infantile form of diffuse brain-sclerosis. *Brain* 1916;**39**:74.

2   Austin JH. Studies in globoid (Krabbe) leukodystrophy. *Neurology* 1969;**19**:1094.

3   Blackwood W, Cummings JN. A histochemical and chemical study of three cases of diffuse cerebral sclerosis. *J Neurol Neurosurg Psychiatry* 1954;**17**:33.

4   Austin J, Lehfeldt D, Maxwell W. Experimental globoid bodies in white matter and chemical analysis in Krabbe's disease. *J Neuropathol Exp Neurol* 1961;**20**:284.

5   Olsson R, Sourander P, Svennerholm L. Experimental studies on the pathogenesis of leucodystrophies. I The effect of intracerebrally injected sphingolipids in the rat brain. *Acta Neuropathol (Berl)* 1966;**6**:153.

6   Suzuki K, Suzuki Y. Globoid cell leucodystrophy (Krabbe's disease): deficiency of galactocerebroside b-galactosidase. *Proc Natl Acad Sci USA* 1970;**66**:302.

7   Austin J, Suzuki K, Armstrong D, *et al.* Studies in globoid (Krabbe) leukodystrophy (GLD). V Controlled enzymatic studies in ten human cases. *Arch Neurol* 1970;**23**:502.

8   Chen YQ, Rafi MA, de Gala G, Wenger DA. Cloning and expression of cDNA encoding human galactocerebrosidase the enzyme deficient in globoid cell leukodystrophy. *Hum Mol Genet* 1993;**2**:1841.

9   Zlotogora J, Charkraborty S, Knowlton RG, Wenger DA. Krabbe disease locus mapped to chromosome 14 by genetic linkage. *Am J Hum Genet* 1990;**47**:37.

10 Oehlmann R, Zlotogora J, Wenger DA, Knowlton RG. Localization of Krabbe disease gene (GALC) on chromosome 14 by multipoint linkage analysis. *Am J Hum Genet* 1993;**53**:1250.

11 Wenger DA, Rafi MA, Luzi P. Molecular genetics of Krabbe disease (globoid cell leukodystrophy): diagnostic and clinical aspects. *Hum Mutat* 1997;**10**:268.

12 Rafi MA, Luzi P, Chen YQ, Wenger DA. A large deletion together with a point mutation in the GALC gene is a common mutant allele in patients with infantile Krabbe disease. *Hum Mol Genet* 1995;**4**:1285.

13 Luzi P, Rafi MA, Wenger DA. Characterization of the large deletion in the GALC gene found in patients with Krabbe disease. *Hum Mol Genet* 1995;**4**:2335.

14 Schochet SS Jr, Hardman JM, Lampert PW, Earle KM. Krabbe's disease (globoid leukodystrophy): electron microscopic observations. *Arch Pathol* 1969;**88**:305.

15 Clarke JTR, Ozere RL, Krause VW. Early infantile variant of globoid cell leukodystrophy with lung involvement. *Arch Dis Child* 1981;**8**:640.

16 Hagberg B, Sourander P, Svennerholm L. Diagnosis of Krabbe's infantile leukodystrophy. *J Neurol Neurosurg Psychiatry* 1963;**26**:195.

17 Hagberg B. The clinical diagnosis of Krabbe's infantile leucodystrophy. *Acta Paediatr Scand* 1963;**52**:213.

18 Suzuki K, Grover WD. Krabbe's leukodystrophy (globoid cell leukodystrophy): an ultrastructural study. *Arch Neurol* 1970;**22**:385.

19 Allen N, de Veyra E. Microchemical and histochemical observations in a case of Krabbe's leukodystrophy. *J Neuropathol Exp Neurol* 1967;**26**:456.

20 Nelson E, Aurebeck G, Osterberg K, *et al.* Ultrastructural and chemical studies on Krabbe's disease. *J Neuropathol Exp Neurol* 1963;**22**:414.

21 Yunis EJ, Lee RE. The ultrastructure of globoid (Krabbe) leukodystrophy. *Lab Invest* 1969;**21**:415.

22 Laxdal T, Hallgrimsson K. Krabbe's globoid cell leucodystrophy with hydrocephalus. *Arch Dis Child* 1974;**49**:23.

23 Moosa A. Peripheral neuropathy and ichtyosis in Krabbe's leukodystrophy. *Arch Dis Child* 1971;**46**:112.

24 Korn-Lubetzki I, Nevo Y. Infantile Krabbe disease. *Arch Neurol* 2003;**60**:1643.

25 Hogan GR, Gutmann L, Chou SM. The peripheral neuropathy of Krabbe's (globoid) leukodystrophy. *Neurology* 1969;**19**:1094.

26 Matsuyama H, Minoshima I, Watanabe I. An autopsy case of leucodystrophy of Krabbe type. *Acta Pathol Jpn* 1963;**13**:195.

27 Lieberman JS, Oshtory M, Taylor RG, Dreyfus PM. Perinatal neuropathy as an early manifestation of Krabbe's disease. *Arch Neurol* 1980;**37**:446.

28 Lyon G, Hagberg B, Evrard PH, *et al.* Symptomatology of late onset Krabbe's leukodystrophy: the European experience. *Dev Neurosci* 1991;**13**:240.

29 Kolodny EH, Raghavan S, Krivit W. Late onset Krabbe disease (globoid cell leukodystrophy): clinical and biochemical features of 15 cases. *Dev Neurosci* 1991;**13**:322.

30 Fiumara A, Pavone L, Siciliano L, *et al.* Late-onset globoid cell leukodystrophy: report on seven new patients. *Childs Nerv Syst* 1990;**6**:194.

31 Crome L, Hanefeld F, Patrick D, Wilson J. Late onset globoid cell leukodystrophy. *Brain* 1973;**96**:84.

32 Hanfeld F, Wilson J, Crome L. Die juvenile form der globoidzell-leukodystrophie. *Monatsschr Kinderheilkd* 1973;**121**:293.

33 Henderson RD, MacMillan JC, Bradfield JM. Adult onset Krabbe disease may mimic motor meurone disease. *J Clin Neurosci* 2003;**10**:638.

34 Grewal RP, Petronas N, Barton NW. Late-onset globoid cell leukodystrophy. *J Neurol Neurosurg Psychiatry* 1991;**54**:1011.

35 Verdru P, Lammens M, Dom R, *et al.* Globoid cell leukodystrophy: a family with both late-infantile and adult type. *Neurology* 1991;**41**:1382.

36 Loonen MCB, Van Diggelen OP, Janse HC, *et al.* Late-onset globoid cell leukodystrophy (Krabbe's disease). Clinical and genetic delineation of two forms and their relation to the early infantile form. *Neuropediatrics* 1985;**16**:137.

37 Kolodny EH, Adams RD, Haller JS, *et al.* Late-onset globoid cell leukodystrophy. *Ann Neurol* 1980;**8**:219.

38 Malone MJ, Szoke MC, Looney GL. Globoid leukodystrophy. I Clinical and enzymatic studies. *Arch Neurol* 1975;**32**:606.

39 Vos AJM, Joosten EMG, Gabreëls-Festem AAWM, Gabreëls FJM. An atypical case of infantile globoid cell leukodystrophy. *Neuropediatrics* 1983;**14**:110.

40 Goebel HH, Harzer K, Ernst JP, *et al.* Late-onset globoid leukodystrophy: unusual ultrastructural pathology and subtotal b-galactocerebrosidase deficiency. *J Child Neurol* 1990;**5**:299.

41 Rolando S, Cremonte M, Leonardi A. Late onset globoid leukodystrophy: unusual clinical and CSF findings. *Ital J Neurol Sci* 1990;**11**:57.

42 Phelps M, Aicardi J, Vanier MT. Late-onset Krabbe's leukodystrophy. A report of four cases. *J Neurol Neurosurg Psychiatry* 1991;**54**:293.

43 Satoh J-I, Tokumoto H, Kurohara K, *et al.* Adult-onset Krabbe disease with homozygous T1853C mutation in the galactocerebrosidase gene. Unusual MRI findings of corticospinal tract demyelination. *Neurology* 1997;**49**:1392.

44 Demaerel P, Wilms G, Verdru P, *et al.* Findings in globoid cell leuko-dystrophy. *Neuroradiology* 1990;**32**:520.

45 Lane B, Carroll BA, Pedley TA. Computerized cranial tomography in cerebral diseases of white matter. *Neurology* 1978;**28**:534.

46 Heinz ER, Drayer BP, Haenggeli CA, *et al.* Computed tomography in white matter disease. *Radiology* 1979;**130**:371.

47 Barnes DM, Enzmann DR. The evolution of white matter disease as seen on computed tomography. *Radiology* 1981;**138**:379.

48 Ieshima A, Eda S, Matsui A, *et al.* Computed tomography in Krabbe's disease: comparison with neuropathology. *Neuroradiology* 1983;**25**:323.

49 Sasaki M, Sakuragawa N, Takashima S, *et al.* MRI and CT findings in Krabbe disease. *Pediatr Neurol* 1991;**7**:283.

50 Korn-Lebutzki I, Dor-Wollman T, Soffer D, *et al.* Early peripheral nervous system manifestations of infantile Krabbe disease. *Pediatr Neurol* 2003;**28**:115.

51 Yamanouchi H, Kasai H, Sakuragawa N, Kurokawa T. Palatal myoclonus in Krabbe disease. *Brain Dev* 1991;**13**:355.

52 Aldosari M, Altuwaijri M, Husain AM. Brain-stem auditory and visual evoked potentials in children with Krabbe disease. *Clin Neurophysiol* 2004;**115**:1653.

53 Wallace BJ, Aronson SM, Volk BW. Histochemical and biochemical studies of globoid cell leucodystrophy (Krabbe's disease). *J Neurochem* 1963;**11**:367.

54 Yunis EJ, Lee RE. Further observations on the fine structure of globoid leukodystrophy: peripheral neuropathy and optic nerve involvement. *Hum Pathol* 1972;**3**:371.

55 Austin JH, Lehfeldt D. Studies in globoid (Krabbe) leukodystrophy. III Significance of experimentally produced globoid-like elements in rat white matter and spleen. *J Neuropathol Exp Neurol* 1965;**24**:265.

56 Hagberg B, Kollberg H, Sourander P, Akesson HO. Infantile globoid cell leukodystrophy (Krabbe's disease). Clinical and genetic studies of 11 Swedish cases 1953–1967. *Neuropediatrics* 1969;**1**:74.

57 Wenger DA, Sattler M, Clark C, McKelvey H. An improved method for the identification of patients and carriers of Krabbe's disease. *Clin Chim Acta* 1974;**56**:199.

58 Suzuki K, Schneider EL, Epstein CJ. *In utero* diagnosis of globoid cell leukodystrophy (Krabbe's disease). *J Pediatr* 1976;**88**:76.

59 Suzuki Y, Suzuki K. Krabbe's globoid cell leukodystrophy: deficiency of galactocerebrosidase in serum leukocytes and fibroblasts. *Science* 1971;**171**:73.

60 Vanier MT, Svennerholm L, MÅnsson JE, *et al*. Prenatal diagnosis of Krabbe disease. *Clin Genet* 1981;**20**:79.

61 Wenger DA, Riccardi VM. Possible misdiagnosis of Krabbe's disease. *J Pediatr* 1976;**88**:76.

62 Li Y, Scott CR, Chamoles NA, *et al*. Direct multiplex assay of lysosomal enzymes in dried blood spots for newborn screening. *Clin Chem* 2004;**50**:1785.

63 Suzuki K, Suzuki K. The twitcher mouse: a model of human globoid cell leukodystrophy (Krabbe's disease). *Am J Pathol* 1983;**111**:394.

64 Sweet H. Twitcher is on Ch 12. *Mouse Newslett* 1986;**75**:30.

65 Kleijer WJ, Keulemans JLM, van der Kraan M, *et al*. Prevalent mutations in the GALC gene of patients with Krabbe disease of Dutch and other European origin. *J Inherit Metab Dis* 1997;**20**:587.

66 Harzer K, Knoblich R, Rolfs A, *et al*. Residual galactosylsphingosine (psychosine) beta-galactosidase activities and associated GALC mutations in late and very late onset Krabbe disease. *Clin Chim Acta* 2002;**317**:77.

67 Scaravilli F, Jacobs JM, Teixeira F. Quantitative and experimental studies on the twitcher mouse: in *Neurological Mutations Affecting Myelination* (ed. N Baumann) Elsevier, Amsterdam;1980:115.

68 Miyatake T, Suzuki K. Globoid cell leukodystrophy: additional deficiency of psychosine galactosidase. *Biochem Biophys Res Commun* 1972;**48**:538.

69 Suzuki K, Tanaka H, Suzuki K. Studies on the pathogenesis of Krabbe's leukodystrophy. Cellular reaction of the brain to exogenous galactosylsphingosine monogalactosyl diglyceride and lactosylceramide: in *Current Trends in Sphingolipidoses and Allied Disorders* (eds BW Volk, L Schneck). Plenum Press, New York;1976:99.

70 Choi KG, Sung JH, Clark HB, Krivit W. Pathology of adult-onset globoid cell leukodystrophy (GLD). *J Neuropathol Exp Neurol* 1991;**50**:336.

71 Krivit W, Whitley CB, Chang P-N, *et al*. Lysosomal storage diseases treated by bone marrow transplantation: review of 21 patients: in *Bone Marrow Transplantation in Children* (eds FL Johnson, C Pochedly). Raven, New York;1990:261.

72 Krivit W, Shapiro EG, Peters C, *et al*. Hematopoietic stem-cell transplantation in globoid-cell leukodystrophy. *N Engl J Med* 1998;**338**:1119.

98

Wolman disease/cholesteryl ester storage disease

MAJOR PHENOTYPIC EXPRESSION

Vomiting, diarrhea, failure to thrive, abdominal distension, hepatosplenomegaly, adrenal calcification, vacuolated peripheral lymphocytes and foam cells in the marrow, storage of cholesterylesters and triglycerides, and deficiency of lysosomal acid lipase.

INTRODUCTION

Wolman and colleagues [1] reported first one, then two more siblings in the same family, in whom the accumulation of cholesterol and triglycerides was associated with abdominal distension, hepatosplenomegaly and calcification of the adrenals. Death occurred within the first 3 months of life. The molecular defect in this disease is the lysosomal acid

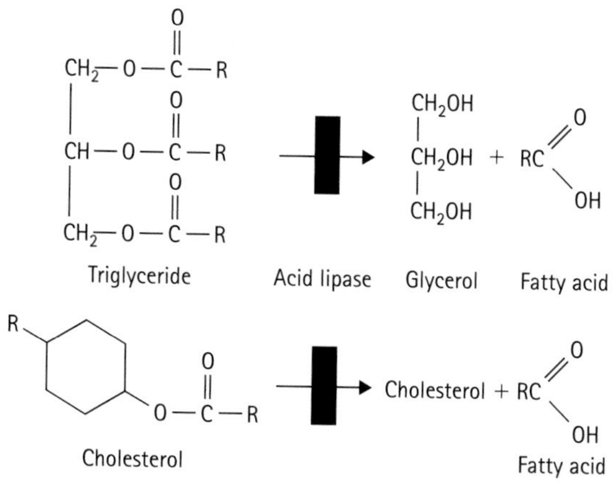

Figure 98.1 *Schematic view of acid lipase, the site of the defect in Wolman and cholesterylester storage diseases. The enzyme catalyzes the release of free fatty acids from triglycerides and from cholesterylesters.*

lipase (EC 3.1.1.13) [2]. This lipase, first demonstrated to be defective in liver and spleen, is a 46 kDa glycoprotein active on both triglycerides and cholesteryl esters (Figure 98.1). This enzyme is also defective in cholesteryl ester storage disease. The two diseases are allelic, caused by mutations at the *LIPA* locus on chromosome 10q23.2-q23.3 [3]. In general the mutations in patients with Wolman disease are major alterations that lead to absence of enzyme activity [4–6]. Most patients with cholesteryl ester storage disease have at least one copy of a single mutant allele, a G934A mutation at the exon 8 splice junction, which leads to exon skipping and the loss of codons 254–277 [7,8].

CLINICAL ABNORMALITIES

Symptoms of Wolman disease begin in the early weeks of life, and most patients have died by 6 months of age; survival as long as 14 months has been observed [2]. Infants appear normal for 2–7 weeks; then they develop diarrhea and vomiting [1,9–11]. This presentation is sufficiently nonspecific that patients are usually thought at first to have gastroenteritis. Stools remain watery and green, and soon failure to thrive is evident (Figure 98.2). In a few infants loose watery stools occur in the first weeks of life [12,13]. As symptoms persist, an intestinal or malabsorption etiology is generally sought. The abdomen regularly becomes impressively distended

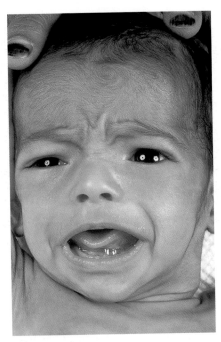

Figure 98.2 *S.I.I.S. a 3-month-old boy with Wolman disease. The emaciation is evident in the face.*

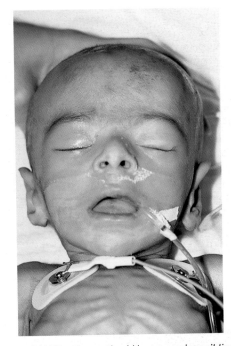

Figure 98.4 *I.M.I.S., a 2-month-old boy, a previous sibling of the boy in Figures 98.1 and 98.2, also with Wolman disease. He was seriously ill, endotracheally intubated, and died 12 days later. He developed watery, green diarrhea and vomiting at 3 weeks of age and was admitted to hospital for abdominal distress at 23 days.*

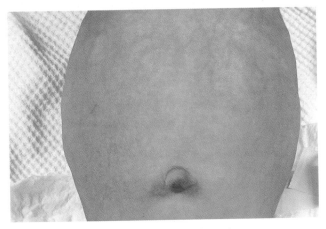

Figure 98.3 *The distended abdomen and prominent venous pattern of the same patient. The liver was enlarged. Enzyme assay of cultured fibroblasts revealed less than five percent of control activity.*

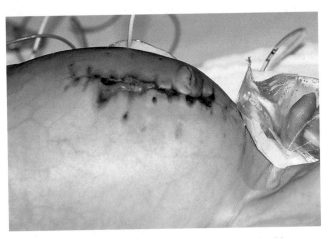

Figure 98.5 *Abdominal distension remained massive in this patient following surgery for what had been thought to be intestinal obstruction and there was dehiscence of the wound. Grossly enlarged and yellow lymph nodes were noted at surgery. Histologic examination revealed lipid storage.*

(Figures 98.3, 98.4). This may lead to laparotomy in a search for intestinal obstruction [14], or for other reasons [9] (Figure 98.5). The diagnosis of a lipid storage disease will usually be evident on laparotomy because of the appearance of the liver and spleen. Biopsy will confirm the presence of lipid storage. Not all patients come to laparotomy; thus other clues to the diagnosis must be sought. Affected patients appear wasted and severely ill (Figures 98.2, 98.4) [9,10,14]. Some patients have jaundice [10,11,15] and some, a low grade fever [1,10]. There is impressive, massive enlargement of the liver and spleen [1,2–14]. Hepatosplenomegaly may be evident as early as the fourth day of life [12] and may be massive.

Calcification of the adrenals is a hallmark feature of this disease [16]. In an infant with the usual clinical manifestations it

should lead to the diagnosis. Calcification may be seen on plain roentgenogram of the abdomen, as fine-stippled or discrete, punctate calcification [9,10]. However, it may be readily missed on routine roentgenograms, especially in the presence of ascites. It is no accident that the most frequently reproduced illustration is of a roentgenogram of adrenals following their removal at autopsy [10]. The calcifications are diffuse, and

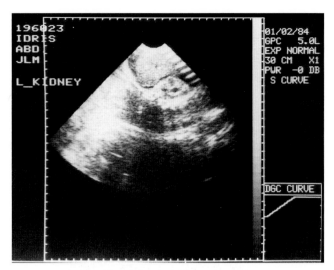

Figure 98.6   *Ultrasound of the left kidney shows a dark acoustic shadow resulting from the calcification in the adrenal.*

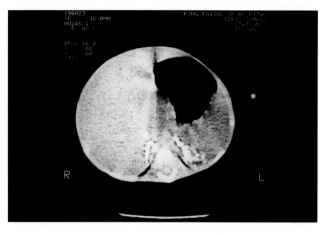

Figure 98.8   *In this view the CT scan clearly shows both adrenals to be densely calcified.*

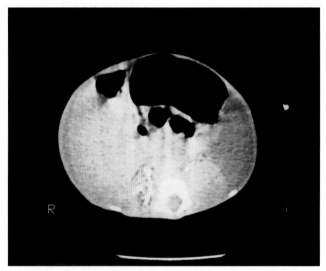

Figure 98.7   *CT scan of the abdomen reveals the calcifications in the left adrenal and enlargement of the right adrenal.*

follow the outline of the glands. This appearance distinguishes these adrenal calcifications from those of adrenal hemorrhage or a neuroblastoma. The earliest appearance may be of enlarged adrenals, which may displace the kidney downward or flatten the superior pole, without deforming the caliceal system or interfering with renal function. Over the next few months of life the adrenals shrink and become increasingly calcified. The calcifications may be found on ultrasonographic examination (Figure 98.6), in which a dark acoustic shadow is evident. The best way to visualize calcified adrenals is with the CT scan (Figures 98.7 and 98.8); various cuts permit an estimation of the size of the adrenals, and the dense calcification is readily evident.

Other roentgenographic features of the disease include the hepatosplenomegaly and/or ascites. The bones are usually

hypodense, and there may be a wide marrow cavity and thin cortex, or poor modeling [10].

Anemia is a prominent early feature of the disease [1,9,10], usually evident by 6 weeks. It worsens progressively and may require transfusion. Acanthocytosis has been reported [17]. Thrombocytopenia is not a feature of the disease. Vacuolated lymphocytes or granulocytes (Figure 98.9) may be found in the peripheral blood. The vacuoles are both intracytoplasmic and intranuclear. In many patients the initial clinical impression is first confirmed by the aspiration of lipid-laden histiocytes from the bone marrow (Figure 98.10). These foam cells are quite similar to those found in Niemann-Pick disease [18] and a number of patients reported as Niemann-Pick disease with adrenal calcifications were probably early examples of Wolman disease. Rarely, phagocytosis of erythrocytes by these cells may be seen [9]. These large, pale, foamy cells may be present in the marrow as early as 40 days. Later they are present in large numbers and may even be seen in the peripheral blood [1]. Electronmicroscopic examination may reveal vacuolation and granular inclusions in circulating granulocytes; vacuoles may be seen on light microscopy. Acanthocytosis has been reported [18].

Psychomotor development appears delayed or to deteriorate, but these patients are so ill that it is difficult to assess whether or not the nervous system is abnormal. Neurologic examination may be normal. Patients are often described as bright and alert but weak [9]. Deep tendon reflexes may by hypoactive or brisk [10], and the plantar response may be extensor, but this may be normal at this age. In one patient [11] deep tendon reflexes were exaggerated and there was ankle clonus, as well as opisthotonos. The electroencephalogram is usually normal [10,11,18].

Plasma cholesterol and lipids may be low or normal [9,17], or the serum may be hyperlipemic in the fasting state [9] and levels of lipids elevated. The lipid is largely triglyceride. The erythrocyte sedimentation rate may be elevated. Liver function tests are usually abnormal [2]. Hypoglycemia may occur as hepatic function deteriorates. Malabsorption

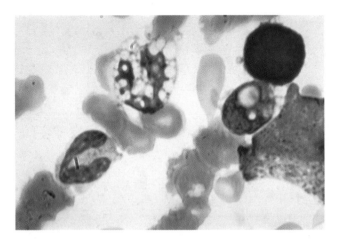

Figure 98.9   *Vacuolation in a peripheral blood granulocyte.*

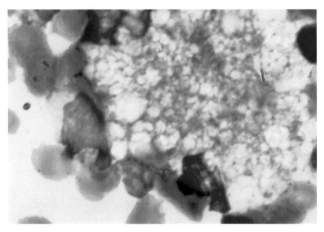

Figure 98.10   *Large foamy histiocyte from an aspirate of bone marrow.*

can be shown using ^{131}I-labeled triolein [18] or unlabeled fat [12] to demonstrate impaired absorption of fat. Administration of adrenocorticotropic hormone (ACTH) may reveal diminished responsiveness of the adrenals [12].

Pathologic examination [1,10,14,19] of material obtained at biopsy or autopsy showed the liver to be yellow or yellow-tan and greasy on its cut surface. Hepatic architecture is distorted, so that only the portal spaces may be recognizable. Foamy macrophages or Kupffer cells are scattered amid large vacuolated hepatocytes. By the time of death periportal fibrosis is the rule, and there may be frank portal cirrhosis [10,12,20]. Electron microscopic examination discloses well-defined fat droplets bound by a trilaminated membrane and, with the exception of hepatocytes, slender crystals [20]. Most fat droplets are within lysosomes [17]. The endoplasmic reticulum may be distended [21]. The adrenals are large and pale or bright yellow. Calcifications may be felt as gritty on cutting. On section it is the outer cortex that is yellow; the central zone is gray. The histologic architecture is preserved, but the cells are large, vacuolated and swollen [9,10,14]. Foam cells contain sudanophilic material; some contain birefringent crystals, and occasionally the Maltese crosses typical

of cholesterol [12,20]. Some foam cells become necrotic and it is in these areas that calcification is prominent. It may be condensed in dense crystalline lumps [9]. There may be extensive fibrosis.

The small bowel may be yellow, thickened and dilated [14,20], and changes are most marked in the proximal small bowel. Pneumatosis has been described in the colon [14]. Infiltration of the small intestine by foamy histiocytes is extensive and the mucosal cells are also foamy. These changes appear to account for the malabsorption [14,21]. In addition, there is infiltration of the ganglion cells of the intestine [14], which may be related to the distension that is so characteristic of these patients. There may also be ileus resulting from potassium losses caused by the chronic diarrhea. The spleen is grossly enlarged, and spleen and lymph nodes are largely comprised of large foamy, vacuolated cells. Clear-cut evidence of storage of lipid in neurons of the brain has been reported [14,22–24]. Swollen glial cells and histiocytes have also been observed. There may be a decrease in the numbers of neurons and retarded myelination [10]. Gliosis of the white matter has been reported [23,24], but this apparent leukodystrophy may be artefactual [25]. Electronmicroscopic examination has documented extensive accumulation of lipid throughout the central and peripheral nervous system. In the brain oligodendrocytes were the major sites of storage.

Cholesteryl ester storage disease

Deficiency of the same lysosomal acid lipase that is defective in Wolman disease is found in cholesteryl ester storage disease [26]. Patients with this disorder have a much more indolent disorder which may present with otherwise asymptomatic hepatomegaly or hepatosplenomegaly in childhood or adulthood [27–33]. Massive splenomegaly and a splenic abscess were reported in one patient [32]. Recurrent abdominal pain has occurred in some patients, and some have had recurrent epistaxis or intestinal bleeding. There may be evidence of cirrhosis on biopsy. Esophageal varices have occasionally been observed [31,34,35]. Acute or chronic hepatic failure has been reported in a few patients [35,36]. Some are icteric. Clotting factors, including prothrombin and factor V, may be reduced. Some patients have hyperlipemia and elevation of the plasma concentration of cholesterol. Hyperlipoproteinemia type IIb is commonly encountered, and some patients have xanthelasma. There may be impressive premature atherosclerosis.

The reduction in activity of the acid lipase is 50- to 100-fold [37] – severely depressed but much less so than in Wolman disease. On the other hand, in most assays the difference in activity seen in cholesteryl ester disease is not appreciably different from that of Wolman disease, and certainly not enough to account for the differences in phenotype [26,38]. However, this is also the case in most attempts to study genetic heterogeneity by enzyme assay in lysates of cells or tissues. Normal amounts of cross-reacting material (CRM) have been found in fibroblasts.

Patients have been described [39] with similar biochemical and histological findings as those in Wolman disease, but a much more benign course. It is likely that considerable heterogeneity and a spectrum of defects in this enzyme will ultimately be evident.

GENETICS AND PATHOGENESIS

Chemical analysis of tissues in both Wolman and cholesteryl ester storage diseases reveals increased quantities of cholesteryl esters and triglycerides [9,10,40,41]. This may be readily demonstrated by thin layer chromatography. A high performance liquid chromatography (HPLC) method for the quantification of lipids is useful in the differentiation of Wolman disease, Niemann-Pick disease and Gaucher disease [42]. It may be used with fibroblasts, lymphocytes or leukocytes, as well as tissue samples. Lipid analysis has most commonly been reported of liver and spleen, where the triglyceride content may be as much as 10 and 350 times the normal value, and the total cholesterol content is always increased [41]. An eight-fold elevation has been reported in adrenal [12]. Storage of cholesteryl ester has also been documented in fibroblasts [40]. Unusual oxygenated steryl esters such as those of 7-α-hydroxycholesterol have been found in tissues [41].

The defective activity in the acid lipase is consistent with the accumulation of these lipids in tissues. The enzymatic defect is demonstrable in a wide variety of tissues [2,43], including leukocytes [44–46] and cultured fibroblasts [26,38,47]. Lysosomal acid lipase may be separated electrophoretically into three isozymes: A, B and C. It is the A isozyme that is defective in Wolman and cholesteryl ester storage diseases [26,48]. Immunochemical studies using antibodies against normal acid lipase revealed cross-reacting material in fibroblasts of patients with both diseases [37]. The amounts of CRM were at the level found in normal cells, while enzyme activity in Wolman disease was reduced 200-fold.

Wolman disease and cholesteryl ester storage disease are caused by allelic recessive genes at the same locus on chromosome 10 [49], causing deficiency of lysosomal acid lipase [34]. Multiple affected siblings of normal parents have been reported in a number of families [11,50], as has consanguinity [1,11,51–53]. Heterozygosity can be detected by assay of acid lipase in leukocytes or cultured fibroblasts [20,35,44–46,54–56]. Levels are about 50 percent of normal. Prenatal diagnosis has been accomplished in Wolman disease by demonstration of the deficiency of acid lipase in cultured amniocytes [57]. In a family in which the mutation is known DNA diagnosis may be employed for heterozygote detection and prenatal diagnosis.

The gene for lysosomal acid lipase has been cloned [28] and localized to chromosome 10q23.3 [3]. The gene has been sequenced and contains 10 exons. A number of mutations has been identified [3,7,8,58,59]. The common G934A mutation in cholesteryl ester storage disease leads to a truncated protein missing 24 amino acids [7,8]. Patients nevertheless have had a variety of levels of enzyme activity. The cholesteryl ester disease phenotype has also been seen in patients with the common mutation in compound with mutations otherwise found in Wolman disease such as L179P [4]. The G934A mutation has not however been found in patients with the Wolman phenotype.

In the first patient with Wolman disease in whom mutations were identified, L179P was in compound with a frameshift mutation at nucleotide 634 (insT) causing a premature stop (Fs178) [4]. A majority of patients with Wolman disease have been homozygotes, and many had truncating mutations [60–62].

TREATMENT

There is no recognized treatment for Wolman disease. The use of HMG CoA reductase inhibitors to reduce cholesterol biosynthesis and apolipoprotein B generation might be prudent in cholesterol ester storage disease [63]. Hepatic transplantation has been employed in hepatic failure [64]. Despite bone marrow transplantation and engraftment one patient died of pulmonary dysfunction, and three others were failures despite successful engrafting in two [65]. However, success has more recently been reported [66].

References

1   Wolman M, Sterk VV, Gatt S, Frenkel M. Primary family xanthomatosis with involvement and calcification of the adrenals. Report of two more cases in siblings of a previously described infant. *Pediatrics* 1961;**28**:742.

2   Patrick AD, Lake BD. Deficiency of an acid lipase in Wolman's disease. *Nature* 1969;**222**:1067.

3   Anderson RA, Rao N, Byrum RS, *et al. In situ* localization of the genetic locus encoding the lysosomal acid lipase/cholesteryl esterase (LIPA) deficient in Wolman disease to chromosome 10q232-233. *Genomics* 1993;**15**:245.

4   Anderson RA, Byrum RS, Coates PM, Sando GN. Mutations at the lysosomal acid cholesteryl ester hydrolase gene locus in Wolman disease. *Proc Natl Acad Sci USA* 1994;**91**:2718.

5   Mayatepek E, Seedorf U, Wiebusch H, *et al.* Fatal genetic defect causing Wolman disease. *J Inherit Metab Dis* 1999;**22**:93.

6   Seedorf U, Guardamagna O, Strobl W, *et al.* Mutation report: Wolman disease. *Hum Genet* 1999;**105**:337.

7   Klima H, Ullrich K, Aslanidis C, *et al.* A splice junction mutation causes deletion of a 72-base exon from the mRNA for lysosomal acid lipase in a patient with cholesteryl ester storage disease. *J Clin Invest* 1993;**92**:2713.

8   Gasche E, Aslanidis C, Kain R, *et al.* A novel variant of lysosomal acid lipase in cholesteryl ester storage disease associated with mild phenotype and improvement on lovastatin. *J Hepatol* 1997;**27**:744.

9   Marshall WC, Ockenden BG, Fosbrooke AS, Cumings JN. Wolman's disease. A rare lipidosis with adrenal calcification. *Arch Dis Child* 1969;**44**:331.

10 Crocker AC, Vawter GF, Neuhauser EBD, Rosowsky A. Wolman's disease: three new patients with a recently described lipidosis. *Pediatrics* 1965;**35**:627.

11 Konno T, Fujii M, Watanuki T, Koizumi K. Wolman's disease: the first case in Japan. *Tohoku J Exp Med* 1966;**90**:375.

12 Lough J, Fawcett JF, Wiegensberg B. Wolman's disease. An electron microscopic histochemical and biochemical study. *Arch Path* 1970;**89**:103.

13 Marks M, Marcus AJ. Wolman's disease. *Can Med Assoc J* 1968;**99**:232.

14 Kahana D, Berant M, Wolman M. Primary familial xanthomatosis with adrenal involvement (Wolman's disease). Report of a further case with nervous system involvement and pathogenetic considerations. *Pediatrics* 1968;**42**:70.

15 Kamalian N, Dudley AW, Beroukhim F. Wolman's disease with jaundice and subarachnoid hemorrhage. *Am J Dis Child* 1973;**126**:671.

16 Abramov A, Schorr S and Wolman M. Generalized xanthomatosis with calcified adrenals. *Amer J Dis Child* 1956;**91**:282.

17 Eto Y, Kitagawa T. Wolman's disease with hypolipoproteinemia and acanthocytosis: clinical and biochemical observations. *J Pediatr* 1970;**77**:862.

18 Neuhauser BD, Kirkpatrick JA, Wientraub B. Wolman's disease: a new lipidosis. *Ann Radiol* 1965;**8**:175.

19 Wallis K, Gross M, Kohn R, Zaidman J. A case of Wolman's disease. *Helv Paediatr Acta* 1971;**26**:98.

20 Schaub J, Janka GE, Christomanou H, *et al*. Wolman's disease: clinical biochemical and ultrastructural studies in an unusual case without striking adrenal calcification. *Eur J Pediatr* 1980;**135**:45.

21 Kamoshita S, Landing BH. Distribution of lesions in myenteric plexus and gastrointestinal mucosa in lipidoses and other neurological disorders of children. *Am J Clin Pathol* 1968;**49**:312.

22 Wolman M. Involvement of nervous tissue in primary familial xanthomatosis with adrenal calcification. *Pathol Eur* 1968;**3**:259.

23 Guazzi GC, Martin JJ, Philippart M, *et al*. Wolman's disease. *Eur Neurol* 1968;**1**:334.

24 Guazzi GC, Martin JJ, Philippart M, *et al*. Wolman's disease: distribution and significance of the central nervous system lesions. *Pathol Eur* 1968;**3**:266.

25 Byrd III JC, Powers JM. Wolman's disease: ultrastructural evidence of lipid accumulation in central and peripheral nervous systems. *Acta Neuropathol* 1979;**45**:37.

26 Cortner JA, Coates PM, Swoboda E, Schnatz JD. Genetic variation of lysosomal acid lipase. *Pediatr Res* 1976;**10**:927.

27 Frederickson DS. Newly recognized disorders of cholesterol metabolism. *Ann Intern Med* 1963;**58**:718.

28 Frederickson DS, Sloan HR, Ferran VJ, Demosky SJ Jr. Cholesteryl ester storage disease: a most unusual manifestation of deficiency of two lysosomal enzyme activities. *Trans Assoc Am Physicians* 1972;**85**:109.

29 Lageron A, Caroli J, Stralin H, Barbier P. Polycorie cholestérolique de l'adulte. 1 Etude clinique électronique histochimique. *Presse Méd (Paris)* 1967;**75**:2785.

30 Partin JC, Schubert WK. Small intestinal mucosa in cholesterol ester storage disease: a light and electron microscope study. *Gastroenterology* 1969;**57**:542.

31 Schiff L, Schubert WK, McAdams AJ, *et al*. Hepatic cholesterol ester storage disease a familial disorder. 1 Clinical aspects. *Am J Med* 1968;**44**:538.

32 Elleder M, Ledvinova J, Cieslar P, Kuhn R. Subclinical course of cholesterol ester storage disease diagnosed in adulthood. Report on two cases with remarks on the nature of the liver storage process. *Virchows Arch [A]* 1990;**416**:357.

33 Edelstein RA, Filling K, Pentschev P, *et al*. Cholesteryl ester storage disease: a patient with massive splenomegaly and splenic abscess. *Am J Gastroenterol* 1988;**83**:687.

34 Wolf H, Hug G, Michaelis R, Nolte K. Seltene angeborene Erkrankung mit Cholesterinester-Speicherung in der Leber. *Helv Paediatr Acta* 1974;**29**:105.

35 Beaudet AL, Ferry GD, Nichols BL, Rosenberg HS. Cholesterol ester storage disease: clinical biochemical and pathological studies. *J Pediatr* 1977;**90**:910.

36 Cagle PT, Gerry GD, Beaudet AL, Hawkins EP. Clinopathologic conference: pulmonary hypertension in an 18-year-old girl with cholesteryl ester storage disease (CESD). *Am J Med Genet* 1986;**24**:711.

37 Burton BK, Reed SP. Acid lipase cross-reacting material in Wolman disease and cholesterol ester storage disease. *Am J Hum Genet* 1981;**33**:203.

38 Guy GJ, Butterworth J. Acid esterase activity in cultured skin fibroblasts and amniotic fluid cells using 4-methylumbelliferyl palmitate. *Clin Chim Acta* 1978;**84**:361.

39 Lake BD, Patrick AD. Wolman's disease: deficiency of 600-resistant acid esterase activity with storage of lipids in lysosomes. *J Pediatr* 1970;**76**:262.

40 Kyriakides EC, Filippone N, Paul B, *et al*. Lipid studies in Wolman's disease. *Pediatrics* 1970;**46**:431.

41 Assmann G, Frederickson DS, Sloan HR, *et al*. Accumulation of oxygenated steryl esters in Wolman's disease. *J Lipid Res* 1975;**16**:28.

42 Markello TC, Guo J, Gahl WA. High-performance liquid chromatography of lipids for the identification of human metabolic disease. *Analyt Biochem* 1991;**198**:368.

43 Sloan HR, Frederickson DS. Enzyme deficiency in cholesteryl ester storage disease. *J Clin Invest* 1972;**51**:1923.

44 Suzuki Y, Kawai S, Kobayashi A, *et al*. Partial deficiency of acid lipase with storage of triglycerides and cholesterol esters in liver. *Clin Chim Acta* 1976;**69**:219.

45 Aubert-Tulkins G, Van Hoaf F. Acid lipase deficiency: clinical and biochemical heterogeneity. *Acta Paediatr Belg* 1979;**32**:239.

46 Young EP, Patrick AD. Deficiency of acid esterase activity in Wolman's disease. *Arch Dis Child* 1970;**45**:664.

47 Burton BK, Emery D, Mueller HW. Lysosomal acid lipase in cultivated fibroblasts: characterization of enzyme activity in normal and enzymatically deficient cell lines. *Clin Chim Acta* 1980;**101**:25.

48 Coates PM, Cortner JA, Hoffman GM, Brown SA. Acid lipase activity of human lymphocytes. *Biochim Biophys Acta* 1979;**572**:225.

49 Koch GA, McAvoy M, Naylor SL, *et al*. Assignment of lipase A (LIPA) to human chromosome 10. *Cytogenet Cell Genet* 1979;**25**:176.

50 Spiegel-Adolf M, Baird HW, McCafferty M. Hematologic studies in Niemann-Pick and Wolman's disease (cytology and electrophoresis). *Confin Neurol* 1966;**28**:399.

51 Raafat R, Hashemian MP, Abrishami MA. Wolman's disease: report of two new cases with a review of the literature. *Am J Clin Pathol* 1973;**59**:490.

52 Uno Y, Taniguchi A, Tanaka E. Histochemical studies in Wolman's disease: report of an autopsy case accompanied with a large amount of milky ascites. *Acta Pathol Jap* 1973;**23**:779.

53 Lajo A, Gracia R, Navarro M, *et al*. Enfermedad de Wolman en su forma aguda infantil. *An Esp Pediatr* 1974;**7**:438.

54 Lake BD. Histochemical detection of the enzyme deficiency in blood films in Wolman's disease. *J Clin Pathol* 1971;**24**:617.

55 Kelly S, Bakhru-Kishore R. Fluorimetric assay of acid lipase in human leucocytes. *Clin Chim Acta* 1979;**97**:239.

56 Orme RLE. Wolman's disease: an unusual presentation. *Proc R Soc Med* 1970;**63**:489.

57 Coates PM, Cortner JA, Mennuti MT, Wheeler JE. Prenatal diagnosis of Wolman disease. *Am J Med Genet* 1978;**2**:407.

58 Redonnet-Vernhet I, Cjatelut M Basile JP, Salvayre R, Levade T. Cholesteryl ester storage disease: relationship between molecular defects and *in situ* activity of lysosomal acid lipase. *Biochem Mol Med* 1997;**62**:42.

59 Anderson RA, Muruguchi Y. Mutations at the lysosomal acid lipase gene locus in patients with Wolman disease and with cholesteryl ester storage disease. *Am J Hum Genet* 1993;**53**:882.

60 Aslanidis C, Ries S, Fehringer P, *et al*. Genetic and biochemical evidence that CESD and Wolman disease are distinguished by residual lysosomal acid lipase activity. *Genomics* 1996;**33**:85.

61 Ries S, Aslanidis C, Fehringer P, *et al.* A new mutation in the gene for lysosomal acid lipase leads to Wolman disease in an African kindred. *J Lipid Res* 1996;**37**:1761.

62 Fujiyama J, Sakuraba H, Kuriyama M, *et al.* A new mutation (LIPA Tyr22X) of lysosomal acid lipase gene in a Japanese patient with Wolman disease. *Hum Mutat* 1996;**8**:377.

63 Ginsberg HN, Le N, Short MP, *et al.* Suppression of apolipoprotein B production during treatment of cholesterol ester storage disease with lovastatin. *J Clin Invest* 1987;**80**:1692.

64 Kelly DR, Hoeg JM, Demosky S, Brewer HB Jr. Characterization of plasma lipids and lipoproteins in cholesteryl ester storage disease. *Biochem Med* 1985;**33**:29.

65 Krivit W, Freese D, Chan KW, Kulkarni R. Wolman's disease: a review of treatment with bone marrow transplantation and considerations for the future. *Bone Marrow Transplant* 1992;**10**:(suppl 1) 97.

66 Krivit W, Peters C, Dusenbery K, *et al.* Wolman disease successfully treated by bone marrow transplantation. *Bone Marrow Transplant* 2000;**26**:567.

Fucosidosis

MAJOR PHENOTYPIC EXPRESSION

Progressive mucopolysaccharidosis-like disease with developmental retardation, shortness of stature, coarse features, hepatosplenomegaly and dysostosis multiplex; increased sweat chloride; angiokeratomas; vacuolated lymphocytes; glycolipid storage and oligosaccharide and glycopeptide excretion; and defective activity of α-fucosidase.

INTRODUCTION

Fucose is a deoxysugar, an aldohexose in which the terminal CH_2OH is replaced by a methyl group (Figure 99.1). It occurs in glycoproteins and glycolipids as a terminal oligosaccharide linked to galactose or N-acetylglucosamine (Figure 99.2). The degradation of glycoproteins takes place sequentially in the lysosomes.

Fucosidosis was described first in 1968 by Durand and colleagues in two brothers [1,2]. The enzyme defect was reported in the same year by Van Hoff and Hers [3]. Heterogeneity was recognized early. Most patients encountered have had the fatal infantile form of fucosidosis, but more indolent phenotypes have been reported with survival even to adulthood [4,5]. There has been a tendency to classify these variants as type II [6] or III, with the infantile as I, but it is increasingly clear that a spectrum of mutation leads to a spectrum of variability in clinical expression [7]. The gene has been mapped to chromosome 1 p34 [8,9]. A number and variety of mutations have been identified. One mutation that causes a premature termination (Q422X) was found in eight families [10,11], but most mutations have been unique to a single family [12,13].

CLINICAL ABNORMALITIES

The classic infantile phenotype (Figures 99.3, 99.4) is Hurler-like in that patients appear normal at birth but during late infancy they develop progressive coarsening of the features, and retardation of linear growth and cognitive development.

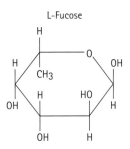

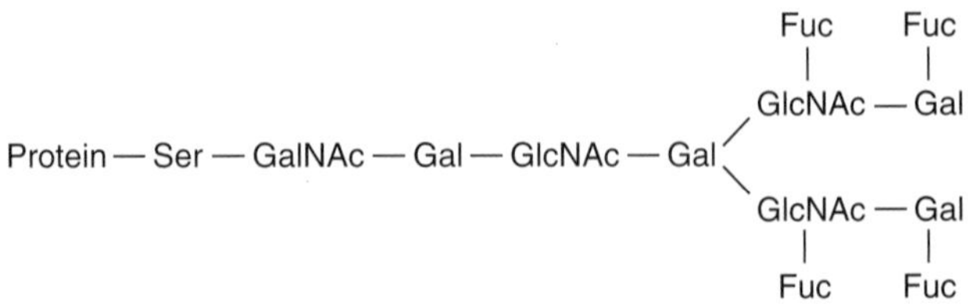

Figure 99.1   *L-Fucose.*

Protein — Ser — GalNAc — Gal — GlcNAc — Gal

with terminal:
```
                              Fuc     Fuc
                               |       |
                            GlcNAc — Gal
```
```
                            GlcNAc — Gal
                               |       |
                              Fuc     Fuc
```

Figure 99.2   *Glycoprotein structure with terminal fucose residues. The N-glycosidic linkage to amino acid could also be to threonine. In addition to the linkage shown there is N-glycosidic linkage to the asparagine residues of proteins by GalNAc. Fuc, fucose; Gal, galactose; GalNAc, N-accetylgalactosamine; GlcNAc, N-acetylglucosamine; Ser, serine.*

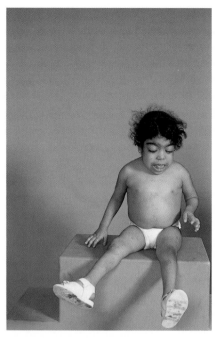

Figure 99.3   *A 5-year-old Saudi girl with fucosidosis. She was mentally retarded and short and had coarse features. The cornea was hazy. Two siblings were affected.*

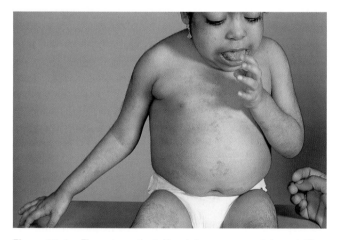

Figure 99.4   *The same patient. Her abdomen was protuberant. The tongue was large. α-Fucosidase activity of cultured fibroblasts was 0.05 percent of control.*

Cerebral degeneration and mental deterioration progress to dementia and spasticity. There is gradual loss of muscle strength and tremor. The protuberant abdomen is a consequence of hepatosplenomegaly. The cornea may be hazy. Roentgenograms reveal the typical appearance of dysostosis multiplex (Chapter 77). Imaging of the central nervous system may reveal atrophy. The concentration of chloride in the sweat is quite high. Respiratory infection may be a problem. An end-stage decerebrate rigidity is usually followed by death within the first decade.

In the more indolent disease [7,14] the first sign may be the development of angiokeratomas (Figure 99.5), which

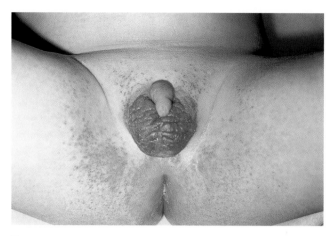

Figure 99.5   *Angiokeratomas may be prominent, as in the inguinal area of this patient. (The illustration was kindly provided by Dr. John Aase of Albuquerque, New Mexico.)*

may be present as early as 6 months to 4 years. By 20 years of age they are seen in 85 percent of patients [7]. They are prominent over the buttocks and genitalia and are indistinguishable from those of Fabry disease (Chapter 89). Red streaks may be noted on the gingivae even earlier, and may be perpendicular to the roots of the teeth. There may be tortuosity of conjunctival vessels [15]. Pigmentary retinopathy has been observed [15]. The skin may appear thickened. With time facial features become coarse, and the eyelids may be puffy. These patients may have normal sweat chloride concentrations, but they may have hypohidrosis. Hepatosplenomegaly is not characteristic. Mental deterioration is slower, and patients may live to adult life. Neurologic features include a stiff broad-based gait, spasticity, increased deep tendon reflexes and positive Babinski responses. Some patients have seizures. One patient had rapidly progressive dystonia [16]. Hearing loss has been observed [7]. Stature is reduced, but head circumference is normal [7]. The skeletal abnormalities are those of a dysostosis multiplex, which may be milder [14,17]. The spine, pelvis and hips may be the most affected. Vertebral bodies are flattened and beaked, and there may be odontoid hypoplasia. There may be clinical kyphoscoliosis. Coxa valga is associated with flattening of the femoral heads and widened, scalloped, sclerotic acetabula. Shafts of the long bones may be wide. Neuroimaging reveals changes in the thalamus, globus pallidus and internal capsule [18,19].

Another phenotype [20] in which α-fucosidase was deficient was that of spondyloepiphyseal metaphyseal dysplasia. Stature was quite short, but mental development was normal. Problems in classification are highlighted by the occurrence of mild and severe presentations in the same sibship [21] and among patients homozygous for the common 422-stop mutation [7]. In addition, a patient with an initial mild appearance went on to a rapidly fatal progression [22].

Vacuolated lymphocytes are visible in the peripheral blood, and histologic examination of the liver reveals foamy cytoplasm and vacuoles, some with lamellar structure [23,24].

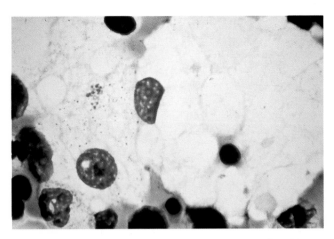

Figure 99.6 *Foam cell in the marrow of a patient with fucosidosis.*

Foam cells are demonstrable in the bone marrow (Figure 99.6). Vacuoles may also be demonstrable in the sweat glands on skin biopsy [14], or in conjunctival cells [25]. The brain was large at autopsy and the adrenals atrophic [26]. Storage vacuoles have also been found in the ultrastructure of the brain [23].

GENETICS AND PATHOGENESIS

Fucosidosis is autosomal recessive. Consanguinity has commonly been noted. The gene for the infantile type is common in Reggio Calabria in southern Italy [27]. In the US the disease has been found in the Southwest (Figure 99.5).

The gene is composed of eight exons spanning 23 kb [28]. Three patterns of mRNA were found [29] in Italian patients: two lacked mRNA; one had reduced amounts of an RNA with a cDNA by hybridization of a pattern indicating loss of a restriction site; and three had mRNA that was normal in size and content. Among mutations defined a deletion of two exons [10] resulted in marked reduction of cross reactive material (CRM) and absence of enzyme activity; a C-to-T transition leading to a TAA stop-codon, Q422X, deleting the carboxyl end of the enzyme [16,30,31]. This mutation causes loss of an *Eco*RI restriction site that is useful for molecular diagnosis [11]. Among other mutations, most have so far not been missense, but deletions, insertions, splice site changes, and other stop codons [10–13,32,33].

Defective activity of the enzyme can be demonstrated in leukocytes and cultured fibroblasts [14,34–37]. Routine assays use artificial substrates and fluorimetric or colorimetric analysis. The different phenotypes cannot be distinguished by enzymatic assay as activity is essentially absent in all. There is fucosidase activity in serum or plasma, but assay is not a reliable method of diagnosis, as some normal individuals have low levels of activity in the fluid [38].

Heterozygotes tend to have activity values intermediate between patients and controls in leukocytes or fibroblasts [14,37,39], but there is sufficient overlap with controls that heterozygote detection and screening for carriers in a high risk population are not reliable. Prenatal diagnosis has been accomplished [39] by assay of the enzyme in cultured amniocytes. In families in which the mutation is known, this is the method of choice for prenatal diagnosis and heterozygote detection [7].

Complementation analysis of cells from patients with the different phenotypes did not yield restoration of activity [37]. Molecular evidence of genetic heterogeneity was provided in a study of 11 patients, in eight of whom there was no detectable enzyme protein; in two patients, normal amounts of the 53 kDa precursor were synthesized, but none of the mature 50 kDa protein; and in one there was a small amount of CRM [35].

A variety of fucose-containing glycolipids and glycoproteins accumulate in patients with fucosidosis. The blood groups H and Lewis are degraded with difficulty and may be present in high concentration. The H antigen glycolipid, Fuc-Gal-GlcNAc-Gal-ceramide, accumulates [40]. A variety of oligosaccharides are found in the urine [41], and this provides an approach to the initial diagnosis, although most request enzymatic analysis in a patient in whom the diagnosis is suspected. Thin layer chromatography and staining with orcinol gives a diagnostic pattern in fucosidosis, mannosidosis, sialidosis and aspartylglycosaminuria. The glycopeptides found in the urine in fucosidosis all have GlcNAc linked to asparagine [42], often with fucose in α-1,6 linkage with GlcNac. In addition the fucosylGlcNAc disaccharide is found. Thin layer chromatography of the urine and staining with ninhydrin, followed by heating to 120°C, yields a bright blue spot in fucosidosis (as in aspartylglycosaminuria) that may be useful in screening [43].

TREATMENT

Only supportive treatment is available. In canine fucosidosis in Springer spaniels bone marrow transplantation led to increased enzyme activity in neural as well as visceral tissues and reduction of storage along with clinical amelioration [44,45]. Bone marrow transplantation in an 8-month-old patient with fucosidosis yielded a much milder degree of developmental delay 18 months later than observed in his affected sibling at the same age [46].

References

1 Durand P, Borrone C, Della Cella G, Philippart M. Fucosidosis. *Lancet* 1968;**1**:1198.

2 Durand P, Rossanna G, Borrone G. Fucosidosis: in *Genetic Errors of Glycoprotein Metabolism* (eds Durand P, O'Brien JS). Springer-Verlag;1982:49.

3 Van Hoff F, Hers HG. Mucopolysaccharidosis by absence of α-fucosidase. *Lancet* 1968;**1**:1198.

4 Patel V, Watanabe I, Zeman W. Deficiency of α-L-fucosidase. *Science* 1972;**176**:426.

5 Ikeda S, Kondo K, Oguchi K, *et al*. Adult fucosidosis: histochemical and ultrastructural studies of rectal mucosa biopsy. *Neurology* 1984;**34**:561.

6   Schoondewaldt HC, Lamers KJB, Leijnen FM, *et al.* Two patients with an unusual form of type II fucosidosis. *Clin Genet* 1980;**18**:348.

7   Willems PJ, Gatti R, Darby JK, *et al.* Fucosidosis revisited: A review of 77 patients. *Am J Med Genet* 1991;**38**:111.

8   Carritt B, King J, Welch HM. Gene order and localization of enzyme loci on the short arm of chromosome 1. *Ann Hum Genet* 1982;**46**:329.

9   Fowler ML, Nakai H, Byers MG, *et al.* Chromosome 1 localization of the human alpha-L-fucosidase structural gene with a homologous site on chromosome 2. *Cytogenet Cell Genet* 1986;**43**:103.

10 Willems PJ, Darby JK, DiCioccio RA, *et al.* Identification of a mutation in the structural α-L-fucosidase gene in fucosidosis. *Am J Hum Genet* 1988;**43**:756.

11 Kretz KA, Darby JK, Willems PJ, O'Brien JS. Characterization of EcoRI mutation in fucosidosis patients: A stop codon in the open reading frame. *J Mol Neurosci* 1989;**1**:177.

12 Seo H-C, Willens PJ, Kretz KA, *et al.* Fucosidosis: Four new mutations and a new polymorphism. *Hum Mol Genet* 1993;**2**:423.

13 Seo HC, Meiheng Y, Kim AH, *et al.* A 66-basepair insertion in exon 6 of the α-L-fucosidase gene of a fucosidosis patient. *Hum Mutat* 1996;**7**:183.

14 Kousseff BG, Beratis NG, Strauss L, *et al.* Fucosidosis Type 2. *Pediatrics* 1976;**57**:205.

15 Snodgrass MB. Ocular findings in a case of fucosidosis. *Br J Ophthalmol* 1976;**60**:508.

16 Gordon BA, Gordon KE, Seo HC, *et al.* Fucosidosis with dystonia. *Neuropediatrics* 1995;**26**:325.

17 Brill PW, Beratis NG, Kousseff BG, Hirschhorn K. Roentgenographic findings in fucosidosis type 2. *Am J Roentgen* 1975;**124**:75.

18 Provenzale JM, Barboriak DP, Sims K. Neuroradiologic findings in fucosidosis a rare lysosomal storage disease. *Am J Neuroradiol* 1995;**16**:809.

19 Terespolsky D, Clarke JTR, Blaser SI. Evolution of the neuroimaging changes in fucosidosis type II. *J Inherit Metab Dis* 1996;**19**:775.

20 Schafer IA, Powell DW, Sullivan JC. Lysosomal bone disease. *Pediatr Res* 1971;**5**:391.

21 Fleming C, Rennie A, Fallowfield M, McHenry PM. Cutaneous manifestations of fucosidosis. *Br J Dermatol* 1997;**136**:594.

22 Bock A, Fang-Kircher S, Braun F, *et al.* Another unusual case of fucosidosis. *J Inherit Metab Dis* 1995;**18**:93.

23 Loeb H, Tondeur M, Jonniaux G, *et al.* Biochemical and ultrastructural studies in a case of mucopolysaccharidosis 'F' (fucosidosis). *Helv Paediatr Acta* 1969;**24**:519.

24 Freitag F, Kuchemann K, Blumcke S. Hepatic ultrastructure in fucosidosis. *Virchows Arch* (B) 1971;**7**:99.

25 Libert J, Van Hoof F, Tondeur M. Fucosidosis: Ultrastructural study of conjunctiva and skin and enzyme analysis of tears. *Invest Ophthalmol* 1976;**15**:626.

26 Larbrisseau A, Brouchu P, Jasmin G. Fucosidose de type I: Etude anatomique. *Arch Fr Pediatr* 1979;**36**:1013.

27 Sangiorgi S, Mochi M, Beretta M, *et al.* Genetic and demographic characterization of a population with high incidence of fucosidosis. *Hum Hered* 1982;**32**:100.

28 Kretz KA, Cripe D, Carson GS, *et al.* Structure and sequence of the human α-L-fucosidase gene and pseudogene. *Genomics* 1992;**12**:276.

29 Guazzi S, Persici P, Gatti R, *et al.* Heterogeneity of mRNA expression in Italian fucosidosis patients. *Hum Genet* 1989;**82**:63.

30 Kretz KA, Darby JK, Willems PJ, *et al.* Heterogeneity of mRNA expression in Italian fucosidosis patients. *Hum Genet* 1989;**82**:63.

31 Yang M, Allen H, DiCioccio RA. Pedigree analysis of α-L-fucosidase gene mutations in a fucosidosis family. *Biochem Biophys Acta* 1993;**1182**:245.

32 Cragg H, Williamson M, Young E, *et al.* Fucosidosis: Genetic and biochemical analysis of eight cases. *J Med Genet* 1997;**34**:105.

33 Seo HC, Yang M, Tonlorenzi R, *et al.* A missense mutation (S63L) in α-L-fucosidase is responsible for fucosidosis in an Italian patient. *Hum Mol Genet* 1994;**3**:2065.

34 Zielke K, Veath ML, O'Brien JS. Fucosidosis: Deficiency of a-L-fucosidase in cultured skin fibroblasts. *J Exp Med* 1972;**136**:197.

35 Johnson K, Dawson G. Molecular defect in processing α-fucosidase in fucosidosis. *Biochem Biophys Res Commun* 1985;**133**:90.

36 Wood S. A sensitive fluorometric assay for a-L-fucosidase. *Clin Chem Acta* 1975;**58**:251.

37 Beratis NG, Turner BM, Labadie G, Hirschhorn K. α-L-Fucosidase in cultured skin fibroblasts from normal subjects and fucosidosis patients. *Pediatr Res* 1977;**11**:862.

38 Wood S. Human a-L-fucosidase: A common polymorphic variant for low serum enzyme activity studies of serum and leukocyte enzyme. *Hum Hered* 1979;**29**:226.

39 Durand P, Gatti R, Borrone C, *et al.* Detection of carriers and prenatal diagnosis for fucosidosis in Calabria. *Hum Genet* 1979;**51**:195.

40 Dawson G, Spranger JW. Fucosidosis: A glycosphingolipidosis. *N Engl J Med* 1971;**285**:122.

41 Holmes EW, O'Brien JS. Separation of glycoprotein-derived oligo-saccharides by thin-layer chromatography. *Anal Biochem* 1979;**93**:167.

42 Yamashita K, Tachibana Y, Takada S, *et al.* Urinary glycopeptides of fucosidosis. *J Biol Chem* 1979;**254**:4820.

43 Simell O, Sipila I, Autio S. Extra heating of TLC plates detects two lysosomal storage diseases aspartylglucosaminuria and fucosidosis during routine urinary amino acid screening. *Clin Chem Acta* 1983;**133**:227.

44 Taylor RM, Farrow BRH, Stewart GH, Healy PJ. Enzyme replacement in nervous tissue after allogeneic bone-marrow transplantation for fucosidosis in dogs. *Lancet* 1986;**II**:772.

45 Taylor RM, Farrow BRH, Stewart GJ. Amelioration of clinical disease following bone marrow transplantation in fucosidase-deficient dogs. *Am J Med Genet* 1992;**42**:628.

46 Vellodi A, Cragg H, Winchester B, *et al.* Allogeneic bone marrow transplantation for fucosidosis. *Bone Marrow Transplant* 1995;**15**:153.

α-Mannosidosis

MAJOR PHENOTYPIC EXPRESSION

Infantile phenotype

Severe mental and motor retardation with deterioration and early death; coarse features; hepatosplenomegaly; dysostosis multiplex; cataracts and corneal opacities; deafness.

Juvenile-adult phenotype

Mental retardation; hearing loss.

Both phenotypes

Storage of mannosylglycoproteins, urinary excretion of mannosyl-oligosaccharides and defective activity of α-mannosidase.

INTRODUCTION

Patients have been increasingly recognized in which the clinical features were those of mucopolysaccharidosis, but there was no mucopolysacchariduria. The recognition of inclusions set out I-cell disease (Chapter 84) as a distinct entity in 1967. In the same year, Öckermann [1] described α-mannosidosis. The enzyme (Figure 100.1) exists in at least two forms, which are immunologically indistinguishable and are coded for by a single gene on chromosome 19 p13–q12 [2]. The gene has been sequenced [3–5]. A mutation, 212A-T, was found in two siblings of a consanguineous mating [6]. A small number of other missense mutations have been reported [7].

CLINICAL ABNORMALITIES

Clinical features in more than 90 patients with the disease have reflected considerable phenotypic diversity [8–17]. Patients

have been classified into the severe infantile of type (I) of disease and a more indolent form (type II). It is already clear that there is a spectrum including a wide variety of expression. Phenotypic heterogeneity within sibships has also been

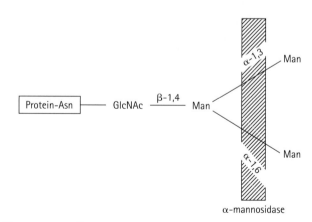

Figure 100.1   *The mannosidase reaction. Abbreviations include: Asn, asparagine; GlcNAc, N-acetylglucosamine; and Man, mannose.*

described [18], which means that there are modifiers of expression and that certainly classification into two forms is simplistic.

The infantile or classic form of mannosidosis is characterized by a very early onset of a disease that resembles a severe mucopolysaccharidosis (Figures 100.2–100.5). Hernias may be among the earliest findings. Facial features are very coarse. The skin may feel thickened, indicating the presence of stored material. Hepatosplenomegaly is prominent. There may be noisy breathing, nasal discharge or frequent respiratory infections. Macrocephaly is present, along with frontal bossing [13]. Mental development is severely retarded. Speech development may be worse – a consequence of impaired hearing. Gait may be broad-based. Dysostosis multiplex is extreme [19]. The sella turcica is J-shaped and the calvaria thickened. Vertebral bodies are hypoplastic and flattened or ovoid with anterior beaking. A gibbus may be present. Proximal metacarpals are tapered and the iliac wings flared. Pulmonary infiltrates are commonly seen. There may be corneal opacities and posterior lenticular cataracts in a spoke-like pattern [20–22]. Deterioration may be rapid, and most patients die between 3 and 10 years-of-age, often of pneumonia.

Other patients may have a more indolent course. Major features are mental retardation and hearing loss [23–26] (Figures

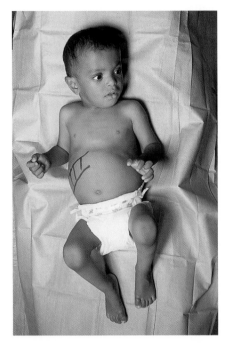

Figure 100.2   A.M.R. A 20-month-old Saudi Arabian boy with mannosidosis. At this age, he could stand and cruise, but did not walk or speak. The activity of α-mannosidase in fibroblasts was 10 percent of control.

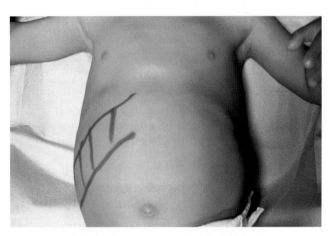

Figure 100.4   A.M.R. The abdomen was protuberant. The hepatomegaly is outlined. The spleen was also enlarged. Bone marrow revealed foamy histiocytes.

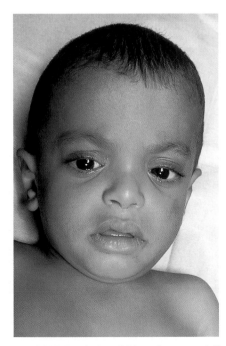

Figure 100.3   A.M.R. The facies of this patient, especially the lips and nose, suggested the presence of storage material.

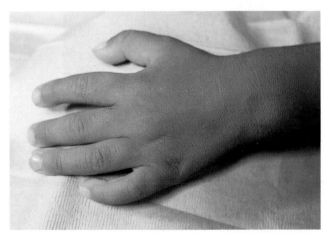

Figure 100.5   A.M.R. He had clinodactyly of the fifth fingers and proximally placed thumbs.

100.6, 100.7). Survival into adulthood is common. Some of these patients have mild dysostosis multiplex, while others do not [24]. Other skeletal problems include kyphoscoliosis (Figure 100.6) and destructive synovitis of the knees [26,27].

Hepatosplenomegaly may be absent, and the eyes are usually clear. Hearing loss is progressive, and storage material has been found in the ear (Figure 100.7). Hydrocephalus has been reported [28] and spastic paraplegia [29]. Hyperphagia has been observed [17]. Magnetic resonance imaging (MRI) findings have included cerebellar atrophy and abnormal signal in the white matter [30]. Cardiovascular abnormality has been observed in premature ventricular contractions and a shortened PR interval on electrocardiogram (EKG) [31].

Hematological evaluation regularly reveals vacuolated lymphocytes in patients with all types of mannosidosis [13,24] (Figure 100.8). Polymorphonuclear leukocytes may also be vacuolated (Figure 100.9), and the bone marrow may reveal foamy

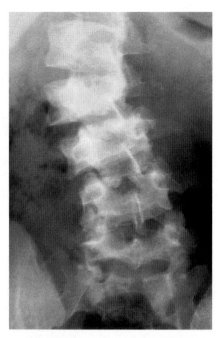

Figure 100.6 *Roentgenogram of the spine of patient with mannosidosis shows scoliosis. There was generalized dysostosis multiplex. (Illustration was kindly provided by Dr. Philip Benson.)*

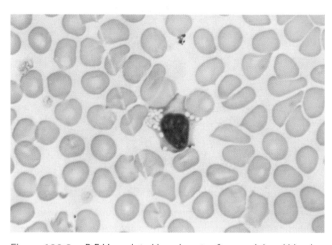

Figure 100.8 *D.F. Vacuolated lymphocytes from peripheral blood.*

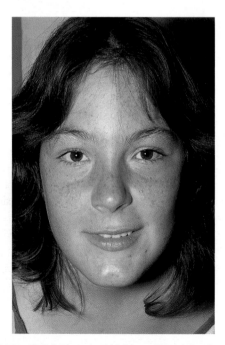

Figure 100.7 *D.F. A 15-year-old with a mild variant of mannosidosis. She had a learning disability from infancy and had an IQ of 78. She had bilateral hearing loss. Surgery on the right middle ear at 19 years revealed extensive deposits of mannoside.*

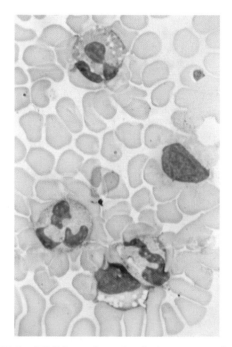

Figure 100.9 *D.F. Polymorphonuclear leukocytes were also vacuolated.*

macrophages. Pancytopenia has been reported [32]. Increased susceptibility to infections, both bacterial and viral, has been documented and associated with a variety of abnormalities in leukocyte function [13,33], including defective response to chemotactic stimulation and slowed phagocytosis. The ability of lymphocytes to undergo transformation was reduced. There may be some reduction in IgG.

Histopathology has revealed foamy, vacuolated hepatocytes [9,13,28,29,34]. Neuronal changes were widespread [13,35], with ballooning and ultrastructural evidence of storage vacuoles.

GENETICS AND PATHOGENESIS

α-Mannosidosis is an autosomal recessive disease, and affected offspring have been of both sexes [8]. The gene has been assigned to chromosome 9 [36] to the central region between p13.2 and q12 [2,37]. It contains 24 exons. The mutation at nucleotide 212 leads to the H71L amino acid change [6]. Two other mutations were recently reported [38] in two homozygous Italian patients with α-mannosidosis, IVS-2A→G and 322-323insA. The first led to skipping of exon 21. The second caused a frame shift with a stop codon at amino acid 160.

The defective enzyme, acid α-mannosidase (Figure 100.1), is lysosomal and is synthesized in a precursor form followed by processing into smaller subunits assembled in human liver into forms which are separable by chromatography and electrophoresis but immunologically indistinguishable [8,13, 39–41]. Residual activity in affected patients usually ranges between three and five percent of control [15,25,42]. Some variant patients have had higher (15–20 percent) residual activity [25,42]. Levels in leukocytes tend to be lower than those in fibroblasts, but the diagnosis can be made with either. The diagnosis has also been evident on assay of the enzyme in plasma, but this is not recommended as reliable [13]. Immunologic cross-reactive material appears to be present in most patients [15,42].

Prenatal diagnosis has been carried out by assay of the enzyme in cultured amniocytes or in chorionic villus material [43–49]. Normal activity in chorionic villi may be considerably less than in amniocytes [47]. Accurate prenatal diagnosis must take into account not only the issue of variant residual activity, but forms of α-mannosidase that are not defective in patients with mannosidosis [41].

Heterozygotes may have intermediate levels of enzyme activity, but they are more often normal [13,15]; therefore, this is not reliable. If the mutation is known, molecular methodology is the choice for both prenatal and heterozygote detection.

The result of the defective enzymatic activity is the storage of a variety of glycoproteins and glycoprotein-derived oligosaccharides. These have been best characterized in the urine

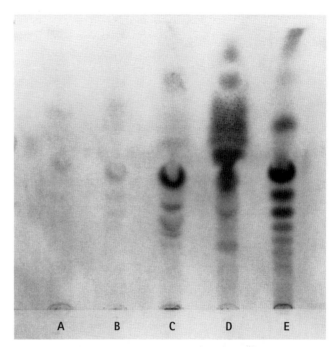

Figure 100.10 *Thin layer chromatogram of urinary oligosaccharides. Lane A was normal urine; Lane B the patient, and Lane C a patient with classic mannosidosis. Lanes D and E were the normal and patient 20x concentrated, indicating the presence in D.F. of smaller concentrations of the oligosaccharides than seen in unconcentrated urine in the more classic mannosidosis phenotype. (This illustration and Figure 100.11 were kindly provided by Dr. Thomas G. Warner and are printed with permission from* Clinical Genetics *1984;25:248.)*

[48–50], and it is by study of the patterns of urinary oligosaccharides (Figures 100.10, 100.11) that the diagnosis has usually been first made chemically, mainly by thin layer chromatography (Figure 100.10) [15,24,51,52]. There are a number of mannosyloligosaccharides in the urine of these patients. The major one is the trisaccharide, Man-α(1,3)Man-β(1,4)GlcNAc [24,53,54] (Figure 100.11).

Affected patients, and those with aspartylglucosaminuria, have been reported to have elevated levels of dolichol in the serum [55,56]. This could prove useful in diagnosis. It may reflect the fact that complex glycoproteins are synthesized by the transfer of oligosaccharide precursor from dolichol to the asparagine of the peptide.

TREATMENT

Effective specific treatment for mannosidosis has not been reported. Bone marrow transplantation has potential utility [57].

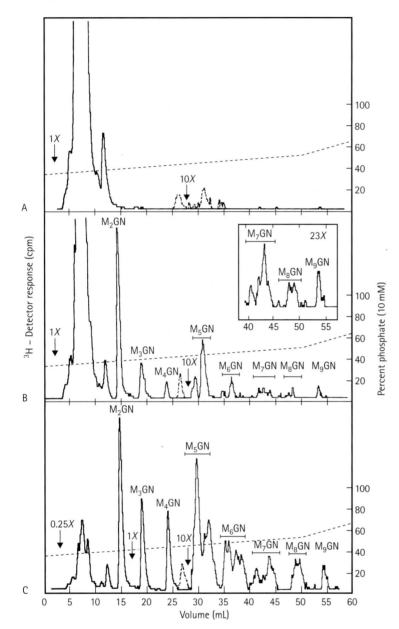

Figure 100.11   *HPLC chromatogram of urinary oligosaccharides as* ^{3}*H-aldols. A was normal urine, B the patient and C half as much urine of the classic patient. The mannose containing fractions were labeled M, e.g., M$_2$GN, the major fraction, was the trisaccharide Man α(1-3)Man β(1-4)GlcNAc.*

References

1   Öckerman P-A. A generalized storage disorder resembling Hurler's syndrome. *Lancet* 1967;**2**:239.

2   Kaneda Y, Hayes H, Uchida T, *et al.* Regional assignment of five genes on human chromosome 19. *Chromosoma* 1987;**95**:8.

3   Liao YF, Lal A, Moreman KW. Cloning expression purification and characterization of the human broad specificity lysosomal acid α-mannosidase. *J Biol Chem* 1996;**271**:28348.

4   Wakamatsu N, Gotoda Y, Saito S, Kawai H. Characterization of the human MANB gene encoding lysosomal α-D-mannosidase. *Gene* 1997;**198**:351.

5   Riise HMF, Berg T, Nilssen O, *et al.* Genomic structure of the human lysosomal α-mannosidase gene (MANB). *Genomics* 1997;**42**:200.

6   Nilssen O, Berg T, Riise HMF, *et al.* α-Mannosidosis: functional cloning of the lysosomal α-mannosidase cDNA and identification of a mutation in two affected siblings. *Hum Mol Genet* 1997;**6**:717.

7   Gotoda Y, Wakamatsu N, Nishida Y, *et al.* Structural organization sequence and mutation analysis of MANB gene encoding the human lysosomal α-mannosidase. *Am J Hum Genet* 1996;**59**:A260.

8   Chester MA, Lundblad A, Öckerman P-A, Autio S. Mannosidosis: in *Genetic Errors of Glycoprotein Metabolism* (eds Durand P, O'Brien JS). Springer-Verlag, Berlin;1982:89.

9   Kjellman B, Gamstorp I, Brun A, *et al.* Mannosidosis: a clinical and histopathologic study. *J Pediatr* 1969;**75**:366.

10 Tsay GC, Dawson G, Matalon R. Excretion of mannose-rich complex carbohydrates by a patient with α-mannosidase deficiency (mannosidosis). *J Pediatr* 1974;**84**:865.

11 Farriaux JP, Legouis I, Humbel R, *et al.* La mannosidose: A propos de 5 observations. *Nouv Presse Med* 1975;**4**:1867.

12 Aylsworth AS, Taylor HA, Stuart CF, Thomas GH. Mannosidosis: phenotype of severely affected child and characterization of α-mannosidase activity in cultured fibroblasts from the patient and his parents. *J Pediatr* 1976;**88**:814.

13 Desnick RJ, Sharp HL, Grabowski GA, *et al*. Mannosidosis: clinical morphologic immunologic and biochemical studies. *Pediatr Res* 1976;**19**:985.

14 Yunis JJ, Lewandowski RC, Sanfilippo SJ, *et al*. Clinical manifestations of mannosidosis – a longitudinal study. *Am J Med* 1976;**61**:841.

15 Warner TG, O'Brien JS. Genetic defects in glycoprotein metabolism. *Ann Rev Genet* 1990;**17**:395.

16 Bennett JK, Dembure PP, Elsas LJ. Clinical and biochemical analysis of two families with type I and type II mannosidosis. *Am J Med Genet* 1995;**55**:21.

17 Owayed A, Clark JTR. Hyperphagia in patients with α-mannosidosis type II. *J Inherit Metab Dis* 1997;**20**:727.

18 Mitchell ML, Erickson RP, Schmid D, *et al*. Mannosidosis: two brothers with different degrees of disease severity. *Clin Genet* 1981;**20**:191.

19 Spranger J, Gehler J, Cantz M. The radiographic features of mannosidosis. *Radiology* 1976;**119**:401.

20 Murphree AL, Beaudet AL, Palmer EA, Nichols BL. Cataract in mannosidosis. *Birth Defects* 1976;**12**:319.

21 Arbisser AL, Murphree AL, Garcia CA, Howell RR. Ocular findings in mannosidosis. *Am J Ophthalmol* 1976;**82**:465.

22 Letson RD, Desnick RJ. Punctate lenticular opacities in type II mannosidosis. *Am J Ophthalmol* 1978;**85**:218.

23 Booth CW, Chen KK, Nadler HL. Mannosidosis: clinical biochemical and ultrastructural studies in a family of affected adolescents and adults. *J Pediatr* 1976;**88**:821.

24 Warner TG, Mock AK, Nyhan WL, O'Brien JS. α-Mannosidosis: analysis of urinary oligosaccharides with high performance liquid chromatography and diagnosis of a case with unusually mild presentation. *Clin Genet* 1984;**25**:248.

25 Bach G, Kohn G, Lasch EE, *et al*. A new variant of mannosidosis with increased residual enzymatic activity and mild clinical manifestation. *Pediatr Res* 1978;**12**:1010.

26 Montgomery TR, Thomas GH, Valle DL. Mannosidosis in an adult. *Johns Hopkins Med J* 1982;**151**:113.

27 Weiss SW, Kelly WD. Bilateral destructive synovitis associated with alpha mannosidase deficiency. *Am J Surg Pathol* 1983;**7**:487.

28 Halperin JL, Landis DMD, Weinstein LA, *et al*. Communicating hydrocephalus and lysosomal inclusions in mannosidosis. *Arch Neurol* 1984;**41**:777.

29 Kawai H, Nishino H, Nishida Y, *et al*. Skeletal muscle pathology of mannosidosis in two siblings with spastic paraplegia. *Acta Neuropathol (Berl)* 1985;**68**:201.

30 Dietemann L, Filippi de la Palavesa MM, Tranchant C, Kastler B. MR findings in mannosidosis. *Neuropathology* 1990;**32**:485.

31 Mehta J, Desnick RJ. Abbreviated PR interval in mannosidosis. *J Pediatr* 1978;**92**:599.

32 Press OW, Fingert H, Lott IT, Dickersin CR. Pancytopenia in mannosidosis. *Arch Intern Med* 1983;**143**:1268.

33 Quie PG, Cates KL. Clinical conditions associated with defective polymorphonuclear leukocyte chemotaxis. *Am J Pathol* 1977;**88**:711.

34 Monus Z, Konyar E, Szabo L. Histomorphologic and histochemical investigations in mannosidosis. *Virchows Arch B Cell Pathol* 1977;**26**:159.

35 Sung JH, Hayano M, Desnick RJ. Mannosidosis: pathology of the nervous system. *J Neuropathol Exp Neurol* 1977;**36**:807.

36 Champion MJ, Shows TB. Mannosidosis: assignment of the lysosomal a-mannosidase B gene to chromosome 19 in man. *Proc Natl Acad Sci USA* 1977;**74**:455.

37 Martinvik F, Ellenbogen A, Hirschhorn K, Hirschhorn R. Further localization of the gene for human acid alpha glucosidase (GAA) peptidase D (PEPD) and α-mannosidase B (MANB) by somatic cell hybridization. *Hum Genet* 1985;**69**:109.

38 Beccari T, Bibi L, Ricci R, *et al*. Two novel mutations in the gene for human α-mannosidase that cause α-mannosidosis. *J Inherit Metab Dis* 2003;**26**:819.

39 Carroll M, Dance N, Masson PK, *et al*. Human mannosidosis – the enzyme defect. *Biochem Biophys Res Commun* 1972;**49**:579.

40 Pohlmann R, Hasilik A, Cheng S, *et al*. Synthesis of lysosomal α-mannosidase in normal and mannosidosis fibroblasts. *Biochem Biophys Res Commun* 1983;**115**:1083.

41 Cheng SH, Malcolm S, Pemble S, Winchester B. Purification and comparison of the structures of human liver acidic α-D-mannosidase A and B. *Biochem J* 1986;**233**:65.

42 Poenaru L, Miranda C, Dreyfus J-C. Residual mannosidase activity in human mannosidosis. Characterization of the mutant enzyme. *Am J Hum Genet* 1980;**32**:354.

43 Maire I, Zabot MT, Mathieu M, Cotte J. Mannosidosis: tissue culture studies in relation to prenatal diagnosis. *J Inherit Metab Dis* 1978;**1**:19.

44 Poenaru L, Girard S, Thepot F, *et al*. Antenatal diagnosis in three pregnancies at risk for mannosidosis. *Clin Genet* 1979;**16**:428.

45 Poenaru L, Kaplan L, Dummies J, Dreyfus JC. Evaluation of possible first trimester prenatal diagnosis in lysosomal diseases by trophoblast biopsy. *Pediatr Res* 1984;**18**:1032.

46 Petushkova NA. First-trimester diagnosis of an unusual case of α-mannosidosis. *Prenat Diagn* 1991;**11**:279.

47 Fukuda M, Tanaka A, Ishiki G. Variation of lysosomal enzyme activity with gestational age in chorionic villi. *J Inherit Metab Dis* 1990;**13**:862.

48 Yamashita K, Tachibana Y, Mihara K, *et al*. Urinary oligosaccharides of mannosidosis. *J Biol Chem* 1979;**255**:5126.

49 Matsuura F, Nunez HA, Grabowski GA, Sweeley CC. Structural studies of urinary oligosaccharides from patients with mannosidosis. *Arch Biochem Biophys* 1981;**207**:337.

50 Kistler JP, Lott IT, Kolodny EH, *et al*. Mannosidosis: new clinical presentation enzyme studies and carbohydrate analysis. *Arch Neurol* 1977;**34**:45.

51 Humbel R, Collart M. Oligosaccharides in urine of patients with glycoprotein storage diseases. *Clin Chim Acta* 1975;**60**:143.

52 Sewell AC. An improved thin layer chromatographic method for urinary oligosaccharide screening. *Clin Chim Acta* 1979;**92**:411.

53 Nordén NE, Lundblad A, Svenson S, Autio S. Characterization of two mannose-containing oligosaccharides isolated from the urine of patients with mannosidosis. *Biochemistry* 1974;**13**:871.

54 Nordén NE, Lundblad A. A mannose-containing trisaccharide isolated from urines of three patients with mannosidosis. *J Biol Chem* 1973;**248**:6210.

55 Salaspuro M, Salmela K, Humaloja K, *et al*. Elevated level of serum dolichol in aspartylglucosaminuria. *Life Sci* 1990;**47**:627.

56 Humaloja K, Roine RP, Salmela K, *et al*. Serum dolichols in different clinical conditions. *Scand J Clin Lab Invest* 1991;**51**:705.

57 Walkley SU, Thrall MA, Dobrenis K, *et al*. Bone marrow transplantation corrects the enzyme defect in neurons of the central nervous system in a lysosomal storage disease. *Proc Natl Acad Sci USA* 1994;**91**:2970.

Galactosialidosis

MAJOR PHENOTYPIC EXPRESSION

Early infantile

Edema, fetal (hydrops fetalis)-neonatal; telangiectases; hepatosplenomegaly; growth failure; psychomotor delay and deterioration; dystosis multiplex; cardiac failure; proteinuria; and death in infancy.

Late infantile

Hepatosplenomegaly; dystosis multiplex; corneal clouding; hernias; valvular cardiac disease; shortness of stature and hearing loss.

Juvenile (adult)

Ataxia; myoclonus; seizures; mental retardation and deterioration; cherry red spots; corneal clouding; angiokeratomas; platyspondyly; and shortness of stature.

Each Type

Coarse facies; cherry red spots; foam cells; defective activity of β-galactosidase and neuraminidase resulting from abnormality in the lysosomal protective protein/cathepsin A (PPCA).

INTRODUCTION

Features of GM_1 gangliosidosis and sialidosis result from defective activity of both β-galactosidase and neuraminidase as a result of fundamental deficiency in the lysosomal PPCA.

Following the discovery in 1968 of β-galactosidase deficiency in generalized GM_1 gangliosidosis [1], a number of patients were reported with atypical features such as cherry red macular spots and an absence of hepatosplenomegaly [2–5]. The combination of features of cerebral lipidosis and mucopolysaccharidosis without mucopolysacchariduria suggested a mucolipidosis. Complementation studies in somatic cell hybrids indicated that two of these patients [4,5] had mutations distinct from or non-allelic with GM_1 gangliosidosis, though

they were clearly deficient in β-galactosidase [6]. Wenger et al. [7] in 1978 reported the coexisting deficiency of neuraminidase and β-galactosidase in leukocytes and fibroblasts of a patient with what had been thought [8] to be a variant form of GM_1 gangliosidosis. Then other patients were reported in whom sialidase deficiency was present [9–12] along with that of β-galactosidase.

That the primary defect was not in sialidase was shown by complementation of the cells of patients with sialidosis by hybridization with cells of patients with the combined defect [11,13]. Further, in the combined defect cells, both enzyme defects could be restored by a glycoprotein corrective factor produced in culture by normal fibroblasts or those of β-galactosidase deficiency indicating the presence of a third protein acting as a corrective factor. The turnover of β-galactosidase in normal fibroblasts was 10 days, while in the cells deficient in both enzymes it was less than one day [14], and in experiments with purified enzyme it was clear that the rapid turnover was caused by proteolytic degradation of the enzyme [15,16]. The disorder was named galactosialidosis in 1981 [17]. The molecular defect was found by D'Azzo and colleagues [16] to be in the protective protein (PPCA), which aggregates with both enzymes to form multimers that resist lysosomal degradation. The gene has been mapped to chromosome 20q13.1 [18,19], and the human cDNA has been cloned [20]. A number of mutations have been discovered [21,22].

CLINICAL ABNORMALITIES

Considerable phenotypic heterogeneity has been observed consistent with different mutations. Nevertheless, it continues to appear useful to distinguish the early infantile and late infantile phenotypes, while the rest, accounting for 70 percent of the patients, have been called the juvenile/adult type and appear to represent quite a broad spectrum of variants.

The early infantile is the most severe form of the disease. Fetal hydrops may lead to stillbirth or early neonatal death [23]; extensive edema may be evident in the neonatal period (Figures 101.1–101.3). Features are coarse [24–30] (Figures 101.4, 101.5), and there is hepatosplenomegaly. Inguinal hernias are common. Psychomotor delay may be global, and deterioration is progressive to death at an average age of 7 months. Dysostosis multiplex is uniformly present; it may be less prominent than in other forms of the disease because of the short interval in which to develop before demise. Telangiectases have been found in the early infantile disease, but angiokeratomas are rarely seen. There may be corneal clouding and cherry red spots [24]. Proteinuria is an early sign of renal dysfunction; renal failure may ensue [28,29]. Infiltration of the heart leads to thickened septa, cardiomegaly, and congestive failure may occur as early as the first week of life [24–26,31]. Recurrent fetal hydrops has been reported in two families [32,33]. Thrombocytopenia with purpura and anemia were reported in a patient with fetal hydrops [34]. Anemia and thrombocytopenia were also found, along with hemophagocytosis in a 7-month-old boy [35].

The late infantile form of the disease may be evident as early as the first month of life. Patients have coarse features, hepatosplenomegaly and dysostosis multiplex with the appearance of mucopolysaccharidosis [5,17,36–38]. Some have had cherry red spots and/or corneal clouding [17,37]; others have not [5,36]. Generalized seizures or petit mal have rarely been observed [5]. Mental retardation in these patients has generally been mild. Neurologic deterioration has not generally been seen [5]. Cardiac involvement is a regular feature of the disease. Valvular involvement has included thickened

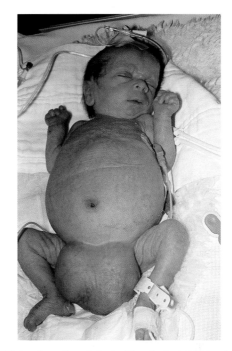

Figure 101.1 *A newborn infant with galactosialidosis who presented with non-immune hydrops fetalis and had extreme edema of the vulva.*

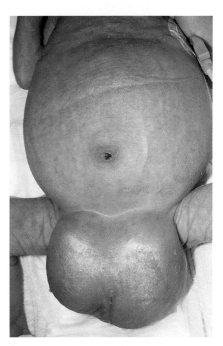

Figure 101.2 *Close-up of the edematous genitalia. A mutation V132M was found by analysis of the DNA by Dr. Suzuki.*

mitral and aortic valves. Hearing loss may be conductive or mixed. Shortness of stature may be a consequence of disease of the spine, and there may be atrophy of the muscles. Angiokeratomas are uncommon.

Patients classified as juvenile/adult have varied considerably in severity. A sizable number have been reported from

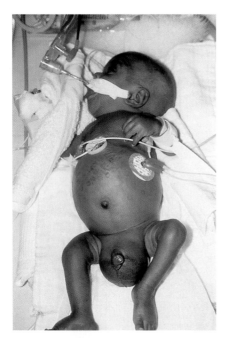

Figure 101.3   *Another infant with hydrops fetalis. (The illustration was kindly provided by Dr. Aida Al Aqeel, Military Hospital, Riyadh, Saudi Arabia.)*

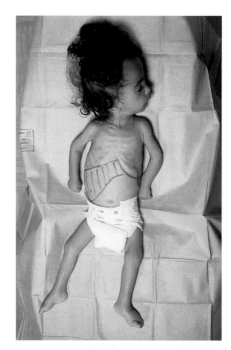

Figure 101.5   *A one-year-old with galactosialidosis. Developmental retardation was global. The liver and spleen were enlarged and there were cherry red macular spots. (The illustration was kindly provided by Dr. Aida Al Aqeel.)*

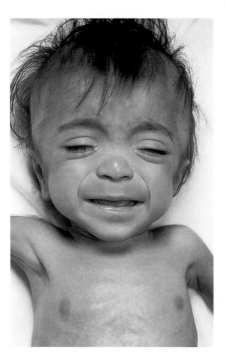

Figure 101.4   *A 7-month-old Omani child with galactosialidosis. The features were quite coarse and the eyebrows abundant. There was a substantial amount of hair on the head despite almost complete absence of subcutaneous tissue. There were cherry red macular spots. (The illustration was kindly provided by Dr. Aida Al Aqeel.)*

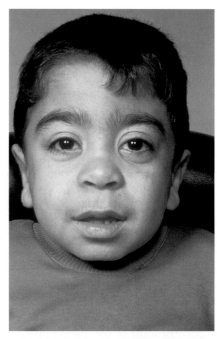

Figure 101.6   *A 5-year-old boy with galactosialidosis. He was mildly retarded and had mildly coarse features and hirsutism. Dr. Suzuki found a seven-nucleotide insertion between exons 13 and 14.*

Japan [12,13,29,39–49]. In a Mexican family with first cousin parents, two boys and a girl had coarse features, dysostosis multiplex, shortness of stature and mental retardation, along with cherry red spots, corneal clouding, seizures and hearing loss,

but no hepatosplenomegaly [2]. Onset of symptoms has been as early as 1 year of age [45] or as late as 40 years [29]. Coarse features are regularly seen, but they may be mild (Figure 101.6). Most patients have platyspondyly, but fully developed dysostosis multiplex is unusual. Hepatosplenomegaly is not common.

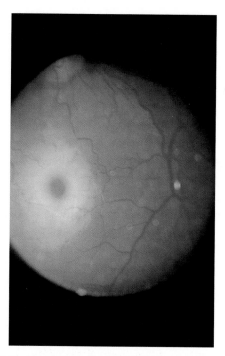

Figure 101.7   *The cherry red spot of the 5-year-old boy.*

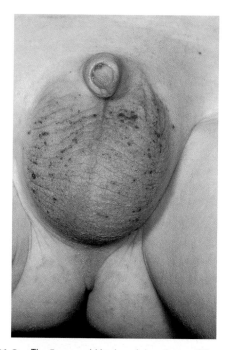

Figure 101.8   *The 5-year-old had angiokeratoma of the scrotum. Histologic analysis was confirmatory.*

Neurologic features include generalized seizures and myoclonus, ataxia and retarded mental development. Deterioration may be progressive. Deep tendon reflexes are brisk [25]. Bilateral cherry red spots are found in most patients (Figure 101.7). There may be corneal clouding, punctate lenticular opacities and loss of visual acuity. Other patients have no neurological abnormalities.

Angiokeratomas are common [29,45] (Figure 101.8). They are found in clusters in a distribution indistinguishable from those of Fabry disease (Chapter 89).

All patients with galactosialidosis have foam cells in the marrow and vacuolated lymphocytes in peripheral blood. Vacuoles may also be seen in Kupfer cells [50]. Pathologic features include macroscopic cerebral atrophy [50]. Membrane-bound inclusions are seen on electron microscopy of lymphocytes or skin [37], brain [51–53], peripheral Schwann cells [48,54,55] and in the myenteric plexus of the rectum [43,48]. Their appearance is similar to those of GM_1 gangliosidosis and sialidosis. They may have lamellar or wavy concentric structure [52,53]. An early infantile patient was reported in which multiple infarctions were found in the brain [56]. In another there were periventricular calcifications [30].

GENETICS AND PATHOGENESIS

The disorder, in all of its variants, is transmitted in an autosomal recessive fashion. Rates of consanguinity have been quite high. Fibroblasts of a parent were shown to have reduced amounts of mRNA for the protective protein, providing chemical evidence of heterozygosity [57]. Enzyme activity attributable to the protective protein also yielded intermediate values in fibroblasts of heterozygotes [58,59].

The molecular defect is in the lysosomal protective protein (PPCA), the existence of which became evident through studies of patients with galactosialidosis [18,60]. This protein is normally synthesized as a 54 kDa precursor, which is modified post-translationally to 32 and 20 KDa polypeptides which proved to be the corrective factor [13,16,61]. Immunoprecipitation demonstrated absence of the 54, 32 and 20 kDa polypeptides in fibroblasts of patients with galactosialidosis [16]. Neuraminidase aggregates normally with β-galactosidase and protective factor in a large multimer that resists proteolytic degradation [61–64]. Neuraminidase requires protective protein for activity. The multimer aggregate correctly routes the two glycosidases to the lysosome and protects them from rapid lysosomal proteolysis. The isolation of the cDNA for the protective protein [57] and its expression in COS cells [58,65] has elucidated the structure, function and physiology of this protein. The sequence begins with a signal peptide that is cleaved, followed by 298 amino acids of the 32 kDa protein, which is followed by the 20 kDa protein; the two make up the 54 kDa precursor. The latter, synthesized in COS cells from the cDNA, is taken up by the fibroblasts of patients with galactosialidosis and restores activity in both enzymes [57].

Once the primary structure of the protein was known, its homology to yeast and plant serine carboxypeptidases became apparent. The protective protein was then shown to have carboxypeptidase activity [66] – and this activity is deficient in galactosialidosis. The properties of this carboxypeptidase are consistent with those of cathepsin A [58]. Site-directed mutagenesis which abolishes cathepsin activity does not interfere with protective activity; so the two functions are distinct [58]. Nevertheless, cathepsin A activity provides a simple test that is useful for heterozygote detection. The fact that the protective function and cathepsin activity are distinct provides an argument for continued diagnostic reliance on the assay of β-galactosidase and neuraminidase in leukocytes or fibroblasts [57,58]. The three enzyme activities, cathepsin, β-galactosidase and neuraminidase copurify [57]. PPCA and galactosidase are found separate from the complex, but all of the neuraminidase is present in the complex [67]. PPCA functions as an intracellular transport protein [68]. It has a mannose-6-phosphate recognition marker [69]. The enzyme also has deamidase and esterase activities, and these activities are deficient in cultured cells of patients [70].

Prenatal diagnosis of an affected fetus has been accomplished by assay of β-galactosidase and neurominidase in cultured amniocytes [32] and also by the detection of sialyloligosaccharides in amniotic fluid [71].

Failure to synthesize immunoprecipitable protective protein was found in fibroblasts of a patient with the early infantile disease [16]. There was no protective protein mRNA [57]. In contrast, in the late infantile disease there was a larger quantity of the 54 kDa precursor protein [71] and a trace amount of the mature 32 kDa protein [72]. In a patient with the juvenile/adult disease [4] a small amount of normal-sized precursor was found [71], while others in this group made precursors of various molecular sizes from 45 to 63 kDa [73]. The gene was mapped to chromosome 20 by somatic cell hybridization [60] and *in situ* hybridization [18]. There are 15 exons over 7 kb of genomic DNA [74].

Japanese patients with adult mild clinical disease were found to have a deletion of exon 7 [29,75]. This resulted from a substitution at the donor splice site of intron 7, which causes aberrant splicing of the precursor mRNA [22]. Patients with the genotype have had relatively more severe disease with juvenile onset. The exon 7 deletion was in compound with point mutations changing glycine 49 to arginine, tryptophan 69 to arginine and tyrosine 395 to cysteine [22,29,76]. Adult, milder phenotype patients with the exon 7 deletion are generally homozygous. Two patients with the late infantile disease [5,36] were found to have mutations for phenylalanine 412 to valine [21]. Expression in COS cells led to a precursor that was to some extent retained in the endoplasmic reticulum, which would be consistent with the finding of increased precursor and shortage of mature protein in this form [71]. A number of Caucasian patients with this form of the disease have been found to have a point mutation changing tyrosine 221 to asparagine [77]. Others had phenylalanine 112 valine 22 [78]. Early infantile patients have been found to have valine 104 methionine, leucine 208 proline and glycine 411 serine [78].

The natures of the enzymatic defects in β-galactosidase and in neuraminidase lead to the accumulation in tissues of these patients of GM_1 ganglioside [43] and other gangliosides, including GM_3, as well as sialylated storage compounds as in sialidosis [79–81]. A variety of sialyloligosaccharides is excreted in the urine. Their detection by thin layer chromatography may be useful in leading to the diagnosis [26,58,82]. These studies must be followed up with enzyme assays to establish the diagnosis, and most often the diagnosis is now made by direct assay of the activities of β-galactosidase and neuraminidase.

TREATMENT

Effective specific therapy has not been devised. The availability of animal models should permit studies on gene transfer as an approach to therapy. Bone marrow transplantation has been successful in PPCA ($-/-$) mice [83].

References

1   Okada S, O'Brien JS. Generalized gangliosidosis β-galactosidase deficiency. *Science* 1968;**160**:1002.
2   Goldberg MF, Cotlier E, Fischenser LG, *et al*. Macular cherry-red spot corneal clouding and β-galactosidase deficiency. *Arch Intern Med* 1971;128:387.
3   O'Brien JS, Ho MW, Veath ML, *et al*. Juvenile GM₁-gangliosidosis clinical pathological chemical and enzymatic studies. *Clin Genet* 1972;**3**:411.
4   Loonen MCB, van der Lugt L, Francke CL. Angiokeratoma corporis diffusum and lysosomal enzyme deficiency. *Lancet* 1974;ii:785.
5   Pinksy L, Miller J, Shanfield B, *et al*. GM₁ gangliosidosis in skin fibroblast culture: enzymatic differences between types 1 and 2 and observations on a third variant. *Am J Hum Genet* 1974;**26**:563.
6   Galjaard H, Hoogeveen AT, Keijzer W, *et al*. Genetic heterogeneity in GM₁-gangliosidosis. *Nature* 1975;**257**:60.
7   Wenger DA, Tarby TJ, Wharton C. Macular cherry-red spots and myoclonus with dementia: coexistent neuraminidase and β-galactosidase deficiencies. *Biochem Biophys Res Commun* 1978;**82**:589.
8   Justice PM, Wenger DA, Naidu S, Rosenthanl IM. Enzymatic studies in a new variant of GM₁-gangliosidosis in an older child. *Pediatr Res* 1977;**11**:407.
9   Thomas GH, Goldberg MF, Miller CS, Reynolds LW. Neuraminidase deficiency in the original patient with the Goldberg syndrome. *Clin Genet* 1979;**16**:323.
10 Lowden JA, O'Brien JS. Sialidosis: a review of human neuraminidase deficiency. *Am J Hum Genet* 1979;**31**:1.
11 Hoogeveen AT, Verheijen FW, d'Azzo A, Galjaard H. Genetic heterogeneity in human neuraminidase deficiency. *Nature* 1980;**285**:500.
12 Okada M, Inui M, Chiyo H. A case of neuraminidase deficiency associated with a partial β-galactosidase defect. Clinical biochemical and radiological studies. *Eur J Pediatr* 1981;**130**:292.
13 Hoogeveen A, d'Azzo A, Brossmer R, Galjaard H. Correction of combined β-galactosidase/neuraminidase deficiency in human fibroblasts. *Biochem Biophys Res Commun* 1981;**103**:292.
14 van Diggelen OP, Schram AW, Sinnot ML, *et al*. Turnover of β-galactosidase in fibroblasts from patients with genetically different types of β-galactosidase deficiency. *Biochem J* 1981;**200**:143.
15 van Diggelen OP, Hoogeveen AT, Smith PJ, *et al*. Enhanced proteolytic degradation of normal β-galactosidase in the lysosomal storage disease with combined β-galactosidase and neuraminidase deficiency. *Biochim Biophys Acta* 1982;**703**:69.

16 d'Azzo A, Hoogeveen A, Reuser AJ, *et al*. Molecular defect in combined β-galactosidase and neuraminidase deficiency in man. *Proc Natl Acad Sci USA* 1982;**79**:4535.

17 Andria G, Strisciuglio P, Pontarelli G, *et al*. Infantile neuraminidase and β-galactosidase deficiencies (galactosialidosis) with mild clinical courses: in *Sialidases and Sialidosis* (eds P Durand, G Tettamanti, S Di Donato). Edi Ermes, Milan;1981:379.

18 Wiegant J, Galjaard NJ, Rapp AK, d'Azzo A. The gene encoding human protective protein (PPGB) is on chromosome 20. *Genomics* 1991;**10**:345.

19 Whitmore T, Day J, Albers J. Localization of the human phospholipid transfer protein gene to chromosome 20q12-q131. *Genomics* 1995;**28**:599.

20 Day J, Albers J, Lofton-Day C, *et al*. Complete cDNA encoding human phospholipid transfer protein from human endothelial cells. *J Biol Chem* 1994;**269**:9388.

21 Zhou XY, Galjart NJ, Willemsen R, *et al*. A mutation in a mild form of galactosialidosis impairs dimerization of the protective protein and renders it unstable. *EMBO J* 1991;**10**:4041.

22 Shimmoto M, Fukuhara Y, Itoh K, *et al*. Protective protein gene mutations in galactosialidosis. *J Clin Invest* 1993;**91**:2393.

23 Stone DL, Sidransky E. Hydrops fetalis: Lysosomal storage disorders in extremis. *Adv Pediatr* 1999;**46**:409.

24 Gravel RA, Lowden JA, Callahan JW, *et al*. Infantile sialidosis. A phenocopy of type 1 GM₁ gangliosidosis distinguished by genetic complementation and urinary oligosaccharides. *Am J Hum Genet* 1979;**31**:669.

25 Suzuki Y, Nanba E, Tsuiji A, *et al*. Clinical and genetic heterogeneity in galactosialidosis. *Brain Dysfunct* 1988;**1**:285.

26 Okada S, Sugino H, Kato T, *et al*. A severe infantile sialidosis (β-galactosidase-α-neuraminidase deficiency) mimicking GM1-gangliosidosis type 1. *Eur J Pediatr* 1983;**140**:295.

27 Yamano T, Dezawa T, Koike M, *et al*. Ultrastructural study on a severe infantile sialidosis (β-galactosidase-α-neuraminidase deficiency). *Neuropediatrics* 1985;**16**:109.

28 Sewell AC, Pontz BF, Weirzel D, Humburg C. Clinical heterogeneity in infantile galactosialidosis. *Eur J Pediatr* 1987;**146**:528.

29 Takano T, Shimmoto M, Fukuhara Y, *et al*. Galactosialidosis: clinical and molecular analysis of 19 Japanese patients. *Brain Dysfunct* 1991;**4**:271.

30 Zammarchi E, Donati MA, Marrone A, *et al*. Early infantile galactsialidosis: clinical biochemical and molecular observations in a new patient. *Am J Med Genet* 1996;**64**:453.

31 Claeys M, Van Der Hoeven M, de Die-Smulders C, *et al*. Early-infantile type of galactosialidosis as a case of heart failure and neonatal ascites. *J Inherit Metab Dis* 1999;**22**:666.

32 Kleijer WJ, Hoogeveen A, Verheijen FW, *et al*. Prenatal diagnosis of sialidosis with combined neuraminidase and β-galactosidase deficiency. *Clin Genet* 1979;**16**:60.

33 Landau D, Zeigler M, Shinwell E, *et al*. Hydrops fetalis in four siblings caused by galactosialidosis. *Isr J Med Sci* 1995;**31**:321.

34 Tekinalp G, Aliefendioglu D, Yuce A, *et al*. A case with early infantile form of galactosialidosis with unusual haematological findings. *J Inherit Metab Dis* 1999;**22**:668.

35 Olcay L, Gumruk F, Boduroglu K, *et al*. Anaemia and thrombocytopenia due to haemophagocytosis in a 7-month-old boy with galactosialidosis. *J Inherit Metab Dis* 1998;**21**:679.

36 Strisciuglio P, Sly W, Dodson WE, *et al*. Combined deficiency of β-galactosidase and neuraminidase: natural history of the disease in the first 18 years of an American patient with late infantile onset form. *Am J Med Genet* 1990;**37**:573.

37 Chitayat D, Applegarth DA, Lewis J, *et al*. Juvenile galactosialidosis in a white male: a new variant. *Am J Med Genet* 1988;**31**:887.

38 Richard C, Tranchemontagne J, Elsliger M, *et al*. Molecular pathology of galactosialidosis in a patient affected with two new frameshift mutations in the cathepsin A/protective protein gene. *Hum Mutat* 1998;**11**:461.

39 Orii T, Minami R, Sukegawa K, *et al*. A new type of mucolipidosis with β-galactosidase deficiency and glyco-peptiduria. *Tohoko J Exp Med* 1972;**107**:303.

40 Yamamoto A, Adachi S, Kawamura S, *et al*. Localized β-galactosidase deficiency. Occurrence in cerebellar ataxia with myoclonus epilepsy and macular cherry red-spot. A new variant of GM₁-gangliosidosis. *Arch Intern Med* 1974;**134**:627.

41 Suzuki Y, Fukuoka K, Sakuraba H. β-Galactosidase neuraminidase deficiency with cerebellar ataxia and myoclonus: in *Spinocerebellar Degenerations* (ed. Sobue I). University of Tokyo, Tokyo;1980: 339.

42 Matsuo T, Egawa I, Okada S, *et al*. Sialidosis type 2 in Japan. Clinical study in two siblings cases and review of literature. *J Neurol Sci* 1983;**58**:45.

43 Yoshino H, Miyashita K, Miyatani N, *et al*. Abnormal glycosphingolipid metabolism in the nervous system of galactosialidosis. *J Neurol Sci* 1990;**97**:53.

44 Tsuiji S, Yamada T, Ariga T, *et al*. Carrier detection of sialidosis with partial β-galactosidase deficiency by the assay of lysosomal sialidase in lymphocytes. *Ann Neurol* 1984;**15**:181.

45 Suzuki Y, Sakuraba H, Yamanaka T, *et al*. Galactosialidosis: a comparative study of clinical and biochemical data on 22 patients: in *The Developing Brain and Its Disorders* (eds M Arima, Y Suzuki, H Yabuuchi). University of Tokyo, Tokyo;1984:161.

46 Suzuki Y, Nakamura N, Fukuoka K, *et al*. β-Galactosidase deficiency in juvenile and adult patients. *Hum Genet* 1977;**36**:219.

47 Tsuji S, Yamada T, Tsutsumi A, Miyatake T. Neuraminidase deficiency and accumulation of sialic acid in lymphocytes in adult type sialidosis with partial β-galactosialidase. *Ann Neurol* 1982;**11**:541.

48 Miyatake T, Atsumi T, Obayashi T, *et al*. Adult type neuronal storage disease with neuraminidase deficiency. *Ann Neurol* 1979;**6**:232.

49 Kuriyama M, Miyatake T, Owada M, Kitagawa T. Neuraminidase activities in sialidosis and mucolipidosis. *J. Neurol Sci* 1982;**54**:181.

50 Berard-Badier M, Adechy-Benkoel L, Chamlian A, *et al*. Etude ultrastructurale du parenchyme hépatique dans les mucopolysaccharidoses. *Path Biol* (Paris) 1970;**18**:117.

51 Giljaard H, Hoogeveen A, Verheijen FW, *et al*. Relationship between clinical, biochemical and genetic heterogeneity in sialidase deficiency: in *Sialidases and Sialidoses* (G Tettamanti, P Durand, S Di Donato eds). Milan: Edi Ermes, 1981:371.

52 Oyanagi K, Ohama E, Miyashita K, *et al*. Galactosialidosis: neuropathological findings in a case of the late-infantile type. *Acta Neuropathol* 1991;**82**:331.

53 Amano N, Yokoi S, Akagi M, *et al*. Neuropathological findings of an autopsy case of adult β-galactosidase and neuraminidase deficiency. *Acta Neuropathol* 1983;**61**:283.

54 Kobayashi T, Ohta M, Goto I, *et al*. Adult type mucolipidosis with β-galactosidase and sialidase deficiency. *J Neurol* 1979;**221**:137.

55 Ishibashi A, Tsuboi R, Shinmei M. β-Galactosidase and neuraminidase deficiency associated with angiokeratoma corporis diffusum. *Arch Dermatol* 1984;**120**:1344.

56 Nordborg C, Kyllerman M, Conradi N, Mansson J. Early infantile galactosialidosis with multiple brain infarctions: morphological neuropathological and neurochemical findings. *Acta Neuropathol* 1997;**93**:24.

57 Galjart NH, Gillemans N, Harris A, *et al*. Expression of cDNA encoding the human 'protective protein' associated with lysosomal β-galactosidase and neura-minidase: homology to yeast proteases. *Cell* 1988;**54**:755.

58 Galjart NH, Morreau H, Willemsen R, *et al*. Human lysosomal protective protein has cathepsin A-like activity distinct from its protective function. *J Biol Chem* 1991;**226**:14754.

59 Itoh K, Takiyama N, Nagao Y, *et al*. Acid carboxypeptidase deficiency in galactosialidosis. *Jpn J Hum Genet* 1991;**36**:171.

60 Mueller OT, Henry WM, Haley LL, *et al*. Sialidosis and galactosialidosis: chromosomal assignment of two genes associated with neuraminidase-deficiency disorders. *Proc Natl Acad Sci USA* 1986;**83**:1817.

61 Hoogeveen AT, Verheijen FW, Galjaard H. The relation between human lysosomal β-galactosidase and its protective protein. *J Biol Chem* 1983;**258**:12143.

62 Suzuki Y, Sakuraba H, Hayashi K, *et al*. β-Galactosidase-neuraminidase deficiency: restoration of β-galactosidase activity by protease inhibitors. *J Biochem* 1981;**90**:271.

63 Verheijen FW, Bossmer R, Galjaard H. Purification of acid β-galactosidase and acid neuraminidase from bovine testis: evidence for an enzyme complex. *Biochem Biophys Res Commun* 1982;**108**:868.

64 Verheijen FW, Palmeri S, Hoogeveen AT, Galjaard H. Human placental neuraminidase activation stabilization and association with β-galactosidase and its protective protein. *Eur J Biochem* 1985;**149**:315.

65 Bonten E, van der Spoel A, Fornerod M, *et al*. Characterization of human lysosomal neuraminidase defines the molecular basis of the metabolic storage disorder sialidosis. *Genes Dev* 1996;**10**:3156.

66 Tranchemontagne J, Michaud L, Potier M. Deficient lysosomal carboxypeptidase activity in galactosialidosis. *Biochem Biophys Res Commun* 1990;**168**:22.

67 Pshezhetsky A, Potier M. Association on N-acetylgalactosamine-6-sulfate sulfatase with the multienzyme lysosomal complex of β-galactosidase cathepsin A and neuraminidase. *J Biol Chem* 1996;**271**:28359.

68 van der Spoel A, Bonten E, d'Azzo A. Transport of human lysosomal neuraminidase to mature lysosomes requires protective protein/cathepsin A. *EMBO J* 1998;**17**:1588.

69 Morreau H, Galjart NJ, Willemsen R, *et al*. Human lysosomal protective protein. Glycosylation intracellular transport and association with β-galactosidase in the endoplasmic reticulum. *J Biol Chem* 1992;**267**:17949.

70 Kase R, Itoh K, Takiyama N, *et al*. Galactosialidosis: simultaneous deficiency of esterase carboxy-terminal deamidase and acid carboxypeptidase activities. *Biochem Biophys Res Commun* 1990;**172**:1175.

71 Sewell AC, Pontz BF. Prenatal diagnosis of galactosialidosis. *Prenat Diagn* 1988;**8**:151.

72 Strisciuglio P, Parenti G, Giudice C, *et al*. The presence of a reduced amount of 32-kd 'protective' protein is a distinct biochemical finding in late infantile galactosialidosis. *Hum Genet* 1988;**80**:304.

73 Nanba ET, Tsuji A, Omura K, Suzuki Y. Galactosialidosis: molecular heterogeneity in biosynthesis and processing of protective protein for b-galactosidase *Hum Genet* 1988;**80**:329.

74 Shimmoto M, Nakahori Y, Matsushita I, *et al*. A human protective protein gene partially overlaps the gene encoding phospholipids transfer protein on the complementary strand of DNA. *Biochem Biophys Res Comm* 1996;**220**:802.

75 Shimmoto M, Takano T, Fukuhara Y, *et al*. Japanese-type adult galactosialidosis. A unique and common splice junction mutation causing exon skipping in the protective protein carboxypeptidase gene. *Proc Jpn Acad* 1990;**66**:217.

76 Fukuhara Y, Takano T, Shimmoto M, *et al*. A new point protection of protective protein gene in two Japanese siblings with juvenile galactosialidosis. *Brain Dysfunct* 1992;**5**:319.

77 Zhou XY, Willemsen R, Gillemans N, *et al*. Common point mutations in four patients with the late infantile form of galactosialidosis. *Am J Hum Genet* 1993;**53**:966A.

78 Zhou XY, van der Spoel A, Rottier R, *et al*. Molecular and biochemical analysis of protective protein/cathepsin A mutations: correlation with clinical severity in galactosialidosis. *Hum Mol Genet* 1996;**5**:1977.

79 van Pelt J, Bakker HD, Kamerling JP, Vliegenthart JFG. A comparative study of sialyloligosaccharides isolated from sialidosis and galactosialidosis in urine. *J Inherit Metab Dis* 1991;**14**:730.

80 van Pelt J, van Kuik JA, Kamerling JP, *et al*. Storage of sialic acid containing carbohydrates in the placenta of a human galactosialidosis fetus. Isolation and structural characterization of 16 sialyloligosaccharides. *Eur J Biochem* 1988;**177**:327.

81 van Pelt J, Kamerling JP, Vliegenthart JFG. A comparative study of the accumulated sialic acid-containing oligosaccharides from cultured human galactosialidosis and sialidosis fibroblasts. *Clin Chim Acta* 1988;**174**:325.

82 Sewell AC. An improved thin layer chromatographic method for urinary oligosaccharide screening. *Clin Chim Acta* 1979;**92**:411.

83 Zhou XY, Morreau H, Rottier R, *et al*. Mouse model for the lysosomal disorder galactosialidosis and correction of the phenotype with over-expressing erythroid precursor cells. *Genes Dev* 1995;**9**:2623.

Metachromatic leukodystrophy

MAJOR PHENOTYPIC EXPRESSION

Delay or deterioration in walking, progressive neurodegenerative disease, optic atrophy and grayish discoloration of the retina, symmetrical decrease in the density of cerebral white matter, elevated cerebrospinal fluid protein, increased excretion of urinary sulfatide and deficient activity of arylsulfatase A.

INTRODUCTION

Metachromatic staining of the brain in neurodegenerative disease was reported as early as 1910 by Perusini and by Alzheimer [1,2] in studies of adults. The classic late infantile form of metachromatic leukodystrophy (MLD) was first reported by Greenfield [3] in 1933. Scholz [4], in 1925, published a detailed clinical pathologic study of juvenile or childhood-onset leukodystrophy, and Peiffer [5], 34 years later, demonstrated that the neural tissues of Scholz's frozen sections stained metachromatically. The metachromasia results from the accumulation of sulfatides, and this was discovered independently in 1958 by Jatzkewitz [6] and Austin [7]. It was Austin [8] and his colleagues who found the defective activity of arylsulfatase A. Mehl and Jatzkewitz [9] demonstrated defective activity against cerebroside sulfate, the material that accumulates in MLD (Figure 102.1).

The sulfatase enzyme is heat labile. A heat stable factor that increases activity several fold is known as saposin B, and in rare instances MLD results from defective activity of this protein, and arylsulfatase activity is normal [10,11]. Deficiency of the heat stable factor carries deficiency of the enzymatic hydrolysis of sulfatide [12–14]. Other variants with clinical MLD have signs of mucopolysaccharidosis and have been found to have multiple sulfatase deficiency (Chapter 103).

The gene for arylsulfatase A has been localized distal to band q13 on chromosome 22 [15], and it has been cloned and sequenced [16]. A number of mutations have been elucidated. In general, patients with late infantile MLD have null mutations leading to absence of enzyme activity and immunoreactive enzyme either in patient cells or when the gene is introduced into animal cell-line expression systems [17]. Mutations which express small amounts of cross-reacting material (CRM) and active enzyme are found on at least one allele in juvenile onset and adult disease.

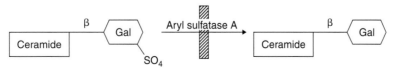

Figure 102.1   *The arylsulfatase A reaction, site of the defect in metachromatic leukodystrophy. Abbreviations include: CER, ceramide; GAL, galactose, and SO$_4$ sulfate. A number of other sulfatides, such as lactosylceramide sulfate, as well as the galactosylceramide sulfate shown are natural substrates for the enzyme.*

The diagnosis of MLD is complicated by the fact that there is a benign pseudodeficiency allele for arylsulfatase A, which in homozygotes leads to absence of arylsulfatase A activity and no clinical abnormalities [18,19]. Thus not only can patients with MLD have normal activity of arylsulfatase A (when the deficiency is in saposin B), but patients with little or no activity of arylsulfatase A may not have MLD (when they have the pseudodeficiency allele in homozygosity).

CLINICAL ABNORMALITIES

MLD has been divided into four or five subgroups on the basis of the age of onset and rapidity of neurologic degeneration. As in the case of many genetic diseases, the advent of molecular biology may make all of these classifications obsolete, but it currently remains useful to distinguish at least the infantile and adult phenotypes. The classic late infantile disease (Figures 102.2, 102.3) begins before 30 months of life and is progressive to death in 1 to 7 years. The first manifestations are loss of acquired motor skills, especially walking, which becomes unsteady. Examination at this time reveals hypotonia, and often a pronounced genu recurvatum. Deep tendon reflexes are diminished or even absent, indicative of neuropathy. In some patients walking is delayed, and some never learn to walk [20,21], but most learn to walk unassisted and to speak short sentences, and then these skills deteriorate. Intercurrent infection may be followed by ataxia and weakness, which may disappear, but reappear later. The initial presentation with hypotonia and reflex changes may suggest a myopathy or peripheral neuropathy [22–24]. There may be intermittent severe pains in the legs [23].

Hagberg [23] has viewed the progression of the disease in four stages, the initial picture representing stage I. In stage II the patient is no longer able to stand, but can sit. There is ataxia, and truncal titubation. Speech deteriorates and is dysarthric or aphasic, and mental function regresses. Muscle tone is increased in the legs, and deep tendon reflexes are exaggerated. Ocular nystagmus develops, and ophthalmoscopy reveals optic atrophy and a grayish discoloration of the retina and macula, sometimes with a central red spot reminiscent of Tay-Sachs disease [24](Chapter 91). In stage III the patient develops spastic quadriplegia and is confined to bed. There may be decerebrate or decorticate rigidity or dystonic movements. Seizures develop in about a third of patients [25]. Pharyngeal muscle coordination is lost, and there is difficulty with feeding and with the airway. Mental deterioration continues, and speech is lost. The child may continue to respond to parents and smile. In stage IV contact is lost. The patient is blind and cannot swallow. Tube feeding is required. Death results usually from pneumonia.

Juvenile MLD has been the designation of patients where initial presentation was between 4 and 16 years-of-age, often with a decrease in school performance in the first or second grade, sometimes with unusual behavior [26]. The patient may

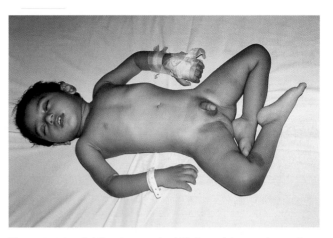

Figure 102.2 *S.A.S., a 24-month-old infant with metachromatic leukodystrophy, was markedly hypotonic and assumed a frog-leg position. He had lost milestones achieved. He had markedly diminished deep tendon reflexes. Arylsulfatase A activity was <0.1 nmol/mg/hr.*

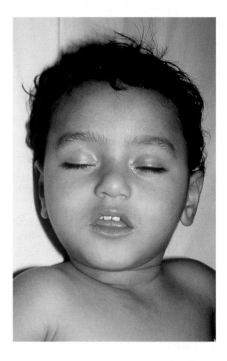

Figure 102.3 *S.A.S. The closed eyelids symbolize loss of contact with surroundings. CSF protein was 80 mg/dL. Nerve conduction velocity was diminished.*

appear confused or to be daydreaming. Some have had dementia, psychosis or emotional illness. Younger patients may present with clumsiness of gait, as in the infantile patients [25]. Muscular rigidity, postural abnormalities and ataxia may occur. Within a year of onset the patient is unable to walk. Urinary incontinence may occur early. Progression is to stages III and IV, as in the late infantile disease. It is clear that patients within this group may have phenotypes overlapping those of younger and older patients; the distinction may be artificial. In fact, instances have been described of siblings in the same family with juvenile and adult disease [27–31]. Some unusual visceral presentations have been with acute cholecystitis [27], chronic hemorrhagic pancreatitis [32], abdominal mass [33] or gastrointestinal bleeding [34].

Adult MLD refers to patients presenting after puberty [35]. Onset may be as young as 15 years-of-age [36] or as late as 62 [37]. Survival may be for five or 10 years or longer. Symptomatology is largely psychiatric. The recognition of these patients is a strong argument for neuroimaging studies in psychiatric patients [38]. Dementia may be manifest in loss of memory or decrease in intellectual ability. Psychotic changes may be those of schizophrenia. There may be emotional lability, anxiety or apathy. Visual-spatial discrimination may be impaired. Auditory hallucinations and delusions were reported in 18 percent and 27 percent of patients, and psychosis in 53 percent [39]. Depression and chronic alcoholism have been observed.

Motor disturbances may develop with clumsiness of gait and dysarthria. Muscle tone increases, and deep tendon reflexes are brisk. Some develop ataxia, and some have Parkinson-like features. In some patients the initial manifestations are those of peripheral neuropathy [40–42]. Dystonic movements may develop. Degeneration progresses to spastic tetraparesis, bulbar involvement and decorticate posturing. Optic atrophy and nystagmus are found. There may be seizures. Ultimately, the patient is blind, mute and unresponsive.

Patients with MLD as a result of deficiency of the cerebroside sulfatase activator, saposin B, have generally presented as juvenile MLD [10,11,43,44]. In one patient onset was at 48 years with intellectual deterioration, apathy and withdrawal [45]. Each was recognized initially on the basis of an MLD phenotype with normal activity of arylsulfatase A [12].

The clinical laboratory evaluation of patients with established MLD is notable for elevation of the concentration of protein in the cerebrospinal fluid. The level may be normal early in infantile disease, but it rises progressively to levels of 100 mg/dL or higher. This is true also for the younger-onset juvenile patients; while later-onset juvenile and adult-onset patients usually have normal levels of protein, though there have been a few with elevated concentrations [40].

The electroencephalograph (EEG) may be abnormal, especially in those with seizures [46–49]. There may be diffuse slowing or spike discharges, often focal. Noise may induce a marked startle response. The EEG tends to be normal in the adult-onset patient [49].

Motor nerve conduction is slowed [25]. These abnormalities have been demonstrated in presymptomatic patients, indicating the presence of peripheral neuropathy well before the onset of symptoms. Delay may be evident in afferent nerves before that of efferent nerves [50–53]. There may also be abnormalities in brainstem auditory evoked responses (BAERs), visual evoked responses or somatosensory responses. Abnormalities in BAER may be evident when peripheral nerve conduction is unimpaired [54]. Biopsy of peripheral nerve reveals the characteristic inclusion bodies (Figure 102.4).

Neuroimaging by computed tomography (CT) or magnetic resonance (MR) is consistent with loss of myelin and increase

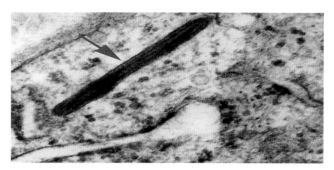

Figure 102.4 *Electron microscopy of biopsied sural nerve indicating the dense inclusion body. These inclusions have been called zebra bodies because of the stripes.*

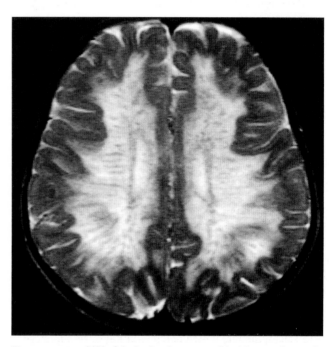

Figure 102.5 *MRI of the brain of a 5-year-old with metachromatic leukodystrophy. There was diffuse high T2 signal throughout the white matter in a sunray appearance. She had regressed developmentally and had diminished deep tendon reflexes.*

in water. Low density on CT and hyperintense T_2 images on magnetic resonance imaging (MRI) are visible in periventricular white matter indicative of leukodystrophy (Figure 102.5) [55–57]. Later there is evident atrophy. Proton MR spectroscopy reveals reduction in N-acetylaspartate and increase of myoinositol, a glial marker [58].

GENETICS AND PATHOGENESIS

MLD is inherited in an autosomal recessive fashion. Multiple affected sibs of both sexes and normal parents have often been observed, and consanguinity was noted early [59]. The incidence of the late infantile form has been estimated at one in 40 000 in Sweden [59]; the juvenile form is about four times less common. An unusually high incidence of late infantile MLD of one in 75 live births was reported in an isolate of Habbanite Jews [60].

The molecular defect is in arylsulfatase A [8], which acts in tissues as the cerebroside sulfatase (Figure 102.1, p. 681). This acidic glycoprotein enzyme is synthesized as a 62 kDa precursor protein, and then translocated via a mannose-6-phosphate receptor to the lysosome as 57 to 62 kDa forms [61]. The deficiency has been demonstrated in many different tissues, including brain, cultured fibroblasts, leukocytes and urine [62–67]. The enzyme activity is usually measured against artificial substrate, such as p-nitrocatechol sulfate; the assay usually reveals some residual activity. Immunochemical studies have revealed CRM positive and CRM negative examples of late infantile MLD [68,69]. There is evidence of rapid degradation of synthesized enzyme in juvenile and adult-onset MLD. Studies of the degradation of cerebroside sulfate in intact fibroblasts have yielded correlations between the effectiveness of the cells in catabolizing sulfatide and the age or sex and severity of the clinical phenotype [28,70]. Arylsulfatase A activity is also defective, along with those of other sulfatases in multiple sulfatase deficiency (Chapter 103).

Arylsulfatase A activity is normal in patients with MLD that results from the activator saposin B [14], but cultured cells from these patients fail to degrade added sulfatide. Addition of purified activator protein corrects this defective behavior, and immunologic study reveals an absence of CRM against saposin B protein [43–45,71,72].

Pseudodeficiency of arylsulfatase A was first identified through the testing of clinically normal relatives of patients with MLD [73–75]. These individuals have a pseudodeficiency gene (pd), which leads to arylsulfatase A activity of 5 to 15 percent of normal [68]. They do not have sulfatiduria or storage of metachromatic material. The protein is kinetically normal, but smaller in size, and it lacks a glycosyl subunit.

The gene for arylsulfatase A is on chromosome 22 and q13 [15,76–78]. The saposin B gene is on chromosome 10 [79,80]. The arylsulfatase A gene consists of eight exons in a small 3.2 kb coding area [81]; the mRNA is 2.1 kb [82]. A large number of mutations has been found for arylsulfatase A [17,82,83]. A common polymorphism leads to an enzyme with perfectly normal activity and a threonine to serine change in exon 7 [17]. In late infantile MLD the mutant alleles are sometime referred to as I-type mutations [17]. More often these are now referred to as null alleles, which code for no enzyme activity. Two splice-site mutations have been identified that lead to this phenotype. They include the G609A transition that destroys the splice donor site of exon 2 by changing the exon-intron boundary from AGgt to AGat [17]. This common mutation in Europeans has also been seen in Arabs. Another was a G2195A transition at the splice-recognition site between exon 7 and the next intron [84]. In addition, an 11 bp deletion in exon 8, which causes a frame shift, was also found in this phenotype [85]. Point mutations have also been found in this phenotype, including a glycine 99 to aspartic acid change in exon 2 [86], common in Japan, and a

glycine 245 to arginine change in exon 4 [87]. Other common mutations among Europeans are Pro426Leu [17] and Ile79Ser [82]. Mutations, such as the G-to-A transition in exon 2 which results in a change from glycine 99 to aspartic acid [88] and the proline 426 change to leucine have been referred to as type A mutations and in the homozygous situation lead to adult-onset MLD. They are now referred to as R alleles, and they code for some residual activity.

Compounds of A-type and I type mutations have been found in juvenile onset patients [17]. The pseudodeficiency enzyme is 2–4 kDa smaller than normal enzyme. This is a result of a point mutation (asparagine to serine) at the C-terminal glycosylation site leading to loss of an oligosaccharide side chain [89]. The Pro426Leu mutation, second most common in Europeans, codes for an enzyme that is synthesized normally and targeted normally to the lysosomes, but there it is promptly degraded [90]. Two R alleles are usually found in the adult-onset disease [17,82,91]. Patients with I179S on one allele usually begin with psychiatric manifestations, while those carrying P426L usually begin with a neurologic picture [92].

The molecular biology of the saposin B activator has also been clarified. A prosaposin precursor gene directs the synthesis of a precursor protein from which the individual saposins are derived [93]. Mutations have been identified including a C-to-T transition leading to a substitution of isoleucine for threonine that eliminates a glycosylation site with a neighboring asparagine [94] in the original family of Shapiro and colleagues [10].

Heterozygote detection has been accomplished by assay of arylsulfatase A activity in leukocytes and fibroblasts [60,68,95]. Overlap with the normal range made the designation of noncarrier less reliable. The pseudodeficiency allele is common [14], and this may even suggest that a relative is affected. Testing with sulfatide-loaded fibroblasts may be required for resolution [95]; molecular detection of the pseudodeficiency pd allele will also resolve this. The pd allele causes two A-to-G mutations, changing arginine 352 to serine, with loss of a glycosylation site, and the change of a polyadenylation signal. In families in which the mutation is known, this information can be used for heterozygote detection. Searching for the most common splice-site mutation in late infantile MLD may be particularly useful.

It may also be employed for prenatal diagnosis. So far, enzyme assay has been employed for this purpose [70,96,97]. Prenatal diagnosis has been accomplished with cultured amniocytes and chorionic villus material. Here, too, the pseudodeficiency allele is a problem that must be recognized and dealt with. Sulfatide loading is usually helpful.

The consequence of cerebroside sulfatase deficiency is the accumulation of sulfatides in tissues, notably the cerebral white matter [6,7,98]. The accumulated sulfatide leads to decreased content of cerebrosides and the other lipid components of myelin. Sulfatide is also found in increased quantity in the urine [99]. The amounts may be 100 to 200 times the normal level [54,100,101]. This property has sometimes been employed to identify patients for testing for saposin B deficiency in those with clinical MLD and normal arylsulfatase A activity. Patients with pseudodeficiency do not have sulfatiduria [102].

The demyelination that characterizes the disease is doubtless a consequence of the accumulated sulfatide. Neuropathologic changes have been seen even in fetuses at the fifth month of presentation. The oligodendroglia and Schwann cells appear particularly to be targeted.

TREATMENT

Treatment of patients with MLD has been largely supportive. Vigabatrin may be useful in reducing spasticity [103].

Bone marrow transplantation has been employed in a number of patients [104–109]. Normal levels of circulating arylsulfatase A have been achieved, and the clinical course has seemed to slow, particularly as compared with that of an affected sibling [105,106]. It appears most useful in presymptomatic or early symptomatic patients. It may even accelerate progression in rapidly deteriorating patients [7,105]. In 10 families in which presymptomatic diagnosis was made because a previous sibling had had disease there was successful engraftment in each [108]. Best results were in juvenile and adolescent forms. Adults with psychiatric disease may benefit from transplantation [108]. Transplantation is currently not recommended for symptomatic early onset forms of the disease [109].

References

1 Perusini G. Uber klinisch und histologisch eigenartige psychische Erkrankungen des spateren Lebensalters. *Nissl-Alzheimer's Histol Histopathol Arb* 1910;**3**:297.

2 Alzheimer A. Beitrage zur Kenntnis der pathologischen Neurologia und ihrer Beziehung zu del Abbau-vorgangen im Nervengewebe. *Nissl-Alzheimer's Histol Histopathol Arb* 1910;**3**:493.

3 Greenfield JG. A form of progressive cerebral sclerosis in infants associated with primary degeneration of the interfascicular glia. *J Neurol Psychopathol* 1933;**13**:289.

4 Scholz W. Klinische, pathologisch-anatomische und erbbiologische Untersucchungen bei familiarer, diffuser Hirnsklerose im Kindesalter. *Z Gestamte Neurol Psychiatr* 1925;**99**:42.

5 Peiffer J. Uber die metachromatischen Leukodystrophien (Typ Scholz). *Arch Psychiatr Nervenkr* 1959;**199**:386.

6 Jatzkewitz H. Zwei Typen von Cerebrosid-schwelfelsauresog. 'Pralipoide' und Speichersubstanzen bei der Leukodystrophie, Typ Scholz (metachromatisch Form der diffusel Sklerose). *Z Physiol Chem* 1958;**311**:279.

7 Austin J. Metachromatic sulfatides in cerebral white matter and kidney. *Proc Soc Exp Biol Med* 1958;**100**:361.

8 Austin JH, Balasubramanian AS, Pattabiraman TN, *et al.* A controlled study of enzymatic activities in three human disorders of glycolipid metabolism. *J Neurochem* 1963;**10**:805.

9 Mehl E, Jatzkewitz H. Evidence for the genetic block in metachromatic leukodystrophy (ML). *Biochem Biophys Res Commun* 1965;**19**:407.

10 Shapiro LJ, Aleck KA, Kaback MM, *et al.* Metachromatic leukodystrophy without arylsulfatase A deficiency. *Pediatr Res* 1979;**13**:1179.

11 Hahn AF, Gordon BA, Feleki V, *et al.* A variant form of metachromatic leukodystrophy without arylsulfatase deficiency. *Ann Neurol* 1989;**12**:33.

12 Stevens RL, Fluharty AL, Kihara H, *et al.* Cerebroside sulfatase activator deficiency induced metachromatic leukodystrophy. *Am J Hum Genet* 1981;**33**:900.

13 Mehl E, Jatzkewitz H. Eine Cerebrosidsulfatase aus Schweineniere. *Hoppe-Seyleros Z Physiol Chem* 1964;**339**:260.

14 Wenger DA, Inui K. Studies on the sphingolipid activator protein for the enzymatic hydrolysis of GM$_1$ ganglioside and sulfatide: in *The Molecular Basis of Lysosomal Storage Disorders*, (eds RO Brady, JA Barranger). Academic Press, New York;1984:61.

15 Geurts van Kessel AHM, Westerveld A, de Groot PG, *et al.* Regional localization of the genes coding for human ACO2, ARSA, and NAGA on chromosome 22. *Cytogenet Cell Genet* 1980;**28**:169.

16 Stein C, Gieselmann V, Kreysing J, *et al.* Cloning and expression of human arylsulfatase A. *Biol Chem* 1989;**264**:1252.

17 Polten A, Fluharty CB, Kappler J, *et al.* Molecular basis of different forms of metachromatic leukodystrophy. *N Engl J Med* 1991;**324**:18.

18 Hohenschutz C, Eich P, Friedl W, *et al.* Pseudodeficiency of arylsulfatase A: a common genetic polymorphism with possible disease implications. *Hum Genet* 1989;**82**:45.

19 Baldinger S, Pierpont ME, Wenger DA. Pseudo deficiency of arylsulfatase A: a counseling dilemma. *Clin Genet* 1987;**31**:70.

20 Kihara H. Metachromatic leukodystrophy, an unusual case with a subtle cerebroside sulfatase defect: in *Brain Mechanisms in Mental Retardation* (eds N Buchwald, MAB Brazier). Academic Press, New York;1975:501.

21 Zlotogora J, Costeff H, Elian E. Early motor development in metachromatic leukodystrophy. *J Neurol Neurosurg Psychiatry* 1973;**36**:30.

22 Desilva KL, Pearce J. Neuropathy of metachromatic leukodystrophy. *J Neurol Neurosurg Psychiatry* 1973;**36**:30.

23 Hagberg B. Clinical symptoms, signs and tests in metachromatic leukodystrophy: in *Brain Lipids and Lipoproteins, and the Leukodystrophies*, (eds J Folch-Pi, H Bauer). Elsevier, Amsterdam;1963:134.

24 Cogan DG, Kuwabara T, Moser H. Metachromatic leukodystrophy. *Ophthalmologia* 1970;**160**:2.

25 MacFaul R, Cavanagh N, Lake BD, *et al.* Metachromatic leukodystrophy: review of 38 cases. *Arch Dis Child* 1982;**57**:168.

26 Balsev T, Cortez MA, Blaser SI, Haslam RHA. Recurrent seizures in metachromatic leukodystrophy. *Pediatr Neurol* 1997;**17**:150.

27 Clarke JTR, Skomorowski MA, Chang PL. Marked clinical difference between two sibs affected with juvenile metachromatic leukodystrophy. *Am J Med Genet* 1989;**33**:10.

28 Kappler J, Von Figura K, Gieselman V. Late-onset metachromatic leukodystrophy: molecular pathology in two siblings. *Ann Neurol* 1992;**31**:256.

29 Percy AK, Kaback MM, Herndon RM. Metachromatic leukodystrophy: comparison of early and late-onset forms. *Neurology* 1977;**27**:933.

30 Manowitz P, Kling A, Kohn H. Clinical course of adult metachromatic leukodystrophy presenting as schizophrenia. *J Nerv Ment Dis* 1978;**166**:500.

31 Alves D, Pires MM, Guimaraes A, Miranda MC. Four cases of late onset metachromatic leukodystrophy in a family: clinical, biochemical and neuropathological studies. *J Neurol Neurosurg Psychiatry* 1986;**49**:1423.

32 Deeg KH, Reif R, Stehr K, *et al.* Chronisch hämmorrhagische Pankreatitis bei Gallenblasenpolyposis als Erstsymptom der metachromatischen Leukodystrophie. *Monatsschr Kinderheilkd* 1986;**134**:272.

33 Tesluk H, Munn RJ, Schwartz MZ, Ruebner BH.Papillomatous transformation of the gallbladder in metachromatic leukodystrophy. *Pediatr Pathol* 1989;**9**:741.

34 Siegel EG, Lucke H, Schauer W, Creutzfeldt W. Repeated upper gastrointestinal hemorrhage caused by metachromatic leukodystrophy of the gall bladder. *Digestion* 1992;**51**:121.

35　Duyff RF, Weinstein HC. Late-presenting metachromatic leukodystrophy. *Lancet* 1996;**348**:1382.

36　Furst W, Sandhoff K. Activator proteins and topology of lysosomal sphingolipid catabolism. *Biochim Biophys Acta* 1992;**1126**:1.

37　Wu C-SC, Lee NM, Loh HH, *et al*. β-Endorphin: formulation of α-helix in lipid solutions. *Proc Natl Acad Sci USA* 1979;**76**:3656.

38　Brismar J. CT and MRI of the brain in inherited neurometabolic disorders. *J Child Neurol* 1992;**7**:(suppl.) S112.

39　Hyde TM, Ziegler JC, Weinberger DR. Psychiatric disturbances in metachromatic leukodystrophy. Insights into the neurobiology of psychosis. *Arch Neurol* 1992;**49**:401.

40　Bosch EP, Hart MN. Late adult-onset metachromatic leukodystrophy: dementia and polyneuropathy in a 63-year-old man. *Arch Neurol* 1978;**35**:475.

41　Fressinaud C, Vallat JM, Mason M, *et al*. Adult-onset metachromatic leukodystrophy presenting as isolated peripheral neuropathy. *Neurology* 1992;**42**:1396.

42　Bateman JB, Philippart M, Isenberg SJ. Ocular features of multiple sulfatase deficiency and a new variant of metachromatic leukodystrophy. *J Pediatr Ophthalmol Strabismus* 1984;**21**:133.

43　Wenger DA, Degala G, Williams C, *et al*. Clinical, pathological and biochemical studies on an infantile case of sulfatide/GM1 activator protein deficiency. *Am J Med Genet* 1989;**33**:255.

44　Scholte W, Harzer K, Christomanou H, *et al*. Sphingolipid activator protein 1 deficiency in metachromatic leukodystrophy with normal arylsulfatase A activity. A clinical morphological, biochemical, and immunological study. *Eur J Pediatr* 1991;**150**:584.

45　Lu-Ning W, Ke-Wei H, Dong-Gang W, Ze-Yan L. Adult metachromatic leukodystrophy without deficiency of arylsulphatase. *Chinese Med J* 1990;**103**:846.

46　Fukumizu M, Matsui K, Hanaoka S, *et al*. Partial seizures in two cases of metachromatic leukodystrophy: electrophysiologic and neuroradiologic findings. *J Child Neurol* 1992;**7**:381.

47　Blom S, Hagberg B. EEG findings in late infantile metachromatic and globoid cell leukodystrophy. *Electroencephalogr Clin Neurophysiol* 1967;**22**:253.

48　Mastropaolo C, Pampiglione G, Stephens R. EEG studies in 22 children with sulfatide lipidosis (metachromatic leukodystrophy). *Dev Med Child Neurol* 1971;**13**:20.

49　Klemm E, Conzelmann E. Adult-onset meta-chromatic leukodystrophy presenting without psychiatric symptoms. *J Neurol* 1989;**236**:427.

50　Clark JR, Miller RG, Vidgoff JM. Juvenile-onset metachromatic leukodystrophy: biochemical and electrophysiologic studies. *Neurology* 1979;**29**:346.

51　Pilz H, Hopf HC. A preclinical case of late adult metachromatic leukodystrophy: neurophysiological findings. *J Neurol Neurosurg Psychiatry* 1972;**35**:360.

52　Wulff CH, Trujaborg W. Adult metachromatic leukodystrophy: neurophysiologic findings. *Neurology* 1985;**35**:1776.

53　Cruz AM, Ferrer MT, Fueyo E, Galadós L. Peripheral neuropathy detected on an electrophysiological study as the manifestation of MLD in infancy. *J Neurol Neurosurg Psychiatry* 1975;**38**:169.

54　Brown FR, Shimizu H, McDonald JM, *et al*. Auditory evoked brainstem response and high-performance liquid chromatography sulfatase assay as early indices of metachromatic leukodystrophy. *Neurology* 1981;**31**:980.

55　Suárez EC, Rodríguez AS, Tapia AG, *et al*. Ichthyosis: the skin manifestation of multiple sulfatase deficiency. *Pediatr Dermatol* 1997;**14**:369.

56　Jayakumar PN, Aroor SR, Jha RK, Arya BYT. Computed tomography (CT) in late infantile metachromatic leukodystrophy. *Acta Neurol Scand* 1989;**79**:23.

57　Kim TS, Kim IO, Kim WS, *et al*. MR of childhood metachromatic leukodystrophy. *Am J Neuroradiol* 1997;**18**:733.

58　Kruse B, Hanefeld F, Christen HJ, *et al*. Alterations of brain metabolites in metachromatic leukodystrophy as detected by localized proton magnetic resonance spectroscopy *in vivo*. *J Neurol* 1993;**241**:68.

59　Gustavson K-H, Hagberg B. The incidence and genetics of metachromatic leukodystrophy in northern Sweden. *Acta Paediatr Scand* 1971;**60**:585.

60　Zlotogora J, Bach G, Barak V, Elian E. Metachromatic leukodystrophy in the Habbanite Jews: high frequency in a genetic isolate and screening for heterozygotes. *Am J Hum Genet* 1980;**32**:663.

61　Fujii T, Kobayashi T, Honke K, *et al*. Proteolytic processing of human lysosomal arylsulfatase A. *Biophys Acta* 1992;**1122**:93.

62　Tonnesen T, Bro PV, Brondum Nielsen K, Lykkelund C. Metachromatic leukodystrophy and pseudoaryl-sulfatase A deficiency in a Danish family. *Acta Paediatr Scand* 1983;**72**:175.

63　Thomas GH, Howell RR. Arylsulfatase A activity in human urine: quantitative studies on patients with lysosomal disorders including metachromatic leukodystrophy. *Clin Chim Acta* 1972;**36**:99.

64　DuBois G, Turpin JC, Georges MC, Bauman N. Arylsulfatase A and B in leukocytes: a comparative statistical study of late infantile and juvenile forms of metachromatic leukodystrophy and controls. *Biomedicine* 1980;**33**:2.

65　Percy AK, Brady RO. Metachromatic leukodystrophy: diagnosis with samples of venous blood. *Science* 1968;**161**:594.

66　Porter MT, Fluharty AL, Kihara H. Metachromatic leukodystrophy: arylsulfatase-A deficiency in skin fibroblast cultures. *Proc Natl Acad Sci USA* 1978;**62**:887.

67　Kaback MM, Howell RR. Infantile metachromatic leukodystrophy: heterozygote detection in skin fibroblasts and possible applications to intrauterine diagnosis. *N Engl J Med* 1970;**282**:1336.

68　Kappler J, Leinekugel P, Conzelmann E, *et al*. Genotype-phenotype relationship in various degrees of arylsulfatase A deficiency. *Hum Genet* 1991;**86**:463.

69　Tamaka A, Higami S, Isshiki G, *et al*. Immunofluorescence staining, and immunological studies of arylsulfatase deficiency (MSD) and metachromatic leukodystrophy (MLD) fibroblasts. *J Inherit Metab Dis* 1983;**6**:21.

70　Porter MT, Fluharty A, Trammell J, Kihara H. A correlation of intracellular cerebroside sulfatase activity in fibroblasts with latency in metachromatic leukodystrophy. *Biochem Biophys Res Commun* 1971;**44**:660.

71　Fujibayashi S, Inui K, Wenger DA. Activator protein-deficient metachromatic leukodystrophy: diagnosis in leukocytes using immunologic methods. *J Pediatr* 1984;**104**:739.

72　Inui K, Emmett M, Wenger DA. Immunological evidence for deficiency in an activator protein for sulfatide sulfatase in a variant form of metachromatic leukodystrophy. *Proc Natl Acad Sci USA* 1983;**80**:3074.

73　DuBois G, Turpin JC, Baumann N. Absence of ASA activity in healthy father of patient with metachromatic leukodystrophy. *N Engl J Med* 1975;**293**:302.

74　Lott IT, Dulalney JT, Milunsky A, *et al*. Apparent biochemical homozygosity in two obligatory heterozygotes for metachromatic leukodystrophy. *J Pediatr* 1976;**89**:438.

75　DuBois G, Harzer K, Baumann N. Very low arylsulfatase A and cerebroside sulfatase activities in leukocytes of healthy members of metachromatic leukodystrophy family. *Am J Hum Genet* 1977;**29**:191.

76　Hors-Cayla MC, Heuertz S, Van Cong N, *et al*. Confirmation of the assignment of the gene for arylsulfatase A to chromosome 22 using somatic cell hybrids. *Hum Genet* 1979;**49**:33.

77　Gustavson K-H, Arancibia W, Eriksson U, Svennerholm L. Deleted ring chromosome 22 in a mentally retarded boy. *Clin Genet* 1986;**29**:337.

78　Phelan MC, Thomas GR, Saul RA, *et al*. Cytogenetic, biochemical and molecular analyses of a 22q13 deletion. *Am J Med Genet* 1992;**43**:872.

79　Inui K, Kao F-T, Fujibayashi S, *et al*. The gene coding for a sphingolipid activator protein, SAP-1, is on human chromosome 10. *Somat Cell Mol Genet* 1985;**69**:197.

80 Kao F-T, Law ML, Hartz J, *et al.* Regional localization of the gene coding for sphingolipid activator protein SAP-1 on human chromosome 10. *Somat Cell Mol Genet* 1987;**13**:685.

81 Kreysing J, Von Figura K, Gieselmann V. Structure of the arylsulfatase A gene. *Eur J Biochem* 1990;**191**:627.

82 Berger J, Loschl B, Bernheimer H, *et al.* Occurrence , distribution, and phenotype of arylsulfatase A mutations in patients with metachromatic leukodystrophy. *Am J Med Genet* 1997;**69**:335.

83 Gieselmann V, Polten A, Kreysing J, *et al.* Molecular genetics of metachromatic leukodystrophy. *Dev Neurosci* 1991;**13**:222.

84 Fluharty AL, Fluharty CB, Bohne W, I. Two new arylsulfatase A (ARSA) mutations in a juvenile metachromatic leukodystrophy (MLD) patient. *Am J Hum Genet* 1991;**49**:1340.

85 Bohne W, Von Figura K, Gieselmann V. An 11-bp deletion in the arylsulfatase A gene of a patient with late infantile metachromatic leukodystrophy. *Hum Genet* 1991;**49**:1340.

86 Kondo R, Wakamatsu N, Yoshino H, *et al.* Identification of a mutation in the arylsulfatase A gene of a patient with adult-type leukodystrophy and Gaucher disease. *Am J Hum Genet* 1991;**48**:971.

87 Eto Y, Kawame H, Hasegawa Y, *et al.* Molecular characteristics in Japanese patients with lipidosis: novel mutations in metachromatic leukodystrophy and Gaucher disease. *Mol Cell Biochem* 1993;**119**:179.

88 Barth ML, Fensom A, Harris A.Prevalence of common mutations in the arylsulphatase A gene in metachromatic leukodystrophy patients diagnosed in Britain. *Hum Genet* 1993 ;**91**:73.

89 Kihara H, Meek WE, Fluharty AL. Attenuated activities and structural alterations of arylsulfatase A in tissues from subjects with pseudo arylsulfatase A deficiency. *Hum Genet* 1986;**74**:59.

90 von Figura K, Steckel F, Hasilik A. Juvenile and adult metachromatic leukodystrophy: partial restoration of arylsulfatase A (cerebroside sulfatase) activity in inhibitors of thiol proteinases. *Proc Natl Acad Sci USA* 1983;**80**:6066.

91 Gieselman V, Zlotogora J, Harris A, *et al.* Molecular genetics of metachromatic leukodystrophy. *Hum Mutat* 1994;**4**:233.

92 Porter MT, Fluharty AL, Harris SE, Kihara H. The accumulation of cerebroside sulfates by fibroblasts in culture from patients with late infantile metachromatic leukodystrophy. *Arch Biochem Biophys* 1970;**138**:646.

93 O'Brien JS, Kishimoto Y.Saposin proteins: structure, function and role in human lysosomal storage disorders. *FASEB J* 1991;**5**:301.

94 Kretz KA, Carson GS, Morimoto S, *et al.* Characterization of a mutation in a family with saposin B deficiency: a glycosylation site defect. *Proc Natl Acad Sci USA* 1990;**87**:2541.

95 Raghavan SS, Gajewski A, Kolodny EH. Leukocyte sulfatidase for the reliable diagnosis of metachromatic leukodystrophy. *J Neurochem* 1981;**36**:724.

96 Eto Y, Tahara T, Koda N, *et al.* Prenatal diagnosis of metachromatic leukodystrophy. A diagnosis by amiotic fluid and its confirmation. *Arch Neurol* 1982;**39**:29.

97 Percy AK, Farrell DF, Kaback MM. Cerebroside sulphate (sulphatide) suphohydrolase: an improved assay method. *J Neurochem* 1972;**19**:233.

98 Svennerholm L. Some aspects of the biochemical changes in leukodystrophy: in *Brain Lipids and Lipoproteins, and the Leucodystrophies,* (eds J Folch-Pi, H Bauer). Elsevier Publishing, Amsterdam;1963:104.

99 Pilz H, Muller D, Linke L. Histochemical and biochemical studies of urinary lipids in metachromatic leukodystrophy and Fabryōs disease. *J Lab Clin Med* 1973;**81**:7.

100 Philippart M, Sarlieve L, Meurant C, Mechler L. Human urinary sulfatides in patients with sulfatidosis (metachromatic leukodystrophy). *J Lipid Res* 1971:**12**:434.

101 Natowicz MR, Prence EM, Chaturvedi P, Newburg DS. Urine sulfatides and the diagnosis of metachromatic leukodystrophy. *Clin Chem* 1996;**42**:232.

102 Lugowska A, Tylki-Symanska A, Berger J, Molzer. Elevated sulfatide excretion in compound heterozygotes of metachromatic leukodystrophy and ASA-pseudodeficiency allele. *Clin Biochem* 1997;**30**:325.

103 Jaeken J, Casaer P, De Cock P, Francois B. Vigabatrin in GABA metabolism disorders. *Lancet* 1989;**1**:1074.

104 Krivit W, Shapiro E, Kennedy W, *et al.* Treatment of late infantile metachromatic leukodystrophy by bone marrow transplantation. *N Engl J Med* 1990;**322**:28.

105 Shapiro E, Lipton ME, Krivit W. White matter dysfunction and its neuro-psychological correlates: a longitudinal study of a case of metachromatic leukodystrophy treated with bone marrow transplant. *J Clin Exper Neuropsychiatry* 1992;**14**:610.

106 Pridjian G, Humbert J, Willis J, Shapiro E. Presymptomatic late-infantile metachromatic leukodystrophy treated with bone marrow transplantation. *J Pediatr* 1994;**125**:755.

107 Krivit W, Shapiro EG. Bone marrow transplantation for storage diseases: in *Treatment of Genetic Disease* (ed. RJ Desnick). Churchill Livingstone, New York;1991:203.

108 Krivit W, Lockman LA, Watkins PA, *et al.* The future for treatment by bone marrow transplantation for adrenoleukodystrophy, metachromatic leukodystrophy, globoid cell leukodystrophy and Hurler syndrome. *J Inherit Metab Dis* 1995;**18**:398.

109 Shapiro EG, Lockman LA, Balthazor M, Krivit W. Neuropsychological outcomes of several storage diseases with and without bone marrow transplantation. *J Inherit Metab Dis* 1995;**18**:413.

Multiple sulfatase deficiency

MAJOR PHENOTYPIC EXPRESSION

Facial and somatic features and dysostosis multiplex of a mucopolysaccharidosis; ichthyosis; neurologic features of a late infantile metachromatic leukodystrophy; mucopolysacchariduria; defective activity of arylsulfatase A, B and C, steroid sulfatase and the mucopolysaccharide sulfatases, including iduronate sulfatase, heparan-N-sulfatase, N-acetylgalactosamine-6-sulfatase and N-acetylglucosamine-6-sulfatase; and defective post-translational change of sulfatase cysteine-69 to aminopropionic acid.

INTRODUCTION

Multiple sulfatase deficiency was reported in 1965 by Austin, Armstrong and Shearer [1,2] as metachromatic leukodystrophy (MLD) in which there were also features of mucopolysaccharidosis. Deficient activity of a number of sulfatases led to the designation of multiple sulfatase deficiency (MSD) [3]. At least seven enzymes are now known to be deficient [2–5].

The deficiency of arylsulfatase A would be consistent with clinical features of MLD. The deficiency of steroid sulfatase would be responsible for the skin lesions of X-linked ichthyosis. Among the enzymes of mucopolysaccharide metabolism: deficiency of iduronate sulfatase would give manifestations of Hunter syndrome; that of heparan sulfatase could yield the mental retardation and cerebral features of Sanfilippo A disease; that of N-acetylglucosamine-6-sulfatase, those of Sanfilippo B disease and that of N-acetylgalactosamine-6-sulfatase could give rise to features of Morquio disease; and deficiency of N-acetylgalactosamine-4-sulfatase, also known as arylsulfatase B, would cause features of Maroteaux-Lamy disease, including corneal clouding. Obviously different degrees of deficiency or amounts of residual enzyme activity would be expected to lead to quite different phenotypes. A number of different forms have been delineated [4] including the classic

late infantile form, a neonatal form, a juvenile form and a Saudi variant.

The fundamental defect [6,7] represents a novel mechanism of disease in which the mutation is in an enzyme responsible for post-translational change of a cysteine moiety of each of the sulfatases, a change that conveys activation of the enzyme (Figure 103.1). This cysteine is conserved in each of the sulfatases (Table 103.1).

It is converted to 2-amino-3-oxopropionic acid (formylglycine) (Figure 103.1). The gene, termed sulfatase modifying

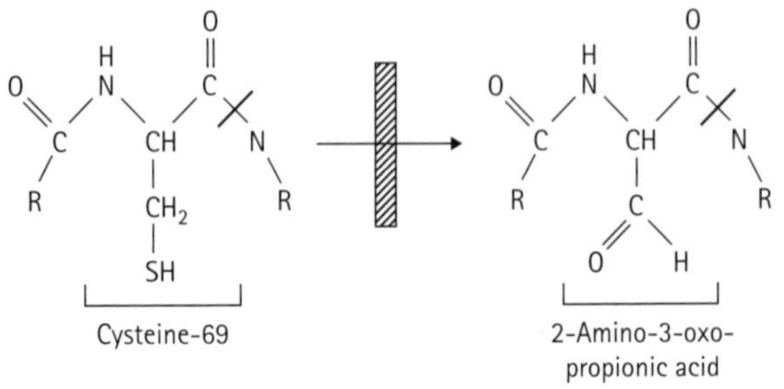

Figure 103.1 *Mechanism of activation of sulfatase enzymes by conversion of a highly conserved cysteine at position 69 in arylsulfatase A to 2-amino-3-oxopropionic acid.*

Table 103.1   *Homology of sulfatase sequences*

Arylsulfatase A	L	C	T	P	S	R
Arylsulfatase B	L	C	T	P	S	R
Steroid sulfatase	L	C	T	P	S	R
N-Acetylglucosamine-6-sulfatase	L	C	C	P	S	R
Iduronate sulfatase	V	C	A	P	S	R
N-Acetylgalactosamine-6-sulfatase	L	C	S	P	S	R
Sea urchin arysulfatase	V	C	T	P	S	R

factor 1 (*SUMF* 1) has been identified, and missense mutations have been discovered which lead to variable loss of function(8).

CLINICAL ABNORMALITIES

The clinical picture of MSD represents a summation of the various enzymatic defects [4,5,7,9]. In its classic form, it presents in late infancy with the symptoms of the progressive degeneration of myelin of MLD [9], or in the neonatal form with a picture of a severe mucopolysaccharidosis [10]. A milder juvenile form with onset at about 5 years-of-age has been reported [6]. At least 50 patients have been reported.

The more commonly described presentation is that of an MLD [5,7,9] with mild features of mucopolysaccharidosis [11–14]. Early development may be normal, and patients may walk and speak at normal times [4], but some may be developmentally delayed early on. During the second or third year, milestones attained are slowly lost. Increased deep tendon reflexes and ankle clonus may be followed by spastic quadriparesis. There may be seizures. Neurodegeneration is progressive to blindness and loss of hearing [9,15], and deafness may be severe. The head becomes microcephalic [9,16,17]. Swallowing becomes difficult, and tube feeding is required. Death may occur at 10 to 18 years, but there has been survival into the third decade.

Mucopolysaccharidosis-like features maybe evident very early in life [10,18] and may well be the first evidence of disease. The diagnosis should be considered in young patients with signs of mucopolysaccharidosis. The facial features are coarse, and there is hirsutism (Figures 103.2–103.5). There may be stertorous breathing, nasal discharge, or hernias. Hepatosplenomegaly may be prominent (Figure 103.6). Joints become stiff, and there may be contractures. The claw hand may be identical to that of Hurler disease (Figures 103.7, 103.8). Virtually all patients have roentgenographic evidence of dysostosis multiplex (Chapter 77). The initial diagnosis may be of Hunter or Sanfilippo disease [5,18]. Cardiac complications have been observed [10]. A few patients do not appear to have recognizable clinical features of mucopolysaccharidosis. Ophthalmologic findings have included optic atrophy, retinal degeneration and nystagmus [5,10,19]. The cornea is usually clear [5,9,18]. Two patients have had a cherry red macula [12,20]. The classic presentation is with ichthyosis (Figure 103.3) [5,16,17].

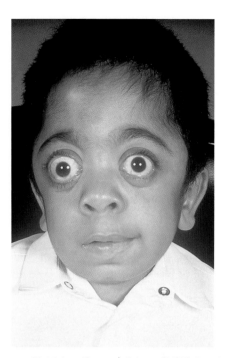

Figure 103.2   *Multiple sulfatase deficiency (MSD). A patient with MSD whose eyes were strikingly proptotic. He also had atlantoaxial dislocation. Sulfatase activities were very low.*

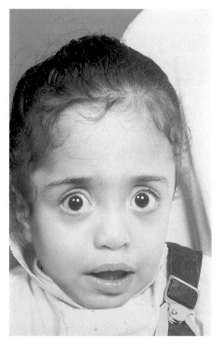

Figure 103.3   *I.Q. This girl with MSD also had strikingly prominent eyes.*

Another neonatal phenotype has been distinguished [4] in which there is presentation at birth with prominent features of mucopolysaccharidosis, severe encephalopathy and early demise [10,15,21]. Hepatosplenomegaly is pronounced. These patients have also had ichthyosis by 2 to 3 years-of-age [10,21]. The neck was short, and there was hypoplasia of the vertebral

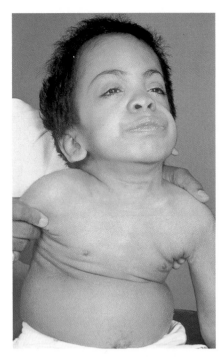

Figure 103.4   *M.M. A boy with MSD. Facial features were coarse, the nasal bridge depressed and the nasal tip tilted, highlighting the abundant nasal subcutaneous tissue. The skin of the legs, as well as the torso illustrated was ichthyotic.*

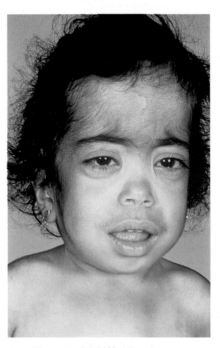

Figure 103.5   *H.Z., a girl with MSD. Hirsutism was very pronounced and the facial features coarse.*

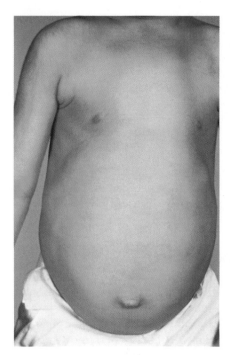

Figure 103.6   *H.Z. The abdomen was protruberant as a consequence of hepatosplenomegaly.*

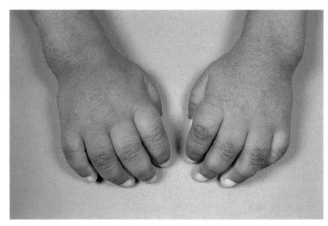

Figure 103.7   *M.M. The hands were just like those of a patient with Hurler disease.*

bodies and epiphyseal dysplasia. Consistent with the severity of the phenotype, enzyme activities of all of the sulfatases tested were very severely depressed [10,21].

A Saudi variant has been distinguished [4] in which there was early infantile onset of severe dysostosis multiplex, appearing as Maroteaux-Lamy syndrome or Morquio disease. There was corneal clouding in six of eight patients. Facial features were coarse. The orbit may appear shallow and the eyes proptotic (Figures 103.2, 103.3, 103.11). Deafness was absent, but one patient had abnormal auditory evoked potentials on one side. Ichthyosis was absent, and in six of seven patients studied the activity of steroid sulfatase was normal [4]. On the other hand, we have since seen ichthyosis in another Saudi patient. Patients had mild to moderate mental retardation, and one patient had a normal cognitive quotient despite motor retardation. There may be macrocephaly (Figures 103.9,103.11) and gingival hyperplasia (Figure 103.10). Most of these patients had retinal changes, but two had lenticular opacities, which have been

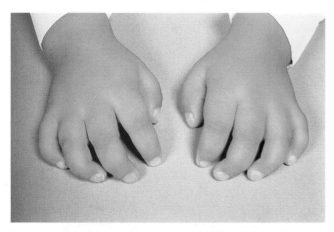

Figure 103.8   *A.A., another patient with MSD and very striking hands. A brother had MSD too.*

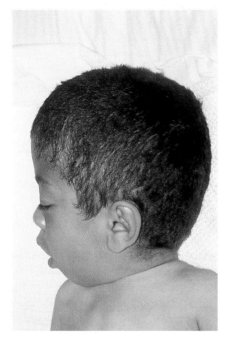

Figure 103.9   *M.M., a patient with MSD who was macrocephalic. Facial features were coarse, and he was hirsute.*

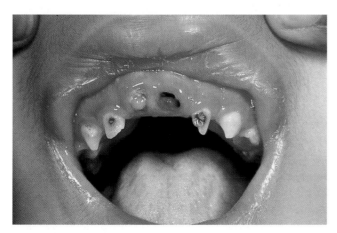

Figure 103.10   *A.A. The gingival hyperplasia was as striking as that seen in I-cell disease (Chapter 84). The teeth were carious.*

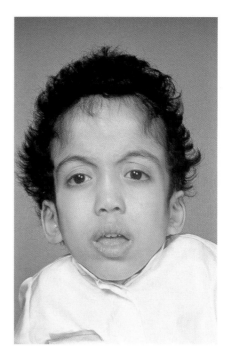

Figure 103.11   *A.R., a patient with MSD had an unusually shaped head and a prominent keel or frontal bridge.*

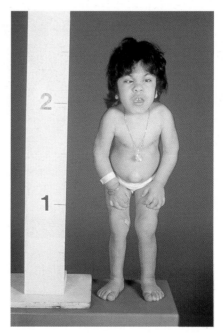

Figure 103.12   *Stature was short and the neck particularly short. Flexion of the hips and knees, as well as the elbows contributed to the Morquio-like appearance.*

seen, but rarely in the classic presentation [5]. Stature was short (Figures 103.12, 103.13), often with a crouch, Morquio-like position because of contractures. Two patients had evidence of cervical cord compression with the development of sudden quadriparesis, followed in one by death.

A juvenile-onset form of MSD was reported by Tanaka [22] in which there was onset at 5 years of a slowly progressive

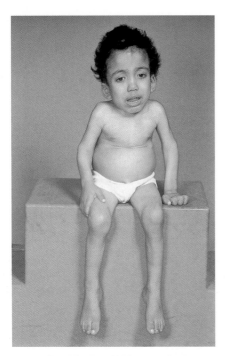

Figure 103.13   *A.Q., who also had Morquio-like habitus.*

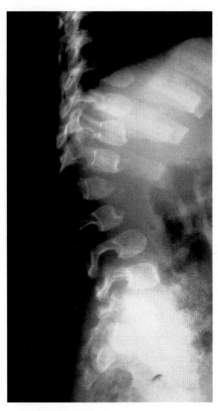

Figure 103.15   *Roentgenogram of the spine of R.I., illustrating advanced dysostosis multiplex. The ribs were broad and spatulate. The vertebrae were ovoid and the lumbar vertebrae had anterior hooks.*

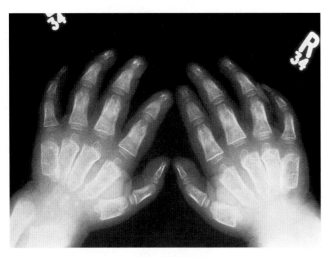

Figure 103.14   *The hands of R.I. (Figure 103.12) illustrated the characteristic broad, short proximally-tapering metacarpals and broad phalanges.*

quadriplegia, retinitis and blindness. There was ataxia and dysarthria. Hepatomegaly was only moderate. Stature was short, and the skin was ichthyotic. Death was at 26 years.

Roentgenograms usually reveal some degree of dysostosis multiplex (Figures 103.14, 103.15). In the Saudi patients' premature synostosis of one or more cranial sutures led to deformities such as trigonocephaly, brachycephaly, or dolichocephaly [4]. Macrocephaly was seen as well as the microcephaly more common in other forms of MSD. Some patients have had a J-shaped sella. Abnormalities of the odontoid have been observed [4]; C1 has been lower than normal. The posterior arch has been anterior, compressing the cord; there has been anterior subluxation of the atlas; and hypoplasia of C2. Nerve conduction may be slowed.

Neuroimaging of the brain by computed tomography (CT) or magnetic resonance imaging (MRI) (Figures 103.16, 103.17) reveals a symmetric decrease in attenuation of white matter, with high T2 signal throughout the white matter. White matter changes were seen in all of the Saudi patients [4]. One had hydrocephalus and one an arachnoid cyst.

Laboratory findings in all of these patients include mucopolysacchariduria (dermatan sulfate and heparan sulfate). Alder-Reilly granules are found in leukocytes of the bone marrow and peripheral blood. The cerebrospinal fluid (CSF) protein concentration may be elevated. Diagnosis is made by confirming the deficiency in the activity of a number of sulfatase enzymes (10).

GENETICS AND PATHOGENESIS

Transmission is autosomal recessive. Both sexes are equally represented, often with more than one affected patient in a sibship. Consanguinity has been documented. Prevalence in Australia has been reported as 1 in 1.4 million (23).

The locus has been shown by complementation studies in somatic cell hybrids to be different from that of MLD. Fusion of MLD and MSD fibroblasts led to correction of arylsulfatase A

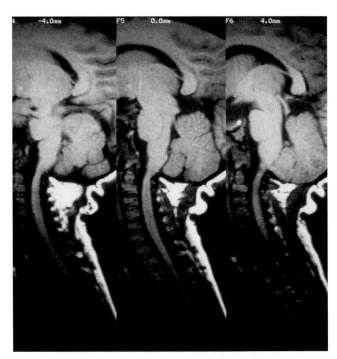

Figure 103.16   *MRI of R.F., a patient with MSD. A localized quite marked constriction of the AP diameter and compression of the cord to about one-half of normal size.*

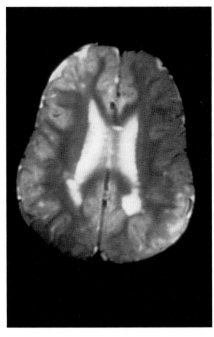

Figure 103.17   *MRI of the brain of S.R., a 4-year-old patient with MSD. Moderately extensive high T2 changes in the subcortical white matter were present bilaterally.*

deficiency [24,25]. Hybridization of cells of the classic and neonatal forms of MSD was not complementary, and enzyme activity was not restored [26,27].

Defective activity of sulfatases can be shown in cultured fibroblasts [18,19,27,28] and in tissues such as kidney, brain

and liver [2,10,29,30]. There has been some correlation of the levels of residual enzyme activity and clinical phenotype [3,27,31,32]. In general classic patients have had severe deficiency [3,33,34], while activity is absent or certainly less than 10 percent of control in the neonatal patients [21,33]. In the Saudi patients activities ranged from 3–10 percent of arylsulfatase A to 20–41 percent of control of the Sanfilippo A enzyme [4].

In the juvenile patients of Tanaka [22], lymphocytes and fibroblasts displayed 20–60 percent of control levels. Cultured fibroblasts of the neonatal patients incorporated significantly greater amounts of ^{35}S-labeled sodium sulfate into acid mucopolysaccharide than did those of cells of classic MSD patients [26]. Prenatal diagnosis has been reported [35] by sulfatase assay of cultured amniocytes or chorionic villus cells. In one patient with MSD a low estriol was recorded in maternal urine [36], and in another with neonatal MSD there was placental hormone deficiency [21]. Heterozygotes have been reported [37] to have intermediate activities of sulfatase in cultured fibroblasts.

As in MLD, urinary excretion of sulfatide is elevated. Sulfatide levels in the CSF are also increased. Accumulation of cholesteryl sulfate has been identified in liver, kidney, plasma and urine. Cerebral gangliosides have been abnormal, as in Hunter disease [10,18,21].

The activity of sulfatases in cultured fibroblasts can be influenced by additions to the medium. Activity may be increased by the substitution of N-2-hydroxymethylpiperazine-N-2-sulfonic acid for bicarbonate buffer [34], and addition of leupeptin, a thiol protease inhibitor, leads to the appearance of arylsulfatase A activity and the ability to degrade labeled sulfatides [38]. These observations are consistent with the concept that the synthesis of the enzymes may be normal but their degradation is rapid [38]. Furthermore, isolated individual sulfatases from MSD material had normal kinetic properties [28,34]. It was postulated that the mutation is an enzyme responsible for co- or post-translational modification of the sulfatase polypeptides [39]. Relevant to this hypothesis are the results of gene transfer of the cDNA for the arylsulfatases into fibroblasts [40]: cDNAs from MSD sources were expressed in normal and MSD cells. In MSD cells mature enzyme proteins were present, but they were less than five percent as active as normal. This would fit with failure of an enzyme responsible for activation through modification.

In an elegant series of experiments, Schmidt *et al.* [6] showed that a cysteine predicted from the cDNA sequence that is conserved among all known sulfatases is replaced by a 2-amino-3-oxopropionic acid in active enzymes, while in sulfatases of MSD cells the cysteine is unchanged (Figure 103.1, p. 688). In arylsulfatase A the cysteine of position 69 was found to be replaced with a compound containing no sulfur and an aldehyde function on tandem mass spectrometry, and the compound was definitely identified as 2-amino-3-oxopropionic acid in both arylsulfatase A and B. In MSD fibroblasts the residue was cysteine. These observations have uncovered a novel modification of enzyme that confers catalytic activity on the protein. It is clearly the enzyme that catalyzes this modification that is defective in MSD.

The gene SUMF1 was cloned independently by Cosma *et al.* [41] and Dierks *et al.* [42] and mapped to chromosome 3p26 [42]. It contains 9 exons spanning 105 kb. Among mutations identified a 4 bp deletion (GTAA) at position 5 of intron 3 leads to loss of the splice donor site for the intron and in frame deletion of exon 3. It has been referred to as IVS 3 + 5-8 del [42] and 519 + 4 del GTAA [41]. One patient had a C to T transversion on the other allele at nucleotide 1076 (S359X) and another had R327Y on the other allele [41,42]. In addition to a 1 bp deletion at 276C, missense mutations identified were: R345C, C218Y, A348P and M1V [41]. Expressions of the SUMF1 genes carrying missense mutations revealed loss of function [8].

TREATMENT

The symptomatic treatment of the leukodystrophy is supportive. Nasogastric or gastrostomy feeding may be required. Surgical fusion to stabilize the upper cervical spine may save the life of a patient or avert disabling quadriparesis. Magnetic resonance imaging is helpful in identifying candidates for surgery. Bone marrow transplantation has met with limited success in MLD and in various mucopolysaccharidoses. Experience is not available in MSD. Enzyme replacement therapy in mucopolysaccharidosis has encouraged the development of other enzymes for this purpose, including the sulfatases. The development of the expressed product of the SUMF1 gene has potential for the treatment of individual sulfatase deficiencies as well as of MSD [8].

References

1   Austin JH, Armstrong D, Shearer L. Metachromatic form of diffuse cerebral sclerosis. V The nature and significance of low sulfatase activity: a controlled study of brain liver and kidney in four patients with metachromatic leukodystrophy (MLD). *Arch Neurol* 1965;**13**:593.

2   Austin J. Studies in metachromatic leukodystrophy. XII Multiple sulfatase deficiency. *Arch Neurol* 1973;**28**:258.

3   Basner R, Von Figura K, Glossl J, *et al.* Multiple deficiency of mucopolysaccharide sulfatases in mucosulfatidosis. *Pediatr Res* 1979;**13**:1316.

4   Al Aqeel A, Ozand PT, Brismar J, *et al.* Saudi variant of multiple sulfatase deficiency. *J Child Neurol* 1992;**7**:(suppl) S12.

5   Bateman JB, Philippart M, Eisenberg SJ. Ocular features of multiple sulfatase deficiency and a new variant of metachromatic leukodystrophy. *J Pediatr Ophthalmol Strabismus* 1984;**21**:133.

6   Schmidt B, Selmer T, Ingendoh A, von Figura K. A novel amino acid modification in sulfatases that is defective in multiple sulfatase deficiency. *Cell* 1995;**82**:271.

7   von Figura K, Schmidt B, Selmer T, Dierks T. A novel protein modification generating an aldehyde group in sulfatases – its role in catalysis and disease. *Bioessays* 1998;**20**:505.

8   Ballabio A, Cosma MP, Pepe S, *et al.* The multiple sulfatase deficiency gene SUMF1 and its therapeutic potential for sulfatase deficiencies. *Am J Human Genet* 2003;**73**:200.

9   Soong B-W, Casamassima AC, Fink JK, *et al.* Multiple sulfatase deficiency. *Neurology* 1988;**38**:1273.

10 Burch M, Fensom AH, Jackson M, *et al.* Multiple sulfatase deficiency presenting at birth. *Clin Genet* 1986;**30**:409.

11 Couchot J, Plout M, Schmauch MA, *et al.* La mucosulfatidose. Etude de trois cas familiaux. *Arch Franc Pediatr* 1974;**31**:775.

12 Hogan K, Matalon R, Berlow S, *et al.* Multiple sulfatase deficiency: clinical radiologic electrophysiologic and biochemical features. *Neurology* 1983;**33**:(suppl 2) 245.

13 Rampini S, Isler W, Baerlocher K, *et al.* Die Kombination von metachromatischer Leukodystrophie und Mukopolysaccharidose als selbstaendiges Krankheitsbild (Mukosulfatidose). *Helv Paediatr Acta* 1970;**25**:436.

14 Lansky LL, Hug G. Enzymatic and structural studies in mucosulfatidosis. *Pediatr Res* 1979;**13**:421.

15 Burk R, Valle D, Thomas G, *et al.* Multiple sulfatase deficiency (MSD): clinical and biochemical studies in two patients. *Am J Hum Genet* 1981;**33**:73A (abstr).

16 Nevsimalova S, Elleder M, Smid F, Zemankova M. Multiple sulfatase deficiency in homozygotic twins. *J Inherit Metab Dis* 1984;**7**:38.

17 Bharrucha BA, Naik G, Sawliwala AS, *et al.* Siblings with the Austin variant of metachromatic leukodystrophy multiple sulfatidosis. *Indian J Pediatr* 1984;**51**:477.

18 Burk RD, Valle D, Thomas GH, *et al.* Early manifestations of multiple sulfatase deficiency. *J Pediatr* 1984;**104**:574.

19 Harbord M, Buncic JR, Chuang SA, *et al.* Multiple sulfatase deficiency with early severe retinal degeneration. *J Child Neurol* 1991;**6**:229.

20 Raynaud EJ, Escourolle R, Baumann N, *et al.* Metachromatic leukodystrophy. Ultrastructural and enzymatic study of a case of variant O form. *Arch Neurol* 1975;**32**:834.

21 Vamos E, Liebaers I, Bousard N, *et al.* Multiple sulfatase deficiency with early onset. *J Inherit Metab Dis* 1981;**4**:103.

22 Tanaka A, Hirabayashi M, Ishii M, *et al.* Complementation studies with clinical and biochemical characterizations of a new variant of multiple sulfatase deficiency. *J Inherit Metab Dis* 1987;**10**:103.

23 Meikle PJ, Hopwood JJ, Clague AE, Carey WF. Prevalence of lysosomal storage disorders. *JAMA* 1999;**281**:249.

24 Horwitz AL. Genetic complementation studies of multiple sulfatase deficiency. *Proc Natl Acad Sci USA* 1979;**76**:6496.

25 Chang PL, Davidson RG. Complementation of arylsulfatase A in somatic hybrids of metachromatic leukodystrophy and multiple sulfatase deficiency disorder fibroblasts. *Proc Natl Acad Sci USA* 1980;**10**:6166.

26 Eto Y, Tokoro T, Liebaers I, Vamos E. Biochemical characterization of neonatal multiple sulfatase deficiency (MSD) disorder cultured skin fibroblasts. *Biochem Biophys Res Commun* 1982;**106**:429.

27 Fedde K, Horwitz AL. Complementation of multiple sulfatase deficiency in somatic cells hybrids. *Am J Hum Genet* 1984;**36**:623.

28 Eto Y, Wiesmann UN, Carson JH, Herschkowitz NN. Multiple sulfatase deficiencies in cultured skin fibroblasts: occurrence in patients with a variant form of metachromatic leukodystrophy. *Arch Neurol* 1974;**30**:153.

29 Murphy JW, Wolfe HJ, Balasz EA, Moser HW. A patient with deficiency of arylsulfatase A B C and steroid sulfatase associated with storage of sulfatide cholesterol sulfate and glycosaminoglycans: in *Lipid Storage Diseases* (eds J Bernsohm, HJ Grossman). Academic Press, New York;1971:67.

30 Eto Y, Rampini A, Wiesmann U, Herschkowitz NN. Enzymic studies of sulphatases in tissues of the normal human and in metachromatic leukodystrophy with multiple sulphatase deficiencies: arylsulfatases in A, B and C cerebroside sulphatase psychosine sulphatase and steroid sulphatases. *J Neurochem* 1974;**23**:1161.

31   Chang PL, Rosa NE, Ballantyne ST, Davidson RG. Biochemical variability of arylsulfatases-A-B and -C in cultured fibroblasts from patients with multiple sulphatase deficiency. *J Inherit Metab Dis* 1983;**6**:167.

32   Steckel F, Hasilik A, Von Figura K. Synthesis and stability of arylsulfatase A and B in fibroblasts from multiple sulfatase deficiency. *Eur J Biochem* 1985;**151**:141.

33   Eto Y, Gomibuchi I, Umezawa F, Tsuda T. Pathochemistry pathogenesis and enzyme replacement in multiple sulfatase deficiency. *Enzyme* 1987;**38**:273.

34   Fluharty AL, Stevens RL, Davis LL, *et al*. Presence of arylsulfatase A (ARSA) in multiple sulfatase deficiency disorder fibroblasts. *Am J Hum Genet* 1978;**30**:249.

35   Patrick AD, Young E, Ellis C, Rodeck CH. Multiple sulphatase deficiency: prenatal diagnosis using chorionic villi. *Prenat Diagn* 1988;**8**:303.

36   Steinmann B, Mieth D, Gitzelmann R. A newly recognized cause of low urinary estriol in pregnancy: multiple sulfatase deficiency of the fetus. *Gynecol Obstet Invest* 1981;**12**:107.

37   Eto Y, Tokoro T, Ito F. Chemical compositions of acid mucopolysaccharides in urine and tissues of patients with multiple sulphatase deficiency. *J Inherit Metab Dis* 1981;**4**:161.

38   Horwitz AL, Warshawsky L, King J, Burns G. Rapid degradation of steroid sulfatase in multiple sulfatase deficiency. *Biochem Biophys Res Commun* 1986;**6**:26.

39   Steckel F, Hasilik A, von Figura K. Multiple sulfatase deficiency: degradation of arylsulfatase A and B after endocytosis in fibroblasts. *Eur J Biochem* 1985;**151**:147.

40   Rommerskirch W, von Figura K. Multiple sulfatase deficiency: catalytically inactive sulfatases are expressed from retrovirally introduced sulfatase cDNAs. *Proc Natl Acad Sci USA* 1992;**89**:2561.

41   Cosma MP, Pepe S, Annunziata I, *et al*. The multiple sulfatase deficiency gene encodes an essential and limiting factor for the activity of sulfatases. *Cell* 2003;**113**:445.

42   Dierks T, Schmidt B, Borissenko LV, *et al*. Multiple sulfatase deficiency is caused by mutations in the gene encoding the human C-alpha-formylglycine generating enzyme. *Cell* 2003;**113**:435.

Miscellaneous

104

Congenital disorders of glycosylation, type Ia

MAJOR PHENOTYPIC EXPRESSION

Infantile failure to thrive, inability to aliment orally, developmental delay, hypotonia, inverted nipples, esotropia, and an unusual lipodystrophy in which a general decrease in subcutaneous fat is associated with accumulated large fat pads in unusual sites, such as above the buttocks; pericardial effusions, hepatic dysfunction and pontocerebellar hypoplasia; in childhood, ataxia and disequilibrium, retinitis pigmentosa and stroke-like episodes; teenage neuropathy, muscular atrophy and secondary skeletal deformities; adult hypogonadism; deficient or absent carbohydrate moieties of secretory glycoproteins, especially serum transferrin; and deficient activity of phosphomannomutase.

INTRODUCTION

Twin girls with retardation of psychomotor development and strabismus were reported in 1978 by Jaeken and colleagues [1] to have decreased amounts of thyroxin-binding globulin (TBG) in the serum and increased activity of serum arylsulfatase A. It was recognized that this unusual association was with two quite different glycoproteins, and heterogeneity was then found in transferrin of serum and cerebrospinal fluid [2]. It was hypothesized that the defect in common was in the carbohydrate moiety. Confirmatory evidence was the demonstration of deficiency of sialic acid, galactose and N-acetylglucosamine in transferrin and in several other serum glycoproteins [3,4].

More than 30 patients had been reported by 1993 [5] and more than twice that number had been identified in Scandinavia alone[6]. At this time, hundreds of patients have been identified worldwide. The disorder was originally described in Belgium [1], but patients have been recognized in Spain [7], Taiwan [8], and the United States [9], including some of African ancestry [10]. Several related disorders of glycosylation have been discovered (Chapter 105). The fundamental biochemical abnormality in type Ia is in the activity of phosphomannomutase-2 (EC 5.4.2.28) [11,12] (Figure 104.1).

CLINICAL ABNORMALITIES

Different phenotypic manifestations characterize this disorder at different ages. They have been differentiated [5] as:

I infantile multisystem stage;
II childhood ataxia-mental retardation stage;
III teenage leg atrophy stage;
IV adult hypogonadal stage.

Most patients have been born at term after an uneventful pregnancy, and birth weight has usually been normal. Some features may be recognized at birth: inversion of the nipples (Figures 104.2, 104.3) is nearly universal [5,6] (Table 104.1) and so is esotropia. Lipoatrophy may be manifest in a general reduction of subcutaneous tissues mass [6], or in lipoatrophic streaks or patches [5]. The most unusual feature is the occurrence of fat pads – collections of subcutaneous tissue in unusual places, most typically over or above the buttocks, but elsewhere too (Figures 104.4–104.7). Patches of thickened skin, especially on the legs, have been described as like tallow or peau d'orange (orange peel) [5]. These features may be absent in the early months, in which the only manifestation may be failure to thrive. Alternatively there may be early neonatal hypotonia, lethargy, edema or cardiac failure [13].

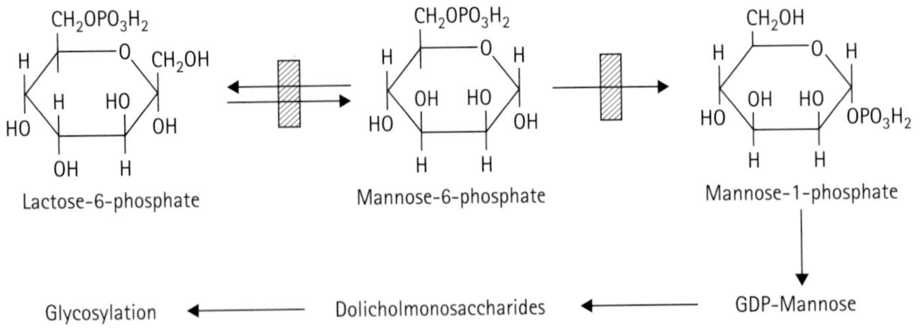

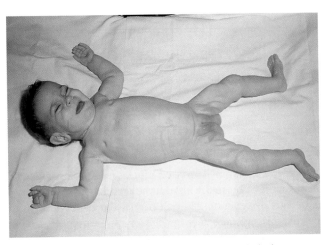

Lactose-6-phosphate   Mannose-6-phosphate   Mannose-1-phosphate

Glycosylation ◄——— Dolicholmonosaccharides ◄——— GDP-Mannose

Figure 104.1   *The phosphomannomutase reactions (PMM) and phosphomannose isomerase (PMI) and its relation to glycosylation.*

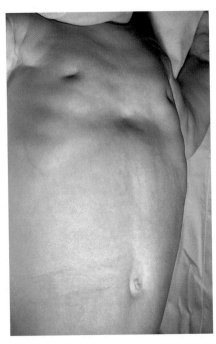

Figure 104.2   *H.S., an 8-month-old infant with carbohydrate-deficient glycoprotein disease. Illustrated are the inverted nipples that constitute an early sign of the syndrome. There were lipoatrophic changes of the lower extremities. (This and the other pictures of patients with this disease kindly provided by Dr. J. Jaeken of the University of Louven, Belgium.)*

Table 104.1   *Inverted nipples – differential diagnosis*

Congenital disorders of glycosylation
Biopterin synthesis disorders
Citrullinemia (Chapter 31)
Isolated autosomal dominant (McKusick No. 163600)
Menkes disease (Chapter 74)
Methylmalonic acidemia (Chapter 3)
Molybdenum cofactor deficiency
Propionic acidemia (Chapter 2)
Pyruvate carboxylase deficiency (Chapter 48)
VLCAD deficiency (Chapter 41)
Weaver syndrome

Difficulties with feeding and failure to thrive regularly characterize the first three months. These infants display little interest in nursing, and nasogastric feedings have been required throughout the first year [6]. Frequent and projectile vomiting has been a problem. At one year most patients have just doubled the weight of birth. Linear growth is also behind. Even older children may not chew, and they may gag and choke on textured or lumpy foods. However, notable exceptions have been observed, and macrosomia may be found [14].

Dysmorphic facial features described have included a high nasal bridge, prominent jaw and large external ears [5], (Figure 104.8). Some have had limitation of joint mobility in the legs. Head circumference at birth is normal, but microcephaly develops in about half of the patients [5].

Hypotonia or floppiness is regularly observed, and developmental delay is obvious early. Head lag may be seen as late as 12 months. In addition, some infants have had stroke-like episodes or episodes of acute deterioration in which developmental landmarks achieved have been lost. A few have had seizures. Ataxia is recognizable as early as 7 months and imaging of the central nervous system reveals cerebellar and pontine atrophy, which may appear, especially after episodes of acute exacerbation. Hepatomegaly is a regular feature. Blood levels of transaminases are increased and levels of albumin and coagulation factors are decreased. There may be intestinal bleeding. Enlarged kidneys may be demonstrated by ultrasound or other forms of imaging.

Recurrent episodes of pericardial effusion have been seen commonly in infancy, and death from cardiac tamponade has been recorded [5]. There may be cardiomyopathy. Serious infections are also common and an infantile and early childhood

Figure 104.3   *H.S. at 8 months – close-up of the inverted nipples.*

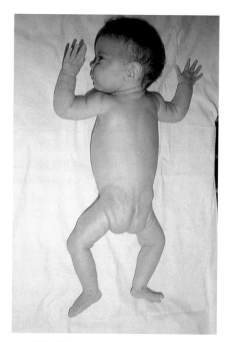

Figure 104.4   *H.S. – illustrates the characteristic fat pads on the buttocks.*

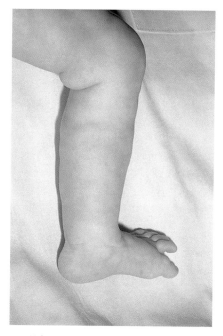

Figure 104.7   *H.S. at 8 months illustrating that fat deposits may occur elsewhere.*

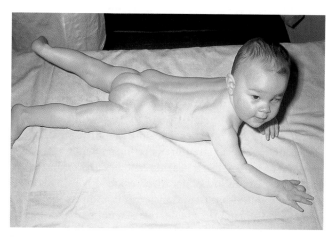

Figure 104.5   *S.F., a 9-month-old patient with the characteristic fat pads over the buttocks.*

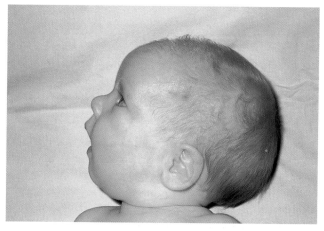

Figure 104.8   *L.A. at 2 months. The face was somewhat dysmorphic, the forehead prominent, the nasal bridge depressed and tip anteverted, and there was some micrognathia. The ears were relatively large.*

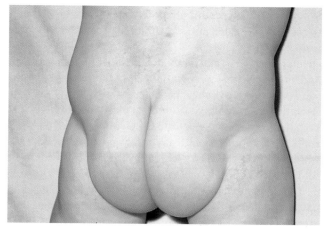

Figure 104.6   *S.F. – close-up of the fat pads.*

mortality of 15–20 percent reflects predominantly infectious disease.

The childhood period from 3 to 12 years-of-age [5,13,15] is characterized by ataxia and mental retardation (Figure 104.9). Some have dyskinetic or choreoathetotic episodes. Only a few patients have learned to walk. Most sit unsupported after 2 years; they ultimately learn to stand on tiptoe because of contractures [16]. Most learn to use a wheelchair. Disequilibrium and impaired coordination are prominent. Motor retardation is uniformly seen but the degree of mental retardation is variable: IQs have ranged from 40 to 60 [5]. Patients understand spoken words but few develop linguistic skills; they speak in staccato fashion. Intellectual regression has not been seen

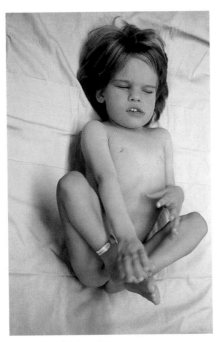

Figure 104.9   *L.A. a 3-year-old female, was developmentally retarded and had motor disability of the lower limbs. Posturing of the left hand is evident. Retinitis pigmentosa leads to loss of vision.*

except following stroke-like episodes. Deep tendon reflexes in the lower extremities disappear at this stage, and peripheral neuropathy becomes evident [16]. Retinal degeneration and retinitis pigmentosa is progressive in most [17]. The stroke-like episodes are more prominent in childhood; there may be stupor or coma, and convulsions, as well as hemiplegia, usually with recovery in hours to days. Permanent hemiplegia has been associated with cerebral infarction. Two patients were blind for months after an episode. One patient had an arterial thrombosis in a hand [18].

The teenage years are dominated by progressive muscle atrophy and weakness, especially of the legs. This appears to be primarily due to lower motor neuron dysfunction. Nerve conduction velocity is reduced. Cerebellar ataxia and poor coordination continue. Skeletal deformities, kyphosis, scoliosis and keel thorax appear to be consequences of muscle atrophy. The unusual fat pads may disappear during this period. Seizures occur in about 50 percent of patients [13], but frequency may decrease in adolescence. Hepatopathy may stabilize or disappear [13].

Hypogonadism may be recognized in this period or in adulthood. This appears especially common in females. It may be hypergonadotrophic [5], but testicular atrophy has been seen in a male. There may be intermittent elevation of prolactin, growth hormone, insulin or follicle stimulating hormone (FSH). Premature ageing may also be seen in young adults [5]. Adults are short, compressed and bent into flexor deformities. Neurologic deficits seem to stabilize in adulthood.

Clinical laboratory evaluation may reveal proteinuria. There is often an intermittent thrombocytosis, with counts up to 800 000 per mm³. There may be hypoprothrombinemia and

diminished factors IX and XI. Elevated transaminases may become normal with age. The serum albumin is usually low, and some have a hypo-β-lipoproteinemia. The stroke-like episodes and thrombotic disease have been associated with decreased levels of antithrombin III and other major inhibitors of coagulation [18]. Thyroxin-binding globulin (TBG) is reduced in 75 percent of patients. Cerebrospinal fluid protein may be elevated. The electroencephalogram (EEG) is usually normal. Nerve conduction velocity is reduced and the deficit increases with age. Histologic examination of the liver reveals some degree of steatosis. There may be lamellar lysosomal inclusions on electron microscopy [19].

GENETICS AND PATHOGENESIS

The biochemical characteristic of this syndrome is the presence of secretory glycoproteins that are deficient in their carbohydrate content. Terminal trisaccharides are characteristically missing. As a result, a number of glycoproteins become abnormal, including transport proteins, enzymes, hormones such as prolactin and FSH, and coagulation factors. In the initial series of patients, serum activity of arylsulfatase A was recognized to be elevated [1]. Because of the abnormal TBG, it would seem that patients should be detected in programs of neonatal screening for hypothyroidism, but that has not been widely encountered.

Among the most used tests for the diagnosis of this condition is the isoelectric focusing of serum transferrin [20,21]. Half of this glycoprotein is found to lack two or four of its terminal sialic acid moieties. The normal transferrin of serum is predominantly tetrasialotransferrin, and there are small amounts of mono-, di-, tri-, penta- and hexa-sialotransferrins; in the disease state, loss of negatively charged sialic acid causes a cathodal shift. Abnormal transferrin is also present in liver and cerebrospinal fluid. Qualitative diagnosis is made by isoelectric focusing and immunofixation of transferrin. Quantitative determination of carbohydrate-deficient transferrin indicated an approximately 10-fold elevation of cathodal transferrin forms [20]. Electrophoresis reveals low molecular weight isoforms of many serum glycoproteins, including α-1 antitrypsin [21]. The diagnostic accuracy may be improved using isoelectric focusing of α-1 antitrypsin and α-1 antichymotrypsin [22], and methodologies such as high performance liquid chromatography (HPLC) [23] and capillary zone electrophoresis [24] may be better suited to automation. Recently, the feasibility of tandem mass spectrometry has been demonstrated to elucidate the glycosylation of transferrin [25], an approach which allows for quantitative results and which offers the specificity to detect variant forms with more subtle differences in glycan processing [26].

The fundamental defect is in the synthesis and transfer of nascent dolichol-linked oligosaccharide precursors, and incorporation of labeled mannose into glycoproteins and the dolichol-linked oligosaccharide precursor is also shown to be deficient [27]. The abnormality in lipid-linked oligosaccharide biosynthesis could lead to failure to glycosylate sites on proteins and to abnormalities in glycoprotein processing or function. Ultrastructural studies of fibroblasts, Schwann cells and hepatocytes have revealed membrane and lamellar, fibrillary and multi-vacuolated inclusions, suggesting a defect in macromolecular catabolism [15]. Furthermore, there is probably a cellular response to unfolded proteins that plays a part in the pathogenesis in this class of disease [28].

Neonatal screening for this disease has not been successfully implemented. While it was reported that the transferrin abnormality may be detectable in dried blood spotted on paper [13], it was not evident in a 19-week fetus [21]. It has been recommended that testing of transferrin glycosylation not be performed before 3 weeks-of-age to avoid false negative results [29]. Of course, the disease is autosomal recessive, and although some heterozygotes may be recognizable chemically, heterozygote detection is not reliable.

The defect in phosphomannomutase [11,12] (Figure 104.1) can be directly assayed in fibroblasts or leukocytes. In 16 patients leukocyte activity ranged from 0.02 to 0.08 mU/mg protein as compared with the control range of 1.6 to 2.3. In fibroblasts the range was 0.1 to 1.4 in patients and 2.2 to 6.4 in controls. The gene for phosphomannose-2 [30], designated PMM2, is localized on chromosome 16p13.3–p13.2, spanning 51.5 kb in 8 exons and coding for 246 amino acids. At this point, more than 76 mutations have been described, including 66 missense mutations. The disease is pan-ethnic, but different populations have their own set of mutations [31]. The most common mutations are R141H and F119L, accounting for approximately 37 percent and 17 percent of alleles, respectively; the R141H mutation is found in more than 75 percent of patients of Caucasian origin [32], and the combination R141H/F119L accounts for about 38 percent of Caucasian patients. The R141H mutation has never been found in a homozygous state, presumably because that condition is incompatible with life. The F119L mutation has a clear founder effect in the Scandanavian population, and the R141H mutation is associated with a specific haplotype which points to a single ancient mutational event. The observed frequency of the R141H allele (1 in 72) in normal populations of Netherlands and Denmark, and the observed frequency of that allele in the compound heterozygous state with other mutations, suggests the frequency of the disease in that population would be expected to be around 1/20 000. The incidence in that population, however, has been estimated to be more on the order of 1/80 000 [33].

TREATMENT

No effective treatment has been reported. Nasogastric feeding and the use of high caloric diets are helpful in infancy, and painstaking approaches to feeding are required through childhood.

References

1 Jaeken J, Van der Schueren-Lodeweyckx M, Casaer P, *et al.* Familial psychomotor retardation with markedly fluctuating serum prolactin, FSH and GH levels, partial TBG deficiency, increased arylsulphatase A and increased CSF protein: a new syndrome? *Pediatr Res* 1980;**14**:179.

2 Jaeken J, van Eijk HG, van der HC, *et al.* Sialic acid-deficient serum and cerebrospinal fluid transferrin in a newly recognized genetic syndrome. *Clin Chim Acta* 1984;**144**:245.

3 Jaeken J, Eggermont E, Stibler H. An apparent homozygous X-linked disorder with carbohydrate-deficient serum glycoproteins. *Lancet* 1987;**2**:1398.

4 Stibler H, Jaeken J. Carbohydrate deficient serum transferrin in a new systemic hereditary syndrome. *Arch Dis Child* 1990;**65**:107.

5 Jaeken J, Stibler H, Hagberg B. The carbohydrate-deficient glycoprotein syndrome. A new inherited multisystemic disease with severe nervous system involvement. *Acta Paediatr Scand Suppl* 1991;**375**:1.

6 Petersen MB, Brostrom K, Stibler H, Skovby F. Early manifestations of the carbohydrate-deficient glycoprotein syndrome. *J Pediatr* 1993;**122**:66.

7 Briones P, Vilaseca MA, Schollen E, *et al.* Biochemical and molecular studies in 26 Spanish patients with congenital disorder of glycosylation type Ia. *J Inherit Metab Dis* 2002;**25**:635.

8 Chu KL, Chien YH, Tsai CE, *et al.* Carbohydrate deficient glycoprotein syndrome type Ia. *J Formos Med Assoc* 2004;**103**:721.

9 Enns GM, Steiner RD, Buist N, *et al.* Clinical and molecular features of congenital disorder of glycosylation in patients with type 1 sialotransferrin pattern and diverse ethnic origins. *J Pediatr* 2002;**141**:695.

10 Tayebi N, Andrews DQ, Park JK, *et al.* A deletion-insertion mutation in the phosphomannomutase 2 gene in an African American patient with congenital disorders of glycosylation-Ia. *Am J Med Genet* 2002;**108**:241.

11 Van Schaftingen E, Jaeken J. Phosphomannomutase deficiency is a cause of carbohydrate-deficient glycoprotein syndrome type I. *FEBS Lett* 1995;**377**:318.

12 Jaeken J, Besley G, Buist N, *et al.* Phosphomannomutase deficiency is the major cause of carbohydrate-deficient glycoprotein syndrome type I. *J Inherit Metab Dis* 1996;**19 Suppl.**:1.

13 Hagberg BA, Blennow G, Kristiansson B, Stibler H. Carbohydrate-deficient glycoprotein syndromes: peculiar group of new disorders. *Pediatr Neurol* 1993;**9**:255.

14 Neumann LM, von Moers A, Kunze J, *et al.* Congenital disorder of glycosylation type 1a in a macrosomic 16-month-old boy with an atypical phenotype and homozygosity of the N216I mutation. *Eur J Pediatr* 2003;**162**:710.

15 Hagberg B, Blennow G, Stibler H. The birth and infancy of a new disease: the carbohydrate-deficient glycoprotein syndrome: in Y Fukuyama, Y Suzuki, S Kamoshita and P Cesaer (eds) *Fetal and Perinatal Neurology.* Basel: Karger, 1992: 314–319.

16 Blennow G, Jaeken J, Wiklund LM. Neurological findings in the carbohydrate-deficient glycoprotein syndrome. *Acta Paediatr Scand* 1991;**51**:385.

17 Stromland K, Hagberg B, Kristiansson B. Ocular pathology in disialotransferrin developmental deficiency syndrome. *Ophthalmic Paediatr Genet* 1990;**11**:309.

18 Iijima K, Murakami F, Nakamura K, *et al.* Hemostatic studies in patients with carbohydrate-deficient glycoprotein syndrome. *Thromb Res* 1994;**76**:193.

19 Conradi N, de Vos R, Jaeken J. Liver pathology in the carbohydrate deficient glycoprotein syndrome. *Acta Paediatr Scand* 1991;**375**:50.

20 Stibler H, Jaeken J, Kristiansson B. Biochemical characteristics and diagnosis of the carbohydrate-deficient glycoprotein syndrome. *Acta Paediatr Scand* 1991;**375**:21.

21   Harrison HH, Miller KL, Harbison MD, Slonim AE. Multiple serum protein abnormalities in carbohydrate-deficient glycoprotein syndrome: pathognomonic finding of two-dimensional electrophoresis? *Clin Chem* 1992;**38**:1390.

22   Fang J, Peters V, Korner C, Hoffmann GF. Improvement of CDG diagnosis by combined examination of several glycoproteins. *J Inherit Metab Dis* 2004;**27**:581.

23   Helander A, Bergstrom J, Freeze HH. Testing for congenital disorders of glycosylation by HPLC measurement of serum transferrin glycoforms. *Clin Chem* 2004;**50**:954.

24   Jaeken J, Carchon H. Congenital disorders of glycosylation: a booming chapter of pediatrics. *Curr Opin Pediatr* 2004;**16**:434.

25   Lacey JM, Bergen HR, Magera MJ, *et al.* Rapid determination of transferrin isoforms by immunoaffinity liquid chromatography and electrospray mass spectrometry. *Clin Chem* 2001;**47**:513.

26   Mills PB, Mills K, Mian N, *et al.* Mass spectrometric analysis of glycans in elucidating the pathogenesis of CDG type IIx. *J Inherit Metab Dis* 2003;**26**:119.

27   Powell LD, Paneerselvam K, Vij R, *et al.* Carbohydrate-deficient glycoprotein syndrome: not an N-linked oligosaccharide processing defect, but an abnormality in lipid-linked oligosaccharide biosynthesis? *J Clin Invest* 1994;**94**:1901.

28   Lecca MR, Wagner U, Patrignani A, *et al.* Genome-wide analysis of the unfolded protein response in fibroblasts from congenital disorders of glycosylation type-I patients. *FASEB J* 2004.

29   Marquardt T, Denecke J. Congenital disorders of glycosylation: review of their molecular bases, clinical presentations and specific therapies. *Eur J Pediatr* 2003;**162**:359.

30   Matthijs G, Schollen E, Pardon E, *et al.* Mutations in PMM2, a phosphomannomutase gene on chromosome 16p13, in carbohydrate-deficient glycoprotein type I syndrome (Jaeken syndrome). *Nat Genet* 1997;**16**:88.

31   Matthijs G, Schollen E, Bjursell C, *et al.* Mutations in PMM2 that cause congenital disorders of glycosylation, type Ia (CDG-Ia). *Hum Mutat* 2000;**16**:386.

32   Schollen E, Kjaergaard S, Legius E, *et al.* Lack of Hardy-Weinberg equilibrium for the most prevalent PMM2 mutation in CDG-Ia (congenital disorders of glycosylation type Ia). *Eur J Hum Genet* 2000;**8**:367.

33   Kristiansson B, Stibler H, Hagberg B, Wahlstrom J. [CDGS-1 – a recently discovered hereditary metabolic disease. Multiple organ manifestations, incidence 1/80 000, difficult to treat]. *Lakartidningen* 1998;**95**:5742.

105

Other forms of congenital disorders of glycosylation

MAJOR PHENOTYPIC EXPRESSION

Type Ib

Congenital hepatic fibrosis; protein-losing enteropathy, associated in some cases with coagulation abnormalities and/or hyperinsulinemic hypoglycaemia, transient elevations of aminotransferases, persistently low albumin; normal mental development.

Type Ic

Psychomotor retardation; elevated serum transaminases during infections; variable dysmorphic features; strabismus.

Type Id

Psychomotor retardation; seizures or hypsarrhythmia; microcephaly; cerebellar atrophy; hypertonia.

Type Ie

Psychomotor retardation; epilepsy; hypotonia; failure to thrive; elevated serum creatine phosphokinase; variable elevation of serum transaminases.

Type If

Severe psychomotor retardation; seizures; failure to thrive; dry, scaling skin with erythroderma; impaired vision.

Type Ig

Psychomotor retardation; hypotonia; failure to thrive; microcephaly.

Type Ih

Ascites, edema, hypoalbuminemia; protein-losing enteropathy; clotting abnormalities; early death.

Type Ii

Psychomotor retardation; seizures; hepatomegaly; coagulopathy; delayed myelination; bilateral colobomas and unilateral cataract at birth in one patient.

Type Ij

Psychomotor retardation; microcephaly; hypotonia; seizures.

Type Ik

Fetal hydrops; cardiomyopathy; refractory seizures; microcephaly; coagulation abnormalities; early death.

Type I*L*

Psychomotor retardation; microcephaly; hypotonia; seizures; hepatomegaly.

Type IIa

Severe psychomotor retardation; epilepsy; stereotypic behaviour.

Type IIb

Dysmorphic features; hypotonia; hypoventilation; seizures; feeding problems; hepatomegaly; early death.

Type IIc

Psychomotor retardation; microcephaly; hypotonia; retarded growth; craniofacial dysmorphy; recurrent infections, with marked leukocytosis during and between the infections; Bombay blood phenotype.

Type IId

Psychomotor retardation; hypotonia; coagulopathy; myopathy with elevated creatinine kinase.

Type IIe

Recurrent infection; cardiac insufficiency; dysmorphic features, including loose, wrinkled skin; hepatospenomegaly; early death.

INTRODUCTION

In addition to the deficiency of phosphomannose mutase which characterises CDG-Ia (Chapter 104), several other steps in the formation of glycoproteins have been identified [1]. For N-linked glycosylation, glycan assembly takes place first on the cytoplasmic side of the endoplasmic reticulum (ER), and then on the lumenal aspect, resulting in the formation of the lipid-linked oligosaccharide dolichylpyrophosphate-$GlcNAc_2Man_9Glc_3$ (Figure 105.1). The oligosaccharide side-chain is then transferred *en bloc* to selected asparagines of nascent proteins. Then the glycan of the newly formed glycoprotein is processed in the ER, where the three glucoses are removed, and then in the Golgi, where the mannose-rich core is removed and replaced, typically with two residues each of N-acetylglucosamine, galactose, and sialic acid (Figure 105.2).

The nomenclature has evolved in recent years. Since 1999 [2], the standard is to refer to these disorders as congenital disorders of glycosylation (CDG), replacing earlier terms such as carbohydrate-deficient glycoproteins syndromes (CDGS) and defects in the steps of N-glycosylation that take place in the cytoplasm or the endoplasmic reticulum as type I disorders. In these conditions, the manifestation is the absence of entire glycan side-chains. Accordingly, there is a distinctive pattern of glycosylation, which can be distinguished in glycoproteins such as transferrin, where the major expressed forms are missing two or four sialic acid residues. In contrast, the type II pattern also shows an increase of the trisialo- and monosialo-fractions, because of the incorporation of truncated or monoantennary sugar chains. Type II disorders arise from abnormalities in the processing of glycans in the Golgi apparatus. The standard in nomenclature [2] has been to sequentially assign letters to different specific enzyme disorders discovered in these pathways (giving, at the time of this writing, CDG-Ia through CDG-I*L* and CDG-IIa through CDG-IIe), and designating individual cases in which the specific defect has not been determined as CDG-Ix or CDG-IIx (Table 105.1).

There is a growing understanding of O-linked glycan metabolism, as well [3]. O-glycan biosynthesis begins in the Golgi apparatus, where GalNAc (or xylose in the case of glycosaminoglycans) is transferred to serine or threonine residues. O-glycans are less branched than most N-glycans, and they are generally found on mucins, but some proteins contain O-glycans either as short chains or as elongated bi-antennary structures [3]. Two categories of disease have been associated with disorders of O-linked glycan synthesis: xylosylprotein-4-β-galactosyltransferase deficiency, which is associated with the progeroid form of Ehler-Danlos syndrome (MIM 130070),

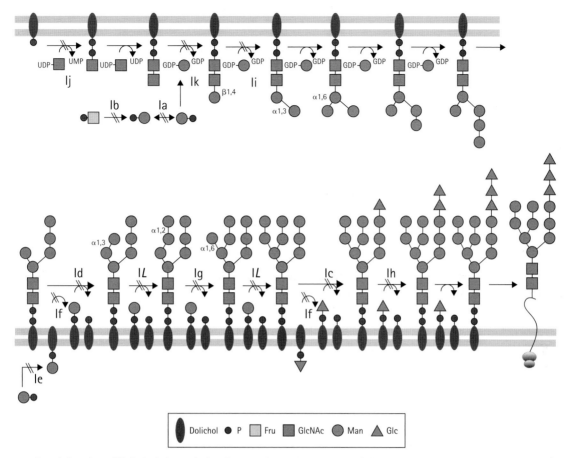

Figure 105.1   *Type I disorders of N-linked glycosylation. Scheme shows the assembly of glycan chains beginning intralumennally (top line) and continuing extraluminally (lower line) until the transfer from the dolichol moiety to a nascent glycoprotein. Symbols for monosaccharides as shown: Man, mannose; Fru, fructose; Glc, glucose.*

and defects in exostosin (EXT1/EXT2 complex) which are associated with multiple hereditary exostoses (MIM 133700, 133701). This chapter, however, deals only with the disorders of N-linked glycan metabolism other than CDG-Ia (Chapter 104), of which at least 16 forms have been discovered.

CLINICAL ABNORMALITIES

Type Ib. Phosphomannose isomerase deficiency (MIM 602579, 154550)

Since this form of CDG was elucidated in 1998 [4], at least 20 patients have been diagnosed [5]. In most, the presenting symptom was hepatic-intestinal disease [6] with liver fibrosis and protein-losing enteropathy, associated in some cases with coagulation abnormalities and/or hyperinsulinemic hypoglycemia [1]. The discovery of underlying defect in this group of patients stemmed from the recognition that the coagulopathy was associated with a profound deficiency of antithrombin III, which was known to be a common feature of CDG-Ia; isoelectric focusing of transferrin showed abnormalities similar to those in phosphomannose mutase (PMM2) deficiency, but

a defect in phosphomannose isomerase (Figure 105.3) was demonstrated [4].

In one consanguineous family with three affected siblings, the main feature was prolonged episodic vomiting, sometimes associated with diarrhea [4,7]. Other notable findings included elevated aminotransferases during attacks and persistently low albumin. In one of those cases there had been an unexplained episode of multiorgan failure at 2 months. All three patients had normal mental and motor development. There are no dysmorphic features in this form of CDG (Figure 105.4). Similar histories and findings have been reported in other cases, but there have also been rather subtler, with episodic hepatic disease in infancy which disappeared after introduction of solid food [6], or a normal woman who had symptoms of hepatic fibrosis and recurrent venous thrombosis in childhood, and whose affected sibling died at age 5, but who was completely asymptomatic at age 33 when she was found to have an abnormal transferrin glycosylation pattern and confirmed PMI mutation [8].

Type Ic. (MIM 603147, 604566)

Approximately 30 patients have been described with this form of CDG [1], originally described in 1998 in four members of

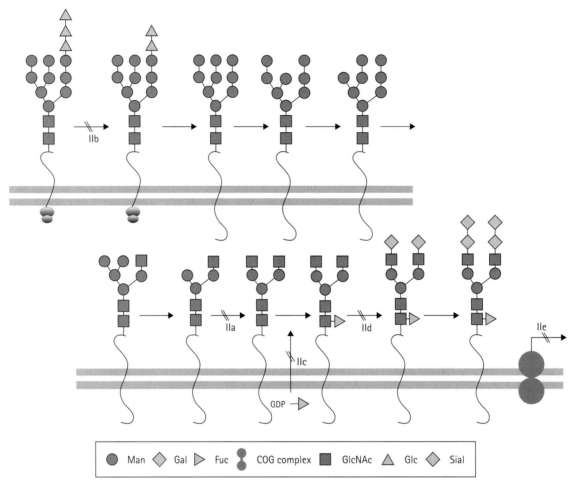

Figure 105.2 *Type II disorders of N-linked glycosylation. Scheme shows the assembly of glycan chains beginning on the nascent glycoprotein in the endoplasmic reticulum and continuing on the protein within the Golgi apparatus. Symbols for monosaccharides as shown: Man, mannose; GlcNAc, N-acetylglucosamine; Gal, galactose; Glc, glucose; Fuc, fucose; Sial, sialic aicd; COG complex, conserved oligomeric Golgi complex.*

a consanguineous Dutch family [9] (and previously designated type CDGS-V) [5]. The clinical presentation has been mainly neurologic, including moderate psychomotor retardation, axial hypotonia, strabismus, epilepsy in most, and ataxia in a few cases. The symptoms are generally milder than in CDG-Ia, and although specific physical findings and cerebellar hypoplasia are not regularly seen, there may be dysmorphic features and some abnormal distribution of fat (Figures 105.5–7). Peripheral neuropathy has not been observed, nor has retinitis pigmentosa. Laboratory findings associated with CDG-Ia are also absent, including hypoalbuminemia and proteinuria. The glycosylation pattern of transferrin is the same as in the other type I conditions, but analysis of the lipid-linked oligosaccharides in fibroblasts reveals accumulation of $Man_9GlcNAc_2$ linked to dolichylpyrophosphate.

Type Id. (MIM 601110)

Two infants were described who were initially classified as Type IV CDGS [10], with clinical features including postnatal microcephaly, atrophy of the brain and corpus callosum,

optic atrophy, iris coloboma, severe epilepsy with hypsarrhythmia, and failure of psychomotor development. There were no signs of liver dysfunction. Several blood glycoproteins demonstrated abnormal isoforms, including transferrin, alpha 1-antitrypsin, antithrombin and thyroxine-binding globulin, and the isoelectric focusing of serum transferrin showed a type 1 pattern but with a deficiency of 1 or 2 sialic acid residues, and without increase of asialotransferrin. Later analysis of lipid-linked oligosaccharide in fibroblasts from one of these patients showed an accumulation of the dolichylpyrophosphate-GIcNAc$_2$Man$_5$ precursor [11].

Type Ie. (MIM 608799, 603503)

Five cases have been reported. Four children from three families were described [12,13] with very profound psychomotor retardation, severe epilepsy, hypotonia, failure to thrive, and mild dysmorphic features including hypertelorism, high arched palate, small hands with dysplastic nails, and inverted nipples in only one case. Brain magnetic resonance imaging (MRI) showed delayed myelination in all, and frontal lobe atrophy

Table 105.1 *Defects in N-linked protein glycosylation*

Group 1: Defects in the generation or transfer of the dolicholpyrophosphate-linked oligosaccharide

Type	Old name	Enzyme defect	Gene	OMIM	
Ia	CDGS Ia	Phosphomannomutase 2	PMM2	212065, 601785	16p13.3-p13.2
Ib	CDGS Ib	Phosphomannose Isomerase	PMI	154550, 602579	15q22-qter
Ic	CDGS V	Dolichyl-P-Glc:Man$_9$GlcNAc$_2$-PP-dolichyl α1,3-Glucosyltransferase	hALG6	603147,604566	1p22.3
Id	CDGS IV	Dolichyl-P-Man:Man$_5$GlcNAc$_2$-PP-dolichyl a1,3-Mannosyltransferase	hALG3	601110	3q27
Ie	CDGS IV	Dolichol-P-Man synthase 1	DPM1	603503	20q13.13
If	–	Dolichol-P-Man Utilization Defect	MPDU1	604041	17p13.1-p12
Ig	–	Dolichyl-P-Man$_7$GlcNAc$_2$-PP-dolichyl α1,6-Mannosyltransferase	hALG12	607143, 607144	22q13.33
Ih	–	Glc$_1$Man$_9$GlcNAc$_2$-PP-dolichyl α3-glucosyltransferase	hALG8	608104, 608103	11q14
Ii	–	GDP-Mannose:Man$_1$GlcNAc$_2$-PP-dolichyl α1,3-Mannosyltransferase	hALG2	607906, 607905	9q22
Ij	–	UDP-GlcNAc:dolichol-P GlcNac-1-phosphate transferase	DPAGT1	608093, 191350	11q23.3
Ik	–	β1,4-mannosyltransferase	hALG1	608540, 605907	16p13.3
IL	–	α1,2-mannosyltransferase	hALG9	608776, 606941	11q23
Ix	–	Unknown genetic basis			

Group II: Defects in processing of N-glycans

Type	Old name	Enzyme defect	Gene	OMIM	
IIa	CDGS II	UDP-GlcNAc:α6-D-mannoside β1,2-GlcNAc transferase II (GnT II)	MGAT2	212066, 602616	14q21
IIb	–	α1,2-Glucosidase I	GCS1	606056, 601336	2p13-p12
IIc	LAD II	GDP-fucose transporter I	FUCT1	266265, 605881	11
IId	–	UDP-Gal:N-acetylglucosamine β-1,4-galactosyltransferase I	B4GALT1	607091, 137060	9p13
IIe	–	Conserved oligomeric Golgi complex subunit 7	COG7	608779, 606978	16p
IIx	–	Unknown genetic basis			

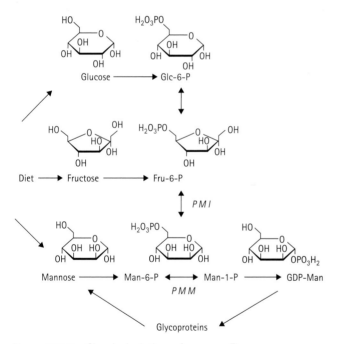

Figure 105.3 *Chemical relations of mannose. The phosphomannose isomerase reaction which is defective in CDG-Ib.*

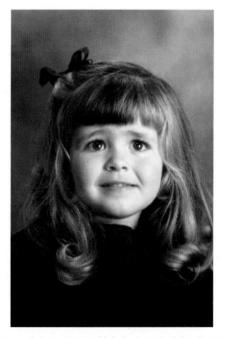

Figure 105.4 *B.J., a girl with CDG-Ib. As typical for these patients, she was cognitively normal and had no dysmorphic features. (Illustration kindly provided by Dr. Hudson Freeze of the Burnham Institute, San Diego.)*

in three, plus cerebellar atrophy in one. A fourth patient was found with milder symptoms [14]; she was a nine year-old girl who had developed simple language and social skills, but exhibited drooling, ataxia, intention tremor and dyscoordination, and a history of a deep vein thrombosis. In that patient,

the MRI showed delayed myelination and transitory hypodensities in the basal ganglia. Serum creatine phosphokinase was mildly to moderately elevated in all five cases, and transaminases were increased in the more severe cases. Isoelectric

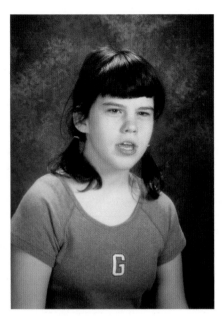

Figure 105.5   *C.M.W., a mildly affected patient with CDG-Ic. (Illustration was kindly provided by Dr. Hudson Freeze of the Burnham Institute, San Diego.)*

focusing of serum transferrin showed a type 1 pattern, but with only little or no increase of asialotransferrin. Only two patients have been identified in the U.S. (Figure 105.8).

Type If. (MIM 604041)

Two reports appearing simultaneously in 2001 presented four patients with this form of CDG. One patient displayed hypotonia and contractures at birth [15], developed nystagmus at 3 months with cortical blindness diagnosed by 6 months, seizures after 5 months, generalized cerebral atrophy, and had a scaling dry erythroderma which was initially hyperkeratotic, and intermittent bouts of vomiting without diarrhea. He developed limited, monosyllabic speech at 2 years, but subsequently lost the ability. At 10 years, he could sit independently but could not stand or walk without support. Coagulation values were normal except for a reduced antithrombin III activity of 50 percent. Transferrin isoelectric focusing gave a typical Type 1 pattern.

The three unrelated patients in the other report [16] had some similar features. One was a boy with intractable seizures from birth and no psychomotor development, who developed a widespread patchy desquamation, and recurrent apnea and ascites progressing to anasarca over the months before his death at age 10 months. Another was a girl with a severe congenital ichthyotic skin disorder, psychomotor retardation, and attacks of hypertonia. At age 16 years, she had severe growth failure, a developmental level of 1 year, and a persistent skin disorder. She also had a low cholesterol level, which was not apparently a feature in the other patients, and electron microscopy of a liver biopsy showed lamellar lysosomal inclusions [1]. The third child was a boy who had severe

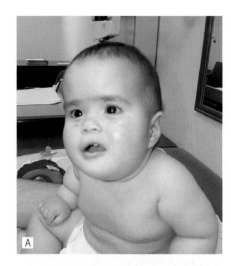

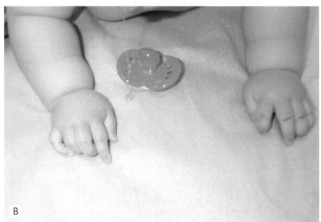

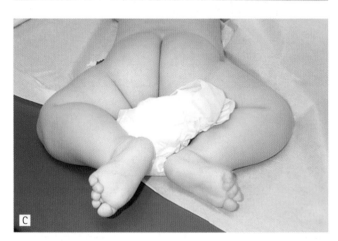

Figure 105.6   *Patient M.T. (CDG-Ic) at 9 months, demonstrating dysmorphic features and abnormal fat distribution. (Photographs kindly provided by Dr. Hudson Freeze of the Burnham Institute, San Diego.)*

psychomotor retardation (developmental age 2.4 at 10 years), but normal somatic growth, and no dermatologic disorder.

Type Ig. (MIM 607143, 607144)

Two cases were described in 2002. A girl born of consanguineous parents presented at birth with generalized hypotonia

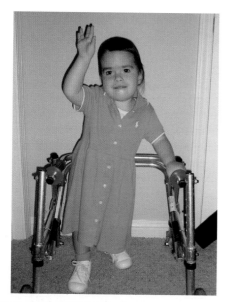

Figure 105.7   *Patient M.T. (CDG-Ic) at age 3 years. She had developed the ability to walk with support, but still had significant ataxia and dyscoordination.*

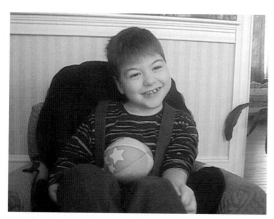

Figure 105.8   *P.Y. (CDG-Ie), at age 8 years. (Illustration was kindly provided by Dr. Hudson Freeze of the Burnham Institute, San Diego.)*

and unspecified facial dysmorphism, and normal routine chemistry results except for hypocalcemia. She exhibited severe developmental delay, major hypotonia, failure to thrive, progressive microcephaly, and frequent upper respiratory infections with low IgG. At 18 months, a gastrostomy was placed, but neuroimaging of the brain was reportedly normal [17]. The other patient [18] was a male child delivered at 34 weeks in a pregnancy notable for HELLP syndrome (hemolysis, elevated liver enzymes, and low platelets), with a neonatal course complicated by respiratory distress, hypoglycaemia, feeding problems and lethargy. At 16 months, CT scan showed evidence of slight frontal atrophy. Developmental retardation and hypotonia were present and at 2.5 years he was unable to sit. Dysmorphic features included inverted nipples, epicanthus, micropenis and cryptorchidism, club foot and wide 'sandal gaps.' Antithrombin-III was low, as were IgA, IgG and IgM levels.

Type Ih. (MIM 608104, 608103)

A female patient was described in 2003 [19] with ascites and edema, severe hypoalbuminemia, diarrhea and protein-losing enteropathy, no dysmorphic features, and normal development through 18 months. A trial of oral mannose was unsuccessful, but diarrhea resolved after 18 months of a low fat diet supplemented with essential fatty acids. Three other patients from two families were reported [20] with severe presentations and early death. A brother and sister had intrauterine growth retardation and reduced fetal movements. The boy was lethargic postnatally, with diarrhea, vomiting, and ascites, and death at 3 months. The girl developed edema and electrolyte abnormalities within hours of birth and expired at 3 days. The third patient had dysmorphic features including an asymmetric skull, large fontanelle, hypertelorism, low-set ears, long philtrum, short neck, cryptorchidism, camptodactyly, clubfeet, bilateral thoracic and pulmonary hypoplasia, perimembranous and trabecular ventricular septal defects, patent ductus arteriosus. Multiple cystic intra- and extra-hepatic bile ducts, cholestasis, and diffuse renal microcysts. He had no diarrhea or vomiting, but developed progressive ascites and died at three months.

Type Ii. (MIM 607906, 607905)

A single patient was described in 2003 [21], a German girl who was found at 2 months-of-age to have bilateral colobomas of the iris and a unilateral cataract. Despite replacement of the affected lens, her vision remained poor and nystagmus developed. Seizures and hypsarrhythmia developed after 4 months, and MRI at 5 months showed delayed myelination, with no progression of myelination by 8 months. Laboratory tests were normal except for prolonged activated partial thromboplastin time and markedly reduced level of factor XI.

Type Ij. (MIM 608093, 191350)

An infant was presented in 2003 [22] who developed infantile spasms within 72 hours of immunization diphtheria Pertussi Tetanus (DPT) at 4 months and went on to display microcephaly, continued intractable seizures, and significant developmental delay, with rudimentary language at 6 years. She also had a few minor dysmorphic features, including a high-arched palate, fifth finger clinodactyly, single palmar creases, and dimples on the upper thighs.

Type Ik. (MIM 608540, 605907)

Three patients were described in 2004. One [23] had intrauterine evidence of nonimmune hydrops and hepatosplenomegaly. He was born at 35 weeks with multiple dysmorphic features, including a large fontanelle, hypertelorism, micrognathia and hypogonadism, and displayed contractures, cardiomyopathy, areflexia, and multifocal epileptic activity. Two others [24] also presented in infancy with severe seizures, microcephaly and cerebral atrophy, and significant coagulation abnormalities. One of these patients developed seizures at 5 months, had frequent unexplained febrile episodes, developed progressive stupor, and expired at 10 months. The other had seizures starting at 2 hours of life, developed a nephrotic syndrome at 1 month, was noted to have a severe paucity of circulating B-cells and no detectable IgG, developed progressive stupor and died of respiratory failure at 11 weeks.

Type IL. (MIM 608776, 606941)

One patient was reported in 2004 [25] with microcephaly, central hypotonia, seizures, developmental delay, hepatomegaly, and bronchial asthma.

Type IIa. (MIM 212066, 602616)

Jaeken and Matthijs [1] summarized the presentation of the first three patients with this form of CDG, characterized by severe mental retardation, dysmorphic features, epilepsy and striking stereotypic behaviour. CDG-IIa was recognized (and initially called CDGS-II) as early as 1991 in an Iranian girl [26] and soon after in a Belgian boy [27], because of lowered serum values of a number of glycoproteins, similar to those with CDG-Ia. However, unlike several defects in the CDG-I group, no lysosomal inclusions were seen on liver biopsy, the appearance of the cerebellum was normal on MRI, and the pattern of transferrin isoelectric focusing was distinctive [28].

Type IIb. (MIM 606056, 601336)

A neonate was identified in 2000 [29], with generalized hypotonia and dysmorphic features including a prominent occiput, short palpebral fissures, long eyelashes, broad nose, retrognathia, high arched palate, and generalized edema, and a course notable for hepatomegaly, hypoventilation, seizures, and death at 74 days.

Type IIc. (MIM 266265, 605881)

Two unrelated Arab children from consanguineous families were reported in 1992 [30], with severe mental retardation, microcephaly, cortical atrophy, seizures, hypotonia, dwarfism, and recurrent infections with neutrophilia. The absence of the sialyl Lewis X (sLeX) ligand for the selectins and the absence of the H antigen in Bombay phenotype both being manifestations of failure of fucosylation, a defect in fucose metabolism was hypothesized. The condition was designated Rambam-Hasharon syndrome, but because of the effects on selectin binding, as had been described the leukocyte adhesion defect (LAD) due to mutation of the integrin β-subunit, this condition was also termed LAD type II. Subsequently, another case

in a patient of Turkish origin was ascertained [31], and two other Arab children were ascertained by the original group [32], with similar clinical features in all cases.

There is no abnormality of isoelectric pattern of transferrin, as sialylation is normal, and delayed separation of the umbilical cord, as seen in LAD type I, is not a regular feature. There were some interesting differences among the patients. The Arab patients had relatively mild infections, with the main manifestation being periodontitis, while the Turkish patient had more severe infections. Also, there was a clinical response to fucose supplementation in the Turkish child, with induction of core fucosylation of serum glycoproteins, disappearance of infections and fevers, and improvement of psychomotor capabilities. There was no apparent response to fucose supplementation in the Arab patients [33].

Type IId. (MIM 607091, 137060)

A single patient was described in 2002 [34], a 16 month-old boy born of nonconsanguineous parents, presenting with hypotonia, myopathy with elevated creatine kinase, developmental delay, and coagulopathy. He also had progressive macrocephaly associated with a Dandy-Walker malformation, which might have been coincidental. The transferrin isoelectric pattern was abnormal, and there was also evidence of reduced sialic acid content of α1-antitrypsin and α1-antichymotrypsin.

Type IIe. (MIM 608779, 606978)

Two consanguineous siblings were described [35] with dysmorphic features including loose, wrinkled skin, low-set dysplastic ears, microagnathia, and short neck; in the male sibling, there was also failure of development of the humeral and tibial epiphyses, and the female sibling had short limbs. There were neurologic abnormalities including generalized hypotonia and seizures. Hepatosplenomegaly and progressive jaundice were observed, and the babies died at 5 and 10 weeks with recurrent infections and cardiac insufficiency.

GENETICS AND PATHOGENESIS

The biochemical characteristic of this syndrome is the presence of secretory glycoproteins which are deficient in their carbohydrate content. As a result, a wide range of glycoproteins become abnormal, including transport proteins, enzymes, hormones such as prolactin and FSH, and coagulation factors such as antithrombin-III and factor XI. Among the most widely used tests for the diagnosis of this condition is the isoelectric focusing of serum transferrin [36]. Secondary abnormalities in which hypoglycosylation of transferrin is found include alcoholism and galactosemia. More refined electrophoretic techniques may be used to reveal lower molecular weight glycoforms of several serum glycoproteins in CDG, including α-1 antitrypsin and α-1 antichymotrypsin [37,38]. Abnormal transferrin glycoforms may also be detected by high performance liquid chromatography (HPLC) [39] or capillary zone electrophoresis [40], techniques which are more suited to automation. Tandem mass spectrometry has been shown to be useful to study the glycosylation of transferrin in clinical samples [41], and that approach allows for quantitative results and can permit detection of subtle variants in glycan processing [42].

All known forms of CDG are autosomal recessive, and while biochemical changes may be discernable in heterozygotes in some cases, carrier detection is not reliable unless by direct testing for mutations. Neonatal screening for these diseases has not been shown to be feasible, and it has been recommended that testing of transferrin glycosylation not be performed before 3 weeks-of-age to avoid false negative results [5].

Type Ib

The human mannose 6-phosphate isomerase (MPI) gene (designated PMI) encodes 423 amino acids in eight exons, spanning only 5 kb [7], and is located on chromosome 15. To date, 16 different mutations have been found in more than 10 families [43,44]. Thirteen of the mutations are missense mutations, mostly affecting conserved amino acids. There is one known case of a one-base insertion, and two nucleotide substitutions at splice sites.

There is no clear explanation for the clinical differences between CDG-Ib (PMI deficiency) and CDG-Ia (PMM2 deficiency), which, though the metabolic steps are consecutive, are strikingly different and particularly intriguing with respect to neurological manifestations. One possible explanation is that brain hexokinase, which can convert mannose to mannose 6-phosphate, has a rather high affinity for mannose, whereas glucokinase, the major hexokinase present in hepatocytes, has a very low affinity for mannose and is thus less efficient in bypassing PMI.

Type Ic

The primary defect is in the dolichylpyrophosphate-GlcNAc2 Man9 α-1,3- glucosyltransferase which adds the first three glucose residues in the lipid-linked oligosaccharide (Figure 105.1, p. 707), first identified in yeast as the ALG6 gene product. Nonglycosylated oligosaccharides are inefficiency transferred to proteins, and accordingly there is accumulation of Man9GlcNAc2 linked to dolichylpyrophosphate in fibroblasts [9]. The human ALG6 gene, hALG6 has 14 exons and spans 55 kb on chromosome 1p22.3 [45]. The 1521 bp open reading frame encodes 507 amino acids. There is a frequent A333V mutation, which was homozygous in four related patients in the first cases [46] and an additional four unrelated patients in a later study [45], which also described a patient who was a compound heterozygote for A333V and an intron 3 5′-splice site transition IVS3C5G > A. A founder effect of the A333V

mutation was demonstrated by haplotype analysis [45]. Four other missense mutations have been described [45,47,48], and it appears that one of those, F304S, may be a frequent polymorphism [1]. Overall, at the time of writing, five missense mutations, one splice site substitution, and two small deletions have been described [44].

Type Id

The defect was determined to involve the endoplasmic reticulum-associated mannosyltransferase that attaches a mannosyl residue from dolicholphosphomannose to Man5GlcNAc2-pyrophosphate-dolichol [11]. The human gene, identified as the Not 56-like protein gene (NOT56L), or the ortholog of the yeast ALG3 gene, codes for 438 amino acids and contains nine exons over 5 kb, and is located on chromosome 3q27. Two missense mutations have been found [11,47], and a silent mutation in exon 1 has also been shown to give rise to an mRNA deletion due to a cryptic splice site [49].

Type Ie

Analysis of the lipid-linked oligosaccharides in the ER of fibroblasts revealed an accumulation of dolichylpyrophosphate-Man5GlcNAc2, consistent with a defect in the dolichol-phosphate-mannose synthase (Figure 105.1, p. 707). The dolichol-phosphate-mannose synthase complex is composed of at least three proteins: a catalytic subunit (DPM1), a membrane-associated anchor (DPM2p), and a stabilizing subunit (DPM3) [50]. DPM is important in the biosynthesis of several glycoconjugates, as it is the donor not only of the last four mannoses in N-linked glycans (Figure 105.1, p. 707), but also all three mannoses in glycosylphosphatidylinositols, and apparently also for some processes of O- and C-linked protein glycosylation. At this point, all of the recognized human defects in dolichol-phosphate-mannose synthase have been found to be in DPM1, a gene of 9 exons spanning 23.6 kbp, which encodes 260 amino acids [13]. Only four patients have been analyzed at the molecular level. One patient was homozygous for the missense mutation R92G [12], two others were compound heterozygous for R92G with either a 13 bp deletion (331-343del13) in exon 4 [12] or a single base deletion (628 delC) in exon 8 [13], and the fourth patient was homozygous for the missense mutation S248P [14].

Type If

Examination of the patients' fibroblast lipid-linked oligosaccharides showed accumulation of truncated forms, including Man5GlcNAc2-, Man9GlcNAc2-, but also of fully assembled Glc3Man9GlcNAc2-linked forms. This indicated a defect in dolichol-phosphate-mannose utilization, and also in dolichol-phosphate-glucose utilization, as had been seen in the CHO-derived Lec35 mutant cells, and mutations were found in the Lec35/MPDU1 (mannose-phosphate-dolichol utilization defect 1) locus, also termed SL15 (suppressor of Lec15). As a result of this defect, there is also an expected deficiency in formation of glysosylphosphoinositols, and there is indirect evidence for defective GPI anchor formation [1]. The MPDU1 locus is found on chromosome 17p13.1–p12, spanning 4.34 kb with 7 exons coding for 247 amino acids. One patient was homozygous for a L119P, another homozygous for a G73E missense mutation, and a third patient [16] was a compound heterozygote for a missense mutation, M1T, affecting the initiating methionine, and a one base frameshift deletion, 511delC. The fourth patient [15] was homozygous for an L74S missense mutation.

Type Ig

The presence of a truncated GlcNAc$_2$Man$_7$ N-linked oligosaccharide [18] suggested that there was a defect in the transfer of the last two mannose residues to the nascent glycan, and as there was no detectable untrimmed GlcNAc$_2$Man$_7$Glc$_3$ species in the presence of the inhibitor castanospermine, the defect was deduced to be in the transfer of the GlcNAc$_2$Man$_7$ substrate to the oligosaccharyltransferase complex (Figure 105.1, p. 707). The human ortholog to the yeast ALG12 gene was identified in silico, and the cDNA sequence documented two amino acid substitutions leading to missense mutations T67M and R146Q in one patient [18], and a homozygous F142V mutation in the other [17]. The human ALG12 gene is localized on chromosome 22q13.33, with 10 exons spanning 15 kb and coding for 488 amino acids.

Type Ih

The pattern of accumulated dolichol-linked oligosaccharides indicated a defect in the glucosyltransferase that adds the second glucose residue [19], the dolichyl-P-glucose: Glc$_1$Man$_9$GlcNAc$_2$-PP-dolichyl α3-glucosyltransferase (ortholog of yeast ALG8). The gene is located on chromosome 11q14 and consists of 13 exons coding for 526 amino acids, with 12 transmembrane domains and an endoplasmic reticulum retention signal. The index case was found to be a compound heterozygote for two frame shift mutations in exon 4: a one base deletion, del413C, and a one base insertion, ins396A. The severely affected patients reported by Schollen et al. in 2004 [20] were compound heterozygotes for a splice site mutation and a missense mutation: in one family the combination was IVS1-2,A>G and T47P, and in the other family the combination was IVS6+4,A>G and G275D.

Type Ii

In addition to the normal dolichol-linked oligosaccharide, Glc$_5$Man$_9$GlcNAc$_2$, which is the normal form, although it was present at a slightly reduced level [21] cells from the index patient accumulated Man$_1$GlcNAc$_2$- and Man$_2$GlcNAc$_2$-PP-dolichol. As predicted, GDP-mannose:Man$_1$GlcNAc$_2$-PP-dolichol α1,3-mannosyltransferase (the enzyme catalyzing the addition of the second mannose, and the ortholog of yeast ALG2) was defective (Figure 105.1, p. 707). The gene is located on chromosome 9q22 and codes for a polypeptide of 416 amino acids. The index patient [21] was a compound heterozygote for a one base deletion, del1040G and a 393G>T substitution.

Type Ij

Metabolic labeling of cultured fibroblasts from the index patient [22] revealed accumulation of the normal GlcNAc$_2$Man$_9$Glc$_2$ product bound to dolichol and to asparagine, but in reduced amounts. A specific assay of microsomal fractions for UDP-GlcNAc:dolichol phosphate N-acetyl-glucosamine-1-phosphate transferase demonstrated a deficiency of that enzyme (designated DPAGT1), which catalyzes the first step in N-linked oligosaccharide synthesis (Figure 105.1, p. 707) and is inhibited by the antibiotic tunicamycin. The gene, located on chromosome 11q23.3, consists of 9 exons spanning 5.13 kb, and codes for 408 amino acids. In the index case [22], a transition in exon 5 leading to the missense mutation Y170C was found on the paternal allele; though no mutation was found on the maternal allele, it produced only 12 percent of the normal amount of mature mRNA, the remainder showing a complex exon-skipping pattern.

Type Ik

To analyze the early intermediates of N-linked glycan synthesis, HPLC was performed with fluorescence detection of 2-amnobenzamide-coupled oligosaccharides [51], and dolichylpyrophosphate-GlcNAc$_2$ was found, suggesting a deficiency of the β1,4-mannosyltransferase homologous with the yeast ALG1, which performs the first mannosylation step (Figure 105.1, p. 707). The gene, located on chromosome 16p13.3, codes for 464 amino acids. A homozygous missense mutation, S258L, was found in two unrelated patients [23,24], and the same mutation was found as one allele in another patient who was a compound heterozygote for E342P [24].

Type IL

Lipid-linked oligosaccharides showed accumulation of GlcNAc$_2$Man$_6$ and GlcNAc$_2$Man$_8$ forms, and N-linked oligosaccharides included an abnormal GlcNAc$_2$Man$_6$ form [25], indicating a defect in the α1,2-mannosyltransferase which adds the seventh and ninth mannose residues on the growing dolichol-linked oligosaccharide (Figure 105.1, p. 707), previously identified in yeast as ALG9. The human ortholog of ALG9 had been described as DIBD1 (disrupted in bipolar disorder 1), a candidate gene associated with bipolar affective disorder, but shown by linkage analysis to have no evidence of a role in susceptibility to bipolar disorder [52]. The mannosyltransferase gene is located on chromosome 11q23, with 15 exons coding 611 amino acids with a multiple membrane spanning motif. An E523K missense mutation was found in the index patient [25].

Type IIa

Isoelectric focusing of serum transferrin showed a type 2 pattern but with nearly absent tetrasialotransferrin, and fine structure analysis of the glycans on serum transferrin revealed that some of the normal, disialo-biantennary N-glycans are replaced by truncated, monosialo-monoantennary N-glycans [27], whose structure indicated that the defect was in UDP-N-acetylglucosamine:alpha-6-D-mannoside-beta-1,2-N-acetyl-glucosaminyltransferase II (GlcNAc-transferase II, GnT II) in the Golgi (Figure 105.2, p. 708). GnT II activity was reduced by over 98 percent in fibroblasts and mononuclear blood cells from patients [1]. The human GnT II gene (designated MGAT2) is located on chromosome 14q21, and the coding region contains only one exon, which encodes a protein of 447 amino acids. Mutation analysis of the GnT II coding sequence (MGAT2 gene) in the first two patients described revealed that they were each homozygous for missense mutations in the C-terminal catalytic domain, S290F and H262R [53]. A third patient [54] was a compound heterozygote for a missense (N318D) and a nonsense (C339X) mutation. A knockout mouse model for GnT II deficiency has been developed [55]. Homozygous knockout mice survive to term, but are born stunted with various congenital abnormalities and die early in the neonatal phase; this severity may explain the rarity with which this disorder is encountered in human cases [9].

Type IIb

Isoelectric focusing of transferrin was normal, but serum hexosaminidase showed a slight cathodal shift. A tetrasaccharide, identified as Glc(α1-2)Glc(α1-3)Glc(α1-3)Man, accumulated in the patient's urine. Electron microscopy showed lamellar intralysosomal inclusions in liver parenchymal cells and macrophages and empty, membrane-bound vacuoles in neurons of the frontal and occipital lobes of the brain. A defect in glucosidase-I, the first step of N-glycan processing (Figure 105.2, p. 708) was demonstrated in liver and cultured fibroblasts [29]. The GCS1 gene is located on chromosome 2p12-p13 and encodes 834 amino acids. The only known patient [29] was found to be a compound heterozygote for two missense mutations, R486T and F652L.

Type IIc

The clinical features arise from hypofucosylation of N- and O-linked glycoproteins. There is no abnormality in the isoelectric pattern of serum transferrin because the normal glycan in transferrin does not contain fucose, and there is no deficiency of sialylation. Cells from a CDG-IIc patient were shown to have decreased transport of GDP-fucose into the Golgi [56], and complementation cloning identified the defect in a GDP-fucose transporter [57,58], which is designated FUCT1. The gene has been assigned to chromosome 11 by radiation hybrid mapping. All of the Arab cases were homozygous for a T308R missense mutation in the predicted ninth membrane-spanning domain [59], consistent with a founder effect, and the Turkish patient was homozygous for R147C mutation in the fourth transmembrane domain [58].

Type IId

The isolectric pattern of transferrin is abnormal [34], with strongly elevated tri-, di-, mono- and asialotransferrin bands (increasing in that order) and a markedly decreased tetrasialotransferrin, and there is also abnormal glycosylation of two other glycoproteins, α1-antotrypsin and α1-antichymotrypsin. The defect was determined [60] to be in the Golgi enzyme UDP-Gal:N-acetylglucosamine β-1,4-galactosyltransferase I (Figure 105.2, p. 708). The gene for this galactosyltransferase, designated B4GALT1, is localized on chromosome 9p13, contains 6 exons spanning more than 50 kb, and encodes a predicted 400 amino acid protein with an N-terminal membrane-anchoring domain [61]. A knock-out mouse model [62]. exhibits growth retardation and semi-lethality, with excessive epithelial cell proliferation of the skin and small intestine, and abnormal differentiation in intestinal villi. Interestingly, the knock-out mice are reported to be deficient in the production of lactose, and the B4GALT1 product appears to be the catalytic subunit of lactose synthase in mammary glands [63], so it appears to have played an important role in mammalian evolution. The mutation in the reported case was found to be a homozygous insertion, ins1031C [34], which leads to premature termination and loss of the C-terminal 50 amino acids [60].

Type IIe

Cells from the affected patient exhibited abnormal glycosylation of transferrin with an equal distribution of zero-, one-, two-, three- and four-sialic acid residues [35]. In addition, there were abnormalities in glycosylation of numerous glycoproteins, and deficient sialylation of surface O-linked glycans. Transport of nucleotide sugars into the Golgi apparatus was defective, and the trafficking of proteins from the endoplasmic reticulum to the Golgi was shown to be defective. The metabolic phenotype was similar to the Chinese hamster cell mutants in the conserved oligomeric Golgi (COG) complex [64], and indirect immunofluorescence [35] indicated that the defect was in the COG7 subunit. The COG7 gene contains 17 exons and is located on chromosome 16p [64], and the index siblings were found to have homozygous mutations in COG7, IVS1+4A>C [35].

TREATMENT

Type Ib

Oral D-mannose administration has been shown to be an effective treatment of PMI deficiency. This is possible because of the ability to convert mannose to mannose 6-phosphate by hexokinases. Doses of 100–150 mg/kg three to six times per day are effective. Symptomatic improvement is expected within weeks, but it may take several months of treatment before the biochemical parameters normalize [65].

Type IIc

Oral fucose supplementation was beneficial in treatment of one patient with CDG-IIc [31] at doses up to nearly 500 mg/kg/day. By contrast, no effect was observed in three of the Arab patients [33], even when using equivalent dosage [32]. It is possible that the difference relates to the observed effects of the mutations, primarily affecting the enzyme's K_m in the responsive form, as opposed to a reduction of the V_{max} in the nonresponsive form [59].

Other types

No effective treatment has been reported.

References

1 Jaeken J, Matthijs G. Congenital disorders of glycosylation. *Annu Rev Genomics Hum Genet* 2001;**2**:129.

2 Aebi M, Helenius A, Schenk B, *et al.* Carbohydrate-deficient glycoprotein syndromes become congenital disorders of glycosylation: an updated nomenclature for CDG. First International Workshop on CDGS. *Glycoconj J* 1999;**16**:669.

3 Van den Steen P, Rudd PM, Dwek RA, Opdenakker G. Concepts and principles of O-linked glycosylation. *Crit Rev Biochem Mol Biol* 1998;**33**:151.

4 de Koning TJ, Dorland L, Van Diggelen OP, *et al.* A novel disorder of N-glycosylation due to phosphomannose isomerase deficiency. *Biochem Biophys Res Commun* 1998;**245**:38.

5 Marquardt T, Denecke J. Congenital disorders of glycosylation: review of their molecular bases, clinical presentations and specific therapies. *Eur J Pediatr* 2003;**162**:359.

6 Jaeken J, Matthijs G, Saudubray JM, *et al.* Phosphomannose isomerase deficiency: a carbohydrate-deficient glycoprotein syndrome with hepatic-intestinal presentation. *Am J Hum Genet* 1998;**62**:1535.

7 Schollen E, Dorland L, de Koning TJ, *et al.* Genomic organization of the human phosphomannose isomerase (MPI) gene and mutation analysis in patients with congenital disorders of glycosylation type Ib (CDG-Ib). *Hum Mutat* 2000;**16**:247.

8 Kjaergaard S, Westphal V, Davis JA, *et al.* Variable outcome and the effect of mannose in congenital disorder of glycosylation Type Ib (CDG-Ib). *J Inherit Metab Dis* 2000;**23** (Suppl 1):184.

9 Burda P, Borsig L, Rijk-van Andel J, *et al.* A novel carbohydrate-deficient glycoprotein syndrome characterized by a deficiency in glucosylation of the dolichol-linked oligosaccharide. *J Clin Invest* 1998;**102**:647.

10 Stibler H, Stephani U, Kutsch U. Carbohydrate-deficient glycoprotein syndrome – a fourth subtype. *Neuropediatrics* 1995;**26**:235.

11 Korner C, Knauer R, Stephani U, *et al.* Carbohydrate deficient glycoprotein syndrome type IV: deficiency of dolichyl-P-Man:Man(5)GlcNAc(2)-PP-dolichyl mannosyltransferase. *EMBO J* 1999;**18**:6816.

12 Kim S, Westphal V, Srikrishna G, *et al.* Dolichol phosphate mannose synthase (DPM1) mutations define congenital disorder of glycosylation Ie (CDG-Ie). *J Clin Invest* 2000;**105**:191.

13 Imbach T, Schenk B, Schollen E, *et al.* Deficiency of dolichol-phosphate-mannose synthase-1 causes congenital disorder of glycosylation type Ie. *J Clin Invest* 2000;**105**:233.

14 Garcia-Silva MT, Matthijs G, Schollen E, *et al.* Congenital disorder of glycosylation (CDG) type Ie. A new patient. *J Inherit Metab Dis* 2004;**27**:591.

15 Kranz C, Denecke J, Lehrman MA, *et al.* A mutation in the human MPDU1 gene causes congenital disorder of glycosylation type If (CDG-If). *J Clin Invest* 2001;**108**:1613.

16 Schenk B, Imbach T, Frank CG, *et al.* MPDU1 mutations underlie a novel human congenital disorder of glycosylation, designated type If. *J Clin Invest* 2001;**108**:1687.

17 Chantret I, Dupre T, Delenda C, *et al.* Congenital disorders of glycosylation type Ig are defined by a deficiency in dolichyl-P-mannose:Man7GlcNAc2-PP-dolichyl mannosyltransferase. *J Biol Chem* 2002;**277**:25815.

18 Grubenmann CE, Frank CG, Kjaergaard S, *et al.* ALG12 mannosyltransferase defect in congenital disorder of glycosylation type Ig. *Hum Mol Genet* 2002;**11**:2331.

19 Chantret I, Dancourt J, Dupre T, *et al.* A deficiency in dolichyl-P-glucose:Glc1Man9GlcNAc2-PP-dolichyl alpha3-glucosyltransferase defines a new subtype of congenital disorders of glycosylation. *J Biol Chem* 2003;**278**:9962.

20 Schollen E, Frank CG, Keldermans L, *et al.* Clinical and molecular features of three patients with congenital disorders of glycosylation type Ih (CDG-Ih) (ALG8 deficiency). *J Med Genet* 2004;**41**:550.

21 Thiel C, Schwarz M, Peng J, *et al.* A new type of congenital disorder of glycosylation (CDG-Ii) provides new insights into the early steps of dolichol-linked oligosaccharide biosynthesis. *J Biol Chem* 2003;**278**:22498.

22 Wu X, Rush JS, Karaoglu D, *et al.* Deficiency of UDP-GlcNAc:dolichol phosphate N-acetylglucosamine-1 phosphate transferase (DPAGT1) causes a novel congenital disorder of glycosylation Type Ij. *Hum Mutat* 2003;**22**:144.

23 Schwarz M, Thiel C, Lubbehusen J, *et al.* Deficiency of GDP-Man:GlcNAc2-PP-dolichol mannosyltransferase causes congenital disorder of glycosylation type Ik. *Am J Hum Genet* 2004;**74**:472.

24 Kranz C, Denecke J, Lehle L, *et al.* Congenital disorder of glycosylation type Ik (CDG-Ik): a defect of mannosyltransferase I. *Am J Hum Genet* 2004;**74**:545.

25 Frank CG, Grubenmann CE, Eyaid W, *et al.* Identification and functional analysis of a defect in the human ALG9 gene: definition of congenital disorder of glycosylation type IL. *Am J Hum Genet* 2004;**75**:146.

26 Ramaekers VT, Stibler H, Kint J, Jaeken J. A new variant of the carbohydrate deficient glycoproteins syndrome. *J Inherit Metab Dis* 1991;**14**:385.

27 Jaeken J, Schachter H, Carchon H, *et al.* Carbohydrate deficient glycoprotein syndrome type II: a deficiency in Golgi localised N-acetyl-glucosaminyltransferase II. *Arch Dis Child* 1994;**71**:123.

28 Schachter H, Jaeken J. Carbohydrate-deficient glycoprotein syndrome type II. *Biochim Biophys Acta* 1999;**1455**:179.

29 De Praeter CM, Gerwig GJ, Bause E, *et al.* A novel disorder caused by defective biosynthesis of N-linked oligosaccharides due to glucosidase I deficiency. *Am J Hum Genet* 2000;**66**:1744.

30 Frydman M, Etzioni A, Eidlitz-Markus T, *et al.* Rambam-Hasharon syndrome of psychomotor retardation, short stature, defective neutrophil motility, and Bombay phenotype. *Am J Med Genet* 1992;**44**:297.

31 Marquardt T, Luhn K, Srikrishna G, *et al.* Correction of leukocyte adhesion deficiency type II with oral fucose. *Blood* 1999;**94**:3976.

32 Etzioni A, Tonetti M. Leukocyte adhesion deficiency II-from A to almost Z. *Immunol Rev* 2000;**178**:138.

33 Etzioni A, Tonetti M. Fucose supplementation in leukocyte adhesion deficiency type II. *Blood* 2000;**95**:3641.

34 Peters V, Penzien JM, Reiter G, *et al.* Congenital disorder of glycosylation IId (CDG-IId) – a new entity: clinical presentation with Dandy-Walker malformation and myopathy. *Neuropediatrics* 2002;**33**:27.

35 Wu X, Steet RA, Bohorov O, *et al.* Mutation of the COG complex subunit gene COG7 causes a lethal congenital disorder. *Nat Med* 2004;**10**:518.

36 Stibler H, Jaeken J, Kristiansson B. Biochemical characteristics and diagnosis of the carbohydrate-deficient glycoprotein syndrome. *Acta Paediatr Scand* 1991;**375**:21.

37 Harrison HH, Miller KL, Harbison MD, Slonim AE. Multiple serum protein abnormalities in carbohydrate-deficient glycoprotein syndrome: pathognomonic finding of two-dimensional electrophoresis? *Clin Chem* 1992;**38**:1390.

38 Fang J, Peters V, Korner C, Hoffmann GF. Improvement of CDG diagnosis by combined examination of several glycoproteins. *J Inherit Metab Dis* 2004;**27**:581.

39 Helander A, Bergstrom J, Freeze HH. Testing for congenital disorders of glycosylation by HPLC measurement of serum transferrin glycoforms. *Clin Chem* 2004;**50**:954.

40 Jaeken J, Carchon H. Congenital disorders of glycosylation: a booming chapter of pediatrics. *Curr Opin Pediatr* 2004;**16**:434.

41 Lacey JM, Bergen HR, Magera MJ, *et al.* Rapid determination of transferrin isoforms by immunoaffinity liquid chromatography and electrospray mass spectrometry. *Clin Chem* 2001;**47**:513.

42 Mills PB, Mills K, Mian N, *et al.* Mass spectrometric analysis of glycans in elucidating the pathogenesis of CDG type IIx. *J Inherit Metab Dis* 2003;**26**:119.

43 Stenson PD, Ball EV, Mort M, *et al.* Human Gene Mutation Database (HGMD): 2003 update. *Hum Mutat* 2003;**21**:577.

44 HGMD: The Human Gene Mutation Database, Cardiff University. http://archive.uwcm.ac.uk/uwcm/mg/hgmd0.html, (accessed 2004).

45 Imbach T, Grunewald S, Schenk B, *et al.* Multi-allelic origin of congenital disorder of glycosylation (CDG)-Ic. *Hum Genet* 2000;**106**:538.

46 Imbach T, Burda P, Kuhnert P, *et al.* A mutation in the human ortholog of the Saccharomyces cerevisiae ALG6 gene causes carbohydrate-deficient glycoprotein syndrome type-Ic. *Proc Natl Acad Sci USA* 1999;**96**:6982.

47 Schollen E, Martens K, Geuzens E, Matthijs G. DHPLC analysis as a platform for molecular diagnosis of congenital disorders of glycosylation (CDG). *Eur J Hum Genet* 2002;**10**:643.

48 de Lonlay P, Seta N, Barrot S, *et al.* A broad spectrum of clinical presentations in congenital disorders of glycosylation I: a series of 26 cases. *J Med Genet* 2001;**38**:14.

49 Denecke J, Kranz C, Kemming D, *et al.* An activated 5' cryptic splice site in the human ALG3 gene generates a premature termination codon insensitive to nonsense-mediated mRNA decay in a new case of congenital disorder of glycosylation type Id (CDG-Id). *Hum Mutat* 2004;**23**:477.

50 Maeda Y, Tanaka S, Hino J, *et al.* Human dolichol-phosphate-mannose synthase consists of three subunits, DPM1, DPM2 and DPM3. *EMBO J* 2000;**19**:2475.

51 Grubenmann CE, Frank CG, Hulsmeier AJ, *et al.* Deficiency of the first mannosylation step in the N-glycosylation pathway causes congenital disorder of glycosylation type Ik. *Hum Mol Genet* 2004;**13**:535.

52 Baysal BE, Willett-Brozick JE, Badner JA, *et al.* A mannosyltransferase gene at 11q23 is disrupted by a translocation breakpoint that co-segregates with bipolar affective disorder in a small family. *Neurogenetics* 2002;**4**:43.

53 Tan J, Dunn J, Jaeken J, Schachter H. Mutations in the MGAT2 gene controlling complex N-glycan synthesis cause carbohydrate-deficient glycoprotein syndrome type II, an autosomal recessive disease with defective brain development. *Am J Hum Genet* 1996;**59**:810.

54 Cormier-Daire V, Amiel J, Vuillaumier-Barrot S, *et al.* Congenital disorders of glycosylation IIa cause growth retardation, mental retardation, and facial dysmorphism. *J Med Genet* 2000;**37**:875.

55 Schachter H. The role of the GlcNAc(beta)1,2Man(alpha)- moiety in mammalian development. Null mutations of the genes encoding UDP-N-acetylglucosamine:alpha-3-D-mannoside beta-1,2-N-acetylglucosaminyltransferase I and UDP-N-acetylglucosamine:alpha-D-mannoside beta-1,2-N-acetylglucosaminyltransferase I.2 cause embryonic lethality and congenital muscular dystrophy in mice and men, respectively. *Biochim Biophys Acta* 2002;**1573**:292.

56 Lubke T, Marquardt T, von Figura K, Korner C. A new type of carbohydrate-deficient glycoprotein syndrome due to a decreased import of GDP-fucose into the golgi. *J Biol Chem* 1999;**274**:25986.

57 Luhn K, Wild MK, Eckhardt M, *et al.* The gene defective in leukocyte adhesion deficiency II encodes a putative GDP-fucose transporter. *Nat Genet* 2001;**28**:69.

58 Lubke T, Marquardt T, Etzioni A, *et al.* Complementation cloning identifies CDG-IIc, a new type of congenital disorders of glycosylation, as a GDP-fucose transporter deficiency. *Nat Genet* 2001;**28**:73.

59 Etzioni A, Sturla L, Antonellis A, *et al.* Leukocyte adhesion deficiency (LAD) type II/carbohydrate deficient glycoprotein (CDG) IIc founder effect and genotype/phenotype correlation. *Am J Med Genet* 2002;**110**:131.

60 Hansske B, Thiel C, Lubke T, *et al.* Deficiency of UDP-galactose: N-acetylglucosamine beta-1,4-galactosyltransferase I causes the congenital disorder of glycosylation type IId. *J Clin Invest* 2002;**109**:725.

61 Masri KA, Appert HE, Fukuda MN. Identification of the full-length coding sequence for human galactosyltransferase (beta-N-acetylglucosaminide: beta 1,4-galactosyltransferase). *Biochem Biophys Res Commun* 1988;**157**:657.

62 Asano M, Furukawa K, Kido M, *et al.* Growth retardation and early death of beta-1,4-galactosyltransferase knockout mice with augmented proliferation and abnormal differentiation of epithelial cells. *EMBO J* 1997;**16**:1850.

63 Ramakrishnan B, Qasba PK. Crystal structure of lactose synthase reveals a large conformational change in its catalytic component, the beta1, 4-galactosyltransferase-I. *J Mol Biol* 2001;**310**:205.

64 Ungar D, Oka T, Brittle EE, *et al.* Characterization of a mammalian Golgi-localized protein complex, COG, that is required for normal Golgi morphology and function. *J Cell Biol.* 2002;**157**:405.

65 Niehues R, Hasilik M, Alton G, *et al.* Carbohydrate-deficient glycoprotein syndrome type Ib. Phosphomannose isomerase deficiency and mannose therapy. *J Clin Invest* 1998;**101**:1414.

α_1-Antitrypsin deficiency

MAJOR PHENOTYPIC EXPRESSION

In infancy and childhood: hepatic disease with conjugated hyperbilirubinemia, hepatocellular damage presenting in a neonatal hepatitis pattern or isolated hepatomegaly. In adulthood: emphysema of early onset. Each has deficiency of α_1-antitrypsin.

INTRODUCTION

α_1-Antitrypsin (AT) deficiency was discovered by Laurell and Eriksson [1] in 1963, when they reported five patients in whom the α_1-globulin band was missing on agarose gel protein electrophoresis. Three had emphysema, and so did nine of 14 other patients with α_1-AT deficiency [2]. The protein itself had been isolated in 1955 by Shultze and colleagues [3], who recognized its function as the major trypsin inhibitor of serum and the major component (90 percent) of the α_1-globulin fraction [4]. It was evident early that partial deficiency was transmitted in an autosomal dominant manner, and that those with severe deficiency were homozygotes [5]. Extensive polymorphism of α_1-AT was recognized first by Fagerhol [6] on electrophoresis on starch gels. The current method of choice is isoelectric focusing on polyacrylamide gel [7], and 75 variants have been recognized. Examination of the DNA for restriction fragment length polymorphism (RFLP) has indicated even greater variation [8,9].

A classification system has been developed [8] in which the variant proteins are designated as PI (protease inhibitor) types. The normal variant was designated PIMM. The classic deficiency phenotype in which serum antitrypsin activity is about 15 percent normal is PIZZ. PIMZ individuals are heterozygotes. PISS is the second most common form of deficiency.

The relationship of α_1-antitrypsin deficiency to hepatic disease in infancy and childhood was discovered by Sharp and colleagues in 1969 [10].

The disease is a model in which an abnormal glycoprotein synthesized in the liver is not released from the hepatocyte into the circulation. The disease provides a model for the understanding of the processing of correctly and incorrectly folded glycoproteins in the endoplasmic reticulum [11]. The gene has been cloned and localized to chromosome 14q32.1 [12]. A number of deficiency mutations has been defined. The Z allele contains a G to A change in exon 5 that changes glutamic acid 342 to lysine (E342K) [13,14].

The relationship of protease and elastin has led to understanding of the pathogenesis of emphysema not only in this common disease, but in other nongenetic forms of emphysema. The gene has been isolated. Recombinant techniques have made abundant supplies of α_1-antitrypsin for protein replacement therapy [15,16], and gene replacement has been done in transgenic animals [17,18]. In addition, the relationship between cigarette smoking and the occurrence of emphysema in individuals that have inherited this susceptibility [19] provides an interesting example of the interaction of genetics and environment, and the development of emphysema in non-α_1-AT deficient smokers has provided a strong scientific argument against smoking [20].

CLINICAL ABNORMALITIES

Hepatic manifestations of α_1-AT deficiency were first recognized by the detection of the deficiency in 14 patients with liver disease [10]. All were PIZZ homozygotes. These patients developed specific manifestations of liver disease in the first year of life with early cholestasis that resolved by 6 months of life, but elevated serum levels of hepatocellular enzymes and hepatomegaly persisted. All but one developed cirrhosis. It has since become evident that most PIZZ individuals do not have severe liver disease. Some 10 percent of PIZZ infants have neonatal cholestasis [21], and about half of PIZZ infants who appear normal have abnormal serum levels of aminotransferases. The most frequent hepatic presentation is with a neonatal hepatitis syndrome [22]. These infants have conjugated hyperbilirubinemia and hepatomegaly. Vomiting may be projectile. Failure to thrive is common; some have low birth weights. Some have splenomegaly. There may be dark urine, indicating the presence of bilirubin. Bilirubinemia is a uniform indicator of cholestatic disease because indirect bilirubin is bound to albumin and not present in urine. Urinary bile acid concentration may be elevated [23].

This disorder is a major cause of the neonatal hepatitis syndrome. It has been found in 14–29 percent of such infants [24]. Bleeding may occur as a result of deficiency of vitamin K. Occasionally in such an infant there are acholic stools and the picture may simulate extrahepatic biliary atresia [25]. The diagnosis of α_1-AT deficiency should obviate the usually demanding work-up for this disorder. In α_1-AT deficiency the jaundice usually clears spontaneously by 7 months-of-age [26].

Another presentation is with transient symptoms of liver disease occurring with intermittent infection or appendicitis at 2 years or later in a previously asymptomatic child [26]. In another group of patients hepatomegaly has been found in childhood without a history of neonatal jaundice. Others may present first in childhood with what appears to be acute hepatitis.

In many patients, once the jaundice has subsided, clinical manifestations of liver disease do not recur and ultimately serum levels of aminotransferases become normal [22]. A small number go on to develop chronic cirrhosis (Figure 106.1). Cirrhosis and early death have been reported in two percent of children with PIZZ and 14 percent of those with hepatic manifestations in infancy [27]. These patients may have spider telangiectases as early as 2 years-of-age. They may develop portal hypertension and esophageal varices. A number have died of this or other complications of cirrhosis during childhood or adolescence, even in infancy, and certainly after the development of cirrhosis. Ascites may be present with or without hypoalbuminemia and edema elsewhere.

We have observed a 10-month-old patient with α_1-AT deficiency who presented with ascites that appeared on paracentesis to be chylous. Its protein content was 4.1 g/dL, and the serum albumin concentration was 3.5 g/dL. This is the so-called pseudochylous ascites in which some patients with chronic

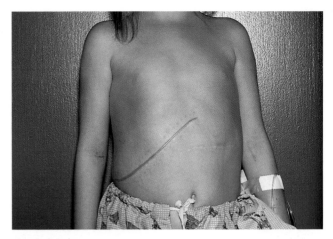

Figure 106.1   *J.P., a 7-year-old girl with α_1-antitrypsin deficiency who presented with hematemesis. She had been found to have hepatomegaly at 2 years-of-age and biopsy revealed cirrhosis. She had two spider telangiectases on the arms and a large healed incision over the liver, which was palpable 3 cm below the costal margin. The spleen was palpated at 8 cm. Endoscopy revealed esophageal varices.*

liver disease have lactescent fluid. Triglyceride content is not high, and this fluid can be distinguished by adding petroleum ether and shaking well, under which circumstances the triglyceride in true chylous fluid dissolves and the fluid becomes clear. Protein content has been used to distinguish exudative from transudative processes, but the range of protein content in liver disease is too great to permit this distinction. Coagulation factors may be reduced, and there may be clinical bleeding, especially gastrointestinal. Pruritis may be present in infancy, or may develop later. We have observed hyperammonemia and hepatic encephalopathy. Cirrhosis has also been observed in a number of adults who had a history of neonatal hepatitis or liver disease in childhood [28]. A few of these patients were found to have hepatomas on biopsy. Levels of α-fetoprotein are not usually elevated in these patients with hepatomas. Hepatocellular carcinoma has been observed.

Pulmonary disease is the most common expression of the PIZZ phenotype [29] (Figure 106.2). As many as 90 percent develop emphysema. It is classically early in onset, occurring at 20–40 years of age in smokers and 55 in nonsmokers [5,30,31]. It is referred to as chronic obstructive pulmonary disease or COPD. The earliest symptom is dyspnea on exertion. Cough develops in about half of the patients, and recurrent pulmonary infections are common. On examination, the patient may be thin, but the diameter of the chest is increased. Breath sounds are diminished, and the chest film reveals hyperinflation, especially in the bases. The diaphragms may be flattened. Pulmonary function tests are typical of severe emphysema consistent with a loss of pulmonary elastic recoil. Total lung capacity is impaired, as is residual volume. Air flow is limited, and diffusion capacity and maximum transpulmonary pressure are reduced. Mild hypoxemia at rest may increase with exercise. Hypocarbia and respiratory alkalosis may be

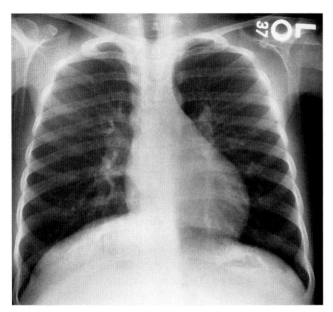

Figure 106.2   *Roentgenogram of the chest of C.T., a 10-year-old girl with α₁-AT deficiency. There were no pulmonary symptoms, but bronchial markings were increased as linear densities, there was hilar prominence, and there was evidence of hyperinflation.*

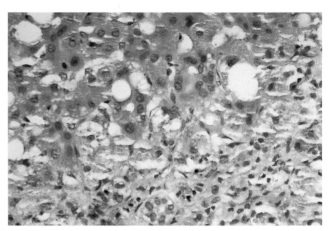

Figure 106.3   *H- and E-stained biopsied liver of a patient with α₁-AT deficiency. Hepatocytes contain eosinophilic globular inclusions. These are especially prominent in periportal areas. In addition, there is fibrosis. (Illustrations in Figures 106.3–106.7 kindly provided by Dr. Henry Krous of the Children's Hospital and Health Center, San Diego, CA.)*

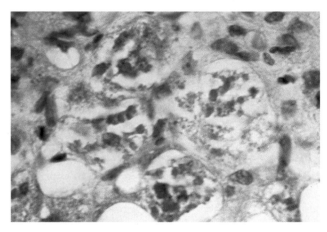

Figure 106.4   *PAS stain after treatment with diastase reveals the bright pink PAS-positive inclusions.*

associated with mild pulmonary hypertension. Electrocardiograms may show chronic strain on the right heart with right axis deviation and right atrial hypertrophy. There may be a right bundle branch block.

The early and more prominent involvement of the lower lobes [31] is in contrast to the preferential involvement of the upper lobes in acquired emphysema. Angiography reveals decreased arborization in the lower lobes in α₁-AT deficiency [32] and radionuclide scanning shows diminished perfusion in these areas [33].

Chronic pulmonary disease in PIZZ children is not common, but some do have clinical or roentgenographic evidence of abnormality (Figure 106.2) [21,22,34], and more have abnormalities detectable by pulmonary function tests. Children with PI null variants may have severe emphysema early in life.

The relationship between smoking and the development of emphysema in this disease has led to the concept of genetic predisposition, in which the defective gene alone is not sufficient to produce the disease, at least by a certain age; noxious elements in the environment combine with the predisposition to yield illness. Smoking influences not only the age of onset of emphysema but the rate of its progression [35–38]. The emphysema is always associated with progressive decrease in lung function. In terms of survival only 18 percent of PIZZ males who smoke are alive at 25 years-of-age, while the figure is 65 percent for nonsmokers. The comparable figures for females are 30 percent and 98 percent [35]. Smoking in adolescence is particularly effective, because maximal pulmonary function is not achieved [39].

The pathology of the lung has indicated that emphysema results from a destructive process involving the alveoli. Electron microscopy reveals extensive destruction of alveolar septal walls with loss of alveolar structure and large air-filled spaces.

The pathology of the liver provided early insights into the molecular pathogenesis of the disease. The distinctive feature is the presence of globules at α₁-AT in the cytoplasm of the hepatocytes [22,40] (Figures 106.3, 106.4). They were present at birth and enlarge with age. They are most prominent in the periportal regions. They stain positively with PAS stain after treatment with diastase (Figure 106.4), and positively with Oil Red O (Figure 106.5). In addition the changes of chronic hepatic disease are nonspecific, but progressive. During the infantile cholestatic stage there is proliferation of bile ducts, fibrosis, some accumulation of fat and occasional giant cells. Later, there is typical cirrhosis. The material has been documented to be α₁-AT by immunofluorescence studies with antibody against α₁-AT (Figure 106.6). In the electron microscopic picture the accumulated amorphous-appearing material is localized to the lumen of the endoplasmic reticulum (Figure 106.7) [22,40].

In addition to disease of the lungs, membranous glomerulonephritis has been observed histopathologically, and some of these patients had signs of renal dysfunction [41]. Some

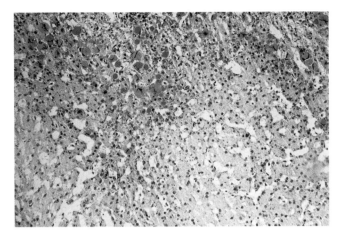

Figure 106.5   *Oil Red O stain indicates some increase in fat.*

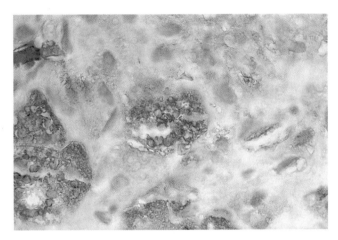

Figure 106.6   *Immunoperoxidase-labeled anti-α_1-antitrypsin antibody identifies the stored material as α_1-antitrypsin.*

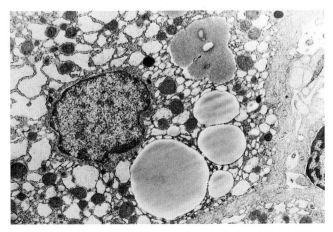

Figure 106.7   *Electron microscopy shows the hepatic inclusions to be membrane-bound.*

evidence of glomerular disease is common at postmortem examination in patients dying of liver disease. Immune complex disease is suggested by immunofluorescent evidence of α_1-AT along with immunoglobulins and C3 on the glomerular basement membrane. A variety of inflammatory disorders have been associated with heterozygosity for the Z allele, including rheumatoid arthritis [42] and uveitis [43]. Severe panniculitis has been reported in 22 homozygotes [44,45].

The diagnosis of α_1-AT deficiency is by quantitative analysis of the content of α_1-AT in serum. Immunologic techniques are the best. The normal range is 20–50 μmol/L, and in the Z variant it is 3–6 μmol/L. Patients with concentrations under 40 percent of normal should be PI typed.

GENETICS AND PATHOGENESIS

The normal α_1-AT phenotype is PIMM, and the classic deficient phenotype is PIZZ [9]. M and Z are codominant autosomal alleles. The heterozygotes are PIMZ. In the PIZZ individual, serum α_1-AT activity is 15 percent of normal. The frequency of the PIZZ phenotype in Sweden, where the disease was discovered, is approximately one in 1500. In the United States, it is one in 6000, and it is more common in those from Europe than from Africa or Asia [20]. The gene frequency for PIZZ in Sweden was reported to be 0.026 [46]. In the United States it is 0.01, while the normal M allele approximates 0.95 [25] and the S allele is 0.03. The PISS homozygote has about 60 percent of normal α_1-AT activity. Among the many other variants [8], most have normal activity. Exceptions are PIII at 68 percent and PIPP at 30 percent of normal [47,48] and the null variants (PI null) in which there is no detectable α_1-AT in serum [8]. Hepatic disease of prenatal origin has been reported in a PIZ null heterozygote [49].

The α_1-AT protein is a glycoprotein with a single polypeptide chain. Its molecular weight is 52 kDa, and its carbohydrate content of 12 percent contains a number of sialic acid residues. The protein synthesized in the liver is longer, containing a signal peptide and an N-terminal methionine [50].

The gene for α_1-AT is located on chromosome 14 at position q32.1 [12,51]. It is 12.2 kb in length and contains 4 exons in a 1434 bp coding region [50]. In classic PIZZ α_1-AT deficiency, a single nucleotide substitution of adenine for guanine codes for a lysine instead of glutamic acid in the M protein (Table 106.1) [13,52]. Oligonucleotide probes have been made which recognize the Z and M sequences and can be used for diagnosis. This is particularly important for prenatal diagnosis, because prior to their development prenatal diagnosis was available only through fetal blood sampling. In the S variant a glutamic

Table 106.1   *Site of the defect in classic α_1-AT deficiency*

PI phenotype	Gene	Protein	Amino acid position
M	GAG	Glutamic acid	342
Z	AAG	Lysine	342

acid at position 264 is changed to valine. Null alleles represent a heterogeneous group of mutations in which a variety of different mechanisms lead to an identical phenotype [53]. Prenatal diagnosis has been carried out in two pregnancies at risk for the ZZ disease by oligonucleotide hybridization to DNA of cultured amniocytes [54]. Both fetuses were found to be MZ heterozygotes. Parental PI typing is essential for prenatal diagnosis to be sure both parents have the Z allele, and that there is no null or rare deficiency allele.

α_1-AT is normally synthesized in the rough endoplasmic reticulum of hepatocytes [8]. Cultured hepatocytes secrete α_1-AT; and *in vivo* α_1-AT is secreted from the liver into the blood. In the Z variant, and other variants in which there is deficiency of α_1-AT, the α_1-AT protein is synthesized normally and levels of mRNA are normal, but the nature of the variant protein is such that it cannot be transported out of the endoplasmic reticulum. The Z variant protein isolated from the liver functions normally [55]. The failure of transport is thought to result from changes in the three-dimensional structures which interfere with normal folding and lead to local aggregation. In the normal protein, the glutamic acid at 342 is thought to form a salt bridge with lysine at 290. The substitution of the lysine at 342 would abolish this salt bridge. Support for this hypothesis was obtained by site-directed mutagenesis in which the lysine 290 in the Z protein was changed to glutamic acid, which would re-establish the salt bridge, and the resultant protein was secreted normally [56]. On the other hand disruption of the salt bridge by changing the wild type lysine 290 to glutamic acid was followed by near normal secretion of the protein, suggesting that tertiary structure is more important than the salt bridge [57]. Aggregation of the Z protein with itself results in the aggregations that form the hepatic inclusions. There is a mobile reactive center loop in the Z protein, which locks into that of another molecule, causing dimerization [58]. This is temperature-sensitive; so an increase in body temperature with fever would be expected to increase aggregation.

The processing of α_1 AT in the endoplasmic reticulum is aided by the transmembrane chaperone calnexin which is involved in the degradation of abnormally folded proteins [59]. Misfolded proteins are dislocated to the cytosol and degraded by the ubiquitin-proteasome system, known as endoplasmic reticulum-associated degradation (ERAD) [11]. A null variant of α_1-AT, Hong Kong, is a substrate for ERAD. Wild type AT was transported to the Golgi, and its carbohydrates were modified into complex glycans. In contrast the stay in the ER of the null protein was prolonged and had protracted interaction with calnexin. Retained incompetent glycoproteins became substrates for the α-mannosidase I that tags ERAD candidates with mannose-8-glycans, which are then subject to accelerated degradation [60].

Introduction of the Z variant human gene into mice led to accumulation of the mutant human protein in mouse liver, and this was followed by hepatic necrosis and inflammation [61].

α_1-AT in the circulation is protective of the lung because it is a very effective inhibitor of elastase and other proteolytic enzymes released from neutrophils and macrophages during the inflammatory process [62,63]. The inactivation of elastase protects the elastic fibers of the lung [63,64]. A growing body of evidence indicates that emphysema represents an imbalance between protease and antiprotease activity in the lung. Elastase itself produces emphysema in experimental animals, as it consumes pulmonary elastin. Furthermore, cigarette smoke inactivates α_1-AT, providing a mechanism for the next most frequent cause of emphysema [65].

TREATMENT

Treatment for hepatic disease is primarily supportive. This includes supplementation with vitamin K and vitamin D. Most patients do not go on to cirrhosis. In those that do cholestyramine may be effective in the management of pruritis. Portacaval or splenorenal shunt may relieve esophageal varices [66]. Transplantation of the liver is curative for advanced hepatic disease [67]. The patient is then left with the prospect of pulmonary disease.

Replacement therapy has been undertaken with intravenous α_1-AT in pharmacological amounts, and protective levels have been obtained in lung fluid as well as serum [68,69]. The product has been licensed in the United States as an Orphan Drug. Recombinant techniques have made available ample quantities [15,16]. Treatment requires weekly intravenous administration, and it is expensive. Analysis of data indicated that the rate of decline of forced expiratory volume was reduced, and so was mortality [38]. Trials were begun with aerosolized α_1-AT [70], because so little intravenously administered protein reaches the lungs. Gene therapy has been accomplished in transgenic mice [17,18].

Avoidance of smoking has been shown to make for an impressive improvement in morbidity and life expectancy [19]. This and the frequency of the gene led to a newborn screening program in Sweden in which 200 000 newborns were screened for α_1-AT deficiency [71,46], but the program was stopped because of unexpected psychological effects. Parents assumed that α_1-AT deficiency posed an immediate serious threat to the health of the child [72], and these negative feelings persisted for 5–7 years [73]. The lesson is that newborn screening requires a considerable effort at public education, and this may be particularly true if the effects of the disease are long delayed. Nevertheless, screening for α_1-AT deficiency combined with a comprehensive program aimed at the avoidance of smoking could markedly decrease morbidity.

References

1 Laurell C-B, Eriksson S. The electrophoretic alpha-1-globulin pattern of serum in alpha-1-antitrypsin deficiency. *Scand J Clin Lab Invest* 1963;**15**:132.

2 Eriksson S. Pulmonary emphysema and alpha-1-antitrypsin deficiency. *Acta Med Scand* 1964;**175**:197.

3 Schultze HE, Gollner I, Heide K, *et al*. Zur Kenntnis der alpha globuline des menschlichen normalserums. *Z Naturforsch* 1955;**10**:463.

4 Schultze HE, Heide K, Haupt H. α_1-Antitrypsin aus humanserum. *Klin Wochenschr* 1962;**40**:427.

5 Eriksson S. Studies in α_1-antitrypsin deficiency. *Acta Med Scand* 1965;**177**:(suppl 432) 5.

6 Fagerhol MK. Serum Pi types in Norwegians. *Acta Pathol Microbiol Scand* 1967;**70**:421.

7 Allen RC, Harley RA, Talamo RC. A new method for determination of alpha-1-antitrypsin phenotypes using isoelectric focusing on polyacrylamide gel slabs. *Am J Clin Pathol* 1974;**62**:732.

8 Fagerhol MK, Cox DW. The Pi polymorphism: genetic biochemical and clinical aspects of human a1-antitrypsin: in *Advances in Human Genetics* (eds H Harris, K Hirschhorn). Plenum Press, New York, London;1981:Vol 11, 1.

9 Fagerhol MK, Laurell CB. The polymorphism of 'prealbumins' and α_1-antitrypsin in human sera. *Clin Chim Acta* 1967;**16**:199.

10 Sharp HL, Bridges RA, Krivit W. Cirrhosis associated with alpha-1-antitrypsin deficiency: a previously unrecognized inherited disorder. *J Lab Clin Med* 1969;**73**:934.

11 Oda Y, Hosokawa N, Wada I, Nagata K. EDEM as an acceptor of terminally misfolded glycoproteins released from calnexin. *Science* 2003;**299**:1394.

12 Schroeder WT, Miller MF, Woo SLC, Saunders GF. Chromosomal localization of the human $\alpha_1\alpha$-antitrypsin gene (PI) to 14q31-32. *Am J Hum Genet* 1985;**37**:868.

13 Jeppsson J-O. Amino acid substitution Gly-Lys in α_1-antitrypsin PiZ. *FEBS Lett* 1976;**65**:195.

14 Yoshida L, Lieberman J, Gaidulis L, Ewing C. Molecular abnormality of human α_1-antitrypsin variant (Pi Z) associated with plasma activity deficiency. *Proc Natl Acad Sci USA* 1976;**73**:1324.

15 George PM, Travis J, Vissers MCM, *et al*. A genetically engineered mutant of α_1-antitrypsin protects connective tissue from neutrophil damage and may be useful in lung disease. *Lancet* 1984;**2**:1426.

16 Courtney M, Buchwalder A, Tessier L-H, *et al*. High-level production of biologically active human α_1-antitrypsin in *Escherichia coli*. *Proc Natl Acad Sci USA* 1984;**81**:669.

17 Sifers RN, Carlson JA, Clift SM, *et al*. Tissue-specific expression of the human alpha-1-antitrypsin gene in transgenic mice. *Nucleic Acids Res* 1987;**15**:1459.

18 Kelsey GD, Povey S, Bygrave AE, Lovell-Badge RH. Species- and tissue-specific expression of human α_1-antitrypsin in transgenic mice. *Genes Dev* 1987;**1**:161.

19 Buist AS. α_1-Antitrypsin deficiency: diagnosis treatment and control: identification of patients. *Lung* 1990;**168**:(suppl) 543.

20 Wulfsberg EA, Hoffman DE, Cohen MC. α_1-Antitrypsin deficiency: impact of genetic discovery on medicine and society. *JAMA* 1994;**271**:217.

21 Sveger T. α_1-Antitrypsin deficiency in early childhood. *Pediatrics* 1978;**62**:22.

22 Moroz SP, Cutz E, Cox DW, Sass-Kortsak A. Liver disease associated with $\alpha_1$antitrypsin deficiency in childhood. *J Pediatr* 1976;**88**:19.

23 Karlaganis G, Nemeth A, Hammarskjold B, *et al*. Urinary excretion of bile alcohols in normal children and patients with α_1-trypsin deficiency during development of liver disease. *Eur J Clin Invest* 1982;**12**:399.

24 Cottrall K, Cook PJL, Mowat AP. Neonatal hepatitis syndrome and alpha-1-antitrypsin deficiency: an epidemiological study in south-east England. *Postgrad Med J* 1974;**50**:376.

25 Latimer JS, Sharp HL. Alpha-1-antitrypsin deficiency in childhood. *Curr Probl Pediatr* 1980;**11**:1.

26 Odiévre M, Martin J-P, Hadchouel M, Alagille D. Alpha-1-antitrypsin deficiency and liver disease in children: phenotypes manifestations and prognosis. *Pediatrics* 1976;**57**:226.

27 Sveger T. Prospective study of children with α_1-antitrypsin deficiency; eight-year-old follow-up. *J Pediatr* 1984;**104**:91.

28 Berg NO, Eriksson S. Liver disease in adults with alpha-1-antitrypsin deficiency. *N Engl J Med* 1972;**287**:1264.

29 Eriksson S. Emphysema before and after 1963. *Ann NY Acad Sci* 1991;**624**:1.

30 Turino GM. Natural history and clinical management of emphysema in patients with and without alpha-1-antitrypsin inhibitor deficiency. *Ann NY Acad Sci* 1991;**624**:18.

31 Guenter CA, Welch MH, Russell TR, *et al*. The pattern of lung disease associated with alpha1-antitrypsin deficiency. *Arch Intern Med* 1968;**122**:254.

32 Stein PD, Leu JD, Welch MH, Guenter CA. Pathophysiology of the pulmonary circulation in emphysema associated with alpha1-antitrypsin deficiency. *Circulation* 1971;**43**:227.

33 Fallat RJ, Powell MR, Kueppers F, Lilker E. 133Xe ventilatory studies in α_1-antitrypsin deficiency. *J Nucl Med* 1972;**14**:5.

34 Talamo RC, Levison H, Lynch MJ, *et al*. Symptomatic pulmonary emphysema in childhood associated with hereditary alpha-1-antitrypsin and elastase inhibitory deficiency. *J Pediatr* 1972;**79**:20.

35 Larsson C. Natural history and life expectancy in severe alpha1-antitrypsin deficiency PiZ. *Acta Med Scand* 1978;**204**:345.

36 Thurlbeck WM, Henderson JA, Fraser RG, Bates DV. Chronic obstructive disease. A comparison between clinical roentgenologic functional and morphologic criteria in chronic bronchitis emphysema asthma and bronchiectasis. *Medicine* 1970;**49**:81.

37 Seersholm N, Kok-Jensen A, Dirksen A. Decline in FEV1 among patients with severe hereditary α_1-antitrypsin deficiency type PiZ. *Am J Respir Crit Care Med* 1995;**152**:1922.

38 α_1-Antitrypsin Deficiency Registry Study Groups: Survival and FEV_1 decline in individuals with severe deficiency of α_1-antitrypsin. *Am J Respir Crit Care Med* 1998;**158**:49.

39 Tager IG, Munoz A, Rosner B, *et al*. Effect of cigarette smoking on the pulmonary function of children and adolescents. *Am Rev Respir Dis* 1985;**131**:752.

40 Sharp HL. α_1-Antitrypsin deficiency. *Hosp Pract* 1971:**55**:83.

41 Moroz SP, Cutz E, Balfe JW. Membranoproliferative glomerulonephritis in childhood cirrhosis associated with alpha-1-antitrypsin deficiency. *Pediatrics* 1976;**57**:232.

42 Cox DW, Huber O. Association of severe rheumatoid arthritis with heterozygosity for α_1-antitrypsin deficiency. *Clin Genet* 1980;**17**:153.

43 Brewerton DA, Webley M, Murphy AH, Milford Ward AM. The α_1-antitrypsin phenotype MZ in acute anterior uveitis. *Lancet* 1978;**1**:1103.

44 Rubinstein HM, Jaffer AM, Kudrna JC, *et al*. α_1-Antitrypsin deficiency with severe panniculitis. *Ann Intern Med* 1977;**86**:742.

45 Breit SN, Clark P, Robinson JP, *et al*. Familial occurrence of α_1-antitrypsin deficiency and Weber-Christian disease. *Arch Dermatol* 1983;**119**:198.z

46 Sveger T. Liver disease in alpha-1-antitrypsin deficiency detected by screening of 200 000 infants. *N Engl J Med* 1976;**294**:1316.

47 Arnaud P, Chapius Cellier C, Vittoz P, Fudenberg H. Genetic polymorphism of serum alpha-1-protease inhibitor (alpha-1-antitrypsin): Pi I a deficient allele of the Pi system. *J Lab Clin Med* 1978;**92**:177.

48 Fagerhol MK, Hauge HE. The PI phenotype MP. Discovery of a ninth allele belonging to the system of inherited variants of serum α_1-antitrypsin. *Vox Sang* 1968;**15**:396.

49 Burn J, Dunger D, Lake B. Liver damage in a neonate with alpha-1-antitrypsin deficiency due to phenotype PiZ Null (Z −). *Arch Dis Child* 1982;**57**:311.

50 Long GI, Chandra T, Woo SLC, *et al*. Complete sequence of the cDNA for human a1-antitrypsin and the gene for the S variant. *Biochemistry* 1984;**23**:4828.

51 Lai EC, Kao F-T, Law ML, Woo SLC. Assignment of the α_1-antitrypsin gene and a sequence-related gene to human chromosome 14 by molecular hybridization. *Am J Hum Genet* 1983;**35**:385.

52 Kidd VJ, Wallace B, Itakura K, Woo SLC. α_1-Antitrypsin deficiency detection by direct analysis of the mutation in the gene. *Nature* 1983;**304**:230.

53 Curiel D, Brantly M, Curiel E, *et al.* α_1-Antitrypsin deficiency caused by the α_1-antitrypsin Null$_{Mattawa}$ gene: An insertion mutation rendering the α_1-antitrypsin gene incapable of producing α_1-antitrypsin. *J Clin Invest* 1989;**83**:1144.

54 Kidd VJ, Golbus MS, Wallace RB, *et al.* Prenatal diagnosis of a-1-antitrypsin deficiency by direct analysis of the mutation site in the gene. *N Engl J Med* 1984;**310**:639.

55 Miller RR, Kuhlenschmidt MS, Coffee CJ, *et al.* Comparison of the chemical physical and survival properties of normal and Z-variant alpha-1-antitrypsins. *J Biol Chem* 1976;**251**:4751.

56 Brantly M, Courtney M, Crystal RG. Repair of the secretion defect in the Z form of a-1-antitrypsin by addition of a second mutation. *Science* 1988;**242**:1700.

57 Foreman RC. Disruption of the Lys 290-Glu 342 salt bridge in human α_1-antitrypsin does not prevent its synthesis and secretion. *FEBS Lett* 1987;**216**:79.

58 Lomas DA, Evans DL, Finch JT, Carrell RW. The mechanism of Z α_1-antitrypsin accumulation in the liver. *Nature* 1992;**357**:605.

59 Qu D, Teckman JH, Omura S, Perlmutter DH. Degradation of a mutant secretory protein α_1-antitrypsin Z in the endoplasmic reticulum requires proteosome activity. *J Biol Chem* 1996;**271**:22791.

60 Molinari M, Calanca V, Galli C, *et al.* Role of EDEM in release of misfolded glycoproteins from the calnexin cycle. *Science* 2003;**299**:1397.

61 Carlson JA, Barton Rogers B, Sifers RN, *et al.* Accumulation of PiZ α_1-antitrypsin causes liver damage in transgenic mice. *J Clin Invest* 1989;**83**:1183.

62 Snider GL, Ciccolella DE, Morris SM, *et al.* Putative role of neutrophil elastase in the pathogenesis of emphysema. *Ann NY Acad Sci* 1991;**624**:45.

63 Gadek JE, Fells GA, Zimmerman RL, *et al.* Antielastases of the human alveolar structures: implications for the protease-anti-protease theory of emphysema. *J Clin Invest* 1981;**68**:889.

64 Gadek JE, Hunninghake GW, Fells GA, *et al.* Evaluation of the protease-antiprotease theory of human destructive lung disease. *Bull Eur Physiopathol Respir* 1980;**16**:27.

65 Gadek JE, Pacht ER. The protease-antiprotease balance within the human lung: implications for the pathogenesis of emphysema. *Lung* 1990;**168**:(suppl) 552.

66 Sotos JF, Cutler EA, Romshe CA, Clatworthy HW Jr. Successful spleno-renal shunt and splenectomy in two patients with alpha-1-antitrypsin deficiency. *J Pediatr Surg* 1981;**16**:12.

67 Hood JM, Koep LJ, Peters RL, *et al.* Liver transplantation for advanced liver disease with alpha-1-antitrypsin deficiency. *N Engl J Med* 1980;**302**:272.

68 Wewers MD, Casolaro MA, Sellers SE, *et al.* Replacement therapy for alpha-1-antitrypsin deficiency associated with emphysema. *N Engl J Med* 1989;**316**:1055.

69 Hubbard RC, Sellers S, Czerski D, *et al.* Biochemical efficacy and safety of monthly augmentation therapy of alpha-1-antitrypsin deficiency. *JAMA* 1988;**260**:1259.

70 Hubbard RC, Crystal RG. Strategies for aerosol therapy of alpha-1-antitrypsin deficiency by the aerosol route. *Lung* 1990;**168**:(suppl) 565.

71 Laurell C-B, Sveger T. Mass screening of newborn Swedish infants for α_1-antitrypsin deficiency. *Am J Hum Genet* 1975;**27**:213.

72 Thelin T, McNeil TJ, Aspegren-Jansson E, Sveger T. Psychological consequences of neonatal screening for alpha-1-antitrypsin deficiency. Parental reactions to the first news of their infants' deficiency. *Acta Paediatr Scand* 1985;**74**:787.

73 Thelin T, McNeil TF, Aspegren-Jansson E, Sveger T. Identifying children at high somatic risk: parents' long-term emotional adjustment to their children's alpha1-antitrypsin deficiency. *Acta Psychiatr Scand* 1985;**72**:323.

Canavan disease/aspartoacylase deficiency

MAJOR PHENOTYPIC EXPRESSION

Hypotonia, delayed development, megalenocephaly, optic atrophy, seizures, neurodegeneration, hypodense white matter, the imaging counterpart of histologic spongy degeneration, N-acetylaspartic aciduria and deficiency of aspartoacylase.

INTRODUCTION

Canavan disease is a progressive neurodegenerative leukodystrophy which is often fatal in the first 10 years of life. It is generally agreed that the definitive delineation of this disorder as a distinct clinical and pathologic entity was that of van Bogaert and Bertrand in 1949 [1,2]. Canavan's report in 1931 [3] was of an infant with a prominently enlarged head and spongy degeneration of white matter of the brain. There was a previous description by Globus and Strauss [4] in 1928. These authors and Canavan referred to these patients as having Schilder disease, but it is clear that this term has been used for a wide variety of conditions and, despite some objections [5], the term Canavan disease is the one by which this disease is known. Eiselberg [6] recognized the genetic nature of the disease. Its prevalence in Ashkenazic Jews [7–9] was recognized by van Bogaert and Bertrand [1,2] but the disorder is panethnic.

The urinary excretion of N-acetylaspartic acid was reported by Kvittingen, Hagenfeldt and their colleagues [10,11]. The former reported aspartoacylase activity (Figure 107.1) as normal [10], while the latter correctly documented the deficiency of this enzyme [11]. However, neither group appreciated

that they were dealing with Canavan disease. The association of aspartoacylase deficiency and N-acetyl-aspartic aciduria with Canavan disease was made by Matalon [12] and Divry [13,14] and their colleagues in 1988. Aspartoacylase (EC 3.5.1.15) catalyzes the hydrolysis of N-acetylaspartic acid to l-aspartic and acetic acids (Figure 107.1). Kaul and his colleagues [15–18] cloned the cDNA for aspartoacylase and localized it to the terminal end of the short arm of chromosome 17. They have identified a number of mutations and in the case of the Ashkenazic Jewish population proposed a founder effect in the basis of the predominance of two mutations [19].

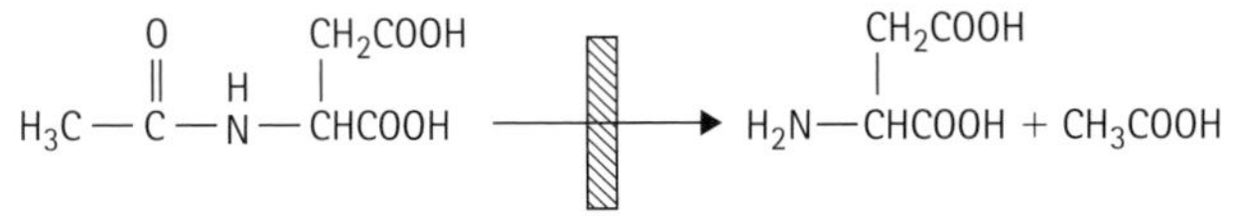

CLINICAL ABNORMALITIES

Patients with this disease usually appear normal at birth and during the first few months. In the classic presentation, axial hypotonia and enlarged head are usually evident by the second to the fourth months [7–9,20–24]. Some infants have been noted to have irritability, poor visual fixation and poor suck from birth [25]. Spontaneous movements are decreased. The disease has been divided [19,22] into congenital, infantile and juvenile forms. The classic infantile form, which accounts for most of the patients, is evident by 6 months; the more aggressive congenital form may be evident in the first weeks of life, and the juvenile by 4 to 5 years [26–29]. The enzyme deficiency has been documented in two juvenile patients [19,29], in two of the congenital forms, and in at

Figure 107.1 *The aspartoacylase reaction.*

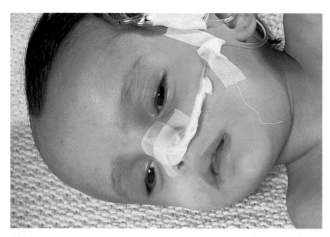

Figure 107.2   H.A., a female infant with Canavan disease. Macrocephaly was already evident.

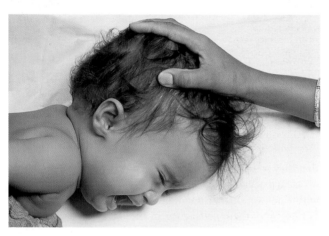

Figure107.3   F.H. This infant with Canavan disease was more strikingly macrocephalic.

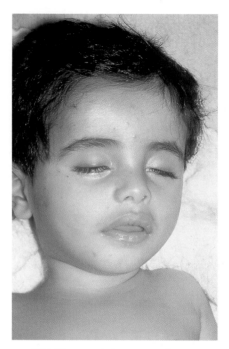

Figure 107.4   N.M. Macrocephaly was prominent.

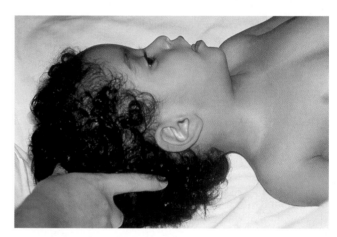

Figure107.5   M.M. A macrocephalic infant with Canavan disease.

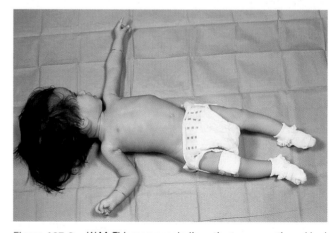

Figure 107.6   W.M. This macrocephalic patient was spastic and had assumed a tonic neck reflex posture.

least 161 infantile patients [19,30–32]. The advent of enzyme analysis and the definition of the nature of mutations may make these classifications obsolete; correlations of phenotype with genotype may emerge.

Macrocephaly is evident by 6 months, and by one year the head circumference is in the 90th percentile or above [33] (Figures 107.2–107.6). There may be delayed closure of the anterior fontanel. The weight of the brain is found to be increased at autopsy, and this is true for at least the first 3 years [34]; brain weight decreases in those dying later. Hypotonia, head lag or poor head control and macrocephaly have been suggested [19] as a diagnostic triad.

With progression, milestones achieved such as smiling and grasping may be lost. The infant becomes inattentive. With time, the hypotonia is replaced by spasticity [5,19,35] (Figures 107.6–107.8), and there may be opisthotonic posturing with tonic extensor spasms, accentuated deep tendon reflexes and positive Babinski responses. Irritability and disturbed sleeping occur. Patients develop early blindness, and optic atrophy (Figure 107.9) is associated with nystagmus [9].

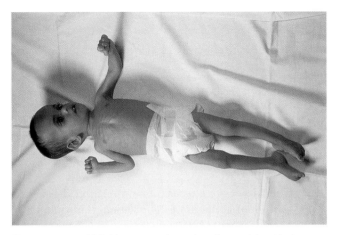

Figure 107.7   *M.S. Also assumed a tonic reflex position. Heel cords already appeared shortened.*

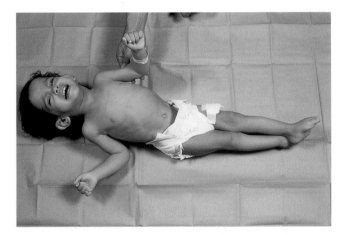

Figure107.8   *A.G. This patient with Canavan disease demonstrated advanced spastic quadriplegia.*

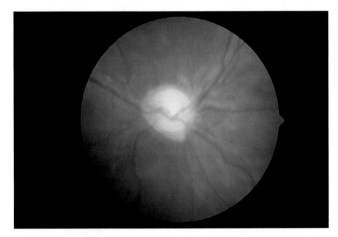

Figure107.9   *M.M. Fundus photograph.*

Seizures, tonic and clonic, develop in the second year of life in about 50 percent of patients. Weight gain falls off, and difficulty with swallowing and gastroesophageal reflux may require gastrostomy. Late findings are decerebrate or decorticate posturing.

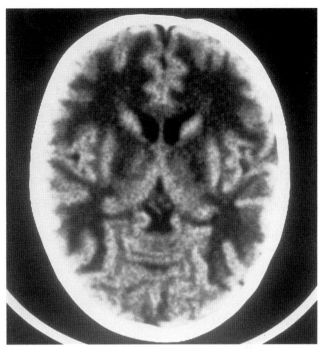

Figure 107.10   *CT scan of the brain revealed diffuse symmetrical disease of the white matter.*

Among patients with the juvenile form of the disease [26–29,36–39] there may be a progressive cerebellar syndrome with dysarthria and tremor leading to spasticity and dementia. There may be optic atrophy and retinal pigmentation. Temperature instability is common, and pneumonia may be the cause of death.

Neuroimaging by computed tomography (CT) (Figure 107.10) or magnetic resonance imaging (MRI) reveals diffuse symmetrical white matter disease [35,39–47]. T2 weighted images on MRI show generalized increase in signal throughout the subcortical cerebral white matter. The cerebellum and brainstem are less markedly involved. Decreased intensity is seen on T1 images and CT and increased signal on T2. Leukodystrophy can also be demonstrated by ultrasound [48]. Changes in white matter may sometimes be absent [29]. Nuclear magnetic resonance (NMR) spectroscopy has been used to demonstrate increased amounts of N-acetylaspartic acid in the brain *in vivo* [42–45,49] or amounts disproportionate to choline and creatine [50].

Electroencephalograph (EEG) changes, such as excessive slow activity and poor sleep spindle formations, have been described in approximately 40 percent of the patients [35]. The EEG may be notable for the lack of epileptiform discharges in patients who had generalized convulsions. In the majority of patients, visual or auditory evoked responses (VER and BAER) were absent, or showed delayed latencies [35].

The histopathology of Canavan disease – the spongy degeneration (Figure 107.11) [1,2,5,22,34,51] – is the characteristic by which this disease was classically defined. The gross character of the white matter is soft or gelatinous. The vacuolization is seen in the subcortical white and lower layers of gray

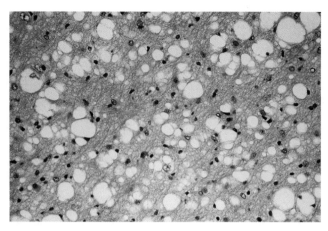

Figure 107.11 *Histopathology of the brain in Canavan disease. This is the classic picture of spongy degeneration with large vacuoles.*

Table 107.1 *Mutations in the aspartoacylase gene in Canavan disease*

Nucleotide change	Protein change	Frequency	
		Jewish	Non-Jewish
854 A to G	285 Glu to Ala	0.836	0.014
693 C to A	231 Tyr to Stop	0.134	0.028
914 C to A	305 Ala to Glu	0.019	

matter. Astrocytes are increased in number. Electron microscopy reveals swollen astrocytes with elongated mitochondria with distorted cristae [26,34,37,51–53]. There are membrane-bound vacuoles within the swollen cytoplasm of the astrocytes. Extensive loss of myelin is mirrored in a decrease in lipid content of the white matter [54,55].

GENETICS AND PATHOGENESIS

Canavan disease is transmitted in an autosomal recessive fashion. Consanguinity has been reported in as many as 23 percent of families [7]. The disease is panethnic in distribution, but it is particularly prevalent in Ashkenazic Jews [7,19]; the disease is also common in Saudi Arabia [56].

The molecular defect is in the activity of aspartoacylase [12–14] (Figure 107.1, p. 725). The enzyme catalyzes the conversion of N-acetylaspartic acid to aspartic acid and acetic acid. The enzyme purified from bovine brain is a 55 kDa monomer [57] and it is particularly abundant in white matter. Immunohistochemical localization of the enzyme in mammalian brain showed abundance in myelin [58]. Activity of enzyme is readily assayed in cultured fibroblasts [11,12,59].

The bovine cDNA was isolated by Matalon and colleagues following purification and partial sequencing of the enzyme [31]. This cDNA was employed in the isolation of the human cDNA [15]. The protein predicted for the cDNA contains 313 amino acids. The gene spans 29 kb, and there are six exons; the human gene is located on chromosome 17p13-pter [18].

Two mutations were found in the Ashkenazic population [16,60] (Table 107.1). The most frequent is a missense mutation at codon 854, which changes glutamic acid 285 to an alanine and accounts for 84 percent of 104 alleles tested [19]. Another missense mutation (Y231X) changing tyrosine to a stop-codon accounted for 13 percent of Jewish alleles [16]. A number of other mutations have been identified, including a splicing mutation in the second intron (433-2A → G) [16].

Among non-Jews, the most common mutation, accounting for 93 percent of alleles in this population, is in codon 914, which changes alanine 305 to glutamic acid [16,61]. A spectrum of mutations has been found in non-Jews [61].

Carrier detection is most readily done by molecular techniques in families in which the mutation is known. It has been employed in the screening of Jewish populations for the two common mutations [19]. Assay of the enzyme for heterozygote detection requires cultured fibroblasts.

Prenatal diagnosis by assay of the enzyme in cultured amniocytes or chorionic villus material is unreliable because the activity is usually so low [62,63]. Prenatal diagnosis has been accomplished by gas chromatography/mass spectrometry (GCMS) analysis for N-acetylaspartic acid in amniotic fluid; isotope dilution internal standard methods are preferable [63,64] because the differences between affected and unaffected values are small. Also concentrations increase in normal amniotic fluid as gestation proceeds. DNA analysis is preferred if the mutation is known; the frequency of the C-854 mutation in Jewish populations makes it particularly useful [19,65]. The mutation creates a restriction enzyme recognition sequence for EagI [15] converting a normal 183 bp fragment to two of 123 and 60 bp.

In the presence of defective activity of aspartoacylase, the major metabolic consequence is the accumulation of N-acetylaspartic acid in body fluids. It is readily detected in the urine (Figure 107.12). The mean level in 95 patients was 1441 ± 873 mmol/mol creatinine [31]. In 53 normal individuals, the mean was 24 ± 16 mmol/mol creatinine. Levels in patients were usually twenty times the upper limit of normal.

The compound is also elevated in the blood and cerebrospinal fluid [12]. The diagnosis is usually made by GCMS analysis of N-acetylaspartic acid in the urine [66,67].

The compound is found in cells only in mammalian nervous tissues [68,69], where its concentration is very high. A level of 8 mmol/g tissue has been reported [19]. This concentration is second only to glutamic acid in brain. The compound is formed from acetylCoA and aspartic acid in a reaction catalyzed by acetylCoA-L-aspartate-N-acetyl transferase [70,71]. It is thought that the synthesis takes place in mitochondria [72]. Synthesis is in the gray matter, where aspartoacylase is undetectable [57,73]. The function of the compound in the metabolism of the brain is not clear. It is possible that toxicity of the compound itself accounts for the neurodegeneration that characterizes the disease.

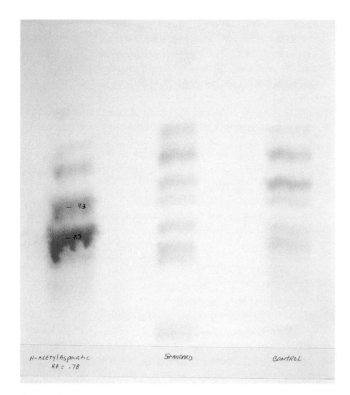

N-ACETYL|ASPARTIC
RF = .78   STANDARD   CONTROL

Figure 107.12 *High voltage electrophoretic pattern of N-acetyl-aspartic acid.*

TREATMENT

Supportive treatment is the only available modality.

References

1 van Bogaert L, Bertrand I. Sur une idiotie familiale avec dégénérescence spongieuse de néuraxe. *Acta Neurol Belg* 1949;**49**:572.

2 van Bogaert L, Bertrand I. *Spongy Degeneration of the Brain: in Infancy.* North Holland Publishing Co, Amsterdam;1967:3.

3 Canavan MM. Schilder's encephalitis periaxialis diffusa. *Arch Neurol Psychiatr* 1931;**25**:299.

4 Globus JH, Strauss I. Progressive degenerative subcortical encephalopathy (Schilder's disease). *Arch Neurol Psychiatr* 1928;**20**:1190.

5 Banker BQ, Robertson JT, Victor M. Spongy degeneration of the central nervous system in infancy. *Neurology* 1964;**14**:981.

6 Eiselberg F. Uber frühkindliche familiääre diffuse Hirnsklerose. *Z Kinderheilk* 1937;**58**:702.

7 Banker BQ, Victor H. Spongy degeneration of infancy: in *Genetic Diseases Among Ashkenazi Jews* (eds RM Goodman, AG Motulsky). Raven Press, New York;1979:201.

8 Goodman RM. *Genetic Disorders Among Jewish People.* Johns Hopkins University Press, Baltimore;1979:109.

9 Ungar M, Goodman RM. Spongy degeneration of the brain in Israel: a retrospective study. *Clin Genet* 1984;**23**:23.

10 Kvittingen EA, Guldal B, Børsting S, *et al.* N-acetylaspartic aciduria in a child with a progressive cerebral atrophy. *Clin Chim Acta* 1986;**158**:217.

11 Hagenfeldt L, Bollgren I, Venizelos N. N-acetyl-aspartic aciduria due to aspartoacylase deficiency – a new aetiology of childhood leukodystrophy. *J Inherit Metab Dis* 1987;**10**:135.

12 Matalon R, Michals K, Sebesta D, *et al.* Asparto-acylase deficiency and N-acetylaspartic aciduria in patients with Canavan Disease. *Am J Med Genet* 1988;**29**:463.

13 Divry P, Vianey-Liaud C, Gay C, *et al.* N-acetyl-aspartic aciduria: report of three new cases in children with a neurological syndrome associated with macrocephaly and leukodystrophy. *J Inherit Metab Dis* 1988;**11**:307.

14 Divry P, Mathieu M. Aspartoacylase deficiency and N-acetylaspartic aciduria in patients with Canavan disease. *Am J Med Genet* 1989;**32**:550.

15 Kaul R, Gao GP, Balamurugan K, Matalon R. Cloning of the human aspartoacylase cDNA and a common missense mutation in Canavan disease. *Nat Genet* 1993;**5**:118.

16 Kaul R, Gao GP, Aloya M, *et al.* Canavan disease: mutations among Jewish and non-Jewish patients. *Am J Hum Genet* 1994;**55**:34.

17 Kaul R, Gao GP, Michals K, *et al.* A novel (cys 152 > arg) missense mutation in an Arab patient with Canavan disease. *Hum Mutat* 1995; **5**:269.

18 Kaul R, Balamurugan K, Gao GP, Matalon R. Canavan disease: genomic organization and localization of human ASPA to 17p13-ter and conservation of the ASPA gene during evolution. *Genomics* 1994;**21**:364.

19 Matalon R, Michals K, Kaul R. Canavan disease: from spongy degeneration to molecular analysis. *J Pediatr* 1995;**127**:511.

20 Buchanan DS, Davis RL. Spongy degeneration of the nervous system: a report of 4 cases with a review of the literature. *Neurology* 1965;**15**:207.

21 Sacks O, Brown WJ, Aguilar MJ. Spongy degeneration of white matter Canavan's sclerosis. *Neurology* 1965;**15**:2165.

22 Adachi M, Schneck L, Cara J, Volk BW. Spongy degeneration of the central nervous system (van Bogaert and Bertrand type; Canavan disease). *Hum Pathol* 1973;**4**:331.

23 Gambetti P, Mellman WJ, Gonatas NK. Familial spongy degeneration of the central nervous system (van Bogaert-Bertrand disease). *Acta Neuropathol* 1969;**12**:103.

24 Hogan GR, Richardson GP Jr. Spongy degeneration of nervous system (Canavan's disease): report of a case in an Irish-American family. *Pediatrics* 1965;**35**:284.

25 Traeger EC, Rapin I. The clinical course of Canavan disease. *Pediatr Neurol* 1998;**18**:207.

26 Goodhue WW Jr, Couch RD, Namiki H. Spongy degeneration of the CNS: an instance of the rare juvenile form. *Arch Neurol* 1979;**36**:481.

27 Bruchner JM, Dom R, Robin A. Dégénérescence spongieuse juvenile du système nerveux centrale. *Rev Neurol (Paris)* 1968;**119**:425.

28 Jellinger K, Seitelberger F. Juvenile form of spongy degeneration of the CNS. *Acta Neuropathol* 1969;13:276.

29 Toft PB, Geiss-Holtorff R, Rolland MO, *et al.* Magnetic resonance imaging in juvenile Canavan disease. *Eur J Pediatr* 1993;**152**:750.

30 Matalon R, Kaul R, Michals K. Canavan disease: in *The Molecular and Genetic Basis of Neurological Disease* (eds RN Rosenberg, SB Prusiner, S DiMauro, *et al*). Butterworth-Heineman, Boston;1993:541.

31 Matalon R, Kaul R, Michals K. Canavan disease: biochemical and molecular studies *J Inherit Metab Dis* 1993;**16**:744.

32 Matalon R, Kaul R, Michals K. Spongy degeneration of the brain: Canavan disease: in *Pediatric Neuropathology* (ed. S Duckett). Williams and Wilkins, Baltimore;1995:625.

33 Ozand PT, Gascon GG, Dhalla M. Aspartoacylase deficiency and Canavan disease in Saudi Arabia. *Am J Med Genet* 1990;**35**:266.

34 Adachi M, Aronson SM. Studies on spongy degeneration of the central metabolism (van Bogaert-Bertrand type): in *Inborn Errors of Sphingolipid Metabolism* (eds SM Aronson, BW Volk). Pergamon Press, Oxford;1967:129.

35 Gascon GG, Ozand PT, Mahdi A, *et al.* Infantile CNS spongy degeneration – 14 cases: clinical update. *Neurology* 1990;**40**:1876.

36 von Moers A, Sperner J, Michael T, *et al.* Variable course of Canavan disease in two boys with early infantile aspartoacylase deficiency. *Dev Med Child Neurol* 1991;**33**:824.

37 Adachi M, Volk BW. Protracted form of spongy degeneration of the central nervous system (van Bogaert and Bertrand type). *Neurology* 1968;**18**:1084.

38 Zelnik N, Luder AS, Elpeleg ON, *et al.* Protracted clinical course for patients with Canavan disease. *Dev Med Child Neurol* 1993;**35**:355.

39 Zafeiriou DI, Kleijer WJ, Maroupoulos G, *et al.* Protracted course of N-acetylaspartic aciduria in two non-Jewish siblings: identical clinical and magnetic resonance imaging findings. *Brain Dev* 1999;**21**:205.

40 Brismar J, Brismar G, Gascon GG, Ozand P. Canavan disease CT and MR imaging of the brain. *Am J Neuroradiol* 1990;**11**:805.

41 Matalon R, Michals J, Kaul R, Mafee M. Spongy degeneration of the brain: Canavan disease. *Int Pediatr* 1990;**5**:121.

42 Grodd W, Krägeloh-Mann I, Petersen D, *et al. In vivo* assessment of N-acetylaspartate in brain in spongy degeneration (Canavan disease) by proton spectroscopy. *Lancet* 1990;**336**:437.

43 Marks HG, Caro PA, Wang ZY, *et al.* Use of computed tomography magnetic resonance imaging and localized 1H magnetic resonance spectroscopy in Canavan's disease: a case report. *Ann Neurol* 1991;**30**:106.

44 Austin SJ, Connelly A, Gadian DG, *et al.* Localized 1H-NMR spectroscopy in Canavan's disease: a report of two cases. *Magn Reson Med* 1991;**19**:439.

45 Grodd W, Krägeloh-Mann I, Klose U, Sauter R. Metabolic and destructive brain disorders in children: findings with localized proton MR spectroscopy. *Radiology* 1991;**181**:173.

46 Boltshauser E, Isher W. Computerized axial tomography in spongy degeneration. *Lancet* 1976;**1**:1123.

47 McAdams HP, Geyer CA, Done SL, *et al.* CT and MR imaging of Canavan disease. *Am J Neuroradiol* 1990;**11**:397.

48 Bührer C, Bassir C, von Moers A, *et al.* Cranial ultrasound findings in aspartoacylase deficiency (Canavan disease). *Pediatr Radiol* 1993;**23**:395.

49 Wittsack H-J, Kugel H, Roth B, Heindel W. Quantitative measurements with localized ^{1}H MR spectroscopy in children with Canavan's disease. *J Magn Reson Imaging* 1996;**6**:889.

50 Barker PB, Bryan RN, Kumar AJ, Naidu S. Proton NMR spectroscopy of Canavan disease. *Neuropediatrics* 1992;**23**:263.

51 Adachi M, Torii J, Schneck L, Volk BW. Electron microscopic and enzyme histochemical studies of the cerebellum in spongy degeneration (van Bogaert and Bertrand type). *Acta Neuropathol* 1972;**20**:22.

52 Adornato BT, O'Brien JS, Lampert PW, *et al.* Cerebral spongy degeneration of infancy: a biochemical and ultrastructural study of affected twins. *Neurology* 1972;**22**:202.

53 Luo Y, Huang K. Spongy degeneration of the CNS in infancy. *Arch Neurol* 1984;**41**:164.

54 Kamoshita S, Rapin I, Suzuki K, Suzuki K. Spongy degeneration of the brain. Neurology 1968;**19**:975.

55 Lees MB, Folch-Pi J. A study of some human brains with pathological changes: in *Chemical Pathology of the Nervous System* (ed. J Folch-Pi). Pergamon Press, Oxford;1961:75.

56 Ozand PT, Devol EB, Gascon GG. Neuro-metabolic diseases at a national referral center: five years' experience at the King Faisal Specialist Hospital and Research Centre. *J Child Neurol* 1992;**7**:(suppl) S4.

57 Kaul RK, Casanova J, Johnson A, *et al.* Purification characterization and localization of aspartoacylase from bovine brain. *J Neurochem* 1991;**56**:129.

58 Johnson A, Kaul R, Casanova J, Matalon R. Aspartoacylase the deficient enzyme in spongy degeneration (Canavan disease) is a myelin-associated enzyme. *J Neuropathol Exp Neurol* 1989;**48**:349 (abstr).

59 Barash V, Flhor D, Morag B, *et al.* A radiometric assay for aspartoacylase activity in fibroblasts: application for the diagnosis of Canavan's disease. *Clin Chim Acta* 1991;**201**:175.

60 Shaag A, Anikster Y, Christensen E, Glustein JZ, *et al.* The molecular basis of Canavan (aspartoacylase deficiency) disease in European non-Jewish patients. *Am J Hum Genet* 1995;**57**:572.

61 Elpeleg ON, Shaag A. The spectrum of mutations of the aspartoacylase gene in Canavan disease in non-Jewish patients. *J Inherit Metab Dis* 1999;**22**:531.

62 Matalon R, Michals K, Gashkoff P, Kaul R. Prenatal diagnosis of Canavan disease *J Inherit Metab Dis* 1992;**15**:392.

63 Bennett MJ, Gibson KM, Sherwood WG, *et al.* Reliable prenatal diagnosis of Canavan disease (asparto-acylase deficiency): comparison of enzymatic and metabolite analysis. *J Inherit Metab Dis* 1993;**16**:831.

64 Kelley RI. Prenatal diagnosis of Canavan disease by measurement of N-acetyl-aspartate in amniotic fluid. *J Inherit Metab Dis* 1993;**16**:918.

65 Elpeleg ON, Shaag A, Anikster Y, Jakobs C. Prenatal detection of Canavan disease (aspartoacylase deficiency) by DNA analysis. *J Inherit Metab Dis* 1994;**17**:664.

66 Jakobs C, ten Brink HJ, Langelaar SA, *et al.* Stable isotope dilution analysis of N-acetylaspartic acid in CSF blood urine and amniotic fluid: accurate postnatal diagnosis and the potential for prenatal diagnosis of Canavan disease. *J Inherit Metab Dis* 1991;**14**:653.

67 Kelley RI, Stamas JN. Quantification of N-acetyl-L-aspartic acid in urine by isotope dilution gas chromatography-mass spectrometry. *J Inherit Metab Dis* 1992;**15**:97.

68 Tallan HH, Moore S, Stein WH. N-Acetyl-l-aspartic acid in brain. *J Biol Chem* 1956;**219**:257.

69 Birken DL, Oldendorf WH. N-Acetylaspartic acid: a literature review of a compound prominent in 1H-NMR spectroscopic studies of brain. *Neurosci Biobehav Rev* 1989;**13**:23.

70 Knizley H Jr. The enzymatic synthesis of N-acetyl-1-aspartic acid by a water-insoluble preparation of a cat brain acetone powder. *J Biol Chem* 1967;**242**:4619.

71 Goldstein FB. Biosynthesis of N-acetyl-1-aspartic acid. *J Biol Chem* 1959;**234**:2702.

72 Patel TB, Clark JB. Synthesis of N-acetyl-l-aspartate by rat brain mitochondria and its involvement in mitochondrial cytosolic carbon transport. *Biochem J* 1979;**184**:539.

73 Truckenmiller ME, Namboodiri MAA, Brownstein MJ, Neale JH. N-Acetylation of 1-aspartate in the nervous system: differential distribution of a specific enzyme. *J Neurochem* 1985;**45**:1658.

Glutamyl-ribose-5-phosphate storage disease/ ADP-ribosyl-protein lyase deficiency

MAJOR PHENOTYPIC EXPRESSION

Progressive neurological degeneration and renal failure, accumulation of glutamyl-ribose-5-phosphate and deficiency of ADP-ribosyl-protein lyase.

INTRODUCTION

Deficiency of ADP-ribosyl-protein lyase leads to a disorder that may be a model for other diseases that affect the central nervous system, in which the small molecule that must be detected to identify the presence of the disease does not get out of the central nervous system. Glutamyl ribose-5-phosphate accumulates in this disorder, but it was found only when brain tissue became available at autopsy [1]. It is now apparent that the compound also accumulates in kidney; so the diagnosis could be made by renal biopsy.

The marker compound was found in lysosomes. It was isolated and its structure was determined to be that of glutamyl-ribose-5-phosphate [2] (Figure 108.1). This represents the linkage region of ADP-ribosyl-histone proteins. Its structure

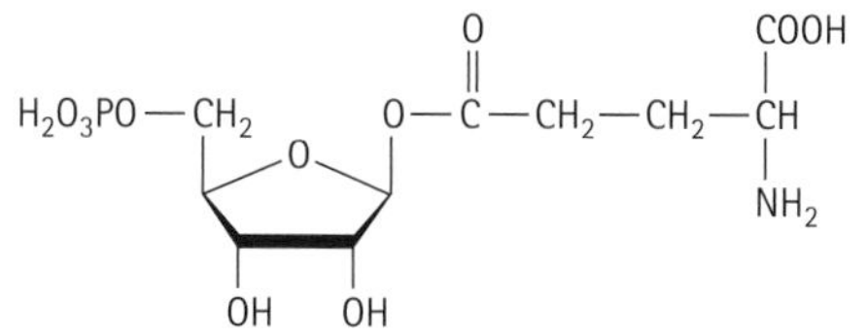

Figure 108.1 *Structure of glutamyl ribose-5-phosphate.*

suggested that the molecular defect was in the enzyme ADP-ribosyl-protein lyase (Figure 108.2). This has now been documented by studies on tissues of the original patient [3]. This was the first reported heritable defect in poly(ADP-ribosyl)ation.

CLINICAL ABNORMALITIES

The disorder has to date been described in a single patient, a boy who died at 8 years after a 6-year period of progressive neurologic deterioration and renal failure.

The patient developed normally until 2 years-of-age, when his speech and language began to deteriorate. At 3 years, he had a febrile grand mal seizure and thereafter had daily akinetic seizures. He developed microcephaly, proteinuria, hypoalbuminemia and biopsy evidence of focal segmental glomerulosclerosis. Developmental delay was evident.

On examination at 5 years, he weighed 4 kg and was 102 cm long. Head circumference was 47.5 cm. His facies was mildly coarse (Figures 108.3, 108.4), and he had optic atrophy, generalized hypotonia, muscular wasting and frequent seizures. Electroencephalogram (EEG) revealed slow waves and multiphasic spikes. The electroretinogram was consistent with degeneration of photoreceptors. The cerebral ventricles

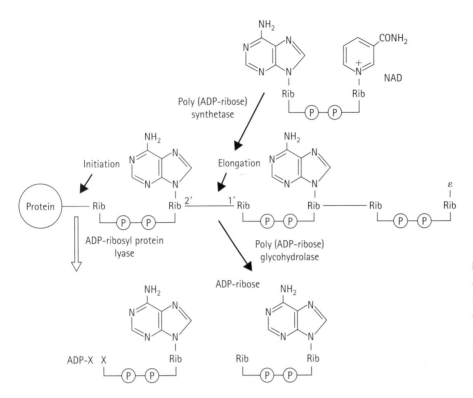

Figure 108.2   *Poly(ADP-ribosyl)protein and its metabolism. Two different sugars have been observed in the position designated X in the product of the lyase reaction, each a deoxypentose. The abbreviation ε, for etc., indicates elongation by the addition of repeating ADP ribose units, including branched structures.*

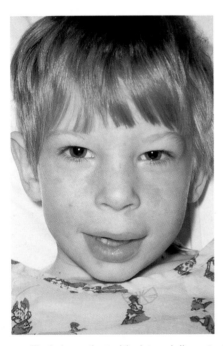

Figure 108.3   *The index patient with glutamyl ribose-5-phosphate storage disease. The facial appearance was somewhat coarse.*

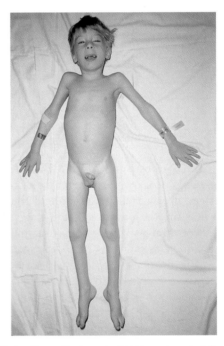

Figure 108.4   *The patient was bedridden and wasted. Deep tendon reflexes were accentuated.*

were dilated. Electron microscopy following conjunctival biopsy revealed lysosomes containing granular and lamellar material.

By 6 years-of-age he could not walk and spoke only single words, and hypotonia had increased. There was severe optic atrophy and granular retinopathy, decreased deep tendon reflexes and nystagmus on lateral gaze. The creatinine was 0.5 mg/dL and the albumin 2.2 g/dL. He excreted 1.7 g of protein in 24 hours and had a generalized amino aciduria. Over the next 2 years, renal and neurological function progressively deteriorated and he died of renal failure. Renal histology revealed focal segmental glomerulosclerosis (Figure 108.5), and localized interstitial fibrosis. On electron microscopy there was effacement of glomerular foot processes. There was evidence of end-stage renal disease, uremic pericarditis and

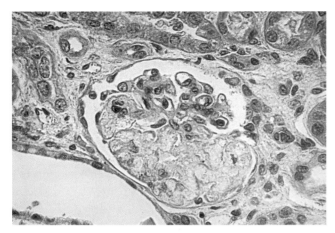

Figure 108.5 *Glomerulus of the biopsied kidney was sclerotic.*

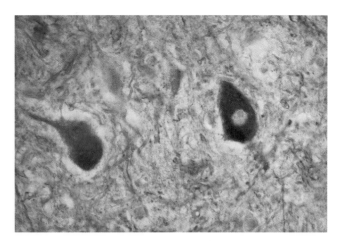

Figure 108.7 *Brain stem neuronal storage with PAS stain.*

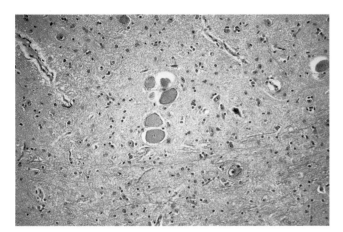

Figure 108.6 *Brain stem neurons contained stored material (H and E stain).*

pancreatitis. The brain was small; it weighed 862 g and displayed diffuse cortical atrophy. There was evidence of widespread neuronal loss. Neurons also revealed evidence of stored material (Figures 108.6, 108.7).

The enzyme (Figure 108.2) plays an important role at a rate-limiting step in the metabolic turnover of poly ADP-ribosyl groups in the cell [4], in which primary ADP-ribosyl groups are removed from acceptor proteins. The enzyme, originally called ADP-ribosyl-histone-splitting enzyme, cleaves the attachment of ADP-ribose to the carboxyl group of histones and nonhistone proteins [5]. ADP-ribosylation is a general post-translational modification of proteins [6]. Poly (ADP-ribosyl)ation takes place in the nucleus and appears to have a role in DNA repair, the cell cycle and cellular differentiation.

GENETICS AND PATHOGENESIS

The history of the original family indicated the disorder to be an X-linked recessive.

TREATMENT

None is yet available.

References

1 Williams JC, Butler IJ, Rosenberg HS, *et al*. Progressive neurologic deterioration and renal failure due to storage of glutamyl ribose-5-phosphate. *N Engl J Med* 1984;**311**:152.

2 Williams JC, Chamber JP, Liehr JG. Glutamyl ribose-5-phosphate storage disease. A hereditary defect in the degradation of poly(ADP-ribosylated) proteins. *J Biol Chem* 1984;**259**:1037.

3 Oka J, Ueda K, Hayaishi O, *et al*. ADP-ribosyl protein lyse. *J Biol Chem* 1984;**259**:986.

4 Wielckens K, Schmidt A, George E, *et al*. DNA fragmentation and NAD depletion. *J Biol Chem* 1982;**257**:12872.

5 Okayama H., Honda M., Hayaishi O. Novel enzyme from rat-liver that cleaves an ADP-ribosyl histone linkage. *Proc Natl Acad Sci USA* 1978;**75**:2254–57

6 Ueda K, Hayaishi O. ADP-ribosylation. *Ann Rev Biochem* 1985;**54**:73.

Ethylmalonic encephalopathy

MAJOR PHENOTYPIC EXPRESSION

Progressive neurodegenerative disease, acrocyanosis, petechial skin lesions, episodic acidosis, neuroimaging and neuropathologic evidence of basal ganglia lesions, lactic academia, ethylmalonic aciduria and mutations in the ETH1 gene.

INTRODUCTION

Ethylmalonic aciduria (Figure 109.1) is most commonly encountered in what has been termed ethylmalonic-adipic aciduria in less severe forms of glutaric aciduria Type II, or multiple acylCoA dehydrogenase deficiency, which is due to deficiency in electron transport flavoprotein (ETF) or ETF dehydrogenase [1–3] (Chapter 45). It is also encountered in short chain acylCoA dehydrogenase (SCAD) deficiency (Figure 109.1) [4]. These patients present with hypoketotic hypoglycemia, myopathic weakness or cardiomyopathy, characteristics of disorders of fatty acid oxidation (Chapter 45).

A different type of disorder in which ethylmalonic aciduria is associated with a very different phenotype and normal oxidation of fatty acids was first reported in 1991 and 1994 [5–7]. It is recognized most readily by the association of encephalopathy, acrocyanosis and petechiae. Death in infancy is also characteristic.

CLINICAL ABNORMALITIES

The most important abnormalities are those involving the central nervous system (Figures 109.2–109.4). Hypotonia, head lag and delayed development have been noted as early as 3–4 months [7,8]. Developmental milestones have failed to be achieved. Generalized tonic-clonic seizures or infantile spasms begin in infancy and may be frequent, and there may be episodes of status epilepticus. Deep tendon reflexes are exaggerated, and there may be ankle clonus and positive Babinski responses. One patient had microcephaly and quadriparesis [7] (Figure 109.4). Neurological deterioration is progressive and may be rapid following diarrhea or other intercurrent illness and leads to terminal coma and death in the first, second or fourth year [7,8].

Manifestations of vascular abnormality are an unusual feature of the disease (Figures 109.2, 109.3, 109.5–109.9). This has been observed in at least 10 patients with this disease [5–8]. Acrocyanosis (Figure 109.5) may be the mildest manifestation, and it may be associated with edema of the extremities. Patients also have episodic showers of petechiae, often associated with infection. One of our patients (Figure 109.2) was originally investigated for meningococcemia before referral to us. There may also be ecchymoses (Figures 109.6–109.8) or hemorrhagic streaks (Figure 109.9).

Dilated tortuous retinal vessels (Figures 109.10, p. 737, 109.11, p. 738) may be seen as early as 3–4 months of life. Five patients had hematuria, and in two erythrocytes were reported in the cerebrospinal fluid (CSF) [7,9]. One patient had an infarct of the basal ganglia. One had a terminal hemoperitoneum. Biopsies of the skin lesions showed nothing but hemorrhage [7]. There was no evidence for an immunologic abnormality. Nor were there abnormalities of bleeding, clotting, or platelets. A markedly elevated level of plasminogen activator inhibitor-1 has been encountered [8]. Terminal

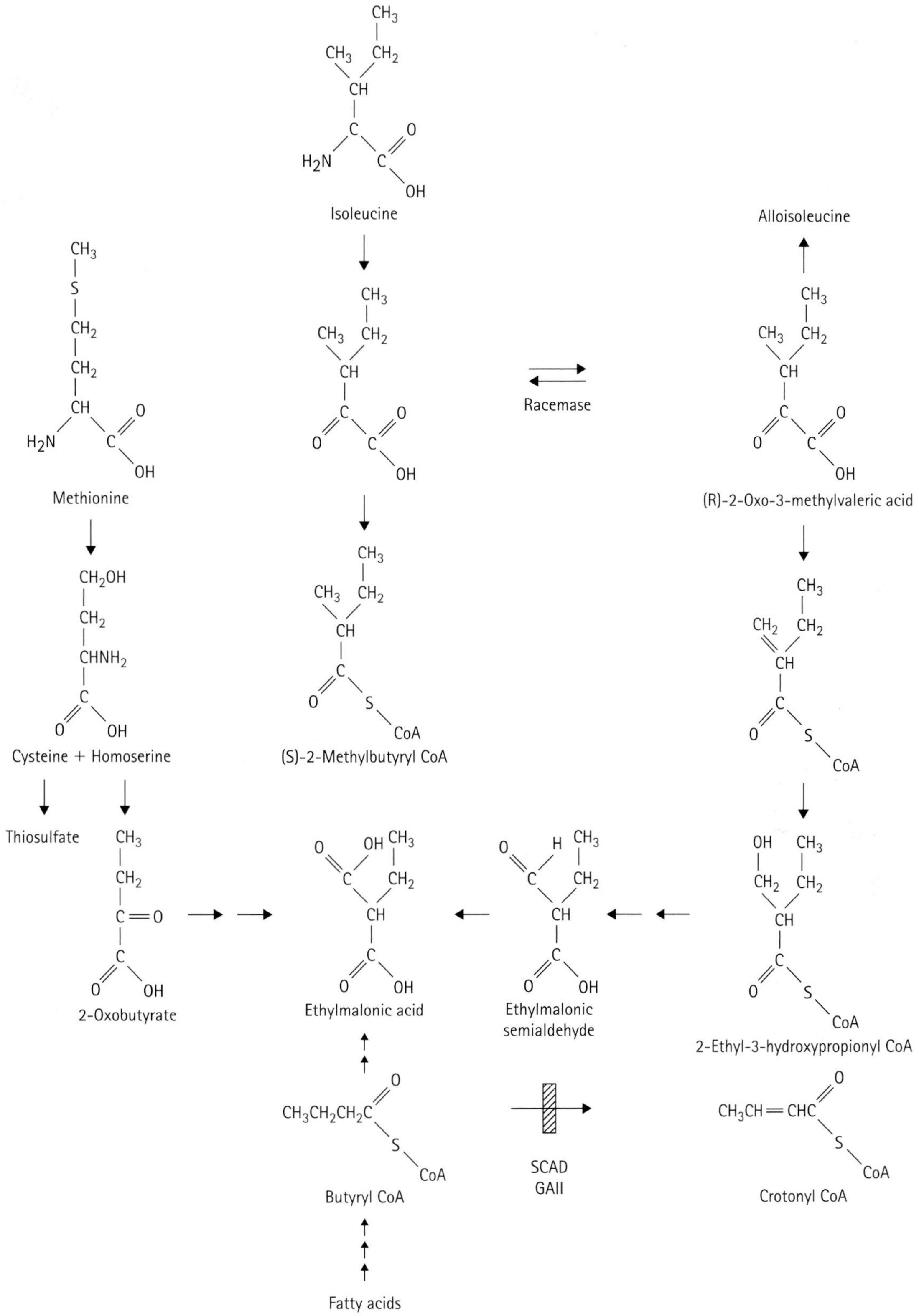

Figure 109.1 *Metabolic pathways in the potential genesis of ethymalonic acid.*

events in two patients appeared to be pulmonary edema, and one had cerebral edema.

Facial features were mildly dysmorphic [7–9] (Figures 109.6, 109.12, p. 738, 109.13, p. 738). The facies of these patients tended to resemble each other. Some had epicanthal folds. In most the nasal bridge was broad and depressed.

Neuroradiological findings (Figures 109.14, 109.15, p. 738) revealed frontotemporal atrophy and delayed myelination. In

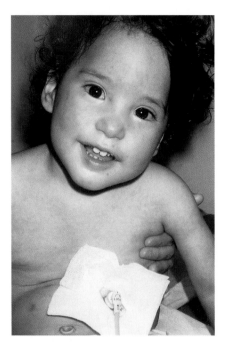

Figure 109.2   *S.P., a 19-month-old Hispanic-American girl with ethylmalonic aciduria. She was hypotonic and had delayed development. Petechial clusters visible in the forehead, cheeks, and chest came and went.*

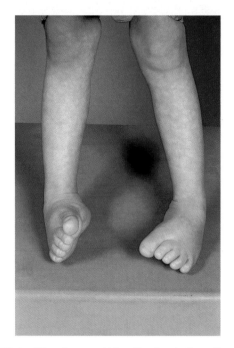

Figure 109.4   *F.E., a 3-year-old Egyptian boy had spastic quadriplegia.*

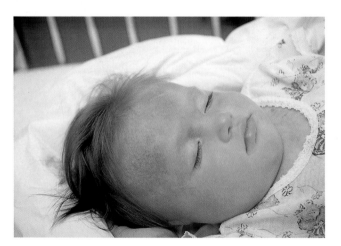

Figure 109.3   *A.P., a 5-month-old girl with ethylmalonic aciduria. The facial appearance and the petechial lesions are illustrated. She was floppy, unresponsive and had virtually constant infantile spasms. She had epicanthal folds, upslanting palpebral fissures, an upturned nose and depressed nasal bridge.*

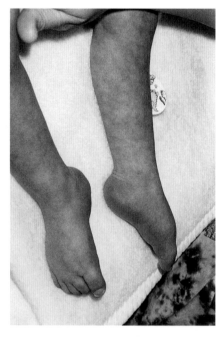

Figure 109.5   *S.P. The feet and lower legs were cold and alternately pale red or blue.*

addition there were areas of high T2 intensity in the heads of the caudate nuclei, putamina and posterior fossa [7,8,10]. Other abnormalities on magnetic resonance imaging (MRI) included cerebral ectopia and a tethered cord [11]. Electroencephalograms (EEGs) were abnormal, revealing multiple focal discharges, or hypsarrhythmia. Studies of nerve conduction indicated sensory neuropathy in the legs [8].

Acute metabolic crises are seen with lactic acidemia and mild hypoglycemia. Between attacks the blood concentrations of

lactate and pyruvate remained high, and metabolic acidosis was compensated. Concentrations of 3.9 to 6.0 mmol/L of lactate and 158 to 230 μmol/L of pyruvate were recorded; while in the acute attack levels of lactate as high as 17 mmol/L were found, and there was severe acidosis with pH values of 7.05 and 7.10, and base excess of −19 without ketosis. Liver

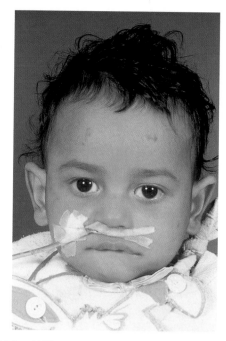

Figure 109.6 *M.M., a 12-month-old Yemeni boy with ethylmalonic aciduria. There were hemorrhagic spots on the forehead. He also had epicanthal folds.*

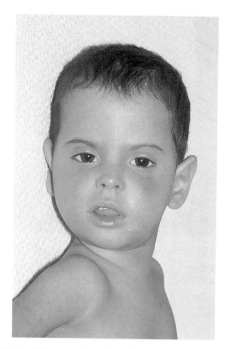

Figure 109.8 *T.M., a 23-month-old Yemeni girl with ethylmalonic aciduria and a large ecchymotic area on the cheek.*

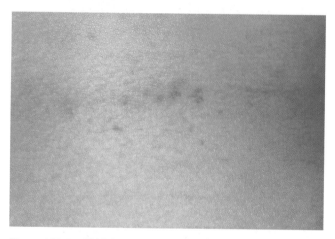

Figure 109.7 *M.M. A mixture of petechiae and hemorrhagic spots.*

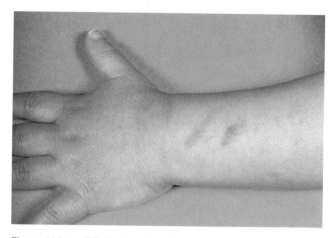

Figure 109.9 *F.E. At 12months-of-age this Egyptian boy had fresh hemorrhagic streaks on his arm.*

function tests may be elevated. Creatine phosphokinase (CPK) may be normal or elevated as high as 2100 IU/L [8]. Blood ammonia is normal.

Muscle biopsy revealed increased droplets of lipid but no ragged red fibers; on electron microscopy, there were mildly increased numbers of pleomorphic subsarcolemmal mitochondria [8]. Neuropathological examination revealed marked capillary proliferation in the substantia nigra, periaqueductal area, putamen, caudate and medial thalamus (Figure 109.16). Endothelial cells were increased in number and size. There was a relative sparing of neurons and pallor of the background parenchyma that was quite prominent in the substantia nigra. There was vascuolization of white matter tracts.

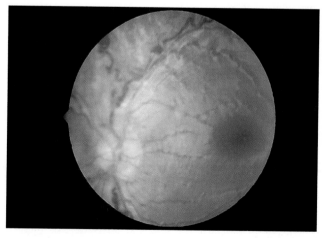

Figure 109.10 *Dilated tortuous vessels in the ocular fundus of the patient in Figure 109.9.*

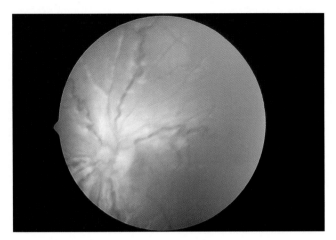

Figure 109.11   *Dilated tortuous vessels in the ocular fundus of the patient in Figure 109.4.*

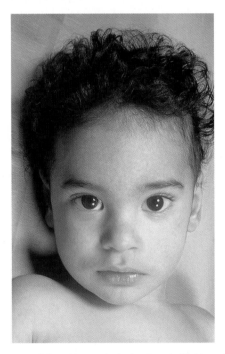

Figure 109.12   *F.E. at 12 months had epicanthal folds and upward-slanting palpebral fissures.*

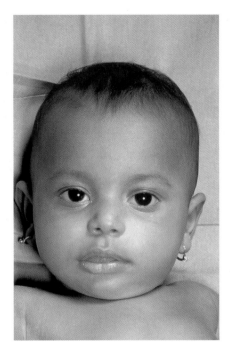

Figure 109.13   *N.S. The nasal bridge was broad, and she had epicanthal folds.*

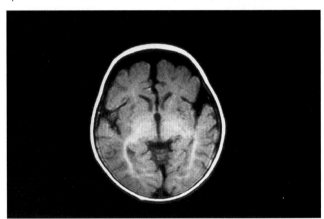

Figure 109.14   *CT scan of the brain of N.S. showed frontotemporal atrophy.*

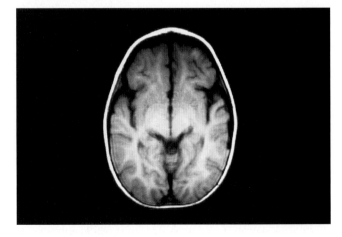

Figure 109.15   *MRI scan of the brain of patient F.E. revealed extensive atrophy, especially frontotemporal.*

GENETICS AND PATHOGENESIS

The disorder is transmitted in an autosomal recessive fashion. Boys and girls have been observed in the same family. In two reports [5,7], the parents were consanguineous. Patients reported have been Yemeni, Italian, Egyptian, Native American and Hispanic-American.

The major metabolic abnormality is the excretion of ethylmalonic acid in the urine. Amounts reported have ranged from 54 to 2270 mmol/mol creatinine (normal <17). In some patients, the excretion of methylsuccinic acid was also elevated, but in others it was not, and levels were as high as 266 mmol/mol creatinine (normal <12) in only one patient.

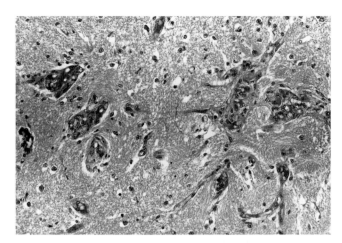

Figure 109.16 *Histologic appearance of the caudate nucleus, of N.P., the brother of the patient shown in Figure 109.3. He died at 8 months. There was marked endothelial proliferation of capillaries and an increase in the number of capillaries. (H and E, 500×) (Reprinted with permission from the* Archive of Neurology *[9].)*

Adipic aciduria was not present, although in one patient a level as high as 334 μmol/mol creatinine was recorded. Tandem mass spectrometry (MS) of the blood and urine showed an elevation in C4 and C5 carnitine esters and excretion increased after treatment with carnitine. Levels of free carnitine in blood and urine are low. Acylglycine excretions, including butyrylglycine and isobutyrylglycine, were increased [6].

In searching for the pathway leading to accumulation of ethylmalonic acid, elevated excretion of this compound and methylsuccinic acid after a load of isoleucine was reported by Malgorzata *et al.* [12], but in our patient loading with isoleucine did not change the excretion of ethylmalonic acid [8]. Malgorzata *et al.* [12] postulated a block at the levels of 2-methylbutyrylCoA dehydrogenase; however, the activity of this enzyme was studied by Burlina *et al.* [6] and found to be normal. Furthermore, Ozand and colleagues [7] found the oxidation of ^{14}C-isoleucine to ^{14}CO$_2$ to be normal in fibroblasts derived from typical patients. In these studies the oxidation of ^{14}C-butyrate was normal, consistent with our findings on triglyceride loading. Normal oxidation of fatty acids was also observed by Burlina *et al.* [6].

It is not clear why results were different following isoleucine administration in our patient and the patient of Malgorzata *et al.* [12], but neither of the siblings reported by their group [11] had petechiae; so they could have been studying a different disease. In our patient loading with methionine was followed by an increase in excretion of ethylmalonic acid of 1.7 times to 648 mmol/mol creatinine, and that of methylsuccinic acid also rose. A relationship between this syndrome and the metabolism of sulfur amino acids was suggested by Duran and colleagues [13] who found increased excretion of inorganic thiosulfite and an absence of detectable sulfite. They also reported two sulfur-containing acidic amino acids s-sulfocysteine and s-sulfothiocysteine, each of which can be formed nonenzymatically from thiosulfate and cysteine. The increase in excretion of ethylmalonic acid in our patient following methionine is consistent with these observations.

Methionine is converted normally to homoserine and cysteine. Homoserine is converted to 2-oxobutyric acid which could be a source of ethylmalonic acid. Cysteine is converted to 2-mercaptopyruvic acid which is metabolized to pyruvic acid and thiosulfate and ultimately sulfate. Ethylmalonic acid can be formed via carboxylation of butyryl CoA (Figure 109.1, p. 735) catalyzed by propionyl CoA carboxylase [14], and this appears to be the source of ethylmalonic acid found in short-chain acylCoA dehydrogenase (SCAD) deficiency and in multiple acylCoA dehydrogenase deficiency. In our patient loading with medium-chain triglyceride did not greatly increase the excretion of ethylmalonic acid. Ethylmalonic acid could be a product of isoleucine metabolism through the R pathway after racemization of 2-oxo-3-methylvaleric acid, the precursor of alloisoleucine, from the S to the R form, which is then convertible to 2-methylbutyryl CoA, 2-ethyl-3-hydroxypropionyl CoA and ethylmalonic semialdehyde and then to ethylmalonic acid.

Ethylhydracrylic acid is a potential source of ethylmalonic acid, but there is evidence that it is first converted to butyryl CoA [15]; furthermore, this compound was not elevated in the urine of these patients [7,8].It has been shown that methylsuccinic acid is formed from ethylmalonic acid in bacteria [16]. Methylsuccinic acid may also be made from 4-hydroxyisovaleric acid, which would account for its presence in glutaric aciduria type II, where isovaleryl CoA dehydrogenase is impaired. The possibility that this disease is a disorder of mitochondrial electron transport has been raised [17], but studies of mitochondrial DNA in blood and muscle and the enzymes of the electron transport chain in muscle and fibroblasts were normal [6–8].

The gene for this disease was found via homozygosity mapping to reside in chromosome 9q13 near the midpoint of the long arm [18]. Physical and functional genomic data and mutational analysis permitted identification of the gene, which has been named *ETHE1*. The protein product whose function is not yet known is targeted to the mitochondria, where it is cleared of a short leader peptide and is internalized into the matrix. It belongs to a super-family of β-lactamases, with similarities to glyoxalyse II, but it differs in the C terminal structure. It is thought to be a thioesterase.

Over 20 mutations have been found in patients with ethylmalonic encephalopathy [18,19]. One patient was homzygous for His79Leu. His79 by sequence comparison with glyoxalase II is thought to be a catalytically active site. It is thought that other mutations affect synthesis, folding or stability of the protein.

TREATMENT

The disease is lethal in infancy or early childhood. Of the patients reported only two were surviving at the time of report [6,7]. Treatment with riboflavin, carnitine, glycine, ascorbic acid and vitamin E were without evident effect.

In our patient [8] a diet restricted in methionine led to a decrease in excretion of ethylmalonic and methylsuccinic acids and normalization of concentrations of lactic acid and bicarbonate, but the disease was relentless, and she died at 11 months of age.

References

1   Nyhan WL. Ethylmalonic aciduria: in *Abnormalities in Amino Acid Metabolism in Clinical Medicine.* Appleton Century Crofts, Norwalk CN;1984:118.

2   Tanaka K, Mantago S, Genel M, *et al.* New defect in fatty-acid metabolism with hypoglycaemia and organic aciduria. *Lancet* 1977;**2**:986.

3   Goodman SI, Frerman FE, Loehr JP. Recent progress in understanding glutaric acidurias. *Enzyme* 1987;**38**:76.

4   Bennet MJ, Gray RGF, Isherwood DM, *et al.* The diagnosis and biochemical investigation of a patient with a short chain fatty acid oxidation defect. *J Inherit Metab Dis* 1985;**8**:135.

5   Burlina AB, Zachello F, Dionisi-Vici C, *et al.* New clinical phenotype of branched-chain acyl-CoA defect. *Lancet* 1991;**338**:1522.

6   Burlina AB, Dionisio-Vici C, Bennett MJ, *et al.* A new syndrome with ethylmalonic aciduria and normal fatty acid oxidation in fibroblasts. *J Pediatr* 1994;**124**:79.

7   Ozand PT, Rashed M, Millington DS, *et al.* Ethylmalonic aciduria: an organic acidemia with CNS involvement and vasculopathy. *Brain Dev* 1994;**16**:12.

8   McGowan KA, Nyhan WL, Barshop BA, *et al.* The role of methionine in ethylmalonic encephalopathy with petechiae. *Arch Neurol* 2004;**61**:570

9   Chen E, Jerucki ER, Rinaldo P, *et al.* Nephrotic syndrome and dysmorphic facial features in a new family of three affected siblings with ethylmalonic encephalopathy. *Am J Hum Genet* 1994;**55**:A2000

10 García-Silva MT, Rives A, Campos Y, *et al.* Syndrome of encephalopathy petechiae and ethylmalonic aciduria. *Pediatr Neurol* 1997;**17**:165.

11 Nowaczyk MJM, Blasser SI, Clarke JTR. Central nervous system malformations in ethylmalonic encephalopathy. *Am J Med Genet* 1998;**75**:292.

12 Malgorzata JM, Nowaczyk JM, Lehotay DC, *et al.* Ethylmalonic and methylsuccinic aciduria in ethylmalonic encephalopathy arise from abnormal isoleucine metabolism. *Metabolism* 1998;**47**:836.

13 Duran M, Dorland L, van den Berg IET, *et al.* The ethylmalonic acid syndrome is associated with deranged sulfur amino acid metabolism leading to urinary excretion of thiosulfate and sulfothiocysteine. *Vienna VIIth International Congress of Inborn Errors of Metabolism.* 1997:Abstract 048.

14 Hegre CS, Halenz DK, Lane MD. The enzymatic carboxylation of butyryl coenzyme A. *J Am Chem Soc* 1959;**81**:6526.

15 Baretz BH, Lollo CP, Tanaka K. Metabolism in rats *in vivo* of *RS*-2-methylbutyrate and *N*-butyrate labelled with stable isotopes at various positions: Mechanism of biosynthesis and degradation of ethylmalonyl semialdehyde and ethylmalonic acid. *J Biol Chem* 1979;**254**:34678.

16 Retey J, Smith E, Zagalak B. Investigation of the mechanism of the methylmalonyl-CoA mutase reaction with the substrate analogue: ethylmalonyl-CoA. *Eur J Biochem* 1978;**83**:437.

17 Garavaglia B, Colamaria V, Carrara F, *et al.* Muscle cytochrome c oxidase deficiency in two Italian patients with ethylmalonic aciduria and peculiar clinical phenotype. *J Inherit Metab Dis* 1994;**17**:301.

18 Zeviani M, Tiranti V, D'Adamo P, *et al.* Ethylmalonic encephalopathy is due to mutations in ETHE1. *J Inherit Metab Dis* 2004;**27**:suppl 1):177-O.

19 Bischoff C, Vang S, Burlina A, *et al.* High levels of EMA in suspected SCAD patients are in certain cases due to defects in the ETHE1 gene. *J Inherit Metab Dis* 2004;**27**:(Suppl 1): 176-P.

Disorders of creatine metabolism

DEBORAH MARSDEN

MAJOR PHENOTYPIC EXPRESSION

Severe delay of expressive speech and language, hypotonia, movement disorder (dystonia, choreoathetosis), mental retardation, seizures, autistic-like behavior, depletion of central nervous system (CNS) creatine (on magnetic resonance spectroscopy [MRS]), increased blood and urine guanidinoacetate (in guanidinoacetatetransferase [GAMT] deficiency), low urine creatine (in arginine:glycine aminotransferase [AGAT]) deficiency and increased urine creatine/creatinine excretion (in creatinetransporter [CRTR]) deficiency.

INTRODUCTION

Creatine and phosphocreatine play an important role in intracellular energy metabolism as a high energy buffering system through the reversible reaction catalyzed by creatine kinase in which creatine and adenosine triphosphate (ATP) form phosphocreatine and adenosine diphosphate (ADP) in the mitochondria. Approximately 95 percent of creatine is found in skeletal muscle, with the rest distributed between the CNS, liver and kidney [1]. Some 50 percent is synthesized *de novo*, primarily in the liver, kidney and pancreas; the rest is from dietary sources. In the biosynthesis of creatine, the rate-limiting step is the conversion of arginine and glycine to guanidinoacetate (GAA) and ornithine by arginine:glycine amidinoacetate (AGAT) in the kidney. GAA is methylated in the liver to creatine by guanidinoacetate methyltransferase (GAMT) with S-adenosylmethionine acting as the methyl donor. Creatine is transported through the blood and taken up into cells against a concentration gradient by a saturable Na^+ and Cl^-dependent creatine transporter (CRTR). Creatine is converted non-enzymatically to creatinine, which is excreted in the urine in amounts approximately equal to the glomerular filtration rate [2].

CLINICAL ABNORMALITIES

Disorders of creatine metabolism represent a recently described group of three known disorders of the synthesis and transport of creatine. Each disorder is characterized by severely reduced or absent creatine in the CNS and neurological manifestations that range from mild to moderate developmental delay to severe hypotonia, movement disorder, autistic-like behavior and mental retardation. Seizures are common in patients with GAMT and CRTR. All patients have severe speech and language delay.

Stockler *et al.* [3] reported the first recognized disorder, GAMT deficiency in 1996. The index patient presented at 22 months with global developmental delay, and severe hypotonia; dystonic movements were noticed from the age of 4–6 months. By 11 months he had lost his ability to roll and was unable to sit or crawl. Seizure-like drop attacks were noted over the next few months, and an electroencephalogram (EEG) showed intermittent high-voltage slow runs with some spikes. Magnetic resonance imaging (MRI) at 12 months showed increased signal bilaterally in the globus pallidus and magnetic resonance spectroscopy (MRS) showed absent creatine and increased guanidinoacetate. GAMT activity in liver homogenate was 1.35 nmol/h. To date, over 10 patients have been reported with GAMT deficiency.

The second disorder, arginine:glycine amidinotransferase deficiency was reported by Bianchi *et al.* in 2000 [4] in two Italian sisters aged 4 and 6 with mild mental retardation and severe expressive speech delay. One sibling had a history of one febrile seizure, but no other seizure activity had occurred. MRS studies showed absent CNS creatine. Plasma creatine was normal. Plasma guanidinoacetate was slightly decreased, and urine creatine excretion was very low. Fibroblast enzyme studies subsequently showed undetectable AGAT activity. A third patient in the same family (the fathers of this patient and the two index patients are first cousins) presented at 2 years-of-age with psychomotor delay, absent language, mild hypotonia and autistic-like behavior, characterized by poor socialization, short attention span and stereotypic hand movements [5]. All three patients had some degree of microcephaly.

In 2001, Salomons *et al.* [6] reported the third disorder, creatine transporter deficiency (CRTR). The index patient presented with hypotonia and developmental delay and a seizure disorder. Mental retardation was diagnosed at 6 years-of-age. His mother and maternal grandmother both had learning disabilities; the mother's sister was normal, but their brother was severely retarded. CNS creatine was absent on MRS. Urine and plasma guanidinoacetate levels were normal, but creatine levels were increased. Further studies of the three female relatives showed increased creatine in the plasma of the mother and aunt and increased urine creatine in all three women; MRS studies of the mother and aunt showed reduced, but detectable, CNS creatine. The presence of more severe symptoms in the male family members suggested X-linked inheritance, which was later confirmed by finding a mutation in the creatine transporter gene (SLC6A8) at Xq28.

In a recent review of 13 patients and 13 female carriers in seven unrelated families [7] the most frequent clinical findings in the families were moderate-severe mental retardation (7/7), expressive speech delay (7/7) and autistic-like behaviors (7/7). Seizures were also common (5/7). Other less frequent symptoms included short stature and gross motor delay. Head circumference was variable. Female carrier patients have had variable degrees of learning disability (6/13). SLC6A8 deficiency has also been found to have a prevalence of at least 2.1 percent in a study of 290 patients with non-syndromic X-linked mental retardation [8].

We have diagnosed two patients with CRTR deficiency [7]. They had severe hypotonia and mental retardation present from birth; both have a severe movement disorder not previously noted in patients with this defect. The first patient was from a consanguineous Middle Eastern family. He presented for evaluation at the age of 30 months with severe hypotonia and developmental delay present since birth and a more recent onset of dystonia and later, choreoathetosis. He had swallowing difficulties. There was no speech development. He was normocephalic and had no dysmorphic features. He also had a history of transient mild elevations of lactic acid and ammonia. MRS studies showed almost complete absence of creatine (Figure 110.1). An MRI showed abnormal increased signal in the periatrial white matter on the T2-weighted images, abnormal signal intensity in bilateral globi pallidi with associated thinning of splenium of the corpus callosum (Figures 110.2–110.4). MRS showed almost complete absence of the creatine peak. Urine guanidinoacetate was elevated at 121.3 mmol/mol creatinine (normal 54 ± 26), but plasma guanidinoacetate was normal at 1.41 µmol/L (normal 1.04 ± 0.4). Urine creatine/creatinine ratio was elevated at 3.67 (normal 0.39 ± 0.29). His mother, older brother and three older sisters were healthy. Fibroblast creatine uptake studies and mutation analysis confirmed the diagnosis. Mutation analysis in his mother was negative.

The second patient presented at the age of 12 months for further evaluation of severe global developmental delay present

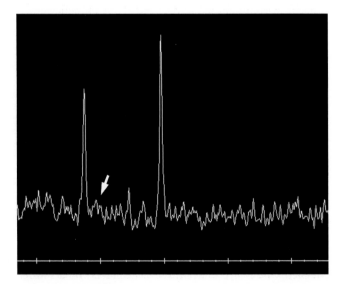

Figure 110.1   *Magnetic resonance spectroscopy (MRS) of the brain of a patient with CRTR deficiency. Single voxel MR spectrum with TE = 144, demonstrating reduction in the creatine peak (arrow).*

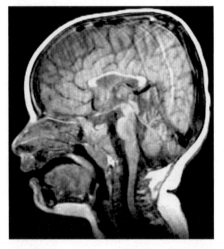

Figure 110.2   *MRI of the brain of a patient with CRTR deficiency. This sagittal T1 image shows marked abnormal thinning of the entire corpus callosum.*

from birth. He also had dystonia and severe truncal hypotonia and swallowing difficulties. Urine organic acid analysis showed large elevation of tricarboxylic acid (TCA) cycle intermediates. He was dysmorphic, with microcephaly, a large cupped ear, deep-set eyes, prominent nasal bridge, high-arched palate and fifth finger clinodactyly. He had bilateral sensorineural hearing loss, visual impairment and retinal dysfunction on electroretinogram studies. A muscle biopsy showed mitochondrial respiratory enzyme deficiencies. A brain MRI at 12 months showed areas of T2 hyperintensity within the globus pallidus bilaterally and delayed myelination of white matter with thinning of the entire corpus callosum. A

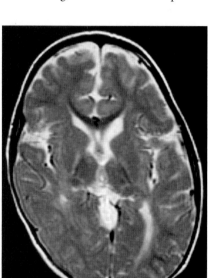

Figure 110.3 *MRI of the brain. This T$_2$ weighted image demonstrates abnormal signal intensity in the periventricular white matter and globus palidus bilaterally.*

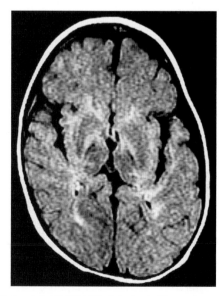

Figure 110.4 *Axial FLAIR MRI of the brain illustrating abnormalities in the periventricular white matter and globus pallidus.*

magnetic resonance spectroscopy study at that time reported absence of a lactate peak, but there was no comment on the creatine spectrum. At 30 months of age a repeat MRI with MRS reported almost complete absence of the creatine peak. Review of the previous MRS also showed absence of creatine peak. There was no significant change in the MRI appearance. Subsequent testing revealed mild elevation of guanidinoacetate excretion in the urine at 168 mmol/mol creatinine (normal 54 ± 26) with elevated creatine/creatinine ratio at 2 (normal 0.39 ± 0.29). Fibroblast creatine uptake studies and mutation analysis confirmed CRTR deficiency. His mother and older sister were healthy; mutation analysis was negative in both.

GENETICS AND PATHOGENESIS

The common biochemical abnormality in all three disorders is depletion of creatine in the CNS, which is likely the primary pathogenic mechanism, possibly involving a resulting effect on mitochondrial energy metabolism, particularly in the genesis of the basal ganglia lesions and movement disorder [9]. Patients with both GAMT and CRTR deficiencies have movement disorder. It has also been suggested that GAA, a known neurotoxin, also plays a significant role, especially as an epileptogenic agent [3], although one of our patients with CRTR (and normal plasma GAA) also presented with status epilepticus. Clinically, all patients have had mental retardation of varying degree, all have had severe expressive language delay; and many have had autistic-like behavior. The precise pathogenic mechanism of these manifestations is not understood.

AGAT and GAMT deficiency are inherited as autosomal recessive disorders. Mutation analysis of the index patient with AGAT deficiency and 26 family members revealed the same homozygous mutation, W149X [5]. In GAMT deficiency, the gene has been mapped to chromosome 19p13.3; four mutations have been reported to date [3,10]. CRTR deficiency is an X-linked disorder, mapped to Xq28. The majority (twelve) of mutations to date are missense, nonsense and single amino acid deletions [7]. Our two patients had large deletions (a 7 exon deletion in the first patient and deletion of the complete coding region of the gene in the other), which likely explains the more severe manifestations in these patients, suggesting some degree of genotype/phenotype correlation. The variable, milder symptoms in female carriers are consistent with varying degrees of Lyonization.

TREATMENT

Treatment with supplemental creatine monohydrate (400 mg/kg/day) has resulted in significant improvement in patients with AGAT and GAMT deficiencies. In the three patients with AGAT, there was rapid improvement in fine-motor skills and the behavioral disorder; these improvements paralleled the increase in brain levels of creatine. Speech and cognition remained significantly impaired. In GAMT deficiency, oral supplementation in the first three reported patients, with creatine monohydrate in doses of 0.35–2.0 g/kg/day resulted in gradual increase in the CNS creatine signal on MRS, but it was still significantly below normal. GAA levels remained high, suggesting the possibility that it may inhibit the transport of creatine into the CNS, thus preventing normalization of the creatine levels. Nevertheless, the index patient showed significant clinical improvement: the movement disorder, swallowing difficulties and seizure disorder resolved. His gross motor function improved, and he was able to walk at the age of 5 years. He continued to have some autistic-like and self-injurious behaviors.

Another patient showed improved psychomotor function and resolution of the seizures and globus pallidus lesions; a third showed no improvement; seizures continued. In one patient, dietary arginine restriction (1.5 g/kg/day) resulted in no long-term benefit [11], but arginine restriction and ornithine supplementation (100 mg/kg/day) with an arginine-free essential amino acid formula (0.4 g/kg/day), resulted in significant reduction of plasma GAA and improvement in seizure activity and EEG [12]. Supplementation of creatinine in doses as high as 750 mg/kg/day has not resulted in any improvement in either the clinical symptoms or MRS creatine signal in patients with CRTR deficiency.

References

1 Walker JB. Creatine: biosynthesis regulation and function. *Adv Enzymol Relat Areas Mol Biol* 1979;**50**:177.

2 Wyss M, Kaddurah-Daouk R. Creatine and creatinine metabolism. *Physiol Rev* 2000;**80**:1107.

3 Stockler S, Isbrandt D, Hanefeld F, et al. Guanidinoacetate methyltransferase deficiency: the first inborn error of creatine metabolism in man. *Am J Hum Gene* 1996;**58**:914.

4 Bianchi MC, Tosetti M, Fornai F, et al. Reversible brain creatine deficiency in two sisters with normal blood creatine level. *Ann Neuro* 2000;**47**:511.

5 Battini R, Leuzzi V, Carducci C, et al. Creatine depletion in a new case with AGAT deficiency: clinical and genetic study in a large pedigree. *Mol Genet Metab* 2002;**77**:326.

6 Salomons GS, van Dooren SJ, Verhoeven NM, et al. X-linked creatine-transporter gene (SLC6A8) defect: a new creatine-deficiency syndrome. *Am J Hum Genet* 2001;**68**:1497.

7 Salomons GS, van Dooren SJ, Verhoeven NM, et al. X-linked creatine transporter defect: an overview. *J Inherit Metab Dis* 2003;**26**:309.

8 Rosenberg EH, Almeida LS, Kleefstra T, et al. High prevalence of SLC6A8 deficiency in X-linked mental retardation. *Am J Hum Genet* 2004;**75**:97.

9 von Figura K, Hanefeld F, Isbrandt D, Stockler-Ipsiroglu S. Guanidinoacetate methyltransferase deficiency: in *The Metabolic and Molecular Bases of Inherited Disease* (eds CR Scriver, AL Beaudet, WS Sly, D Valle). 8th ed. McGraw-Hill, New York;2001.

10 Carducci C, Leuzzi V, Carducci C, et al. Two new severe mutations causing guanidinoacetate methyltransferase deficiency. *Mol Genet Metab* 2000;**71**:633.

11 Schulze A, Mayatepek E ,Bachert B, et al. Therapeutic trial of arginine restriction in creatine deficiency syndrome. *Eur J Pediatr* 1998;**157**:606.

12 Schulze A, Ebinger F, Rating D, Mayatepek E. Improving treatment of guanidinoacetate methyltransferase deficiency: reduction of guanidinoacetic acid in body fluids by arginine restriction and ornithine supplementation. *Mol Genet Metab* 2001;**74**:413.

Sanjad-Sakati syndrome

MAJOR PHENOTYPIC EXPRESSION

Hypoparathyroidism, growth failure, developmental retardation, characteristic facial appearance and deficiency of tubulin specific chaperone E(TBCE).

INTRODUCTION

Sanjad, Sakati and colleagues [1] reported in 1991 a syndrome of hypothyroidism, growth failure and minor anomalies in 12 Saudi Arabian children [2]. Each had developmental retardation, low levels of parathyroid hormone, and hypocalcemic neonatal tetany. All but one of 13 Saudi families were consanguineous. A similar clinical picture was described in eight Kuwaiti children and in six reported from Israel [3]. An additional finding of medullary sclerosis of the long bones and T-cell abnormality was observed in the Kuwaiti families [2]. This bony picture, along with diaphyseal cortical thickening was also reported along with hypoparathyroidism and intrauterine growth retardation in the Kenny-Caffey syndrome [4].

The gene for both syndromes was mapped by homozygosity and linkage disequilibrium to a 1 cM interval on chromosome 1q42–45[5,6], and it became clear that the Sanjad-Sakati and Kenny-Caffey syndromes were allelic, sharing an ancestral haplotype [7]. Mutational analysis revealed a 12bp deletion in all of the Middle Eastern families in the tubulin-specific chaperone E(TBCE)] gene [8]. This cytosolic chaperone is required for proper folding of the α-tubulin subunit and its heterodimerization with the β subunit. This chaperone mutation causes disruption of the organization of microtubules.

CLINICAL ABNORMALITIES

The presenting manifestations are those of neonatal hypocalcemic tetany [1,2]. This is virtually always manifest clinically with generalized seizures. In our patient, hypocalcemia responded nicely to oral calcium supplementation, but the treatment was stopped after two weeks when the concentration of calcium became normal, and at 5 months she again developed seizures, and was found to have a calcium concentration in serum of 5.6 mg/dL. The phosphorus was 9.5 mg/dL and the alkaline phosphatase 316 IU/L. This is the classic presentation. All have had low levels of parathyroid hormone. In our patient [2] the intact parathyroid hormone (PTH) was 3 pg/mL [nl 10.55], and the mid molecule PTH was undetectable with a concurrent calcium of 7.8 mg/dL. Infusion of PTH, 3 mL/kg [100 USP units/mL] was followed by a normal rise of cyclic AMP to 15 nmol/dL and phosphorus to 30 mg/dL in the urine. This is the picture of primary hypoparathyroidism, excluding end organ unresponsiveness. The parathyroids appear normal on magnetic resonance imaging (MRI) [2].

Growth failure may be evident at birth, and postnatal deficiency of growth is profound [1]. The index patient weighed 1500 g at term birth. At 4 years 10 months our patient [Figure 111.1] weighed 8.1 kg [50th percentile for 7½ months;] her length was 79.5 cm [50th percentile for 8½ months.] At 2½ years her bone age was 1½ years. At 4 years 10 months it was

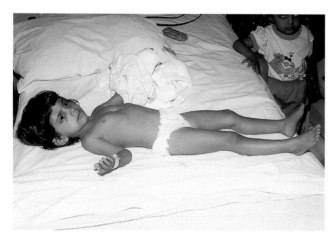

Figure 111.1   *A.J., a 4 years, one month old girl with Sanjad-Sakati syndrome. She was tiny, no larger than a 7–8-month-old infant.*

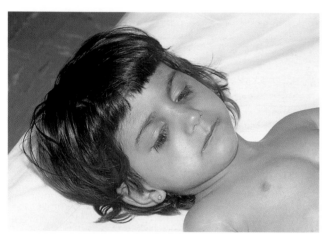

Figure 111.2   *Close-up of the face illustrating the characteristic facies. The jaw was small. The nasal bridge was depressed and the eyes deeply set. The philtrum was long and the upper lip thin.*

2½ years. A 15-year-old patient was 99 cm in height [9]. Concentrations of growth hormone may be normal [1]. In our patient levels ranged from 2.3 to 3.9 mg/mL. Following stimulation with arginine and with L-DOPA, there was a rise only to 5.8 and a fall to 1.2 ng/mL respectively [normal rise to 10 ng/mL]. After clonidine stimulation there was a rise to 15 ng/mL, but only after 120 minutes. In contrast, infusion of growth hormone releasing hormone (GHRH) led to a rise to 22 ng/mL in 75 minutes. The data indicate a hypothalamic origin of the failure to grow.

The facial characteristics of these patients are very similar [Figure 111.2]. They have deep-set eyes, long eyelashes, thin lips, a long philtrum and micrognathia. The nasal bridge is depressed and the nose beaked. The Kuwaiti patients were described [10] as having floppy ear lobes. They also had medullary stenosis of the long bones, as did patients with the Kenny-Caffey syndrome [4,11,12]. Patients with the Kenny-Caffey syndrome also have microcephaly and ocular refractive errors. The Saudi patients have all had a characteristic nasal 'bird-like' voice [9].

Developmental delay has been observed in all of the Middle Eastern patients. Formal developmental assessment in our patient revealed moderate delay at 4 years 4 months, with receptive language skills better than expressive. The Kuwaiti patients [10] were much more severely retarded than the Saudi patients. Only one of eight was able to walk or talk. Patients with the Kenny-Caffey syndrome were described as cognitively normal [11,12].

Hypogonadism, cryptorchidism and micropenis have been observed in males [1,9]. Infections have been common, even fatal, but immunologic status has appeared normal; reduced numbers of T cells were observed in four of four tested by Richardson and Kirk [10].

GENETICS AND PATHOGENESIS

The elucidation of the fundamental nature of this disorder is an example of the power of technology that has been made possible by the information from the human genome project. The first step was the mapping of the gene to chromosome 1q42–43 [5,6]. Homozygosity and linkage disequilibrium mapping narrowed the gene to a 1 cm region of the chromosome. Next was the establishment that the Kenny-Caffey syndrome was allelic with the Sanjad-Sakati syndrome; they shared a haplotype, and it appeared that there was a common founder mutation [7]. Haplotype analysis using new polymorphic markers and bacterial artificial chromosome (BAC) and P1-derived artificial chromosome (PAC) clones established in the human gene project narrowed the critical region to 230 to bp [8]. Exons found in this area included geranylgeranylpyro phosphate synthase 1, TBCE and parts of two other genes. Mutation analysis was carried out on all four of these genes in the Middle Eastern families and the 12 bp deletion (155–166 del) was found in TBCE in all of them. In a Belgian pedigree with two affected siblings there was compound heterozygosity of two mutations in the same gene, a 2 bpAG deletion at 66 and 67 and a nonsense T1113A mutation in exon 12.

Tubulin is a heterodimer with α and β subunits whose proper folding requires the cytosolic chaperonin and a group of five tubulin specific chaperones (A to E). TBCE is required for the folding of α and its heterodimerization to β. Tubulin molecules, once assembled, polymerize to form microtubules in a polar fashion nucleating at the MTOC (microtubule organizing center).

The TBCE protein contains two known functional motifs, a cytoskeletal associated protein (CAP) which is rich in glycine (CAP-Gly) which binds α-tubulin, and a series of leucine-rich repeats which mediate protein-protein interactions.

The 12 bp Middle Eastern deletion removed four amino acid residues (52–55) including a highly conserved glycine in the CAP-Gly domain.

The Belgium mutations caused a frame shift after amino acid 22 and termination at amino acid 48 [Val23fs48X] and truncation of the protein after 370[Cys371X]. The big 22 bp deletion and the Cys371X were overexpressed and found to be stable; so they could have some activity *in vivo*.

Northern analysis indicated normal expression of the mRNA for tubulin, but there was a decrease in the amount of α-tubulin incorporated into microtubules. Immunofluorescence studies with antibody against α-tubulin revealed disruption in mutant cells of the radial pattern polarity and perinuclear organization seen in controls.

This represents the first example of a human disease resulting from mutations that induce defective folding and assembly of the building blocks of microtubules. It illustrates the power of technology made possible by the elucidation of the human genome. The pleiotropic manifestations of disease appear logical in tissues, with abundant microtubules, such as brain and testis. The specific absence of parathyroids in the presence of normal thyroid and other branchial derivatives is more difficult to understand, as is the occurrence of osteosclerosis in some patients.

An animal model of mutation in the *Tbce* gene; a Trp524Gly that leads to an unstable protein, produces an autosomal recessive progressive motor neuropathy (pmn) [13]. Descending motor neurons degenerate leading to death at 6 weeks resulting from loss of function of the phrenic nerve. Sensory neurons are spared. These *pmn* mice have brains that weigh 40 percent of that of normal mice, and their body weight 60 percent of control and spermatogenesis is defective [14], which are similar to the microcephaly, growth failure and hypogonadism of the Sanjad-Sakati syndrome. Furthermore, it has not yet been reported, but the Saudi patients have begun to die of pulmonary failure in which ventilation is inefficient and pCO_2 levels very high [9].

TREATMENT

The hypocalcemia and its consequences can be successfully managed by the administration of 1 α-cholecalciferol. Vitamin D (calciferol) and supplemental calcium has also been effective [1].

In our patient [2] treatment with human growth hormone 0.05 mg/kg 6 times a week was followed by a substantial increase in height (5 cm in 1 month); as growth velocity slowed the dose was doubled.

References

1 Sanjad SA, Sakati NA, Abu-Osba YK, *et al*. A new syndrome of congenital hypoparathyroidism, severe growth failure, and dysmorphic features. *Arch Dis Child* 1991;**66**:193.

2 Marsden D, Nyhan WL, Sakati NO. Syndrome of hypoparathyroidism growth hormone deficiency, and multiple minor anomalies. *Am J Med Genet* 1994;**52**:334.

3 Hershkovitz E, Shalitin S, Levy J, *et al*. The new syndrome of congenital hypoparathyroidism associated with dysmorphisms, growth retardation, and developmental delay – a report of six patients. *Isr J Med Sci* 1995;**31**:293.

4 Khan S, Tahseen K, Uma R, *et al*. Kenny-Caffey syndrome in six Bedouin sibships: autosomal recessive inheritance is confirmed. *Am J Med Genet* 1997;**69**:126.

5 Parvari R, Hershkovitz E, Kanis A, *et al*. Homozygosity and linkage-disequilibrium mapping of the syndrome of congenital hypoparathyroidism, growth and mental retardation and dysmorphisms to a 1 cM interval on chromosome 1q42–43. *Am J Hum Genet* 1998;**63**:163.

6 Diaz GA, Khan KT, Gelb BD. The autosomal recessive Kenny-Caffey syndrome locus maps to chromosome 1q42–q43. *Genomics* 1998;**54**:13.

7 Diaz GA, Gelb BD, Ali F, *et al*. Sanjad-Sakati and autosomal recessive Kenny-Caffey syndromes are allelic: evidence for an ancestral founder mutation and locus refinement. *Am J Med Genet* 1999;**85**:48.

8 Parvari R, Herskovitz E, Grossman N, *et al*. Mutation of TBCE causes hypoparathyroidism – retardation – dysmorphisms and autosomal recessive Kenny-Caffey syndrome. *Nat Genet* 2002;**32**:448, letter.

9 Sakati HO. personal communication.

10 Richardson RJ, Kirk JMW. Short stature, mental retardation, and hypoparathyroidism: a new syndrome. *Arch Dis in Child* 1990;**65**:1113.

11 Kenny FM, Linarelli L. Dwarfism and cortical thickening of tubular bones. *Am J Dis Child* 1966;**111**:201.

12 Lee WK, Vargas A, Barnes J, Root AW. The Kenny-Caffey syndrome: growth retardation and hypocalcemia in a young boy. *Am J Med Genet* 1983;**14**:773.

13 Martin N, Jaubert J, Gounon P, *et al*. A Missense mutation in Tbce causes progressive neuronopathy in mice. *Nat Genet* 2002;**32**:443.

14 Schmalbruch H, Jensen HJ, Bjaerg M, *et al*. A new mouse mutant with progressive motor neuronopathy. *J Neuropathol Exp Neurol* 1991;**50**:192.

Al Aqeel-Sewairi syndrome – multicentric osteolysis, nodulosis, arthropathy (MONA) – MMP-2 deficiency

AIDA I AL AQEEL

MAJOR PHENOTYPIC EXPRESSION

An autosomal recessive, multicentric osteolysis in Saudi Arabian families with distal arthropathy of the metacarpal, metatarsal and interphalangeal joints, with ultimate progression to the proximal joints and ankylosis and generalized osteopenia; large, painful to touch palmar and plantar pads; hirsutism and mild dysmorphic facial features including proptosis, a narrow nasal bridge, bulbous nose and micrognathia; and mutations in the matrix metalloproteinase 2 (MMP-2) gene.

INTRODUCTION

The multicentric osteolysis disorders, sometimes called vanishing bones syndromes are a group of inherited disorders of bone characterized by progressive destruction of bones and joints leading to skeletal deformities and functional impairment. Inheritance may be autosomal recessive or dominant, and there may or may not be associated nephropathy or mental retardation [1]. The disorders have been classified by the international skeletal dysplasia society into four groups (Table 112.1) [2]. They are notable for erosions in the interphalangeal joints that mimic severe juvenile rheumatoid arthritis (OMIM 166300, 259600, 259610, and 277950).

Al Aqeel-Sewairi syndrome (OMIM 605156) is a distinctive multicentric osteolysis in which crippling arthritis is associated with carpal and tarsal resorption, severe osteoporosis, distinctive facies, and palmar and plantar subcutaneous nodules [3,4]. Its occurrence in a number of consanguineous Saudi Arabian families permitted localization of the gene to chromosome 16q12–21, and haplotype analysis narrowed the critical region to 1.2 cm, which contained the MMP-2 gene [5]. Molecular analysis of candidate genes in this area identified all affected Saudi patients as lacking the MMP-2 gelatinolytic activity as a consequence of inactivating mutations. Some affected individuals were homoallelic for a nonsense mutation (TCA > TAA) in codon 244 of exon 5, predicting the replacement of a tyrosine residue by a stop codon in the first fibronectin type II domain (Y244X). Other affected members had a missense mutation in exon 2 replacing arginine 101 with histidine (R101H).

The development of a multicellular organism is dependent upon an extracellular matrix (ECM), which facilitates the organization of cells into tissues and organs [6]. The turnover of ECM is carried out by specialized proteinases. Among these are matrix metalloproteinases (MMPs) [7]. MMPs are a

Table 112.1 *Classification of the multicentric osteolysis disorders*

	Mode of inheritance	OMIM	Present at birth	Chromosomal locus
Multicentric predominantly carpal and tarsal in the hand				
Multicentric carpal-tarsal osteolysis with and without nephropathy	AD	166300		
Shinohara carpal-tarsal osteolysis				
Multicentric predominantly carpal-tarsal and interphalangeal				
Francois syndrome	AR	221800		
Winchester syndrome	AR	277950		
Torg syndrome	AR	259600		
Whyte Hemingway carpal-tarsal phalangeal osteolysis	AD			
Al-Aqeel	AR	605156		16q12–21
Predominantly distal phalanges				
Hadju-Cheney syndrome	AD	102500		
Giacci familial neurogenic acroosteolyses	AR	201300		
Mandibuloacral syndrome	AR			
Predominantly involving diaphyses and metaphyses	AD	174810	+	18q21.1–22
Familial expansile osteolysis	AR	228600		
Juvenile hyaline fibromatosis				

AD, autosomal dominant; AR, autosomal recessive

family of zinc- and calcium-dependent endopeptidases that are active at neutral pH, and they also degrade nonmatrix proteins [8,9]. Disruption of their activity has been implicated in many disease processes in which there is increased or decreased removal of matrix, such as arthritis [10,11], tumor invasion and metastasis [12], and angiogenesis [13]. The MMP2 gene encodes a member of the MMPs that degrades matrix proteins; the gene product has gelatinase activity [14], and it is involved in hydrolysis of gelatin and type IV collagen, the major structural component of the basement membrane, as well as elastin, laminin, fibronectin, aggrecan and fibrillin [14]. It is believed to be involved in normal collagen turnover [14] and tumor cell invasiveness [15]. MMP-2 increased activity has been implicated in many disease processes. The identification of the unique molecular defect in the MMP2 gene represents the first genetic disease caused by mutation in an MMP. The fact that defective proteolysis of the ECM results in osteolysis, nodulosis and arthropathy provides insights into the roles of MMP-2 and the ECM in the pathophysiology of bone and joint development.

CLINICAL ABNORMALITIES

Two patients were reported [3,4] who developed symptoms in the first year of life. They were members of a highly consanguineous Saudi Arabian family in which there were six affected members in three branches of the family, in each of which the parents were first cousins. Five other patients were reported from other Saudi Arabian families in which parents were also first cousins [16]. All of the patients developed symptoms in the first two years of life with progressive painful swelling of the interphalangeal joints of the hands and feet. Two patients began walking with difficulty and walked on the lateral aspects of their feet. The more proximal joints were involved with increasing age. There was decreased range of movement and deformities of the hands, feet, wrists and other joints [3,4,16] (Figures 112.1, 112.2) (Table 112.2). Wrists were tender, and there was fusiform swelling and tenderness of the fingers. There were flexion contractures of the interphalangeal joints (Figure 112.1). Ankles were markedly restricted in motion. The sibling (Figure 112.2), a 20-year-old woman, was short (127 cm). Elbows were fixed in flexion and wrists had flexion and ulnar deviation deformities (Figure 112.2). Knees were stiff and fixed in hyperextension. The feet were varus, had absent fifth digits and fixed abducted halluces.

The patients have mildly dysmorphic features characterized by proptosis, bulbous nose, narrow nasal bridge and hypertelorism. In one family [4] generalized hirsutism (Figure 112.1) was described. These patients had normal intelligence, but in other families some patients were mildly mentally retarded [16].

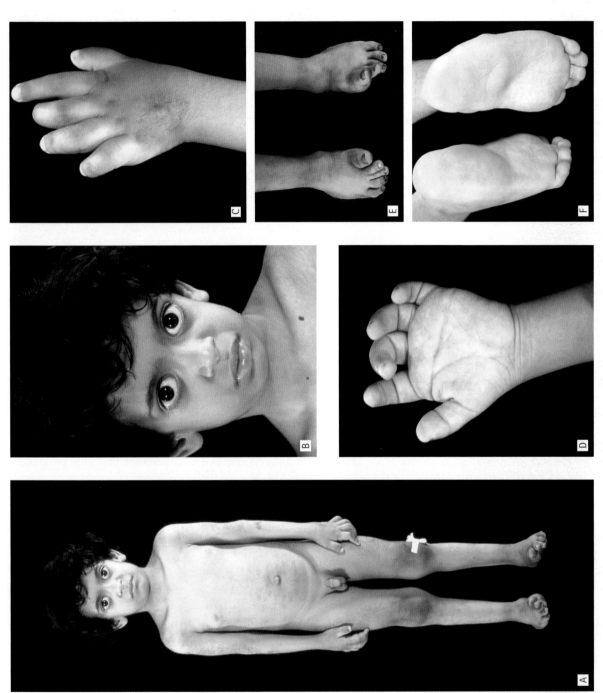

Figure 112.1   Patient A at 4 years-of-age. A. Whole body, which shows thin wasted body habitus. There was a generalized hirsutism involving the forehead, shoulders, arms and legs. B. Bilateral proptosis, bulbous nose, narrow nasal bridge, and small chin. C. Fusiform swelling of fingers with hyperextension of metacarpophalangeal joints and flexion of interphalangeal joints. A scar on the dorsum of the hand is evident at the site of a nodule biopsy. D. Subcutaneous painful nodules covered the entire palm of the hand. E. The feet displayed planovarus deformity and fixed hyperextension of the halluces. Hirsutism of the legs is evident. F. Hard painful plantar subcutaneous nodules.

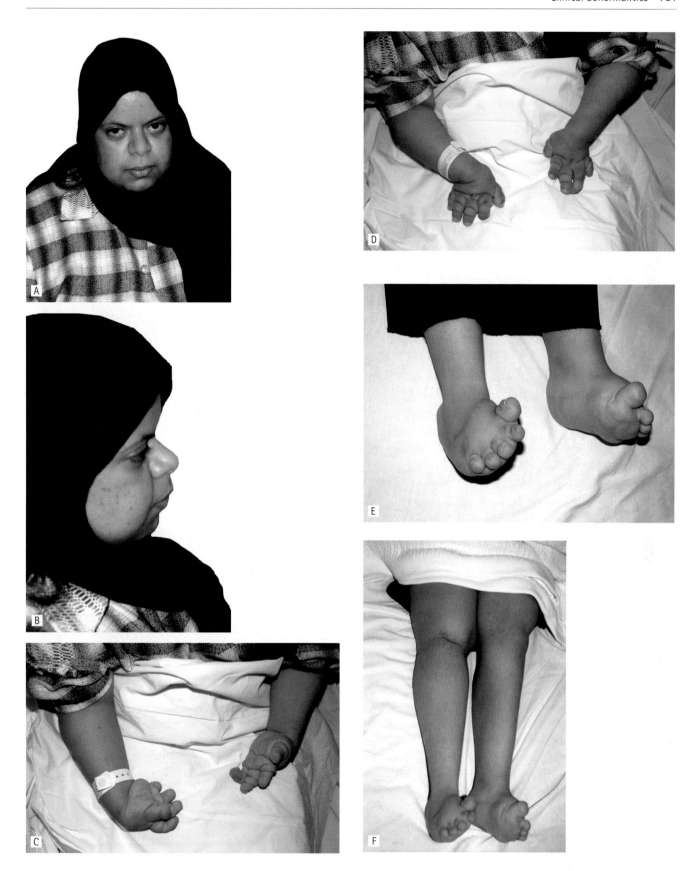

Figure 112.2   *Patient H at 20 years-of-age. A. Anterior view of patient displayed full cheeks and a bulbous nose. B. Lateral view of face also showed mild proptosis, and a small chin. C,D. Elbows and wrists were distorted and deformed with fixed flexion at the elbows and foreshortening of all of the fingers. Palms had subcutaneous nodules. E. Deformed feet with foreshortening of all of the toes, and there were subcutaneous nodules on the soles. F. Knees were fixed in hyperextension. Left knee had a scar from previous surgical corrective procedure.*

Table 112.2 *Comparison of the present report with previous reports of autosomal recessive multicentric osteolysis*

	Al-Aqeel	Torg	Winchester	Francois
Clinical features				
Face				
Corneal opacities	−	+/−	+	+
Proptosis/exophthalmos	+	+	−	−
Bulbous nose	+	−	+	−
Maxillary hypoplasia	+	+	−	
Macrognathia	+	+	−	
Gum hypertrophy	−	−	+	
Subcutaneous nodules	+	+	+	+
Nodule biopsy	Fibrofatty	Fibrofatty		
Hyperpigmented lesions	−	+	−	
Swelling of digits	+	+	+	
Deformity of hands and feet	+	+	+	
Contracture and ankylosis of joints	+	+	−	
Nephropathy	−	+/−	−	−
Hirsutism	+	−	−	−
Inheritance	AR	AR	AR	AR
Radiologic findings				
Osteolysis				
Carpal and tarsal	+++	++	+++	
Metacarpal and metatarsal	+	+	+	
Interphalangeal and phalangeal	+	+/−	+	
Other joints	+	+	+	
Spine	−	+/−	+	
Osteopenia	+++	++	+++	

−, absent; +, present; +/−, variable; ++, mild; +++, severe.

A striking feature of the syndrome was the development of large painful subcutaneous pads on the hands and feet which progressively increased in size. Magnetic resonance imaging (MRI) of these nodules showed rim enhancement near the margins (Figure 112.3) which suggested a fibrocollagenous nature (4).

Laboratory evaluation including complete blood count, serum chemistries, kidney, liver, bone, rheumatology panels, serum and urine metabolic studies, including enzyme studies for Farber lipogranulomatosis, were all normal [4]. Proteinuria was absent in a 24-hour urine collection, and creatinine clearance and urinary electrolytes were normal, as were renal ultrasound and diethylenetriamiacpentacetic acid (DTPA) scans.

Radiological evaluation (Figures 112.4, 112.5) has revealed generalized osteopenia, fusiform swelling of fingers with hyperextension of metacarpal phalangeal joints and flexion of interphalangeal joints, osteolysis of carpal and tarsal bones, which progressively led to the destruction of metacarpal, metartarsal, phalangeal and interphalangeal joints, as well as ankylosis of other joints. Cortical thinning and epiphyseal enlargement were evident and there was loss of joint space and pelvic distortion [4]. Joint biopsy revealed normal synovium with no evidence of inflammation.

Biopsy of the nodule showed fibrous fatty tissue [4] (Figure 112.6, p. 756).

GENETICS AND PATHOGENESIS

Inherited multicentric, osteolysis, nodulosis and arthropathy is an autosomal recessive disorder that was recently identified by two independent groups in eleven affected offspring of six consanguineous Saudi Arabian Families [3,4,16].

A genomewide search for homozygosity by descent was performed using polymerase chain reaction (PCR)-based microsatellite markers in three affected Saudi Arabian families. The disease gene was localized to chromosome 16q12, with a maximum lod score of 4.59 for marker D16S3253. Haplotype analysis narrowed the critical region to a 13 cM interval between markers D16S3396 and GATA67G11. Further haplotype analysis narrowed the critical region to 1.2 cM region that spans the gene encoding MMP-2 [5,17,18].

In one family, all affected individuals were homoallelic for a nonsense mutation (TCA → TAA) in codon 244 of exon 5 of the gene, predicting the replacement of a tyrosine residue

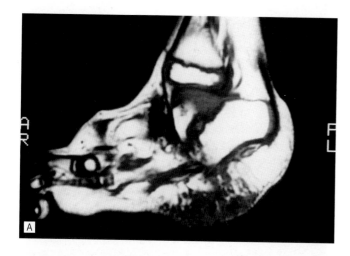

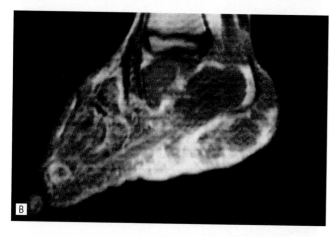

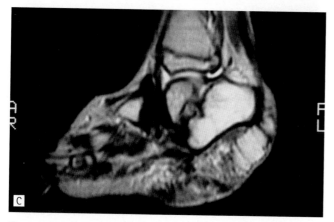

Figure 112.3   *MRI of the left foot. A. Large subcutaneous lesions, markedly hypointense on T1 sequences. B. A rim of enhancement extended all around the nodules in the immediate subcutaneous layer. C. The subcutaneous lesion is of intermediate to low signal intensity on T2 sequences.*

by a stop codon (Y244X) [4,5,17,18]. In a second family a G →A transition was found in codon 10 of exon 2, predicting the replacement of an arginine with histidine (R101H) [5,16]. In the third family no inactivating mutations were found in the exonic sequences of the gene. A mutation might be present in the promotor or intrinsic sequences. A non-pathogenic homoallelic G →T polymorphism resulted in the substitution of an aspartate with tyrosine residue (D210Y), which was also present in 50 unaffected members of the tribe [5,16]. All of the affected members had no MMP-2 gelatinolytic activity in serum or fibroblasts, while parents and heterozygous siblings had half normal levels of activity [5,17,18]. (Figure 112.7, p. 756) This absence of MMP-2 enzyme activity was characteristic of serum and fibroblasts of all of the Saudi families studied.

The matrix metalloproteinases (MMPs), also called matrixins, represent a family of zinc and calcium-dependent and membrane-associated endopeptidases that are active at neutral pH. Each member has specificity for a subset of extracellular matrix (ECM) molecules; collectively they catalyze the proteolysis of all components of the ECM [6], as well as other extracellular non-matrix proteins [19]. To date 22 MMPs have been identified [19,20].

The development of a multicellular organism is dependent upon an extracellular matrix, which facilitates the organization of cells into a more complex functional unit, such as tissues and organs. The extracellular matrix is the glue that holds cells together and provides texture, strength and integrity to the tissues. Diversity in tissue function depends not only upon diversity in cell types but also upon diversity in the composition of the ECM. Bone, for example, is comprised of one type of ECM; that of lung and brain is quite different. It has become increasingly apparent that the ECM harbors informational cues that direct cell behavior. In fact, the interaction of a cell with its ECM regulates some of the most fundamental cellular processes, such as growth, survival, differentiation, motility, signal transduction and changing shape [21].

MMPs participate in many normal biological processes including embryonic development, blastocyst implantation, organ morphogenesis, nerve growth, ovulation, cervical dilatation, postpartum uterine involution, endometrial cycling, hair follicle cycling, bone remodeling, wound healing, angiogenesis and apoptosis [12,13,19,22–24]. They also are involved in pathological processes, such as arthritis, cancer, cardiovascular disease, nephritis, neurological disease, periodontal disease, ulceration of the skin, cornea and muscle, fibrosis of the liver and lung [12,19,20,22,25,26].

MMPs are synthesized as pre-pro-enzymes and secreted as active pro-MMPs [20,27,19], which are activated by membrane type matrix metalloproteinases (MT-MMPs). Inhibition of MMPs is by endogenous tissue inhibitors (TIMPS) [28]. Four MMPs are known. MT1-MMP is a membrane-associated matrix metalloproteinase that is highly expressed in osteocartilagenous and muscolotendinous structure [29] and may function as a pericellular activator of MMP-2 in a trimeric complex with TIMP-2 and MMP-2 [30–32] (Figure 112.8, p. 757).

MMP-2 is thought to regulate the activity of a critical growth factor, transforming growth factor-beta (TGF-β).

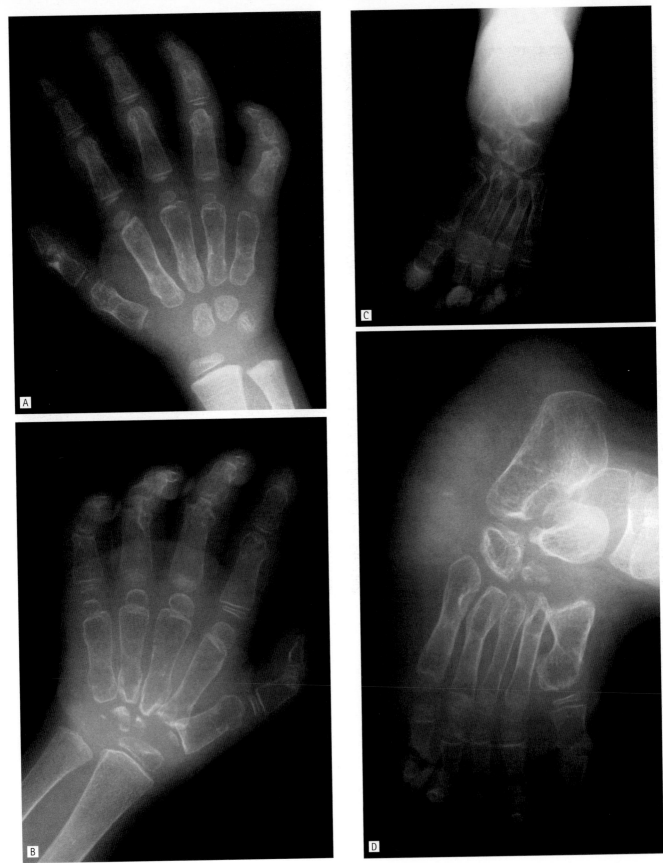

Figure 112.4 *Roentgenograms of the hand and feet of patient A. A. Hands at age 2 years display osteopenia, fusiform swelling of fingers, and osteolysis of interphalangeal joints. B. At 4 years-of-age there was further destruction of the carpal bones. Progressive involvement of the metacarpal bones had occurred with proximal tapering and bilateral distal notching in addition to severe cortical thinning and undermineralization, with seeming increase in the caliber of the metacarpals and phalanges. Shadowing by the subcutaneous palmar nodule is evident. C. Feet at age 4 years displayed marked tarsal osteolysis. D. Subcutaneous plantar nodule over the sole of the feet.*

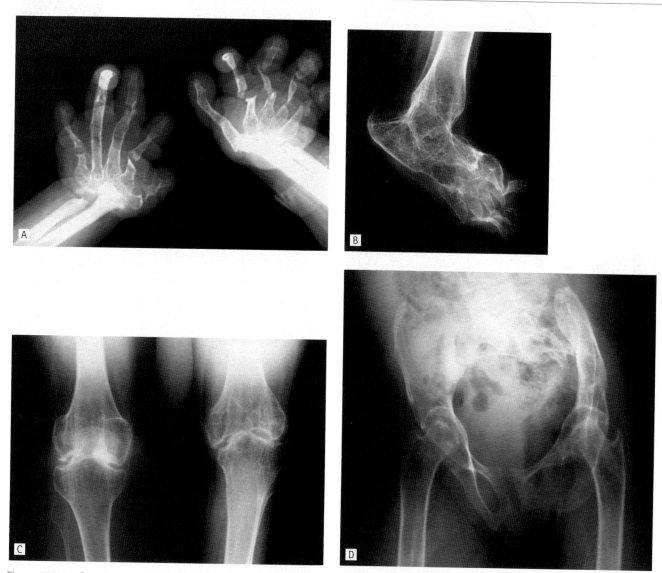

Figure 112.5 *Roentgenographic features of patient H. A. Film of the hands reveals complete chaotic destruction and loss of all of the carpal bones, marked destruction of metacarpals and phalanges and ankylosis of the remaining bones. B. Feet were markedly distorted. There was complete anklyosis of the ankle joint, distal tapering of the metacarpals and loss of the fifth digits. The osteopenia involved the tibia and fibula. There was thickening of subcutaneous tissue with nodular irregularities. C. Knees were markedly osteopenic and had cortical thinning, epiphyseal enlargement, and reduced joint spaces. No obvious erosive changes were seen. D. Pelvis was markedly distorted in configuration. Both hips were osteopenic and had irregularity of the femoral heads and protruding acetabuli, but no erosive changes.*

TGF-β-signalling mediates the coupling of the reciprocal activities of bone formation and resorption by influencing the maturation of osteocytes and enhancing the activity of osteoclasts [6]. Physiologically TGF-β may coordinate osteoclast activity by recruiting osteoclasts to the existing site of resorption. Pathologically TGF-β-induced osteoclast recruitment may be critical for expansion of primary and metastatic tumors in bone [33]. Plasmin, elastase, MMP-9 and MMP-2 activate TGF-β by proteolytically cleaving the latent-associated peptide, latent TGF-beta-binding protein (LTBp1) to produce the 125-165-kDa fragment, providing the mechanism for the release of active TGF-β from ECM-bound stores

[34,35]. Lack of MMP-2 may therefore affect bone formation and homeostasis through modulating the level of active TGF-β (Figure 112.8).

ECM remodeling is important for morphogenesis and homeostasis. The balancing act of ECM deposition and break down is very critical; therefore deficiency of MMP-2 may lead to an imbalance between the breakdown and deposition of the ECM [6]. Although MMP-2 null mice have no developmental defects [36] (which may reflect genetic redundancy), mice with targeted inactivation of the MT1-MMP gene have many of the same features as people with multicentric osteolysis and arthritis syndrome [36]. As MT1-MMP activates

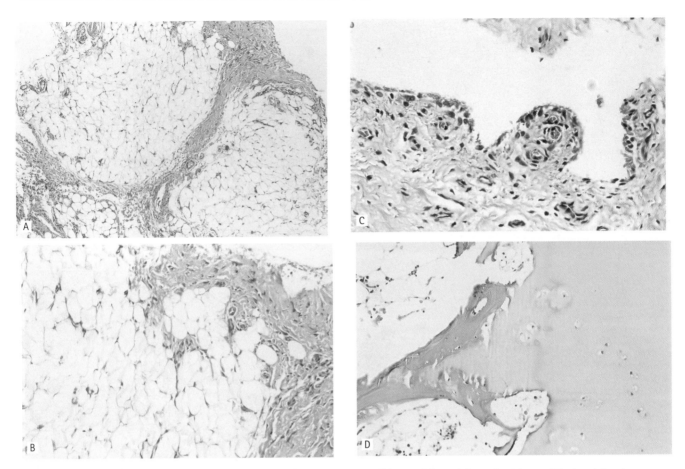

Figure 112.6   *Biopsy of fibrocollagenous nodule. A. Low magnification view of biopsy of the nodule on the dorsum of the hand showing fibrofatty tissue. B. Higher magnification showed clear fatty infiltration with fibrous bands layered between. C,D. Biopsy of the metacarpal phalangeal joint showing normal synovium containing normal mesothelial cells, cartilage and bone.*

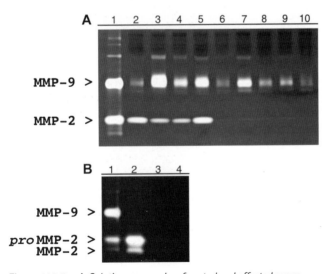

Figure 112.7   *A. Gelatin zymography of control and affected serum samples. Lane 1, MMP2 and MMP9 zymography standards (Chemicon International); 2, serum from an unaffected, unrelated individual; 3–5, sera from unaffected parents and siblings; 6–10, sera from affected children. B. Gelatin zymography of control and patient fibroblast conditioned medium. Lane 1, mixture of MMP2 and MMP9 zymogram standards; 2, unrelated, unaffected individual; 3 and 4, two affected members.*

MMP-2, it is not surprising that deficiency in either of these enzymes, even in different species, can result in similar defects. Deficiency of MTI in mice results in a decrease of collagen breakdown by fibroblasts in the skin and osteoblasts, decrease in bone formation, and increase in the number of osteoclasts, especially at ectopic sites. Tissue fibrosis may therefore be attributed to impaired function of fibroblasts; arthritis and osteolysis to increased osteoclastic activity; and craniofacial dysmorphism and osteopenia to impaired function of osteoblasts (Figure 112.8).

TREATMENT

There is no specific treatment available for the multicentric osteolysis. Our patients responded well to prednisolone 5–10 mg a day and methotrexate 5 mg weekly with improvement in joint pain, contractures, nodulosis and growth. Osteolysis did not improve but was nonprogressive. Osteopenia responded to pamidronate 2 mg/kg in bimonthly infusions. However, some patients reported bone pains, which resulted in discontinuation of treatment.

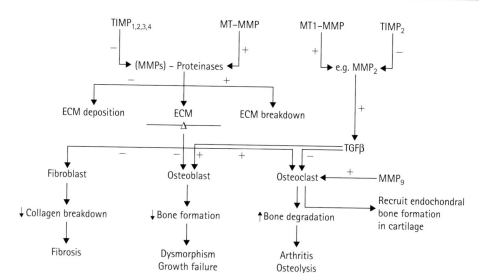

Figure 112.8 *Matrix metalloproteinase regulation and extracellular matrix (ECM) balance. (Reproduced with permission from* Nature Genetics *2001;28:202–4.)*

References

1 Urlus M, Roosen P, Lammens J, *et al.* Carpotarsal osteolysis. Case report and review of the literature. *Genet Couns* 1993;**4**:25.

2 Lachman RS. International nomenclature and classification of the osteochondrodysplasias. *Pediatr Radiol* 1997;**28**:737.

3 Al Aqeel A, Sewairi W. Al Aqeel-Sewairi Syndrome: An autosomal recessive syndrome with nodular arthropathy and acrolysis. *Am J Hum Genet* 1999;**65**:A140.

4 Al Aqeel A, Sewairi W, Edress B, *et al.* Inherited multicentric osteolysis with arthritis: A variant resembling Torg Syndrome in a Saudi family. *Am J Med Genet* 2000;**93**:11.

5 Martignetti JA, Al Aqeel A, Sewairi W, *et al.* Mutation of the matrix metalloproteinase 2 gene (MMP2) causes a multicentric osteolysis and arthritis syndrome. *Nat Genet* 2001;**28**:261.

6 Vu TH. Don't mess with the matrix. *Nat Genet* 2001;**28**:202.

7 Yu AE, Murphy AN, Stetler-Stevenson WG in: Mutation of the matrix metalloproteinase 2 gene (MMP2) causes a multicentric osteolysis and arthritis syndrome. WC Parks, RP Mecham (eds) *Matrix Metalloproteinases.* San Diego: Academic Press, 1999;85–133.

8 Agnihortri R, Crawford HC, Haro H, *et al.* Osteopontin, a novel substrate for matrix metalloproteinase-3 (stromelysin-1) and matrix metalloproteinase-7 (matrilysin). *J Biol Chem* 2001;**276**:28261.

9 McCawley LJ, Matrisian LM. Matrix metalloproteinases: They're not just for matrix anymore! *Curr Opin Cell Biol* 2001;**13**:534.

10 Brinkerhoff CE. Joint destruction in arthritis: Metalloproteinases in the spotlight. *Arthritis Rheum* 1991;**34**:1073.

11 Glegg PD, Carter SD. Matrix metalloproteinase-2 and -9 activated in joint diseases. *Equine Vet J* 1999;**31**:324.

12 Stetler-Stevenson WG. The role of matrix metalloproteinases in tumor invasion, metastasis and angiogenesis. *Surg Oncol Clin N Am* 2001;**10**:383.

13 Sang QX. Complex role of matrix metalloproteinases in angiogenesis. *Cell Res* 1998;**8**:171.

14 Creemers LB, Jansen ID, Docherty AJ, *et al.* Gelatinase A (MMP-2) and cysteine proteinases are essential for the degradation of collagen in soft connective tissue. *Matrix Biol* 1998;**17**:35.

15 Chen WT. Proteases associated with invadopodia, and their role in degradation of extracellular matrix. *Enzyme Protein* 1996;**49**:59.

16 Al Mayouf SM, Majeed M, Hugosson C, Bahabri S. New form of idiopathic osteolysis: Nodulosis, arthropathy and osteolysis (NAO) syndrome. *Am J Med Genet* 2000;**93**:5.

17 Al-Aqeel AI, Al Sewairi WM, Desnick RJ. Al Aqeel-Sewairi Syndrome, a new autosomal recessive disorder with multicentric osteolysis and arthritis with a novel mutation of matrix metalloproteinase 2 gene (MMP-2). *Am J Hum Genet* 2001;**69**:592.

18 Martignetti JA, Al Aqeel AI, Al Sewairi W *et al.* The first matrix metalloproteinase disease: MMP-2 deficiency results in a multicentric osteolysis syndrome. *Am J Hum Genet* 2001;**69**:189.

19 Morgunova E, Tuuttila A, Bergmann U, *et al.* Structure of human pro-matrix metalloproteinase-2: Activation mechanism revealed. *Science* 1999;**284**:1667.

20 Woessner JF. *Matrix Metalloproteinases and TIMPs.* New York: Oxford University Press, 2000.

21 Werb Z, Chin JR. Extracellular matrix remodeling during morphogenesis. *Ann N Y Acad Sci* 1998;**857**:101.

22 Schnaper HW, Grant DS, Stetler-Stevenson WG, *et al.* Type IV collagenase(s) and TIMPs modulate endothelial cell morphogenesis *in vitro. J Cell Physiol* 1993;**156**:235.

23 Pilcher BK, Wang M, Qin XJ, *et al.* Role of matrix metalloproteinases and their inhibition in cutaneous wound healing and allergic contact hypersensitivity. *Ann N Y Acad Sci* 1999;**878**:12.

24 Bord S, Horner A, Hembry RM, Compston JE. Stromelysin-1 (MMP-3) and stromelysin-2 (MMP-10) expression in developing human bone: Potential roles in skeletal development. *Bone* 1998;**23**:7.

25 Birkedal-Hansen H. Role of matrix metalloproteinases in human periodontal diseases. *J Periodontol* 1993;**64**:474.

26 Cockett MI, Murphy G, Birch ML, *et al.* Matrix metalloproteinases and metastatic cancer. *Biochem Soc Symp* 1998;**63**:295.

27 Van Wart HE, Birkedal-Hansen H. The cysteine switch: A principle of regulation of metalloproteinase activity with potential applicability to the entire matrix metalloproteinase gene family. *Proc Natl Acad Sci USA* 1990;**87**:5578.

28 Brew K, Dinakarpandian D, Nagasae H. Tissue inhibitors of metalloproteinases: Evolution, structure and function. *Biochim Biophys Acta* 2000;**1477**:267.

29 Stetler-Stevenson WG, Krutzsch HC, Liotta LA. Tissue inhibitor of metalloproteinase (TIMP-2): A new member of the metalloproteinase inhibitor family. *J Biol Chem* 1989;**264**:17374.

30   Butler GS, Will H, Atkinson SJ, Murphy G. Membrane-type-2 matrix metalloproteinase can initiate the processing of progelatinase A and is regulated by the tissue inhibitors of metalloproteinases. *Eur J Biochem* 1997;**244**:653.

31   Strongin AY. Mechanism of cell surface activation of 72kDA type IV collagenase. Isolation of the activated form of the membrane metalloproteinase. *J Biol Chem* 1995;**270**:5331.

32   Butler GS. The TIMP2 membrane type 1 metalloproteinase 'receptor' regulates the concentration and efficient activation of progelatinase A. A kinetic study. *J Biol Chem* 1998;**273**:871.

33   Pilkington MF, Sims SM, Dixon SJ. Transforming growth factor-beta induces osteoclast ruffling and chemotaxis: Potential role in osteoclast recruitment. *J Bone Miner Res* 2001;7:1237.

34   Dallas SL, Rosser JL, Mundy GR, Bonewald LF. Proteolysis of latent transforming growth factor-beta (TGF-beta) –binding protein-1 by osteocolasts. A cellular mechanism for release of TGF-beta from bone matrix. *J Biol Chem* 2002; **277**:21352.

35   Yu Q, Stamenkovic I. Cell surface-localized matrix metalloproteinase-9 activates TGF-beta and promotes tumor invasion and angiogenesis. *Genes Dev* 2000;**14**:163.

36   Holmbeck K, Bianco P, Caterina J, *et al.* MT1-MMP-deficient mice develop dwarfism, osteopenia, arthritis and connective tissue disease due to inadequate collagen turnover. *Cell* 1999;**99**:81.

Appendix: Differential diagnosis of clinical phenotypes

ACIDOSIS, HYPERCHLOREMIC

Diarrhea

Acrodermatitis, enteropathic
Infectious
Lactase deficiency
Sucrase deficiency

Renal tubular acidosis (RTA)

Cystinosis
Fanconi syndrome
Galactosemia
Glucose, galactose malabsorption
Hepatorenal tyrosinemia
Mitochondrial electron transport defect
Osteopetrosis and RTA
Topamax

ALOPECIA

An(hypo)hidrotic ectodermal dysplasia
Biotin deficiency
Cartilage hair hypoplasia
Conradi-Hünermann syndrome
Multiple carboxylase deficiency – holocarboxylase synthetase
    and biotinidase deficiencies
Trichorrhexis nodosa-argininosuccinic aciduria
Vitamin D-dependent rickets-receptor abnormalities

ANGIOKERATOMAS

Fabry disease
Fucosidosis
Galactosialidosis
GM_1 gangliosidosis
Sialidosis

APPARENT ACUTE ENCEPHALITIS

Glutaric aciduria type I
NARP
Propionic acidemia

ARTHRITIS

Alkaptonuria
Farber disease

Gaucher type I
Gout-HPRT deficiency; PRPP overactivity
Homocystinuria
I cell disease
Lesch-Nyhan disease
Mucolipidosis III
Mucopolysaccharidosis I S; IIS

BLEEDING TENDENCY

Abetalipoproteinemia
α_1-Antitrypsin deficiency
Congenital disorders of glycosylation (CDG)
Chediak-Higashi syndrome
Fructose intolerance
Gaucher disease
Glycogenoses types I and IV
Hermansky-Pudlak syndrome
Peroxisomal disorder
Tyrosinemia type 1

CALCIFICATION OF BASAL GANGLIA

Albright syndrome
Bilateral striato-pallido-dentate calcinosis
Carbonic anhydrase II deficiency
Cockayne syndrome
Down syndrome
Familial progressive encephalopathy with calcification of the
    basal ganglia (Aicardi-Goutieres syndrome)
GM_1-gangliosidosis
Hallervorden-Spatz disease
Krabbe leukodystrophy
Lipoid proteinosis
Microcephaly and intracranial calcification
Mitochondrial cytopathies
Molybdenum cofactor deficiency
Neurofibromatosis
Pterin defects
– Dihydropteridine reductase deficiency
– GTP cyclohydrolase I deficiency
– 6-pyruvoyletetrahydropterin synthase deficiency
– Sepiapterin reductase deficiency
Spondyloepiphyseal dysplasia

CARDIOMYOPATHY

Congenital muscular dystrophy
Disorders of fatty acid oxidation
Electron transport chain abnormalities
Glycogenosis type III

Hemochromatosis
D-2-Hydroxyglutaric aciduria
3-Methylglutaconic aciduria
Mucopolysaccharidosis
Pompe disease

CATARACTS – LENTICULAR OPACITY

Cerebrotendinous xanthomatosis
Electron transport chain disorders
Fabry disease
Galactokinase deficiency
Galactosemia
Homocystinuria
Hyperferritinemia-cataract syndrome
Hyperornithinemia (ornithine aminotransferase
  deficiency)
Lowe syndrome
Lysinuric protein intolerance
Mannosidosis
Mevalonic aciduria
Multiple sulfatase deficiency
Neonatal carnitine palmitoyl transferase (CPT) II
  deficiency)
Δ^1 Pyrroline-5-carboxylate synthase deficiency
Peroxisomal disorders
Smith-Lemli-Opitz (lethal)
Zellweger syndrome

CEREBRAL CALCIFICATION

Abnormalities of folate metabolism
Adrenoleukodystrophy
Aicardi-Goutiere syndrome
Biopterin abnormalities
Biotinidase deficiency
Cockayne syndrome
GM_2 gangliosidosis
Hypoparathyroidism
Kearns-Sayre syndrome
Krabbe disease
MELAS
Osteopetrosis and renal tubular acidosis (carbonic
  anhydrase II deficiency)
L-2-Hydroxyglutaric aciduria
Mitochondrial disorders

CEREBRAL VASCULAR DISEASE

Fabry disease
Familial hypocholesterolemia
Homocystinuria

Menkes disease
Methylene tetrahydrofolate reductase deficiency
Myocardial infarction

CEREBROSPINAL FLUID LYMPHOCYTOSIS

Aicardi-Goutieres syndrome

CHERRY RED MACULAR SPOTS

Galactosialidosis
GM_1 gangliosidosis
Mucolipidosis I
Multiple sulfatase deficiency
Niemann-Pick disease
Sandhoff disease
Sialidosis
Tay-Sachs disease

CHOLESTATIC JAUNDICE

α_1-Antitrypsin deficiency
Byler disease (progressive familial intrahepatic cholestasis)
Citrin deficiency (citrullinemia type II)
Cystic fibrosis
Dubin-Johnson syndrome
Hepatorenal tyrosinemia
LCHAD deficiency
Mevalonic aciduria
Niemann-Pick disease
Niemann-Pick type C disease
Peroxisomal biogenesis disorders
Rotor syndrome
Tyrosinemia, hepatorenal

CHONDRODYSPLASIA PHENOTYPES

Conradi-Hünermann syndrome
Peroxisomal disorders
Warfarin embryopathy

CHRONIC PANCREATITIS

Heriditary (dominant) (with or without lysinuria
  (cystinuria)): with or without pancreatic lithiasis or
  portal vein thrombosis
With hyperparathyroidism in multiple endocrine
  adenomatosus syndrome
MELAS

Organic acidemia
Pearson syndrome
Regional enteritis (Crohn)
Trauma – pseudocyst

CIRRHOSIS OF THE LIVER

α_1-Antitrypsin deficiency
Cystic fibrosis
Defects of bile acid synthesis
Galactosemia
Glycogen storage disease type IV
Hemochromatosis
Hepatorenal tyrosinemia
Niemann-Pick type C
Wilson disease

CORNEAL OPACITY

Cystinosis
Fabry
Fish eye disease
Galactosialidosis
GM1 gangliosidosis
Hurler disease (MPS I)
I-cell disease
Mannosidosis
Mucolipidosis III
Multiple sulfatase deficiency

CORPUS CALLOSUM AGENESIS

Adrenocorticotrophic hormone (ACTH) deficiency
Aicardi syndrome
Mitochondrial disorders (especially pyruvate dehydrogenase
  deficiency)
Nonketotic hyperglycinemia
Peroxisomal disorders

CREATINE KINASE – ELEVATED

Carnitine palmitoyl transferase II deficiency
Disorders of fatty acid oxidation
Drugs – toxins, alcohol, statins
Glutaric acidemia (I)
Glycogenosis – III
Glycogenosis – V – McArdle
Glycogenosis – posphofructokinase
D-2-Hydroxyglutaric aciduria
Inflammatory myopathy – dermatomyositis, polymyositis

Infectious myositis
3-Oxothiolase deficiency
Mevalonic aciduria
Myoadenylate deaminase
Muscular dystrophy – Duchenne, Becker
3-Oxothiolase deficiency
Oxphos abnormalities
Traumatic muscle injury

DERMATOSIS

Acrodermatitic enteropathica
Biotinidase deficiency
Holocarboxylase synthetase deficiency

DIABETES MELLITUS – ERRONEOUS DIAGNOSIS

Congenital disorders of glycosylation
Isovaleric acidemia
Methylmalonic acidemia
3-Oxothiolase deficiency
Propionic acidemia

DIARRHEA

Abetalipoproteinemia
Congenital chloride diarrhea
Electron transport disorders
Enterokinase deficiency
Glucose galactose malabsorption
Johanson-Blizzard syndrome
Lactase deficiency
Lysinuric protein intolerance
Pearson syndrome
Schwachman syndrome
Sucrase deficiency
Wolman disease

DYSOSTOSIS MULTIPLEX

Galactosialidosis
Generalized GM_1 gangliosidosis
Hurler, Hurler-Scheie disease
Hunter disease
Maroteaux-Lamy disease
Mucolipidosis II, I-cell disease
Mucolipidosis III
Multiple sulfatase deficiency
Sanfilippo disease
Sly disease

ECTOPIA LENTIS (DISLOCATION OF THE LENS)

Homocystinuria
Marfan syndrome
Molybdenum cofactor deficiency
Sulfite oxidase deficiency
Weill-Marchesani syndrome

EEG BURST SUPPRESSION PATTERN

Anesthesia-deep stages
Anoxia, cerebral hypoperfusion
Drug overdose (e.g., Phenobarbital)
Molybdenum cofactor deficiency
Nonketotic hyperglycinemia
Organic acidemia (neonatal encephalopathy-propionic acidemia

ELEVATED CEREBROSPINAL FLUID PROTEIN

Carbohydrate deficient glycoprotein disease
Congenital disorders of glycosylation
Kearns-Sayre
Krabbe disease
MELAS – Mitochondrial encephalomyopathy, lactic acidemia, and stroke-like episodes
MERFF – Myoclonic epilepsy with ragged-red fibers
Metachromatic leukodystrophy
Multiple sulfatase deficiency
Neonatal adrenoleukodystrophy
Refsum disease

EXERCISE INTOLERANCE

Defects of glycogenolysis
Disorders of fatty acid oxidation
3-Oxothiolase deficiency
Mitochondrial disorders
Myoadenylate deaminase deficiency

GLYCOSURIA

Cystinosis
Diabetes mellitus
Hepatorenal tyrosinemia
Fanconi-Bickel syndrome – GLUT-2 mutations
Glycogen synthase deficiency
Pearson syndrome
Renal Fanconi syndrome
Wilson disease

HAIR ABNORMALITIES

Argininosuccinic aciduria
Kinky hair, photosensitivity, and mental retardation
Menkes disease (pili torti, trichorrhexis nodosa, monilethrix)
Pili torti: isolated, MIM 261900
Pili torti with deafness or with dental enamel hypoplasia (Bjornstad syndrome)
Trichothiodystrophy: trichorrhexis nodosa, ichthyosis, and neurological abnormalities (Pollit syndrome)

HEMOLYTIC ANEMIA

Defects of glycolysis
5-Oxoprolinuria
Purine and primidine disorders
Wilson disease

HEMOPHAGOCYTOSIS (ERYTHROPHAGOCYTOSIS)

Carnitine palmitoyl transferase I
Hemochromatosis
Lysinuric protein intolerance
Propionic acidemia
Wolman disease

HEPATIC CARCINOMA

α_1-Antitrypsin deficiency
Galactosemia
Glycogen storage disease types I and IV
Hemochromatosis
Hepatorenal tyrosinemia
Progressive intrahepatic cholestasis
Thalassemia
Wilson disease

HEPATIC CIRRHOSIS

α_1-Antitrypsin deficiency
Cholesterylester storage disease
Cystic fibrosis
Electron transport disorders
Fructose intolerance
Galactosemia
Gaucher disease
Glycogenosis types I and IV
Hematochromatosis
Hepatorenal tyrosinemia

Hypermethioninemia
Mitochondrial DNA depletion
Niemann-Pick disease
Phosphoenolpyruvate carboxykinase deficiency
Progressive intrahepatic cholestasis
Thalassemia
Wilson disease
Wolman disease

HEPATIC FAILURE – ACUTE

α_1-Antitrypsin deficiency
Fatty acid oxidation disorders
Galactosemia
Hepatorenal tyrosinemia
Hereditary fructose intolerance
Neonatal hemochromatosis
Niemann-Pick types B and C
Wilson disease

HYDROPS FETALIS

Carnitine transporter deficiency
Congenital disorders of glycosylation
Farber disease (disseminated lipogranulomatosis)
Galactosialidosis
GM_1 gangliosidosis
Gaucher disease
Infantile free sialic acid storage disease (ISSD)
Mucolipidosis II – I-cell disease
Neonatal hemochromatosis
Neimann-Pick disease
Neimann-Pick disease type C
Pearson syndrome (anemia)
Sialidosis
Sly disease-β-glucuronidase deficiency
Wolman disease

HYPERAMMONEMIA

Argininemia
Arginiosuccinic aciduria
Carbamyl phosphate synthetase deficiency
Citrullinemia
HHH syndrome
LCAD
MCAD deficiency
Methylmalonic acidemia
Multiple carboxylase deficiency
Ornithine transcarbamylase deficiency
Pyruvate dehydrogenase complex deficiency
Propionic acidemia

HYPERTYROSINEMIA

Deficiency of 4-hydroxyphenylpyruvate
  dioxygenase
Drug – toxin
Hepatic infection
Hepatorenal tyrosinemia
Hyperthyroidism
Oculocutaneous tyrosinemia
Postprandial
Scurvy
Transient tyrosinemia of the newborn
Treatment with NTBC
Tyrosinemia type III

HYPOKETOTIC HYPOGLYCINEMIA

Carnitine transporter deficiency
CPT I deficiency
HMG CoA lyase deficiency
LCAD
LCHAD
MCAD
VLCAD

HYPOPHOSPHATEMIA

Fanconi syndrome
Hyperparathyroidism
MELAS
Pearson
X-linked hypophosphatemic rickets

HYPOURICEMIA

Fanconi syndrome, cystinosis
Isolated renal tubular defect (Dalmatian dog
  model)
Molybdenum cofactor deficiency
Phosphoribosyl pyrophosphate synthetase deficiency
Purine nucleoside phosphorylase deficiency
Wilson disease
Xanthine oxidase deficiency

ICHTHYOSIS

CHILD syndrome (congenital hemidysplasia ichthyosis and
  limb defects)
CDG (Congenital Disorders of Glycosylation) Type 1f

Gaucher disease
Krabbe disease
Multiple sulfatase deficiency
Refsum disease
Sjogren-Larsson syndrome
X-linked ichthyosis – steroid sulfatase deficiency

ICHTHYOSIS AND RETINAL DISEASE

Refsum syndrome
Sjogren-Larrson syndrome

INVERTED NIPPLES

Biopterin synthesis disorders
Citrullinemia
Congenital disorders of glycosylation
Isolated – dominant (MIM163610)
Menkes disease
Methylmalonic acidemia
Molybdenum cofactor deficiency
Propionic acidemia
Pyruvate carboxylase deficiency
VLCAD deficiency
Weaver syndrome

ISOLATED DEFICIENCY OF SPEECH AS PRESENTATION IN METABOLIC DISEASE

Ethylmalonic aciduria
D-Glyceric aciduria
Histidinemia
3-Methylglutaconyl CoA hydratase

KERATODERMA, PALMS AND SOLES

Oculocutaneous tyrosinemia
Papillon-Lefevie syndrome

LEIGH SYNDROME

Biotinidase deficiency
Electron transport chain abnormalities
Fumarase deficiency
   NARP 3-Methylglutaconic aciduria
Pyruvate carboxylase deficiency
Pyruvate dehydrogenase complex deficiency
Sulfite oxidase deficiency

LEUKOPENIA WITH OR WITHOUT THROMBOPENIA AND ANEMIA

Abnormalities of folate metabolism
Isovaleric acidemia
Johansson-Blizzard syndrome
Methylmalonic acidemia
3-Oxothiolase deficiency
Pearson syndrome
Propionic acidemia
Schwachman syndrome
Transcobalamin II deficiency

MACROCEPHALY

Bannyan-Ruvalcalba-Riley syndrome
Canavan disease
Glutaric aciduria type I
Hurler disease
4-Hydroxybutyric aciduria
3-Hydroxy-3-methylglutaric aciduria
L-2-Hydroxyglutaric aciduria
Krabbe disease
Mannosidosis
Multiple acylCoA dehydrogenase deficiency
Multiple sulfatase deficiency
Neonatal adrenoleukodystrophy
Pyruvate carboxylase deficiency
Tay-Sachs disease

MEGALOBLASTIC ANEMIA

Cobalamin metabolic errors-methylmalonic acidemia and
   homocystinuria-Cbl C and D
Folate metabolism, abnormalities of B12 deficiency – vegan
   or breast-fed infant of vegan mother
CblF cobalamin lysosomal transporter deficiency
Dietary folate deficiency
Folate malabsorption - hereditary
Intestinal B12 transport deficiency – Immerslund-
   Grasbeck-Cubilin deficiency
Mevalonic aciduria
Orotic aciduria
Pearson syndrome
Pernicious anemia – intrinsic factor deficiency
Transcobalamin II deficiency

METABOLIC ACIDOSIS AND KETOSIS

Isovaleric acidemia
Methylcrotonyl CoA carboxylase deficiency

Methylmalonic acidemia
Multiple carboxylase deficiency
Oxothiolase deficiency
Propionic acidemia
SCHAD deficiency

MYOCARDIAL INFARCTION-CEREBRAL VASCULAR DISEASE

Fabry disease
Familial hypercholesterolemia
Homocystinuria
Menkes disease

NEONATAL HEPATIC PRESENTATIONS IN METABOLIC DISEASES

α_1-Antitrypsin deficiency
Cystic fibrosis
Fructose intolerance
Galactosemia
Hemochromatosis
Hepatorenal tyrosinemia
Long-chain hydroxy-acylCoA dehydrogenase deficiency
Mitochondrial DNA depletion syndromes
Niemann-Pick type C disease
Wilson disease
Wolman disease
Sly disease

ODD OR UNUSUAL ODOR

Dimethylglycinuria
Glutaric aciduria type II
Hepatorenal tyrosinemia
Isovaleric acidemia
Maple syrup urine disease
Phenylketonuria
Trimethylaminuria
Treatment of urea cycle disorder with phenylacetate

OPTIC ATROPHY

ADP-ribosyl protein lyase deficiency
Adrenoleukodystrophy (ALD)
Biotinidase deficiency
Canavan disease
GM_1 gangliosidosis
Homocystinuria

Krabbe disease
Menkes disease
MERRF
Metachromatic leukodystrophy
3-Methylglutaconic aciduria, type III (Costeff)
Mevalonic aciduria
Mitochondrial energy metabolism, defects in – including Leber hereditary optic neuropathy (LHON)
Multiple sulfatase deficiency
NARP
Neonatal adrenoleukodystrophy
Sandhoff disease
Tay-Sachs disease

OSTEOPOROSIS AND FRACTURES

Adenosine deaminase deficiency
Gaucher disease
Glycogenesis I
Homocystinuria
I-cell disease
Infantile Refsum disease
Lysinuric protein intolerance
Menkes disease
Methylmalonic acidemia
Propionic acidemia

PAIN AND ELEVATED ERYTHROCYTE SEDIMENTATION RATE

Fabry disease
Familial hypercholesterolemia
Gaucher disease

PANCREATITIS

Cytochrome c oxidase deficiency
Glycogenosis type I
Hereditary dominant, with or without lysinuria; with or without pancreatic lithiasis or portal vein thrombosis
Homocystinuria
Hydroxymethylglutaryl CoA lyase deficiency
Hyperlipoproteinemia Type IV
Isovaleric acidemia
Lipoprotein lipase deficiency, also type IV
Lysinuric protein intolerance
Maple syrup urine disease
MELAS
Methylmalonic acidemia
Ornithine transcobamylase deficiency
Pearson syndrome
Propionic acidemia
Regional enteritis (Crohn)

Trauma - pseudocyst
With hyperparathyroidism in multiple endocrine
  adenomatosus syndrome

PARALYSIS OF UPWARD GAZE

Leigh; Kearns-Sayre syndromes
Neimann-Pick type C
Peripheral neuropathy

PHOTOPHOBIA

Cystinosis
Oculocutaneous tyrosinemia

POLYCYSTIC KIDNEYS

Congenital disorders of glycosylation
Glutaric aciduria type II
Zellweger syndrome

PSYCHOTIC BEHAVIOR

Carbamyl phosphate synthetase deficiency
Cbl Disease
Ceroid lipofucosidosis
Citrullinemia
Hartnup disease
Homocystinuria
Hurler-Schie, Schie disease
Krabbe disease
Lysinuric protein intolerance
Maple syrup urine disease
MeFH4 reductase deficiency
Metachromatic leukodystrophy
Mitochondrial disease (MELAS)
Niemann-Pick type C disease
Ornithine transcarbamylase deficiency
Porphyria
San Filippo disease
Tay-Sachs, Sandhoff late onset
Wilson disease

PTOSIS

Kearn-Sayre syndrome
MNGIE (mitochondrial neurogastrointestinal
  encephalomyelopathy)

RAGGED RED FIBERS

Menkes disease
Mitochondrial DNA mutations

RAYNAUD SYNDROME

Fabry disease

RENAL CALCULI

APRT (adenosine phosphoribosyltransferase) deficiency
Cystinuria
HPRT deficiency-Lesch-Nyhan disease
Oxaluria
PRPP synthetase abnormalities
Wilson disease
Xanthine oxidase deficiency

RENAL FANCONI SYNDROME

Cystinosis
Electron transport defects
Galactosemia
Glycogenosis I and III
Hepatorenal tyrosinemia
Idiopathic
Lowe syndrome
Lysinuric protein intolerance
Wilson disease

RENAL TUBULAR ACIDOSIS (RTA)

Cystinosis
Fanconi syndrome
Galactosemia
Hepatorenal tyrosinemia
Mitochondrial electron transport defect
Osteopetrosis and RTA
Topamax

RETINITIS PIGMENTOSA

Abetalipoproteinemia
Congenital disorders of glycosylation
Ceroid lipofuscinosis
Hunter disease
Kearns-Sayre
LCHAD deficiency
Mevalonic aciduria

NARP
Peroxisomal biosynthesis disorders
Primary retinitis pigmentosa
Refsum disease
Sjogren-Larsson syndrome (fatty alcohol oxidoreductase
  deficiency)

Kearns-Sayre syndrome and other electron transport
  chain disorders
Peroxisomal disorders
PRPP synthetase abnormality
Refsum disease

REYE SYNDROME PRESENTATION

Gluconeogenesis, abnormalities of
  Fatty acid oxidation, disorders of
  Urea cycle, disorders of
  Electron transport chain abnormalities
Fructose intolerance
Organic acidemias

RHABDOMYOLYSIS

Disorders of fatty acid oxidation
– LCHAD
– CPTII
Glutaric acidemia
Glycogenosis
– V – McArdle – myophosphorylase
– VII – Tarui – phosphofructokinase
Glycolysis
– phosphoglycerate kinase
– phosphoglyceromutase
Infection – myositis
Ischemic injury
Mitochondrial DNA deletions (multiple)
Mitochondrial point mutations (MELAS)
Overexertion
Oxphos defects – Complex I, Complex II
Quail ingestion – coturnism
Toxin-tetanus, snake venom, alcohol, cocaine

RHABDOMYOLYSIS – COLD-INDUCED

Carnitine palmitoyl transferase II deficiency

SCOLIOSIS

CDG
Homocystinuria

SENSORINEURAL DEAFNESS

Biotinidase deficiency
Canavan disease

SPASTIC PARAPARESIS

Argininemia
Biotinidase deficiency
HHH syndrome
Metachromatic leukodystrophy
Pyroglutamic aciduria
Sjögren-Larsson syndrome

STROKE-LIKE EPISODES

Carbamyl phosphate synthetase deficiency
Chediak-Higashi syndrome
Congenital disorders of glycosylation
Ethylmalonic aciduria
Fabry disease
Glutaric aciduria type I
Homocystinuria
Isovaleric acidemia
MELAS
Menkes disease
Methylcrotonyl CoA carboxylase deficiency
Methylmalonic acidemia
3-Methylene FH4 reductase deficiency
Ornithine transcarbamylase deficiency
Propionic acidemia
Purine nucleoside phosphorylase deficiency

SUBDURAL EFFUSIONS

Dihydropyrimidine dehydrogenase deficiency
Glutaric aciduria (I)
D-2-Hydroxyglutaric aciduria
Menkes disease
Pyruvate carboxylase deficiency

VOMITING AND ERRONEOUS DIAGNOSIS OF PYLORIC STENOSIS

Ethylmalonic-adipic aciduria
Galactosemia
HMG CoA lyase deficiency

4-Hydroxybutyric aciduria
D-2-Hydroxyglutaric aciduria
Isovaleric acidemia
Methylmalonic acidemia
3-Oxothiolase deficiency
Phenylketonuria
Propionic acidemia

Lipoprotein lipase deficiency
Niemann-Pick disease
Sitosterolemia

XANTHOMAS

Cerebrotendinous xanthomatosis
Familial hypercholesterolemia

Index of disorders

Page numbers appearing in *italics* refer to tables and numbers appearing in **bold** refer to figures.

Index of signs and symptoms

Page numbers appearing in *italics* refer to tables and numbers appearing in **bold** refer to figures.

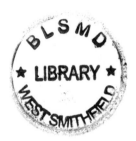